CLINICAL GYNECOLOGIC ONCOLOGY

Fifth Edition

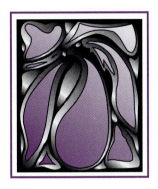

Philip J. DiSaia, M.D.

The Dorothy Marsh Chair in Reproductive Biology
Professor, Department of Obstetrics and Gynecology
University of California, Irvine
College of Medicine; Irvine, California
UCI Medical Center; Orange, California

William T. Creasman, M.D.

Sims-Hester Professor and Chairman
Department of Obstetrics and Gynecology
Medical University of South Carolina
Charleston, South Carolina

with 473 illustrations

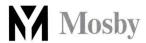

St. Louis Baltimore Boston Carlsbad Chicago Naples New York Philadelphia Portland
London Madrid Mexico City Singapore Sydney Tokyo Toronto Wiesbaden

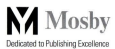
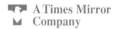

Dedicated to Publishing Excellence

A Times Mirror
Company

Publisher: Anne S. Patterson
Developmental Editor: Ellen Baker Geisel
Manufacturing Manager: Karen Lewis
Project Manager: Carol Sullivan Weis
Manuscript Editor: Florence Achenbach
Designer: Jen Marmarinos

Fifth Edition
Copyright © 1997 by Mosby-Year Book, Inc.

A Mosby imprint of Mosby-Year Book, Inc.

Previous editions copyrighted 1981, 1984, 1989, 1993

Printed in the United States of America
Composition by Graphic World, Inc.
Lithography/color Film by Graphic World, Inc.
Printing/binding by Von Hoffman Press

Mosby-Year Book, Inc.
11830 Westline Industrial Drive
St. Louis, Missouri 64146

Library of Congress Cataloging in Publication Data

DiSaia, Philip J., 1937-
　　Clinical gynecologic oncology / Philip J. DiSaia, William T. Creasman.—5th ed.
　　　　p.　　cm.
　　Includes bibliographical references and index.
　　ISBN 0-8151-2506-2
　　1. Generative organs, Female—Cancer.　I. Creasman, William T., 1934-　　. II. Title.
　　[DNLM: 1. Genital Neoplasms, Female.　　WP 145 D611c 1997]
　RC280.G5D46　　1997
　616.99′465—dc21
　DNLM/DLC
　for Library of Congress　　　　　　　　　　　97-11272
　　　　　　　　　　　　　　　　　　　　　　　　CIP

97　98　99　00　01　/　9　8　7　6　5　4　3　2　1

Dedication

Cognizant of our major sources of support and comfort, we wish to dedicate this work to our loving wives Patti DiSaia and Erble Creasman and our children John DiSaia, Steven DiSaia, Dominic DiSaia, Vincent DiSaia, Valrie Creasman-Duke, and Scott Creasman.

Also, a note of deepest gratitude to all the women, past and present, who have trusted us with their care. These women nurtured the tree of knowledge contained in this book. The roots of this tree have been founded on the courage of these women and intertwined with their lives.

Preface

The first four editions of this book were stimulated by a recognized need for a readable text on gynecologic cancer and related subjects, addressed primarily to the community physician, resident, and other students involved with these patients. The practical aspects of the clinical presentation and management of these problems were heavily emphasized in the first four editions and we have continued that style in this text. As in every other textbook, the authors interjected their own biases on many topics, especially in those areas where more than one approach to management has been utilized. On the other hand, most major topics are treated in depth and supplemented with ample references to current literature so that the text can provide a comprehensive resource for study by the resident, fellow, or student of gynecologic oncology and serve as a source of review material for oral and written examinations.

We continued the practice of placing an outline on the first page of each chapter as a reference to the content of that section. The reader will notice that we included areas not discussed in the former editions and expanded areas previously introduced. Some of these areas include new staging guidelines for cervical and vulvar cancer, current management and reporting guidelines for breast cancer, expanded discussion on the management of early invasive cancer of the vulva, the basic principles of genetic alterations in cancer, and new information on breast and colon cancer screening and detection. Much more information is included to make the text as practical as possible for the practicing gynecologist. In addition, key points are highlighted for easy review.

Fortunately, many of the gynecologic malignancies have a high "cure" rate. This relatively impressive success rate with gynecologic cancers can be attributed in great part to the development of diagnostic techniques that can identify precancerous conditions, the ability to apply highly effective therapeutic modalities that are more restrictive elsewhere in the body, a better understanding of the disease spread patterns, and the development of more sophisticated and effective treatment in cancers that previously had very poor prognoses. As a result, today a patient with a gynecologic cancer may look toward more successful treatment and longer survival than at any other time. This optimism should be realistically transferred to the patient and her family. Patient denial must be tolerated until the patient decides that a frank conversation is required. When the prognosis is discussed, some element of hope should always be introduced within the limits of reality and possibility.

The physician must be prepared to treat the malignancy in light of today's knowledge and to deal with the patient and her family in a compassionate and honest manner. The gynecologic cancer patient needs to feel that her physician is confident and goal oriented. Although, unfortunately, some gynecologic cancers still kill many individuals, it is hoped that the information collected in this book will help increase the survival rate of these patients by bringing current practical knowledge to the attention of the primary care and specialized physician.

Our ideas are only intellectual instruments which we use to break into phenomena; we must change them when they have served their purpose, as we change a blunt lancet that we have used long enough.

Claude Bernard (1813-1878)

Philip J. DiSaia
William T. Creasman

Acknowledgements

We wish to acknowledge the advice given and contributions made by several colleagues, including Drs. Elizabeth Grosen, Erle Henriksen, A. Robert Kagan, Roy T. Parker, James Reynolds, and Felix N. Rutledge. Special thanks to Lucy Diguiuseppe, Diane Roberts, and Barbara Tamsberg for their diligent administrative support in preparing the manuscript and to David F. Baker, M.A., Carol Beckerman, Richard Crippen, Susan Stokskopf, and David Wyer for their excellent and creative contributions to many of the illustrations created for this book.

We are grateful to the sincere and diligent efforts of Susie Baxter, Ellen Baker Geisel, Carol Weis, Florence Achenbach, Karen Lewis, and Jennifer Marmarinos from Mosby in bringing this book to fruition. Through their deliberate illumination and clearing of our path, this material has traversed the far distance between mere concept to a compelling reference book.

We would like to extend our deepest appreciation to Ms. Ladan Hariri for her astute editorial assistance, her dedicated and detailed review of the manuscript, and her suggestions and comments in enhancing the text.

Contents

Appendices

CLINICAL GYNECOLOGIC ONCOLOGY

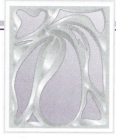

Preinvasive Disease of the Cervix

CERVICAL INTRAEPITHELIAL NEOPLASIA
Clinical Profile

The unique accessibility of the cervix to cell and tissue study and to direct physical examination has permitted intensive investigation of the nature of malignant lesions of the cervix. Although our knowledge is incomplete, investigations have shown that most of these tumors have a gradual, rather than an explosive, onset. Their preinvasive precursors may exist in a reversible phase of surface or in situ disease for some years, although this may be changing, at least in some patients.

According to data from the Third National Cancer Survey, published by Cramer and Cutler, the mean age of patients with carcinoma in situ was 15.6 years younger than that of patients with invasive squamous cell carcinoma, exceeding the 10-year difference found by others. This difference is, at best, a rough approximation of the duration of intraepithelial carcinoma in its assumed progression to clinical invasive cancer. Data such as these serve to emphasize the essential nature of cytologic screening programs, even when performed on less than an annual basis.

Although these early phases may be asymptomatic, they are detectable by currently available methods. This concept of development of cervical malignancy has convinced many that the control of this disease is well within grasp in the foreseeable future. It is possible to eradicate most deaths resulting from cervical cancer by using the diagnostic and therapeutic techniques now available.

There is convincing evidence that cytologic screening programs are effective in reducing mortality from carcinoma of the cervix. The extent of the reduction in mortality achieved is directly related to the proportion of the population that has been screened. In fact, all studies worldwide show that screening for cancer not only decreases mortality but also probably does so by decreasing the incidence. There has been no decrease in the incidence of cervical cancer without a screening program being implemented.

There have been numerous papers and lengthy discussions concerning the optimal screening interval. Unfortunately, numerous recommendations during the last decade and a half have resulted in a confused public and dissatisfied professionals. In 1988 the American College of Obstetricians and Gynecologists and the American Cancer Society agreed on the following recommendation, which has subsequently been accepted by other organizations. It states:

All women who are or who have been sexually active, or who have reached age 18, should undergo an annual Pap test and pelvic examination. After a woman has had three or more consecutive, satisfactory annual examinations with normal findings, the Pap smear may be performed less frequently at the discretion of her physician.

It is generally accepted by many that this recommendation advocates yearly Pap smears, since most women do not satisfy the conditions for less frequent screening. Information from many studies worldwide suggests this to be a reasonable recommendation for American women. Not only has screening decreased the incidence and death rate from cervical cancer, it has also identified a larger number of women with preinvasive neoplasia (which is the role of screening, not to diagnose cancer). It is estimated that as many as 600,000 women per year are identified with CIN in the United States. In addition, women who have been screened but subsequently developed cervical cancer usually have an earlier staged lesion. In the United States, death rates from cervical cancer have dropped from number 1 among all cancers to number 8. In 1995, 15,800 new cervical and 4800 cancer deaths will occur in the United States. About 55,000 new carcinoma in situ will be also diagnosed. Although it has not been proven in a prospective randomized study, all investigators credit screening as a major contributor to this fall in death rate. In contrast to the industrialized world, cancer of the cervix remains the number 1 cancer killer in women in the third-world countries. It is estimated that 500,000 cervical cancers will be diagnosed this year worldwide, representing 12% of all cancers diagnosed in women, and almost half will die from their cancer. Because this is a poor woman's disease, not much political pressure has been brought to bear to improve the situation for this group.

Several comments are appropriate in connection with these recommendations. The high risk woman, it is generally recognized, is an individual who becomes sexually active in the mid-adolescent years and has a tendency to have multiple sexual partners. All would agree that a woman should be screened for CIN shortly after becoming sexually active. It is believed that if an individual is virginal by the time she reaches 18 years of age, cervical cytologic testing should begin. Evidence suggests that there is an increased incidence of adenocarcinoma of the cervix, but the epidemiologic aspects of this disease have not been developed. It should be emphasized that the purpose of cytologic screening of the cervix is to identify the patient who has an intraepithelial lesion and not the one who has invasive cancer. The latter patient probably will be symptomatic, and in many instances her diagnosis will be made because of investigation of her symptoms. The fact that a significant number of women will develop intraepithelial disease within a short time after commencement of sexual activity speaks to the propriety of these recommendations. Although invasive carcinoma of the cervix is not as common in younger women as it is in their older counterparts, an increasing number of patients with invasive cancer are in their twenties and thirties. It is interesting to note that in England and Wales in the mid-1960s a political decision was made not to pay for Pap smears in women under the age of 35 unless they had three or more children. During the ensuing decade, there was a doubling of deaths resulting from carcinoma of the cervix in women of that age group.

Subsequent data from England now suggest that there is an increasing mortality in patients age 45 years and less. These authors feel that current indications suggest that during the next 25 years most of the predicted increase in incidence and mortality will occur among women less than 50 years old. In 1981 women under the age of 50 accounted for one third of new cancer cases and one fifth of the deaths, but by the year 2001 as many as two thirds of new cancers and as many as one half of deaths may occur in women less than 50 years old. Since 1986, invasive cancer incidence has increased about 3% per year in white women under 50 years of age whereas the rates are still declining in African-American women. This is probably related to screening practice, as noted below.

Studies have shown that the older patient is at increased risk for cervical cancer. Mandelblatt reported that 25% of all cervical cancers and 41% of all cancer deaths occurred in women more than 65 years of age. The prevalence of abnormal Pap smears is high in this group (16/1000). The chance of developing an invasive cancer is not necessarily related to prior screening habits in this age group. A recent study noted that increasing age is associated with more advanced disease, yet when stage of disease was controlled, there was no effect of age on disease-free survival. Screening of the patient over 65 years of age would benefit most, with a 63% improvement of 5-year mortality. As a result, Pap smear screening should continue for a lifetime.

A recent study from Connecticut reviewed all invasive cancers diagnosed in the state between 1985 and 1990. The purpose of the study, patterned after the puerperal deaths investigation of the 1930s, was to assess the reason why the cancer was not detected before it became invasive. Even though cervical cytologic screening has been with us for several decades, some very important facts became apparent and others need reemphasis. Over one fourth of patients had never had a Pap smear and almost one fourth had their last Pap smear over five years before cervical cancer diagnosis. The average age of women who were never screened was almost 20 years older (65 vs 46) than the screened cancer patients. This suggests that a large number of older women are not being screened with cervical cytology. Several studies have noted that many physicians may not comply with existing cancer screening guidelines. Of the previous normal Pap smears available for review after cancer diagnosis, about one fifth were re-read as abnormal. This includes those with a premalignant diagnosis. About 10% of women had incomplete evaluation after one or more abnormal smears. Adenocarcinomas were seen about twice as often in women who developed cancer within three years of a satisfactory negative Pap smear compared with the total study group. About one fourth of women had a Pap smear within three years; 77% had normal re-read Pap smears suggesting these patients may be in the category of having rapidly progressive disease.

Demographic studies suggest that 9% of women over age 18 have never had a Pap smear. This translates to over one million women in the United States. Of those screened, 62% did not have a Pap smear in the past year. The group not having a Pap smear in the last year was one of older patients. More than 91% of women 65 years or older and living below the poverty level had not had a Pap smear in the last year. It is estimated that about 11 million white women aged 65 or older in the United States did not have a Pap smear in the past year.

A National Omnibus survey was conducted to ascertain women's knowledge, attitudes, and behavior toward Pap screening. Of women 18 years or older, 82% believed the Pap smear is very important. Among women who felt Pap smear was important, 82% stated it was to identify cancer. Among those age 18-24, only 61% understood that the Pap smear was to detect cancer. Thirty-five percent of this same age group believed the Pap smear was important to detect vaginal infections and STDs. Over one fourth of those who felt Pap smears were important did not have a Pap test during the last year. The older and lower-income women were less likely than others to say that Pap smears are very important, yet they had regular physical examinations. Only 51% of women stated Pap smears identified cervical and endometrial cancers. Seven percent believed breast cancer was found on Pap smear. Risk factors for cervical cancer were poorly understood. About two thirds of women identified a family history as a cervical cancer risk factor. One in five women could not name any risk factors for cervical cancer. Women felt physicians did not sufficiently explain the reasons for Pap smears and the results from these tests. The need for better communication between physicians and women should be obvious.

Screening patterns to some degree appear to be changing, although some habits apparently do not. The number of women who had health insurance, a higher level of education, and current employment were related to Pap smear usage. Of interest is that recently, black women have substantially increased the use of the Pap smear, with rates now exceeding those of white women. This is age-related: screening is similar for blacks and whites to age 29; but from 30 to 49 years, blacks are significantly more compliant. Among those over 70 years old, compliance among white women is greater. Although screening rates appear to be higher in black women, the mortality is lower for whites. Age is also important in that younger women are more compliant than older women. The highest-risk group in the United States appears to be Hispanics, particularly if they speak only Spanish. It is estimated that there are 1.6 million unscreened Hispanics in the United States. This is the fastest growing segment of our population, which may explain why they are not screened. Reasons for noncompliance include these: it was unnecessary, no problems, procrastination, physi-

cians nonrecommendation, having a hysterectomy, and costs. One study noted that 72% of all females had a Pap smear within the last year. Yet nearly 80% of women who have not had a Pap smear reported contact with medical facilities during the past two years, while more than 90% reported a contact during the last 5 years. Obviously there needs to be an educational effort in this regard among health professionals.

Another important consideration is that there is a relatively high false negative Pap smear rate in the United States. Several studies in this country and abroad have shown that a significant number of patients were found to have invasive carcinoma of the cervix within a relatively short time after a reportedly normal Pap smear. A study from Seattle indicates that 27% of patients with stage I carcinoma of the cervix had a normal Pap smear within 1 year of the time of diagnosis. Berman noted that after 3 years from last screen, women who develop cervical cancer have the same incidence of advanced disease as women who have never been screened. The false negative rate of Pap smears is really unknown. Cerviography and colposcopic studies have suggested that the majority of women identified with CIN by these two techniques had normal Pap smears at the time of diagnosis.

There are, therefore, several concerns in determining optimal screening for cervical neoplasia. Although the transit time from carcinoma in situ to invasive cancer is said to require 8, 10, or possibly 20 years, some patients make this transition in a short time. It must be remembered that CIN does not necessarily progress in an orderly fashion to invasive cancer; an earlier CIN lesion can progress directly to invasive cancer. The inaccuracy of the Pap smear must also be taken into consideration. It must be remembered and emphasized that the purpose of screening is to identify preinvasive disease early, when the cost of treatment is considerably less than it is after the patient has developed invasive disease. Cost effectiveness is an important consideration in any screening program; however, multiple factors go into the determination of optimal screening. Essentially all investigators suggest yearly screening for the high risk patient, and it must be remembered that a substantial number of women in the United States are at high risk. The annual Pap smear has routinely led to evaluation of the patient in regard to other malignancies and medical conditions, and it would appear that this is an important consideration in the health care of American women. It has been estimated that annual Pap smear testing reduces a woman's chance of dying of cervical cancer from 4/1000 to about 5/10,000—a difference of almost 90%.

Epidemiology

Numerous epidemiologic studies reported in the literature have established a positive association between cancer of the cervix and multiple, interdependent social factors. A greater incidence of cervical cancer is observed among blacks and Mexican-Americans, and this is undoubtedly related to their lower socioeconomic status. Increased occurrence of cancer of the cervix in multiparous women is probably related to other factors, such as age at first marriage and age at first pregnancy. These facts, combined with the high incidence of the disease in prostitutes, lead to a firm conclusion that first coitus at an early age and multiple sexual partners increase the probability of developing CIN. Even socioeconomic status is interrelated, since an association has long been noted between relative poverty and early marriage and youthful childbearing. The final common factors appear to be onset of regular sexual activity as a teenager and continued exposure to multiple sexual partners. Indeed, cervical cancer is rare in celibate groups such as nuns, and many have labeled cancer of the cervix a "venereal disease."

Much has been made about the sexual activity of a woman as it may affect her risk for developing CIN. Increasing data suggest that a woman may also be placed at increased risk by her sexual partner, even though she does not satisfy the requirements of early intercourse and multiple partners. The sexual history of her partner may be as important as hers. In a study by Zunzunegui, patients with cervical cancer were compared with selected controls. Both populations came from a low socioeconomic group of recent Hispanic migrants to California. All were married. Sexual histories were obtained from both sexes. Among the women the age of first coitus was earlier among the cases than among the controls (19.5 years vs. 21.7 years). The average number of lifetime sexual partners did not differ between cases and controls. Interestingly, case husbands had more sexual partners than control husbands, had first intercourse at an earlier age, and had a much greater history of venereal diseases. Visits to prostitutes were equal between the two groups, but the case husbands tended to have frequented prostitutes more often than control husbands. Case husbands smoked more than control husbands. If the number of sexual partners of the husband was greater than 20, the risk of cervical cancer increased in the wife 5 times more than that of a woman whose husband had fewer than 20 sexual partners. This may be related to the "infectious" agent obtained by the husband and, in turn, to the duration of exposure by the woman. (Note following section on HPV and male factor.)

It is known that the carcinogen has to be transmitted via coitus. It appears that certain men are more "carcinogenic" than others and that the carcinogenesis is related to the occupation of the man. As previously noted, most women from the lower socioeconomic class seem to be at a higher risk for developing cervical cancer. Cervical cancer mortality shows a strong social class gradient. Beral developed mortality ratios for cervical cancer based on social class and the husband's occupation, and a straight-line correlation was established. Kessler attempted to further evaluate the role of the man in cervical carcinogenesis with an epidemiologic study. His method involved direct observation of two large groups of women: one group married to men who previously had wives who sustained cervical cancer and another group married to men without such a history. In the group married to men who had had other wives with cancer, he found 14 with cervical cancer compared with only 4 among the control group. Only nine of these lesions were frankly invasive, several were intraepithelial disease or showed microinvasion, and two were adenocarcinoma. It is also known that the wives of men with penile cancers have more cervical cancers.

Even if the carcinogen is identified, its interaction with the cervix depends on the specific woman at risk. The epidemiologic data strongly suggest that the adolescent is at risk. The probable reason is that active metaplasia is occurring. Since there is active proliferation of cellular transformation from columnar to metaplastic to squamoid epithelium, the potential for interaction between the carcinogen and the cervix is increased. Once this process of metaplasia is complete, it appears that the cervix may no longer be at high risk, although CIN certainly can occur in patients who are virginal until after this process has been completed. Smoking is now considered a high risk factor for carcinoma of the cervix, and this observation correlates with distribution of other smoking-related cancers. It appears that there is an increased, excess risk to preinvasive and invasive disease among smokers, particularly current, long-term users, high risk intensity smokers, and users of nonfiltered cigarettes. Smoking appears to be an independent risk factor, even after controlling for sexual factors. In a case-control study the risk of HGSIL increased with increasing years and pack-years of exposure. The association is for squamous cell cancers only, and no relationship with adenocarcinomas has been noted. Studies have found mutagens in cervical mucus, some many times higher than in blood.

A recent study evaluated whether smoking caused DNA modification (addicts) in cervical epithelium. Smokers had a higher level of DNA addicts than nonsmokers. Women with abnormal Pap smears had a significantly higher number of DNA addicts than those with normal Pap smears. Women with a higher proportion of addicts may have an increased susceptibility to cervical cancer. This suggests direct biochemical evidence of smoking as a cause of cervical cancer.

It has been suggested that vitamin deficiency may have a role in certain malignancies, including cervical cancer. Butterworth evaluated 294 patients with dysplasia and 170 controls defined by cytology and colposcopy. Multiple known risk factors for cervical neoplasia were evaluated along with 12 nutritional indices on nonfasting blood specimens. Plasma nutrient levels were generally not associated with risks; however, red blood cell folate levels at or below 660 nmol/L interacted with HPV-16 infections. Chemoprevention with vitamin A may prevent some cancers. Vitamin A derivatives, particularly retinoids in vitro and in vivo, modulate the growth of normal epithelial cells, usually by inhibiting proliferation and allowing differentiation and maturation of cells to occur. Meyskens, in a randomized prospective study, treated a group of patients with CIN II and III with all-transretinoic acid or a like placebo delivered directly to the cervix. Retinoic acid patients with CIN II had a complete histologic regression of 43% vs 27% for the placebo group (p = 0.041). No treatment difference was noted for the CIN III patients. The results of this study, as well as others, suggest a chemoprevention role in the prevention of cervical neoplasia.

Human Papilloma Virus (HPV)

Epidemiologic studies have identified the association of cervical neoplasia with sexual activity. The initial study suggests this relationship is over 150 years old. The sexually transmitted agent that could be related to the initiation and/or promotion of cervical neoplasia has been sought for many years. Essentially every substance found in the genital tract has been implicated over the years. These have included sperm, smegma, spirochetes, *Trichomonas*, fungus, and more recently herpes simplex virus type II (HSV-2) and human papilloma virus (HPV). During the 1970s, HSV-2 was studied extensively in an attempt to develop a possible etiologic link. These endeavors mainly used case-control studies, which showed a significant higher prevalence of HSV-2 in cancer cases compared to controls. These studies encountered problems with cross-reactivity between HSV-1 and HSV-2 and standardization of assays. It could not be determined if the infection with the virus preceded the cancer. When controlled for high-risk factors, many studies found no difference between patients and controls in the prevalence of HSV-2 antibody. Most investigators today do not consider HSV-2 a serious candidate as an etiologic agent for cervical neoplasia, although some have postulated that it may in some way be a cofactor.

Since the mid-1970s, there has been an explosion of information concerning HPV. It was actually in the mid-1970s when zur Hausen suggested that HPV was a likely candidate as a sexually transmitted agent that may result in genital tract neoplasias. Later in that decade, Meisel published a series of articles that described a new virus-induced condylomatous lesion of the cervix. Although koilocytosis had previously been described, these workers noted the presence of intranuclear HPV in koilocytotic cells associated with CIN. In contrast to the long-identified typical cauliflower condyloma, it was noted that HPV also produced a flat, white lesion, best recognized colposcopically, that was thought to be a precursor of cervical neoplasia. The development of immunoperoxidase techniques that can identify the HPV confirmed these original observations. Subsequently HPV has been isolated from genital lesions, and with the use of hybridization techniques the HPV DNA can be typed.

To date over 70 different types of HPV have been isolated and characterized (Table 1-1). The identity of a new subtype has usually been based on the description of the DNA genome in comparison to known HPV prototypes. A new type must share less than 50% DNA homology to any known HPV. Classification depends on the DNA composition. Out of the 70 different HPV types, 20 have been associated with lesions in the anogenital tract. So-called low risk types (6,11,42,43,44) are mostly associated with benign lesion such as condylomas, which rarely progress to a malignancy. The high risk types (16,18,31,33,35,39,45,51,52,56,58) are detected in intraepithelial and invasive cancers. It is said that more than 85% of all cervical cancers contain high risk HPV sequences. In benign precursor lesions, the HPV DNA is episomal (has extra chromosomal replication). In cancers

Table 1-1   Gynecologic lesions associated with HPV

Type	Lesion
6a-f	Condylomata acuminata
	CIN I, II, III
	VIN I, II, III
11 a,b	Condylomata acuminata
	CIN I, II, III
16	Condylomata acuminata
	CIN I, II, III
	VIN I, II, III
	Bowenoid papulosis
	Carcinoma of cervix
18	Carcinoma of cervix
30	CIN
31	CIN
	Carcinoma of cervix
33	Bowenoid papulosis
	CIN
	Carcinoma of cervix
34	Bowenoid papulosis
35	CIN
	Carcinoma of cervix
39	CIN
	Carcinoma of cervix
40	CIN
42	CIN
43	CIN
44	CIN
45	CIN
	Carcinoma of cervix
51	CIN
	Carcinoma of cervix
52	Carcinoma of cervix
56	CIN
58	Carcinoma of cervix

From de Villiers EM: Heterogeneity of the human papilloma virus group, *J Virol* 63:4898, 1989.

the DNA is integrated into the human genome. All HPVs contain at least seven early genes (E1-7) and two late genes (L1 and 2).

The integration usually occurs in the E1/E2 region, resulting in disrupting gene integrity and expression. These open reading frames encode DNA binding proteins that regulate viral transcription and replication. With HPV 16 and 18, the E2 protein repress the promoter from which the E6 and E7 genes are transcribed. Because of integration, the E6 and E7 genes are expressed in HPV positive cervical cancer. It appears that E6 and E7 are the only viral factors necessary for immortalization of human genital epithelial cells. These two oncoproteins form complexes with host regulatory proteins such as p53 and pRB (retroblastoma susceptibility gene). High risk HPV E6 upon binding with p53 caused rapid degration of the protein, thereby preventing p53 normal function of responding to DNA damage induced by radiation or chemical mutagens. Without this binding, increased levels of p53 growth arrest of cells may occur, which allows repair of damaged DNA to take place or apoptosis (programmed cell death) to occur. E7 protein may bind to several cellular proteins, including pRB. This interaction may inactivate pRB and push the cell cycle into S phase and induce DNA synthesis. Other regulatory genes such as c-myc may also be involved. Other factors obviously are important because only a small percentage of women infected with high risk HPV develop cancer. HPV immortalized human keratinocyte cell lines will only be manifest in nude mice, for instance, after transfection with additional oncogenes such as ras. In humans, the immunologic response may contribute to this very complicated scenario.

HPVs carry their genetic information within a cellular double-stranded DNA molecule. Infections caused by these viruses are usually not systemic but result in local infections manifest as warty papillary condylomatous lesions. HPV-infected cells contain both the fully formed viral particles and their DNA. Replication of the virus occurs only in the cell nuclei, in which DNA synthesis is low. Mature HPV particles are never found in replicating basal or parabasal cells but are found in the koilocytotic cells in the superficial layer. HPV, like HSV-2, may also have a latent intranuclear form in which only fragments of the viral DNA are expressed.

Characterizations of the HPV types identify 7 out of 22 primary genital types to be most frequently associated with benign or malignant lesions. These appear to be sexually transmitted. Initial evaluation noted that HPV 6/11 were associated with genital condyloma and the minor CIN groups, while HPV 16/18 were most commonly associated with cervical cancer and the more significant CIN lesions (Figure 1-1). Other types were seen less commonly but were also noted in invasive cancers. More recently, other types have also been identified in CIN and invasive cancer. This division

between "benign" and "malignant" types of HPV has been promoted in the literature with the suggestion that when the malignant types (mainly 16/18) were identified without cervical neoplasia, the patient was at high risk for developing disease. If these types were present in early CIN, then there was a greater chance of progression to more significant CIN or even invasive cancer.

Reeves reported one of the largest studies of both cervical cancer and controls, and HPV 16/18 were seen in 62% of 759 cancer patients, while HPV 6/11 were identified in 17%. More interesting is that only 7% of 1467 randomly selected, age-matched controls were found to have HPV 6/11 while 32% of controls were positive for HPV 16/18. The crude and adjusted relative risk of cervical cancer associated with HPV 16/18 or HPV 6/11 were similar. Other studies suggest that HPV 16/18 may be present in as many as 80% of the normal population. This proportion of HPV positivity in the normal population does vary depending on geographical area evaluated. Meanwell in evaluating 47 cancer patients, 66% contained HPV 16, compared to 35% of 26 controls. After controlling for age, he found no significant difference between cases and controls in regard to the frequency HPV 16 was identified.

Initially it was suggested that in all cancers the HPV DNA was integrated, whereas in CIN lesions the HPV DNA was episomal. This suggested the role of a more virulent type of HPV (i.e., 16/18). More recently, an increased number of cancers with episomal HPV DNA have been reported. Integration has been noted in CIN lesions, therefore it appears that integration is not a constant finding in cancers. Although integration of HPV 16 has been demonstrated, the importance of this finding in the development of cancer has not been determined.

An interesting study from Greenland and Denmark evaluated the incidence of HPV and HSV-2 in the normal population of these two countries. The cumulative incidence rate of cervical cancer in Greenland is 5.6 times higher than it is in Denmark. A total of 586 women in Greenland and 661 from Denmark were investigated. The total HPV 16/18 rate was 13% in Denmark, compared to 8.8% in Greenland; and the age-adjusted prevalence rate in Greenland was only 67% of Denmark's. HPV 6/11 prevalence was similar in the two populations (6.7% and 7.5%). The authors noted a much higher proportion of women in Greenland with HSV-2 antibodies than of those from Denmark (68.2% vs. 30.9%). They also noted a higher number of sexual partners in Greenland (22% with 40 or more) compared to Denmark (0.3%). Cancer screening was similar in the two areas. Although the authors suggested that these data should be interpreted with caution and that other, similar studies need to be done, the observed HPV 16/18 infection rate in Greenland (compared with the cancer incidence in Greenland as contrasted to Denmark) is not consistent with the etiologic role of these viruses in cervical neoplasia.

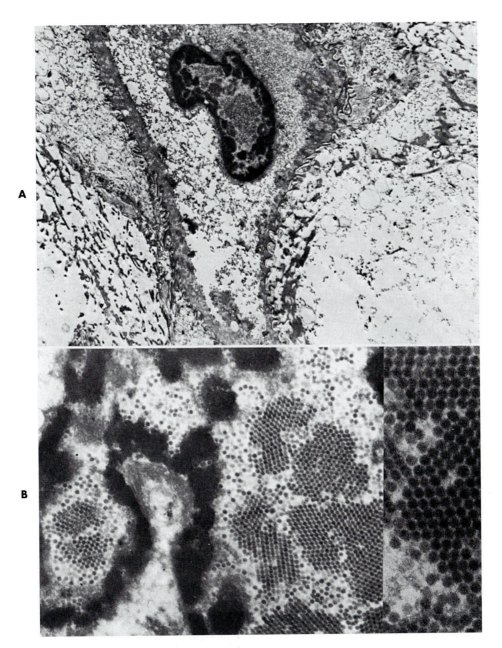

Figure 1-1 A, Koilocytotic cells with intranuclear virions (×6900). **B,** Human papillomavirus particles. Note intranuclear crystalline array ("honeycomb") arrangement of virions (×20,500). Insert (×80,000). (Courtesy Dr. Alex Ferenczy, Montreal.)

It has been suggested that HPV 18 may be more virulent than HPV 16 and may be a prognostic factor. Kurman et al. noted a deficit of HPV 18 in CIN compared to cancer, while there was no significant difference in the distribution of HPV 16 in CIN compared to cancer. These authors postulated that this deficit of HPV 18 in CIN could represent a rapid transit time through the preinvasive phase. Obviously, this is conjecture at this time. Walker did note that those patients with cervical cancer and HPV 18 had a worse prognosis than similar-staged patients with HPV 16 type. One other study noted that prognosis was worse in patients with cervical cancer if no

HPV subtype was identified than if any HPV type was present. All these data appear too preliminary to be of use for clinical management.

Over the last several years, many studies worldwide attempted to characterize HPV DNA in regards to specific types and correlate these findings with the cervical neoplastic process. Although the laboratory evidence of the role of HPV DNA in the carcinogenesis was being established, the epidermologic studies were lacking. Many studies using appropriate testing of the day performed just a few years ago, today are considered inadequate because of the test's insensitivity in light of current technology. For many years, the Southern blot analysis for HPV DNA was considered the gold standard. Because it is very laboratory and personnel intense, as well as difficult to replicate between different laboratories, other techniques were developed. The filter in situ hybridization and dot blot test were developed, the latter used in the commercially available Vira-Pap/Vira-type kits. Both techniques were insensitive. The HPV Profile kit was developed to increase the number of HPV types tested (from 7 to 14) but is labor intense and uses radiolabeling. This was introduced in 1993 but was replaced by Hybrid Capture, which is said to have greater sensitivity, requires less time, and uses a chemicaluminescence substrate instead of radiolabeling. Results of large studies using the Profile or Hybrid Capture are lacking. The PCR test is the most sensitive because of its amplification technique. Even with its increased sensitivity, procedures to increase sensitivity with L1 primers and using semi-quantitative PCR have been suggested. Unfortunately, tests have not been fully standardized and are subject to significant inter-laboratory variations.

With our current knowledge, should HPV typing be offered or suggested as part of our routine screening or even as a triage? This question implies that we know the answer to several other questions; i.e., what is incidence or prevalence in the "normal" population, what affects positive rate, which technique is considered the gold standard, can HPV DNA detection predict future cervical neoplasia, to list a few. It has been stated by some investigators that HPV DNA is ubiquitous and endemic. The most common means of transmittal appears to be sexual; however, nonsexual transfer is not rare. Jenison found 28%-65% of children younger than 10 years old had antibodies HPV 6, 16 or 18 fusion proteins, and 20% had PCR detection of HPV 6 or 16 in oral mucosa. The prevalence of HPV DNA detection appears to increase during pregnancy, and mother to child transmission during delivery is accepted as a possible transfer mechanism. Although the prevalence of HPV DNA does appear to be related to sexual activity, detection of the DNA has been found in coed virgins. It appears that HPV DNA is detected most frequently in women without evidence of CIN in the 15-25 age range. The one-time prevalence of HPV DNA depends on the assay used. One study of adolescents and young women using the dot blot hybridization technique found 9%-11% positive, while another study of similar women using PCR found HPV DNA in 33%. Studies of sexually active adolescents noted detection of HPV DNA varied from 15% to 38%. HPV detection rate usually was higher in women with more sexual partners; however, one study noted the rate decreased significantly as the number of sexual partners increased (more than 10 partners). Rate of detection did not correlate with years of sexual activity. These usually decreased with age when other factors were controlled.

There is limited data on longitudinal studies of HPV DNA detection. deVillier found about 9% of women of all ages with normal cytology to have HPV DNA present on first testing. This increased to 26% if repeat testing was done over a 5-year period. The actual rate is probably higher as they used a less sensitive technique (filter in-situ hybridization).

Moscicki followed a small group of HPV DNA-positive women for over two years with several visits in which HPV DNA using both PCR and dot blot technique were tested. Twelve of 27 were positive for HPV 16/18. Over half of the women became negative spontaneously (defined as two or more negative tests) for the original HPV type detected at first visit. The data suggested the number of virons decreased over a relatively short period and the infection was presumed terminated. When a new HPV type was identified, most reported acquiring a new sexual partner since the last visit. This probably reflects a new infection and not reactivation. Rosenfeld found that over 50% of young urban patients tested positive for HPV at either an initial visit or at follow up 6-36 months later using the Southern blot test. Therefore the prevalence and incidence of HPV DNA appears extremely variable, depending on age, sexual activity, number of times tested and laboratory technique used. It is estimated that over one million in the United States seek medical attention each year because of virus-induced lesions. It therefore appears that finding HPV DNA in the female genital tract is quite high. It is also clear that even with the high risk HPV types, infections commonly cause only mild transient cytologic changes and rarely leads to significant CIN or invasive cancer. Therefore the use of routine screening utilizing HPV DNA probes does not appear to be clinically indicated and is not cost effective, and currently available kits are relatively insensitive when compared to PCR techniques.

It has been suggested that in patients with an abnormality, HPV DNA typing may be used as a triage method to determine who may need further investigation. This is particularly true for patients with ASCUS or LGSIL, as those with HGSIL will most always be evaluated with colposcopy. Goff evaluated the Vira Type kit in patients with ASCUS. Of 171 patients, 19% had detectable HPV DNA and 85% were of the high risk HPV types. Only 6 of 28 patients with atypia and high risk HPV types had CIN; none had CIN III. The authors felt available HPV typing was not clinically useful in identifying patients that should be colposcoped. Sedlacek reached similar conclusions in 334 women referred for evaluation of abnormal cytology. He could not demonstrate a relationship between HPV type and high grade biopsy proven CIN using the Southern blot technique. On the other hand, using PCR with consensus primers or semi-quantitative PCR suggests a significant correlation of high risk HPV types with CIN II and III. These are supposedly new highly accurate methods that are research tools and not available as commercial kits. It has been suggested that the newest of the available kits (Hybrid Capture) may be a useful triage test. Hatch evaluated this kit in 311 patients referred for evaluation of abnormal cytology. Fifty percent of LGSIL, 26% of HGSIL, and 44% of those with invasive cancers were HPV-DNA negative. The test missed one third of histologic LGSIL and HGSIL in those patients with LGSIL on cytology. In the ASCUS group, the ability of the test to identify histologic HGSIL noted a sensitivity of 60%, specificity of 68%, and positive predicative value of 35%. With these results, most clinicians would not want to rely on this test to predict which patient may have significant cervical neoplasia, particularly invasive disease.

The use of HPV typing to predict progression of CIN has been suggested. In a study by Gaarenstoom, HPV 16 presence was significantly related to progression, 29% vs 0% in HPV negative lesions. All patients had colposcopically directed biopsies but were followed without treatment. PCR with a primer was used to identify HPV. Experience with commercially available kits is lacking.

In 1993, a diagnostic and therapeutic technology assessment (DATTA) was performed by the American Medical Association. Three questions were asked. Is HPV DNA testing an effective method of guiding therapy in (l) women with atypical Pap smears, (2) LGSIL, or (3) in a condylomatous cervical lesion identified at colposcopy whose histologic diagnosis is undeterminate? The scientific literature was reviewed and a panel from the obstetrical-gynecologic, pathology, oncology, infectious disease, and preventive medicine community was asked to answer the three questions. Sixty percent, 62%, and 55% respectively felt that HPV DNA testing was investigational in regard to the three questions posed. Only 22%, 15%, and 17% felt HPV DNA testing may be "promising," with a similar group noting that it had "doubtful" effectiveness. Since there does not appear to be a highly accurate commercial kit currently available, the use of HPV DNA typing in patients with ASCUS or LGSIL does not appear to be warranted. Continued investigation with PCR techniques is encouraged and further results are anxiously anticipated.

It has been suggested that the sexual partners of women with CIN and HPV infection should be treated to control the infectious process among women. Campion evaluated 140 females presenting for treatment of biopsy-proven CIN. As a control group, 280 females matched for age and disease severity (two control patients for each study patient) were identified. HPV typing was performed on each control and case. The atypical T-Z was destroyed with the laser in each. Repeat HPV typing was done at 6 months. In the study group, the current sexual partners were evaluated and all HPV lesions were treated. The male partners of the control group were not treated. The

primary-cure rate of CIN was the same in the two groups (92% study vs. 94% control group). The importance of controlling disease in the male sexual partner may be overemphasized.

It is now generally accepted that the virus itself cannot be eliminated with any known therapy. Therefore is there any benefit from knowing HPV subtypes that relates to clinical management? There probably is not. Not only is HPV commonly found in as many as 80% of normal (non-CIN) patients, but after treatment for CIN, HPV was found in 100% of 20 females with CIN who were successfully treated with laser.

Riva and associates treated 25 women with koilocytotic atypia, CIN, VAIN, or VIN. All patients had laser therapy of the cervix, vagina, and vulva in continuity. Morbidity was significant. Histologic persistence of subclinical HPV infection was documented in 88% of patients posttreatment. Neither treatment of male sexual consorts nor sexual abstinence significantly improved treatment outcome.

HIV and Cervical Neoplasia

Human immunodeficiency virus (HIV) infection is an ever increasing disease affecting all our citizenry. Initially thought to be limited to homosexual males and IV drug users, more and more women are being diagnosed with HIV and AIDS. By July 1993, 25,680 cases of AIDS in women were reported to the Centers for Disease Control (CDC). Eighty percent of women who contract AIDS are in the reproductive age group. About 25% acquire these infections during adolescence, and about one third of female cases in 1988 were contracted by heterosexual transmission. In women, early manifestations of the disease are often gynecologic, such as chronic yeast infections, pelvic inflammatory disease, genital warts, and herpes. On January 1, 1993, the CDC expanded the case definition of AIDS to include HIV positive women with invasive cervical cancer. This inclusion remains controversial because it apparently was based on preliminary data suggesting that in HIV positive patients there was a high incidence of CIN, Pap smears were unreliable, and that other diagnostic procedures, i.e., colposcopy, should be part of routine evaluation of these patients.

It is well recognized that immunodeficiency predisposed to development of neoplasia in congenital disorders such as Wiskott-Aldrich syndrome the incidence of cancer may be increased 10,000-fold. Renal transplant patients appear to be at increased risk for lower genital tract neoplasia. Cervical neoplasia has been reported to range from 5% to 40% and anogenital neoplasia is reported 9 to 14 times greater in these patient compared to controls. It is not surprising therefore to see an increased incidence of cancers in HIV positive patients. Kaposi sarcoma and non Hodgkin's lymphoma are the most commonly seen cancers in AIDS patients. Recently squamous cell carcinoma of the anogenital tract and oral cavity have been reported with increased frequency.

Spinillo noted in 75 HIV positive women that 22 (29%) had CIN. Sun evaluated in a cross-sectional study, 344 HIV positive and 325 HIV negative women. HIV positive women were more likely to have HPV-DNA of any type, HPV 16 or 18, or more than one HPV type than HIV negative patients. The HIV positive patients with HPV DNA were more likely to have CIN than HPV infected, HIV negative women. Essentially, all studies noted a much higher rate (up to tenfold) of CIN in HIV positive women compared to controls. Maiman noted that 39% of HIV positive patients but with normal cytology had CIN. He suggested in these women that Pap smears should be done every six months and have routine baseline colposcopy or cervicography. Subsequently, several large studies representing several hundred patients noted only a false negative Pap smear rate of 10%-19%. Wright noted that the Pap smear failed to detect abnormalities in only 0.8% of 398 HIV positive women who actually had high grade CIN. The CDC currently recommends that all HIV positive women have a Pap smear (see box below). If normal, repeat in six months then yearly thereafter as long as the Pap is normal. If the first Pap has severe inflammation with reactive squamous cells, the smear should be repeated in three months. In patients with ASCUS or any degree of SIL, further evaluation (colposcopy) appears warranted.

Not only are HIV positive patients at greater risk for CIN, severity of disease appears related to T-cell function. HIV positive patients with CIN have absolute T-cell counts and T4:T8 ratios of about one half of those positive patients without CIN. Wright noted in evaluation for 398 HIV positive and 357 HIV negative patients that CIN was independently associated with HPV infections (OR 9.8), HIV infection (OR 3.5), CD4$^+$ T-lymphocyte count less than 200 (OR 2.7) and age greater than 34 years (OR 2.0). Johnson noted that half of patients with CD4 T-cell counts less than 200/μL were infected with HPV 18 and HPV 18 was detected in 19% of all HIV positive patients.

Treatment of CIN in HIV positive patients appears to have a high failure rate regardless of modality used.

CDC GUIDELINES IN HIV$^+$ PATIENT

1. All HIV$^+$ patients should be encouraged to have PAP
2. If first PAP negative, repeat in six months and then yearly if normal
3. If first PAP has severe inflammation with reactive squamous cells, repeat in three months

Further suggestions
For ASCUS and all SIL, perform colposcopy

Cryosurgery is reported to have a 48%-78% failure rate, although cold knife cone has also reported a 50% failure. LEEP in one study noted a 56% failure.

Recurrence was associated with CD4 and T-lymphocyte counts but not grade of CIN. Possibly HPV 18 may account for the high failure rate. The AIDS Clinical Trial Group is currently investigating the use of topical 5-FU maintenance therapy as prophylaxis against recurrent CIN after initial therapy.

Data collected by the CDC for the first six months of 1993 noted 36,627 new AIDS cases and 89 were signaled by the presence of cervical cancer. Palefsky noted HIV positive women are at a higher risk of progression to invasive disease. Maiman found in women with cervical cancer and who were HIV positive to have more advanced cancer: high grade tumors with lymph node involvement. Prognosis was poor and most deaths were from cervical cancer and not AIDS. Although the potential for this epidemic may be present and all should be aware of the potential, to date there has not been an increase in the death rate from cervical cancer in young patients.

Natural History

The average age of patients with carcinoma in situ reproducibly is 10 to 15 years less than the average age of patients with invasive cancer of the cervix. However, there are many exceptions, and in the past two decades carcinoma in situ and invasive disease have been reported in an increasing number of patients in their late teens and early twenties. Whether all invasive carcinomas begin as in situ lesions is unknown, but Peterson reported that in one third of 127 untreated patients, invasive carcinoma developed subsequent to carcinoma in situ at the end of 9 years. Masterson found that 28% of 25 untreated patients demonstrated invasive carcinoma at the end of 5 years.

Carcinoma in situ is usually asymptomatic, and on routine examination the lesion is frequently not observed. Recognition of the lesion is assisted considerably by the use of cytologic testing and colposcopy. The mucous membrane sometimes bleeds easily on contact and erosions or a superficial defect of the ectocervix is relatively common in patients with carcinoma in situ, but these findings are not pathognomonic. The diagnosis must always be confirmed by histologic sections of a biopsy specimen.

What happens to a patient with early CIN in regard to its natural history is important because it relates to management. A review of the literature of the last 40 years suggests that more advanced lesions (CIN III) are more likely to persist or progress than CIN I. It is appreciated that CIN III can regress spontaneously, but more important, it is suggested that progression to cancer occurs more than 15% of the time, whereas CIN I progresses to cancer only 1% of the time. It does appear that the regression and persistence of CIN I and II are similar. If the eventual outcome of a given patient with an abnormal Pap smear could be predicted, the problem of management would be greatly simplified. Certainly, not all patients with abnormal cervical cells develop cancer of the cervix or even progression of CIN. Therefore any patient with any degree of dysplasia should be evaluated further.

Unfortunately, most of the studies performed on the natural history of this disease were carried out in the absence of today's diagnostic techniques, namely, colposcopy. Most studies used cytologic tests or biopsy as the diagnostic tools, resulting in varying progression/regression rates. Kessler reviewed many of the studies on the biologic behavior of cervical dysplasia. The occurrence of progression of CIN lesions to either a more severe form or invasive cancer ranges from 1.4% to 60%. Of interest is that the two most variant studies used cytologic tests alone to follow patients. The problems of definitive diagnosis using this technique have been studied in detail, and considerable variation has been noted even in the best of hands. When biopsies are performed, particularly if the lesion is small, the natural history of the disease may be disrupted, further complicating the evaluation of this entity. Even studies on the biologic behavior of cervical carcinoma in situ are varied, with progression to invasive cancer being reported in up to 50% of cases. The differences in these findings may very well be a result of the length of follow-up once the diagnosis of carcinoma in situ was established. Some patients with CIN develop invasive cancer, whereas others, even though followed for many years, do not progress either to a more severe form of CIN or to invasive cancer.

It has become apparent from recent studies that CIN is being diagnosed at a much younger age. In our material the median age for carcinoma in situ of the cervix has decreased from approximately 40 to 28 years of age. This may reflect only that screening of high risk patients is done at an earlier time, resulting in diagnosis at a younger age. Since the majority of these women desire children and in many instances have not started families, preservation of the integrity of the cervix and the uterus is of utmost importance. In an analysis of approximately 800 CIN patients at the Duke University Medical Center, it was noted that 30% were 20 years of age or younger at the time the diagnosis was established. Nulliparity was seen in about one fourth of the population, with 60% having one child or none. More than 95% of the patients had had intercourse by the age of 20, and one half had become sexually active by 16 years of age. More than one half of these patients had three or more sexual partners. About one half of these patients had the diagnosis of CIN established within 5 years of the beginning of their sexual activity. Screening these patients early, when they seek contraception or other medical attention, is extremely important and should be done on a routine basis. This screening probably explains why the diagnosis is being made at a much earlier age.

Table 1-2   Transition time of CIN

Stages	Mean years
Normal to mild-moderate dysplasia	1.62
Normal to moderate-severe dysplasia	2.20
Normal to carcinoma in situ	4.51

Certainly it is not at all unusual to see patients in their teens or early twenties with carcinoma in situ of the cervix. Therefore the lesion may be identified early in the spectrum of disease, and a patient may continue with CIN for a prolonged period, even after reaching the level of a CIN III lesion. Table 1-2 presents the transition time of CIN in our patients. Those patients who progress to carcinoma in situ do so within a very short interval. After that level of abnormality is reached, stabilization may occur in many of the patients. To date, there is no method for predicting which patient will remain within the CIN category, which will progress to a more severe form of CIN or to invasive cancer, and in what time frame this transition will take place.

Cytology

As has already been noted, genital cytology has had a major impact on the incidence of and death rate from cervical cancer. Despite general agreement about this finding, the problems with cervical cytology, particularly as it relates to the false negative rate and to so-called "Pap-mills," has received considerable publicity among laymen and in the medical community. A major concern of clinicians has been the ever-changing terminology used, which has resulted in a lack of meaning in regard to clinical relevance. The Papanicolaou classification has been changed so many times that the numbers have no constant meaning. Many cytologists changed to a descriptive term (*dysplasia* or, more recently, *CIN*) to indicate their diagnostic impression of the smear. In most instances, this terminology was clinically useful; however, there was an increasing tendency to use terms such as *inflammatory atypia*, squamous atypia but not dysplasia, which did not necessarily convey any clinical implications. In an attempt to clarify the varied terminology, the Bethesda System was developed in 1988. Although this new system was subsequently used in an increasing number of cytology laboratories, mainly because of federal mandates, many have asked whether it is an improvement over the older descriptive system (see box on next page). Several of the recommendations of the Bethesda System have a major effect on clinical management:

1. Statement on adequacy of the specimen for diagnostic evaluation. As a generalization, this is good new

COMPARISON OF DIFFERENT CYTOLOGY NOMENCLATURE

Dysplasia/CIS	CIN	Bethesda
Normal	Normal	Within normal limits
Benign atypia	Inflammatory atypia (organism)	Benign cellular changes
		infection—specified
		reactive changes
		inflammation
		atrophy
		radiation, etc
		Squamous cell abnormalities
Atypical cells	Squamous atypia	ASCUS

Mild dysplasia	CIN I	Low grade SIL
		  HPV
		  CIN I

Moderate dysplasia	CIN II	High grade SIL
Severe (marked) dysplasia	CIN III	CIN II
Carcinoma-in-situ (CIS)		CIN III
Adenocarcinoma and CIS		Glandular cell abnormalities

CIN, Cervical Intraepitheal Neoplasia
SIL, Squamous Intraepitheal Lesion
ASCUS, Atypical Squamous Cells of Undetermined Significance

information. If there is a lack of cells (scant cellularity) or foreign material present on the slide that makes it unsatisfactory for interpretation, the clinician should be so informed.

2. Infections. The Bethesda System lists the infections whose presence can be suggested by cytologic examination. Apparently this is a major item for cytology reporting as required by federal legislation.

3. Epithelial cell abnormalities. The Bethesda system has developed new guidelines in regard to these criteria.

   a. Atypias. This designation, used properly, will be of great benefit to clinicians. The term *atypical* is used only when the cytologic findings are of undetermined significance (ASCUS). This terminology should not be used as a diagnosis for defined entities. The report should include a recommendation for action that may help to determine the significance (such as atrophy due to hormonal deprivation) of the atypical cells.

   b. Squamous Intraepithelial Lesions (SIL). The Bethesda System designates two new diagnostic terms within this category.

      (1) Low grade SIL includes those with cellular changes associated with HPV and those with mild dysplasia (CIN I).

      (2) High grade SIL includes those with cellular changes suggestive of moderate or severe dysplasia, as well as carcinoma in situ (CIN II and III).

This new terminology was presented and adopted in hopes of eliminating some of the confusion with previous classifications. New questions, however, have been raised. Some have been addressed in the recent Bethesda II Conference, yet some decisions have been made on less than definitive data and have led to further clinical dilemmas. The following are some of the authors' concerns:

1. Terms such as *unsatisfactory* are very subjective and really meaningless. One of the reasons for an unsatisfactory specimen is the lack of an endocervical component on the slide of a premenopausal woman who has a cervix. This probably represents the largest reason for labeling a smear less than satisfactory. The recent literature contains numerous articles noting that the endocervical brush will increase the endocervical cellular component on a Pap smear over other techniques. Therefore, the recommendation is to use an endocervical brush along with a spatula. Even with a brush, there may be some slides without an endocervical component. What should a clinician do if a report is unsatisfactory because the smear had no endocervical component? Should the patient be recalled; and if so, in what time frame? It is interesting to note that few of the articles suggesting an improvement of the endocervical component through use of a brush address the question whether this increased endocervical component identifies an increased num-

ber of CINs if they are present. One recent study noted that although there were an increased number of endocervical cells on the smear when an endocervical brush was used rather than a regular Pap (spatula and moistened cotton-tip endocervical swab), more CIN lesions were picked up by the regular Pap than by the brush (22% vs. 4%). What was disturbing in this study was that 80 patients (23%) with CIN had normal Pap results when a brush was used. A large longitudinal study of 20,222 women was reported from England. They had both an "entry" smear in 1987 and an "exit" smear in 1989. The authors compared the relationship of endocervical cells with the diagnosis of CIN. This study did not demonstrate a subsequent higher incidence of CIN in those women with negative smears but no endocervical component compared to those with negative smears and an endocervical component. Interestingly, it was noted that with the use of the brush the endocervical component has increased substantially but the rate of CIN has decreased. The authors feel there is no scientific evidence to recommend an immediate or early repeat Pap smear if the first smear is reported as normal but an endocervical component is not present. These authors agree. Two other large studies have shown similar findings. Fortunately, changes were made following the Bethesda II Conference and the phrase "less than optimal" has been eliminated. The presence or lack of endocervical cells no longer determines adequacy of the specimen.

2. As noted above, the Bethesda System makes a point about identifying and reporting infections whose presence may be suggested by cytologic examination. In a study by Roongpisuthipone and associates, it was noted that in their review of the literature on this subject, correlation between Pap smear reporting of infection and verification was extremely poor. The authors felt the Pap smear should not be used to diagnose sexually transmitted disease and that treatment should not be based on cytologic findings alone. Although a general recommendation is to treat the infection and repeat the Pap smear, data do not substantiate that advice.

3. Under the category of epithelial abnormalities, several questions arise. What to do with a relatively large number of "atypical cells" reported without qualifiers remains a problem. This represents the old class II designation. In a small study of ASCUS, 30% were found to have CIN, which is considerably higher than noted with patients who had koilocytosis only or inflammatory atypia on their Pap smears. Another study of 139 patients with atypia without CIN on their cytology noted 25% to have CIN when colposcoped and biopsied. The new

designation of SIL has generated the most discussion about this new system. First of all, it equates HPV changes alone with CIN I. Many have suggested that these are one and the same, although data is lacking. Others have suggested that they are distinct entities and connotate different histology. A recent study by Lonky would add credence to the latter position. They evaluated 782 with cytology diagnosis of ASCUS, 355 with LGSIL determined by HPV alone, and 317 women with LGSIL determined by cytologic evidence of mild dysplasia (CIN I). Colposcopy and/or biopsies were performed. ASCUS and LGSIL with HPV only found no lesions in 61.8% and 64.2% respectively. Only 29.7% of LGSIL CIN I were negative or without lesions. Patients with ASCUS and LGSIL with HPV only had CIN and HGSIL lesions 18% and 14.9% respectively (HGSIL 4.8% and 5%) compared to 42.9% (17% HGSIL) for those with cytology indicative of LGSIL-CIN I. It would appear from this study that low-grade Pap smears have a poor correlation with histology. From this study, one could conclude that patients with Pap smears indicative of ASCUS and LGSIL-HPV only may be conservatively managed while those with LGSIL-CIN I probably need further evaluation besides repeat Pap smears. Other studies have also noted appreciable cervical pathology when CIN I is noted on cytology. It should be remembered that the Bethesda system was adapted and implemented without any evaluation data as to its validity as a guide for clinical management (see section on evaluation of abnormal cervical smear).

The authors of the Bethesda System state that koilocytosis is a descriptive term and not diagnostic. The CIN or dysplasia/CIS nomenclature has been used as a diagnostic term. Should a Pap smear suggestive only of koilocytosis be managed in the same way as one with CIN I? If all patients with Pap smears suggestive of koilocytosis were colposcoped, the cost would increase considerably; and some have suggested that many patients would be overmanaged and overtreated. This dilemma has resulted in several "clinical opinions" published in the literature. Unfortunately, this situation remains debatable and unresolved.

The proponents of this system suggest that since CIN II cannot be distinguished from CIN III with any degree of assurity the two should be included in high-grade SIL. Can CIN I either cytologically or histologically be differentiated with any degree of assurance from CIN II? The data in the literature suggest it cannot.

If CIN I is to be evaluated in the same manner as CIN II and III, why is there a two-tier designation of SIL? This seems to be an extra categorization of a disease process that is well understood by the practicing obstetrician-gynecologist. The low-grade category may connote to these physicians outside the OB-GYN field a less serious process and may delay proper evaluation. Since the cervical epithelium is only 0.25 mm thick, this separation of low- and high-grade SIL really represents a splitting of cells.

Previous cytologic terminology attempted initially or by convention to correlate cytology with histology. The Bethesda system was proposed for cytologic reporting only although the implication is a histologic correlation, i.e., HGSIL is CIN II or III. The authors of the Bethesda system have made the point that the terminology is used as a "descriptive" diagnosis. Clinicians have continued this cross reference of cytology and histology; however, confusion has been increased particularly with the designation of ASCUS and LGSIL.

Pathology

Cervical intraepithelial neoplasia (CIN) is the term now used to encompass all epithelial abnormalities of the cervix. The epithelial cells are malignant but confined to the epithelium. The older terminology using dysplasia and carcinoma in situ connotes a two-tier disease process that, at least in the past, has influenced therapy. That is, if only dysplasia was present, no or limited treatment was needed. If carcinoma in situ was diagnosed, in many instances a hysterectomy was recommended. This concept is inappropriate, particularly when the cervical epithelium may be no thicker than 0.25 mm. Although CIN has been arbitrarily divided into three subdivisions, it does suggest that CIN is a single neoplastic continuum. The histologic criteria for a CIN diagnosis depend on the findings of nuclear aneuploidy, abnormal mitotic figures, and a loss of normal maturation of the epithelium (Figure 1-2). CIN is divided into grade I, II, or III, depending on the extent of cellular stratification aberration within the epithelium. In CIN I the upper two thirds of the epithelium, although showing some nuclear abnormalities, has undergone cytoplasmic differentiation. The cells in the lower one third lack evidence of cytoplasmic differentiation or normal maturation (loss of polarity of the cells). Mitotic figures are few and, if present, are normal. In CIN II the abnormal changes of CIN I involve the lower two thirds of the epithelium. The CIN III lesions have full thickness changes with undifferentiated nonstratified cells. Nuclear pleomorphism is common, and mitotic figures are abnormal. On the basis of nuclear DNA studies, some investigators have suggested that most lesions diagnosed as CIN I are, in fact, flat condylomas that contain human papilloma viruses 6/11 (groups). It should be remembered that HPV 16/18 are more frequently found in CIN I than other subtypes, including HPV 6/11. The impression is that these lesions, by and large, are not of significance relative to this neoplastic process and have a very low risk for progressing to cancer compared with lesions containing HPV 16/18. As the epithelium becomes more involved with this intraepithelial neoplasia, there is a greater probability for HPV 16/18

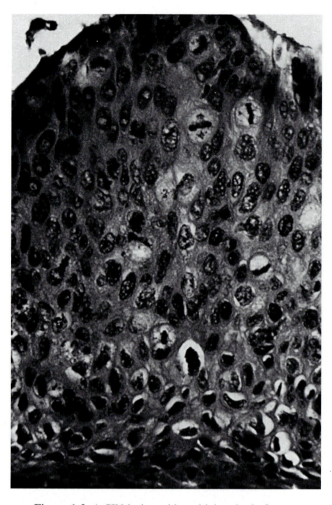

Figure 1-2 A CIN lesion with multiple mitotic figures.

identified with potential for invasion. It should be remembered that HPV 16/18 can be present in CIN I and HPV 6/11 in higher grade CIN.

Evaluation of an Abnormal Cervical Cytology

To fully understand our recommendations for the management of an abnormal cervical smear, the following points should be noted:

1. The cervical cytologic Pap smear, or Pap test, is not a diagnostic tool but a screening mechanism. Diagnosis rests with a tissue biopsy.
2. The Pap test is valid only for screening CIN. Malignant conditions of the corpus, tubes, or ovaries are infrequently associated with positive cervical cytologic findings.
3. The Pap test must be performed with care to yield optimal accuracy. The transformation zone of the cervix must be sampled where most lesions apparently originate. In the postmenopausal woman this area may lie high within the endocervical canal. The sampling for every cervical smear should evaluate the epithelium of the portio of the cervix by scraping it (usually using a wood or plastic spatula) and the epithelium of the endocervix by placing a

---

CAUSES OF ABNORMAL PAP SMEARS

Invasive cancer	Regeneration after injury (metaplasia)
Cervical intraepithelial neoplasia	Vaginal cancer
Atrophic changes	Vulvar cancer
Flat condyloma	Upper genital tract cancer (endometrium, fallopian tube,
Inflammation, especially trichomoniasis and chronic	ovary)
cervicitis	Previous radiation therapy

---

brush or similar cellular sampling device into the canal or aspirating the contents of the canal with a bulb pipette. Both samples can be placed on the same glass slide, thus minimizing handling costs.

4. All possible explanations for the abnormal cytologic findings should be considered (see box above).

With the adoption of the essentially mandated Bethesda system, considerable confusion was initiated by clinicians in regard to management based on the descriptive diagnosis. Since it is estimated that 50 million Pap smears are obtained each year in the United States with 2.5 million women with LGSIL, this management dilemma is a major concern. It has been estimated that the cost of colposcopic and interventional therapy in an attempt to eliminate the LGSIL would be six billion dollars annually.

Since guidelines of management had not been addressed after the introduction of the Bethesda system in 1988 or with revision in 1991, the Early Detection Branch of the National Cancer Institute invited experts to participate in a workshop in 1992 to address this issue. "Interim" guidelines were published in 1994. The participants felt this should be interim in nature because many questions remained unanswered. The guidelines offer clinicians aids in management of patients with abnormal cytology.

ASCUS: This designation should *not* replace the previous category of Class II or atypia. It is limited to epithelial abnormalities that are of uncertain significance. A diagnosis of ASCUS should be no more than 5% of Pap findings. ASCUS in a screened population may be two to three times the rate of SIL. Unless a practice is limited to a high-risk population, a higher rate of ASCUS may represent overuse of that diagnosis. The chance of identifying patients with SIL who have a Pap smear of ASCUS depends on the number (percent) of ASCUS reported by the lab and therefore may determine management schema. In one study, HGSIL was identified in 13% of ASCUS diagnosis when the percent Pap smears was 5%. When the ASCUS rate went to 10%, only 4% had HGSIL.

1. ASCUS Pap smears may be followed without colposcopy. Pap smears are repeated every 4-6

months for two years until there have been three consecutive negative smears. At that point, the patient can be monitored routinely. If second ASCUS appears during the two years, colposcopy should be considered.

2. ASCUS with severe inflammation should be re-evaluated in 2-3 months. Specific infections if identified should be treated and re-evaluation with Pap smears done. In absence of specific diagnosis, nonspecific vaginal treatment is not indicated.

3. In a postmenopausal woman with ASCUS and not on hormone replacement, a course of local estrogen may be helpful in management. If after estrogen ASCUS remains, colposcopy should be considered.

4. If the cytologist favors a neoplastic process as a qualifier with ASCUS, further evaluation should be considered.

5. ASCUS in a high-risk patient such as a previous abnormal Pap warrants colposcopy consideration.

6. Other triage techniques such as HPV typing and cervicography may be helpful. Because of the rapidly changing technology of HPV typing, this should be used only by physicians who understand its limitation (see HPV section).

Low grade SIL

1. The same follow up as noted in number 1 under ASCUS may be an option. If repeated smears show persistent abnormalities, colposcopy and directed biopsy are indicated.

2. Colposcopy, endocervical curettage, and directed biopsy of any abnormalities on the ectocervix is another appropriate option.

   "Routine electroexcision of the T-Z of nonstaining area as a method of evaluating a positive Pap smear diagnosed as LGSIL or ASCUS is not recommended."

3. The use of Ancillary screening techniques as noted in number 6 under ASCUS also apply to LGSIL.

Therapeutic options after histologic diagnosis of LGSIL include the following:

1. Local excision

2. No treatment for compliant patients, since 60% of LGSIL regress spontaneously.

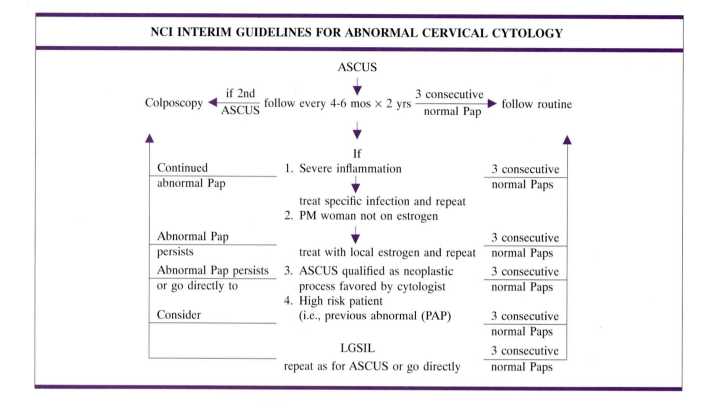

NCI INTERIM GUIDELINES FOR ABNORMAL CERVICAL CYTOLOGY

3. "Ablation without histologic confirmation of the diagnosis is inappropriate and unacceptable."

High grade SIL
1. Colposcopy with directed biopsy (see box above).

Atypical glandular cells of undetermined significance
1. These cells should be further subdivided into reactive or neoplastic.
2. If suspicious of adenocarcinoma in situ, the endocervix should be evaluated probably with a conization.

As one can tell from the above, particularly for ASCUS and LGSIL, many options are present, probably indicating a lack of knowledge in regard to natural history and biologic activity of various early lesions.

CERVICAL GLANDULAR CELL ABNORMALITIES

Cervical glandular cell abnormalities are being identified cytologically as well as histologically in increasing numbers. In 1979, Chrisopherson, based on a large population based series, estimated a 1:239 ratio of cervical adenocarcinoma in situ to squamous cell CIS. Since then the incidence of adenocarcinoma of the cervix has been increasing in relationship to squamous cancers. Most likely, the preinvasive glandular abnormalities are also increasing. Adenocarinoma-in-situ (adenoCIS) is

frequently associated with CIN. Most data would suggest 50% or more of adenoCIS are seen with CIN. Although the entire endocervical canal may be involved, over 95% of adenoCIS occur at the squamocolumnar junction. Several studies suggest abnormal glandular elements are associated with HPV18. This includes adenoCIS and adenocarcinoma. Whether epidemiologic factors associated with squamous CIN are the same for adenoCIS is suggested but unknown. When cytology indicative of glandular abnormalities is present, the canal needs to be evaluated. A patient with atypical glandular cells of undetermined significance (AGUS) may want to be evaluated with repeat Pap before other procedures are done. It should be remembered that a normal second smear may be false negative. Cytology should include the canal with a brush or similar device. Even though AGUS may be present, a considerable number of patients will have more significant disease on histologic evaluation. Although colposcopic findings may not be classic and subtle changes can be missed, most suggest that this is a worthwhile procedure. Colposcopic findings may include areas of whitened villi lying within immature metaplasia. The villi are thicker and more blunt than normal. Long unbranched horizontal vessels may be present. Invasive disease, either adenocarcinoma or squamous, may be suspect and confirmed with biopsies. The findings on ECC may help in the diagnosis and this procedure is encouraged. Most investigators feel conization is the diagnostic technique of choice, unless invasion is proven earlier in the workup.

Increasing data suggest that conization of the cervix may be adequate therapy for adenoCIS or less particularly if surgical margins are free. Muntz found one twelfth of women with uninvolved margins and seven tenths of women with positive margins to have residual disease in the hysterectomy specimen. They followed 18 women for a median interval of three years (1.5-5) who had uninvolved cone margins and none recurred. Other data from the literature notes the same findings. Hitchcock followed 21 patients with cervical glandular atypia, including adenoCIS, after conization with cytology and pelvic exams. After 13 years, none developed abnormal cytology or invasive carcinoma even though 13 conizations contained abnormalities that appeared to be incompletely ressected. Others have, however, sounded a more pessimistic note. Poynor evaluated 28 patients with a diagnosis of adenoCIS made by conization. Only 9 (43%) had a glandular lesion diagnosed on ECC prior to conization. Four of 10 patients with negative cone margins were found to have residual adenoCIS either in the hysterectomy or repeat cone specimens. Four of 8 patients with positive cone margins had residual disease in the second surgical specimen (3 with adenoCIS and 1 with invasive adenocarcinoma). Seven of 15 patients managed conservatively with close follow-up or repeat cone have had a recurrence; two patients with invasive adenocarcinoma. There is an increasing amount of data suggesting that patients who desire future fertility may in fact be managed with cold knife conization only if surgical margins are not involved. There appears to be about 8% persistence rate in these circumstances in contrast to as high as 60% persistence if margins are involved. In situations where fertility is desired and positive margins are present, reconization may be considered. It appears that in patients suspected of having ACIS that the cold knife conization is a better procedure than LLETZ, because the latter tends to have a larger number with positive margins and a higher recurrence rate. In patients who are not interested in future fertility, a simple hysterectomy is suggested as definitive therapy for adenoCIS by many.

Current practice mandates further evaluation of an abnormal Pap smear (dysplasia or CIN), initially with colposcopy biopsies and endocervical curettage (ECC). Further evaluation (conization) may be indicated, depending on these preliminary results.

Colposcopy

With the advent of colposcopy, a conservative schema and treatment plan for the patient with an abnormal Pap test has been generally accepted (Figure 1-3). This schema is safe only if the steps are rigorously followed. This is particularly critical when the endocervical curettage (ECC) findings are positive, even though the lesion is completely seen. In this situation, only an expert colposcopist should proceed with local treatment; otherwise a diagnostic conization must be performed. The possibility of a coexisting unsuspected endocervical adenocarcinoma must also be considered. Omission of any of the diagnostic procedures in the evaluation may lead to the tragedy that results when invasive cancer is missed. A report by Sevin et al. of eight such cases, out of which three patients died, emphasizes the hazards of a less than optimal workup of patients before cryotherapy. Colposcopy was introduced by Hans Hinselman in 1925 (Hamburg, Germany) as a result of his efforts to devise a

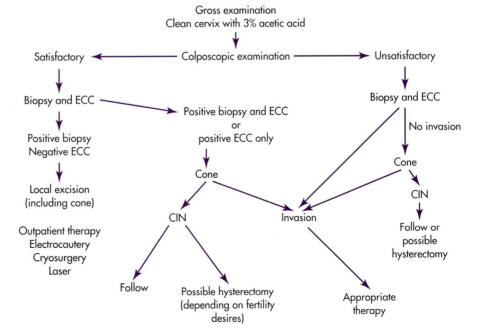

Figure 1-3 Evaluation and management schema for patient with abnormal Pap smear.

practical method of more minute and comprehensive examination of the cervix. He and others of his era believed that cervical cancer began as miniature nodules on the surface epithelium and that with increased magnification and illumination these lesions would be detectable. The meticulous examination of thousands of cases enabled him to clearly define the multiple physiologic and benign changes in the cervix, as well as to correlate atypical changes with preinvasive and early invasive cancer. Unfortunately, Hinselman was primarily a clinician with very little pathology background, and this, in conjunction with the encumbrance of the tumor nodule theory, led to the development of confusing concepts and terminology associated with the use of the colposcope.

In the early 1930s initial efforts were made to introduce colposcopy in the United States as a method of early cervical cancer detection. Because of the cumbersome terminology present at that time, the method was generally ignored; and with the introduction of reliable cytologic testing in the 1940s, North American physicians lost interest in colposcopy. The interest was renewed in the 1950s and early 1960s, but acceptance was slow because of the competitive nature of cytologic examinations, which were more economical and easier to perform and had, for the novice, a lower false negative rate. Over the last two decades the technique has gained a long-awaited popularity and has been recognized as an adjunctive technique to cytologic testing in the investigation of genital tract epithelium. The recent popularity of colposcopy has been enhanced by the discovery of a scientific basis for most morphologic changes and the acceptance of a logical and simplified terminology for these changes.

The colposcope consists, in general, of a stereoscopic, binocular microscope with low magnification. It is provided with a center illuminating device and mounted on an adjustable stand with a transformer in the base. Several levels of magnification are available, the most useful being between 8 × and 18 ×. A green filter is placed between the light source and the tissue to accentuate the vascular patterns and color tone differences between normal and abnormal patterns. Examination of the epithelium of the female genital tract by colposcopy takes no more than a few minutes in the usual case.

Colposcopy is based on study of the transformation zone (Figure 1-4). The transformation zone is that area of the cervix and vagina that was initially covered by columnar epithelium and, through a process referred to as metaplasia, has undergone replacement by squamous epithelium. The wide range and variation in the colposcopic features of this tissue make up the science of colposcopy. The inheritance of variable vascular patterns, as well as the fate of residual columnar glands and clefts, determines the great variety of patterns in this zone. It had been generally taught that the cervix was normally covered by squamous epithelium and that the presence of endocervical columnar epithelium on the ectocervix portio was an abnormal finding. Studies by Coppleson and his associates have established that columnar tissue can initially exist on the ectocervix in at least 70% of young women and extend into the vaginal fornix in an additional 5%. This process of transition from columnar to squamous epithelium probably occurs throughout a woman's lifetime. However, it has been demonstrated that this normal physiologic transformation zone is most active during three periods of a woman's life, that is, fetal development, adolescence, and her first pregnancy. It is known that the process is enhanced by an acid pH environment and is considerably influenced by estrogen and progesterone levels.

The classification of colposcopic findings has been improved and simplified (see box below), facilitating the recognition of abnormal patterns: white epithelium (Figure 1-5), mosaic structure (Figure 1-6), punctation (Figure 1-7), and atypical vessels (Figure 1-8). The term *leukoplakia* is generally reserved for the heavy, thick, white lesion that can frequently be seen with the naked eye. White epithelium, mosaic structure, and punctation herald atypical epithelium (CIN) and provide the target for directed biopsies. The pattern of atypical vessels is most often associated with invasive cancer, and biopsies should be performed liberally in areas with these findings. Although the abnormal colposcopic patterns reflect cytologic and histologic alterations, they are not specific enough for final diagnosis, and biopsy is necessary. The greatest value of the colposcope is in directing the biopsy to the area that is most likely to yield the most significant histologic pattern.

When colposcopy is performed, a standard procedure is followed. First, the cervix is sampled for cytologic screening, and then it is cleansed with a 3% acetic acid solution to remove the excess mucous and cellular debris. The acetic acid also accentuates the difference between normal and abnormal colposcopic patterns. The colposcope is focused on the cervix and the transformation zone, including the squamocolumnar junction, and the area is inspected in a clockwise fashion. In most instances the entire lesion can be outlined, and the most atypical area can be selected for biopsy. If the lesion extends up

---

ABNORMAL COLPOSCOPIC FINDINGS

A. Atypical transformation zone
  1. Keratosis
  2. Aceto—white epithelium
  3. Punctation
  4. Mosaicism
  5. Atypical vessels
B. Suspect frank invasive carcinoma
C. Unsatisfactory colposcopic findings

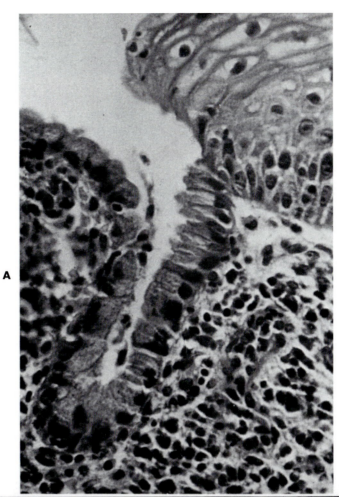

Figure 1-4 A, Squamocolumnar junction (transformation zone). **B,** Large transformation zone.

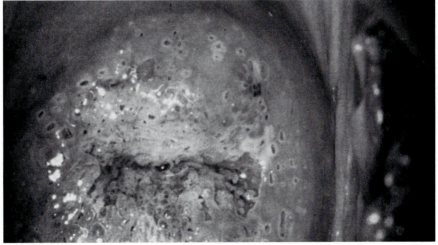

the canal beyond the vision of the colposcopist, the patient will require a diagnostic conization to define the disease. ECC is performed whether or not the lesion extends up the canal, and if invasive cancer is found at any time, plans for a cone biopsy are, of course, abandoned. This plan of investigation, which is outlined in Figure 1-3, is based on the assumption that there are no areas of CIN higher up in the canal if indeed the upper limits of the lesion can be seen colposcopically. In other words, CIN begins in the transformation zone and extends contiguously to other areas of the cervix such that if the upper limits can be seen, one can be assured that additional disease is not present higher in the canal. The colposcope can only suggest an abnormality; final diagnosis must rest on a tissue examination by a pathologist. Selected spot biopsies in the areas showing atypical colposcopic patterns, under direct colposcopic guidance and in combination with cytologic testing, give the highest possible accuracy

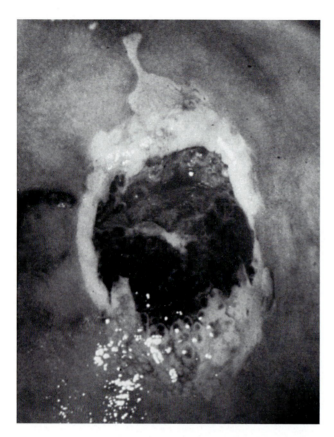

Figure 1-5 White epithelium at cervical os (colposcopic view).

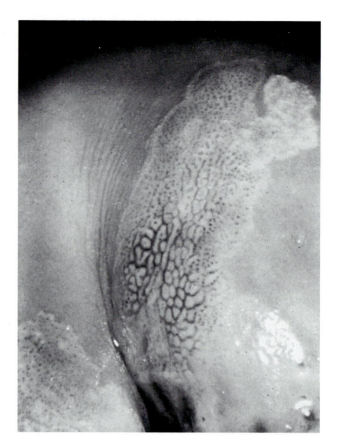

Figure 1-6 Punctation pattern clearly seen above a mosaic structure (colposcopic view).

in the diagnosis and evaluation of the cervix. Probably the greatest value of colposcopy is that in most instances a skilled colposcopist can establish and differentiate invasive cancer from CIN by direct biopsy and thus avoid the necessity of surgical conization of the cervix. This is especially valuable in the young nulliparous woman desirous of childbearing for whom cone biopsy of the cervix may result in problems of impaired fertility. The avoidance of conization also is valuable in reducing the risk to the patient from anesthesia and the additional surgical procedure with its prolonged hospitalization.

In all patients undergoing colposcopic examination, unless they are pregnant, an ECC should be performed, even if the entire lesion is seen. This gives objective proof of the absence of disease in the endocervical canal. It is believed that if the ECC had been done in several of the patients who had been reported in the literature as having invasive cancer diagnosed after outpatient therapy, the cancer would have been identified at an earlier time, and inappropriate therapy would not have been given.

ECC is performed from the internal os to the external os. The external os is the structure that is created by the opening of the bivalve speculum. A speculum as large as can be tolerated should be used to evaluate the patient with an abnormal Pap smear. During curettage it is best to curette the entire circumference of the canal without

removing the curette. This is done twice. Short, firm motions in a circumferential pattern are the most satisfactory. Patients will experience some discomfort early in the procedure, but rarely does the physician have to stop because of discomfort. It is desirable to obtain endocervical stroma in the specimen if possible. On completion of the curettage, all blood, mucous, and cellular debris must be collected and placed on a 2×2 absorbent paper towel. The material is then folded into a mound and, along with the absorbent paper towel, placed into fixative. If any neoplastic tissue is found by the pathologist in the curettings, the results are considered positive. Directed punch biopsies of the cervix are done after the curettage. Using the colposcopic findings as a guide, the physician obtains punch biopsy specimens with a Kervorkian-Younge cervical biopsy instrument (or a similar tool that contains a basket in which the biopsy specimen may be collected). Biopsy specimens also should be placed on a small piece of paper towel with proper orientation to minimize tangential sectioning of the specimen.

The goal of any evaluation of a patient with abnormal cervical cytologic findings is to rule out invasive cancer. Diagnostic studies may be done using outpatient facilities or may require hospitalization. No single diagnostic technique can effectively rule out invasive cancer in all

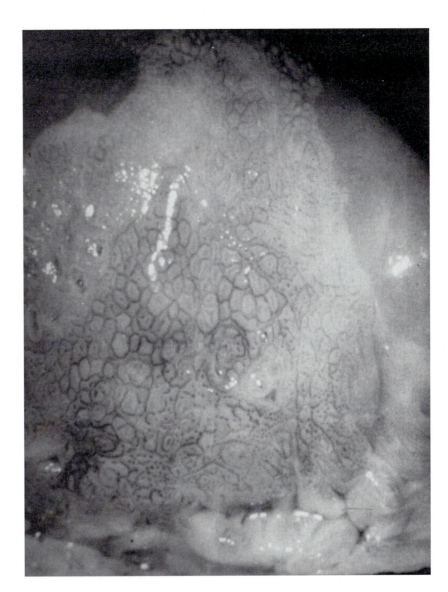

Figure 1-7 Large anterior lip lesion with white epithelium punctation and mosaic patterns.

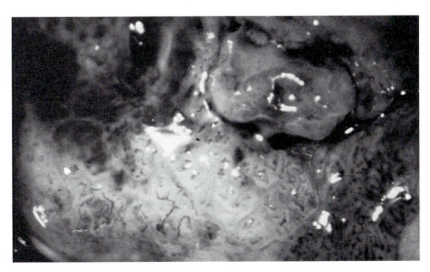

Figure 1-8 Many atypical ("corkscrew, hairpin") vessels indicative of early invasive cancer. (Courtesy Dr. Kenneth Hatch, Tucson, Arizona.)

patients but with multiple diagnostic procedures the risk of missing invasive cancer is essentially eliminated. Even conization of the cervix by itself can miss an invasive cancer. Therefore, cytologic screening, colposcopy, colposcopically directed biopsies, ECC, and pelvic examination must *all* rule out invasive cancer.

Under certain circumstances, conization is indicated, even after the full outpatient evaluation has been performed. Most important, if invasive cancer has not been ruled out by the outpatient evaluation, conization must be performed. Patients who have a positive ECC also require conization. If cytologic testing, biopsies, or colposcopic examination indicates microinvasive carcinoma of the cervix, conization must be performed to fully evaluate the extent of the invasion, which in turn determines appropriate therapy. The postmenopausal patient with abnormal cytologic findings frequently will require conization of the cervix because her lesion is usually located within the endocervical canal and cannot be adequately evaluated with outpatient techniques. The use of local estrogen for several days before colposcopy and biopsy in the postmenopausal patient will augment these diagnostic procedures tremendously.

In patients in whom conization must be done, colposcopy can aid in tailoring the conization to the individual's specific need. If the lesion extends widely onto the portio, the lateral extensions might be missed with a "standard" cone but would be included if colposcopically directed. Occasionally the disease will extend into the vaginal fornix, and colposcopy can identify this patient so that appropriate margins may be obtained. If, however, the concern is the endocervical canal, and the portio is clean, a narrow conization can be done to remove the endocervical canal only. The use of Lugol solution as a substitute for colposcopy to determine the extent of the disease on the cervix is inappropriate and can be misleading. Both false positive and false negative staining with Lugol solution can occur in identifying CIN. The application of Lugol solution may be helpful to evaluate the cervix and vagina before conization. The colposcopic lesion and the nonstaining area of the Lugol solution should match. Failure of matching indicates that appropriate adjustments must be made at the time of conization.

This evaluation schema permits triage of patients based on the colposcopic findings (plus the results of the colposcopically directed biopsies) and ECC findings. If the results of curettage of the canal are negative and only preinvasive neoplasia is found on directed biopsy, the patient has been adequately evaluated and treatment can begin. The method of therapy chosen depends on the patient's age, desire for fertility, and reliability for follow-up and on the histologic appearance and extent of her lesion. Cryosurgery using the double-freeze technique or destruction of the lesion with a laser beam can be performed in some patients who wish to retain their childbearing capacity but who have disease that is more extensive than can adequately be treated with a simple excisional biopsy in the office. Hysterectomy, either simple vaginal or abdominal, without preceding conization may be recommended for patients who desire sterilization. No effort is made in the performance of the hysterectomy to excise additional vaginal cuff unless there is evidence of abnormal epithelium extending to the vagina; this occurs in less than 3% of patients. A final possibility for treatment is to perform a shallow conization or ring biopsy of the cervix (see Figure 1-3).

As noted in the schema we have presented for evaluation of the abnormal Pap smear, ECC is performed on all nonpregnant patients. Diagnostic conization must be done when ECC shows malignant cells or when colposcopic examination is unsatisfactory (the entire lesion is not seen). Since curettage is performed from the internal os to the external os, the lesion that extends only slightly into the canal is often picked up by the curette, resulting in a number of false positive ECC results. Nonetheless, ECC should be performed on all patients unless they are pregnant; if errors are made, they should be made on the side of conization. Some physicians do not routinely perform ECC when the entire lesion is visible on the ectocervix. Although omitting this procedure may be appropriate for a few experienced colposcopists, its inclusion as a routine step will further reduce the chances of missing a lesion in the endocervix. On occasion a previously unsuspected adenocarcinoma of the endocervix will be diagnosed but even more frequently an early invasive squamous cell carcinoma will be uncovered.

In individuals in whom ECC findings are positive and the upper limits cannot be visualized, diagnostic conization must be performed to exclude or confirm invasive cancer. Care should be taken in performing conization to include a sufficient portion of the endocervical canal to rule out occult invasive disease high in the canal.

Colposcopic evaluation of the cervix in the patient with an abnormal cervical smear has dramatically altered the management of the patient afflicted during pregnancy. The schema previously outlined is closely followed in pregnancy, when the transformation zone is everted, making visualization of the entire lesion almost a certainty. Cone biopsy is rarely indicated during pregnancy. If punch biopsy suggests microinvasion, further evaluation is needed. In many instances, a "wedge" resection of the suspicious area will confirm the diagnosis of microinvasion, and conization is not necessary. If not, then cone biopsy to allow proper management should be seriously considered. Pregnant patients with a firm diagnosis of preinvasive or microinvasive disease of the cervix should be allowed to deliver vaginally, and further therapy can be tailored to their needs after delivery. The cervix is very vascular during pregnancy, so that avoiding cone biopsy is in the best interest of both mother and fetus. *Small* biopsies of the *most* colposcopically abnormal areas are recommended in an effort to minimize

---

TREATMENT OPTIONS FOR CIN	
Observations	Laser
Local excision	Cold coagulation
Electrocautery	LEEP
Cryosurgery	Conization
	Hysterectomy

---

bleeding in the diagnostic evaluation. When a patient is in the second or third trimester and colposcopic examination is negative for any suspicion of invasion, many colposcopists will defer all biopsies to the postpartum period. Lurain and Gallup reported on 131 pregnant patients with abnormal Pap smears managed in this manner with excellent results and no invasive cancers missed.

Treatment Options

Many treatment options are available to the patient today (see box above). Essentially all of these should be considered definitive. Decisions about the choice of therapy for CIN depend on many factors, including the patient's desire and the experiences of the physician involved. Probably the most compelling reasons for choosing an outpatient modality over inpatient surgery are the patient's age and desire for subsequent fertility. The recommendation that carcinoma in situ in a teenager or woman in her early twenties must be treated with a hysterectomy is outdated. Unfortunately, this type of therapy is the recommended treatment, and other alternatives, although quite effective, may not be explained to the patient. No therapy is 100% effective; the benefit/risk ratio to the patient should be explained so that she is fully informed, and a reasonable decision can be made concerning her therapy and well-being.

Observation in selected, highly individualized patients may be an option, particularly if the lesion is small and histologically of ASCUS and LGSIL. (See management schema in evaluation of abnormal smear section.) There are also patients who have a small lesion that may be completely removed with the biopsy forceps. Elimination of the disease with this technique has occurred in some patients, although there are some investigators who feel that the entire transformation zone should be destroyed. Obviously, the use of observation and local excision can be made only by the experienced physician and must be highly individualized, depending on the patient's needs, desires, and ability to be followed appropriately.

Outpatient management

Electrocautery. Several modalities of treatment for the CIN patient can be performed on an outpatient basis. If in fact these modalities are as effective as a surgical procedure accomplished in the operating room, the cost-effectiveness is of considerable importance. Electrocautery has been used for many years to eradicate cervical epithelium. It was fashionable historically to destroy the "abnormal" tissue found on the cervix after delivery. Actually, this was columnar epithelium, or the transformation zone of the cervix. Some uncontrolled studies suggest that electrocautery decreased the appearance of CIN lesions in patients so treated. Electrocautery has been shown to be effective in the treatment of CIN. The popularity of this treatment is more apparent in Europe and Australia than in the United States. In a small controlled study Wilbanks et al. showed that electrocautery was effective in destroying early CIN as compared with tetracycline vaginal suppositories with a control group of patients. Ortiz, Newton, and Tsai treated all forms of CIN with electrocautery. In CIN I and II lesions, no failures were noted. In CIN III disease, the failure rate was approximately 13%. Of interest is that the failure rate in patients with carcinoma in situ did not differ whether the glands were involved or not. All the patients were treated on an outpatient basis. Chanen and Rome have used this technique extensively in Australia. Table 1-3 illustrates the excellent results they reported. They treated more than 1700 patients, with a failure rate of only 3%. Cervical stenosis has not been a problem. Dilation and curettage (D&C) is done at the same time the electrocautery is performed. The patient is admitted to the hospital, and with her under anesthesia, electrocautery is performed in the operating room to burn the tissue deep enough to destroy disease that might be present in glands. Chanen and Rome believe this is necessary to obtain excellent results. Electrocautery, of course, is painful if the tissue is burned deeply. If a patient needs to be anesthetized to obtain these results, this negates any benefits that a lesser procedure than conization would obtain. The cost of hospitalization, even on an ambulatory service, would be considerably higher than outpatient treatment.

Cryosurgery. Considerable experience with cryosurgery has been obtained in the treatment of CIN. The side

Table 1-3   Conservative treatment for CIN

Method (based on single treatment)	Failures
Electrocoagulation*	47/1734 (2.7%)
Cryosurgery†	540/6143 (8.7%)
Laser‡	119/2130 (5.6%)
Cold coagulator§ (CIN III)	110/1628 (6.8%)
LEEP‖	95/2185 (4.3%)

*Chanen and Rome
†Richart and Townsend, Benedet et al.
‡Parashevadis
§Duncan
‖Bigrigg, Murdoch, and Luesky

effects of electrocautery, mainly pain during treatment, are not present with cryosurgery and thus it is an ideal outpatient modality as far as patient comfort is concerned.

Ample experience with cryosurgery has now been reported in the literature. In 1980 Charles and Savage reviewed the literature and reported the experience of 16 authors with approximately 3000 patients. The success rate was noted to be between 27% and 96%. Many factors accounted for the wide variation and results, including the experience of the operator, the number of patients treated, criteria established to determine a cure, as well as freezing techniques, equipment, and the refrigerant used. Subsequently, there have been several studies in the literature (see Table 1-3). Total failure for the entire group irrespective of the histologic grade was 8%. Results of cryosurgery are essentially the same as those reported for electrocautery, the advantage being that cryosurgery is essentially pain-free and is effectively performed on an outpatient basis.

Ample experience has been obtained in the long-term follow-up of patients who have been treated with cryosurgery. Richart et al. noted that the recurrence rate was less than 1% in almost 3000 patients with CIN who were treated with cryosurgery and followed for 5 years or longer. Almost half the recurrences were noted within the first year after cryosurgery and to a certain degree probably represent persistence and not true recurrence. No cases of invasive cancer have developed in these patients. The initial failure rate can be reduced even further by a "recycling" of the patient and appropriate retreatment with cryosurgery or some other outpatient modality. Townsend states that all of the failures in the CIN I category were re-treated successfully with cryosurgery, and the failure rate for the re-treated patients who failed the first treatment lowered the overall failure rate to 3% for CIN II and 7% for CIN III. Although the techniques of cryosurgery are simple, several important technical points must be kept in mind to have an optimal freeze. Carbon dioxide or nitrous oxide can be used as a refrigerant for cryosurgery. The larger "D" tank is preferred over the narrow "E" tank, particularly if cryosurgery is performed on several patients over a short time interval. The pressure in the smaller tank can drop because of the cooling in the gas even though there may be adequate volume within the tank. Pressure is of extreme importance in obtaining a satisfactory freeze. If the pressure drops below 40 kg/cm^2 during the freezing process, the treatment should be stopped, tanks changed, and the treatment begun again. A thin layer of water-soluble lubricant over the tip of the probe will allow a more uniform and rapid freeze of the cervix. This allows a better heat transfer mechanism to take place between the probe and cervix. This is particularly important in the woman who may have an irregular cervix, which is common in the parous patient. The probe chosen should cover the entire lesion, and a 4 to 5 mm ice-ball around

---

CRYOSURGERY TECHNIQUE

1. N$_2$O or CO$_2$
2. K-Y jelly on probe
3. Double freeze
   a. 4-5 mm ice-ball
   b. Thaw
   c. 4-5 mm ice-ball

---

the probe is required for an adequate freeze. This should be obtained within 1½ to 2 minutes with most cryosurgery units today. If the 4 to 5 mm ice-ball is not obtained within this time, equipment probably is functioning incorrectly and the problem needs to be identified. We prefer the double-freeze technique: the cervix is allowed to thaw for 4 to 5 minutes and is then refrozen using the same technique (see box above). There is usually a watery discharge for 10 to 14 days. The patient is instructed to refrain from intercourse and to use an external pad if necessary during the time of the watery discharge. She is then seen in 4 months for reevaluation with a Pap smear. If the Pap smear is positive, the abnormality may be a result of the healing process, and the Pap smear is then repeated in 4 to 6 weeks. If cytologic findings remain abnormal 6 months after cryosurgery, it must be considered that the cryosurgery was a failure and the patient should be reevaluated and re-treated.

Attention has been drawn to the fact that several patients have been reported to have invasive carcinoma of the cervix after cryosurgery. A report from Miami details eight patients who were treated by cryosurgery for various indications and subsequently were found to have invasive cancer. Only five of the patients had abnormal cervical cytologic findings, three had colposcopic examinations, two had colposcopically directed biopsies, and only one had endocervical curettage.

Townsend et al. reported on 66 similar patients of members of the Society of Gynecologic Oncologists. Again, inappropriate precryosurgery evaluation was noted in the majority of these patients. Invasive cancer has also been reported in patients treated with other outpatient modalities, again emphasizing the importance of proper evaluation before outpatient therapy, as has been previously stated and should be apparent.

Laser surgery. The term *laser* is an acronym for "*l*ight *a*mplification by *s*timulated *e*mission of *r*adiation." The carbon dioxide laser beam is invisible and is usually guided by a second laser that emits visible light. The energy of the laser is absorbed by water with a high degree of efficiency, and the tissue is destroyed principally by vaporization. The laser is mounted on a colposcope and the laser beam is directed under colposcopic control. Most instruments have a considerable power range and operate by pulse or continuous mode. The spot size may be fixed but usually can be varied. The amount of power delivered to the tissue depends on the spot size and the wattage. Since there is a high-efficiency laser beam absorption by the tissue, as well as the opportunity to precisely direct the beam, the laser is unique. It also has the ability to control the depth of destruction. Since the tissue is destroyed by vaporization, the base of destruction is clean, with little necrotic tissue and rapid healing. As experience is gained with this modality, changes in technique take place. Since the laser can precisely direct the beam, at first it was thought that only the abnormal area needed to be destroyed with the laser. This prevented the destruction of normal cervical tissue. With this technique, the failure rate was excessive, and, as a result, it was suggested that the entire transformation zone be destroyed. Masterson et al. noted that their change in technique from destroying the lesion to ablating the entire transformation zone did not appreciably increase their success rate. The depth of destruction appears to be important in that the failure rate was considerable when only minimal destruction (1 to 2 mm) was achieved. As the depth of destruction increased, the number of failures decreased. Most lasers now advocate the destruction to a depth of 5 to 7 mm. Burke, Lovell, and Antoniolo concluded that successful treatment was not related to the severity of the histologic grade or to the size of the lesion. A continuous beam gave a better result than an intermittent beam. The depth of destruction was important and must include the lamina propria. Involvement of the endocervical crypt did not preclude success (Table 1-4). Certain precautions must be taken while using the carbon dioxide laser to avoid the use of flammable agents, to protect the eyes with appropriate glasses, and to use nonreflective surfaces. As the beam is transferred, the tissue vaporizes, filling the vagina with smoke and steam, which are evacuated by a suction tube attached to the speculum. Complications with the laser include pain, which is greater than with cryosurgery but usually tolerable. Bleeding can be a problem, although spotting is more frequent than significant bleeding. Bleeding does increase as the depth of tissue destruction increases, and larger vessels may be reached with the laser beam. Since 5 to 7 mm of tissue is destroyed, increased bleeding probably will become more frequent.

Experience suggests two disadvantages to the laser that have not been experienced with cryosurgery. First, the process is more painful for the office patient than cryosurgery, and second, the destruction of all but the smallest of lesions requires much more time for both the patient and the physician. Although the data suggest that the laser is effective in destroying CIN, it appears to be no better than other available outpatient methods, and one must question the cost effectiveness of this modality in comparison to cryosurgery.

In 1983 Townsend and Richart reported a study by alternating cases randomly, insofar as possible, on the

---

Table 1-4 CO_2 laser vaporization—cervix

Instruments	CO_2 laser, colposcope, micro-manipulator
Power output	20-25 W
Power density	800-1400 W/CM^2
Spot size	1.5-2 mm diameter
Operating mode	Continuous
Depth of destruction	6-7 mm measured
Width of destruction	4-5 mm beyond visible lesion
Bleeding control	Defocus, power density: 800 W/CM^2
Anesthesia	May need paracervical block
Analgesia	Antiprostaglandins

---

basis of CIN histologic grade and lesion size to compare the efficacy of cryotherapy and carbon dioxide laser therapy. In their study 100 patients were treated with laser therapy and 100 patients were treated with cryotherapy. There were seven failures in the cryotherapy group and 11 failures in the group treated with carbon dioxide laser therapy. These authors found no significant differences in the cure rates between the two modalities. They did feel that "if the therapeutic results are equivalent, it is logical to choose the modality that provides an equivalent grade of care for the least possible cost, and, at least in an office setting, this would seem to favor cryotherapy over laser therapy."

In an evaluation by Parashevadis et al. of 2130 patients treated by laser, they noted failures were higher in women over 40 years of age and in those with CIN III. CIN III lesions accounted for 75% of the failures, whereas only 7% were originally CIN I. Three cases of invasive cancer were diagnosed within two years of laser therapy. There were 119 (5.6%) treatment failures. Of the failures, 18% had a second lesion detected colposcopically in the presence of negative cytology after laser therapy.

Cold coagulator. Duncan has reported experience with a SEMM cold coagulator in the treatment of CIN III. Over a 14-year period, 1628 women were treated, and the primary success rate was 95% at one year and 92% at five years, similar for all age groups. There were 226 pregnancies following therapy, and the rates for miscarriage, preterm, or operative delivery were not increased.

The cold coagulator essentially coagulates at a lower temperature (100° C). Therapy is performed by overlapping applications of the thermal probe so that the transformation zone and lower endocervix are destroyed. In most instances, 2 to 5 applications were required, taking less than 2 minutes (about 20 seconds per application).

The exact depth of destruction is difficult to accurately ascertain. Several investigators found destruction up to 4 mm. Certainly these data suggest that this depth of destruction is adequate in patients with CIN III lesions. If this is the case, one wonders why 6 to 7 mm of destruction is required for adequate therapy when laser therapy is used. Even in the hands of an experienced colposcopist, subsequent carcinomas were noted in this series, as with every other treatment used in outpatient management. Microinvasion was found in two patients, and invasive cancer was found in four. This technique is inexpensive, quick, and essentially pain-free, with very few side effects. Efficacy is excellent (see Table 1-3). One wonders why this technique has not been evaluated and used in the United States.

Loop electrosurgical excision procedure (LEEP). A new approach to an old instrument has come into recent vogue. If cryosurgery was the "in" treatment of the 1970s and laser surgery was the "in" treatment of the 1980s, it appears that the loop electrosurgical excision procedure (LEEP) will be the instrument of the 1990s (see box below). LEEP has gained a tremendous experience within a short time. After colposcopy and if the entire transformation zone is identified, it is excised with a low-voltage diathermy loop under local anesthesia. Usually less than 10 cc of local anesthesia, with epinephrine or vasopressin added to help decrease blood loss, is injected into the cervix at 12, 3, 6, and 9 o'clock. After 3 to 5 minutes, excision can be performed with a loop size that will excise the lesion in total.

An electrosurgical generator is used with wattage set at 25-50, depending on loop size (the larger the loop, the higher the wattage) and blended cut or coagulated. A disposable grounding plate is used, as in the O.R. The cutting loop consists of an insulated shaft with a wire loop attached. The sterilized steel wire is 0.2 mm in diameter and comes in various sizes. LEEP can be performed under colposcopy or after Lugol's application (and if it matches colposcopy findings) as a guide for excision. If Lugol's is used, saline should be applied to the cervix before LEEP, since Lugol's tends to dehydrate the tissue. Care should be taken to avoid the vaginal walls with the loop. A smoke

evacuator, used as with laser, is recommended. In some instances, the 1.5 cm loop is too small to remove the entire lesion and an additional "pass" or two is required to remove the remaining abnormal epithelium. Depth of the excised tissue varies, but 5-8 mm is the usual depth. This allows tissue for adequate evaluation. The base of the excised tissue is then coagulated with a ball electrode and Monsel's paste is applied.

There are several advantages to this technique. The procedure can be done on an outpatient basis. Tissue is available for study. Diagnosis and therapy are all done at one time and during the same visit. In essentially all large studies reported to date, several early invasive lesions were identified that had not been recognized on colposcopy examination. This technique tends to negate this inherent problem of destructive techniques.

Side effects mainly are secondary hemorrhage (initially reported at 10% but with experience found to be in the 1% to 2% range). Long-term effects such as those on pregnancy are not known; but one report noted 48 pregnancies in 1000 after LEEP. From this limited experience, it appears that pregnancies after LEEP are similar to those following laser vaporization or electrocoagulation.

Results of one large study of 1000 patients noted that 897 women were managed with only one visit. The other 103 required more than one visit, including nine women who had microinvasion or invasion. Cervical cytology at 4 months after treatment was performed in 969 women, and 41 (4.1%) were found to be abnormal. Of the nine women with invasion, only four were suspected on cervical smear and colposcopy (see Table 1-3).

LEEP appears to be the current treatment of choice even with very limited follow up for patients with abnormal cytology. It has been estimated that over 30,000 LEEPs have been performed in the United States. Several comments are probably in order. See, diagnose, and treat at one time has been popularized by some, particularly our European colleagues. In some instances, the LEEP has been used before colposcopy or other diagnostic procedures. As previously noted in its guidelines for management of abnormal cervical cytology, the NCI sponsored workshop stated "Routine electroexcision of the TZ of nonstaining areas as a method of evaluating a positive Pap smear diagnosed as LSIL or ASCUS is not recommended." The indiscriminate use of LEEP should not be condoned. In essentially all studies that have addressed the subject, as many as half of LEEP specimens show no epithelial abnormalities (most studies 15%-25% with negative histology). It appears that many patients with ASCUS or LGSIL on cytology are having LEEPs done that do not appear warranted. The see and treat fashion for patients with these degrees of abnormalities on Pap smears should not be encouraged.

Initially, it was said that LEEP caused stenosis, occurring in about 1% of cases. More recent data suggests

---

LEEP TECHNIQUE

1. Cervix colposcopied and lesion outlined
2. Patient grounded with pad return electrode
3. Inject anesthetic solution just beneath and lateral to the lesion (at excision site)
4. Turn on machine and set cut/blend to 25-50 watts (the larger the loop the higher wattage needed)
5. Set coagulation to 60 watts for ball electrode use
6. After adequate time for anesthesia to take effect, excise lesion using the LEEP
7. Coagulate base of cone even if no apparent bleeding
8. Place ferric subsulfate paste on base

that stenosis may be present four times greater than preliminary data suggested. This is still a low figure (comparable to cryosurgery and laser). LEEP does not appear to have an adverse affect on fertility or pregnancy outcome.

Preliminary data on large series suggested a low persistence/recurrence rate but follow-up was short—only 4 months in many patients. Bigrigg has subsequently reported a longer follow-up period in 250 women out of the original 1000 treated with LEEP. These patients during follow-up required 68 second treatments because of persistence or recurrence during their follow-up period.

Thermal artifact, although reported in series to be of minimal concern, in general practice is reported as about 10% of specimens as unreadable, and 20% to 40% have significant coagulation artifact. This is probably related to equipment power setting and technical problems such as "stalling." Bleeding is reported to occur in about 5% of cases mostly posttreatment. Strict adherence to protocol decreases this problem. LEEP done when significant vaginal infection is present will increase the chances of bleeding. In almost all large series, unanticipated microinvasive cancers have been diagnosed when the histologic specimen was evaluated. This has led some authors to suggest that LEEP could be used in place of cold knife conization for evaluation of patients in which cancer has not been ruled out. Murdoch noted that 44 of 1143 of LEEP specimens contained invasive cancer (18 stage IA, 17 stage IB, and 9 with stage IB adenocarcinoma). Thirty three (75%) of the patients had unsatisfactory or suspicious for cancer colposcopy. Two recent patients with invasion on their LEEP histology were treated with radical hysterectomies and lymphadenectomies because the LEEP histology was inadequate to guide less radical therapy. One of the patients had no evidence of cancer in the hysterectomy specimen. These authors feel that the LEEP should not be used in place of conization for this purpose.

Conization of the cervix. After the extent of involvement of epithelium on the ectocervix has been clearly demarcated by colposcopy, the limits of the base of the cone biopsy on the cervix can be determined. An incision that is certain to include all the abnormal areas is made into the mucous membrane of the ectocervix. Many believe that blood loss can be lessened by injecting a dilute solution of phenylephrine (Neo-Synephrine) or pitressin into the line of incision before beginning the procedure. This incision need not be circular but should accommodate excision of all atypical epithelium. The depth of the incision as it tapers toward the endocervical canal should be determined by the length of the cervical canal and the suspected depth of involvement (Figure 1-9). Many times the entire limits of the lesion have been visualized, and a very shallow conization is sufficient (Figure 1-10). Cervical conization need not be a fixed technical procedure for all patients but it should always be

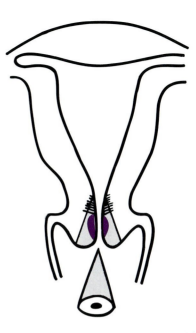

Figure 1-9 Cone biopsy for endocervical disease. Limits of the lesion were not seen colposcopically.

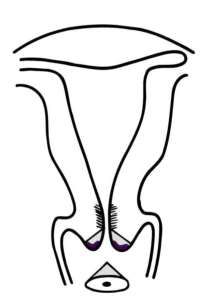

Figure 1-10 Cone biopsy for CIN of the exocervix. Limits of the lesion were identified colposcopically.

an adequate excision of all involved areas. Bleeding from the cone bed can usually be controlled by electrocauterization and placing Monsel on the base. The use of Sturmdorf sutures are probably unnecessary in most cases. Significant cervical stenosis, cervical incompetence, or infertility with a cervical factor are rare complications (Table 1-5) and are functions of the amount of endocervix removed. Several physicians advocate the use of the laser as a cervical tool instead of the knife in conization of the cervix (Table 1-6).

Table 1-5   Major complications of conization

Immediate	Delayed
Hemorrhage	Bleeding (10-14 days after operation)
Uterine perforation	Cervical stenosis
Anesthetic risk	Infertility
In pregnancy:	Incompetent cervix
Rupture of membranes	Increased preterm delivery (low birth weight)
Premature labor	

Table 1-6   CO$_2$ laser conization

Instruments	CO$_2$ laser, colposcope, micro-manipulator
Power output	25-30 W
Power density	1400 W/CM^2
Spot size	0.5 mm
Operating mode	Continuous
Lateral margins	5 mm beyond lesion
Endocervical margin	Surgically cut
Hemostasis	Lateral sutures, Pitressin infiltration
Anesthesia	General, local

Several studies have now shown that blood loss, infection, and stenosis in laser conization are essentially equal to those occurring in cold knife conization. Some have suggested there is less dysmenorrhea after laser conization. Complication rates, at least in one study, were equal when laser vaporization was compared to laser conization. Complications after an open cone procedure appear to be similar to those managed with a closed cone procedure (Sturmdorf or other suturing). Although it has been stated that laser does not distort the cervical margins in regard to pathological evaluation, a recent article suggests this is not the case. The authors reviewed 77 laser conizations, and 28 (36%) showed extensive epithelial denudization, 10 (13%) contained coagulation artifact that made recognition of CIN extremely difficult or impossible, and 11 (14%) showed laser artifacts that made assessment of margins extremely difficult or impossible.

As has already been indicated, in the United States conization of the cervix is used primarily as a diagnostic tool and secondarily as therapy for patients who are young and desire further fertility. However, in other countries conization is used as definitive therapy. Extensive experience has been obtained with this operative modality, particularly in the treatment of severe CIN.

In Europe (especially Scandinavia) conization has been widely used to treat patients with CIN, and some

Table 1-7   Conization and hysterectomy as treatment for CIS

	Persistence CIS	or	Recurrence cancer
Conization (N = 3103)	6.3%		0.6%
Hysterectomy (N = 3729)	0.9%		0.3%

From Boyes, Creasman, Kolstad, Bjerre.

interesting data have been published. Bjerre et al. reported on 2099 cases of women with abnormal vaginal smears in whom conization of the cervix had been performed. The frequency of complications was considered low, and cervical carcinoma in situ was diagnosed in 1500 cases. Conization appeared to be curative in 87% of these 1500 cases. Failure was related to whether the margins of resection were free of pathologic epithelium. If Pap smears were repeatedly negative for the first year after conization, subsequent abnormal smears were found in only 0.4% of the cases. Kolstad and Klem reported on a series of 1121 patients with carcinoma in situ who had been followed for 5 to 25 years. Therapeutic conization had been performed on 795 of these patients, of which 19 (2.3%) had recurrent carcinoma in situ and 7 (0.9%) developed invasive cancer. The corresponding figures for 238 patients treated by hysterectomy were, respectively, 3 (1.2%) and 5 (2.1%). The invasive lesions noted appeared several years later, and the type of initial procedure had no significant influence. Kolstad and Klem stressed that women who have had carcinoma in situ of the cervix will always be at some risk and therefore should be carefully followed for a much longer period than the conventional 5 years (Table 1-7).

If conization has ruled out invasive cancer, those with free surgical margins have almost a 100% disease-free follow-up. The question frequently asked is what should management be post cone if surgical margins, particularly the endocervical, has disease present? Considerable data in the literature suggest the vast majority will have normal cytology post cone and no further treatment is necessary. Anderson noted 58 patients with positive surgical margins and only three (5%) had persistent disease. Lopes noted in 75 similar patients that nine 9 (12%) had residual disease. Grundsell found 3 of 21 patients with positive margins with residual disease. Our practice is to follow up all post cone patients with cytology only irrespective of surgical margin status and intervene only if cytology is abnormal.

Hysterectomy. Traditionally in the United States a vaginal hysterectomy has been the treatment of choice for patients with carcinoma in situ. This was particularly true before the establishment of reliable outpatient diagnostic techniques. Hysterectomy remains a popular and accepted method of management. It is an appropriate method of treatment for the CIN patient who has completed her childbearing, is interested in permanent sterilization, and has other pathology in which hysterectomy is indicated. This decision must be made jointly by the patient, her family, and the physician. For many years the removal of the upper part of the vagina has been advocated in the treatment of carcinoma in situ, yet there is no basis for this recommendation. In a study by Creasman and Rutledge, the recurrence rate for carcinoma in situ of the cervix did not depend on the amount of vagina removed with the

uterus. Unless vaginal extension of disease can be identified colposcopically (this occurrence is less than 5%), there is no reason for routine removal of the upper vagina. There appears to be no reason for so-called modified radical hysterectomy in the management of patients with CIN. It must be remembered, however, that even though hysterectomy is considered definitive therapy, patients must be followed in essentially the same manner as patients chosen for outpatient management. Although the chance of subsequent recurrence of invasive disease is small, recurrence can occur, and these patients must be followed indefinitely.

BIBLIOGRAPHY

Epidemiology and natural history

Ashley DJB: The biological status of carcinoma in situ of the uterine cervix, *J Obstet Gynaecol Br Commonw* 73:372, 1966.

Bauer HM, Ting Y, Greer CE et al: Genital human papilloma virus infection in female university studies as determined by a PCR-based method, *JAMA* 265:472, 1991.

Beral V: Cancer of the cervix; a sexually transmitted infection? *Lancet* 1:1037, 1974.

Bower M: Women's knowledge, attitudes and behavior toward Pap screening, National Omnibus Survey Findings, *The Female Patient* 18:21, 1993.

Brinton LA, Fraumeni JF: Epidemiology of uterine cervical cancer, *J Chron Dis* 39:1051, 1986.

Butterworth CE, Hatch KD, Macaluso M et al: Folate deficiency and cervical dysplasia, *JAMA 267-528, 1992.*

Catalano LW Jr, Johnson LD: Herpesvirus antibody and carcinoma in situ of the cervix, *JAMA* 217:447, 1971.

CDC: Sexually transmitted disease guidelines, *MMWR* 42:90, 1993.

Champion MJ et al: Increased risk of cervical neoplasia in consorts: men with penile condyloma accuminata, *Lancet* 1:943, 1985.

Champion MJ et al: Progressive potential of mild cervical atypia: perspective cytologic, colposcopic and virological studies, *Lancet* 2:273, 1986.

Cohen AL, Rosenberg AJ, McCann MF: Active and passive cigerette smoke exposure and cervical neoplasia, *Ca Epid Biomark and Prev* 1:349, 1992.

Coppleson LW, Brown B: Observations on a model of the biology of carcinoma of the cervix: a poor fit between observation and theory, *Am J Obstet Gynecol* 122:127, 1975.

Coppleson LW, Brown B: The prevention of carcinoma of the cervix, *Am J Obstet Gynecol* 125:153, 1976.

Coppleson M, Pixley E, Reid B: *Colposcopy: a scientific and practical approach to the cervix in health and disease,* Springfield, Ill, 1971, Charles C Thomas.

Coppleson M, Reid B: The etiology of squamous carcinoma of the cervix, *Obstet Gynecol* 32:432, 1968 (editorial).

Cramer DW, Cutler SJ: Incidence and histopathology of malignancies of the female genital organs in the United States, *Am J Obstet Gynecol* 118:443, 1974.

Diagnostic and Therapeutic Technology Assessment (DATTA), *JAMA* 270-2975, 1993.

Fenoglio CM: Viruses in the pathogenesis of cervical neoplasia: an update, *Hum Pathol* 13:785, 1982.

Fenoglio CM, Ferenczy A: Etiologic factors in cervical neoplasia, *Sem Oncol* 9:349, 1982.

Fenoglio CM et al: Herpes simplex virus and cervical neoplasia. In Fenoglio CM, Wolff M, editors: *Progress in Surgical Pathology,* vol 45, New York, 1981, Masson.

Fletcher A: Screening for cancer of the cervix in elderly women, *Lancet* 335:97, 1990.

Fluhmann CF: Carcinoma in situ and the transitional zone of the cervix uteri, *Obstet Gynecol* 16:424, 1960.

Gaarenstoom KN, Melkert P, Walboomers JMM et al: Human papillomavirus DNA and genotypes: prognostic factors for progression of CIN, *Int J Gynecol Cancer* 4:73, 1994.

Gagnon F: The lack of occurrence of cervical carcinoma in nuns, *Proc Second Natl Cancer Conf* 1:625, 1952.

Goff BA, Muntz HG, Bell DA et al: Human papillomavirus typing in patients with Pap smears showing squamous atypia, *Gynecol Onc* 48:384, 1993.

Grussendorf-Conen EI, de Villiers EM, Gissmann L: Human papilloma virus genomes in penile smears of healthy men, *Lancet* 2:1092, 1986.

Harlan LC, Bernstein AB, Kessler LG: Cervical cancer screening: who is not screened and why? *Am J Pub Health* 81:885, 1991.

Hatch KD, Schneider A, Abdel-Nour MW: An evaluation of HPV testing for intermediate and high-risk types as triage before colposcopy, *Am J Obstet Gynecol* 172-1150, 1995.

Jenison SA, Yu X, Valentine JM et al: Evidence of prevalent genital-type human papillomavirus infection in adults and children, *J Infect Dis* 162:60, 1990.

Johnson JC, Burnett AF, Willet GD et al: High frequency of latent and clinical HPV cervical infections in immunocompromised HIV infected women, *Obstet Gynecol* 79:321, 1992.

Kessis TD, Siebos RJ, Nelson WG: Human papillomavirus 16 E6 expression disrupts the p-53 mediated cellular response to DNA damage, *Proc Natl Acad Sci USA* 90:3988, 1993.

Kessler II: Cervical cancer epidemiology in historical perspective, *J Reprod Med* 12:173, 1974.

Kjaer SK, deVilliers EM, Haugaard BJ et al: Human papillomavirus, herpes simplex virus and cervical cancer incidence in Greenland and Denmark: a population-based cross-sectional study, *Int J Cancer* 41:518, 1988.

Knox EG: Ages and frequencies for cervical cancer screening, *Br J Cancer* 34:444, 1976.

Kurman RJ, Schiffman MH, Lancaster WED et al: Analysis of individual human papillomavirus types in cervical neoplasia: a possible role for type 18 in rapid progression, *Am J Obstet Gynecol* 159:293, 1988.

Ley C, Bauer HM, Reingold A et al: Determinants of genital human papillomavirus infection in young women, *J Natl Cancer Inst* 83:997, 1991.

Maiman M: Cervical neoplasia in women with HIV infection, *Oncol* 8:83, 1994.

Meanwell CA, Cox MF, Blackledge GB et al: HPV 16 DNA in normal and malignant cervical epithelium: implications for the aetiology and behaviour of cervical neoplasia, *Lancet* 1:266, 1987.

Meyskens FL, Surrvit E, Moon TE et al: Enhancement of regression of CIN II with topically applied all-transretinoic acid, *J Natl Cancer Inst* 86:539, 1994.

Mitchell H, Drake N, Medley G: Prospective evaluation of risks of cervical cancer after cytologic evidence of human papilloma virus infection, *Lancet* 1:573, 1986.

Moscicki AB, Palefsky J, Smith et al: Variability of human papillomavirus DNA testing in a longitudinal cohort of young women, *Obstet Gynecol* 82:578, 1993.

Munger K, Scheffra M, Huibregtse JM et al: Interaction of HPV E6 and E7 with tumor suppressor gene products, *Cancer Surv* 12:197, 1992.

Munoz N, Bosch X, Kaldor JM: Does human papillomavirus cause cervical cancer? The state of the epidemiological evidence, *Br J Cancer* 57:1, 1988.

Murphy WM, Coleman SA: The long-term course of carcinoma in situ of the uterine cervix, *Cancer* 38:957, 1976.

Ng A: Presidential address, *Acta Cytol* 22:121, 1978.

Ng A: Current status of practice and training in cytology. I. A survey of the practice of cytology in anatomic pathology laboratories, *Am J Clin Pathol* 73:202, 1980.

Okagaki T Tase T, Twiggs LB et al: Histogenesis of cervical adenocarcinoma with reference to HPV 18 as a carcinogen, *J Reprod Med* 34: 639, 1989.

Palefsky JM: Human papillomavirus-associated anogenital neoplasia and other solid tumors in HIV infected individuals, *Curr Opin Oncol* 3:881, 1991.

Peterson O: Spontaneous course of cervical precancerous conditions, *Am J Obstet Gynecol* 72:1063, 1956.

Pinion SB, Kennedy JH, Miller RW et al: Oncogene expression in cervical intraepithelial neoplasia and invasive cancer of cervix, *Lancet* 337:819, 1991.

Rahan T, Mann V, McLaughlin J et al: PCR-detected genital papillomavirus infection: prevalence and association with risk factors for cervical cancer, *Int J Cancer* 49:856, 1991.

Rawls WE et al: Herpesvirus type cryosurgery: association with carcinoma of the cervix, *Science* 161:1255, 1968.

Reeves WC, Brinton LA, Garcia M et al: Human papillomavirus infection and cervical cancer in Latin America, *N Eng J Med* 320:1437, 1989.

Reeves WC, Rawls WE, Brinton LA: Epidemiology of genital papillomaviruses and cervical cancer, *Rev of Inf Diseases* 11:426, 1989.

Reid BL et al: Sperm basic proteins in cervical carcinogenesis: correlation with socioeconomic class, *Lancet* 2:60, 1978.

Richart RM: Natural history of cervical intraepithelial neoplasia, *Clin Obstet Gynecol* 10:748, 1968.

Rosenfeld WD, Rose E, Vermund SH et al: Follow up evaluation of cervicovaginal human papillomavirus in adolescents, *J Pediatrics* 121:307, 1992.

Sedlacek TV, Sedlacek AE, Neff DK et al: Clinical role of human papillomavirus typing, *Gynecol Onc* 42:222, 1991.

Simmons AM, Phillips DH, Coleman DV: Damage to DNA in cervical epithelium related to smoking tobacco, *Brit Med J* 306:1444, 1993.

Spinillo A, Tenti P, Zappatoe R et al: Prevalence, diagnosis, and treatment of lower genital neoplasia in women with HIV infection, *Eur J Obstet Gynecol Reprod Biol* 43:235, 1992.

Sun XW, Ellerbrock TV, Lungu O et al: Human papillomavirus infections in HIV seropositive women, *Obstet Gynecol* 85:680, 1995.

Tidy JA, Parry GCN, Ward P et al: High rate of human papillomavirus type 16 infection in cytologically normal cervices, *Lancet* 1:434, 1989.

Trevathan E, Loyde P, Webster LA et al: Cigarette smoking and dysplasia in carcinoma in situ of the uterine cervix, *JAMA* 250:499, 1983.

de Villiers EM: Heterogeneity of the human papillomavirus group, *J Virol* 63:4898, 1989.

de Villiers EM, Wagner D, Schneider A et al: Human papilloma virus DNA in women without and with cytological abnormalities: results of a five-year follow up study, *Gynecol Oncol* 44:33, 1992.

Vonka V, Kanka J, Hirsch I et al: Perspective study on the relationship between cervical neoplasia and herpes simplex type II virus. II. Herpes simplex type II antibody present in serum taken at enrollment, *Int J Cancer* 33:61, 1984.

Walker J, Bloss JD, Liao SY et al: Human papillomavirus genotype as a prognostic indicator in carcinoma of the uterine cervix, *Obstet Gynecol* 74:781, 1989.

Wright TC, Ellerbrock TV, Chiasson MA et al: CIN in women infected with HIV; prevalence, risk factors, and validity of Pap smears, *Obstet Gynecol* 84:591, 1994.

Zunzunegui MV, King MC, Coria CF et al: Male influence on cervical cancer risks, *Am J Epidemiol* 123:302, 1986.

zur Hausen H: Human papillomaviruses in the pathogenesis of anogenital cancers, *Virology* 184:9, 1991.

zur Hausen H, Meinhof W, Scheiber Wand Born Kamm EW: Attempts to detect virus-specific DNA in human tumors. I. Nucleic acid hybridizations with complementary RNA of human wart virus, *Int J Cancer* 13:650, 1974.

Screening and diagnosis

Bethesda Workshop: The revised Bethesda System for reporting cervical/vaginal cytologic diagnosis: report of the 1991 Bethesda Workshop, *J Reprod Med* 37:383, 1992.

Calle EE, Flander D, Thun MJ: Demographic predictors of mammography and Pap smear screening in US women, *Am J Pub Health* 83:53, 1993.

Coppleson LW, Brown B: Estimation of the screening error rate from the observed detection rates in repeated cervical cytology, *Am J Obstet Gynecol* 119:953, 1974.

Coppleson M, Pixley E, Reid B: *Colposcopy: a scientific and practical approach to the cervix in health and disease*, Springfield, Ill, 1971 Charles C Thomas.

Davis GL, Hernandez E, Davis JL et al: Atypical squamous cells in Papanicolaou smears, *Obstet Gynecol* 69:43, 1987.

Delgado G, Smith JP: Diagnosis of cervical neoplasia by the nonspecialized colposcopist, *Gynecol Oncol* 3:114, 1975.

DePetrillo AD et al: Colposcopic evaluation of the abnormal Papanicolaou test in pregnancy, *Am J Obstet Gynecol* 121:441, 1975.

Ferenczy A: Screening for cervical cancer: a renewed plea for annual smears, *Contemporary Ob/Gyn* 93, 1986.

Gad C, Koch F: The limitation of screening effect; a review of cervical disorders in previously screened women, *Acta Cytol* 21:719, 1978.

Galliher HP: *Optimal ages for Pap smear using a multistrains model for cervical cancer*, Detroit, 1977, Michigan Cancer Foundation.

Gray LA, Christopherson WM: Treatment of cervical dysplasia, *Gynecol Oncol* 3:149, 1975.

Harlan LC, Bernstein AB, Kessler LE: Cervical cancer screening: who is not and why? *Am J Pub Health* 81:885, 1991.

Himmelstein LR: Evaluation of inflammatory atypia: a literature review, *J Reprod Med* 34:634, 1989.

Hoffman MS, Hill DA, Gordy LW et al: Comparing the yield of the standard Papanicolaou brush smears, *J Reprod Med* 36:267, 1991.

Janerich DT, Hadjimichael O, Schwartz PE: The screening histories of women with invasive cervical cancer, Connecticut, *Am J Pub health* 85:791, 1995.

Kaminski PE, Stevens CW, Wheelock JB: Squamous atypia on cytology: the influence of age, *J Reprod Med* 9:617, 1989.

Kohan S et al: Colposcopy and the management of cervical intraepithelial neoplasia, *Gynecol Oncol* 5:27, 1977.

Kolstad P, Klem V: Long-term followup of 1121 cases of carcinoma in situ, *Obstet Gynecol* 48:125, 1976.

Kristensen GB, Jensen LK, Holund B: A randomized trial comparing two methods of cold knife conization with laser conization, *Obstet Gynecol* 76:1009, 1990.

Larsson G, Gullberg BO, Grundsell H: A comparison of complications of laser and cold knife conization, *Obstet Gynecol* 62:213, 1983.

Maier RC, Schultenover SJ: Evaluation of the atypical squamous cell Papanicolaou smear, *Int J Gynecol Pathol* 5:242, 1986.

Mandelblatt J, Gopaul FNP, Wistreich M: Gynecological care of elderly women, *JAMA* 256:367, 1986.

Mitchell H, Medley G: Longitudinal study of women with negative cervical smears according to endocervical status, *Lancet* 337:265, 1991.

Morrison BW, Erickson ER, Doshi N et al: The significance of atypical cervical smears, *J Reprod Med* 35:809, 1988.

NCI Workshop: The 1988 Bethesda System for reporting cervical/vaginal cytological diagnoses, *JAMA* 262:931, 1989.

Reiter RC: Management of initial atypical cervical cytology: a randomized prospective study, *Obstet Gynecol* 68:237, 1986.

Roongpisuthipone A, Grimes DA, Hodges A: Is the Papanicolaou smear useful for diagnosing sexually transmitted disease? *Obstet Gynecol* 69:820, 1987.

Shingleton HM, Gore H, Austin JM Jr: Outpatient evaluation of patients with atypical Papanicolaou smears; contribution of endocervical curettage, *Am J Obstet Gynecol* 126:122, 1976.

Spitzer M, Krumholz BA, Chernys AE et al: Comparative utility of repeat Papanicolaou smears, cervicography, and colposcopy in the evaluation of atypical Papanicolaou smears, *Obstet Gynecol* 69:731, 1987.

Stafl A, Mattingly RF: Colposcopic diagnosis of cervical neoplasia, *Obstet Gynecol* 41:168, 1973.

Urcuyo R, Rome RM, Nelson J: Some observations on the value of endocervical curettage performed as an integral part of colposcopic examination of patients with abnormal cervical cytology, *Obstet Gynecol* 128:787, 1977.

Walton RJ: The task force on cervical cancer screening programs, editorial, *Can Med Assoc J* 114:981, 1976.

Walton RJ (Chairman): Cervical cancer screening programs: summary of the 1982 Canadian Task Force Report, *Can Med Assoc J* 127:581, 1982.

Wilbanks GD et al: Treatment of cervical dysplasia with electro-cautery and tetracycline suppositories, *Am J Obstet Gynecol* 117:460, 1973.

Worth A: The Walton report and its subsequent impact on cervical cancer screening programs in Canada, *Obstet Gynecol* 63:135, 1984.

Pathology and cytology

Al-Nafassi AI, Calquhoun MK, Williams ARW: Accuracy of cervical smear in predicting the grade of cervical intraepithelial neoplasia, *Int J Gynecol Cancer* 3:89, 1993.

Bellina JH, Seto YJ: Pathological and physical investigations into CO_2 laser-tissue interactions with specific emphasis of cervical intraepithelial neoplasia, *Lasers Surg Med* 1:47, 1980.

Coppleson LW, Brown B: Estimation of the screening error rate from the observed detection rates in repeated cervical cytology, *Am J Obstet Gynecol* 119:953, 1974.

Cramer DW, Cutler SJ: Incidence and histopathology of malignancies of the female genital organs in the United States, *Am J Obstet Gynecol* 118:443, 1974.

Fluhmann CF: Carcinoma in situ and the transitional zone of the cervix uteri, *Obstet Gynecol* 16:424, 1960.

Friedell GH, Hertig AT, Younge PA: *Carcinoma in situ of the uterine cervix,* Springfield, Ill, 1960, Charles C Thomas.

Kurman RJ, Henson DE, Herbst AL et al: Interim guidelines for management of abnormal cervical cytology, *JAMA* 271:1866, 1994.

Lonky NM, Navarre EL, Saunder S et al: Lowgrade Pap smears and The Bethesda System: a prospective cytohistopathologic analysis, *Obstet Gynecol* 85:716, 1995.

Roongpisuthipone A, Grimes DA, Hodges A: Is the Papanicolaou smear useful for diagnosing sexually transmitted disease? *Obstet Gynecol* 69:820, 1987.

Shingleton HM, Gore H, Austin JM Jr: Outpatient evaluation of patients with atypical Papanicolaou smears; contribution of endocervical curettage, *Am J Obstet Gynecol* 126:122, 1976.

Taylor RR, Guerrieri JP, Nash JD et al: Atypical cervical cytology, *J Reprod Med* 38:443, 1993.

Wright TC, Sun XLO, Koulos J: Comparison of management algorithms for the evaluation of women with low-grade cytologic abnormalities, *Obstet Gynecol* 85:202, 1995.

Management

Ahlgren M et al: Conization as treatment of carcinoma in situ of the uterine cervix, *Obstet Gynecol* 46:135, 1975.

Anderson B: Management of early cervical neoplasia, *Clin Obstet Gynecol* 20:815, 1977.

Anderson ES, Nielson K, Larsen G: Laser conization: follow up in patients with CIN in the cone margin, *Gynecol Onc* 39:328, 1990.

Anderson MC: Treatment of cervical intraepithelial neoplasia with the carbon dioxide laser: report of 543 patients, *Obstet Gynecol* 59:720, 1982.

Baggish MS: High-power density carbon dioxide laser therapy for early cervical neoplasia, *Am J Obstet Gynecol* 136:117, 1980.

Baggish MS: Management of cervical intraepithelial neoplasia by carbon dioxide laser, *Obstet Gynecol* 60:378, 1992.

Baggish MS, Barash F, Noel Y et al: Comparison of thermal injury zones in loop electrical and laser cervical excisional conization, *Am J Obstet Gynecol* 166:545, 1991.

Bellina JH, Seto YJ: Pathological and physical investigations into CO_2 laser-tissue interactions with specific emphasis on cervical intraepithelial neoplasia, *Lasers Surg Med* 1:47, 1980.

Bellina JH et al: Carbon dioxide laser management of cervical intraepithelial neoplasia, *Am J Obstet Gynecol* 141:828, 1981.

Benedet JL, Nickerson KG, Anderson GH: Cryotherapy in the treatment of cervical intraepithelial neoplasia, *Obstet Gynecol* 58:72, 1981.

Berget A, Andreasson B, Bock JE: Laser and cryosurgery for CIN, *Acta Obstet Gynecol Scand* 70:231, 1991.

Bigrigg MA, Haffenden DK, Sheehan AL et al: Efficacy and safety of large-loop excision of the TZ, *Lancet* 343:32, 1994.

Bigrigg MA, Codling BW, Pearson P et al: Colposcopic diagnosis and treatment of cervical dysplasia at a single clinic visit, *Lancet* 336:229, 1990.

Bigrigg MA, Codling BW, Pearson P et al: Pregnancy after cervical loop diathermy, *Lancet* 337:119, 1991.

Bjerre B et al: Conization as only treatment of carcinoma in situ of the uterine cervix, *Am J Obstet Gynecol* 125:143, 1976.

Boyes DA, Worth AS, Fidler HK: The results of treatment of 4389 cases of preclinical squamous carcinoma, *J Obstet Gynaecol BR Commonw* 77:769, 1970.

Burke H, Lovell L, Antoniolo D: Carbon dioxide laser therapy of cervical intraepithelial neoplasia: factors determining success rate, *Lasers Surg Med* 1:113, 1980.

Burke L: The use of the carbon dioxide laser in the therapy of cervical intraepithelial neoplasia, *Am J Obstet Gynecol* 144:337, 1982.

Campion FM, diPaola ML, Campion MM et al: Cervical intraepithelial neoplasia—should we treat the male partner? *The Colposcopist* 23:5, 1991.

Carter R et al: Treatment of CIN with the CO_2 laser beam, *Am J Obstet Gynecol* 131:831, 1979.

Chanen W, Hollyock VE: Colposcopy and the conservative management of cervical dysplasias and carcinoma in situ, *Obstet Gynecol* 43:527, 1974.

Chanen W, Rome RM: Electrocoagulation diathermy for cervical dysplasia and carcinoma in situ: a 15-year survey, *Obstet Gynecol* 61:673, 1983.

Charles EH, Savage EW: Cryosurgical treatment of CIN, *Obstet Gynecol Surg* 35:539, 1980.

Coppleson M, Reid B: *Preclinical carcinoma of the cervis uteri: its nature, origin, and mangement,* New York, 1967, Pergamon Press.

Creasman WT, Clarke-Pearson DL, Weed JC Jr: Results of outpatient therapy of cervical intraepithelial neoplasia, *Gynecol Oncol* 12:S-306, 1981.

Creasman WT, Parker RT: Management of early cervical neoplasia, *Clin Obstet Gynecol* 18:233, 1975.

Creasman WT, Rutledge F: Carcinoma in situ of the cervix: an analysis of 861 patients, *Obstet Gynecol* 39:373, 1972.

Creasman WT, Weed JC Jr: Conservative management of cervical intraepithelial neoplasia, *Clin Obstet Gynecol* 43:281, 1980.

Creasman WT et al: Efficacy of cryosurgical treatment of severe cervical intraepithelial neoplasia, *Obstet Gynecol* 41:501, 1973.

DiSaia PJ, Townsend DE, Morrow CP: The rationale for less than radical treatment for gynecologic malignancy in early reproductive years, *Obstet Gynecol Surv* 29:581, 1974.

Gordon HK, Duncan ID: Effective destruction of cervical intraepithelial neoplasia (CIN)3 at 100° C using the Semm cold coagulator: 14 years experience, *Br J Obstet Gynaecol* 98:14, 1991.

Gray LA, Christopherson WM: Treatment of cervical dysplasia, *Gynecol Oncol* 3:149, 1975.

Grundsell H, Alan P, Larson G: Cure rates after laser conization for early cervical neoplasia, *Ann Chir Gynecol* 72:218, 1983.

Hal R, Hammond R, Pryse-Davies J: Histologic reliability of laser cone biopsy of the cervix, *Obstet Gynecol* 77:905, 1991.

Hitchcock A, Johnson J, McDowell K et al: A retrospective study into the occurrence of cervical glandular atypia in cone specimen from 1977-78 with clinical follow up, *Int J Gynecol Cancer* 3:164, 1993.

Javaheri G, Balin M, Meltzer RM: Role of cryosurgery in the treatment of intraepithelial neoplasia of the uterine cervix, *Obstet Gynecol* 58:83, 1981.

Kaufman RH, Irwin JF: The cryosurgical therapy of cervical intraepithelial neoplasia, *Am J Obstet Gynecol* 131:381, 1978.

Kolstad P, Klem V: Long-term followup of 1121 cases of carcinoma in situ, *Obstet Gynecol* 48:125, 1976.

Lopes A, Morgan P, Murdoch J et al: The case of conservative management of "incomplete excision" of CIN after laser conization, *Gynecol Onc* 49:247, 1993.

Luesky DM, Cullimore J, Redman CWE et al: Loop diathermy excision of the cervical transformation zone in patients with abnormal cervical smears, *Br Med J* 300:1090, 1990.

Lurain JR, Gallup DG: Management of abnormal Papanicolaou smears in pregnancy, *Obstet Gynecol* 53:484, 1979.

Maiman M, Tarricone N, Vieria J et al: Colposcopic evaluation of human immunity virus seropositive women, *Obstet Gynecol* 78:84, 1991.

Masterson BJ et al: The carbon dioxide laser in cervical intraepithelial neoplasia: a five-year experience in treating 230 patients, *Am J Obstet Gynecol* 139:565, 1981.

Masterson JG: Analysis of untreated intraepithelial carcinoma of the cervix, *Proceedings of the Third National Cancer Conference*, Philadelphia, 1957, JB Lippincott.

Muntz HG: Can ACIS be satisfactorily managed by conization alone? *Gynecol Oncol* 61:303, l996.

Muntz HG, Bell DA, Loge JM et al: Adenocarinoma in situ of the uterine cervix, *Obstet Gynecol* 80:935, 1992.

Murdoch JB, Gishane RN, Monaghan JM: Loop diathermy excision of the abnormal cervical transformation zone, *Int J Gynecol Cancer* 1:1105, 1991.

Murdoch JB, Grimshaw RN, Morgan PR et al: The impact of loop diathermy on management of early invasive cervical cancer, *Int J Gynecol Cancer* 2:129, 1992.

Mylotte M, Allen J, Jordan J: Regeneration of cervical epithelium following laser destruction of CIN. Paper presented at the International Symposium on Gynecologic Oncology, Monaco, 1978.

Nichols F, Hallen MR, West J et al: LLETZ as an alternative to both local ablative and cone biopsy treatment, *J Gynecol Surg* 9:77, 1993.

Ortiz R, Newton M, Tsai A: Electrocautery treatment of cervical intraepithelial neoplasia, *Obstet Gynecol* 41:113, 1973.

Ostergard DR: Cryosurgical treatment of cervical intraepithelial neoplasia, *Obstet Gynecol* 56:233, 1980.

Parashevadis E, Jandial L, Mann EMF et al: Patterns of treatment failure following laser for cervical intraepithelial neoplasia: implications for follow up protocol, *Obstet Gynecol* 78:80, 1991.

Popkin DR, Scali V, Ahmed MN: Cryosurgery for treatment of cervical intraepithelial neoplasia, *Am J Obstet Gynecol* 130:551, 1978.

Poyner EA, Barakat RR, Haskins WJ: Management and follow up of patients with adenocarcinoma in situ of the uterine cervix, *Gynecol Oncol* 57:158, 1995.

Richart RM, Sciarra JJ: Treatment of cervical dysplasia by outpatient electrocauterization, *Am J Obstet Gynecol* 101:200, 1968.

Richart RM et al: An analysis of "long-term" follow-up results in patients with cervical intraepithelial neoplasia treated by cryosurgery, *Am J Obstet Gynecol* 137:823, 1980.

Riva JM, Sedlacek TV, Cunnane ME et al: Extended carbon dioxide laser vaporization in treatment for subclinical papillomavirus infection of the lower genital tract, *Obstet Gynecol* 73:25, 1989.

Saidi MH, White AJ, Weinberg PC: The hazard of cryosurgery for treatment of cervical dysplasia, *J Reprod Med* 19:70, 1977.

Semm K: New apparatus for the "cold coagulation" of benign cervical lesions, *Am J Obstet Gynecol* 95:963, 1966.

Sevin BU et al: Invasive cancer of the cervix after cryosurgery: pitfalls of conservative management, *Obstet Gynecol* 53:465, 1979.

Silbar EL, Woodruff JD: Evaluations of biopsy, cone and hysterectomy sequence in intraepithelial carcinoma of the cervix, *Obstet Gynecol* 27:89, 1966.

Stafl A, Wilkinson EJ, Mattingly RS: Laser treatment of cervical and vaginal neoplasia, *Am J Obstet Gynecol* 128:128, 1977.

Townsend DE: Cryosurgery for CIN, *Obstet Gynecol Surv* 34:838, 1979.

Townsend DE, Ostergard DR: Cryocauterization for preinvasive cervical neoplasia, *J Reprod Med* 6:171, 1971.

Townsend DE, Richart RM: Cryotherapy and carbon dioxide laser management of cervical intraepithelial neoplasia: a controlled comparison, *Obstet Gynecol* 61:75, 1983.

Tredway DR et al: Colposcopy and cryosurgery in cervical intraepithelial neoplasia, *Am J Obstet Gynecol* 114:1020, 1972.

Underwood PB, Lutz MH, Fletcher RV Jr: Cryosurgery, *Cancer* 38:546, 1976.

Urcuyo R, Rome RM, Nelson J: Some observations on the value of endocervical curettage performed as an integral part of colposcopic examination of patients with abnormal cervical cytology, *Obstet Gynecol* 128:787, 1977.

Vedel P, Jakobsen H, Boggsen N et al: Five year follow up of patients with CIN in cone margins after conization, *Europ J Obstet Gynecol Reprod Biol* 50:71, 1993.

Widrich T, Kennedy A, Myers TM et al: Adenocarcinoma in situ of the unterine cervix: management and outcome, *Gynecol Oncol* 61:304-8, 1996.

Wiener JJ, Sweetnam PM, Jones JM: Long-term follow up of women after hysterectomy with a history of preinvasive cancer of the cervix, *Brit J Obstet Gynecol* 99:907, 1992.

Wilbanks GD et al: Treatment of cervical dysplasia with electro-cautery and tetracycline suppositories, *Am J Obstet Gynecol* 117:460, 1973.

Wright JC, Davies EM: The conservative management of cervical intraepithelial neoplasia: the use of cryosurgery and the carbon dioxide laser, *Br J Obstet Gynaecol* 88:663, 1981.

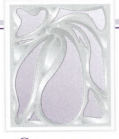

Preinvasive Disease of the Vagina and Vulva

INTRAEPITHELIAL NEOPLASIA OF THE VAGINA

Clinical Profile

Carcinoma in situ of the vagina has been reported sporadically in the last four decades, particularly in patients previously treated for cervical carcinoma in situ. The first report was apparently by Graham and Meigs in 1952. They reported on three patients with carcinoma of the vagina, two intraepithelial and one invasive, that were discovered 6, 7, and 10 years after total hysterectomy for carcinoma in situ of the cervix. Other reports have described multiple primary cancers of the vagina, cervix, and vulva. Several authors have commented on the "field response" of the cervix, vagina, and vulva, which suggests that the squamous epithelium of the lower genital tract may be affected in multiple sites by a similar carcinogenic trigger. Apparent extension of invasive carcinoma of the cervix to the vagina and vestibule may represent simultaneous carcinomas at sites affected by a constant carcinogenic stimulus of several end organs in the genital tract.

Carcinoma in situ of the vagina is much less common than that of the cervix or vulva. Isolated lesions can usually be recognized colposcopically (Figure 2-1) as white epithelium, mosaicism, and punctation, although some authors have described a "pink blush" appearance or a slightly granular texture. The diagnosis is usually confirmed by biopsy, and the limits of the lesion can be identified with the colposcope or with iodine staining (Schiller stain). Almost all lesions are asymptomatic, although an occasional patient will have postcoital staining. An abnormal Pap smear usually initiates the diagnostic survey. Patients with abnormal squamous cytologic findings in the absence of a cervix or not explained by an adequate investigation of the cervix should be subjected to a careful examination of the vaginal epithelium. In most series, the upper third of the vagina is most frequently involved (as is the invasive variety), and this in part relates to the association with the more common cervical lesions. First TeLinde, then Gusberg and Marshall, and later Parker et al. indicated that 2%, 1.9%, and 0.9%, respectively, had vaginal recurrences after hysterectomy for a similar lesion in the cervix. On the other hand, Ferguson and Maclure reported positive cytologic findings in 151 (20.3%) of 633 previously treated patients. This large group included invasive and in situ cancers of the cervix, which were treated by irradiation or hysterectomy. Although the long-term recurrence rate for carcinoma in situ of the vagina is uncertain, it is sufficient to merit continued careful follow-up. Incomplete excision of sufficient vaginal cuff with hysterectomy for carcinoma in situ may

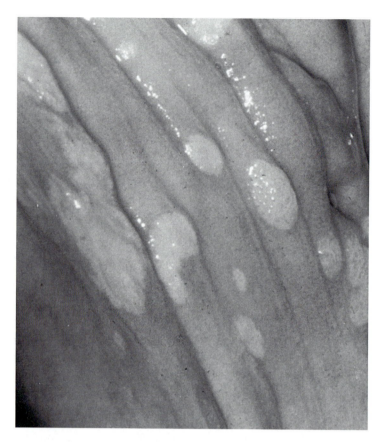

Figure 2-1 Carcinoma in situ of the vagina (colposcopic view).

explain an early recurrence. The finding of carcinoma in situ in the vaginal cuff area less than 1 year after hysterectomy makes this explanation likely. It is therefore important to perform a preoperative evaluation of the upper vagina by Schiller tests or colposcopy at the time of hysterectomy for carcinoma in situ of the cervix. This will allow the surgeon to determine accurately the amount of upper vagina necessary to remove. It is also apparent that both carcinoma in situ and dysplasia may develop in the vagina as primary lesions. Still other preinvasive lesions of the vagina may appear after irradiation therapy for invasive carcinoma of the cervix. Data from the MD Anderson Hospital suggest that these postradiation lesions are truly premalignant and can progress to invasive cancer if untreated. Without therapy, approximately 25% of the patients in this series progressed to the invasive state over varying periods of follow-up. Local therapy must be executed with care because of the previous irradiation.

Patients with vaginal intraepithelial neoplasia (VAIN) tend to have either an antecedent or coexistent neoplasia in the lower genital tract. This is the usual situation in at least one half to two thirds of all patients with VAIN. In patients who have been treated for disease in the cervix or vulva, VAIN can appear many years later, necessitating long-term follow-up.

Diagnosis

Colposcopic examination of the vagina can be difficult to perform. The largest possible speculum should be used and repositioned frequently to allow inspection of all surfaces. Colposcopic findings are similar to those described for the cervix. Our technique calls for the examination of the four walls from apex to introitus as separate and sequential steps. Biopsy specimens are taken with Kevorkian-Younge alligator-jaw forceps, sometimes using a sterilized skin-hook for traction at the biopsy site. Most patients can tolerate these biopsies without local anesthesia. Lugol solution may be helpful in delineating lesions of the vagina. In the postmenopausal patient, local use of estrogen creams for several weeks will help bring out the abnormal areas for identification by colposcopy.

In contrast to CIN, VAIN tends to be multifocal; and even if a lesion is identified, one must search the entire vaginal tube for coexisting multiple lesions. Although typically the lesion is more common in the apex, disease-free skip areas may be encountered with additional VAIN in the lower vagina. In hard-to-locate lesions, selective cytologic methods, obtaining Pap smears from different locations in the vagina, often can pinpoint the area of abnormality so that attention can be paid specifically to the area of highest suspicion.

Management

Local excision of the involved area has been the mainstay of therapy. In many instances a single isolated lesion can be removed easily in the office with biopsy forceps. If larger areas are involved, an upper colpectomy may be necessary if the lesion is to be removed by surgery. The use of a dilute solution of phenylephrine (Neo-Synephrine), which is injected submucosally at the time of surgery, will facilitate the vaginectomy tremendously.

As in CIN, outpatient modalities of therapy have been investigated for VAIN. The topical application of 5-fluorouracil (5-FU) cream has been advocated by some investigators for the last decade or so. Results have varied; however, studies by Petrilli et al. and Caglar, Hurtzog, and Hreshchyshyn indicate that this modality can be effective. One of the problems with 5-FU is the selection of the best mode of application, dosage, and length of treatment. Some advocate the use of a tampon or a diaphragm to keep the 5-FU cream in place. Several techniques have been suggested with equivalent results. One-quarter applicator of 5% 5-FU is inserted high in the vagina each night after the patient is in bed. This is done every night for 7 to 10 days, followed by a 10-day to 2-week rest period, and then the application cycle is repeated. This usually allows an adequate treatment time without having the patient experience the tremendous local reaction that can occur with prolonged use. Treatment can be repeated if not successful after the first cycle. Weekly insertions of 5-FU cream, approximately 1.5 gm (one third of an applicator), deep into the vagina once a week at bedtime for ten consecutive weeks has also been shown to be efficacious. Placement of cotton balls at the introitus will prevent 5-FU contamination of the perineum with resultant skin irritation. Douching the next morning as advocated by some is unnecessary with the weekly instillation. We prefer the latter technique because compliance is high and toxicity is low.

A recent report by Dungar and Wilkinson noted an interesting finding in the vagina after 5-FU therapy which we also have noted. Post treatment, a reddened area suggestive of a lack of squamous epithelium may be present. They found that this represented columnar epithelium consistent with a metaplastic process in which squamous epithelium is replaced with columnar epithelium. They called this finding "acquired vaginal adenosis." These changes are usually found in the upper one third of the vagina but may extend into the mid one third. The columnar epithelium was of a low cuboidal or mucus secreting endocervical type. In some cases, squamous epithelium was noted overlying the glandular elements. Marked superficial chronic inflammation was also present. This has also been noted in the vagina after laser therapy.

Cryosurgery has been used in the treatment of some patients with VAIN, but it has been found not nearly as successful as it is in the treatment of CIN. This is probably attributable to the flaccidity of the vaginal wall and the lack of good freezing contact. Also, the possibility of vesical and rectovaginal fistulae has discouraged some individuals from trying this therapy. At present, there appears to be no enthusiasm for this particular modality in the treatment of VAIN. Benedet evaluated 56 patients who ranged from 22 to 84 years of age. Over half had a prior history of CIN. Measurement of the epithelium was performed of involved as well as uninvolved tissue. The involved epithelium had a mean thickness of 0.46 mm (range 0.1 to 1.4 mm). Uninvolved was thinner with a mean thickness of 0.28 mm. Of interest is that there was no statistical difference in thickness of the involved epithelium in the pre- and postmenopausal patient; however, the uninvolved epithelium was thinner in the postmenopausal patient compared to the premenopausal patient (0.25 vs 0.37 mm). Although this latter figure is statistically significant, it certainly is not clinically significant. Although Benedet did not give treatment results, the study was performed to give guidance as to the depth of vaginal destruction by the laser. Based on this study, the authors felt that destruction of 1.0-1.5 mm would destroy the epithelium without damage to underlying structures. Several authors have suggested that laser therapy is effective.

Over a 6-year period, Townsend et al. treated 36 patients from two large referral hospitals with the laser. These numbers do confirm the apparent rarity of this lesion. In 92% of the patients, the lesions were completely removed by the laser without significant side effects. Almost one fourth of the patients, however, required more than one treatment session. Pain and bleeding have been the main complications but appear to be minimal. Healing is excellent, and sexual dysfunction has not been a problem. The optimal technique of laser therapy for vaginal lesions has yet to be determined. Whereas some investigators suggest removing only the identified lesions, others advocate treating the entire vaginal tube. Schellhas reported two patients treated for VAIN with the laser who subsequently developed invasive disease in the vagina. A thorough diagnostic investigation of the vagina to rule out invasive cancer can be quite difficult, but it is obviously mandatory. Multiple focal lesions particularly post hysterectomy with deep vaginal angles may be difficult to treat with the laser. Small skin hooks and dental mirrors have been suggested as adjuncts to successful laser therapy. Krebs treated 22 patients with topical 5-FU and 37 patients with laser. Success rate was similar between the two treatments. Particularly in multifocal lesions we prefer 5-FU treatment.

Some have advocated surface irradiation using an intravaginal applicator; however, our experience with this method of therapy has been discouraging, with a high recurrence rate and marked vaginal stenosis, making follow-up therapy extremely difficult. At present it appears that local excision is the treatment of choice. Total vaginectomy, with vaginal reconstruction using a split-thickness skin graft, should be reserved for the patient who has failed more conservative therapy.

DES-Related Genital Tract Anomalies
Embryology

In any brief review of the early development of the reproductive tract, it is necessary to discuss the urinary tract, since some components of the urinary tract later become functional portions of the reproductive tract, namely the ducts. In the development of the mammalian excretory system, three successive paired kidneys are formed. The first, the pronephros, probably does not function in the human being. The second kidney, the mesonephros, begins to replace the pronephros in its subdiaphragmatic location in the fourth week. It is composed of tubules similar to those of its predecessor, but instead of elaborating a duct of its own it appropriates the pronephric duct, which thereafter is known as the mesonephric duct, or by the more familiar eponym, the wolffian duct. The definitive kidney, the metanephros, supplants it. The tubules of this final excretory organ form a little lower in the abdominal cavity than those of the kidneys that first appear in the sixth or seventh week. Its duct originates as an outpouching of the lower end of the mesonephric duct, and ureteric bud, which grows upward, eventually invaginating the metanephros and connecting with the metanephric tubules. The connection of the ureter with the mesonephric duct is interrupted at an early stage by differential growth processes that give the two ducts separate entrances to the ureterogenital sinus. It is important to emphasize the close association between the definitive urinary tract and those parts of the reproductive tract that are derived from the mesonephric duct. The common origin of their lining epithelium is shown in Figure 2-2.

The female reproductive tract, the paramesonephric or mullerian duct, originates during the sexually indifferent period, early in the sixth week, and is therefore present in the future male as well as the future female. In the male it degenerates about the tenth week, at approximately the time when the mesonephric duct is degenerating in the female. The mullerian duct originates as an invagination of coelomic epithelium lateral to the upper end of the mesonephric duct. The epithelium at the base of this small pit proliferates to form a solid blind cord that grows downward toward the pelvis. This later becomes canalized. This mechanism, which results in a lining of coelomic epithelium, contrasts with the bulging of the gonads into the body cavity, which produces a covering of coelomic epithelium. The mullerian ducts on either side grow toward each other, crossing over the wolffian duct anteriorly to meet and fuse in the midline in the ninth week. The medial walls of the fused ducts gradually disappear, producing a single uterovaginal cavity (see Figure 2-2). The upper portions of the ducts, which do not fuse, remain as the paired uterine, or fallopian, tubes. When the lower end of the fused mullerian ducts makes contact with the urogenital sinus, the cell cords are still solid. They merge with the endodermal cells growing back from the sinus to form a temporary barrier between the ureterovaginal cavity and the ureterogenital sinus, the mullerian tubercle. The mesonephric ducts enter the ureterogenital sinus immediately lateral to the tubercle. Between the openings of the mesonephric (wolffian) ducts and the mullerian tubercle, the proliferation of sinus cells occurs, producing the dorsolateral (sinovaginal) bulbs. At the same time, the simple columnar epithelium

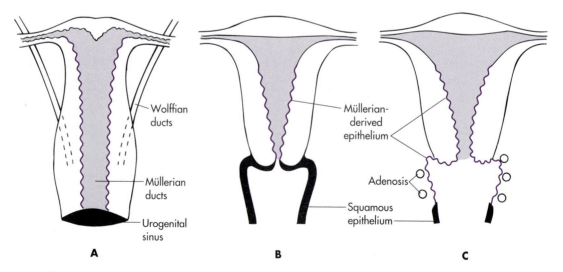

A   Wolffian ducts   Müllerian ducts   Urogenital sinus

B   Müllerian-derived epithelium   Squamous epithelium

C   Müllerian-derived epithelium   Adenosis   Squamous epithelium

Figure 2-2 Schematic representations of the embryologic development of the vagina in unexposed and DES-exposed women. (Reproduced, with permission, from Stillman RJ: In utero exposure to diethylstilbestrol: adverse effects on the reproductive tract and reproductive performance in male and female offspring, *Am J Obstet Gynecol 142(7):905, 1982.*)

that lines the vaginal portion of the ureterovaginal canal begins to undergo transformation into stratified epithelium of polygonal cells. This transformation proceeds cranially until it reaches the columnar epithelium of the future endocervical canal. The vagina, which is initially lined by simple columnar epithelium of mullerian origin, now has acquired a stratified mullerian epithelium. The base of the sinovaginal bulbs proliferates, producing a central mass with lateral wings that sweep cranially to the central mass. This entire structure, the vaginal plate, advances in a caudal-cranial direction, obliterating the existing vaginal lumen. By caudal cavitation of the vaginal plate, a new lumen is formed, and the stratified mullerian epithelium is replaced by a stratified squamous epithelium, probably of sinus origin. Local proliferation of the vaginal plate in the region of the cervicovaginal junction produces the circumferential enlargement of the vagina known as the vaginal fornices, which surround the vaginal part of the cervix. The administration of DES through the eighteenth week of gestation apparently can result in the disruption of the transformation of columnar epithelium of mullerian origin to the stratified squamous successor. This retention of mullerian epithelium gives rise to adenosis. Adenosis may be present in any of the following forms: as a replacement, with glandular cells in place of the normal squamous lining of the vagina; as glandular cells hidden beneath an intact squamous lining; or mixed with squamous metaplasia as new squamous cells attempt to replace glandular cells.

Vaginal adenosis has been observed in patients without a history of DES exposure but rarely to a clinically significant degree. Sandberg sectioned 35 vaginas obtained at autopsy; 22 were from postpubertal women, and

in 9 of these (41%) he demonstrated occult glands. None of the 13 prepubertal specimens examined contained glands. However, Kurman and Scully noted 6 cases of vaginal adenosis among 73 prepubertal vaginal specimens obtained at autopsy. Robboy reported on 41 women born before the DES era who had adenosis confirmed pathologically and noted that the microscopic appearances of adenosis in women born before the DES era were identical to those encountered in young women exposed in utero to DES. Adenosis is more common in patients whose mothers began DES treatment early in pregnancy, and its frequency is not at all increased if DES administration began after the eighteenth week of gestation. At least 20% of females exposed to DES show an anatomic deformity of the upper vagina and cervix. This has been variously described as transverse vaginal and cervical ridge, cervical collar, vaginal hood, and cockscomb cervix. The transverse ridges and anatomic deformities found in one fifth of DES-exposed females make ascertainment of the boundaries of the vagina and cervix difficult. The cervical eversion causes the cervix grossly to have a red appearance. This coloration is caused by the numerous normal-appearing blood vessels in the submucosa. By using a colposcope and applying 3% acetic acid solution, one may recognize involved areas covered with numerous papillae ("grapes") of columnar epithelium similar to those seen in the native columnar epithelium of the endocervix. The hood (Figure 2-3) is a fold of mucous membrane surrounding the portio of the cervix; it very often disappears if the portio is pulled down with a tenaculum or is displaced by the speculum. The cockscomb is an atypical peaked appearance of the anterior lip of the cervix, whereas vaginal ridges are

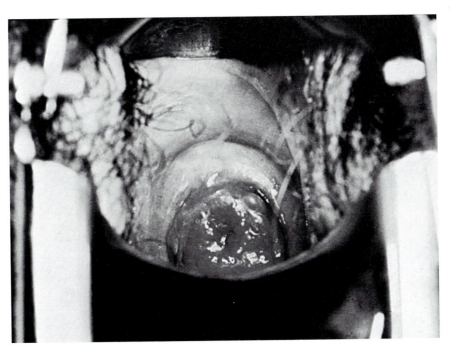

Figure 2-3 Hood surrounding the small DES-exposed cervix, which is completely covered by columnar epithelium (pseudopolyp).

protruding circumferential bands in the upper vagina that may hide the cervix. A pseudopolyp formation (see Figure 2-3) has been described that occurs when the portio of the cervix is rather small and protrudes through a wide cervical hood.

The striking occurrence of vaginal adenosis among young women whose mothers took nonsteroidal estrogens during pregnancy logically points to an occurrence during embryonic development for an explanation. The development of the mullerian system depends on and follows formation of the wolffian, or mesonephric, system. The emergence of the mullerian system as the dominant structure appears unaffected by intrauterine exposure to DES when studied in animal systems. However, it is apparent that steroidal and nonsteroidal estrogens, when administered during the proper stage of vaginal embryogenesis in mice, can permanently prevent the transformation of mullerian epithelium into the adult type of vaginal epithelium, thus creating a situation like adenosis. The colposcopic and histologic features of vaginal adenosis strongly support the concept of persistent, untransformed mullerian columnar epithelia in the vagina as being the explanation of adenosis.

EXAMINATION AND TREATMENT OF THE FEMALE EXPOSED TO DES

Systematic examination of the female offspring exposed to DES (see box below) has disclosed that at least 60% have vaginal adenosis, that is, presence of cervical-like epithelium in the vagina; a smaller portion have minor

---

EXAMINATION OF THE DES-EXPOSED FEMALE OFFSPRING

1. Inspect the introitus and hymen to assess the patency of the vagina.
2. Palpate the vaginal membrane with the index finger (especially noting non-Lugol-staining areas), noting areas of induration or exophytic lesions, which should be considered for biopsy.
3. Perform speculum examination with the largest speculum that can be comfortably inserted (virginal-type speculums are often necessary). Adenosis will usually appear red and granular (strawberry surface).
4. Obtain cytologic specimens from (1) the cervical os and (2) the walls of the upper one third of the vagina.
5. Perform colposcopic examination and/or Lugol staining on the initial visit.
6. Do a biopsy of (1) indurated or exophytic areas and (2) colposcopically abnormal areas with dysplastic Pap smear.
7. Perform bimanual rectovaginal examination.

---

anomalies of the cervix and vagina. Although the origin of clear cell adenocarcinoma from adenosis remains to be established, these patients warrant careful observation. Some authors have suggested that DES-exposed offspring may also have an increased risk of developing squamous neoplasia because of the large number of transformation zones inherent in this condition. Although a few cases of dysplasia and carcinoma in situ associated with adenosis have been reported, the risk of developing squamous lesions remains uncertain at this time, since few DES-exposed offspring have entered the age group in which squamous cell carcinoma is more prevalent.

Fowler et al. reported an increased occurrence of cervical intraepithelial neoplasia (CIN) in women with in utero exposure to DES; among 335 exposed women he found a 15% incidence of CIN. In a DESAD report, an incidence of 15.7/1000 in the exposed persons compared with 7.9/1000 persons per year of follow-up in the unexposed was noted. A 1984 report from the same group reverses this opinion and reports an incidence of 15.7/1000 in the exposed persons, compared with 7.9/1000 persons per year of follow-up in the unexposed. This same report found an unexplained difference between the two groups in the frequency of history of genital herpes. Since human papilloma virus (HPV) infections are often found in the same patient population as herpes, and since HPV has been associated with an increased incidence of dysplasia in the cervix, one wonders about the true significance of the later report from the DESAD project.

All DES-exposed females should have a gynecologic examination on an annual basis beginning at age 14 or at menarche, whichever occurs first. In general, examinations of prepubertal individuals are not recommended, but they should be performed (usually under anesthesia) if any unusual symptoms, such as abnormal bleeding or discharge, develop. Mothers should be encouraged to instruct their daughters in the use of vaginal tampons during menses, since this will facilitate the physician's examination. Examination should include careful inspection of the cervix and of any suspicious area in the vagina. Careful digital palpation of the vagina must be performed. The role of colposcopy remains in the examination of suspicious areas where biopsy may be indicated. Lugol solution may be helpful in delineating abnormal areas. The purpose of regular examination is to permit detection of adenocarcinoma and squamous neoplasia during the earliest stages of development. Although many therapies have been attempted, at the present time no recommended treatment plan for vaginal adenosis exists. Some physicians have advised the use of jellies or foam to lower the vaginal pH and assist the reepithelialization of the mucous membrane. No published studies indicate that such a practice is valid. The use of local progesterone in the vagina has been advocated by others as therapy for vaginal adenosis, but good data are similarly lacking. In most instances the area of adenosis is physiologically transformed into squamous epithelium during varying periods of observation, and no therapy is necessary.

It is anticipated that the vast majority of DES-exposed associated adenocarcinomas have been identified (see Chapter 3). The past history of DES exposure is important in the follow-up of these patients because adenocarcinoma could appear in the future. It is probably more important not to be concerned by adenosis and treat an entity that usually disappears with time. Whether these individuals will be at high risk for VAIN only time will tell. Certainly routine screening with cytology should be continued for the life of the patient.

It has been postulated that squamous cell cancers may arise in the metaplastic tissue that is so extensively found in DES-exposed females. Evidence for an increase in squamous cell carcinoma does not exist at present, but this possibility provides an additional reason for close follow-up of the group. Colposcopic examination of these patients is hampered by the abnormal patterns (Figure 2-4) seen with squamous metaplasia, which can be confused with neoplastic lesions, especially by the inexperienced observer. Careful histologic confirmation is essential before any treatment is undertaken. Marked mosaic (Figure 2-5) and punctation patterns that normally herald intraepithelial neoplasia are commonly seen in the vagina of a DES-exposed female as a result of widespread metaplasia.

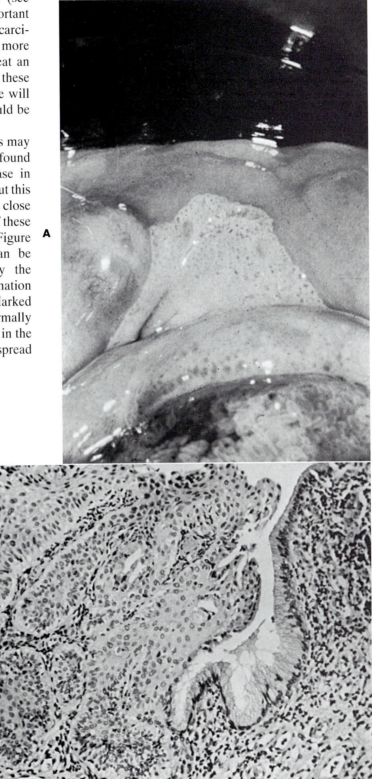

Figure 2-4 A, Area of white epithelium of squamous metaplasia. **B,** Histologic section of the area in **A** showing metaplasia to the left partially covering the adenosis (columnar epithelium) to the right.

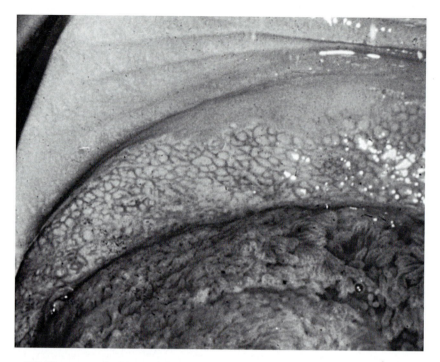

Figure 2-5 Heavy mosaic pattern (histologically proven metaplasia) in a hood surrounding the cervix of a DES-exposed offspring.

INTRAEPITHELIAL NEOPLASIA OF THE VULVA

Nonneoplastic Epithelial Disorders

Nonneoplastic epithelial disorders of the vulvar skin and mucosa are frequently seen in clinical practice and were previously categorized as vulvar dystrophies. In 1987, at a meeting of the International Society for the Study of Vulvar Disease (ISSVD), a new classification of these disorders was adopted (Table 2-1). The new classification was developed to improve a scheme that would be accepted by gynecologists, dermatologists, and pathologists. This would encourage the standardization and comparability of vulvar pathology on an international and interdisciplinary basis.

The old terminology of "dystrophies" was replaced by "nonneoplastic epithelial disorders of skin and mucosa." Not only was the category changed but the specific classification: squamous cell hyperplasia, lichen sclerosus and other dermatoses (see box below). Many previously used terms should be discarded (see box

---

Table 2-1   Vulvar nonneoplastic epithelial disorders

Terminology	Treatment
Lichen sclerosis	Topical 2% testosterone
Squamous cell hyperplasia (formerly hyperplastic dystrophy)	Topical corticosteroids
Other dermatoses	

NONNEOPLASTIC EPITHELIAL DISORDERS OF THE VULVAR SKIN AND MUCOSA

I.   Squamous cell hyperplasia (formerly hyperplastic dystrophy)
II. Lichen sclerosus
III. Other dermatoses

DELETED TERMS

- Lichen sclerosus et atrophicus
- Leukoplakia
- Neurodermatitis
- Leukeratosis
- Bowen's disease
- Carcinoma simplex
- Leukoplakic vulvitis
- Hyperplastic vulvitis
- Kraurosis vulvae
- Erythroplasia of Queyrat

---

above). It was recognized that differences in the appearance of vulvar skin was not due necessarily to separate diseases but rather, they were environmentally conditioned reactions to adverse agents. In support of this suggestion, evidence has been cited that, if the involved vulvar skin is excised and normal skin is transplanted from a site not ordinarily subject to lesions characteristic of the vulvar area, the grafted epithelium may undergo the same changes that occur in the original vulvar skin before its removal. The unique appearance of many of the dystrophies of the vulvar skin is a product of the warm moist environment of this organ.

The new classification clearly separates the nonneoplastic epithelial disorders. Lesions demonstrating atypia do not belong within the classification of nonneoplastic epithelial disorders, since their natural history is entirely different. Unlike the prior classification, which was based purely on histopathologic features of the lesions being studied, the new classification is based on a combination of gross and histopathological changes. Mixed disorders can occur, but both conditions should be reported; i.e., lichen sclerosus with associated squamous cell hyperplasia (which was formerly called mixed dystrophies) should be reported as lichen sclerosus with squamous cell hyperplasia. Squamous cell hyperplasia terminology is used when the hyperplasia cannot be attributable to more specific process. If squamous cell hyperplasia is associated with VIN (vulvar intraepithelial neoplasia), then the diagnosis should be reported as VIN.

Squamous cell hyperplasia

Squamous cell hyperplasia includes lesions with no known cause. Most hyperplastic lesions represent lichen simplex chronicus. The age of the patient may vary, involving the reproductive and postmenopausal years. Pruritus is the most common symptom and the status of the skin usually relates to the amount of scratching. Although these lesions are associated with epithelial thickening and hyperkeratosis, their appearance is highly variable. Moisture, scratching, and medications may cause variations in the appearance of these lesions even in the same patient. The areas of the vulva most frequently involved include the labia majora, intralabial folds, outer aspects of the labia minor, and the clitoris. Changes can also extend to the lateral surfaces of the labia majora or beyond. Areas of squamous cell hyperplasia are often localized, elevated, and well delineated; however, these lesions may be extensive and sometimes poorly defined. The vulva often has a dusky-red appearance when the degree of hyperkeratosis is slight. At other times, well defined, white patches may be seen, or a combination of red and white areas may be observed in different locations. Thickening, fissures, and excoriations require careful evaluation, since carcinoma may be exhibited by these same features.

Biopsy will reveal a variable increase in the thickness of the horny layer (hyperkeratosis) and irregular thickening of the Malpighian layer (acanthosis). This latter process produces a thickened epithelium, as well as lengthening and distortion of the rete pegs. Parakeratosis may also be present. The granular layer of the epithelium is usually prominent. An inflammatory reaction is often present within the dermis with varying numbers of lymphocytes and plasma cells.

Lichen sclerosus

Lichen sclerosus was often termed in the past as kraurosis vulvae or atrophic leukoplakia. Lichen sclerosus represents a specific disease and can be found in nongenital sites. Children and young women may be affected but most patients are postmenopausal. Although not seen initially, pruritus is present in essentially all lesions leading to scratching, which can lead to ecchymosis and ulceration. Studies have suggested that the epithelium in lichen sclerosus is metabolically active and non atrophic. In a well-developed classic lesion, the skin of the vulva is crinkled ("cigarette-paper") or parchment-like in appearance. Often the process extends around the anal region in a figure eight or key hole configuration. At other times, the changes are localized, especially in the periclitoral area or the perineum. Clitoral involvement is usually associated with edema of the foreskin, which may obscure the glands clitoris. Phimosis of the clitoris is often seen late in the course of the disease. The labia minora also completely disappears as a result of atrophy. Synechiae often develop between the edges of the skin in these locations, causing pain and limited physical activity. Fissures also develop in the natural folds of the skin and especially in the posterior fourchette. The introitus may become stenosed to a point where intercourse is impossible. In a study by Dalziel, 44 women with lichen sclerosus were evaluated for sexual dysfunction. Apareunia had been experienced by 19 women at some point. Dyspareunia and decreased frequency were noted by 80%. Orgasm was altered and relationships were affected by half. Local steroids improved sexual function in two thirds of patients. The microscopic features of lichen sclerosus include hyperkeratosis, epithelial thickening with flattening of the rete pegs, cytoplasmic vacuolization of the basal layer of cells, and follicular plugging. Beneath the epidermis is a zone of homogenized, pink-staining, collagenous-appearing tissue that is relatively acellular. Edema is occasionally seen in this area. There is an absence of elastic fibers. Immediately below this zone lies a band of inflammatory cells consistent of lymphocytes and some plasma cells. Lichen sclerosus is often associated with foci of both hyperplastic epithelium and thin epithelium (formerly mixed dystrophy). Squamous cell hyperplasia has been found in 27%-35% of women with lichen sclerosus following microscopic study of vulvar specimens. Approximately 5% of patients with lichen sclerosus were found also to have intraepithelial neoplasia. The etiology of this condition is unknown. Wallace found that only 12/290 (4%) of women with lichen sclerosus, who were followed for an average of 12.5 years, developed vulvar cancer.

Other Dermatosis

The term *"other dermatoses"* applies to the entire range of skin disorders that can affect this area of the body (Table 2-2). In reality, only a few lesions are routinely encountered in an average gynecologic practice. The new classification system gives vulvar dermatoses dermatologic names. This should help to better define the natural history, differential diagnosis, and treatment of the major skin disease. Primary lesions are the basic descriptors: muscle, papule, plaque, nodule, tumor, vesicle, bulla, pustule, weal, telangiectasis, comedone, burrow, or cyst. These generic nouns describe the skin change that results from an underlying pathologic process. When primary lesions are altered by external factors the resulting lesion is a secondary change. Terms describing secondary changes include: *scale, crust, fissure, erosion, ulcer, excoriation, atrophy,* and *scar*. Descriptions of the skin lesions should include 1) primary lesion form, 2) arrangement or pattern of lesions, and 3) distribution on anatomic sites.

Treatment

Before any treatment is given long term, biopsies should be performed from representative areas to assure the correct diagnosis. These biopsies should concentrate on sites of fissuring, ulceration, induration, and thick plaques. Hygienic measures for keeping the vulva clean and dry should be recommended. Anxiety is frequently a factor and should be investigated. Vulvar pruritus is often seen in women with stress and all of this promotes scratching and leads to further secondary skin changes. After lesions with malignant potential have been ruled out, local measures for control of symptoms, primarily pruritus, can be instituted. If an eczematous type of vulvitis is present as the result of infected excoriations or inappropriate medications, wet dressings with agents such as aluminum acetate (Burrow's) solution applied frequently are beneficial. Lotions and creams containing corticosteroids produce a rapid response and are more convenient to apply than wet dressings. Squamous cell hyperplasia is best treated with local application of corticosteroids. The use of moderate and strong topical steroids two to three times daily will relieve pruritus and inflammation. Most dermatologists recommended that fluorinated steroid substances not be used for long periods of time, since they may theoretically result in atrophy of treated tissues. That has not been the authors' experience where prolonged use has often been necessary to keep the vulvar skin asymptomatic. A position of compromise would be to utilize fluorinated steroids until the pruritus is under control and then replace them with medications containing only hydrocortisone. Friedrich has suggested a combination of Eurax (3 parts) and betamethasone valerate (7 parts) because the antipuritic effect of the steroid is enhanced with the Eurax. Treatment twice a day is usually adequate, with results expected in a couple of weeks, although longer therapy may be necessary, particularly if a thickened hyperplastic lesion is present. After the skin returns to normal appearance, therapy can be stopped.

Table 2-2   Other dermatoses

Disorders	Lesions	Genital	Other locations
Seborrheic dermatitis	Erythema with mild scale oval plaques	Mild scaling, also "inverse" type	Central face, neck, scalp, chest, back
Psoriasis	Annular scaly plaques bleed easily	Red plaques with grey-white scale	Scalp, elbows, knees, sacrum
Tinea	Annular plaques with central cleaning	Common	Skin folds or single "ringworm" lesion
LSC: lichen simplex chronicus	Lichenified plaques, some dermatitic	Scrotum or labia majora	Nape of neck, ankle, forearm, antecubital and popliteal lossae
LP: lichen planus	Flat-topped lilac papules and plaques	White network, erosive vaginitis	Volar wrists, shins, buccal mucosa

Traditionally, topical testosterone has been the treatment of choice for lichen sclerosus, improving both gross and histopathologic changes. Testosterone propionate or cypropionate 2% in petrolatum or Aquaphor is easily prepared by a pharmacist. The medication is usually applied at bed time for at least 3-6 months or until pruritus is relieved. Thereafter, the frequency of application is gradually reduced until a maintenance level of once or twice per week is reached. Virilizing side effects can occur and the patient must be monitored closely. In the presence of severe pruritus, a mixture of 1% or 2.5% hydrocortisone in a petrolatum base with testosterone can be utilized. In patients in which local testosterone has not been effective, a new potent steroid (clobetasol propionate) has been effective in eliminating the symptoms. A recent study by Bracco evaluated 79 patients using four different treatment regimens. A three-month course of testosterone (2%), progesterone (2%), clobetasol propionate (0.05%) and a cream base preparation were used in a prospective randomized study. Patients treated with clobetasol had a better response rate in regard to relief of symptoms (75% vs 20% for testosterone and 10% for other preparations). The clobetasol group was the only treatment in which the gross and histologic evaluation improved after treatment. The authors used the steroid b.i.d. for one month, then daily for two months. They noted that symptomatic relief is often dramatic. Recurrences after stopping the steroid occurred but symptoms were relieved when therapy was reinstituted. It appears that clobetasol propionate may be the new treatment of choice for lichen sclerosus.

Occasionally, vulvar pruritus is so persistent that it cannot be relieved by topical measures. In such cases, intradermal injection of steroids has been reported to be effective. Others have reported subcutaneous injection of absolute alcohol to relieve symptoms. Aliquots of 0.1 mg of the alcohol are injected subcutaneously at 1 cm intervals after the vulvar has been carefully mapped out, and the vulvar area is thoroughly massaged to disperse the alcohol evenly. Vulvar burning is sometimes intense following alcohol injection and occasionally urinary retention occurs. Posttreatment surveillance should be thus appropriate. Alcohol injection has been reported to produce significant symptomatic relief of pruritus but is of little value for vulvar burning.

Clinical Profile

VIN has been considered a problem of postmenopausal women in their fifties and sixties but it can develop at any age. Its frequency appears to be increasing among younger women. Today the average age for VIN is said to be about 40 years. During the last two decades the incidence of VIN has almost doubled to 2.1 per 100,000 women years. The incidence has nearly tripled in white women younger than 35 years old. Of interest is, during this time the incidence of vulvar cancer has not increased. Neither age nor parity appears to be a risk factor in the development of intraepithelial neoplasia of the vulva. The disease is asymptomatic in more than 50% of cases. In the remainder of cases, the predominant symptom is pruritus. Presence of a distinct mass, bleeding, or discharge strongly suggests invasive cancer. The most productive diagnostic technique is careful inspection of the vulva in bright light during routine pelvic examination followed by biopsy of suspicious lesions.

Physicians should be familiar with the various premalignant conditions of the vulva. As shown in the box below, they range from dysplasia (VIN I) that is biologically and histologically similar to dysplasia of the cervix or vagina to the more aggressive carcinoma in situ (VIN III). Whether or not these lesions carry the same connotation as their counterparts in the cervix in regard to progression to invasion is unknown. Certainly an invasive lesion can be associated with VIN and the risk of invasive cancer has been reported to be as high as 30%. In other situations the invasive lesion may have arisen de novo.

The acceptance of the new classification of vulvar intraepithelial neoplasia terminology by the ISSVD has undoubtedly clarified much of the confusion that resulted because several other terms were previously used for this disease process. This VIN-dysplasia designation replaced the previously used atypia terms. Other terms, such as *bowenoid papulosis*, *Bowen's disease*, or *erythroplasia of Queyrat*, should not be used for intraepithelial neoplasia diagnosis.

Many of the squamous intraepithelial lesions of the vulva are associated with HPV, particularly type 16/18, 31, 33, 35, and 51. HPV DNA has been found in 80%-90% of VIN but the incidence decreases with age. The incidence of HPV DNA in vulvar cancers also decreases with age. HPV DNA in vulvar cancers also seems to be related to the type of cancers, such as the warty or condylomatous carcinoma and basoloid types that tend to occur in the younger patient.

The ISSVD states that "VIN is characterized by a loss of epithelial cell maturation with associated nuclear hyperchromosis and pleomorphism, cellular crowding, and abnormal mitosis." The thickness of the epithelial abnormality would designate further characterizations of the lesion (VIN I, II, III). VIN III would suggest full

---

CLASSIFICATION OF VIN

VIN I (mild dysplasia)—formerly mild atypia
VIN II (moderate dysplasia)—formerly moderate atypia
VIN III (severe dysplasia, CIS)—formerly severe atypia

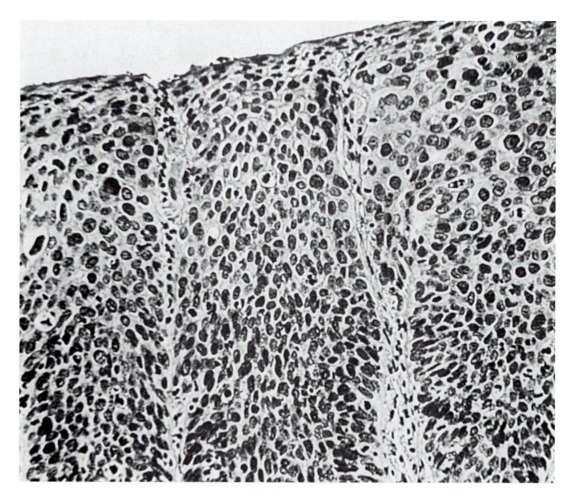

Figure 2-6 Histologic section of carcinoma in situ of the vulva.

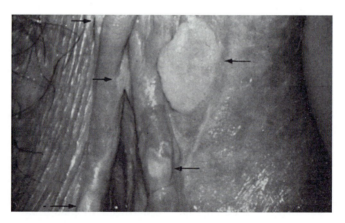

Figure 2-7 Multiple white lesions of the vulva (VIN).

thickness changes (Figure 2-6). The milder forms of VIN first appear clinically as pale areas varying in density. More severe forms are seen as papules or macules, coalescent or discrete, single or multiple. Lesions on the cutaneous surface of the vulva usually have the appearance of lichenified or hyperkeratotic plaques, that is, white epithelium (Figure 2-7). By contrast, lesions of mucous membranes are usually macular and pink or red.

Vulvar lesions are hyperpigmented in 10% to 15% of patients (Figure 2-8). These lesions range from mahogany to dark brown, and they stand out sharply when observed solely with the naked eye.

Diagnosis

The value of careful inspection of the vulva during routine gynecologic examinations cannot be overstated; this

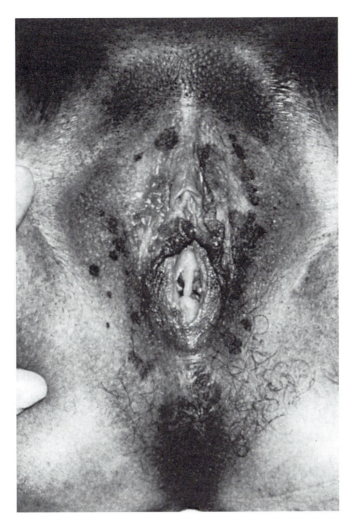

Figure 2-8 Hyperpigmented lesions of vulvar carcinoma in situ.

remains the most productive diagnostic technique. The entire vulva, perineum, and perianal area must be evaluated for multifocal lesions. It is not uncommon to find intraepithelial lesions on hemorrhoid tags. The use of acetic acid is very helpful in identifying subtle lesions. It should be remembered that in contrast to the cervix, the vulva requires application of acetic acid for 5 minutes or longer before many lesions are apparent. Placing many soaked cotton balls on the vulva for the desired length of time is an effective method. After a lesion has been diagnosed, colposcopic examination of the entire vulva and perianal area should follow to rule out multicentric lesions. In general, multifocal lesions are more common in premenopausal patients, whereas postmenopausal patients have a higher rate of unifocal disease.

Some investigators prefer to use toluidine blue to identify vulvar lesions; a 1% aqueous solution of the dye is applied to the external genital area, and after drying for 2 to 3 minutes, the region is washed with 1% to 2% acetic acid solution. Suspicious foci of increased nuclear activity become deeply stained (royal blue), whereas normal skin accepts little or none of the dye. Regrettably, hyperkeratotic lesions, even though neoplastic, are only lightly stained, whereas benign excoriations are often brilliant, an observation that accounts for the high false positive and false negative rates.

It should be emphasized that the diagnosis of VIN can be subtle. To avoid delay, the physician must exercise a high degree of suspicion. Vulvar biopsy should be used liberally. It is best accomplished under local anesthesia with a Keyes dermatologic punch (4 to 6 mm size). This instrument allows removal of an adequate tissue sample and orientation for future sectioning. After obtaining the biopsy specimen, we use the Keyes punch to cut out a piece of Gelfoam; this is positioned in the skin defect and kept in place with a small dressing for at least 24 hours.

Adequate biopsy specimens are also obtainable with a sharp alligator-jaw instrument if one has proper traction on the skin. The problem with ordinary knife biopsies is that only superficial epithelium can be reached. If this technique is employed, one must be careful to sample deeper layers.

There have been few reports on untreated VIN. Jones and McClean observed five of five untreated VIN lesions progress to invasive cancer in 2-3 years. All had multiple focal lesions. Barbero noted 3 of 55 treated VIN patients progressed to carcinoma 14 months to 15 years. These three patients were 58 to 74 years of age. Adequate diagnosis is important. Chafe noted that 19% of women who were thoroughly evaluated and felt to have only VIN had invasive cancer on the vulvectomy specimen.

Pigmented Lesions

Pigmented lesions of the vulva are, for the most part, intraepithelial, with the exception of melanoma, which is covered in Chapter 8. Pigmented lesions probably account for 10% of all vulvar disease. The most common pigmented lesion is a lentigo, which is a concentration of melanocytes in the basal layer of cells. It can have the clinical appearance of a freckle. Confusion with a nevus is common. The borders are fuzzy, but it is not a raised lesion. A lentigo is benign and the diagnosis is usually made microscopically. If there is doubt, a biopsy is performed.

Vulvar intraepithelial neoplasia (VIN) may appear as a pigmented lesion. Friedrich found carcinoma in situ of the vulva more frequent in pigmented lesions even than in nevi. Characteristic raised hyperkeratotic pigmented lesions are suggestive of carcinoma in situ and should be biopsied.

A new term associated with pigmented lesions has recently crept into the gynecologic literature. *Bowenoid papulosis* is a variant of pigmented lesions that dermatologists have noted for some time. These are small pigmented papules that develop and spread rapidly. According to dermatologists, these papules frequently regress spontaneously. Histologically, at least on the vulva, these are squamous cell carcinomas in situ. These lesions have recently been reported to have an aneuploid DNA pattern. Many authorities have not found bowenoid papulosis of the vulva to spontaneously regress. Regardless of the clinical characteristics, if VIN is present histologically, we would treat accordingly.

The management of nevi can be conservative. Many times a nevus can be detected only microscopically. Unfortunately, a simple nevus and an early melanoma cannot be differentiated on clinical evaluation. Excisional biopsy of these raised, smooth, pigmented areas can be done easily in the office. Certainly, if the nevus changes in color, size, and shape, it should be removed for diagnostic purposes. After a nevus is removed, no further therapy is needed regardless of whether it is a compound, an intradermal, or a junctional type.

Management

Surgical excision has been the mainstay of therapy. An important advantage is that excision allows for complete histologic assessment; lesions with early invasion can

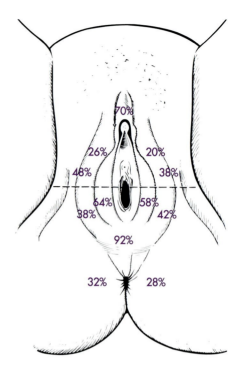

Figure 2-9 Plot of lesion locations in 36 patients treated for multifocal carcinoma in situ of the vulva.

thus be found. Most localized lesions are managed very effectively by wide local excision (a disease-free border of at least 5 mm) with end-to-end approximation of the defect. The vulvar skin and mucous membrane usually have a good deal of elasticity, and cosmetic results are satisfactory after uncomplicated healing.

With multicentric lesions (Figure 2-9), we usually excise the involved skin and substitute a split-thickness skin graft taken from the buttocks or the inner aspect of the thigh. This is the skinning vulvectomy and skin graft procedure introduced by Rutledge and Sinclair in 1968 (Figure 2-10). Its purpose is to replace the skin at risk in the vulvar site with ectopic epidermis from a donor site. We modified the procedure in that the clitoris is always preserved and any lesions on the glans are scraped off with a scalpel blade; the epithelium of the glans regenerates without loss of sensation. Some recent reports have questioned this approach on the grounds that, at least in cases of vulvar dystrophy, the donated skin might be susceptible to a similar dystrophic process. In our experience, lesions have developed outside the grafted area in preserved vulvar skin but rarely in the graft itself. This suggests that the neoplastic potential is inherent in the original vulvar skin and does not translate to skin from other parts of the body placed at the vulvar site.

The skinning vulvectomy and skin graft procedure preserves the subcutaneous tissue of the vulva, giving an optimal cosmetic and functional result. In more than 50 patients treated to date, we have had no complaints of dyspareunia or diminished sexual responsiveness. In the

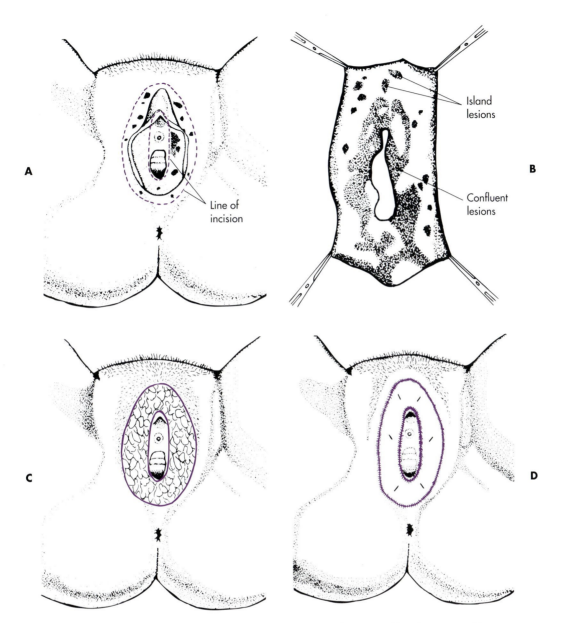

Figure 2-10 Skinning vulvectomy and skin graft. **A,** Excise all areas of involvement en bloc. **B,** Lesions may be isolated or confluent. **C,** Preserve all subcutaneous tissue as the graft bed. **D,** Suture to graft bed.

elderly patient, simple vulvectomy may be preferred, because the skinning vulvectomy and skin graft operation requires prolonged bed rest (6 to 7 days) whereas the split-thickness graft adheres to the graft bed. Thus the potential for morbidity is increased. The wishes of the patient concerning cosmetic results and sexual function must, of course, be taken into account regardless of age (Figure 2-11).

An alternative to excision of a vulvar lesion is to destroy it, principally by hot cautery, laser surgery, or cryosurgery. The disadvantage of destructive therapy is that a necrotic ulcer on the vulva may result and wound healing may be slow. Complete healing following cryo-

surgery may take up to 3 months. The treated area is often very painful for much of that time.

Laser in the management of VIN has evolved into the treatment of choice by many, particularly for multifocal extensive disease. Townsend et al. treated 33 patients with the laser and were said to be successful in 31 (94%); however, 14 of the patients required two or more treatments, with 2 patients requiring five laser treatments. Baggish and Dorsey's results were much the same, in that 32 of 35 patients were believed to have been cured from their disease; however, 26 of the 35 patients required three or more treatments, and 2 women had six treatments. Pain, which has been severe in some patients, has been the

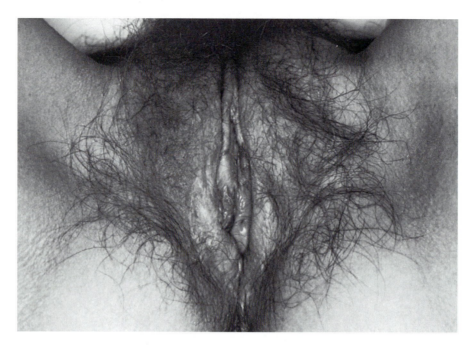

Figure 2-11 After superficial vulvectomy and skin graft for VIN. Excellent cosmetic results are present.

main complication with the laser. Most therapists will treat only a small portion of the vulva on an outpatient basis. Patients require general anesthesia if large areas of the vulva are to be treated at one time. Pain after therapy can be severe in some patients. Bleeding and infection also have been reported. The cosmetic results appear to be excellent. It appears that the laser may be an acceptable treatment modality; however, patients must be evaluated carefully before treatment and invasive carcinoma must be ruled out (Table 2-3). It should be remembered that a greater expertise with the laser is required for this therapy than is needed for cervical vaporization. The depth of destruction must be controlled. Too deep a wound can result in long-term ulcers, which may take some time to heal and cause considerable discomfort. Benedet evaluated 165 women with VIN. Of the 122 with VIN III, the mean thickness of the epithelium was 0.52 mm (range 0.1-1.9). In patients with hair follicles involved with VIN, the mean depth of involvement was 1.9 mm (range 1.0-3.4). Only 19 patients had appendageal involvement. Age did not seem to affect the thickness of involved epithelium. Koilocytosis was present in 74% of VIN I but present in only 19% of VIN III lesions. Multifocal lesions were present in 64% of all patients. The most common sites were the labia minora, posterior fourchette, and perineum. Based on this study, the authors believe that 1.0 mm destruction of nonhair-bearing epithelium is adequate treatment. If skin appendages are involved, 2.5-3.0 mm is required (Figure 2-12).

Reid has defined surgical planes in the vulva as a guide to laser therapy. The first plane is the surface epithelium only, which includes the basement membrane. Opalescent

Table 2-3	CO$_2$ laser vaporization—vulva
Instrument	CO$_2$ laser, colposcopic, micro-manipulator
Power density	600-1000 W/CM^2
Depth of destruction	
non-hairy areas	<1 mm
hairy areas	3 mm
Lateral margins	"Brush"
Anesthesia	General, local
Analgesia	Significant postlaser pain—narcotics

cell debris is noted through the heat char. Healing is rapid with good cosmetic results. The second plane involves the dermal papillae with necrosis extending to the deep papillary area. The appearance is a homogenous yellow color resembling a chamois cloth. Again healing is rapid with good cosmoses. The third plane effects the upper and mid reticular area where the pilosebaceous ducts are located. Some hypertrophy may appear in this area during the healing process. The fourth plane affects the deep reticular area, and "sand grains" can be visualized. Healing is slow and usually by granulation from the sides. Skin grafting may be required. Destruction to the third plane is adequate for hair-bearing tissue; plane one to two is depth needed for non hair-bearing skin. Post laser therapy the vulva is covered with topical steroids. Sitz baths and rinsing of vulva with water after urination and defecation is important. A hair dryer is then used to dry the area. Repeat application of steroids is used after each

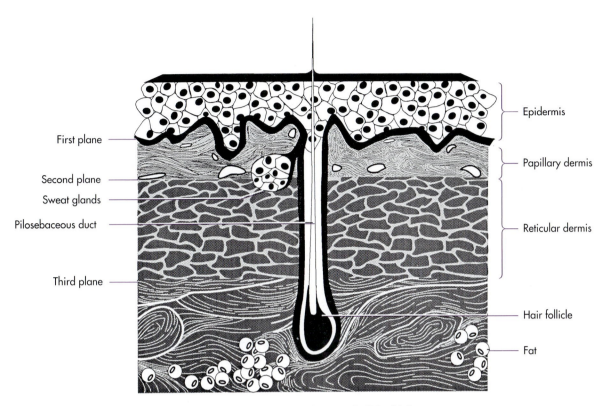

First plane

Second plane

Sweat glands

Pilosebaceous duct

Third plane

Epidermis

Papillary dermis

Reticular dermis

Hair follicle

Fat

Figure 2-12 "Planes" for therapy of VIN with laser.

washing and drying. A local anesthetic can be applied for mild to moderate pain control. Oral pain medication, including narcotics, may be necessary. The most severe pain is usually not evident until 3-4 days after the laser therapy.

Early invasive carcinoma can be very subtle. The group at the University of Florida has routinely treated carcinoma in situ of the vulva with simple vulvectomy. They noted that in 13 of 69 (19%) patients who had been evaluated with multiple biopsies, invasive cancer was noted in vulvectomy specimens. These were unknown cancers prior to vulvectomy. The temptation to preserve vulvar anatomy and prevent possible sexual dysfunction must be tempered with the necessity to rule out invasive disease. A simple vulvectomy may be the treatment of

choice in such an individual and certainly a consideration in the older patient.

In summary it is important to remember that quite often these lesions develop in young women who remain asymptomatic. It has been suggested that women should be taught vulvar self-examination to identify early lesions. This could lead to successful therapy that could also be less radical. Early diagnosis depends on careful vulvar examination under bright light at regular intervals. Biopsy must be done on any suspicious lesions, and if the histologic report confirms intraepithelial neoplasia, an examination for multicentric foci should follow. The therapy selected depends on the extent of disease, the location of the lesions, and, not least of all, the personal desires of the patient.

BIBLIOGRAPHY

Intraepithelial neoplasia of the vagina

Benedet JL, Wilson PS, Matisic JP: Epidermal thickness measurements in VAIN, *J Reprod Med* 37:809, 1992.

Blumberg JM, Ober WB: Carcinoma in situ of the cervix: recurrence in the vaginal vault, *Am J Obstet Gynecol* 66:421, 1952.

Caglar H, Hurtzog RW, Hreshchyshyn MM: Topical 5-FU treatment of vaginal intraepithelial neoplasia, *Obstet Gynecol* 58:580, 1981.

Capen CV et al: Laser therapy of vaginal intraepithelial neoplasia, *Am J Obstet Gynecol* 142:973, 1982.

Carter ER, Salvaggio AT, Jarkowski TL: Squamous cell carcinoma of the vagina following vaginal hysterectomy of intraepithelial carcinoma of the cervix, *Am J Obstet Gynecol* 82:401, 1961.

Copenhaver EH, Salzman FA, Wright KA: Carcinoma in situ of the vagina, *Am J Obstet Gynecol* 89:962, 1964.

Cromer JK: Invasive squamous-cell carcinoma of the vagina following surgery for carcinoma in situ of the cervix, *Med Ann DC* 34:115, 1965.

Dungar CF, Wilkinson EJ: Vaginal columnar cell metaplasia: an acquired adenosis associated with topical 5-FU therapy, *J reprod Med* 40:361, 1995.

Ferguson JH, Maclure JG: Intraepithelial carcinoma, dysplasia, and exfoliation of cancer cells in the vaginal mucosa, *Am J Obstet Gynecol* 87:326, 1963.

Graham JB, Meigs JV: Recurrence of tumor after total hysterectomy for carcinoma in situ. *Am J Obstet Gynecol* 64:1159, 1952.

Gusberg SB, Marshall D: Intraepithelial carcinoma of the cervix: a clinical reappraisal, *Obstet Gynecol* 19:713, l962.

Koss LG, Melamed MR, Daniel WW: In situ epidermoid carcinoma of the cervix and vagina following radiotherapy for cervical cancer, *Cancer* 14:353, 1961.

Marcus SL: Multiple squamous cell carcinoma involving the cervix, vagina, and vulva: the theory of multicentric origin, *Am J Obstet Gynecol* 80:801, 1961.

Margulis RR, Dustin RW, Daugherty GD: Carcinoma in situ of the cervix with genital tract extension, *Mich Med* 64:251, 1965.

McPherson HA et al: Epidermoid carcinoma of cervix, vagina, and vulva: a regional disease, *Obstet Gynecol* 21:145, 1963.

Moran JP, Robinson HJ: Primary carcinoma in situ of the vagina, *Obstet Gynecol* 20:405, 1962.

Mussey E, Soule EH: Carcinoma in situ of the cervix: a clinical review of 842 cases, *Am J Obstet Gynecol* 77:957, 1959.

Newman W, Cromer JK: The multicentric origin of carcinoma of the female anogenital tract, *Surg Gynecol Obstet* 108:273, 1959.

Ostergard DR, Morton DG: Multifocal carcinoma of the female genitals, *Am J Obstet Gynecol* 99:1006, 1967.

Parker RT et al: Intraepithelial cancer of the cervix, *Am J Obstet Gynecol* 80:693, 1961.

Petrilli ES et al: Vaginal intraepithelial neoplasias: biologic aspects and treatment with topical 5-fluorouracil and the carbon dioxide laser, *Am J Obstet Gynecol* 138:321, 1980.

Rutledge F: Cancer of the vagina, *Am J Obstet Gynecol* 97:635, 1967.

Samuels B, Bradburn DM, Johnson CG: Primary carcinoma in situ of the vagina, *Am J Obstet Gynecol* 82:393, 1961.

Schellhas HF: Personal communication, 1982.

TeLinde RW: Carcinoma in situ of the cervix, *Postgrad Med* 29:458, 1961.

Townsend DE et al: Treatment of vaginal carcinoma in situ with carbon dioxide laser, *Am J Obstet Gynecol* 143:565, 1982.

Woodruff JD: Treatment of recurrent carcinoma in situ in the lower genital canal, *Clin Obstet Gynecol* 8:757, 1965.

DES-related genital tract anomalies

Fowler WC et al: Risks of cervical intraepithelial neoplasia among DES-exposed women, *Obstet Gynecol* 38:720, 1981.

Herbst AL, Scully RE, Robboy SJ: Problems in examination of the DES-exposed female, *Obstet Gynecol* 46:353, 1975.

Kurman RJ, Scully RE: The incidence and histogenesis of vaginal adenosis: an autopsy study, *Hum Pathol* 5:265, 1974.

Ng ABP et al: Natural history of vaginal adenosis in women exposed to diethylstilbestrol in utero, *J Reprod Med* 18:1, 1977.

O'Brien PC et al: Vaginal epithelial changes in young women enrolled in the National Cooperative Diethylstilbestrol Adenosis (DESAD) project, *Obstet Gynecol* 53:300, 1979.

Report of the Committee on Terminology: New nomenclature for vulvar disease, *Am J Obstet Gynecol* 160:769, l989.

Robboy SJ et al: Increased incidence of cervical and vaginal dysplasia in 3,980 diethylstilbestrol-exposed young women, *JAMA* 252:2979, 1984.

Ulfelder H, Robboy SJ: The embryologic development of the human vagina, *Am J Obstet Gynecol* 126:769, 1976.

Wilkinson EJ, Kneale B, Lynch PJ: Report of the ISSVD terminology committee, *J Reprod Med* 31:973, 1986.

Intraepithelial neoplasia of the vulva

Abell MR, Gosling JR: Intraepithelial and infiltrative carcinoma of vulva, Bowen's type, *Cancer* 14:318, 1961.

Baggish MS, Dorsey HJ: CO_2 laser for treatment of vulvar carcinoma in situ, *Obstet Gynecol* 57:371, 1981.

Barbero M, Micheletti L, Preti M et al: Biologic behavior of vulvar intraepithelial neoplasia, *J Reprod Med* 38:108, l993.

Benedet JL, Wilson PS, Matisic J: Epidermal thickness and skin appendage involvement in VIN, *J Reprod Med* 36:608, 1991.

Bowen JT: Precancerous dermatoses, *J Cutan Dis* 30:241, 1912.

Carson TE, Hoskins WJ, Wurzel JF: Topical 5-fluorouracil in the treatment of carcinoma in situ of the vulva, *Obstet Gynecol* 47(suppl):59, 1976.

Chafe W, Richards A, Morgan L et al: Unrecognized invasive carcinoma in VIN, *Gynecol Oncol* 31:154,1988.

Collin CG: A clinical stain for use in selecting biopsy sites in patients with vulvar diseases, *Obstet Gynecol* 28:158, 1966.

Crum CP et al: Vulvar intraepithelial neoplasia: correlation of nuclear DNA content in the presence of human papilloma virus (HPV) structural antigen, *Cancer* 49:468, 1982.

Friedrich EG Jr: Reversible vulvar atypia, *Obstet Gynecol* 39:173, 1972.

Friedrich EG Jr: Vulvar carcinoma in situ in identical twins—an occupational hazard, *Obstet Gynecol* 39:837, 1972.

Higgins RV, Van Nagell JR Jr, Donaldson ES et al: The efficacy of laser therapy in the treatment of cervical intraepithelial neoplasia, *Gynecol Oncol* 36:79, 1990.

Jones RW, McLean MR: CIS of vulva: a review of 31 treated and 5 untreated cases, *Obstet Gynecol* 68:499, l986.

Jones RW, Park JS, McLean MR et al.: Human papilloma virus in women with VIN III, *J Reprod Med* 35:1124, 1990.

Kaufman RH, Dreesman GR, Burek J: Herpes-induced antigen in squamous cell carcinoma in situ of the vulva, *N Engl J Med* 305:483, 1981.

Krupp PJ, Bohm JW: 5-fluorouracil topical treatment of in situ vulvar cancer, *Obstet Gynecol* 51:702, 1978.

Litwin MS et al: Topical chemotherapy of lentigo maligna with 5-fluorouracil cream, *J Surg Oncol* 35:721, 1975.

Raaf JH et al: Treatment of Bowen's disease with topical dinitrochlorobenzene and 5-fluorouracil, *Cancer* 37:1633, 1976.

Reid R: Superficial laser vulvectomy, *Am J Obstet Gynecol* 152:504, l985.

Richart RM: A clinical staining test for the in vivo delineation of dysplasia and carcinoma in situ, *Am J Obstet Gynecol* 86:703, 1963.

Rutledge F, Sinclair M: Treatment of intraepithelial carcinoma of the vulva by skin excision and graft, *Am J Obstet Gynecol* 102:806, 1968.

Simonsen EF: CO_2 laser used for carcinoma in situ/Bowen's disease (VIN) and lichen sclerosus in the vulvar region, *Acta Obstet Gynecol Scand* 68:551, 1989.

Sturgeon SS, Brinton LA, Devesa SS et al: In situ and invasive vulvar cancer incidence trends (l973 to l987), *Am J Obstet Gynecol* 166:1482, l992.

Townsend DE et al: Management of vulvar intraepithelial neoplasia by carbon dioxide laser, *Obstet Gynecol* 60:49, 1982.

Woodruff JD, Hildebrandt EE: Carcinoma in situ of the vulva, *Obstet Gynecol* 12:414, l958.

Woodruff JD et al: The contemporary challenge of carcinoma in situ of the vulva, *Am J Obstet Gynecol* 115:677, 1973.

Non-metastatic epithelial disorders of the vulva

Bracco EL, Carli P, Sonni L et al: Clinical and hispotlogic effects of topical treatment of vulval lichen sclerosus, *J Reprod Med* 38:37, l993.

Dalziel KL: Effect of lichen sclerosus on sexual function and parturition, *J Reprod Med* 40:35l, 1995.

Friedrich EG, Julian CG, Woodruff JD: Acridine orange fluorescence in vulvar dysplasia, *Am J Obstet Gynecol* 90:1281, 1964

Friedrich EG Jr: Vulvar distrophy, *Clin Obstet Gynecol* 28:178, l985.

Friedrich EG Jr, Kalra PS: Serum levels of sex hormones in vulvar lichen sclerosus, and the effect of topical testosterone, *N Engl J Med* 310:488, 1984.

Harrington CI, Dunsmore JR: An investigation into the incidence of auto-immune disorders in patients with lichen sclerosus et atrophicus, *Br J Dermatol* 104:563, l981.

Hart WR, Norris HJ, Helwig EB: Relation of lichen sclerosus et atrophicus of vulva to the development of carcinoma, *Obstet Gynecol* 45:369, 1975.

International Society of Vulvar Disease (ISSVD), *Am J Obstet Gynecol* 160:769, 1989.

Jeffcoat TNA: The dermatology of the vulva, *J Obstet Gynaecol Br Comm* 69:888, l962.

Jeffcoat TNA Chronic vulva dystrophies, *Am J Obstet Gynecol* 95:61, l966.

Kaufman RH, Gardener HL, Brown D Jr, Beyth Y: Vulvar dystrophies: an evaluation, *Am J Obstet Gynecol* 120:363, 1974.

Wallace HJ: Lichen sclerosus et atrophicus, *Trans St. Julius Hosp Dermatol Soc* 57:9, 1971.

Woodruff JD, Borkowf HI, Holzman GB et al: Metabolic activity in normal and abnormal vulvar epithelia, *Am J Obstet Gynecol* 91:809, l965.

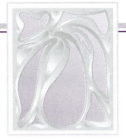

Invasive Cervical Cancer

GENERAL OBSERVATIONS

The uterine cervix is of major interest and importance to almost every obstetrician and gynecologist. To the gynecologic oncologist it represents a common focus for the development of malignant tissue. To the obstetrician it represents the primary barometer in the process of labor and delivery. No other organ is as accessible to the obstetrician and gynecologist in terms of both diagnosis and therapy. Its accessibility led to the great strides made possible by the Pap smear, resulting in complete reversal of the prognosis in cancer of this organ. Easy access to the cervix led also to the skillful application of radiation techniques, which have resulted in some of the best overall cure rates for any malignancy found in humans.

The cause of cervical cancer is unknown but its development seems related to multiple insults and injuries sustained by the cervix. Squamous cell carcinoma of the cervix is virtually nonexistent in a celibate population: only one case has been reported in the literature. It is more prevalent in women of lower socioeconomic groups and is correlated with first coitus at an early age and with multiple sexual partners. There is no correlation with the frequency of sexual intercourse. However, studies have shown that husbands of women with cervical cancer reported significantly more sexual partners than husbands of controls. Husbands of women who had cervical cancer were also more likely to report histories of various genital conditions, including genital warts, gonorrhea, and genital herpes.

Currently, greater attention is being paid to the human papillomavirus (HPV) infection of the cervix as a link to etiology. The power, consistency, and specificity of the association between subclinical papillomavirus infection and cervical neoplasia raise the strong possibility that this relationship may be causal. The biologic plausibility of this is supported by evidence that this sexually transmitted oncogenic virus often produces persistent subdural infection of metaplastic epithelium in the cervical transformation zone. The postulate that cervical neoplasia may arise by mutagenesis within papillomavirus-infected cells at the squamocolumnar junction is discussed with other corollaries in Chapter 1.

The cervix (L. *cervix*, neck) is a narrow, cylindric segment of the uterus; it enters the vagina through the anterior vaginal wall and lies, in most instances, at right angles to it. In the average patient it measures 2 to 4 cm in length and is contiguous with the inferior aspect of the uterine corpus. The point of juncture of the uterus and the cervix is known as the isthmus; this area is marked by slight constriction of the lumen. Anteriorly, the cervix is separated from the bladder by fatty tissue and is connected laterally to the broad ligament and parametrium (through which it obtains its blood supply). The lower intravaginal portion of the cervix, a free segment that projects into the vault of the vagina, is covered with mucous membrane; the cervix opens into the vaginal cavity through the external os. The cervical canal extends from the anatomic external os to the internal os, where it joins the uterine cavity. The histologic internal os is where there is a transition from endocervical to endometrial glands. The intravaginal portion of the cervix (portio vaginalis, exocervix) is covered with stratified squamous epithelium that is essentially identical to the epithelium of the vagina. The endocervical mucosa is arranged in branching folds (plicae palmatae) and is lined by cylindric epithelium. The stroma of the cervix is composed of connective tissue with stratified muscle fibers and elastic tissue. The elastic tissue is found primarily around the walls of the larger blood vessels.

The stratified squamous epithelium of the portio vaginalis is composed of several layers conventionally described as basal, parabasal, intermediate, and superficial. The basal layer consists of a single row of cells and rests on a thin basement membrane. This is the layer in which active mitosis occurs. The parabasal and intermediate layers together constitute the prickle-cell layer, which is analogous to the same layer in the epidermis. The superficial layer varies in thickness, depending on the degree of estrogen stimulation. It consists primarily of flattened cells that show an increasing degree of cytoplasmic acidophilia toward the surface. The thickness and the glycogen content of the epithelium increase following estrogen stimulation, accounting for the therapeutic effect of estrogens in atrophic vaginitis. The staining of glycogen in the normal epithelium of the portio vaginalis is the basis of Schiller test.

MICROINVASIVE CARCINOMA OF THE CERVIX

There is probably no more an area of controversy in gynecologic oncology than the diagnosis and mangement of microinvasive carcinoma of the cervix. The evolution and sometimes revolution concerning the diagnosis and management have occurred since Mestwerdt, in 1947, observed that invasive cervical cancer diagnosed only microscopically could be cured by nonradical surgery. During the last three decades, definitions and treatment plans have changed dramatically. It is hoped that most of these changes occurred as new data became available and changes were therefore logical. Much of the confusion can be related to the fact that FIGO has changed the criteria for early stage invasive carcinoma of the cervix at least five or six times since 1960. These changes were made as additional information in regard to this disease process became available. Other influences, however, also contributed to the confusion. Over the years as many as 20 different definitions have been proposed and as many as 27 terms have been applied to this entity. The recommended therapy has also changed, going from radical surgery with any invasion to being more conservative with various depths of invasion.

In 1971, FIGO designated stage Ia carcinoma of the cervix as those cases of pre-clinical carcinoma. It is obvious that pre-clinical invasive cancer may be only a mm or two in depth or 10 mm or greater (Figure 3-1). In 1973, the Society of Gynecologic Oncologists (SGO) accepted the following statement concerning the definition of microinvasive carcinoma of the cervix: "1) Cases of intraepithelial carcinoma with questionable invasion should be regarded as intraepithelial carcinoma and 2) a microinvasive lesion should be defined as one in which a neoplastic epithelium invaded the stroma in one or more places to the depth of 3 mm or less below the base of the epithelium (Figure 3-2) and in which lymphatic or vascular involvement is not demonstrated." This definition was not agreed to unanimously by the SGO; nevertheless, in the United States it became the most quantifiable definition for this entity at that time. It subsequently was used as a guide for therapy by many physicians. FIGO has consistently stated that staging of all cancers are for comparison purposes and not as the guide for therapy. In 1979, the Japanese Society of Obstetrics and Gynecology essentially adopted the SGO definition, except cases with confluent patterns were excluded and were considered to belong to stage Ib. In 1985, for the first time, FIGO attempted to quantify the histological definition of stage Ia carcinoma of the cervix. Stage Ia was defined as the earliest forms of invasion in which minute foci of invasion are visible only microscopically. Stage Ia2 is a macroscopically measurable micro carcinoma that should not exceed 5 mm in depth and 7 mm in width. Vascular space involvement, either venous or lymphatic, should not alter staging. This definition has been criticized for several reasons. Although the upper limits of invasion for depth and width were stated, upper limits for measurement for stage Ia1 were not defined. It was therefore difficult to quantify patients in the two subgroups. Other areas of criticism

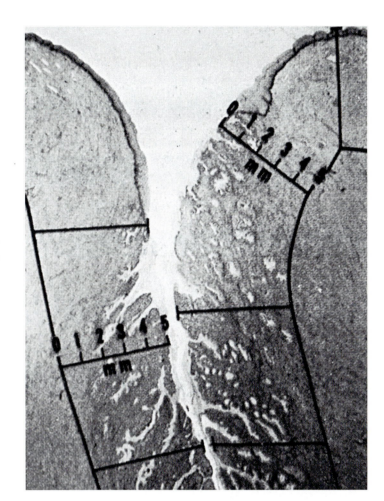

Figure 3-1 Five-millimeter rule on a histologic section of a normal squamo-columnar junction. (Courtesy Dr. Hervy Averette, Miami, Florida.)

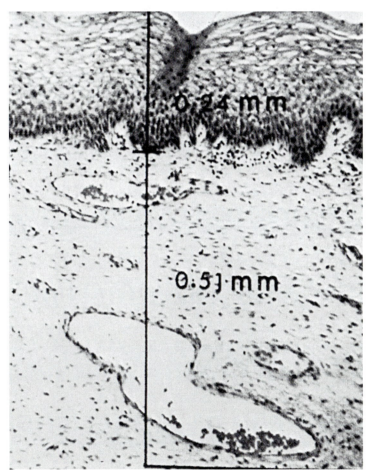

Figure 3-2 Vascular channels within 0.5 mm of the surface epithelium shown on histologic section of a normal cervix. (Courtesy Dr. Hervy Averette, Miami, Florida.)

were aimed at the fact that the FIGO definition could not be used as a guide for treatment and it included patients with vascular lymphatic channel involvement. These variations illustrate the problem with specific definition.

Authors have suggested various levels of invasion for this diagnosis and over the years have varied from 1 to 3 to 5 and even greater depth of invasion. The width of the lesion has only recently been addressed and is included only in the FIGO definition. Some authors have even suggested that volume of tumor should be used as a defining point. In most countries, this is impractical due to cost of that determination. Some authorities exclude patients with confluent growth, although this is usually ill defined. Investigators have looked at tumor grade as an independent prognostic variable, and it is generally agreed that this has no importance. As mentioned earlier, probably the most controversial aspect of the definition is whether or not patients with capillary-like space involvement (vascular lymphatic channel) should be included in the definition. FIGO does not exclude it; however, the SGO and the Japanese society do.

In 1994, FIGO, in an attempt to better qualify the definition of microinvasive carcinoma of the cervix, adopted the following definition for microinvasive carcinoma of the cervix (see box below). Stage Ia1 cancers would be those with stromal invasion up to 3 mm in depth and no greater than 7 mm. Stage Ia2 would be when invasion is present at 3-5 mm in depth and no greater than 7 mm. Lymphatic vascular space involvement would not exclude a patient from this definition. It was appreciated that the recurrence rate of patients in these two substages would probably be no more than 1%-2%. Survival of stage Ia1 would approach 99% and stage Ia2, would approach 97%-98%. This new definition will allow further evaluation of what might be appropriate therapy for the different substages, particularly stage Ia2 cancers.

Vascular space involvement was not excluded from the FIGO definition for several reasons. There is disagreement among pathologists as to the reproducibility of this entity. At least in one study, the number of slides prepared from the cervix depended on the incidence of capillary-like space involvement. Shrinkage artifact can lead to an over diagnosis and verification has been suggested with special staining to verify true capillary-like space involvement. In one study in which immunoperoxidase staining with Ulex Europaeus agglutin 1 lectin (UEAI) was used 10 of 32 cases of vascular space involvement were excluded in which involvement was initially thought to exist.

As greater experience is obtained, the tendency has been toward conservative management; i.e., conization of the cervix or simple hysterectomy for more superficial invasion (0-3 mm) and even in some patients with 3-5 mm of invasion. In 1978, Lohe reported on 285 patients with early stromal invasion and 134 patients with micro carcinoma. He defined early stromal invasion as only isolated, variably-shaped projections with true signs of infiltration present; whereas, micro carcinomas' true confluent carcinomatosis masses were present. Tumor length and depth were 10 mm and 5 mm. He stated that the three-dimensional definition of the size of the tumor is essential to the microscopic diagnosis of early stromal invasion and of micro carcinoma. In his series, 72% with early stromal invasion and 41% with micro carcinoma were treated with conservative surgery (conization or simple hysterectomy). After long-term follow-up, no patients with early stromal invasion died. Three patients with micro carcinomas have recurred and died. In a larger collected series of 435 patients with micro carcinoma, 24 (5.5%) had recurrence of disease. Using his criteria, Lohe predicted less than 1% incidence of lymph node metastasis in micro carcinoma and essentially none in early stromal invasion. Boyce has reported a large series with both "microscopic foci" of invasion (360 cases) and "occult invasion" (390 cases). Most (283) of the patients with microscopic foci invasion were treated with simple hysterectomy and only 14 with conization. After 5-15 years follow-up, only one patient is dead of disease. The majority (262) of the patients with occult invasion received irradiation therapy. Most of these lesions were greater than 5 mm in depth and all were characterized by confluent masses of neoplastic cells. Twenty-four of the 390 patients with occult invasion are dead of disease in five years. Benedet reported on 180 patients with microinvasion and occult invasive squamous cell carcinoma of the cervix who were examined by colposcopy during a 10-year period. Colposcopy led to the correct management in 90% of patients with occult invasive carcinoma and in 84% of patients with microinvasive cancer. Colposcopy appeared to be less sensitive in detecting microinvasive lesions than in detecting occult carcinoma. Atypical vessels indicative of early invasive cancer many times are subtle and difficult to identify. They are best visualized when the cervix has been bathed

---

STAGE Ia CANCER OF THE CERVIX

Stage Ia: Cancer invasion identified only microscopically. All gross lesions, even with superficial invasion, are stage Ib cancers. Measured stromal invasion with maximum depth of 5.0 mm and no wider than 7.0 mm.*

    Stage Ia1: Measured invasion of stroma up to 3.0 mm.

    Stage Ia2: Measured invasion of stroma of 3-5 mm and no wider than 7 mm.

*The depth of invasion should not be more than 5 mm taken from the base of the epithelium; either surface or glandular, from which it originates. Vascular space involvement, either venous or lymphatic, should not alter the staging.

in normal saline. Acetic acid in many instances can cover atypical vessels by enhancing white epithelium that obscures the vessels. Östör in Australia has recently made an extensive review on this subject of the literature published since 1976. As a pathologist, he has critically reviewed many of the parameters that have historically been suggested as important prognostic factors.

0-3 mm Invasion

Östör identified 3683 patients from the literature with less than 1 mm of invasion. Four patients had lymph node metastasis. With the incidence of lymph node metastasis in this group essentially 0, it would certainly appear that there is no place for lymphadenectomy in this group of patients. There were 17 invasive recurrences and 16 cancer-related deaths. In several cases that resulted in death, patients refused further therapy or follow-up. Therefore the death rate in this group of patients would appear to be less than 0.1%, with invasive recurrences being approximately 0.4% (Table 3-1). Östör identified 1324 patients who had invasion of 1-3 mm. Of these, 333 definitely had lymphadenectomies with seven nodal metastasis. At least two of these probably had greater than 3 mm of stromal invasion. The incidence based on these figures suggests that lymph node metastasis would be approximately 1%. There were 26 invasive recurrences and 6 deaths! Some of these patients probably had greater than 3 mm of invasion and also included some patients with "microinvasive adenocarcinoma." In a review of reports over the last 15 years with most occurring within the last decade, Creasman identified 1704 patients who had an invasion of 0-3 mm and 17 (1%) recurred. Only 3 (0.17%) died from their cancer. These were in patients with squamous lesions.

It appears that the management of early invasive lesions (0-3 mm of invasion, Figure 3-3, *A-C*) has generally been agreed to by the gynecologic oncology community. Patients with FIGO stage Ia1 and SGO criteria for microinvasion could be treated conservatively with simple hysterectomy, or if continued fertility is desired conization only, provided surgical margins are free of cancer. Most of the data in the literature concerning patients with 0-3 mm of invasion is based on conservative therapy, although some have had lymphadenectomies. From collected series it would therefore appear that the role of vascular space involvement in this group of patients does not predict lymph node metastasis nor recurrence. Although still in dispute, it appears that a growing number of investigators do not use capillary-like space involvement as an exclusion criterion for this stage.

3-5 mm Invasion

Östör identified 674 patients in this category of which 221 definitely had lymphadenectomies, 6% having nodal metastasis. If most or all of the other patients had lymphadenectomy, which is certainly possible, and all of the nodes were negative, the figure would be close to 2%. Twenty-five (4%) patients developed an invasive recurrence, and 13 (2%) died from their disease. Of interest is the fact that 23% of the patients were said to have had capillary-like space involvement. Creasman identified from the literature 264 patients with 3-5 mm invasion who had lymphadenectomy and in which vascular space involvement was specifically evaluated. In those patients with vascular space involvement, 2 of 83 (2.4%) and 7 of 181 (3.8%) without vascular space involvement had lymph node metastasis. In the recent literature, 488 patients with 3-5 mm were identified and 15 (3%) developed a recurrence with 9 (1.8%) dying of cancer deaths. The recurrence and death rates in patients with 3-5 mm certainly approaches those with 0-3 mm invasion. It should be noted that most, but not all, of patients treated for 3-5 mm invasion were managed with radical hysterectomy and pelvic lymphadenectomy. There are patients, however, in this category who have been managed only with conization. In the 3-5 mm range, vascular space status does not appear to correlate with lymph node metastasis. There is limited experience with patients with these clinical lesions but patients with limited invasion of 3-5 mm have a much greater incidence of lymph node metastasis (7%) and should be treated as a stage Ib cancer.

The data on patients with 3-5 mm invasion still remains fairly limited. With an extremely low incidence of lymph node metastasis (2%-3%), it seems reasonable to evaluate the role of more conservative therapy in this group of patients. This may be done after consultation with the pathologist and gynecologic oncologist. If one is concerned about the 3% incidence of lymph node metastasis, these nodes can be evaluated with laparoscopy or retroperitoneal lymphadenectomy. If there is no evidence

---

Table 3-1   Lymph node metastases, recurrences, and deaths in stage Ia carcinoma of the cervix

Invasion depth (mm)	Number of patients	Invasion recurrence	Died of cancer	Number with CLSI*	Number with positive nodes
0-3	5007	35 (0.7%)	10 (0.2%)	182 (3.6%)	8/666 (1.2%)
3-5	674	25 (4.0%)	13 (2.0%)	124 (18.4%)	14/221 (6.3%)

*CLSI: Capillary-like Space Involvement.
Modified from Östör AG, *Annual Pathology*, 1995.

of extrauterine disease via these procedures, simple hysterectomy or even conization may be reasonable. Twenty years ago, it was not unusual for investigators to suggest radical hysterectomy and pelvic lymphadenectomy for any degree of stromal invasion. With increased experience, more conservative therapy was found to be just as efficacious as radical therapy. It appears that we are now in the same arena for 3-5 mm today as we were for 0-3 mm two decades ago. Although vascular space involvement does not appear to predict lymph node metastasis with 3-5 mm invasion, there have been anecdotal reports in the literature suggesting that recurrences are higher in patients with capillary-like space involvement but without metastasis in the lymph nodes. Östör noted in his review that 496 (14%) of 3597 patients who had capillary-like space involvement did not have an invasive recurrence. Hopefully, this question will be resolved in the future as more data is accumulated.

Conservative management for stage Ia2 carcinoma of the cervix does not seem unreasonable in light of the fact that some investigators have suggested that conservative therapy might be feasible for patients with "small stage Ib" cervical cancers. Girardi from Graz reported on a series of 69 patients with small stage Ib carcinomas of the cervix. Treatment consisted of conization or simple hysterectomy in 27, radical hysterectomy with lymphadenectomy in 25, radical vaginal hysterectomy in 13, and conization followed by radiotherapy in 4. No patient developed a recurrence during the ensuing 2 to 35 years. Two of the 25 patients with lymphadenectomy had one positive lymph node each. This study comes from a group of investigators who over the years have meticulously evaluated pathologic specimens and traditionally have been surgically aggressive. Östör recently reviewed the literature since 1976 with regard to conization as definitive therapy for stage Ia cancers. He has identified 655 patients with 0-5 mm invasion treated with conization resulting in 12 invasive recurrences and one death.

CLINICAL PROFILE OF INVASIVE CANCER

A substantial and well-publicized screening program is needed to make the public and the profession more aware of *cervical* cancer as the possible cause of even minimal gynecologic symptoms. All public education should emphasize the prevention and cure of cancer, and a more

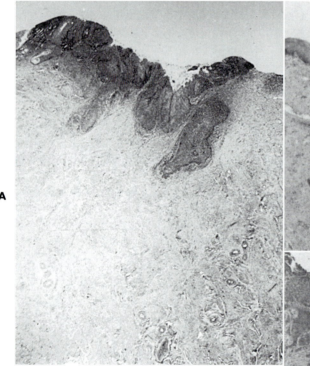

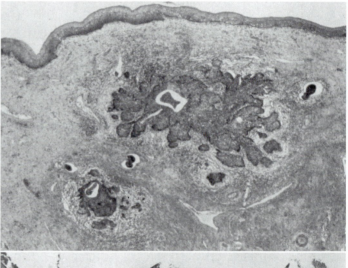

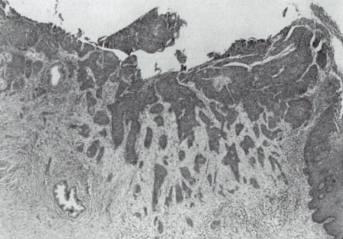

Figure 3-3 A, Microinvasion (stage Ia1) squamous cell carcinoma of the cervix. Invasion of less than 1 mm, no confluency or vascular space involvement; true microinvasion. **B,** Micro carcinoma with less than 3 mm of invasion, but with vascular space involvement. **C,** Micro carcinoma—"spray" type—with less than 1 mm of invasion.

optimistic attitude would help motivate patients and physicians to seek appropriate action. The need for early diagnosis rests on the incontrovertible fact that definite cure, in actuarial terms, is readily achieved when cervical cancer is minimal but nearly impossible if the tumor is given time to grow and spread to the pelvic wall or into adjacent structures such as the bladder and rectum. The gradient of percentage curability from early invasive cancer to late, grossly invasive disease is such a steep one that even a moderate reduction in tumor size could not fail to create a substantial improvement in curability. It is true, of course, as with other cancers, that some carcinomas of the cervix grow more rapidly than others. The basis for this difference in growth rate is still beyond our knowledge, but it is not beyond our capability to prevent undue growing time. Even the relatively slow-growing malignancy, if given enough time, will become incurable; and the most rapid-growing tumor, if diagnosed while of still moderate dimension, is definitely curable. The earlier most tumors are detected and treated, the better the chances of cure. Pap smear from a patient with early invasive squamous cell carcinoma illustrating a typical multinucleated "Tad pole" cell (Figure 3-4). Cytology and colposcopy are valuable tools in the eradication of cervical cancer. Every opportunity should be taken to disseminate modern concepts of cancer control to schools of nursing and other paramedical organizations because there is still a need for more coordinated effort in these fields. The burden should not be left with the physician alone.

The frequency with which invasive cervical cancer occurs In the United States is not known exactly, but the best incidence data indicate a rate of approximately 8 to 10/100,000/year (Figure 3-5). The incidence appears to change from one locality to another and is less frequent in rural areas than in metropolitan areas. The occurrence of cancer of the cervix is apparently less frequent in Norway and Sweden than in the United States. However, in the underdeveloped areas of the world its frequency is more noteworthy, relative to their overall cancer problem, especially when compared to the United States (Table 3-2) and Western Europe. In point of fact, in many South American and Asian countries cervical cancer accounts for the largest percentage of cancer deaths in women. One wonders whether nutritional deficiencies in these underdeveloped nations play a role in cervical cancer etiology. Orr reported abnormal vitamin levels were more commonly present in patients with cervical cancer. When compared with control values, levels of plasma folate,

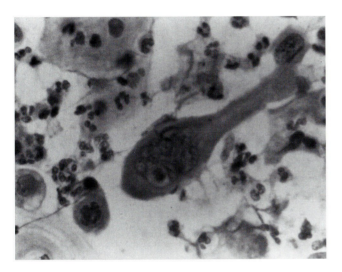

Figure 3-4 Multinucleated "tadpole" cell—early invasive squamous cell carcinoma.

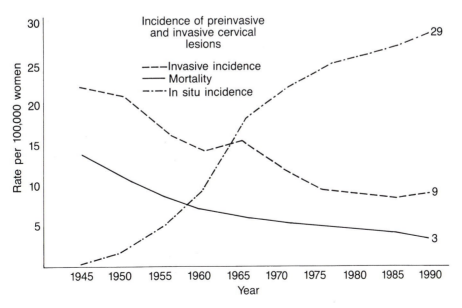

Figure 3-5 American Cancer Society figures for 1991. Cervical cancer incidence and mortality.

Table 3-2 ACS/1995/USA

	Cases	Deaths
Breast	182,000	46,000
Colorectal	67,500	28,000
Corpus	32,800	5,900
Ovary	26,600	14,500
Cervix	15,800	4,800
Lung	73,900	62,000
Melanoma	15,400	2,700

American Cancer Society, *Cancer J. Clin* 45(1):8-30, 1995.

MALIGNANT TUMORS OF THE CERVIX

I. Tumors of epithelium
  A. Squamous cell carcinoma
    1. Large cell nonkeratinizing
    2. Large cell keratinizing
    3. Small cell
    4. Verrucous carcinoma
  B. Adenocarcinoma
    1. Common pattern
    2. Adenoma malignum (minimal deviation adenocarcinoma)
    3. Mucinous
    4. Papillary
    5. Endometroid
    6. Clear cell
    7. Adenoid cystic
  C. Adenosquamous carcinoma
  D. Stem cell carcinoma (glassy cell carcinoma)
II. Tumors of mesenchymal tissue
  A. Endocervical stromal sarcoma
  B. Carcinosarcoma
  C. Adenosarcoma
  D. Leiomyosarcoma
  E. Embryonal rhabdomyosarcoma (of infants)
III. Tumor of Gartner duct (true mesonephroma)
IV. Others
  A. Metastatic tumors
  B. Lymphomas
  C. Melanoma
  D. Carcinoid

---

beta carotene, and vitamin C were significantly lower in patients with cervical cancer. Personal cigarette smoking and exposure to passive smoke as risk factors for cervical carcinoma have been examined in case control studies. Personal cigarette smoking increases the risk of cervical cancer after adjustment for age, educational level, church attendance, and sexual activity. The adjusted risk estimate associated with being a current smoker was 3.42; for having smoked for five or more pack years, it was 2.81; and for having smoked at least 100 lifetime cigarettes, it was 2.21. The adjusted risk estimate associated with passive smoke exposure for three or more hours per day was 2.96. This study, reported by Slattery in 1989, has been confirmed by others, confirming a strong association of smoking and increased risk of squamous cell carcinoma of the cervix.

Some studies suggest that cancer of the cervix is more frequent among oral contraceptive users; however, these studies may be influenced by confounding factors such as early onset of sexual activity after puberty, multiple sexual partners, and previous history of sexually transmitted diseases. Ursin reported a twofold greater risk of adenocarcinoma of the cervix especially among those who used oral contraceptives for 12 years or more.

Because of the cervix's sensitivity to hormonal influences, it may be considered biologically plausible that oral contraceptives could induce or promote cervical carcinoma. Piver reviewed a large number of early investigations of this issue and failed to show a consistent association. Moreover these data are based on exposure to oral contraceptive preparations that contained high doses of estrogen and progestin and are no longer available today.

In most large series, about 85% to 90% of malignant lesions of the cervix are squamous cell, but other lesions are possible (see the box top right). Most information regarding etiology and epidemiology is pertinent only to the more common squamous cell lesions.

Symptoms

A typical patient with clinically obvious cervical cancer is a multiparous woman between 45 and 55 years (Figure 3-6) who married and delivered her first child at an early age, usually before 20. Probably the first symptom of early cancer of the cervix is a thin, watery, blood-tinged vaginal discharge that frequently goes unrecognized by the patient. The classic symptom is intermittent, painless metrorrhagia or spotting only postcoitally or after douching. As the malignancy enlarges, the bleeding episodes become heavier, more frequent, and of longer duration. The patient may also describe what seems to her to be an increase in the amount and duration of her regular menstrual flow; ultimately the bleeding becomes essentially continuous. In the postmenopausal woman, the bleeding is more likely to prompt early medical attention.

Late symptoms or indicators of more advanced disease include the development of pain referred to the flank, or leg, which is usually secondary to the involvement of the ureters, pelvic wall, and/or sciatic nerve routes. Many patients complain of dysuria, hematuria, rectal bleeding, or obstipation resulting from bladder or rectal invasion. Distant metastasis and persistent edema of one or both lower extremities as a result of lymphatic and venous blockage by extensive pelvic wall disease are late manifestations of primary disease and frequent manifestations of recurrent disease. Massive hemorrhage and

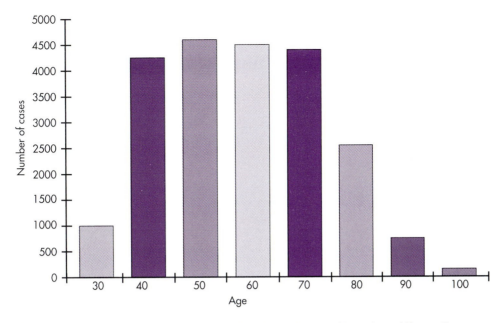

Figure 3-6 Carcinoma of the uterine cervix. Distribution by age. (From *Annual Report Gynecological Cancer, FIGO* 22, 1994.)

development of uremia with profound inanition may also occur as preterminal events.

Gross Appearance

The gross clinical appearance of carcinoma of the cervix varies considerably and depends on the regional mode of involvement and the nature of the particular lesion's growth pattern. Three categories of gross lesions have traditionally been described. The most common is the exophytic lesion, which usually arises on the ectocervix and often grows to form a large, friable, polypoid mass that can bleed profusely. These exophytic lesions sometimes arise within the endocervical canal and distend the cervix and the endocervical canal, creating the so-called barrel-shaped lesion. A second type of cervical carcinoma is created by an infiltrating tumor that tends to show little visible ulceration or exophytic mass but is initially seen as a stone-hard cervix that regresses slowly with radiation therapy. A third category of lesion is the ulcerative tumor (Figure 3-7), which usually erodes a portion of the cervix, often replacing the cervix and a portion of the upper vaginal vault with a large crater associated with local infection and seropurulent discharge.

Routes of Spread

The main routes of spread of carcinoma of the cervix are (1) into the vaginal mucosa, extending microscopically down beyond visible or palpable disease; (2) into the myometrium of the lower uterine segment and corpus, particularly with lesions originating in the endocervix; (3) into the paracervical lymphatics and from there to the most commonly involved lymph nodes (i.e., the obturator, hypogastric, and external iliac nodes); and (4) direct extension into adjacent structures or parametria, which

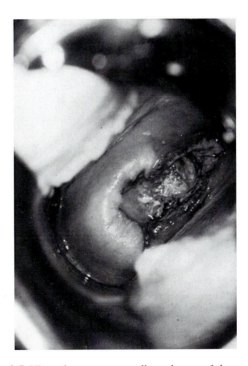

Figure 3-7 Ulcerative squamous cell carcinoma of the cervix.

may reach to the obturator fascia and the wall of the true pelvis. Extension of the disease to involve the bladder or rectum can result with or without the occurrence of a vesicovaginal or rectovaginal fistula.

The prevalence of lymph node disease correlated well with the stage of the malignancy in several anatomic studies. Lymph node involvement in stage I is between 15% and 20% and in stage II between 25% and 40%; in stage III it is assumed that at least 50% have positive nodes. Variations are sometimes seen with different

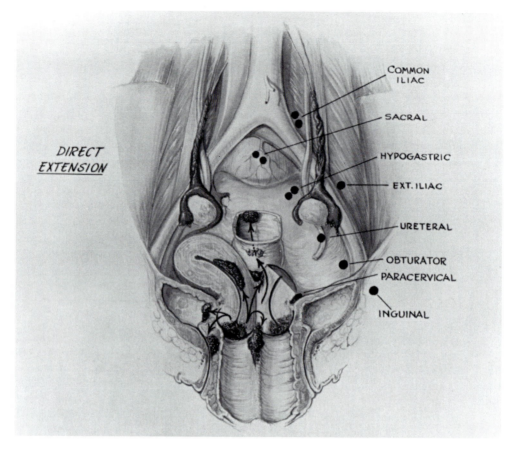

DIRECT EXTENSION

COMMON ILIAC
SACRAL
HYPOGASTRIC
EXT. ILIAC
URETERAL
OBTURATOR
PARACERVICAL
INGUINAL

Figure 3-8 Lymph node chains draining the cervix. (From Henriksen E: *Am J Obstet Gynecol* 58:924, 1949.)

material. The best study of lymph node involvement in cervical cancer was done by Henriksen (Figure 3-8). The nodal groups described by Henriksen follow:

Primary group

1. The parametrial nodes, which are the small lymph nodes traversing the parametria
2. The paracervical or ureteral nodes, located above the uterine artery where it crosses the ureter
3. The obturator or hypogastric nodes surrounding the obturator vessels and nerves
4. The hypogastric nodes, which course along the hypogastric vein near its junction with the external iliac vein
5. The external iliac nodes, which are a group of from six to eight nodes that tend to be uniformly larger than the nodes of the other iliac groups
6. The sacral nodes, which were originally included in the secondary group

Secondary group

1. The common iliac nodes
2. The inguinal nodes, which consist of the deep and superficial femoral lymph nodes
3. The periaortic nodes

In his autopsy studies, Henriksen plotted the percentage of nodal involvement for treated and untreated patients (Figures 3-9 and 3-10). Distribution is as one would expect, with a greater number of involved nodes found in the region of the cervix than in distant metastases. Although the series was an autopsy study, Henriksen found that only 27% had metastasis above the aortic chain. Cervical cancer kills by local extension with ureteral obstruction in a high percentage of patients.

In 1980 the Gynecologic Oncology Group reported the results of a series of 545 patients with cancer of the cervix who were surgically staged within their institutions. This study was prompted because traditional ports of radiation therapy were destined to treatment failure when the disease extended to the periaortic nodes (Figure 3-11). They found periaortic node involvement in 18.2% of patients with stage IIa disease and up to 33.3% in patients with stage IVa disease (Table 3-3). Piver correlated the size of the cervical lesion with the incidence of lymph node metastasis in stage I disease (Table 3-4).

When clinical staging was compared with surgical staging, inaccuracies were found of the magnitude of a 22.9% misstaged occurrence in stage IIb disease and a 64.4% misstaged occurrence in stage IIIb disease. These data raise the question of whether knowing that disease

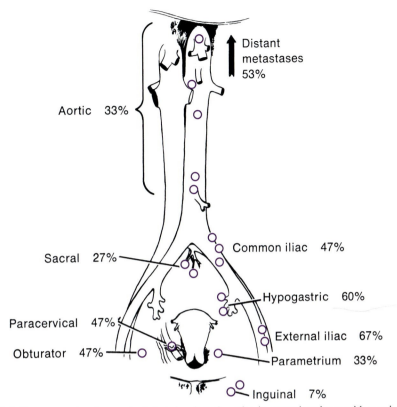

Figure 3-9 Percentage involvement of draining lymph nodes in treated patients with cervical cancer. (From Henriksen E: *Am J Obstet Gynecol* 58:924, 1949.)

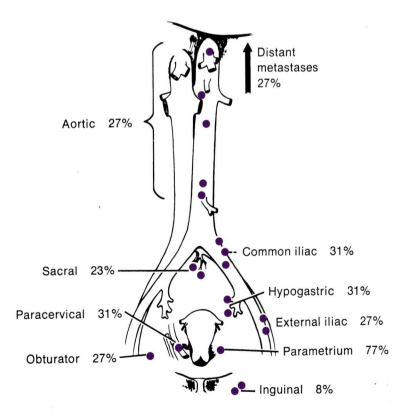

Figure 3-10 Percentage involvement of draining lymph nodes in untreated patients with cervical cancer. (From Henriksen E: *Am J Obstet Gynecol* 58:924, 1949.)

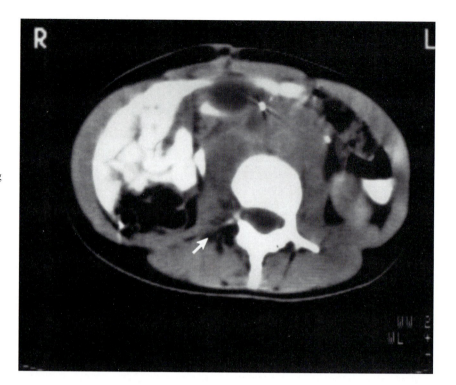

Figure 3-11 CT scan of abdomen illustrating periaortic nodes that are very enlarged and have eroded a portion of the vertebral bone on the right.

Table 3-3 Percentage incidence of pelvic and periaortic node metastasis by clinical stage

Clinical stage	Positive pelvic nodes	Positive periaortic nodes
I	15.4	6.3
II	28.6	16.5
III	47.0	28.6

Table 3-4 Size of cervical lesion and lymph node metastasis in Stage Ib cervical cancer

Site (cm)	No. of patients	No. with metastasis	Percent	
≤1	22	4	18.1	
2-3	72	16	22.1	}21.1
4-5	45	16	35.5	
≥6	6	3	50.0	}35.2
TOTAL	145	39	26.9	

20% of 436 patients (stages IIb through IVa) were found to have metastatic disease to periaortic nodes. He also reported that 25% of these patients, or 5% of those surgically staged, demonstrated a 3-year, disease-free survival. The majority of the patients with known periaortic node involvement received extended postoperative field irradiation.

Cumulative results from many studies utilizing lymphadenectomy in the surgical staging of cervix cancer has resulted in frequency of positive pelvic nodes as shown in Table 3-3.

ADENOCARCINOMA OF THE CERVIX

Some 85% to 90% of cervical cancers are squamous cell, and the majority of the remaining 10% to 15% are adenocarcinomas. There appears to be an increase in the frequency of cervical adenocarcinomas, but this may be a result of the decrease in the incidence of invasive squamous cell lesions. Adenocarcinoma arises from the endocervical mucus-producing gland cells; and because of its origin within the cervix, it may be present for a considerable time before it becomes clinically evident. These lesions are characteristically bulky neoplasms that expand the cervical canal and create the so-called barrel-shaped lesions of the cervix. The spread pattern of these lesions is similar to that of squamous cell cancer, with direct extension accompanied by metastases to regional pelvic nodes as the primary routes of dissemination. Local recurrence is more common in these lesions, and this has resulted in the commonly held belief that they are more radioresistant than their squamous counterpart.

has spread to the periaortic area enables the clinician to institute therapeutic modalities that can result in increased salvage. In other words, does the treatment of patients with spread of disease beyond the pelvis result in more cures? Berman, reporting the Gynecologic Oncology Group experience with staging laparotomy, indicated that

It seems more likely, however, that the bulky, expansive nature of these endocervical lesions, rather than a differential in radiosensitivity, accounts for the local recurrence. This problem has led many oncologists to advocate combined radiotherapy and surgery for optimal control of the central lesion.

No clear definition of "microinvasive" adenocarcinoma of the cervix has been put forward, and many authries doubt its existence. The endocervical epithelium, unlike the squamous epithelium, has no clear basement membrane from which measurements can be made. In Addition, adenocarcinoma is often multifocal. Thus parameters for conservative therapy following conization revealing early invasive adenocarcinoma are not currently established.

Kjorstad investigated the metastatic potential and patterns of dissemination in 150 patients with stage Ib adenocarcinoma of the cervix treated during a 20-year period from 1956 to 1977. All cases were treated with a combination of intracavitary radium followed by radical hysterectomy with pelvic lymph node dissection. It was found that the incidence of pelvic metastases and distant recurrences and the survival rates were the same as those given in previously published reports for squamous cell carcinoma treated in the same manner. In one respect, the adenocarcinomas showed a significant difference from the squamous cell cancers. The incidence of residual tumor in the hysterectomy specimens after intracavitary treatment was much higher (30% versus 11%). Kjorstad considered this a strong argument for surgical treatment of patients with early stages of adenocarcinoma of the cervix.

Berek reported on 100 patients with primary adenocarcinoma of the uterine cervix. Of 48 stage I patients, 13 were treated with radical surgery, 16 with radiation alone, and 19 with combination therapy. Analysis of stage I patients by Berek showed no significant difference in survival for those treated with radical surgery or combination therapy. However, both of these groups had a greater 5-year survival ($p > 0.05$) than those treated with radiation alone. Higher tumor grade was associated with poorer survival for each stage regardless of treatment. More complications were associated with radiation therapy than with radical therapy. Radiation therapy alone did not appear to be sufficient therapy for patients with stage I or stage II disease.

Moberg reported on 251 patients at Radiumhemmet in Stockholm with adenocarcinoma of the uterine cervix. The 5-year survival rate was compared with that in the total of cervical epithelial malignancies, and the rate was lower in the adenocarcinoma cases, with respective crude 5-year survival rates of 84%, 50%, and 9% in stages I, II, and III. Combined treatment consisting of two intracavitary radium treatments with an interval of 3 weeks followed by a radical hysterectomy with pelvic lymphadenectomy done within 3 months gave improved 5-year survival in a nonrandomized series. Prempree also suggested combined therapy for stage II lesions or those greater than 4 cm.

A large series of 367 cases of adenocarcinoma of the cervix was reported by Eifel et al. Their conclusions were that the central control of adenocarcinomas with radiation therapy is comparable to that achieved for squamous cell carcinomas of comparable bulk. They found no evidence that combined treatment (radiation therapy plus hysterectomy) improved local regional control or survival. In their study, radiation therapy alone was as effective a treatment for most patients with stage I disease. They noted, as others have, that patients with bulky stage I (greater than 6 cm), stage II or stage III disease, particularly with poorly differentiated lesions or evidence of nodal spread, had a very high rate of extrapelvic disease spread.

Eifel reported the results of 160 patients with adenocarcinoma of the cervix; 84 were treated with radiation therapy alone, 20 were treated with external and intracavitary radiation followed by hysterectomy, and 56 were treated with radical hysterectomy. Survival was strongly correlated with tumor size and grade. There was a 90% survival rate for lesions ≤3 cm. After 5 years, 45% of the patients treated with radical hysterectomy had a recurrence. These recurrences were stongly correlated with lymph/vascular space invasion and poorly differentiated lesions, as well as larger tumor size.

NEUROENDOCRINE SMALL-CELL AND GLASSY CELL CARCINOMA OF THE CERVIX

Neuroendocrine small-cell cervical cancers (Figure 3-12), which occur infrequently, provide a diagnostic dilemma for the pathologist and a therapeutic challenge for the clinician. The pathologist's dilemma results from the large number of pathological entities all described as "small-cell cancers," including fully differentiated small-cell nonkeratinizing squamous cell carcinoma, reserved-cell carcinoma, and neuroendocrine (oat cell) carcinoma. Neuroendocrine carcinomas, which can be identified by characteristic light and electron microscopic criteria, are indistinguishable from oat cell cancers of the lung. In addition, they appear to have the poorest prognosis of the various "small-cell" cancers. Therefore, it is important to distinguish this particular subtype of cancer from the rest and to consider innovative approaches to treatment. True neuroendocrine small-cell cervical carcinoma has a very poor prognosis. Abeler reported on 26 cases. The 5-year survival was 14% despite aggressive therapy including surgery, radiation, and chemotherapy. In our experience with 14 patients in stage Ib or IIa treated by radical hysterectomy with postoperative radiation therapy, all 14 have experienced recurrence, 12 before the thirty-first month following therapy. Innovative approaches to

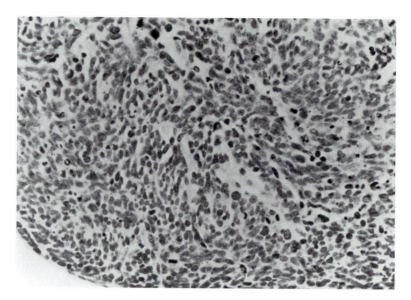

Figure 3-12 Small cell carcinoma.

treating this subset of unfortunate patients are under study.

Glassy cell carcinoma of the cervix has also been classically regarded as a poorly differentiated adenosquamous carcinoma, infrequently diagnosed and associated with a poor outcome regardless of the modality of therapy. Many recurrences occur in the first year following therapy, and most have occurred by 24 months. Reported survival rates are more encouraging than those associated with neuroendocrine carcinomas, rates as high as 50% being reported for stage I disease in some series. Lotocki reported 32 cases, which accounted for 5% of all cervical carcinomas in his series. The mean age was 10 years younger than other histologic subtypes. The 5-year survival for Ib lesions was 45% when treated with radical hysterectomy as compared to 90% for squamous cell carcinoma and 78% for adenocarcinoma.

STAGING

The staging of cancer of the cervix is a clinical appraisal, preferably confirmed with the patient under anesthesia; it cannot be changed later if findings at operation or subsequent treatment reveal further advancement of the disease.

International classification of cancer of the cervix
(Figure 3-13)

Stage 0	Carcinoma in situ, intraepithelial carcinoma
Stage I	The carcinoma is strictly confined to the cervix (extension to the corpus should be disregarded)
Stage Ia	Invasive cancer identified only microscopically; all gross lesions even with superficial invasion are stage Ib cancers Invasion is limited to measured stromal invasion with maximum depth of 5.0 mm and no wider than 7.0 mm
Stage Ia1	Measured invasion of stroma no greater than 3.0 mm in depth and no wider than 7.0 mm
Stage Ia2	Measured invasion of stroma greater than 3 mm and no greater than 5 mm and no wider than 7 mm. The depth of invasion should not be more than 5 mm taken from the base of the epithelium, surface or glandular, from which it originates. Vascular space involvement, venous or lymphatic, should not alter the staging.
Stage Ib	Clinical lesions confined to the cervix or preclinical lesions greater than stage Ia
Stage Ib1	Clinical lesions no greater than 4.0 cm in size
Stage Ib2	Clinical lesions greater than 4 cm in size
Stage II	Involvement of the vagina but not the lower third, or infiltration of the parametria but not out to the sidewall
Stage IIa	Involvement of the vagina but no evidence of parametrial involvement
Stage IIb	Infiltration of the parametria but not out to the sidewall
Stage III	Involvement of the lower third of the vagina or extension to the pelvic sidewall; all cases with a hydronephrosis or nonfunctioning kidney should be included, unless they are known to be attributable to other cause
Stage IIIa	Involvement of the lower third of the vagina but not out to the pelvic sidewall if the parametria are involved
Stage IIIb	Extension onto the pelvic sidewall and/or hydronephrosis or nonfunctional kidney
Stage IV	Extension outside the reproductive tract
Stage IVa	Involvement of the mucosa of the bladder or rectum
Stage IVb	Distant metastasis or disease outside the true pelvis

The following diagnostic aids are acceptable for determining a staging classification: physical examination,

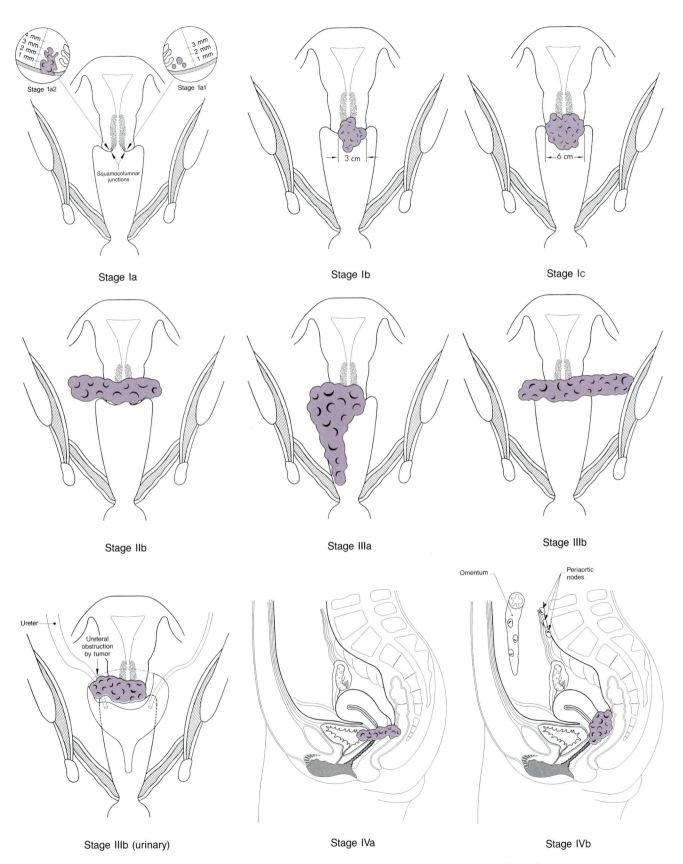

Figure 3-13 FIGO stagings and classification of cancer of the cervix. (From DiSaia PJ: Stagins and surgical therapy of uterine malignancies, *Adv Oncol* 8(2):15, 1992.)

routine radiographs, colposcopy, cystoscopy, proctosigmoidoscopy, IVP, and barium studies of the lower colon and rectum. Other examinations, such as lymphography, CT scans, MRI examinations, arteriography, venography, laparoscopy, and hysteroscopy, are not recommended for staging, since they are not uniformly available from institution to institution. It is important to stress that staging is a means of communicating between one institution and another. Probably more important, however, staging is a means of evaluating the treatment plans used within one institution. For these reasons, the method of staging should remain fairly constant. Staging does not limit the treatment plan, and therapy can be tailored to the architecture of the malignancy in each patient. Findings uncovered by CT scan or MRI examinations can be used in the planning of therapy but should not influence the initial clinical staging of the lesion. Unfortunately, clinical staging is only a rough value in prognosis, since diseases of wide variability are often included under one subheading. This is particularly true in stage Ib2, where a clinically obvious 3 cm lesion carries the same stage as a 7 cm lesion confined to the uterus. Clinical staging is enhanced with the liberal use of rectovaginal examinations (Figure 3-14) in that this type of pelvic examination allows more complete palpation of the parametria and cul-de-sac.

The role of laparoscopic lymphadenectomy is investigational at this time. The ability to perform pelvic and para-aortic lymphadenectomy in skilled hands allows for a more complete surgical staging of cancers of the cervix but no conclusive data exists supporting an advantage to this approach.

Some gynecological oncologists feel that limited staging procedures are warranted on paitents with advanced stage cervical cancer to place patients on institutional or national group protocols. The status of periaortic nodes should be known before initiation of treatment in such cases to plan appropriate modalities, such as the extent of the radiation field or concomitant chemotherapy. An extraperitoneal approach for removal of the periaortic nodes is preferred by many clinicians in an effort to reduce morbidity from the procedure. More advanced lesions have been investigated with a retroperitoneal lymphadenectomy to determine the extent of disease prior to planning radiotherapy fields (Figure 3-15). The following is an explanation of one such approach (Figure 3-16, A-J):

TREATMENT

After the diagnosis of invasive cervical cancer is established, the question is how to best treat the patient. Specific therapeutic measures are usually governed by the age and general health of the patient, by the extent of the cancer, and by the presence and nature of any complicating abnormalities. It is thus essential to carry out a complete and careful investigation of the patient (see the box on p. 69), and then a joint decision regarding treatment should be made by the radiotherapist and gynecologist. The choice of treatment demands clinical judgment, but apart from the occasional patient for whom only symptomatic treatment may be best, this choice lies between surgery and radiotherapy. In most institutions the initial method of treatment for locally advanced disease is radiotherapy, both intracavitary (cesium or radium) and external x-ray therapy. The controversy between surgery and radio-therapy has existed for decades and essentially surrounds the treatment of stage I and stage IIa cervical cancer. For the most part, all stages above stage I and stage IIa are treated with radiotherapy. The 5-year survival figures from two large series, one treated with

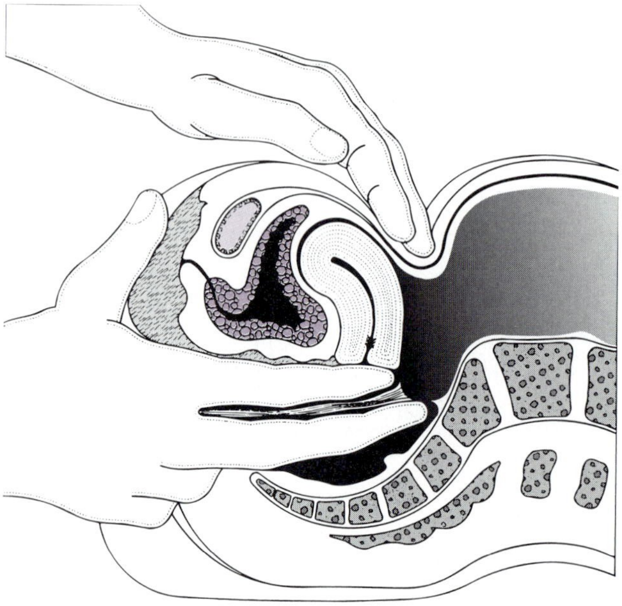

Figure 3-14 Technique of rectovaginal examination.

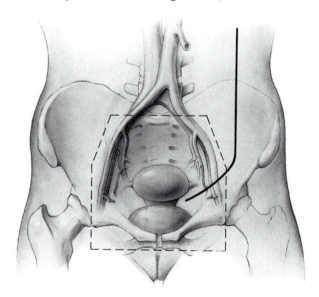

Figure 3-15 Pelvic diagram. The dashed line indicates the radiation field and the position of the uterus and cervix within the field. The bold line indicates the "J" incision path relative to the field and to the major vessels.

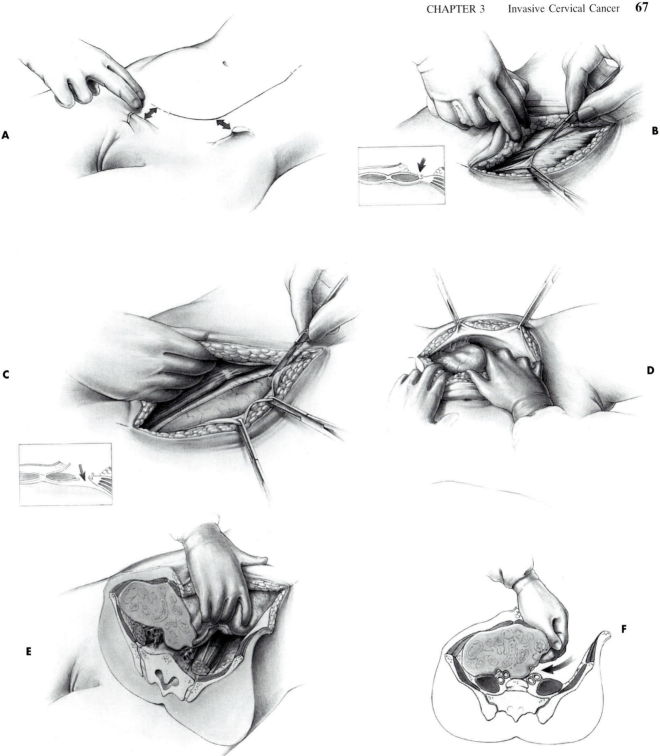

Figure 3-16 A, Path of incision. First measurement of 2-3 cm (two fingerwidths) above pubic symphysis, second measurement 2-3 cm medial to anterior superior iliac spine. Diagonal line connecting these points. Vertical line drawn superiorly to 3-4 cm above level of umbilicus. Incision begins at lateral margin of rectus muscle. **B,** Division of external sheath of rectus and cross section. After initial incision through skin, lateral margin of sheath is divided with bovie along length of muscle. Cross-section arrow points to ideal point of separation. **C,** Division of internal sheath of rectus and cross-section. Rectus muscle mobilized medially. Internal sheath divided with care to preserve underlying exposed peritoneum. **D,** Blunt dissection. Blunt dissection with hand following the plane of the peritoneum and separating it from transversalis fascia. **E,** Blunt dissection (cont.: perspective cross-section). Dissection along peritoneum until contact is made with left ureter. Ureter is preserved with peritoneum and mobilized medially as dissection continues. Psoas muscle and common iliac vessels are exposed. **F,** Cross section. Proper pathway of dissection along peritoneum over psoas.   *Continued.*

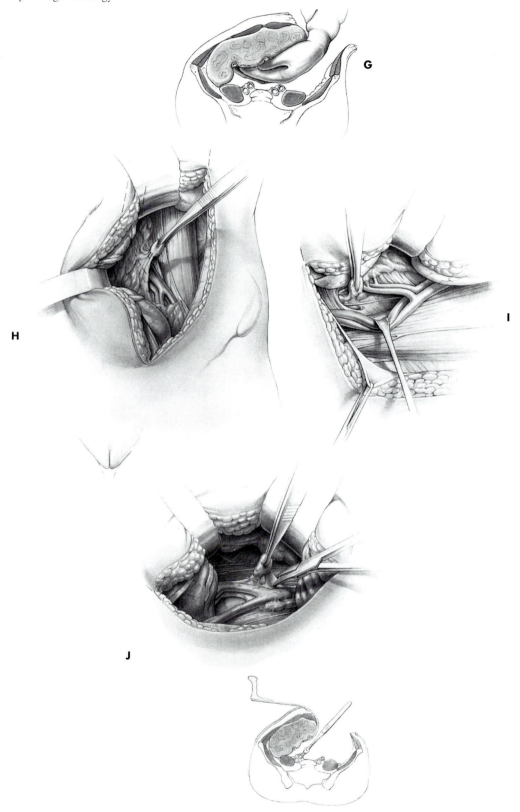

Figure 3-16, cont'd. G, Cross-section of deep dissection. Exposure of left and right common iliac vessels underneath peritoneum at about the level of L5-S1. CAUTION: Avoid damage to inferior mesenteric artery. **H,** Lymphadenectomy begins along left common iliac vessels. After medial and superior retraction of mesentery and beginning about the bifurcation of internal and external iliac vessels, lymph nodes are removed along the length of left common iliac to junction with aorta. **I,** Obturator nodes. Lateral mobilization of external iliac vessels with vein retractor. Obturator nerve is identified and nodes are removed. **J,** Right common iliac. Right common and para-aortic lymph nodes are clipped and removed. Diagram shows deep access to right common iliac nodes.

PRETREATMENT EVALUATION OF CARCINOMA OF THE UTERINE CERVIX

1. History, physical examination, and routine blood studies
2. Radiologic studies
   a. Chest film
   b. IVP or CT scan with IV contrast
   c. Barium enema (adenocarcinomas, advanced stages, or where otherwise clinically indicated, as in a patient with lower bowel symptoms)
3. Cystoscopy (very low yield in stage I)
4. Rectosigmoidoscopy (same indications as barium enema)

---

radiotherapy alone and the other with surgery, are included here. Currie reported the results of 552 radical operations for cancer of the cervix:

Stage I	189 cases	86.3%
Stage IIa	103 cases	75.0%
Stage IIb	78 cases	58.9%
Other stages	41 cases	34.1%

Some of these patients with positive nodes received postoperative radiotherapy.

In 1981 Zander reported results of a 20-year cooperative study from Germany dealing with 1092 patients with stages Ib and II cancer of the cervix treated with radical hysterectomy of the Meigs type and bilateral pelvic lymphadenopathy. Of the 1092 patients, 50.6% had surgery only, with a 5-year survival rate of 84.5% in stage Ib and 71.1% in stage II (most were stage IIa). This correlates well with the figures reported by Currie and Falk. The rest of the patients reported by Zander received postoperative whole-pelvis irradiation therapy. No significant difference could be observed in the survival rates of patients undergoing only surgery as compared with those of patients undergoing adjuvant postoperative radiation. In fact, in 199 patients with lymph node involvement, the difference in survival rates of those undergoing only surgery and those undergoing additional postoperative radiation therapy was statistically insignificant.

Of 2000 patients treated with radiotherapy at MD Anderson Hospital and Tumor Institute, Fletcher reports the following 5-year cure rates:

Stage I	91.5%
Stage IIa	83.5%
Stage IIb	66.5%
Stage IIIa	45.0%
Stage IIIb	36.0%
Stage IV	14.0%

Two later reports give very similar 5-year survivals for radiotherapy alone. Perez reported 87% for stage Ib, 73% for IIa, 68% for IIb, and 44% for stage III. Montana reported 76% for IIa, 62% for IIb, and 33% for stage III.

In general, in early stages, comparable survival rates result from both treatment techniques. The advantage of radiotherapy is that it is applicable to virtually all patients, whereas radical surgery of necessity excludes certain medically inoperable patients. The possible occurrence of immediate serious morbidity must be kept in mind when this treatment plan is selected. In many institutions surgery for stage I and stage IIa disease is reserved for young patients in whom preservation of ovarian function is desired and improved vaginal preservation is expected. The modern operative mortality and the postoperative ureterovaginal fistula rate both have been recently reported at far less than 1%, making an objective decision for therapy even more difficult. Other reasons given for the selection of radical surgery over radiation include cervical cancer in pregnancy, concomitant inflammatory disease of the bowel, previous irradiation therapy for other disease, presence of pelvic inflammatory disease or an adnexal neoplasm along with the malignancy, as well as patient preference. Among the disadvantages of radiation therapy, one must consider the permanent injury to the tissues of the normal organ bed of the neoplasm and the possibility of second malignancies developing in this bed.

Surgical Management

The use of radical hysterectomy in the United States was initiated by Joe V. Meigs at Harvard University in 1944, and shortly thereafter the radical hysterectomy with pelvic lymphadenopathy was adopted by many clinics in the United States because of dissatisfaction with the limitations of radiotherapy. Some had found that many lesions were not radiosensitive, and some patients had metastatic disease in regional lymph nodes that were alleged to be radioresistant. Radiation injuries had been reported, and one of the overriding points in favor of surgery was that gynecologists were surgeons rather than radiotherapists and thus felt more comfortable with this treatment. At the time of the popularization of this procedure, modern techniques of surgery, anesthesia, antibiotics, and electrolyte balance had emerged, reducing the enormous morbidity that once attended major operative procedures in the abdomen.

Radical hysterectomy is a procedure that must be performed by a skilled technician with sufficient experience to make the morbidity acceptable (1% to 5%). The procedure involves removal of the uterus, the upper 25% of the vagina, the entire uterosacral and uterovesical ligaments (Figure 3-17), and all of the parametrium on each side, along with pelvic node dissection encompassing the four major pelvic lymph node chains: ureteral, obturator, hypogastric, and iliac. Metastatic lesions to the ovaries are rare, and preservation of these structures is acceptable, especially in young women. The procedure is complex because the tissues removed are in close proximity to many vital structures such as the bowel, bladder, ureters (Figure 3-18), and great vessels of the pelvis. The object of the dissection is to preserve the

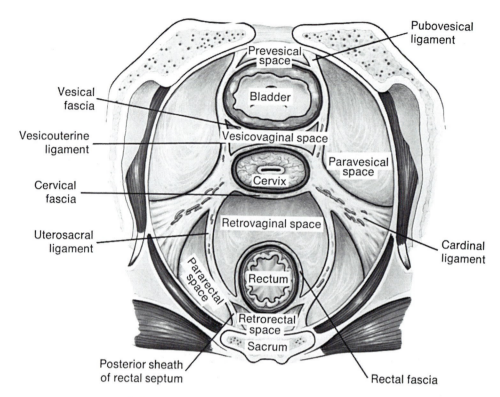

Figure 3-17 Cross section of the pelvis at the level of the cervix.

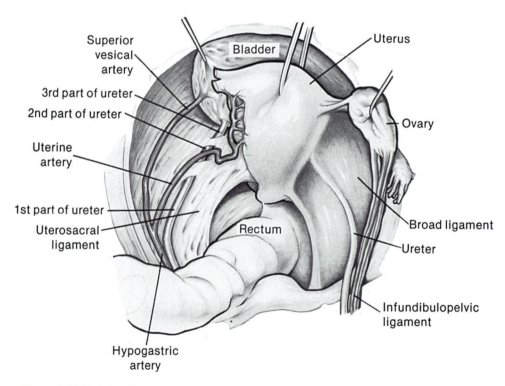

Figure 3-18 Relationship of the ureter to the uterosacral ligaments, uterine artery, infundibulopelvic ligament, and uterus.

bladder, rectum, and ureters without injury but to remove as much of the remaining tissue of the pelvis as is feasible.

There is no doubt that in stage I, as well as the more restricted stage II cases, surgical removal of the disease is feasible. The addition of pelvic lymphadenectomy to the operative procedure caused considerable controversy in the early part of the century. Wertheim removed nodes only if they were enlarged and then not systematically. He believed that when accessible regional nodes were involved, the inaccessible distant nodes were also involved, and removal of suspicious nodes was more for prognostic than for therapeutic value. He thought that node involvement was a measure of the lethal quality of the tumor and not merely a mechanical extension of the disease. The operative procedure popularized by Meigs included meticulous pelvic lymphadenectomy. Indeed, Meigs demonstrated a 42% 5-year survival rate in another series of patients with positive nodes. Lymphadenectomy is now an established part of the operative procedure for any patient with disease greater than stage Ia1. There has been some interest in combining a radical vaginal operation with a retroperitoneal lymphadenectomy, and the results reported by Mitra, Navratil and Kastner, and McCall are surprisingly good. The survival rate in patients with negative nodes is usually in the range of 90% or more.

Patients with positive pelvic nodes usually receive postoperative whole-pelvis irradiation, although scientific evidence that this improves outcome is lacking. A small multi-institutional retrospective survey conducted by SGO in 1979 and reported by Morrow revealed an unaltered incidence of recurrence with the addition of pelvic irradiation (Table 3-5). The lower incidence of pelvic recurrence in the irradiated group was countered by an increased incidence of distant metastases in the unirradiated group. A large study is needed before firm conclusions can be reached. Evidence for the potentially curative role of adjuvant pelvic radiotherapy is at this time intuitive, but some facts suggest benefit. Pelvic relapses after surgery are salvaged in 15% to 45% of the cases with the use of radiotherapy. Pelvic radiotherapy appears to effectively reduce the relapse risk when surgical margins are close or positive. The expected frequency of lymph node positivity encountered at surgery is apparently reduced by the use of preoperative external pelvic radiotherapy. These and other observations have led many, including these authors, to continue to recommend postoperative radiotherapy in patients with multiple positive pelvic nodes following surgical therapy.

Techniques

In 1974 Piver, Rutledge, and Smith reported on the five classes or types of extended hysterectomy (Table 3-6) devised by Rutledge and used in treating women with cervical cancer at the MD Anderson Hospital. They suggested that the term *radical hysterectomy* is not adequate to record and communicate the different amounts of therapy attempted and the subsequent risk of complications when different surgeons report their re-

Table 3-5   Stage Ib squamous cell carcinoma of the cervix with positive pelvic nodes following radical hysterectomy pelvic lymphadenectomy

Site of recurrence	Radiotherapy		No radiotherapy	
	N	% Total	N	% Total
Pelvis	5	(10.6)	27	(18.5)
Central	3	(6.4)	8	(5.5)
Pelvic wall	2	(4.2)	19	(13.0)
Distant metastases	9	(19.1)	9	(6.2)
Both	4	(8.5)	21	(14.4)
TOTAL	18/47	(38.3)	57/146	(39.0)

Table 3-6   Rutledge classification of extended hysterectomy

Class	Description	Indication
I	Extrafascial hysterectomy; pubocervical ligament is incised, allowing lateral deflection of ureter	CIN, early stromal invasion
II	Removal of medial half of cardinal and uterosacral ligaments; upper third of vagina removed	Microcarcinoma postirradiation
III	Removal of entire cardinal and uterosacral ligaments; upper third of vagina removed	Stage Ib and IIa lesions
IV	Removal of all periureteral tissue, superior vesical artery, and three fourths of vagina	Anteriorly occurring central recurrences where preservation of the bladder is still possible
V	Removal of portions of distal ureter and bladder	Central recurrent cancer involving portions of the distal ureter or bladder

From Piver MS, Rutledge FN, Smith PJ. Reprinted with permission from The American College of Obstetricians and Gynecologists (*Obstetrics and Gynecology*, 44:265, 1974).

sults. These authors believed that describing the technical features of five operations enabled them to evaluate more accurately their results *and* provided a better understanding of the need to tailor each patient's treatment by using an operation that was adequate but not excessive.

The goal of the class I hysterectomy was to ensure removal of all cervical tissue. Reflection and retraction of the ureters laterally without actual dissection from the ureteral bed allows one to clamp the adjacent paracervical tissue without cutting into the side of the cervical tissue itself. Class I operations are advocated primarily for in situ and true microinvasive carcinomas of the cervix. A class I procedure is also performed after preoperative radiation in adenocarcinoma of the cervix or after preoperative radiation in the so-called barrel-shaped endocervical squamous cell carcinoma. The operation described is essentially the extrafascial hysterectomy employed routinely at the MD Anderson Hospital.

Class II extended hysterectomy is described as a moderately extended radical hysterectomy. The purpose of the class II hysterectomy is to remove more paracervical tissue (Figure 3-19) while still preserving most of the blood supply to the distal ureters and bladder. The ureters are freed from their paracervical position but are not dissected out of the pubovesical ligament. The uterine artery is ligated just medial to the ureter as it lies in "the tunnel," ensuring preservation of the distal ureteral supply. The uterosacral ligaments are transected midway between the uterus and their sacral attachments (Figure 3-20). The medial halves of both cardinal ligaments are removed, as well as the upper 25% of the vagina. A pelvic lymphadenectomy is usually performed with a class II hysterectomy. A class II operation is reported to be suitable for the following conditions: (1) microinvasive carcinomas in which the depth of invasion is considered greater than early stromal invasion and (2) small postirradiation recurrences limited to the cervix.

The class III procedure is a wide radical excision of the parametrial and paravaginal tissues in addition to the removal of the pelvic lymphatic tissue. The uterine artery is ligated at its origin on the internal iliac artery. In the dissection of the ureter from the pubovesical ligament (between the lower end of the ureter and the superior vesical artery) care is taken to preserve the ligament, maintaining some additional blood supply to the distal ureter. The hazard of fistula formation is decreased by preservation of the superior vesical artery, along with a portion of the associated pubovesical ligament. The uterosacral ligaments are resected at the pelvic sidewall. The upper 25% of the vagina is removed (Figure 3-21),

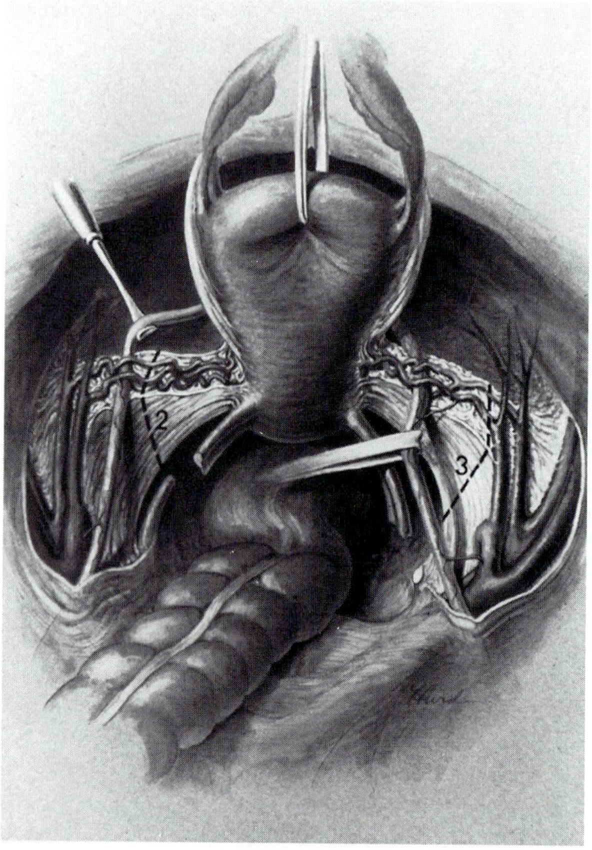

Figure 3-19 Broken lines identify the point of transection of the cardinal ligaments in class II and class III radical hysterectomy. (Courtesy Dr. Gregorio Delgado.)

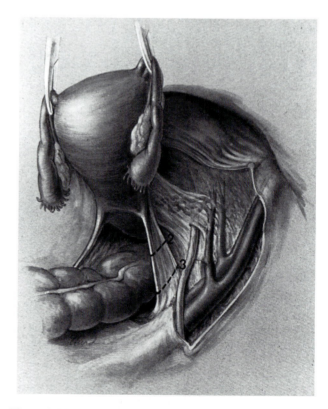

Figure 3-20 Broken lines identify the point of transection of the uterosacral ligaments in class II and class III radical hysterectomy. (Courtesy Dr. Gregorio Delgado.)

and a pelvic lymphadenectomy is routinely performed. This operation is primarily for the patient with stage I or IIa carcinoma of the cervix with or withou preservation of ovarian function.

The aim of the class IV radical hysterectomy is complete removal of all periureteral tissue, a more extensive excision of the paravaginal tissues, and, when indicated, excision of the internal iliac vessels along an involved portion of the medial pelvic wall tissue. This differs from the class III operation in three respects: (1) the ureter is completely dissected from the pubovesical ligament, (2) the superior vesical artery is sacrificed, and (3) 50% of the vagina is removed. This procedure is used primarily for more extensive anteriorly occurring central recurrences when preservation of the bladder is seemingly still possible. Extension of the dissection laterally is needed when the disease has focally involved the medial parametrium. Sacrificing blood vessels to the bladder is unfavorable because the risk of fistula formation increases significantly. In most instances these patients are more appropriately treated with an anterior exenteration.

The purpose of the class V hysterectomy is to remove a central recurrent cancer involving portions of the distal ureter or bladder. It is different from a class IV operation because the disease involves a portion of the distal ureter or bladder, or both, which is removed with the disease. A reimplantation of the ureter into the bladder, often as a ureteroneocystostomy, is then performed. This procedure has a rare application to a small, specifically located recurrence when exenteration is considered unnecessary or has been refused by the patient.

The modified Rutledge classification of extended hysterectomies has considerable practical value. It once again underlines the necessity for the surgeon to tailor the operative procedure to the disease extent. The patient with a stage Ia2 lesion does not need an operative procedure as radical as the patient with a large IIa lesion. This is particularly pertinent in the decision between a class II and class III radical hysterectomy. In many countries the class II radical hysterectomy (called a modified radical hysterectomy) is combined with a bilateral pelvic lymphadenectomy as standard therapy for early stage cervical cancer. Indeed, the class III type of radical hysterectomy is a phenomenon of particular prevalence in the Western hemisphere and the Orient because of the dual influences of Meigs and Okabayashi. The class III or Meigs-Okabayashi procedure is a derivative of the halstedian principle that a lesion should be removed en bloc with its draining lymphatics; thus, the class III radical hysterectomy calls for removal of all the parametria at the pelvic sidewall and transection of the uterosacral ligaments at the sacrum. Advocates of the modified radical hysterectomy or class II procedure with pelvic lymphadenectomy for stages I and IIa lesions suggest that the intervening lymphatics are not at risk in an early cancer of the cervix. Indeed, spread from the primary lesion to the draining pelvic wall nodes probably occurs as an embolic phenomenon. One virtually never finds a tumor in lymphatics except surrounding the primary lesions. My personal experience (P.J.D.) with radical hysterectomy has supported this concept. Over the last several years, my colleagues and I have urged our pathologist to take several sections of the most distal portion of the parametria

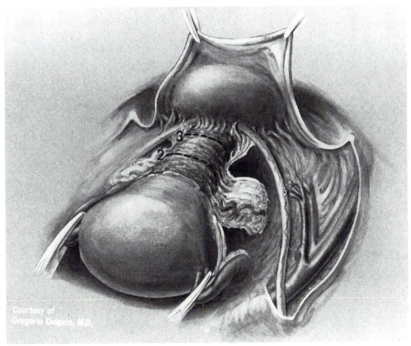

Figure 3-21 Broken lines illustrate level of vaginal removal of class II and class III radical hysterectomy. (Courtesy Dr. Gregorio Delgado.)

following a class III radical hysterectomy for stage I or IIa cervical cancer in an effort to determine the presence or absence of malignant cells in lymphatics distant from the primary lesion. To date, we have not found any evidence that plugs of malignant cells are trapped in these channels in the distal portion of the parametria. This has prompted us to become less radical with early lesions, especially with microscopic invasive disease. In the presence of a bulky central lesion, the need for an adequate surgical margin of resection often mandates a more extensive procedure than the typical class II radical hysterectomy. However, preservation of any portion of the lateral parametria appears to be associated with a greatly diminished incidence of bladder atony. Forney reported on 22 women extensively studied after undergoing radical hysterectomy; in 11 women, the cardinal ligaments had been divided completely, and in the other 11, the inferior 1 to 2 cm of these ligaments had been spared. Satisfactory voiding occurred significantly earlier (20 versus 51 days) in women who had had an incomplete transection. In a similar manner, preservation of a portion of the uterosacral ligaments appears to be associated with fewer complaints of postoperative obstipation. Undoubtedly, the preserved tissue contains intact nerve tracts, which avoid the extensive denervation associated with the typical class III type or radical hysterectomy.

Complications

Undoubtedly, the major complication following radical surgery for invasive cancer of the cervix is postoperative bladder dysfunction. Reports in the literature by Seski and Carenza, Nobili, and Giacobini suggest that bladder dysfunction is a direct result of injury to the sensory and motor nerve supply to the detrusor muscle of the bladder. The more radical the surgery, the greater the extent of damage and the more likely postoperative bladder dysfunction will result. This dysfunction is usually manifested in the patient by a loss of the sense of urgency to void and an inability to empty the bladder completely without a Credê maneuver. Although most patients learn to compensate for the sensory and motor loss and return to near normal function, patients occasionally need to be taught intermittent self-catheterization, or long periods of constant bladder drainage may be necessary postoperatively. Sophisticated urodynamic studies have shown that a residual hypertonicity in the bladder detrusor muscle and urethral sphincter mechanism sometimes produces dysuria and stress incontinence. Treatment is symptomatic with near total recovery in most patients. Limitation of the extent and radicality of surgery, especially in patients with early lesions, can minimize this morbidity. Bandy reported on the long-term effects on bladder function following radical hysterectomy (class III) with and without postoperative radiation. In his study, the necessity for bladder drainage of 30 or more days after surgery in 30% of patients was associated with significantly worse long-term residual and other bladder dysfunction. Adjunctive pelvic radiation was associated with significantly more contracted and unstable bladder.

Drainage of the retroperitoneal space with continuous suction catheters can be used to help reduce the particularly troublesome complication of the lymphocyst formation. Two studies testing the hypothesis that avoiding reperitonealization of the pelvic peritoneum obviates the need for such drainage have been reported; both studies suggest that drainage is not necessary if the peritoneum is left open over the surgical site. Ligation of the lymphatics entering the obturator fossa under the external iliac vein helps reduce the flow of lymph into this area, where lymphocyst formation is prevalent. Lymphocysts, if present, rarely cause injury and are usually reabsorbed if given enough time. Choo reports that cysts less than 4 to 5 cm usually resolve within 2 months and only observation is necessary. Surgical intervention is necessary when there is some evidence of significant ureteral obstruction. During laparotomy the surgeon should unroof the lymphocyst and prevent reformation by suturing a tongue of omentum into the cavity (internal marsupialization). Percutaneous aspiration of the cyst, which is often associated with subsequent infection, should be utilized cautiously.

Pulmonary embolism is the one complication most likely to cause mortality in the period surrounding the operative therapy of cervical cancer. This must be kept in mind at all times, and particular care must be exercised during and after surgery to avoid this devastating complication. The operative period is certainly the most dangerous period for the formation of a thrombus in the leg or pelvic veins. Care should be taken to ensure that a constriction of veins in the leg does not occur during the operative procedure, and careful dissection of the pelvic veins should lead to minimal thrombus formation in those structures. In 1975 Kakkar reported on the use of subcutaneous heparin, 5000 IU given 2 hours preoperatively and every 8 hours thereafter for 7 days or until the patient was walking well. After a multicenter prospective randomized trial, he showed that prophylactic low-dose heparin will reduce the incidence of fatal postoperative embolism without evidence of serious bleeding during surgery. Although most of his patients were not undergoing radical surgical procedures, our experience is that this type of therapy is safe and that increased bleeding is minimal even with radical surgery. Our practice has been to consider this so-called minidose heparin therapy for patients with a history of thromboembolic disease or severe venous varicosities and for others, when we suspect that they may be at increased risk for a postoperative embolus. At present, all our patients wear pneumatic compression stockings during major operative procedures and continue to wear them for several days into the postoperative period.

Soisson reported on 43 women undergoing radical hysterectomy for early stage cervical cancer. All patients had a body weight at least 25% greater than their ideal

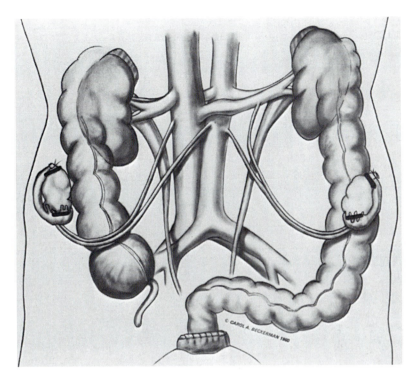

Figure 3-22 Diagram illustrating location of transposed adnexae to a non-pelvic site where they can be spared postoperative pelvic irradiation. (From DiSaia PJ: *Cancer* 48:548, 1981.)

weight. Survival was not compromised, and the incidence of serious complications was not increased in obese patients when compared to a control group. Operative technique is more difficult; the procedure lasts longer, and surgery is associated with greater blood loss.

Preservation of ovarian function is often desirable for patients who must undergo a surgical procedure for invasive cancer of the cervix. Many times, after a careful histologic examination of the operative specimen, including the pelvic lymph nodes, a postoperative recommendation for pelvic radiation is indicated. For example, our experience has shown that patients with deep invasion of the cervical stroma, even with negative nodes, are at higher risk for recurrence and should be considered for postoperative pelvic irradiation. Standard pelvic placement of preserved ovaries will result in postirradiation ovarian failure; therefore, a procedure for transposition of the ovaries to an extrapelvic site (Figure 3-22) has been devised. Shielding during postoperative pelvic irradiation is possible with the ovaries so placed. The ovaries receive some radiation but not usually enough to prevent continued steroid production. Husseinzadeh reported only a 17% incidence of ovarian failure in women whose ovaries had been transposed and shielded during postoperative pelvic irradiation therapy. A word of caution has been interjected by Mann and others regarding the rare occurrence of occult metastases to the ovary in patients with adenocarcinoma of the cervix. The two largest studies suggest that the incidence is between 0.6% and 1.3%, respectively. Most patients with metastatic disease in the ovary are postmenopausal or have had gross adnexal pathology or positive pelvic lymph nodes. These guidelines can be helpful in identifying patients for whom

preservation of ovarian tissue is unwise. The incidence of occult metastasis to the ovary from squamous cell carcinoma of the cervix (stage I and IIa) is so rare that preservation of ovarian tissue does not carry the same concerns.

Recurrent disease can be expected in 10% to 20% of patients treated with radical hysterectomy and bilateral lymphadenectomy. A tumor is likely to regrow from viable cancer cells left behind at the time of radical surgery. Recurrences cause rather dismal prognoses, leading to death in more than 85% of cases. Krebs et al. reported on 40 patients with recurrence following radical surgery for early invasive cancer of the cervix; 58% of the recurrences were found within the first 12 months after surgery and 83% within the first 2 years. The site of recurrence was found to influence diagnosis, symptoms, clinical findings, prognosis, cause of death, and therapy. Prognosis for patients with recurrent cervical cancer was poor, with only five patients (13%) surviving free of disease 5 years after recognition of the occurrence. Krebs et al. suggested radiation therapy as the treatment of choice for patients with pelvic recurrences who did not have prior radiation therapy. The survival rate in that group of patients in their study was 25%. Of their patients, 35% had recurrences outside the pelvis. The authors stressed the importance of close follow-up of patients after radical hysterectomy and bilateral node dissection, with monthly examinations during the first year and bimonthly examinations during the second and third years. Early recognition of a recurrent lesion centrally located appears to give the best prognosis for salvage.

The major complications of radical hysterectomy are formation of ureteral fistulae and lymphocysts, pelvic

Table 3-7 Complications of radical hysterectomy with approximate incidences (%)

Vesicovaginal fistula	1%
Ureterovaginal fistula	2%
Severe bladder atony	4%
Bowel obstruction (requiring surgery)	1%
Lymphocyst (requiring drainage)	3%
Thrombophlebitis	2%
Pulmonary embolus	1%

infection, and hemorrhage. All these complications are preventable, and the incidence is decreasing steadily (Table 3-7). Ureteral fistulae are now infrequent (0% to 3%), primarily as a result of the improvement in techniques, such as avoiding excess damage to the structure itself and preserving alternate routes of blood supply. Retroperitoneal drainage of the lymphadenectomy sites by means of suction catheters and/or avoiding reapproximation of the pelvic peritoneum has considerably reduced the incidence of lymphocysts and pelvic infection. The use of electrocautery and hemoclips has assisted the surgeon immensely with hemostasis, and postoperative hemorrhage is rare. The wide spectrum of antibiotics available today is invaluable in the prevention of pelvic infection, which had contributed significantly to fistula formation, adhesions, and bowel complications. Full dose irradiation to the pelvis before radical hysterectomy will result in a significant increase in complications, particularly urinary tract fistulae and ureteral obstruction caused by fibrosis, or more frequent lymphocyst formation.

Radiotherapy

Over the past half century radiotherapy has emerged as a notable alternative to radical surgery, primarily because of improvements in technique. The number of radiation-resistant lesions was discovered to be small, and skilled radiologists limit radiation injury, especially with the moderate dosages used for early disease. Much evidence has been presented recently that proves that radiotherapy can destroy disease in lymph nodes and in the primary lesion. Over the past two decades, radical hysterectomy has been reserved in many institutions for patients who are relatively young, lean, and in otherwise good health. In other areas of the United States, radiotherapy or surgery is used alone when the alternate modality is not available. The relative safety of both treatment modalities, as well as the high curability for stages I and IIa lesions, gives physician and patient a true option for therapy.

Radiotherapy for cancer of the cervix was begun in 1903 in New York by Margaret Cleaves. In 1913 Abbe was able to report an 8-year cure. The Stockholm method was established in 1914, the Paris method in 1919, and the

Manchester method in 1938. Radium was the first element used; it has always been the most important element in radiotherapy of this lesion. External irradiation was used to treat the lymphatic drainage areas in the pelvis lateral to the cervix and the paracervical tissues.

Successful radiation therapy depends on the following:
1. Greater sensitivity of the cancer cell, as compared with the cells of the normal tissue bed, to ionizing radiation
2. Greater ability of normal tissue to recuperate after irradiation
3. A patient in reasonably good physical condition

The maximal effect of ionizing radiation on cancer is obtained in the presence of a good and intact circulation and adequate cellular oxygenation. Preparation of the patient for a radical course of irradiation therapy should be as careful as the preparation for radical surgery. The patient's general condition should be as well maintained as possible with a diet high in proteins, vitamins, and calories. Excessive blood loss should be controlled and hemoglobin maintained well above 10 g.

Some consideration must be given to the tolerance of normal tissues of the pelvis, which are likely to receive relatively high doses during the course of treatment of cervical malignancy. The vaginal mucosa in the area of the vault tolerates between 20,000 and 25,000 cGy.* The rectovaginal septum is said to tolerate approximately 6000 cGy over 4 to 6 weeks without difficulty. The bladder mucosa can accept a maximal dose of 7000 cGy. The colon and rectum will tolerate approximately 5000 to 6000 cGy, but small bowel loops are less tolerant and are said to accept a maximal dose of between 4000 and 4200 cGy. This of course pertains to small bowel loops within the pelvis; the tolerance of the small bowel when the entire abdomen is irradiated is limited to 2500 cGy. One of the basic principles of radiotherapy is implied here: the normal tissue tolerance of any organ is inversely related to the volume of the organ receiving irradiation.

External irradiation and intracavitary radium therapy must be used in various combinations (Table 3-8). Treatment plans must be tailored to each patient and her particular lesion. The size and distribution of the cancer, not the stage, should be treated. Success in curing cancer of the cervix depends on the ability of the therapy team to evaluate the lesion (as well as the geometry of the pelvis) during treatment and then make indicated changes in therapy as necessary. Intracavitary radium therapy is ideally suited to the treatment of early tumors because of the accessibility of the portio of the cervix and the cervical canal. It is possible to place radium or cesium in close proximity to the lesion and thus deliver surface doses that approach 15,000 to 20,000 cGy. In addition, normal cervical and vaginal tissue has a particularly high tolerance to irradiation. One thus has an ideal situation for the treatment of cancer in that there are accessible lesions

---

* 1 cGy equals 1 rad of absorbed dose (see Appendix G, p. 619).

Table 3-8 Suggested therapy for cervical cancer

Stage	Whole pelvis (cGy)	Brachytherapy (mg-hr)	Surgery
Ia1 true micro-invasive			Extrafascial hysterectomy
Ia2	2000 (2000 parametrial)	8000 (2 applications)	Radical hysterectomy with bilateral pelvic lymphadenectomy as option
Ib		6000 (2 applications)	
IIa	4000	6000 (2 applications)	
	4000		
IIb	4000-5000*	5000-6000 (2 applications)	Consider pelvic exenteration for tumor persistence
IIIa	5000-6000*	2000-3000 and/or interstitial implant	
IIIb	5000-6000*	4000 (1 application), 5000 (2 applications)†	
IVa	6000	4000 (1 application), 5000 (2 applications)†	
IVb	500-1000 pulse 2-4 times 1 week apart	Palliative	

*Patients with larger lesions or poor vaginal geometry merit the higher dose of external radiation.
†Two applications are suggested following whole-pelvis radiation with larger lesions or when the first application has less than optimum dosimetry.

that lie in a bed of normal tissue (cervix and vagina) that is highly radioresistant.

Radium/cesium therapy

Radium is the isotope that traditionally has been used in the treatment of cancer of the cervix. Its greatest value is that its half-life is some 1620 years, and therefore it provides a very stable, durable element for therapy. In recent years both cesium and cobalt have been used for intracavitary therapy. Cesium has a half-life of 30 years, and with present-day technology it provides a very adequate substitute for radium. Four major technologies for the application of radium in the treatment of cervical cancer have found continuing favor among gynecologists. Three are intracavitary techniques using specially designed applicators, and the fourth technique involves the application of radium in the form of needles directly into the tumor. The variations between the three techniques of intracavitary brachytherapy are found in the Stockholm, Paris, and Manchester schools of treatment (Figure 3-23). The differences are largely in the number and length of time of applications, the size and placement of the vaginal colpostats, and radium loading. In the United States the tendency has been to use fixed radium applicators with the intrauterine tandem and vaginal colpostats originally attached to each other. Over the last three decades a flexible afterloading system, Fletcher-Suit, has gained increasing popularity because it provides flexibility and the safety of afterloading techniques.

The Paris method originally employed a daily insertion of 66.66 mg of radium divided equally between the uterus and the vagina. The radium remained in place for 12 to 14 hours, and the period of treatment varied from 5 to 7 days. An essential feature of the Paris method, and a part of the modification of this technique, is the vaginal colpostat, consisting of two hollow corks that serve as radium containers joined together by a steel spring that separates them into the lateral vaginal wall.

The Stockholm technique uses a tandem in the uterine cavity surrounded by a square radium plaque applied to the vaginal wall and portio vaginalis of the cervix. No radium is placed in the lower cervical canal, and vaginal sources are used to cover the cervical lesion. The uterine tandem and vaginal plaque are immobilized by packing and left in place for 12 to 36 hours. Two to three identical applications are made at weekly intervals.

The Manchester system is designed to yield constant isodose patterns regardless of the size of the uterus and vagina. The source placed in the neighborhood of the cervical canal is considered the unit strength. The remaining sources in the corpus and vagina are applied as multiples of this unit and are selected and arranged to produce equivalent isodose curves in each case and an optimal dose at preselected points in the pelvis. The applicator is shaped to allow an isodose curve that delivers radiation to the cervix in a uniform amount. The Fletcher-Suit system (Figure 3-24) previously mentioned is a variation of the Manchester technique.

An effort is made in the two radium insertions to administer approximately 7000 cGy to the paracervical tissues as the sum of the dose from both external and intracavitary irradiation. The isodose distribution around a Manchester system is pear-shaped (Figure 3-25). The maximal total dose delivered by the two radium insertions is a function of the sum dose to the bladder and rectum. The total dose received by the rectal mucosa from both radium applications usually ranges between 4000 and 6000 cGy. The nearest bladder mucosa may receive

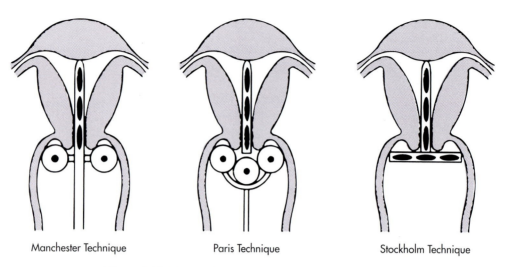

Manchester Technique   Paris Technique   Stockholm Technique

Figure 3-23 Three techniques of intracavitary brachytherapy.

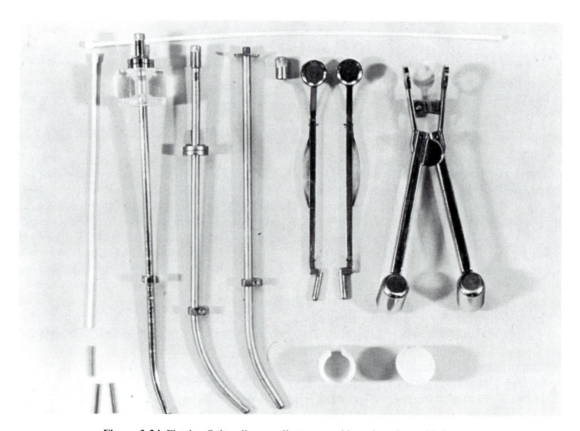

Figure 3-24 Fletcher-Suit radium applicators: ovoids and tandem with inserts.

between 5000 and 7000 cGy. When whole-pelvis irradiation is used, the radium dose must be reduced to keep the total dose to the bladder and rectum within acceptable limits.

In conjunction with the development of a system of radium distribution, British workers have defined two anatomic areas of the parametria (see Figure 3-25) where dose designation can be correlated with clinical effect. These are situated in the proximal parametria adjacent to the cervix at the level of the internal os and in the distal parametria in the area of the iliac lymph nodes and are designated point A and point B. The description states that point A is located 2 cm from the midline of the cervical canal and 2 cm superior to the lateral vaginal fornix. The dose at point A is representative of the dose to the paracervical triangle that correlates well with the incidence of sequelae and with the 5-year control rate in many studies. Point B is 3 cm lateral to point A. This point,

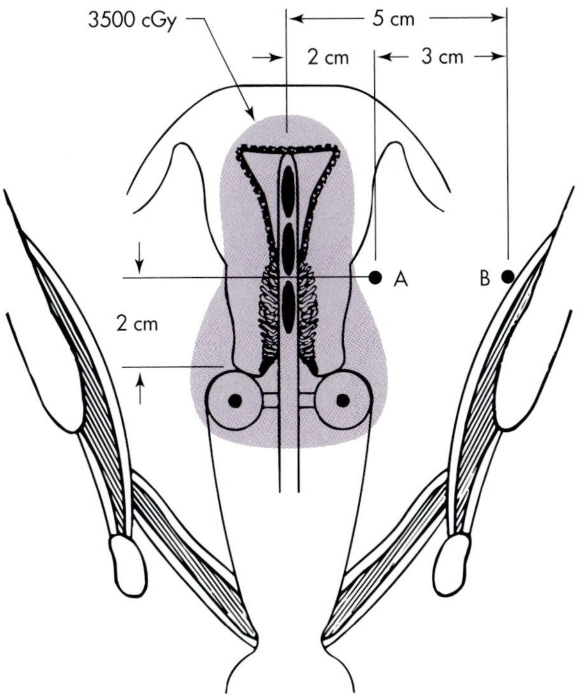

Figure 3-25 Pear-shaped distribution of radiation delivered to tissues surrounding a typical radium application with the Manchester type applicators. Points A and B are noted as reference points.

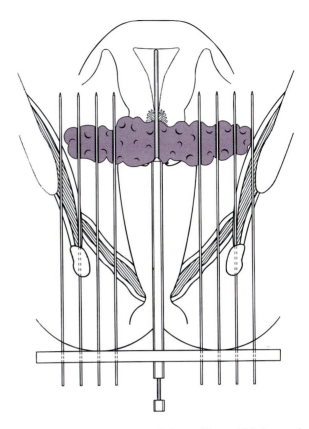

Figure 3-26 Diagram of the technique of interstitial therapy for advanced cervical cancer using Syed-Noblett template.

together with the tissue superior to it, is of significance in considering the dose to the node-bearing tissue. It is clear from what has been said relative to points A and B that they can represent important points on a curve describing the dose gradient from the radium sources to the lateral pelvic wall. This gradient is different for the various techniques. In a comparison of the physical characteristics of radio techniques the ratio of the dose at point A to the dose at point B should help define physical differences. In addition, determining the dose at point A relative to the calculated dose at points identified as bladder trigone and rectal mucosa provides a means of assessing the relative safety of one application over another. The concepts of points A and B have been questioned by many authors, including Fletcher. They remain as imaginary points but seem to provide a framework in which therapy is planned. Again, the distribution of the disease must be the primary guide in planning therapy, and the total dose to either point A or point B is relative only to their position with regard to the disease distribution.

Whole-pelvis irradiation is usually administered in conjunction with brachytherapy (e.g., intracavitary radium or cesium) in a dose range of 4000 to 5000 cGy. Megavoltage machines such as cobalt, linear accelerators, and the betatron have the distinct advantage of giving greater homogeneity of dose to the pelvis. In addition, the hard, short rays of megavoltage pass through the skin without much absorption and cause very little injury, allowing virtually unlimited amounts of radiation to be delivered to pelvic depths with little if any skin irritation. Orthovoltage, because of its relatively long wavelength and low energy, has the disadvantage that doses to the skin are particularly high and, in delivering the required amount of radiation to the pelvis, may cause temporary and permanent skin changes. Thus, for pelvis irradiation, high-energy megavoltage equipment has definite advantages over orthovoltage and even low-energy megavoltage equipment.

Interstitial therapy

In advanced carcinoma of the cervix, the associated obliteration of the fornices or contracture of the vagina may interfere with accurate placement of conventional intracavitary applicators. Poorly placed applicators fail to irradiate the lesion and the pelvis homogeneously. Syed and Feder have revived a solution to this problem by advocating transvaginal and transperineal implants. The technique employs a template to guide the insertion of a group of 18-gauge hollow steel needles into the parametria transperineally (Figure 3-26). These hollow needles are subsequently "afterloaded" with iridium wires when the patient has returned to her hospital room. Theoretically this technique locates a pair of paravaginal interstitial colpostats in both parametria. This approach holds great promise, but long-term studies illustrating improved survival rate and reasonable morbidity are not available. Also, there is no report reflecting, prospectively, the effectiveness, in comparable groups of patients, of the interstitial technique versus the standard intracavitary approach.

Interstitial therapy may have particular value in the treatment of carcinoma of the cervical stump. Although carcinoma of the cervical stump has become a relatively rare disease, accounting for less than 1% of all gynecologic malignancies, it does create difficult problems in terms of optimal geometry for delivery of effective irradiation therapy. In some series of cervical cancer, the incidence of carcinoma of the cervical stump approaches 10%. Prempree, Patanaphan, and Scott reported excellent results with absolute survival rates of 83.3% for stage I, 75% for stage IIa, and 62.5% for stage IIb using radiation therapy with an emphasis on parametrial interstitial implants in the more advanced diseases. Similar results have been obtained by Puthawala et al.

Extended field irradiation therapy

Over the past two decades, attempts have been made to salvage more patients with advanced cervical cancer by identifying the presence of periaortic lymph node metastases and applying extended field irradiation to the area (Figure 3-27). The en bloc pelvic and periaortic portals extend superiorly as far as the level of the dome of the diaphragm and inferiorly to the obturator foramen. The width of the periaortic portion of the field is usually 8 to 10 cm, and the usual dose delivered is between 4000 and 5000 cGy in 4 to 6 weeks. A boost of 1000 cGy is often given to the pelvic field alone. Identification of periaortic lymph node involvement was initially attempted by use of lymphangiography, but this technique did not find general acceptance because of varied accuracy from institution to institution and from radiologist to radiologist. Surgical localization of periaortic involvement has been more satisfactory.

Several reports have discussed survival and complications in patients with carcinoma of the cervix and periaortic metastases who received extended field irradiation (Table 3-9). Piver and Barlow of Roswell Park Memorial Institute, Buffalo, reported on 20 women with previously untreated cervical cancer who received radical irradiation to the periaortic lymph nodes and pelvis after the diagnosis of periaortic lymph node metastases had been established by surgical staging. They noted that 90% of these patients received 6000 cGy to the periaortic nodes and pelvis in 8 weeks using a split-course technique. A later report shows that 30% died of complications of this therapy and 45% of recurrent disease. Only 25% of patients survived disease-free for 16, 18, 24, and 36 months. The criticism may be that the dose is too high, yet a lesser dose might be ineffective, and four patients did survive. It is obvious that a safe yet

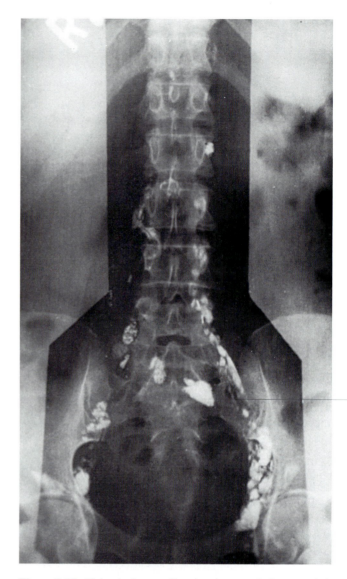

Figure 3-27 Abdominal x-ray film showing portals for extended field irradiation in cervical cancer.

Table 3-9 Late complications of radiation therapy with approximate incidence (%)

Sigmoiditis	3%
Rectovaginal fistula	1%
Rectal Stricture	1%
Small bowel obstruction	1%
(with extended fields)	20%
Vesicovaginal fistula	1%
Ureteral stricture	1%

effective dosage level for extended field irradiation therapy has not yet been established.

Wharton et al. of the MD Anderson Hospital reported on 120 women treated with preirradiation celiotomy. Of these patients, 32 had severe bowel complications and 20

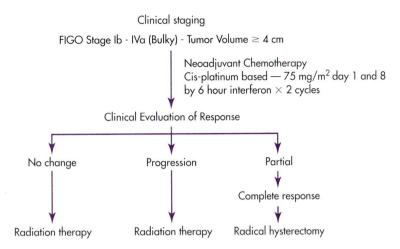

Clinical staging

FIGO Stage Ib - IVa (Bulky) - Tumor Volume ≥ 4 cm

Neoadjuvant Chemotherapy
Cis-platinum based — 75 mg/m² day 1 and 8
by 6 hour interferon × 2 cycles

Clinical Evaluation of Response

No change   Progression   Partial

Complete response

Radiation therapy   Radiation therapy   Radical hysterectomy

Figure 3-28 Neoadjuvant chemotherapy for cervical cancer.

(16.6%) eventually died as a result of the surgery or of the surgery and irradiation. Four of these patients died immediately as a result of the surgical procedure. Of 64 patients with positive nodes who were irradiated, 17% were alive 13 to 38 months after treatment. No patient had survived for 5 years. Wharton et al. further reported that in 36 women with positive nodes it was possible to accurately determine the failure sites after completion of the full course of irradiation therapy. In 25 of these patients, distant metastases were the first evidence of treatment failure; 11 had disease or developed recurrence within the treatment fields; disease of the pelvic wall was found in only 2 patients.

Experience has shown that doses of about 4500 cGy, particularly when administered in daily fractions of 150 to 180 cGy, are safely tolerated by the organs in the periaortic treatment volume, and a complication rate of 5% is to be expected. Extraperitoneal surgery appears to be associated with less postradiation morbidity, probably because of reduced bowel adhesions. The issues of the utility of periaortic radiation and surgical staging in the management of cervical carcinoma are closely intertwined. Although many hypotheses have been raised to support or reject the use of surgical staging, it is clear that some patients with biopsy-proven periaortic node metastases can be cured with radiotherapy employing extended fields. About 20% of patients who receive extended-field radiotherapy survive cervical cancer metastatic to the periaortic lymph nodes. Rubin had a 50% survival in a group of Ib patients with documented periaortic lymph node involvement. In many reports, the true value of extended field radiation is clouded because patients with periaortic node involvement often have advanced disease in which any node or regional therapy may have little effect on long-term survival.

Neoadjuvant Chemotherapy

Neoadjuvant therapy for advanced squamous cell carcinoma of the cervix has attracted several investigations

throughout the world. This is a new approach in the management of carcinoma of the uterine cervix, its goal being better therapeutic results in locally advanced cases. Chemotherapy, which has hitherto been reserved for patients with metastasis or recurrence after irradiation therapy, is used initially for patients with bulk disease. Various regimens have been used. Most of the regimens have been platinum-based combinations, often including bleomycin and vincristine. Dramatic reductions in the size of the neoplasm have been documented after as little as three courses or three weeks of therapy. The response of unirradiated lesions has been in sharp contrast to the poor response of recurrent cervix cancer in irradiated pelvis. Several authors (Sardi) have demonstrated complete disappearance of the neoplasm on pathological review of the surgical specimen following neoadjuvant chemotherapy. Some clinicians have utilized irradiation therapy and others radical surgery following neoadjuvant chemotherapy. Others have utilized radical surgery for good responders (Figure 3-28) and irradiation therapy for poor responders. Toxicity appears to be acceptable, but no prospective randomized studies have been reported. It has yet to be learned whether this technique eventuates in better survivals or is yet another technique that demonstrates good responses but offers no improved outcome.

Cancer of the Cervix in Pregnancy

Carcinoma of the cervix complicates pregnancy in approximately 0.01% of patients. In deciding on therapy for these malignant neoplasms, one must consider the extent of the disease and the duration of the pregnancy. A detrimental effect of pregnancy on cancer of the cervix has not been demonstrated, anecdotal evidence to the contrary. The hypothesis found in previous literature that pregnancy accelerates the growth of the tumor has not been substantiated. It was once thought that parturition was capable of squeezing viable cells into the vascular system and increasing the incidence of metastatic spread, but this has not been substantiated by recent studies.

Several studies have shown that, stage for stage, the outcome for the pregnant patient with cervical cancer is roughly the same as that for the nonpregnant patient.

The construction of a treatment plan for the pregnant patient with cervical cancer (see Figure 16-5) depends on several factors, including stage of disease, duration of pregnancy, religious conviction of patient and family, desire of the mother for the child, and background of the physician, in addition to the medical problem itself. For stage I and early stage II lesions, a radical surgical procedure (radical hysterectomy) is acceptable therapy during any trimester. If preservation of the pregnancy is desired, a waiting period of several weeks may be required to ensure reasonable viability of the fetus. It is generally recommended that patients in the first and second trimesters not be allowed to await fetal viability; interruption of the pregnancy is usually advised. Exceptions have been made in cases of early invasive disease in which the central lesion has been thoroughly analyzed by an excisional biopsy and found to be limited (e.g., stage Ia1).

Radiation therapy is acceptable also for patients before 24 weeks' gestation. The pregnancy is disregarded, and the patient is started on whole-pelvis irradiation. If abortion does not occur, excision of the remaining neoplasm by means of a modified radical hysterectomy (class II) or surgical evacuation of the uterus must follow completion of the external irradiation. Once the uterus is evacuated, radiotherapy can resume. If the uterus has been removed, vaginal vault irradiation may be all that is necessary. In the event that a hysterotomy with evacuation of the uterus has been performed, standard radium techniques are applicable to the postoperative uterus and upper vagina after a 4-week waiting period.

For the patient at 24 weeks gestation or more, therapy is usually delayed until fetal viability is reached. Cesarean section is performed when appropriate on the basis of pediatric and obstetric criteria. If a radical hysterectomy with pelvic lymphadenectomy is not performed at the time of cesarean section, whole-pelvis irradiation begins immediately after the abdominal incision has healed. Intracavitary irradiation can follow completion of the whole-pelvis irradiation. The basic treatment plan used for cancer of the cervix in a nonpregnant patient can generally be used for those patients in whom only cesarean section has been performed.

Suboptimal Treatment Situations

There are several situations in which patients with invasive cancer of the cervix receive suboptimal treatment: (1) cancer in a cervical stump, (2) inadequate surgery, and (3) poor vaginal geometry for radium.

Cancer that occurs in a cervical stump is fortunately a diminishing problem, since supracervical hysterectomies are performed less frequently. Carcinoma occurring in a cervical stump presents a special problem, since often an optimal dose of intracavitary radium cannot be applied

because there is insufficient place to insert the central tandem, which contributes significantly to the radiation dose to the central tumor and to the pelvic sidewall. Radical surgery is also more difficult; the bladder and rectum firmly adhere to the stump and may adhere to each other. Also, the ureters are more difficult to dissect cleanly from the parametrial tissue because of fibrosis from the previous surgery. The net result is an increase in the risk of significant surgical complications involving the ureters, bladder, and rectum. In modern gynecologic surgery, supracervical hysterectomy is rarely indicated, and only under exceptional circumstances encountered at the operating table would supracervical hysterectomy be acceptable.

In a report of the MD Anderson experience with 263 patients with carcinoma of the cervical stump, Miller noted a 30% complication rate following full therapy with radiation. Urinary and bowel complications result from postsurgical adhesions, the absence of the uterus, which acts as a shield, and a tendency to emphasize external radiation therapy. We have had a similar experience, resulting in a preference for radical cervicectomy in cervical-stump patients in whom stage and medical conditions allow. The increased technical difficulty of performing such a procedure seems to be outweighed by the low complication rate and comparable survivals.

Inadequate surgery usually results when a simple hysterectomy is performed and frank invasive cervical cancer is subsequently discovered. This situation may occur because of poor preoperative evaluation or because the surgery was performed under emergency conditions without an adequate preoperative cervical evaluation. Such a situation may occur in a patient presenting with acute abdomen from ruptured tubo-ovarian abscesses. In any event, if an extensive cancer is found in the cervix, the prognosis is poor because optimal irradiation cannot be given with the cervix and uterus absent. An even more ominous situation occurs when a hysterectomy is performed with a "cut through" of the cancer; that is, the hysterectomy dissection passes through the cancer. The prognosis is uniformly poor in this event. In the examples just given, surgical cures are not obtained, and the probability of curative radiotherapy is greatly diminished.

In 1968, Durrance reported survival rates of 92% to 100% using postoperative radiation therapy in selected patients with presumed stage I or II disease following suboptimal surgery. Excellent survivals were also reported by Andras in 148 patients who had invasive cervical carcinoma found incidentally in the hysterectomy specimen. Of these patients, 126 were treated with postoperative radiation therapy. Patients with microscopic disease confined to the cervix had a 96% 5-year survival rate. Those with gross tumor confined to the cervix had an 84% 5-year survival. Patients with tumor cut through at the margins of surgical resection, but with no obvious residual cancer, had a 5-year survival rate of

87%. Patients with obvious residual pelvic tumor had a 47% 5-year survival rate. In 1986 Heller reviewed the literature and reported equivalent survivals in 35 patients also treated mostly with radiation.

Orr and his colleagues have preferred radical parametrectomy, upper vaginectomy, and lymphadenectomy as the treatment of choice following simple hysterectomy. We have also preferred this approach, particularly since many of these patients are young and desirous of preserving optimal sexual function. We are also concerned about postoperative small bowel adhesions and the difficulty of delivering effective irradiation to the medial parametria in the absence of a uterus. Survival rates with either approach appear to be exceptionally good; undoubtedly this clinical situation creates a bias for smaller lesions that may be easier to eradicate.

The incidence of pelvic recurrence following irradiation alone for stages Ib, IIa, and IIb carcinomas of the cervix increases with increasing tumor diameter. Data from the MD Anderson Hospital showed an improved pelvic control rate, as well as a small increase in survival, when patients with the bulky, so-called barrel-shaped lesions were treated with preoperative irradiation followed by extrafascial hysterectomy. The subject continues to be controversial with conflicting studies in the literature. Gallion reported on 75 patients with "bulky, barrel-shaped" stage Ib cervical cancer; 32 received radiation alone and 43 were treated with radiation followed by extrafascial hysterectomy. The incidence of pelvic recurrence was reduced from 19% to 2% and extrapelvic recurrence from 16% to 7% in patients treated by combination therapy, which produced no increase in treatment-related complications. On the other hand, Weems described 123 such patients treated from two different eras at his institution. Examination of pelvic control rates, as well as disease-free survival, showed no significant advantage in pelvic control, disease-free survival, or absolute survival for either treatment group when compared by stage and tumor size. Unfortunately, there is no large prospective randomized study, and that would be necessary to clarify this issue.

Adequate radiotherapy is also compromised in patients who have a vagina or cervix that cannot accommodate a complete radium application. This situation is encountered with atrophic stenotic pelvic structures. These patients are treated by inserting the tandem and ovoids in a compromised manner, such as insertion of the ovoids singly or independently of the central tandem. In any event standard optimal doses are usually not obtained, and the possibility of sustaining a radiation injury is increased.

SURVIVAL RESULTS AND PROGNOSTIC FACTORS

Review of the annual reports on results of treatment of carcinoma of the uterus reveals a wide dispersion of 5-year recovery rates among several stages of carcinoma of the cervix. One can find data supporting any stand one wishes to take with regard to therapy. The overall cure rate in a cumulative series of 22,428 patients from 1987 to 1989 (Twenty-second FIGO report on gynecologic cancer, l993) with stage I cancer of the cervix was 85% in the U.S. (Figure 3-29). In addition, the 5-year survival rates for stage II and III disease were 66% and 39%,

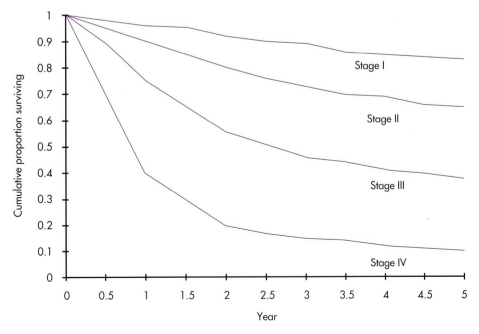

Figure 3-29 Carcinoma of the uterine cervix. Actuarial survival by stage. (From *Annual Report Gynecological Cancer* FIGO 22:1994.)

respectively. The individual institutions reported 5-year cure rates for stage I disease from 69% to 90% with surgery alone and from 60% to 93% with radiotherapy alone. Results may imply that one form of therapy has advantages over the other, but considering the rather wide dispersion that, in fact, may be unrelated to treatment, we must maintain collective open-mindedness about the efficacy of individual therapeutic regimens. The best available figures for the two methods give results that are nearly identical, and because the presence of other factors affect the samples being compared, large differences would be necessary to be significant. Individual physicians will probably continue to decide on the basis of personal preferences and comparison of complications and later disabilities.

The recovery rates of patients with operative squamous cell carcinoma of the cervix depend on many factors, including the histologically documented extent of the carcinoma. Baltzer et al. studied 718 surgical specimens of patients with squamous cell carcinoma of the cervix. Lymphatic and blood vessel invasion significantly influenced survival, blood vessel invasion being much more ominous. In their study, 70% of the patients who demonstrated blood vessel invasion succumbed to the disease, whereas 31% of the patients demonstrating only lymphatic invasion succumbed to the disease process. Other studies have not found prognostic significance for vascular invasion. A definite linkage was noted between the size of the carcinomas and the frequency of metastases. Fuller et al. drew similar conclusions. In their study of 431 patients who underwent radical hysterectomy for stages Ib or IIa carcinoma of the cervix at Memorial Sloan-Kettering Cancer Center, they found 71 patients who had nodal spread that correlated closely with increased primary tumor size, extracervical extension of tumor, and the presence of adenocarcinoma. Although these factors were recognized as having prognostic significance, the authors were not able to demonstrate that these detrimental effects could be overcome by postoperative pelvic radiation. Patients receiving postoperative irradiation therapy seemed to have some better local control, but the problem of systemic spread of disease resulted in little overall improvement in survival. In a similar study Abdulhayogu et al. reported on a series of patients with negative lymph nodes at the time of radical hysterectomy who subsequently developed recurrent disease. They too pointed out the histologic architecture of invasion as an important prognostic indicator. Recurrence was more likely in patients who had deep invasion of the cervical stroma, especially when it extended to the serosal surface, even when the parametria were not involved. Once again the volume of tumor correlated with the eventual prognosis for the patient. They suggested that these patients were in need of postoperative therapy, and radiation therapy for local control was recommended in the absence of any other demonstrated effective adjuvant

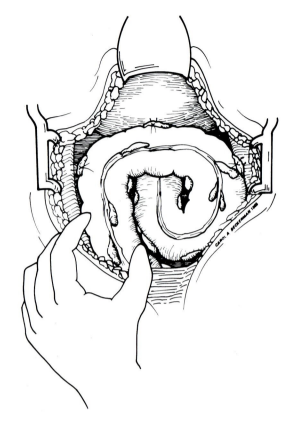

Figure 3-30 Technique of filling pelvic basin with redundant rectosigmoid. (From DiSaia PJ: *Cancer* 48:548, 1981.)

modality for this set of circumstances. Gauthier had similar results, and in a multifactorial analysis of clinical and pathologic factors, demonstrated that the depth of stromal invasion is the single most important determinant of survival.

We have practiced a philosophy that patients with positive pelvic nodes have manifested aggressive disease, and postoperative pelvic radiation therapy should destroy microscopic residual disease in the pelvis following surgery and thereby improve survival. Future prospective studies may influence this policy. To reduce possible bowel injuries as a result of postoperative radiation to the pelvis, we have also followed a practice of filling the pelvic basin with the redundant rectosigmoid (Figure 3-30) so that small bowel loops are prevented from adhering to the operative site where they could be seriously injured by subsequent irradiation therapy.

Rutledge and others have investigated the prognosis of young women with cervical cancer. In the report by Rutledge, young patients with advanced disease do poorly (stages IIb and IIIb), but those with high volume stage Ib do better. On the other hand, Orlandi has reported on 264 patients with stage Ib and IIIa cervical squamous cancer, all treated with radical hysterectomy and pelvic lymphadenectomy. The 65 patients under age 35 had a higher incidence of lymph node metastases (46% vs 24%) and lower 5-year survival (65% vs 76%) than the older group (n=199). Although the conclusions are at variance, the subject matter appears to be worthy of further study.

Sexual function after therapy for cervical cancer is a frequently ignored subject. Many patients never regain pretreatment sexual function. Andersen studied sexual behavior, level of sexual responsiveness, and presence of sexual dysfunction of 41 women with uterine cancer compared with a matched group of healthy women. The two groups were similar until the onset of disease signs, sometimes long before diagnosis, at which time the cancer patients began experiencing significant sexual dysfunction. Sexual morbidity, therefore, begins actually in the prediagnosis period for many patients. Seibel reported on 46 patients who were interviewed more than a year after treatment for carcinoma of the cervix to establish the effects of radiation therapy and of surgical therapy on sexual feelings and performance. The irradiated patients experienced statistically significant decreases in sexual enjoyment, opportunity, and sexual dreams. The surgically treated group had no significant change in sexual function after treatment. Both groups experienced a change in self-image but did not feel that their partners or family viewed them differently. Myths about cancer and the actual effects of pelvic irradiation were found to have disrupted the sexual marital relationships of many women. Therapeutic programs with counseling and vaginal rehabilitation with the use of estrogen vaginal creams and possibly the use of dilators may be beneficial.

RECURRENT AND ADVANCED CARCINOMA OF THE CERVIX
Clinical Profile

In the United States the mortality from cervical cancer in 1945 was 15/100,000 female population. This had declined to approximately 4.6/100,000 by 1986 and 3.4/100,000 by 1991. It is not clear whether the mortality from cervical cancer is falling as a result of cervical cytologic screening and intervention at the in situ stage or cervical screening has caused an increase in the proportion of early stage cancer at diagnosis and registration. Following therapy for invasive disease, adequate follow-up is the key to early detection of recurrence (Table 3-10). The yield of examinations such as IVP, CT scan, and chest x-ray in patients with initial early disease (stages I to IIa) is so low that many have discontinued their routine use. However, frequent Pap tests from the vaginal apex/cervix are recommended.

West studied the age of registration and the age of death of women with cervical cancer in South Wales. He found that the observed age at death was very close to 59 years regardless of stage and age at diagnosis. Although the 5-year survival rate of women with localized (early stage) cervical cancer was much higher than that of women with nonlocalized (late stage) cancer, the women

Table 3-10   Optimal interval evaluation of cervical cancer following radiotherapy/surgery (asymptomatic patient*)

Year	Frequency	Examination
1	3 months	Pelvic examination, Pap smear
	6 months	Chest film, CBC, BUN, creatinine
	1 year	IVP or CT scan with contrast
2	4 months	Pelvic examination, Pap smear
	1 year	Chest films, CBC, BUN, creatinine IVP or CT scan with contrast
3-5	6 months	Pelvic examination, Pap smear

*Symptomatic patients should have appropriate examinations where indicated.

with localized cancer tended to be younger than those with advanced cancer. Calculations of expected age at death of the whole population suggest that more than half the advantage in survival rate shown by women with early stage cancers is a result of the diagnosis of the former in younger women.

Christopherson et al. reported that the percentage of patients diagnosed as having stage I disease increased by 78%, in the population studied, from 1953 to 1965. The increase was most remarkable in younger women. The authors concluded that the major problem in cervical cancer control was the screening of older women. Older women had higher incidence rates, the percentage with stage I disease also decreased with each decade, reaching a low of 15% for those 70 years of age and older. These older women with cervical cancer rarely are screened and contribute heavily to the death rate. Initial advanced stage contributes heavily to the patient population with advanced recurrent cervical cancer. These patients, therefore, deserve very close posttreatment observation in an effort to detect a recurrence in its earliest possible form.

It is estimated that approximately 35% of patients with invasive cervical cancer will have recurrent or persistent disease following therapy. The diagnosis of recurrent cervical cancer is often difficult to establish (see the box on p. 86). The optimal radiation therapy that most patients receive makes cervical cytologic findings difficult to evaluate. This is especially true immediately following completion of radiation therapy. Suit and Gallagher, using mammary carcinomas in C_3H mice, demonstrated that persistence of histologically intact cancer cells in irradiated tissue was not indicative of regrowth of tumor. Radiobiologically, a viable cell is one with the capacity for sustained proliferation. A cell would be classified as nonviable if it had lost its reproductive integrity, although it could carry out diverse metabolic activities. This reproductive integrity was demonstrated by the transplantation "take" rate when histologically viable tumor cells were transplanted into a suitable recipient. It was evident

<table>
<tr><td>

SIGNS AND SYMPTOMS OF RECURRENT CERVICAL CANCER

Weight loss (unexplained) Leg edema (excessive and often unilateral)
Pelvic and/or thigh-buttock pain
Serosanguineous vaginal discharge
Progressive ureteral obstruction
Supraclavicular lymph node enlargement (usually left side)
Cough
Hemoptysis
Chest pain

</td></tr>
</table>

from these experiments in mice that relatively normal-appearing cancer cells can persist for several months following radiation therapy but that these cells are "biologically doomed." Thus cytologic evaluation of a patient immediately after radiation therapy may erroneously lead to the supposition that persistent disease exists. In addition, subsequent evaluation of the irradiated cervix is also difficult because of the distortion produced in the exfoliated cells, often called *radiation effect*. Thus histologic confirmation of recurrent cancer is essential. This can be accomplished by punch or needle biopsy of suspected areas of malignancy when they are accessible. An interval of at least 3 months should elapse following completion of radiation therapy. The clinical presentation of recurrent cervical cancer is varied and often insidious. Many patients develop a wasting syndrome with severe loss of appetite and gradual weight loss over a period of weeks to months. This is often preceded by a period of general good health following completion of radiation therapy. Since most recurrences of cancer occur within 2 years following therapy, the period of good health rarely lasts more than a year before the symptoms of cachexia become evident. Diagnostic evaluation at this time of suspected recurrence should include a chest film and CT scan, CBC, BUN, creatinine clearance, and liver function tests.

Autopsy studies of the location of advanced recurrent and/or persistent disease have been reported (Figures 3-31 and 3-32). Following radical hysterectomy, about one fourth of recurrences occur locally in the upper part of the vagina or the area previously occupied by the cervix. The location of recurrence after radiation therapy showed a 27% occurrence in the cervix, uterus, or upper vagina; 6% in the lower two thirds of the vagina; 43% in the parametrial area, including the pelvic wall, 16% distant, and 8% unknown.

Often one will note the development of ureteral obstruction in a patient who had a normal urinary tract before therapy. Although ureteral obstruction can be caused by radiation fibrosis, this is relatively rare, and

95% of the obstructions are caused by progressive tumor. Central disease may not be evident, and in the absence of other findings, a patient with ureteral obstruction and a negative evaluation for metastatic disease following therapy should undergo exploratory laparotomy and selected biopsies to confirm the diagnosis of recurrence. Patients with ureteral obstruction in the absence of recurrent malignancy should be considered for urinary diversion or internal antegrade ureteral stents.

The definition of primary healing after radiation therapy is a cervix covered with normal epithelium or an obliteration of the vaginal vault without evidence of ulceration or discharge. On rectovaginal examination, the residual induration is smooth with no nodularity. The cervix is no greater than 2.5 cm in width, and there is no evidence of distant metastasis. The definition of persistent disease after radiation therapy is (1) evidence of a portion of the tumor that was clinically present before treatment or (2) development of a new demonstrable tumor in the pelvis within the treatment period. The definition of recurrence after radiation therapy is a regrowth of tumor in the pelvis or distally, noted after complete healing of the cervix and vagina.

Recurrence after surgery is defined as evidence of a tumor mass after all gross tumor was removed and the margins of the specimen were free of disease. Persistent disease after surgery is defined as persistence of gross tumor in the operative field or local recurrence of tumor within 1 year of initial surgery. A new cancer of the cervix would be a lesion that occurs locally at least 10 years after primary therapy.

The triad of weight loss accompanied by leg edema and pelvic pain is ominous. Leg edema is usually the result of progressive lymphatic obstruction, occlusion of the iliofemoral vein system, or both. The clinician should consider the possibility of thrombophlebitis, but recurrent cancer is more likely. Patients characteristically describe pain that radiates into the upper thigh either to the anterior medial aspect of the thigh or posteriorly into the buttock. Other patients describe pain in the groin or deep-seated central pelvic pain. The appearance of vaginal bleeding or watery, foul, vaginal discharge strongly suggests central recurrence. These lesions are among the more readily detectable recurrent cervical cancers, and histologic confirmation is easily obtained.

Less than 15% of patients with recurrent cervical cancer will develop pulmonary metastasis. When this does occur, patients will complain of cough, hemoptysis, and occasionally chest pain. In many instances there will be enlargement of supraclavicular lymph nodes, especially on the left side. Needle aspiration of enlarged lymph nodes can be accomplished easily and avoids the necessity for an open biopsy of the area.

In almost every instance, the diagnosis of recurrent cervical cancer must be confirmed histologically. CT-directed needle biopsies have provided us with a tool that

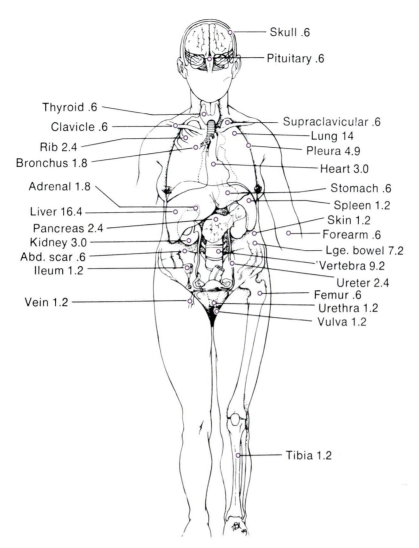

Skull .6
Pituitary .6
Thyroid .6
Clavicle .6
Rib 2.4
Bronchus 1.8
Adrenal 1.8
Liver 16.4
Pancreas 2.4
Kidney 3.0
Abd. scar .6
Ileum 1.2
Vein 1.2
Supraclavicular .6
Lung 14
Pleura 4.9
Heart 3.0
Stomach .6
Spleen 1.2
Skin 1.2
Forearm .6
Lge. bowel 7.2
Vertebra 9.2
Ureter 2.4
Femur .6
Urethra 1.2
Vulva 1.2
Tibia 1.2

Figure 3-31 Metastatic sites of treated patients with cervical cancer and percentage of involvement. (From Henriksen E: *Am J Obstet Gynecol* 58:924, 1949.)

avoids the necessity of more elaborate operative procedures. In addition to the standard roentgenographic evaluations, such as IVP and chest film, the clinician may find more sophisticated studies such as lymphangiography and MRI helpful in localizing deep-seated areas of recurrent cervical cancer.

Bony metastases presenting clinically are particularly rare. In a study of 644 patients with invasive cervical carcinoma, Peeples et al. were able to find only 29 cases of remote metastases. Of these, 15 were to the lungs, and only 12 were to the bone, an incidence of 1.8%. No bony metastases were found at initial staging and diagnosis. The earliest discovery of bone metastasis came 8 months after diagnosis. Therefore a bone survey was not recommended as part of the staging examination for cervical cancer.

Blythe et al. reported on 55 patients treated for cervical carcinoma who developed bony metastases. Roentgenograms were diagnostic in all but 2 of the patients. In 15 patients a combination of radioactive scans and roentgenograms was used to establish the diagnosis. The most common mechanism of bony involvement from carcinoma of the cervix was extension of the neoplasia from periaortic nodes, with involvement of the adjacent vertebral bodies. The longest interval from the primary diagnosis until the discovery of bony metastases was 13 years. Sixty-nine percent of the patients were diagnosed within 30 months of initial therapy, and 96% died within 18 months. Of the 36 patients treated with radiation therapy, 4 received complete relief of symptoms, 24 gained some relief, and 8 received no relief.

Van Herik et al. examined the records of 2107 cases of cervical cancer for recurrence after 10 years. Sixteen patients, or 0.7%, had recurrence 10 to 26 years after initial therapy. Of these patients, 25% had bony metastasis or extension of the recurrence into bone. The finding of metastasis after 10 years correlates with the findings of Paunier et al., who indicated that 92.5% of deaths

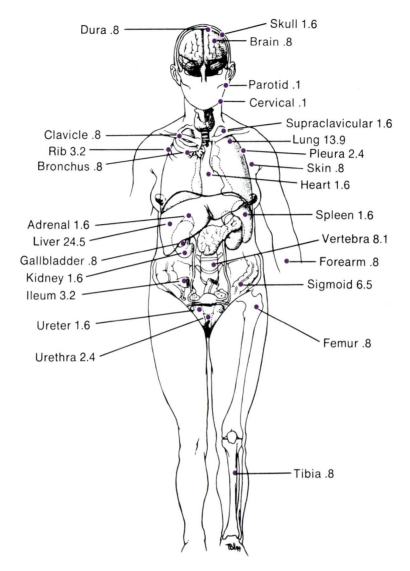

Figure 3-32 Metastatic sites of untreated patients with cervical cancer and percentage of involvement. (From Henriksen E: *Am J Obstet Gynecol* 58:924, 1949.)

resulting from carcinoma of the cervix occur in the first 5 years after diagnosis. In addition, their cumulative death rate curve was flat after 10 years.

Deaths resulting from cancer of the cervix occur most frequently in the first year of observation and decrease thereafter. About half of all the deaths occur in the first year after therapy, 25% in the second year, and 15% in the third year, for a total of 85% by the end of the third year.

Since more than three fourths of the recurrences are clinically evident in the first 2 years after initial therapy, posttreatment evaluation done at frequent intervals during this critical period is mandatory. The patient should be examined every 3 to 4 months, and cervical cytologic testing should be done at these visits. In addition, particular attention should be paid to the parametria on rectovaginal examination to detect evidence of progressive disease. For several months after the completion of radiation therapy, the examiner may observe a progressive

fibrosis in the parametria, creating the so-called horseshoe fibrosis. The amount of fibrosis may at times be alarming, but smoothness of the induration should be reassuring when compared with the nodular presentation of recurrent parametrial malignancy. Parametrial needle biopsies, with the patient under anesthesia, may be helpful when the palpatory findings are equivocal. Generous use of endocervical curettage at these follow-up visits is recommended, especially when central failure is suspected following radiation therapy. An IVP or CT scan and chest film should be obtained annually in the asymptomatic patient and more frequently when pelvic recurrence is suspected. Every follow-up examination should include a careful palpation of the abdomen for evidence of periaortic enlargement, hepatomegaly, and unexplained masses. Every follow-up examination should begin with a careful palpation of the supraclavicular areas for evidence of nodal enlargement. This frequently omitted portion of the examination will sometimes reveal the only evidence of recurrent disease.

The prognosis for the patient with recurrent or advanced cervical cancer depends of course on the location of the disease. Of those patients with recurrent cervical cancer, the most favorable for therapy following primary irradiation are those with a central recurrence. These patients are candidates for curative radical pelvic surgery, including pelvic exenteration. There will be further discussion of this group of patients later in this chapter. With the advent of sophisticated methods of radiation therapy, including improved methods of brachytherapy and supervoltage external irradiation therapy, patients with pure central recurrence have become a rarity.

Isolated lung metastases from pelvic malignancies have responded in very selected cases to lobectomy. Gallousis reported metastases to the lung from cervical cancer in 1.5% of 5614 cases reviewed, with solitary nodules present in 25% of the cases. A surgical attack for isolated pulmonary recurrence should be considered, especially if the latent period has been greater than 3 years.

Other patients who deserve serious consideration are those with radiation bowel injury. Over the past decade the limits of human tolerance to radiation therapy have been reached, with treatment techniques for advanced disease that include large extended fields to the periaortic area. Many patients with advanced stage primary lesions have been treated with large doses of pelvic radiation (6000 to 7000 cGy), often following intra-abdominal surgery. These techniques, as well as standard radiation therapy, can lead to a small but significant number of patients with chronic radiation injury to the large or small bowel. These patients frequently develop cachexia indistinguishable from the clinical presentation of recurrent and progressive malignancy. All too often these patients are quickly and superficially diagnosed as having recurrent disease, and no further investigation is initiated. Careful investigation of these patients reveals a history of postprandial crampy abdominal pain causing anorexia and weight loss. The diagnostic evaluations discussed previously reveal no conclusive evidence of persistent malignancy. In most instances, these patients can be returned to health with appropriate bowel surgery, including internal bypass procedures. In every patient suspected of recurrent malignancy, an effort should be made to confirm this suspicion by biopsy (histologic confirmation), and patients without recurrence who have radiation bowel injury should be identified.

Management
Prognosis

Persistent or recurrent carcinoma of the cervix is a discouraging clinical entity for the clinician, with a 1-year survival rate between 10% and 15%. Treatment failures

are, as expected, much more common in more advanced stages of the disease, and therefore most patients are not likely candidates for a second curative approach with radical pelvic surgery. Cases of curative therapy applied to isolated lung metastases or lower vaginal recurrences are reported but rare. Unfortunately, most recurrences are suitable for palliative management only.

Radical hysterectomy

Radical hysterectomy has been reported as therapy for patients with a small recurrent cervical carcinoma following radiation. Coleman's series of 50 patients from MD Anderson Cancer Center were treated with radical hysterectomy (type II or type III). Severe postoperative complications occurred in 42% of these patients. Twenty eight percent developed urinary tract injury. Survival was 90% at 5 years for patients with lesions less than 2 cm as opposed to 64% in patients with larger lesions. Excessive mordibity can be limited if an omental pedicle is placed at the operative site at the end of the procedure, bringing in a new blood suppy to the operative field that has undergone previous radiation therapy.

Irradiation therapy

With recurrent disease outside the initial treatment field, irradiation is frequently successful in providing local control and symptomatic relief. External irradiation in moderate and easily delivered doses is usually effective in relieving pain from bone metastases. A dose of 3000 cGy delivered in a 2- to 3-week period is often sufficient to relieve pain from vertebral column or long-bone metastases.

Reirradiation of pelvic recurrences of cervical cancer occurring within the previously treated field is a subject of some controversy. The results following reirradiation of patients with recurrent cervical malignancy have varied considerably. Truelsen reported a 3-year cure rate of 1.7%. Murphy and Schmitz reported a 9% salvage rate in 1956, and Nolan et al. reported on the use of cobalt 60 teleradiation with a 25% salvage rate. At the Roswell Park Memorial Institute, Murphy adopted the policy of reirradiating patients with recurrence, delivering a full or near-full course for a second time. Among the highly selected series of 46 patients, 9% to 10% were living and well at the end of 5 years. Only 7 patients had biopsy-proven recurrences before treatment. Others have shown that the results of reirradiation depend on many factors, including site of recurrence, initial clinical stage, and initial dose of radiation therapy.

Careful perusal of these reports suggests that most patients who benefited from reirradiation were those who received far less than optimal radiation during initial therapy. This set of circumstances has become rare in recent times, when more sophisticated radiotherapy is being delivered in many areas of the United States. Therefore, reirradiation for recurrent disease is usually not a worthwhile consideration. Indeed, the potential for necrosis and fistula formation with even moderate doses of reirradiation in the pelvis by external or interstitial sources can give very unfavorable results.

Chemotherapy

The management of disseminated cervical cancer has not improved significantly with the progress of modern chemotherapy (Table 3-11). Some explanations for this are worth noting. First, a large percentage of patients with recurrent disease develop tumor in a previously irradiated area, and the malignant tissue is encased in a fibrotic and avascular capsule. It is therefore difficult to obtain high blood and tissue concentrations of drug in the neoplasm to create the optimal situation for response. In addition, squamous cell carcinoma (constituting 85% to 90% of cervical cancers) generally has been one of the histologic varieties least responsive to most chemotherapeutic agents. Further, many drugs are nephrotoxic and have limited usefulness because of the frequent occurrence of ureteral obstruction in patients with recurrent cervical cancer. Combination chemotherapy in cervical cancer has usually involved bleomycin, cyclophosphamide, adria-

mycin, cisplatin, and methotrexate. The combinations have usually been used on patients failing surgery or radiotherapy. There have been more than 40 reports of various drug regimens used in treating this disease.

The Gynecologic Oncology Group initially reported on 34 patients with advanced or recurrent squamous cell carcinoma of the cervix no longer amenable to control with surgery or radiation therapy who were treated with cisplatin at a dose rate of 50 mg/m^2 intravenously every 3 weeks. Among 22 patients who had received no prior chemotherapy, three complete and eight partial responses were observed (a response rate of 50%), whereas only two partial responses were observed among 12 patients who had received prior chemotherapy. The overall frequency of response was 38% (13/34). Responses were observed in those with pelvic (7/20) and extrapelvic (6/14) disease.

Also reported by GOG (Thigpen et al) was the largest experience with cisplatin in the treatment of recurrent cervical cancer. In this study more than 300 patients were treated to define the optimal dose and schedule of cisplatin. The size of this trial and the care with which it was conducted make it the definitive cisplatin study in cervical cancer. The response rate was 17% to 18% for all dose schedules (Table 3-12), with a 4-month median response duration and 6½ month median survival. Despite such low response rates, cisplatin alone remains as effective as any other drug or combination reported and confirmed in a large series.

Alberts et al. reported on a combination chemotherapy regimen containing mitomycin C (10 mg/m^2, day 2), vincristine (0.5 mg/m^2, days 1 and 4), bleomycin (30 U/day, days 1 through 4 as a continuous IV infusion during courses 1 and 2 only), and cisplatin (50 mg/m^2, days 1 and 22) administered every 6 weeks to 14 evaluable patients with advanced or recurrent squamous cell carcinoma of the cervix. Four patients (29%) achieved a complete response, lasting 8, 9½, 17, and 21 months. Three of these patients had a complete disappearance of their pulmonary metastasis, and one has had resolution of a large left-sided pelvic wall mass. Subsequent studies utilizing this same combination have not reported such encouraging results.

Table 3-11 Cervical cancer single-agent chemotherapy

Drug	Response rate
Antimetabolites	
5-Fluorouracil	23%
Methotrexate	20%
Alkylating agents	
Cyclophosphamide	16%
Melphalan	20%
Ifosfamide	15%-30%
Antibiotics	
Adriamycin	16%
Mitomycin-C	22%
Bleomycin	10%
Cisplatin	17%-38%

Table 3-12 Frequency of response by regimen

Response category	Treatment		
	Rapid infusion (%) 50 mg/m^2 IV at 1 mg/min every 3 weeks	Continuous infusion (%) 50 mg/m^2 IV over 24 hr every 3 weeks	Total (%)
Complete response	10 (6%)	9 (6%)	19 (6%)
Partial response	18 (11%)	19 (12%)	37 (12%)
Stable disease	90 (55%)	92 (59%)	182 (57%)
Progressive disease	46 (28%)	36 (23%)	82 (26%)
Total	164 (100%)	156 (100%)	320 (100%)

From Thigpen T et al: *Gynecol Oncol,* 32(2):198, 1989.

Sutton has reported an overall response rate of 16% with ifosfamide (1.2 gm/m^2) in women with recurrent squamous lesions. The GOG is currently comparing cisplatin alone versus cisplatin plus ifosfamide versus cisplatin plus Dibromodulcitol in large scale randomized trials.

Several factors continue to influence chemotherapeutic response. First is the fact that carcinoma of the cervix has limited sensitivity to cytotoxic agents, especially when it recurs in the irradiated pelvis. Second, the median of response is usually only 3 to 7 months (although there are a few cases of complete response with a reasonable duration of remission). Third, there is a difficulty in showing a meaningful increase in survival of the patient population as a whole. Last, there is an impressive refractoriness among patients who have failed any prior chemotherapy. Thus, to the clinician, chemotherapy is beneficial to a small percentage of patients. Combination therapy with cisplatin continues to show the best results. Whether other drugs add to the effectiveness of cisplatin alone has yet to be demonstrated conclusively.

The approach to the patient should involve the following considerations. First, that a histological review of the specimen confirms the diagnosis of squamous or adenocarcinoma of the cervix. Second, the possibility of therapy by exenteration must be excluded. Relief of pain is a main indication of the use of chemotherapy. The presence of isolated painful metastatic sites that might lend themselves to regional irradiation therapy should promote consultation with a radiation oncologist. The pain of pelvic recurrence is a difficult problem requiring a multifaceted approach, including the use of designated pain consultants. Patients should also have acceptable hematological and renal function for chemotherapy to be considered. Careful attention must be paid to the side-effects of therapy, particularly nausea and vomiting, to avoid making a patient's limited life expectancy less tolerable than it would be without therapy.

Intra-arterial infusion for pelvic recurrence

Morrow et al reported on a series of 20 patients from five institutions in the Gynecologic Oncology Group who were treated with continuous pelvic arterial infusion of bleomycin for squamous cell carcinoma of the cervix recurrent after radiation therapy. All patients had documented unresectability and life expectancy of greater than 8 weeks. Bleomycin was infused through a femoral arterial catheter introduced percutaneously and threaded into the lower aorta to a position between the inferior mesenteric artery and the aortic bifurcation. A few patients were treated via bilateral hypogastric artery catheters inserted at the time of exploratory laparotomy. A continuous infusion of bleomycin (20 mg/m^2/week) for a minimum of 10 weeks or a total cumulative dose of 300 mg was given by means of low-flow portable infusion pumps. Infusion was discontinued if evidence of pulmonary toxicity appeared. Of the 20 patients studied, 10 had

toxicity of moderate to severe degree. There were 16 evaluable patients available and no complete responses. Only two partial responses were noted among 20 patients. The mean survival time was 7 months, with a range from 1 to 19 months. The 2 patients exhibiting partial tumor responses survived 5 and 8 months, respectively. The authors concluded that continuous arterial infusion of bleomycin is not helpful in the management of squamous cell carcinoma of the cervix recurrent in the pelvis after radiation therapy.

Lifshitz et al. reported on 14 patients with histologically confirmed recurrent pelvic malignancy treated with 44 courses of intr-arterial pelvic infusion of methotrexate or vincristine. Tumor regression was observed in 3 of 14 patients (21.4%). In 5 patients there were major complications related to 28 intra-arterial catheter placements. The authors concluded that the value of intra-arterial infusion chemotherapy in gynecologic cancer is limited.

Intra-arterial infusion for pelvic recurrence has also been attempted with cisplatin with very discouraging results. Explanations for these failures of pelvic infusion have varied. Some believe that the malignant cells are protected in a cocoon of fibrosis, whereas others feel that those cells that have survived initial radiation therapy are resistant to chemotherapy delivered by any route. Intra-arterial infusion for large primary lesions that are considered too large for cure by radiation alone may have value as initial therapy, shrinking the tumor for improved presentation to the radiotherapist.

MANAGEMENT OF BILATERAL URETERAL OBSTRUCTION

The patient with bilateral ureteral obstruction and uremia secondary to the extension of cervical cancer presents a serious dilemma for the clinician. Management should be divided into two subsets of patients: 1) those who have received no prior radiation therapy and 2) those who have recurrent disease after pelvic irradiation.

The patient who has bilateral ureteral obstruction from untreated cervical cancer or from recurrent pelvic disease after surgical therapy should be seriously considered for urinary diversion followed by appropriate radiation therapy. The salvage rate among this group of patients is low but realistic. Placement of antegrade ureteral stents should be attempted. When this is not possible, our preference has been to make a urinary conduit, anastomosing both ureters into an isolated loop of ileum (Bricker procedure) or creating one of a variety of continent pouches from a segment of bowel. We have also used these procedures in patients who had vesicovaginal fistulae secondary to untreated cervical malignancies. The ease with which pelvic radiation therapy can be optimally delivered is facilitated when the urinary diversion is performed before the irradiation is begun. In our experience, placement of urinary stents cystoscopically as an interim relief of the obstruction has been associated with multiple problems, leading us to favor the complete urinary diversion or antegrade ureteral stents. The traditional retrograde urinary stents are difficult to place bilaterally, and their presence in the ureter and bladder during the weeks to months of radiation therapy invariably leads to acute and chronic urinary tract infections. Interventional radiology with the use of percutaneous nephrostomy has created a reasonable option for these patients. Coddington and others have reported acceptable results after placement of internal ureteral stents via percutaneous nephrostomy. Patients require only local anesthesia for this procedure. Our experience has been favorable also, and an attempt at placement of these antegrade stents seems appropriate in patients with obstruction only and no vesicovaginal fistula before resorting to a urinary diversion.

The patient with bilateral ureteral obstruction (Figure 3-33) following a full dose of pelvic radiation therapy is an even more complicated problem. Less than 5% of these patients will have obstruction caused by radiation fibrosis, and often this group is difficult to identify. However, simple diversion of the urinary stream in this subset of patients is lifesaving, and therefore all patients must be considered as possibly belonging to this category until recurrent malignancy is found. When the presence of recurrent disease has been unequivocally established, the decision process becomes difficult and somewhat philosophical. Numerous studies suggest that "useful life" is not achieved by urinary diversion in this subset of patients. Brin et al. reported on 47 cases (5 with cervical cancer) of ureteral obstruction secondary to advanced pelvic malignancy. The results of this report are discouraging; the average survival time was 5.3 months, with only 50% of the patients alive at 3 months and only 22.7% alive at 6 months. After the diversion 63.8% of the survival time was spent in the hospital. Delgato also reported on a group of patients with recurrent pelvic cancer and renal failure who underwent urinary conduit diversion. His results showed no significant increase in survival time.

It has been suggested that these patients should never undergo urinary diversion, since a more preferable method of expiration (uremia) is thereby eliminated from the patient's future. It is obvious that these decisions should be made in consultation with the family and even with the patient if possible. The decision must be heavily shared by the physician, but the attitudes of patient and family must serve as a guide. These attitudes can, in most instances, be perceived without transferring the decision-making process entirely to the family or the patient. As more sophisticated methods of chemotherapy evolve, the option for diversion may become more suitable. There are patients who need additional time to settle personal matters, and diversion with effective chemotherapy may result in a reasonable extension of life. However, in most instances the avoidance of uremia results in an accentuation of the other clinical manifestations of recurrent pelvic cancer (i.e., severe pelvic pain, repeated infections, and hemorrhage). Pain control and progressive cachexia plague the physician and the patient. Episodes of massive pelvic hemorrhage are associated with difficult decisions for transfusion. An extension of the inpatient hospital stay is inevitable, and the financial impact that this may have on the patient and her family should also be a consideration.

Newer techniques, where placement of permanent ureteral stents via both the cystoscope and percutaneous insertion, have resulted in new options for this difficult clinical problem. Percutaneous placement of double J tubes with one end in the bladder and one end in the renal pelvis is now possible in many patients. As stated previously, this is especially advantageous in patients who have bilateral ureteral obstruction before any therapy, when radiation therapy may be very useful as a palliative procedure.

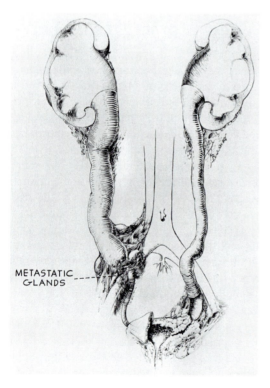

METASTATIC GLANDS

Figure 3-33 Hydroureters bilaterally secondary to a side wall recurrence on the patient's right and a parametrial recurrence on her left.

PELVIC RECURRENCE AFTER SUBOPTIMAL SURGERY

A small percentage of patients who have been treated by inadequate surgery or radical hysterectomy will have isolated pelvic recurrences. These patients are candidates for radiation therapy, and this should consist of external irradiation followed by appropriate vaginal or interstitial therapy. In recent years vaginal recurrences have been more successfully approached by use of interstitial irradiation following optimal external irradiation. The geometry of the postsurgical vagina with recurrence is such that standard vaginal applicators often are not suitable for optimal therapy. These patients are, of course, at higher risk for radiation injury because of the antecedent radical surgery. An open implant procedure, as described in Chapter 9, is often prudent.

PELVIC EXENTERATION

Extended or ultraradical surgery in the treatment of advanced and recurrent pelvic cancer is an American invention made possible by advances in the ancillary sciences that support the surgical team. The natural history of many pelvic cancers is that they may be locally advanced but still limited to the pelvis. They thus lend themselves to radical resection, unlike most other malignancies. In 1948 Brunschwig introduced the operation of pelvic exenteration for cancer of the cervix (Figure 3-34).

Since that time, extensive experience with pelvic exenteration has been accumulated, and the techniques as well as patient selection have steadily improved so that now, 44-50 years later, this procedure has attained an important role in the treatment of gynecologic malignancies. Although pelvic exenterative surgery was subjected to severe initial criticism, it is now accepted as a respectable procedure that can offer life to selected patients when no other possibility of cure exists. The criticism of this procedure has been lessened by steadily improving mortality and morbidity and a gratifying 5-year survival record. Most important, however, it has been shown that patients who survive this procedure can be rehabilitated to a useful and healthful existence.

Although pelvic exenteration has been used for various pelvic malignancies, its greatest and most important role is in the treatment of advanced or recurrent carcinoma of the cervix. Total exenteration (Figure 3-35) with removal of the pelvic viscera, including the bladder and rectosigmoid, is the procedure of choice for carcinoma of the cervix recurrent or persistent within the pelvis after irradiation. In very selected cases the procedure may be limited to anterior exenteration (Figure 3-36) with removal of the bladder and preservation of the rectosigmoid or posterior exenteration (Figure 3-37) with removal of the rectosigmoid and preservation of the bladder. Cogent objections have been raised regarding these limited operations, especially in patients with carcinoma of the cervix recurrent after irradiation, because of the increased risk of an incomplete resection. In addition, those patients in whom the bladder or rectum is preserved often have multiple complications and malfunctioning of the preserved organ. Consequently, some surgeons have

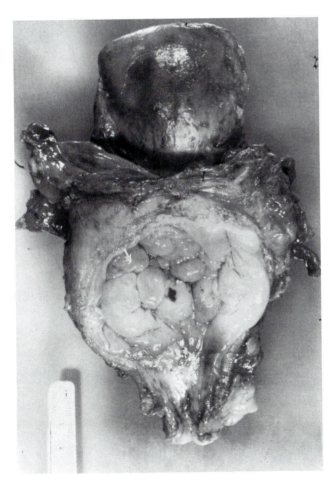

Figure 3-34 Specimen from an anterior exenteration done for recurrent cervical carcinoma; specimen consists of uterus, vagina, and bladder (anterior wall has been opened to expose bullous edema of the trigone [arrow]).

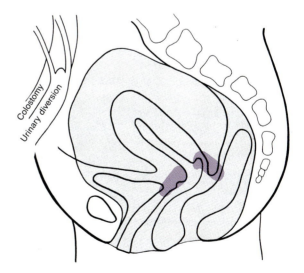

Figure 3-35 Total exenteration with removal of all pelvic viscera. Fecal stream is diverted via colostomy, and urinary diversion is via an ileal or sigmoid conduit or a continent pouch. (From DiSaia PJ, Morrow CP: *Calif Med* 118:13, Feb., 1973.)

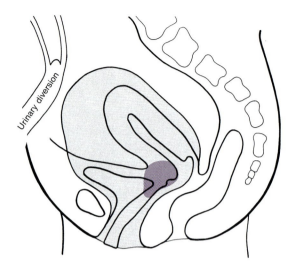

Figure 3-36 Anterior exenteration with removal of all pelvic viscera except the rectosigmoid. Urinary stream is diverted into an ileal or sigmoid conduit or a continent pouch. (From DiSaia PJ, Morrow CP: *Calif Med* 118:13, Feb., 1973.)

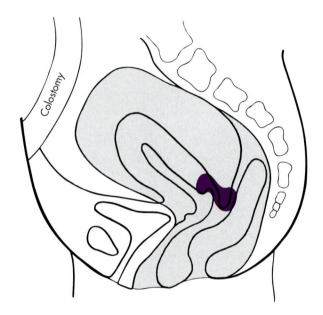

Figure 3-37 Posterior exenteration with removal of all pelvic viscera except the bladder. Fecal stream is diverted via colostomy. (From DiSaia PJ, Morrow CP: *Calif Med* 118:13, Feb., 1973.)

completely abandoned subtotal exenterations, and most oncologists use them very selectively.

One of the greatest technical advances in the evolution of pelvic exenteration is the intestinal conduit for diversion of the urinary stream. Originally Brunschwig transplanted the ureters into the left colon just proximal to the colostomy, creating the so-called wet colostomy. The complication rate from this procedure, especially electrolyte imbalance and severe urinary tract infections, was unacceptable. We are indebted to Bricker for popularizing the use of an ileal segment conduit for

urinary diversion. More recent developments have resulted in several techniques for creation of a continent reservoir, again utilizing a segment of bowel (Figure 3-38). The incidence of both postoperative pyelonephritis and hypochloremic acidosis has been greatly reduced. Furthermore, the patients are dry and comfortable and therefore more easily rehabilitated. Some surgeons have used a segment of sigmoid colon as a urinary conduit rather than small bowel in selected cases. This technique offers the additional advantage of avoiding a small-bowel anastomosis and the threat of fistula formation and obstruction attending any such procedure. Still other surgeons have preferred transverse colon as the segment of bowel for the conduit because it is usually out of the previous irradiation field. This technique may avoid some of the problems that can be associated with utilizing irradiated segment of bowel for reconstructive surgery.

Patient Selection

Only a small portion of the patients with recurrent cancer of the cervix are suitable for this operation (Table 3-13). Metastases outside the pelvis, whether manifested preoperatively or discovered at laparotomy, are an absolute contraindication to pelvic exenteration. The triad of unilateral leg edema, sciatic pain, and ureteral obstruction is pathognomonic of recurrent and unresectable disease in the pelvis. The triad must be complete, however, to be entirely reliable. Weight loss, cough, anemia, and other aberrations suggestive of advanced disease are not sufficient justification by themselves to discontinue efforts toward surgical management. Obesity, advanced age, and systemic disease may interdict extensive surgery in direct relation to the severity of these factors. Some patients are unsuitable because of psychologic reasons, and a number of women, otherwise candidates for pelvic exenteration, elect to accept the fate of unresected recurrence.

Although the pelvic examination plays a key role in the preoperative assessment of the patient, the examiner's impression of resectability must be tempered by the knowledge that errors are common. A small central lesion with freely mobile parametria reliably demonstrates resectability; however, immobility can be caused by radiation fibrosis and/or pelvic inflammatory disease (e.g., old salpingitis, inflammation from uterine perforation). Consequently, even when the disease seems inoperable on pelvic examination, if other factors are favorable, one should proceed with the investigation and exploratory laparotomy to avoid the error of a premature decision. Obviously, in many cases the finest clinical judgment must be used to avoid rejection of a potentially curable patient and also to prevent, as often as possible, subjection of an unsuitable patient to the anguish, fears, and false hopes of prolonged preparation for a fruitless operation.

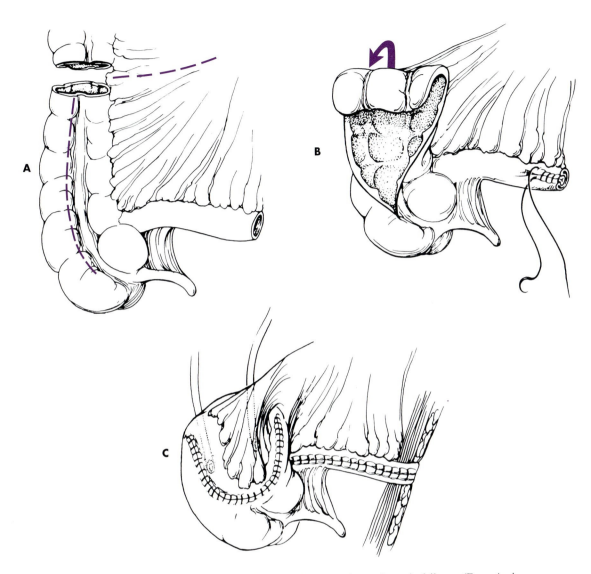

Figure 3-38 A-C, Construction of Indiana pouch from colon and terminal ileum. (From Amis ES et al: *Radiology* 168:398, 1988.)

Table 3-13 MD Anderson Hospital central recurrence rate for carcinoma of the cervix following treatment with radiation therapy	
Stage I	1.5%
Stage IIb	5.0%
Stage IIIa	7.5%
Stage IIIb	17.0%

Evaluation studies before surgery include chest film, CT scan of the abdomen and pelvis with intravenous contrast, creatinine clearance, liver function tests, and assessment of the patient's hemostatic mechanism. Any suspected disease outside the pelvis noted on any of the diagnostic studies should prompt an attempt at confirmation using a fine needle biopsy technique. Bilateral lower extremity lymphography has been found useful by some surgeons. Bone survey and liver scan are not part of the "routine" evaluation. A blind scalene node biopsy has been advocated by Ketcham and, if positive, would be a contraindication to further surgery.

Preparation for pelvic exenteration is often traumatic to patients with recurrent cervical cancer, especially when the procedure is aborted. The increased use of CT-directed fine needle aspirants has contributed greatly to lowering the fraction of patients explored who are found to be unexenterable. In a study by Miller, patients who underwent an aborted exploration were younger (median age 49 years) than patients undergoing exenteration (median age 54 years). On the other hand, the ratio of exenteration to aborted procedures was 1.57 among patients between the age of 30 and 39 to 3.26 in the age range 60 to 69. The reason for aborting the exenteration was the persistence of peritoneal tumor spread in 42% of the patients. Peritoneal cytology was predictive of peritoneal disease only in patients with adenocarcinoma. The procedure was aborted for nodal disease in 41% of patients. Parametrial fixation and other reasons for aborting the surgery made up the remaining 17%.

At laparotomy the entire abdomen and pelvis are explored for evidence of metastatic and intraperitoneal cancer (Figure 3-39). The liver should be carefully inspected visually and by palpation. The lymph nodes surrounding the lower aorta are the first to be sampled if the exploration of the abdomen has revealed no evidence of disease. If a lymphangiogram has been obtained before laparotomy, it may be helpful in directing the surgeon to suspicious nodes in the periaortic and pelvic area. If the lower aortic area findings are negative, a bilateral pelvic lymphadenectomy is performed. There have been virtually no survivors among those patients who have undergone pelvic exenteration with multiple grossly positive pelvic wall nodes. Therefore immediate frozen section analysis of the pelvic wall nodes is necessary to determine whether the resection should continue.

In a series of approximately 200 patients undergoing pelvic lymphadenectomy, Ketcham et al. found a positive pelvic lymph node after radiation therapy in only one 5-year survivor. In a similar series by Barber from Memorial Hospital, 148 patients with radiation failures undergoing pelvic exenteration were found to have positive nodes at the time of surgery, and only four of these patients were 5-year survivors. Creasman and Rutledge suggested a slightly more optimistic view of patients with positive lymph nodes who had undergone pelvic exenteration for recurrent cervical cancer following pelvic irradiation. However, in their series most survivors with positive nodes had only microscopic disease in the nodes. Furthermore, in nearly every case in the literature reported in detail of survival following exenteration for recurrent squamous cell carcinoma of the cervix in which there was a positive pelvic node, the nodal disease was not only microscopic but also unilateral.

Strenuous efforts have been made to decrease the permanent morbidity and increase patient acceptance of pelvic exenteration by tailoring the procedure to the known extent of the patient's disease. Although it is rarely justifiable to salvage the bladder because of its natural anatomic association with the cervix, the rectosigmoid occasionally may be preserved, and at times it is feasible to perform a lower segmental resection of the rectosigmoid and reanastomosis. A temporary diverting colos-

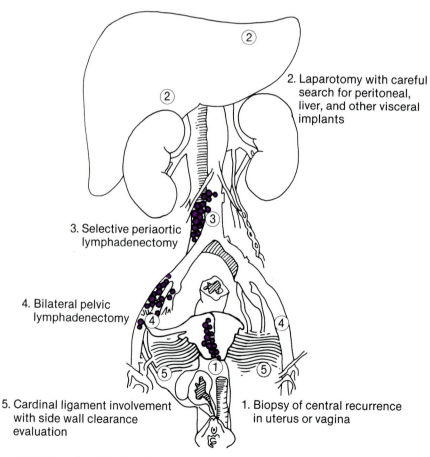

Figure 3-39 Steps in evaluation of patient for an exenterative procedure. (Courtesy Dr. A Robert Kagan, Los Angeles.)

tomy to protect the low anastomosis has been one practice, but with the current staple-gun anastomosis more patients can be considered for no colostomy if the surgeon feels confident of the water-tightness and viability of the reanastomosis. In most patients the possibility of constructing a neovagina from a split-thickness skin graft or from an isolated segment of bowel at the time of initial surgery should also be considered. Others have advocated rectus abdominis or gracilis myocutaneous grafts to re-create the vaginal canal. With these modifications, exenteration for pelvic malignancy frequently can be performed today, leaving the patient with but one stoma and a functional vagina. In the experience of the author, these neovaginas are seldom used postoperatively. This unfortunate fact has made the author prefer the more simple procedure requiring less time in what is already a very lengthy operative procedure.

Morbidity and Mortality

Most of the morbidity and mortality directly related to exenteration occur within the first 18 months following the procedure. Many of the complications can be sequelae to any major surgery. These include cardiopulmonary catastrophes such as pulmonary embolism, pulmonary edema, myocardial infarction, and cerebrovascular accidents. The length of these surgical procedures and the magnitude of blood loss definitely increase the incidence of cardiovascular complications. This category of complications usually occurs within the first week after the procedure. Then there is a period when sepsis is the greatest threat to the patient's health and life. This sepsis usually originates in the pelvic cavity with occurrence of a pelvic abscess or, more common, diffuse pelvic cellulitis.

One of the most serious postoperative complications of exenteration is small-bowel obstruction related to the denuded pelvic floor. In the last decade several techniques have been employed in an effort to avoid the adherence of small bowel to this large raw surface, including mobilization of omentum or abdominal wall peritoneum to cover the pelvic floor (Figure 3-40). When small-bowel obstruction does occur, it is appropriately treated with conservative therapy. However, half these patients come to reoperation, and the mortality of this group approaches 50% in some series. The risk of bowel obstruction is increased by the presence of pelvic infection, and both conditions predispose to the development of small-bowel fistulae, which always require reoperation and frequently are fatal. Lichtinger reports a 53% mortality in patients developing a small-bowel fistula following pelvic exenteration. In general, complications are far more common in patients who have recurrence after radiation therapy. Irradiated tissue is less likely to give good wound healing, and the formation of granulation tissue is severely retarded. The tendency toward fistula formation

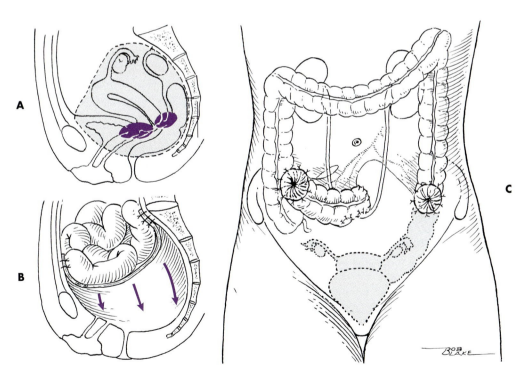

Figure 3-40 A, Lateral view of recurrent cancer involving cervix and upper vagina with extension into bladder and rectum. Stippled area is tissue to be removed by exenteration. **B,** Lateral view after pelvic viscera have been removed. Omental "carpet" is used to keep intestines out of pelvis during immediate postoperative period. With time, omental "carpet" will descend into pelvis and "carpet" will adhere to pelvic floor. **C,** Urinary conduit and colostomy diversion after exenteration. Dotted areas of sigmoid, bladder, and internal genitalia have been removed.

is markedly increased. Since surgical dissection is usually more difficult in the irradiated patient, longer operating times and increased blood loss often result. Both these factors are associated with higher morbidity and mortality. Thus the patient who has had previous radiation therapy is at much greater risk for serious complications than the nonirradiated patient and is less capable of a competent physiologic response.

The long-term morbidity from exenteration is predominantly related to urinary diversion. Once the period of susceptibility to sepsis has passed, urinary obstruction and infection become the major nonneoplastic life-threatening complications. Recurrent cancer is forever the most likely long-term life-threatening situation following the operative procedure, but the more preventable complications of the ileal conduit deserve primary attention. Many believe that these patients should be managed with long-term urinary antisepsis, perhaps for life. Pyelonephritis is common and should be treated promptly and vigorously. Periodic IVPs must be obtained to assess the collecting system for hydronephrosis. A mild degree of obstruction is frequently retained following construction of an ileal conduit, but progressive hydronephrosis will require correction to salvage renal function. It is tragic to lose a patient after exenteration because of resulting, but perhaps treatable renal disease when there is no residual carcinoma.

Orr et al. reported on 115 urinary diversions at the time of pelvic exenteration. An ileal segment was used as a conduit in 97 patients, and a segment of transverse colon was used in 16 patients. Two patients had sigmoid colon conduits. Eighty-five patients (73.9%) had the intestinal anastomosis and conduit constructed with a gastrointestinal stapler. Fourteen patients (12.2%) required a second operation for non-cancer-related urinary complications. Complications included ureteral strictures, conduit stoma stenosis or prolapse, and renal calculi. Sixty-one percent of the patients required rehospitalization for nonmalignant indications involving the urinary tract. Late pyelonephritis was the most common reason for rehospitalization. The incidence of complications appeared to be less in those patients in whom an unirradiated portion of bowel had been used for construction of the conduit.

Averette reported on 88 patients who had urinary diversion at the time of pelvic exenteration. Urinary fistulae developed in 12% of these, with a 45% mortality on surgical correction. Also, 16% of the 92 patients who had bowel surgery at the time of pelvic exenteration developed gastrointestinal fistulae, and of these there was a 40% operative mortality associated with correction. In an effort to avoid reoperation and its associated high mortality, we first attempt conservative management of these fistulae, including drainage and hyperalimentation, if sepsis is not present. Many of the fistulae will close when satisfactory patency of the bowel or ureter is achieved.

The morbidity and mortality from radical surgery can be minimized by careful selection of patients. This, however, implies a system in which some patients who may be resectable are denied an opportunity for resection in order to keep the morbidity low. This becomes a philosophic question that each physician must answer. However, the outcome of recurrent carcinoma of the cervix in a patient who is given no further treatment is clear.

Walton published a comprehensive review of the factors involved in the stress reaction of the patient after radical pelvic surgery, calling attention to the biochemical, psychological, gastrointestinal, hepatic, and cardiac effects. He concluded that with total care, the occurrence of these stress reactions will decrease but will not disappear, since the human organism reacts in such a complex manner, and derangement would occur in the weakest adaptive link to the surrounding environment.

Survival Results

The 5-year cumulative survival rate after pelvic exenteration varies in the literature from 20% to 62% (Table 3-14). Reported survival rates depend greatly on the circumstances of patient selection for exenteration. For instance, patients who undergo pelvic exenteration as a primary procedure have a 5-year survival rate 20% to 25% higher than a similar group of patients with recurrence following irradiation. (Pelvic exenteration may be performed as a primary procedure for carcinoma of the vulva extending up the vagina and into the bladder but not out to the pelvic sidewalls.) Survival rates can be improved by excluding the elderly, the obese, the heavily irradiated, and other high-risk patients. Cumulative survival rates are always improved when no patient is exenterated who has a positive pelvic node following pelvic irradiation. In general, however, both morbidity and mortality and the 5-year survival rate have steadily improved over the last two decades. Mortality in most centers is now well below 5%, and morbidity has been similarly lowered.

The survival prognosis for many patients is related to well-defined preoperative findings. The MD Anderson Hospital series reported that 47% of the patients whose recurrences were symptomatic (pain or edema) but who were found resectable at the time of surgery survived 2 years. However, 73% of the patients who were symptom free at the time of laparotomy survived 2 years. Of the patients who had a normal IVP at the time of laparotomy, 59% survived 2 years, whereas only 34% of the patients who had some IVP abnormality before laparotomy survived 2 years. Forty-six percent of the patients who had recurrence within 2 years of their primary treatment survived 2 years or more after treatment. Such factors as the status of the IVP, the presence or absence of symptoms, and the interval between primary treatment and recurrence should be considered in the preoperative assessment of the patient. One can improve the cumulative survival rate by excluding patients who have these deleterious characteristics; however, in so doing, one may

Table 3-14   Pelvic exenteration

Author	Institution	Number of patients treated	Number of operative deaths	Number surviving 5 years*
Douglas and Sweeney (1957)	New York Hospital	23	1 (4.3%)	5 (22%)
Parsons and Friedell (1964)	Harvard University	112	24 (21.4%)	24 (21.4%)
Brunschwig (1965)	Memorial Hospital	535	86 (16%)	108 (20.1%)
Bricker (1967)	Washington University	153	15 (10%)	53 (34.6%)
Krieger and Embree (1969)	Cleveland Clinics	35	4 (11%)	13 (37%)
Ketcham et al. (1970)	National Cancer Institute	162	12 (7.4%)	62 (38.2%)
Symmonds et al. (1975)	Mayo Clinic	198	16 (8%)	64 (32.3%)
Morley and Lindenauer (1976)	University of Michigan	34	1 (2.9%)	21 (62%)
Rutledge et al. (1977)	MD Anderson Hospital	296	40 (13.5%)	99 (33.4%)
Averette et al. (1984)	University of Miami			
	1966-1971	14	4 (28.5%)	5 (36%)
	1971-1976	45	15 (33.3%)	10 (22%)
	1976-1981	33	4 (12.1%)	19 (58%)
Lawhead et al. (1989)	Memorial Hospital	65	6 (9.2%)	15 (23%)
	1972-1981			
Soper et al. (1989)	Duke University	69	5 (7.2%)	28 (40.5%)
Shingleton et al. (1989)	University of Alabama	143	9 (6.3%)	71 (50%)
TOTAL		1917	242 (12.6%)	647 (33.8%)

*In almost every series the operative death rate and the 5-year survival rate were dramatically improved in the latter years of each series.

be excluding some patients who are resectable and therefore curable.

Although lesions other than carcinoma of the cervix may be cured by pelvic exenteration, cervical cancer is numerically of greatest importance. This procedure offers the only possibility for cure in patients who have pelvic recurrence after receiving optimal amounts of irradiation. With improved radiotherapy techniques, the number of patients with isolated central failure is steadily diminishing, but there remain a number of patients with recurrent cancer of the cervix after radiation therapy for whom the procedure offers the only chance for life. For the mortality and morbidity to be acceptable, the surgery should be done in medical centers by experienced surgical teams who are knowledgeable in the multidisciplinary approach to cancer therapy and can tailor the management to each patient's needs. These ultraradical surgical procedures should be done only by those individuals with adequate training and background who are willing to take on the responsibility of long-term postoperative care and rehabilitation. Each patient must be assessed individually with the risks of the procedure weighed against the possible benefits. It is encouraging that technical advances continue to reduce the operative mortality and ameliorate the postoperative morbidity associated with pelvic exenteration. Many patients can be not only cured but also rehabilitated to functional and comfortable lives; no patient should be deprived of this opportunity.

Advanced age was once considered a relative contraindication to ultraradical exenterative surgery. Matthews, however, reviewed the outcome of 63 patients,

age 65 or more, who underwent pelvic exenteration between 1960 and 1991 at the University of Texas MD Anderson Cancer Center. Although 63% of the patients had preexisting medical illnesses, tolerance of the surgery was quite good. Whereas 60% of the patients experienced one or more infectious complications, including pyelonephritis, wound infection, sepsis, and flap necrosis accounting for the largest category of complications, 24% experienced no complications. Operative mortality was 11%; multisystem failure was the most frequent cause of death. Within a mean follow-up of 12 years following exenteration, 22 of the 63 patients were alive and without clinical evidence of disease. The 5-year survival for the group was 46%. It appears that the morbidity and mortality of pelvic exenteration in elderly patients are similar to those noted in previous studies of younger patients, with a similar 5-year survival rate. Therefore, age should not be considered an absolute contraindication to exenteration.

SARCOMA, LYMPHOMA, AND MELANOMA OF THE CERVIX

In the SEER report of 6549 cases of cervical carcinoma from 1973 to 1977, there were only 36 cases of cervical sarcoma, an incidence of 0.55%. Cervical leiomyosarcomas are rare tumors with poor prognosis regardless of the mode of therapy. Cervical stromal sarcomas arise from the basic paramesonephric stroma (mesoderm). These tumors may be homologous or combined with an epithelial element, mixed mesodermal tumor, or carcinosarcoma. Embryonal rhabdomyosarcoma or sarcoma botryoides of the cervix usually occurs in women during their reproductive years. Although the role of adjuvant chemotherapy such as that used for children with perineal rhabdomyosarcoma has not been investigated in this group of patients, it appears to be worthy of serious consideration in patients with large lesions. Ninety-six cases of cervical sarcoma were reviewed by Rotmensch, and no clear statement could be made regarding management, although surgery was consistently utilized for early stage lesions. Lymphangiomas and lymphosarcomas of the reticulum cell variety are also seen rarely. Identification of these lesions requires differentiation from anaplastic carcinoma, with which they can be readily confused. These lesions are usually metastatic, and further investigation of the patient reveals multiple foci.

Perren reviewed 77 cases of the reticuloendothelial neoplasia who presented with disease apparently limited to the cervix or upper vagina. The most common clinical feature at presentation was abnormal vaginal bleeding (54%). Other presentations included vaginal mass (12%) and dyspareunia (5%). An abnormal cervical smear was noted in only two cases. The conclusion is that lymphomas of the genital tract have an unpredictable prognosis.

There is no evidence that radical gynecological surgery is advantageous and patients are best treated as for other lymphomas with radiation therapy and combination chemotherapy.

Malignant melanoma of the uterine cervix is a very rare manifestation, and neither prospective nor retrospective studies on this disease have been published. There are approximately 25 published case reports recently collated in an attempt to clarify the origin, presenting symptoms, macroscopic appearance, and staging of this lesion. It is often difficult to ascertain whether the lesion is of primary or metastatic origin. A careful survey should be done of the patient's skin and mucous membrane for a possible primary site. Almost 90% of the patients are asymptomatic, vaginal bleeding being the main complaint. While primary cervical malignancies usually afflict women in the 40- to 50-year age range, melanoma of the cervix generally manifests in patients between 60 and 70 years of age. The vast majority of lesions present as an exophytic polypoid cervical mass with obvious coloring. Nearly all patients diagnosed are stage I or II, and preferred therapy has been radical hysterectomy. The 5-year survival is very poor, not exceeding 40% of stage I and 14% of stage II.

BIBLIOGRAPHY

General observations

Andersen B et al: Sexual dysfunction and signs of gynecologic cancer, *Cancer* 57:1880, 1986.

Boon ME et al: Efficacy of screening for cervical squamous and adenocarcinoma: the Dutch experience, *Cancer* 59:862, 1987.

Coppleson M, Reid B: The etiology of squamous carcinoma of the cervix, *Obstet Gynecol* 32:432, 1968 (editorial).

Hildesheim A, Brinton LA, Mallin K, Lehman HF et al: Barrier and spermicidal contraceptive methods and risk of invasive cervical cancer (see comments), *Epidemiology* 1 (4):266, 1990.

Piper JM: Oral contraceptives and cervical cancer, *Gynecol Oncol* 22:1, 1985.

Reid R et al: Genital warts and cervical cancer, *Cancer* 50:377, 1982.

Seibel MM, Freeman MG, Graves WL: Carcinoma of the cervix and sexual function, *Obstet Gynecol* 55:484, 1980.

Weijmar Schultz WCM, Van De Wiel HBM, Bouma J: Psychosexual functioning after treatment for cancer of the cervix: a comparative and longitudinal study, *Int J Gynecol Cancer* 1:37, 1991.

Wentz WB et al: Induction of uterine cancer with inactivated herpes simplex virus, types 1 and 2, *Cancer* 48:1783, 1981.

West RR: Cervical Cancer: age at registration and age at death, *Br J Cancer* 35:236, 1977.

Microinvasive carcinoma of the cervix

Benedet JL, Anderson GH, Boyes DA: Colposcopic accuracy in the diagnosis of microinvasive and occult invasive carcinoma of the cervix, *Obstet Gynecol* 65:557, 1985.

Boutselis JG, Ullery JC, Charmer L: Diagnosis and management of stage Ia (microinvasive) carcinoma of the cervix, *Am J Obstet Gynecol* 110:984, 1971.

Boyce DA, Worth AJ: Treatment of early cervical neoplasia: definition and management of preclinical invasive carcinoma, *Gynecol Oncol* 12:317, 1981.

Boyce DA, Worth AJ, Fidler HK: The results of treatment of 4389 cases of preclinical cervical squamous carcinoma, *J Obstet Gynaecol Br Commonw* 77:769, 1970.

Burghardt E, Girardi F, Lahousen M et al: Microinvasive carcinoma of the uterine cervix, *Cancer* 67:1037, 1991.

Copeland LJ, Silva EE, Gershenson DM, Morris M et al: Superficially invasive squamous cell carcinoma of the cervix, *Gynecol Oncol* 45:307, 1992.

Creasman WT, Fetter BF, Clarke-Pearson DL et al: Management of stage Ia carcinoma of the cervix, *Am J Obstet Gynecol* 153:164, 1985.

Creasman WT, Parker RT: Microinvasive carcinoma of the cervix, *Clin Obstet Gynecol* 16:261, 1973.

Girardi F, Burghardt E, Pickel H: Small stage Ib cervical cancer, *Gynecol Onc* 55:427, 1994.

Halzer E: Microinvasive carcinoma of the cervix—clinical aspects, treatment, and follow-up. In Burghardt E, Halzer E, eds: *Minimal Invasive Cancer*, London: W.B. Saunders Co Ltd, 1982, p.315.

Hasumi K, Sakamoto A, Sugano H: Microinvasive carcinoma of the uterine cervix, *Cancer* 45:928, 1980.

Hopkins MP, Morley GW: Squamous cell carcinoma of the cervix: clinical pathological features related to survival, *Am J Obstet Gynecol* 164:1520, 1991.

Hopkins MP, Morley GW: Squamous cell cancer of the cervix: prognostic factors related to survival, *Int J Gynecol Cancer* 1:173, 1991.

Kolstad P: Follow-up study of 232 patients with stage Ia1 and 411 patients with stage Ia2 squamous cell carcinoma of the cervix (microinvasive carcinoma), *Gynecol Oncol* 33:265, 1989.

Leman MH, Benson WL, Kurman RJ et al: Microinvasive carcinoma of the cervix, *Obstet Gynecol* 48:571, 1976.

Lohe KJ: Early squamous cell carcinoma of the uterine cervix I, *Gynecol Oncol* 6:10, 1978.

Lohe KJ: Early squamous cell carcinoma of the uterine cervix III, *Gynecol Oncol* 6:51, 1978.

Lohe KJ et al: Early squamous cell carcinoma of the uterine cervix II, *Gynecol Oncol* 6:31, 1979.

Maiman MA: Superficially invasive squamous cell carcinoma of the cervix, *Obstet Gynecol* 72 (3, pt. 1):399, 1988.

Mussey E, Soule EH, Welch JS: Microinvasive carcinoma of the cervix: late results of operative treatment in 91 cases, *Am J Obstet Gynecol* 104:738, 1969.

Ng AB, Reagan JW: Microinvasive carcinoma of the uterine cervix, *Am J Clin Pathol* 52:511, 1969.

Östör AG, Rome RM: Microinvasive squamous cell carcinoma of the cervix: a clinicopathologic-pathologic study of 200 cases with long term follow up, *Int J Gynecol Cancer* 4:257, 1994.

Roche WD, Norris HJ: Microinvasive carcinoma of the cervix: the significance of lymphatic invasion and confluent patterns of stromal growth, *Cancer* 180, July, 1985.

Sedlis A, Gall S, Tsukoda Y et al: Microinvasive carcinoma of the uterine cervix: a clinical pathologic study, *Am J Obstet Gynecol* 133:67, 1979.

Seski JC, Abell MR, Morley GW: Microinvasive squamous carcinoma of the cervix, *Obstet Gynecol* 50:410, 1977.

Sevin BU, Nadji M, Averette HE et al: Microinvasive carcinoma of the cervix, *Cancer* 70:2121, 1992.

Simon NL, Gore H, Shingleton HM: Study of superficially invasive carcinoma of the cervix, *Obstet Gynecol* 68:19, 1986.

Tsukamoto N, Kaku T, Matsukuma K et al: The problem of stage Ia (FIGO 1985) carcinoma of the uterine cervix, *Gynecol Oncol* 34:1, 1989.

Van Nagell Jr, Greenwell N, Powell DF et al: Microinvasive carcinoma of the cervix, *Am J Obstet Gynecol* 145:982, 1983.

Yasgashi N, Sata S, Inque Y et al: Comparative surgical treatment in cervical cancer with 3-5 mm stromal invasion in the absence of confluent invasion and lymph-vascular pace involvement, *Gynecol Onc* 54:333, 1994.

Clinical profile of invasive cancer

Acs J et al: Regional distribution of human papillomavirus DNA and other risk factors for invasive cervical cancer in Panama, *Cancer Res* 49:5725, 1989.

Barron BA, Richart RM: A statistical model of the natural history of cervical carcinoma based on a prospective study of 557 cases, *J Natl Ca Inst* 41:1343, 1968.

Berman ML et al: Survival and patterns of recurrence in cervical cancer metastatic to periaortic lymph nodes, *Gynecol Oncol* 19:8, 1984.

Brinton LA: Epidemiology of cervical cancer—overview, *IARC* 3:1993.

Brinton LA: Oral contraceptives and cervical neoplasia, *Contraception* 43:581, 1991.

Burger MPM et al: Cigarette smoking and human papillomavirus in patients with reported cervical cytological abnormality, *Br Med J* 306:749, 1993.

Chu J, White E: Decreasing incidence of invasive cervical cancer in young women, *Am J Obstet Gynecol* 157:1105, 1987.

Creadick RH: Carcinoma of the cervical stump, *Am J Obstet Gynecol* 75:565, 1958.

Daling JR et al: Cigarette smoking and the risk of anogenital cancer, *Am J Epidemiol* 135:180, 1992.

Delgato G et al: A prospective surgical pathological study of stage I squamous carcinoma of the cervix: a Gynecologic Oncology Group study, *Gynecol Oncol* 35:314, 1989.

Gagnon F: The lack of occurrence of cervical carcinoma in nuns, *Proc Second Natl Cancer Conf* 1:625, 1952.

Henriksen E: The lymphatic spread of carcinoma of the cervix and of the body of the uterus: a study of 420 necropsies, *Am J Obstet Gynecol* 58:924, 1949.

Henriksen E: The dispersion of cancer of the cervix, *Radiology* 54:812, 1950.

Henriksen E: Distribution of metastases in stage I carcinoma of the cervix, *Am J Obstet Gynecol* 80:919, 1960.

Hopkins MP, Morlay GW: Squamous cell carcinoma of the cervix: clinical pathological features related to survival, *Am J Obstet Gynecol* 164:1520, 1991.

Mvula M et al: Detection of human papillomavirus types 16 and 18 in primary and metastatic lesions of cervical carcinomas, *Gynecol Oncol* 53:156, 1994.

Reeves WC et al: Human papillomavirus infection and cervical cancer in Latin America, *N Eng J* Med 320:1437, 1989.

Simons AM, Philips DH, Coleman DV: Damage to DNA in cervical epithelium related to smoking tobacco, *Br Med J* 306:1444, 1993.

Slattery ML et al: Cigarette smoking and exposure to passive smoke are risk factors for cervical cancer, *JAMA* 261:1593, 1989.

Ursin G et al: Oral contraceptive use and adenocarcinoma of cervix, *Lancet* 344:1390, 1994.

Adenocarcinoma of the cervix

Angel C, Dubeshter B, Lin JY: Clinical presentation and management of stage I cervical adenocarcinoma: a 25-year experience, *Gynecol* Oncol 44:71, 1992.

Anton-Culver H et al: Comparison of adenocarcinoma and squamous cell carcinoma of the uterine cervix: a population based epidemiologic study, *Am J Obstet Gynecol* 166:1507, 1992.

Berek JS et al: Adenocarcinoma of the uterine cervix, *Cancer* 48:2734, 1981.

Boon ME et al: Adenocarcinoma in situ of the cervix, *Cancer* 48:768, 1981.

Brand E, Berek JS, Hacker NF: Controversies in the management of cervical adenocarcinoma, *Obstet Gynecol* 71:261, 1988.

Davidson SE, Symonds RP, Lamont D et al: Does adenocarcinoma of uterine cervix have a worse prognosis than squamous carcinoma when treated by radiotherapy? *Gynecol Oncol* 33:23, 1989.

Duk JM et al: Tumor markers CA 125, squamous cell carcinoma antigen, and carcinoembryonic antigen in patients with adenocarcinoma of the uterine cervix, *Obstet Gynecol* 73:661, 1989.

Eifel PJ, Burke TW, Delclos L et al: Early stage I adenocarcinoma of the uterine cervix: treatment results in patients with tumors <4 cm in diameter, *Obstet Gynecol* 41:199, 1991.

Eifel PJ et al: Adenocarcinoma of the uterine cervix, *Cancer* 65:2507, 1990.

Eifel PJ et al: Early stage I adenocarcinoma of the uterine cervix: treatment results in patients with tumors ≤4 cm in diameter, *Gynecol Oncol* 41:199, 1991.

Hopkins MP, Morlay GW: Comparison of adenocarcinoma and squamous cell carcinoma of the cervix, *Obstet Gynecol* 77:912, 1991.

Hopkins MP et al: The prognosis and treatment of stage I adenocarcinoma of the cervix, *Obstet Gynecol* 72:915, 1988.

Kilgore LC et al: Analysis of prognostic features in adenocarcinoma of the cervix, *Gynecol Oncol* 31:137, 1988.

Kjorstad KE, Bond B: Stage Ib adenocarcinoma of the cervix: metastatic potential and patterns of dissemination, *Am J Obstet Gynecol* 150:297, 1984.

Kleine W et al: Prognosis of the adenocarcinoma of the cervix uteri: a comparative study, *Gynecol Oncol* 35:145, 1989.

Matthews CA et al: Stage I cervical adenocarcinoma: prognostic evaluation of sugically treated patients, *Gynecol Oncol* 49:19, 1993.

Moberg PJ et al: Adenocarcinoma of the uterine cervix, *Cancer* 57:407, 1986.

Parazzin IF, LaVecchia C: Epidemiology of adenocarcinoma of the cervix, *Gynecol Oncol* 39:4, 1990.

Prempree T, Amornmarn R, Wizenberg MJ: A therapeutic approach to primary adenocarcinoma of the cervix, *Cancer* 56:1264, 1985.

Raju KS, Kjorstad KE, Abeler V: Prognostic factors in the treatment of stage 1b adenocarcinoma of the cervix, *Int J Gynecol Cancer* 1:69, 1991.

Rose PG, Reale FR: Case Report: Serous papillary carcinoma of the cervix, *Gynecol Oncol* 50:361, 1993.

Rutledge FN, Gutierrez AG, Fletcher GH: Management of stage I and II adenocarcinomas of the uterine cervix on intact uterus, *AJR* 102:161, 1968.

Yamakawa Y et al: Human papillomavirus DNA in adenocarcinoma and adenosquamous carcinoma of the uterine cervix detected by polymerase chain reaction (PCR), *Gynecol Oncol* 53:190, 1994.

Young RH, Scully RE: Invasive adenocarcinoma and related tumors of the urterine cervix, *Semin Diagn Pathol* 7:205, 1990.

Neuroendocrine small-cell and glassy cell carcinoma of the cervix

Abeler VM, Holm R, Nesland JM, Kjorstad KE: Small cell carcinoma of the cervix, *Cancer* 73:672, 1994.

Barrett RJ, Davos I, Leuchter RS et al: Neuroendocrine features in poorly differentiated and undifferentiated carcinomas of the cervix, *Cancer* 60:1089, 1987.

Hoskins PJ et al: Small cell carcinoma of the cervix treated with concurrent radiotherapy, cisplatin, and etoposide, *Gynecol Oncol* 56:218, 1995.

Lewandowski GS, Copeland LJ: Case report: a potential role for intensive chemotherapy in the treatment of small cell neuroendocrine tumors of the cervix, *Gynecol Oncol* 48:127, 1993.

Lotocki RJ et al: Glassy cell carcinoma of the cervix: a bimodal treatment strategy, *Gynecol Oncol* 44:254, 1992.

Morris M et al: Treatment of small cell carcinoma of the cervix with cisplatin, doxorubicin, and etoposide, *Gynecol Oncol* 47:62, 1992.

Pazdur R et al: Neuroendocrine carcinoma of the cervix: implications for staging and therapy, *Gynecol Oncol* 12:120, 1981.

Sheets EE, Berman ML, Hrountas CK et al: Surgically treated, early-stage neuroendocrine small-cell cervical carcinoma, *Obstet Gynecol* 71:10, 1988.

Stoler MH, Mills SE, Gersell DJ et al: Small-cell neuroendocrine carcinoma of the cervix, *Am J Surg Pathol* 15 (1):28, 1991.

Tamimi HK et al: Glassy cell carcinoma of the cervix redefined, *Obstet Gynecol* 71:837, 1988.

Staging

Belenson JL, Goldberg MI, Averette HE: Paraaortic lymphadenectomy in gynecologic cancer, *Gynecol Oncol* 7:188, 1979.

Brenner DE et al: An evaluation of the computed tomographic scanner for the staging of carcinoma of the cervix, *Cancer* 50:2323, 1982.

Buchsbaum HJ: Extrapelvic lymph node metastases in cervical carcinoma, *Am J Obstet Gynecol* 133:814, 1979.

Burke TW et al: Evaluation of the scalene lymph nodes in primary and recurrent cervical carcinoma, *Gynecol Oncol* 28:312, 1987.

Childers JM, Hatch K Surwitt EA: The role of paparoscopic lymphadenectomy in the management of cervical carcinoma, *Gynecol Oncol* 47:38, 1992.

Childers JM, Hatch K, Tran AN, Surwitt EA: Laparoscopic para-aortic lymphadenectomy in gynecologic malignancies, *Obstet Gynecol* 82:741, 1993.

Dargent D: Laparoscopic surgery and gynecologic cancer, *Curr Opin Obstet Gynecol* 5:294, 1993.

Delgato G, Smith JP, Ballantyne AJ: Scalene node biopsy in carcinoma of the cervix; pelvic and paraaortic lymphadenectomy, *Cancer* 35:784, 1975.

Lagasse LD et al: Results and complications of operative staging in cervical cancer: experience of the Gynecologic Oncology Group, *Gynecol Oncol* 9:90, 1980.

Lanciano RM, Won M, Hanks GE: A reappraisal of the international federation of gynecology and obstetrics staging system for cervical cancer, *Cancer* 69: 482, 1992.

Nelson JH Jr et al: The incidence and significance of para-aortic lymph node metastases in late invasive carcinoma of the cervix, *Am J Obstet Gyneco* 118:749, 1974.

Patish RA et al: The impact of extra-peritoneal surgical staging on morbidity and tumor recurrence following radiotherapy for cervical carcinoma, *Am J Clin Oncol* 7:245, 1984.

Schellhaus HF: Extraperitoneal para-aortic dissection through an upper abdominal incision, *Obstet Gynecol* 46:444, 1975.

Treatment

Abbe R: The use of radium in malignant disease, *Lancet* 2:524, 1913.

Alberts DS, Garcia D, Mason-Liddil N: Cisplatin in advanced cancer of the cervix: an update, *Sem Oncol* 18 (1):11, 1991.

Alberts DS et al: Mitomycin C, bleomycin, vincristine, and cis-platinum in the treatment of advanced recurrent squamous cell carcinoma of the cervix, *Cancer Clin Trials* 4:313, 1981.

Ampil F, Datta R, Datta S: Elective postoperative external radiotherapy after hysterectomy in early-stage carcinoma of the cervix: is additional vaginal cuff irradiation necessary? *Cancer* 60:280, 1987.

Anderson B, LaPolla J, Turner D, Chapman G, Buller R: Ovarian transposition in cervical cancer, *Gynecol Oncol* 49:206, 1993.

Andras EJ, Fletcher GH, Rutledge F: Radiotheraphy of carcinoma of the cervix following simple hysterectomy, *Am J Obstet Gynecol* 115:647, 1973.

Artman LE et al: Radical hysterectomy and pelvic lymphadenectomy for stage IB carcinoma of the cervix: 21 years experience, *Gynecol Oncol* 28:8, 1987.

Bandy LC, et al: Long-term effects on bladder function following radical hysterectomy with and without postoperative radiation, *Gynecol Oncol* 26:160, 1987.

Barnes W et al: Manometric characterization of rectal dysfunction following radical hysterectomy, *Gynecol Oncol* 42:116, 1991.

Barton DPJ et al: Radical hysterectomy for treatment of cervical cancer: a prospective study of two methods of closed-suction drainage, *Am J Obstet Gynecol* 166:533, 1992.

Bianchi UA et al: Treatment of primary invasive cervical cancer; considerations on 997 consecutive cases, *Eur J Gynaecol Oncol* 9(1):47, 1988.

Bloss JD et al: Bulky stage IB cervical carcinoma managed by primary radical hysterectomy followed by tailored radiotherapy, *Gynecol Oncol* 47:21, 1992.

Bloss JD et al: A phase II trial of neoadjuvant chemotherapy prior to radical hysterectomy +/or radiation therapy in the management of advanced carcinoma of the cervix. Presented at meeting of the Society of Gynecologic Oncologists — San Francisco, CA 1995.

Bonfiglio M: The pathology of fracture of the femoral neck following irradiation, *AJR* 70:449, 1953.

Bosch A, Marcial VA: Carcinoma of the uterine cervix associated with pregnancy, *AJR* 96:92, 1966.

Brack CB, Everett HC, Dickson R: Irradiation therapy for carcinoma of the cervix: its effect on urinary tract, *Obstet Gynecol* 7:196, 1956.

Bremer GL et al: Early stage cervical cancer: aborted versus completed radical hysterectomy, *Euro J Obstet Gynecol Reprod Biol* 47:147, 1992.

Brenner DE et al: Simultaneous radiation and chemotherapy for advanced carcinoma of the cervix, *Gynecol Oncol* 26:381, 1987.

Brookland RK, Rubin S, Danoff BF: Extended field irradiation in the treatment of patients with cervical carcinoma involving biopsy-proven para-aortic nodes, *Rad Oncol Biol Phys* 10:1875, 1984.

Brown JV, Fu YS, Berek JS: Ovarian metastases are rare in stage I adenocarcinoma of the cervix, *Obstet Gynecol* 76:623, 1990.

Carenza L, Nobili F, Giacobini S: Voiding disorders after radical hysterectomy, *Gynecol Oncol* 13:213, 1982.

Chambers SK et al: Sequelae of lateral ovarian transposition in unirradiated cervical cancer patients, *Gynecol Oncol* 39:155, 1990.

Chapman JA, Mannel RS, DiSaia PJ et al: Surgical treatment of unexpected invasive cervical cancer found at total hysterectomy, *Obstet Gynecol* 80:931, 1992.

Chism SE, Park RC, Keys HM: Prospects for paraaortic irradiation in treatment of cancer of the cervix, *Cancer* 35:1505, 1975.

Choo YC: Chemotherapy in advanced primary and recurrent cervical carcinoma, *Int J Gynaecol Obstet* 20:417, 1982.

Choo YC et al: The management of intractable lymphocyst following radical hysterectomy, *Gynecol Oncol* 24:309, 1986.

Corn BW et al: Technically accurate intracavitary insertions improve pelvic control and survival among patients with locally advanced carcinoma of the uterine cervix, *Gynecol Oncol* 53:294, 1994.

Creasman WT, Super JT, Clarke-Pearson D: Radical hysterectomy as therapy for early carcinoma of the cervix, *Am J Obstet Gynecol* 155:964, 1986.

Currie DW: Operative treatment of carcinoma of the cervix, *J Obstet Gynaecol Br Commonw* 78:385, 1971.

Czesnin K, Wronkowski Z: Second malignancies of the irradiated area in patients treated for uterine cervix cancer, *Gynecol Oncol* 6:309, 1978.

Delgato G, Caglar H, Walker P: Survival and complications in cervical cancer treated by pelvic and extended field radiation after paraaortic lymphadenectomy, *AJR* 130:141, 1978.

DiSaia PJ: Surgical aspects of cervical carcinoma, *Cancer* 48:548, 1981.

DiSaia PJ: The case against the surgical concept of en bloc dissection for malignancies of the reproductive tract, *Cancer* 60:2025, 1987.

DiSaia PJ et al: Phase III study on the treatment of women with cervical cancer, stage IIb, IIIb, and IVa (confined to the pelvis and/or periaortic nodes), with radiotherapy alone versus radiotherapy plus immunotherapy with intravenous *Corynebacterium parvum*: a Gynecologic Oncology Group study, *Gynecol Oncol* 26:386, 1987.

Dottino PR et al: Induction chemotherapy followed by radical surgery in cervical cancer, *Gynecol Oncol* 40:7, 1991.

Durrance Fy: Radiotherapy following simple hysterectomy in patients with states I and II carcinoma of the cervix, *Am J Roent Radium Ther Nuc Med* 102:165, 1968.

Falk V et al: Primary surgical treatment of carcinoma stage I of the uterine cervix, *Acta Obstet Gynecol Scand* 61:481, 1982.

Feder BH, Syed AMN, Neblett D: Treatment of extensive carcinoma of the cervix with the "transperineal parametrial butterfly," *Int J Radiat Oncol Biol Phys* 4:735, 1978.

Fletcher GH, Rutledge FN: Extended field technique in the management of the cancers of the uterine cervix, *AJR* 114:116, 1972.

Forney JP: The effect of radical hysterectomy on bladder physiology, *Am J Obstet Gynecol* 138:374, 1980.

Gallion HH et al: Combined radiation therapy and extrafascial hysterectomy in the treatment of stage IB barrel-shaped cervical cancer, *Cancer* 56:262, 1985.

Giaroli A et al: Lymph node metastases in carcinoma of the cervix uteri: response to neoadjuvant chemotherapy and its impact on survival, *Gynecol Oncol* 39:34, 1990.

Gilinsky WH et al: The natural history of radiation-induced proctosigmoiditis: an analysis of 88 patients, *Q J Med* 205:40, 1983.

Gutherie RT et al: Para-aortic lymph node irradiation in carcinoma of the uterine cervix, *Cancer* 34:166, 1974.

Hatch KD et al: Ureteral strictures and fistulae following radical hysterectomy, *Gynecol Oncol* 19:17, 1984.

Heaton D et al: Treatment of 29 patients with bulky squamous cell carcinoma of the cervix with simultaneous cisplatin, 5-fluorouracil, and split-course hyperfractionated radiation therapy, *Gynecol Oncol* 338:323, 1990.

Heller PB, Barnhill DR, Mayer AR: Cervical carcinoma found incidentally in a uterus removed for benign indications, *Obstet Gynecol* 67:187, 1986.

Hodel K et al: The role of ovarian transposition in conservation of ovarian function in radical hysterectomy followed by pelvic irradiation, *Gynecol Oncol* 13:195, 1982.

Hoffman MS, et al: A phase II evaluation of cisplatin, bleomycin, and mitomycin-C in patients with recurrent squamous cell carcinoma of the cervix, *Gynecol Oncol* 40:144, 1991.

Hopkins MP, Morley GW: Radical hysterectomy verus radiation therapy for stage IB squamous cell cancer of the cervix, *Cancer* 68:272, 1991.

Hreschyshn MM et al: Hydroxyurea or placebo combined with radiation to treat stages IIIb and IV cervical cancer confined to the pelvis, *Int J Radiat Oncol Biol Phys* 5:317, 1979.

Husseinzadeh N, Van Aken ML, Aron B: Ovarian transposition in young patients with invasive cervical cancer receiving radiation therapy, *Int J Gynecol Cancer* 4:61, 1994.

Husseinzadeh N et al: The preservation of ovarian function in young women undergoing pelvic radiation therapy, *Gynecol Oncol* 18:373, 1984.

Inoue T, Morita K: 5-year results of postoperative extended-field irradiation on 76 patients with nodal metastases from cervical carcinoma stages Ib to IIIb, *Cancer* 61:2009, 1988.

Jakobsen A et al: Is radical hysterectomy always necessary in early cervical cancer? *Gynecol Oncol* 39:80, 1990.

Johnston CM et al: Case report: recurrent cervical squamous cell carcinoma in an ovary following ovarian conservation and radical hysterectomy, *Gynecol Oncol* 41:64, 1991.

Jolles CJ et al: Complications of extended-field therapy for cervical carcinoma without prior surgery, *Rad Oncol Biol Phys* 12:179, 1986.

Kagan AR et al: A new staging system for irradiation injuries following treatment for cancer of the cervix uteri, *Gynecol Oncol* 7:166, 1979.

Khorram O, Stern JL: Case report: bleomycin sclerotherapy of an intractable inguinal lymphocyst, *Gynecol Oncol* 50:244, 1993.

Kim DS et al: Preoperative adjuvant chemotherapy in the treatment of cervical cancer stage Ib, IIa, and IIb with bulky tumor, *Gynecol Oncol* 29:321, 1988.

Kim RY: Radiotherapeutic management in carcinoma of the uterine cervix: current status, *Int J Gynecol Cancer* 3:337, 1993.

Kinney WK, Alvarez RD, Reid GC et al: Value of adjuvant whole-pelvis irradiation after Wertheim hysterectomy for early-stage squamous carcinoma of the cervix with pelvic nodal metastasis: a matched-control study, *Gynecol Oncol* 34:258, 1989.

Kinney WK, Egorshin EV, Ballard DJ, Podratz KC: Long-term survival and sequelae after surgical management of invasive cervical carcinoma diagnosed at the time of simple hysterectomy, *Gynecol Oncol* 44:24, 1992.

Kirsten F et al: Combination chemotherapy followed by surgery or radiotherapy in patients with locally advanced cervical cancer, *Br J Obstet Gynaecol* 94:583, 1987.

Kramer C et al: Radiation treatment of FIGO stage IVa carcinoma of the cervix, *Gynecol Oncol* 32:323, 1989.

Krebs HB et al: Recurrent cancer of the cervix following hysterectomy and pelvic node dissection, *Obstet Gynecol* 59:422, 1982.

Larson DM, Malone JM, Copeland LJ et al: Ureteral assessment after radical hysterectomy, *Obstet Gynecol* 69:612, 1987.

Larson DM, Stringer CA, Copeland LJ et al: Stage Ib cervical carcinoma treated with radical hysterectomy and pelvic lymphadenectomy: role of adjuvant radiotherapy, *Obstet Gynecol* 69:378, 1987.

Lee Y et al: Radical hysterectomy with pelvic lymph node dissection for treatment of cervical cancer: a clinical review of 954 cases, *Gynecol Oncol* 32:135, 1989.

Liu W, Meigs JW: Radical hysterectomy and pelvic lymphadenectomy, *Am J Obstet Gynecol* 69:1, 1955.

Madhu J et al: Preliminary results of concomitant radiotherapy and chemotherapy in advanced cervical carcinoma, *Gynecol Oncol* 28:101, 1987.

Mann WJ et al: Ovarian metastases from stage Ib adenocarcinoma of the cervix, *Cancer* 60:1123, 1987.

Mann WJ et al: Management of lymphocysts after radical gynecologic surgery, *Gynecol Oncol* 33:248, 1989.

Maruyama Y et al: Specimen findings and survival after preoperative[252] Cf Neutron brachytherapy for stage II cevical carcinoma, *Gynecol Oncol* 43:252, 1991.

Massi G, Savino L, Susini T: Schauta-Amreich vaginal hysterectomy and Wertheim-Meigs abdominal hysterectomy in the treatment of cervical cancer: a retrospective analysis, *Am J Obstet Gynecol* 168:928, 1993.

McIntyre JF, Eifel PJ, Levenback C, Oswald MJ: Ureteral stricture as a late complication of radiotherapy for stage IB carcinoma of the uterine cervix: *Cancer* 75:837, 1995.

Miller BE et al: Carcinoma of the cervical stump, *Gynecol Oncol* 18:100, 1984.

Monk BJ et al: Extent of disease as an indication for pelvic radiation following radical hysterectomy and bilateral pelvic lymph node dissection in the treatment of stage IB and IIA cervical carinoma, *Gynecol Oncol* 54:4, 1994.

Montana GS et al: Carcinoma of the cervix, stage III, *Cancer* 57:148, 1986.

Morrow CP: Is pelvic radiation beneficial in the postoperative management of stage Ib squamous cell carcinoma of the cervix with pelvic node metastasis treated by radical hysterectomy and pelvic lymphadenectomy? *Gynecol Oncol* 10:105, 1980.

Muss HB et al: Neoadjuvant therapy for advanced squamous cell carcinoma of the cervix: cisplatin followed by radiation therapy—a pilot study of the Gynecologic Oncology Group, *Gynecol Oncol* 26:35, 1987.

Nolan JF, Anson JH, Steward M: A radium applicator for use in the treatment of cancer of the uterine cervix, *AJR* 79:36, 1958.

Orr JW, Wilson K, Bodiford C: Corpus and cervix cancer: a nutritional comparison, *Am J Obstet Gynecol* 153:775, 1985.

Owens S et al: Ovarian management at the time of radical hysterectomy for cancer of the cervix, *Gynecol Oncol* 35:349, 1989.

Panici PB, Greggi S, Scambia G et al: High-dose cisplatin and bleomycin neoadjuvant chemotherapy plus radical surgery in locally advanced cervical carcinoma: a preliminary report, *Gynecol Oncol* 41:212, 1991.

Panici PB, Scambia G, Baiocchi G et al: Neoadjuvant chemotherapy and radical surgery in locally advanced cervical cancer: prognostic factors for response and survival, *Cancer* 67:372, 1991.

Panici P et al: Neoadjuvant chemotherapy and radical surgery in locally advanced cervical carcinoma: a pilot study, *Obstet Gynecol* 71:344, 1988.

Park TK, Choi DH, Kim SN et al: Role of induction chemotherapy in invasive cervical cancer, *Gynecol Oncol* 41:1007, 1991.

Park TK et al: Combined chemotherapy and radiation for bulky stages I-II cervical cancer: comparison of concurrent and sequential regimens, *Gynecol Oncol* 50:196, 1993.

Patsner B: Closed-suction drainage versus no drainage following radical abdominal hysterectomy with pelvic lymphadenectomy for stage IB cervical cancer, *Gynecol Oncol* 57:232, 1995.

Patsner B, Sedlacek TV, Lovecchio JL: Para-aortic node sampling in small (3-cm or less) stage IB invasive cervical cancer, *Gynecol Oncol* 44:53, 1992.

Perez CA et al: Correlation between radiation dose and tumor recurrence and complications in carcinoma of the uterine cervix: stages I and IIa, *Int J Radiat Oncol Biol Phys* 5:373, 1979.

Perez CA et al: Irradiation alone or in combination with surgery in stages Ib and IIa carcinoma of the uterine cervix: a nonrandomized comparison, *Cancer* 43:1062, 1979.

Petersen LK, Mamsen A, Jakobsen A: Carcinoma of the cervical stump, *Gynecol Oncol* 46:199, 1992.

Photopulos GJ, Van der Zwaag R: Class II radical hysterectomy shows less morbidity and good treatment efficacy compared to class III, *Gynecol Oncol* 40:21, 1991.

Photopulos GJ et al: Vaginal radiation brachytherapy to reduce central recurrence after radical hysterectomy for cervical carcinoma, *Gynecol Oncol* 38:187, 1990.

Piver MS: Extended field irradiation in the treatment of patients with cervical carcinoma involving biopsy proven para-aortic nodes, *Int J Radiat Oncol Biol Phys* 10:1993, 1984.

Piver MS, Barlow JJ: High dose irradiation to biopsy-confirmed aortic node metastases from carcinoma of the uterine cervix, *Cancer* 39:1243, 1977.

Piver MS, Rutledge FN, Smith PJ: Five classes of extended hysterectomy of women with cervical cancer, *Obstet Gynecol* 44:265, 1974.

Potish R et al: The morbidity and utility of periaortic radiotherapy in cervical carcinoma. *Gynecol Oncol* 15:1, 1983.

Puthawala A et al: Integrated external and interstitial radiation therapy for primary carcinoma of the vagina, *Obstet Gynecol* 62:367, 1983.

Rabinovich MG, Focaccia G, Ferreyra R et al: Neoadjuvant chemotherapy for cervical carcinoma, *Obstet Gynecol* 78:685, 1991.

Remy JC, DiMaio T, Fruchter RG et al: Adjunctive radiation after radical hysterectomy in stage Ib squamous cell carcinoma of the cervix, *Gynecol Oncol* 38:161, 1990.

Rettenmaier MA, Casanova DM, Micha JP et al: Radical hysterectomy and tailored postoperative radiation therapy in the management of bulky stage Ib cervical cancer, *Cancer* 63:2220, 1989.

Roman LD et al: Prognostic factors for patients undergoing simple hysterectomy in the presence of invasive cancer of the cervix, *Gynecol Oncol* 50:179, 1993.

Rubin SC et al: Para-aortic nodal metastases in early cervical carcinoma: long-term survival following extended field radiotherapy, *Gynecol Oncol* 18:213, 1984.

Russell AH: Comtemporary radiation treatment planning for patients with cancer of the unterine cervix, *Sem Oncol* 21:30, 1994.

Rutledge FN, Wharton JT, Fletcher GH: Clinical studies with adjunctive surgery and irradiation therapy in the treatment of carcinoma of the cervix, *Cancer* 38:596, 1976.

Sardi J: Neoadjuvant chemotherapy in locally advanced carcinoma of the cervix-uterus, *Gynecol Oncol* 38:486, 1990.

Sardi JE et al: A possible new trend in the management of the carcinoma of the cervix uteri, *Gynecol Oncol* 25:139, 1986.

Seibel M, Freeman MG, Graves WL: Sexual function after surgical and radiation therapy for cervical carcinoma, *South Med J* 75:1195, 1982.

Sekiba K: Radical hysterectomy for cancer of the uterine cervix, *Sem Surg Oncol* 1:95, 1985.

Seski JC, Dioknoac N: Bladder dysfunction after radical hysterectomy, *Am J Obstet Gynecol* 128:6, 1977.

Slater JD, Slater JM, Wahlen S: The potential for proton beam therapy in locally advanced carcinoma of the cervix, *Int J Radiation Oncology Biol Phys* 22:343, 1991.

Soisson AP, Soper JT, Berchuck A, Dodge R, Clarke-Pearson D: Radical hysterectomy in obese women, *Obstet Gynecol* 80:940, 1992.

Soisson AP, Soper JT, Clarke-Pearson DL et al: Adjuvant radiotherapy following radical hysterectomy for patients with stage Ib and IIa cervical cancer, *Gynecol Oncol* 37:390, 1990.

Stallworthy J: Radical surgery following radiation treatment for cervical carcinoma, *Ann R Coll Surg Eng* 34:161, 1964.

Stehman FB et al: Carcinoma of the cervix treated with radiation therapy. I. A multi-variate analysis of prognostic variables in the Gynecologic Oncology Group, *Cancer* 67:2776, 1991.

Surwit EA et al: Interstitial thermo radiotherapy in recurrent gynecologic malignancies, *Gynecol Oncol* 15:95, 1983.

Syed AMN, Feder BH: Technique of afterloading interstitial implant, *Radiol Clin* 46:458, 1977.

Tabata M et al: Incidence of ovarian metastasis in patients with cancer of the uterine cervix, *Gynecol Oncol* 28:255, 1987.

Thigpen T et al: A randomized comparison of rapid versus prolonged (24-hour) infusion of cisplatin in therapy of squamous cell carcinoma of the uterine cervix, *Gynecol Oncol* 32:198, 1989.

Thomas GM, Dembo AJ: Is there a role for adjuvant pelvic radiotherapy after radical hysterectomy in early stage cervical cancer? *Int J Gynecol Cancer* 1:1, 1991.

Weems DH et al: Carcinoma of the intact uterine cervix, stages Ib-IIa-b, ≥6 cm in diameter: irradiation alone vs. preoperative irradiation and surgery, *Rad Oncol Biol Phys* 11:1911, 1985.

Wharton JT et al: Pre-irradiation celiotomy and extended field irradiation for invasive carcinoma of the cervix, *Am J Obstet* Gynecol 118:749, 1974.

Yabuki Y, Asamoto A, Hoshiba T et al: Dissection of the cardinal ligament in radical hysterectomy for cervical cancer with emphasis on the lateral ligament, *Am J Obstet Gynecol* 164:7, 1991.

Zander J et al: Carcinoma of the cervix: an attempt to individualize treatment; results of a 20-year cooperative study, *Am J Obstet Gynecol* 139:752, 1981.

Survival results and prognostic factors

Abdulhayogu G et al: Selective radiation therapy in stage Ib uterine cervical carcinoma following radical pelvic surgery, *Gynecol Oncol* 10:84, 1980.

Adcock L et al: Carcinoma of the uterine cervix FIGO stage Ib, *Gynecol Oncol* 14:199, 1982.

Alvarez RD et al: Identification of prognostic factors and risk groups in patients found to have nodal metastasis at the time of radical hysterectomy for early-stage squamous carcinoma of the cervix, *Gynecol Oncol* 35:130, 1989.

Baltzer J et al: Histological criteria for prognosis in patients with operative squamous cell carcinoma of the cervix, *Gynecol Oncol* 13:184, 1982.

Barber HRK, Brunschwig A: Gynecologic cancer complicating pregnancy, *Am J Obstet Gynecol* 85:156, 1963.

Berman ML, Bergen S, Salazar H: Influence of histological features and treatment on the prognosis of patients with cervical cancer metastatic to pelvic lymph nodes, *Gynecol Oncol* 39:127, 1990.

Burghardt E, Baltzer J, Tulusan AH, Haas J: Results of surgical treatment of 1028 cervical cancers studied with volumetry, *Cancer* 70:648, 1992.

Burke TW et al: Prognostic factors associated with radical hysterectomy failure, *Gynecol Oncol* 26:153, 1987.

Delgato G: Prospective surgical pathological study of disease free interval in patients with stage Ib carcinoma of the cervix: a GOG study, *Gynecol Oncol* 38:352, 1990.

Fiorica JV, Roberts WS, Greenberg H et al: Morbidity and survival patterns in patients after radical hysterectomy and postoperative adjuvant pelvic radiotherapy, *Gynecol Oncol* 36:343, 1990.

Fuller AF et al: Lymph node metastasis from carcinoma of the cervix, stages Ib and IIa: implications for prognosis and treatment, *Gynecol Oncol* 13:165, 1982.

Gauthier P et al: Identification of histopathologic risk groups in stage Ib squamous cell carcinoma of the cervix, *Obstet Gynecol* 66:569, 1985.

Gusberg SB, Yannopoulos K, Cohen CJ: Viruleance indices and lymph nodes in cancer of the cervix, *AJR* 111:273, 1971.

Hopkins MP, Morley GW: Squamous cell cancer of the cervix: prognostic factors related to survival, *Int J Gynecol Cancer* 1:173, 1991.

Hopkins MP, Morley GW: Stage IB squamous cell cancer of the cervix: clinicopathologic feature related to survival, *AM J Obstet Gynecol* 164:1520, 1991.

Inoue T, Morita K: The prognostic significance of number of positive nodes in cervical carcinoma stages Ib, IIa, and IIb, *Cancer* 65:1923, 1990.

Lanciano RM, Martz K, Montant GS, Hanks GE: Influence of age, prior abdominal surgery, fraction size, and dose on complications after radiation therapy for squamous cell cancer of the uterine cervix, *Cancer* 69:2124, 1992.

Lovecchio JL et al: 5-year survival of patients with periaortic nodal metastases in clinical stage Ib and IIa cervical carcinoma, *Gynecol Oncol* 34:43, 1989.

Manetta A et al: The significance of paraaortic node status in carcinoma of the cervix and endometrium, *Gynecol Oncol* 23:284, 1986.

Montana GS et al: Analysis of results of radiation therapy for state II carcinoma of the cervix, *Cancer* 55:956, l985.

Orlandi C, Costa S, Terzano P: Lymph-node metastases in women aged 35 or younger with invasive squamous cell carcinoma of the cervix. Presented at the Felix Rutledge Society meeting 6/1/95 in Houston, Texas.

Perez CA et al: Effect of tumor size on the prognosis of carcinoma of the uterine cervix treated with irradiation alone, *Cancer* 69:2796, 1992.

Perez CA et al: Radiation therapy alone in the treatment of carcinoma of uterine cervix, *Cancer* 51:1393, 1983.

Pettersson F: Annual report on the results of treatment in gynecological cancer, Twenty-second volume, Statements of results obtained in patients treated in 1987 to 1989, inclusive actuarial survival up to 1993, International Federation of Gynecology and Obstetrics.

Prempree T, Patanaphan V, Scott R: Radiation management of carcinoma of the cervical stump, *Cancer* 43:1262, 1979.

Rutledge FN et al: Youth as a prognostic factor in carcinoma of the cervix: a matched analysis, *Gynecol Oncol* 44:123, 1992.

Sardi JE et al: Results of a phase II trial with neoadjuvant chemotherapy in carcinoma of the cervix uteri, *Gynecol Oncol* 31:256, 1988.

Thomassen LV, Warshaw J, Lawhead RA, Unger ER: Invasive cervical cancer in young women, *J Repro Medicine* 37:901, 1992.

Tinga DJ, Timmer PR, Bouma J: Prognostic significance of single vs. multiple lymph node metastases in cervical carcinoma stage Ib, *Gynecol Oncol* 39:175, 1990.

Ulfelder H, Smith CJ, Costello JB: Invasive carcinoma of the cervix during pregnancy, *Am J Obstet Gynecol* 98:424, 1967.

Zaino RJ et al: Histopathologic predictors of the behavior of surgically treated stage IB squamous cell carcinoma of the cervix, A Gynecologic Oncology Group Study, *Cancer* 69:1750,1992.

Recurrent and advanced carcinoma of the cervix

Alberts DS, Garcia D, Mason-Liddil N: Cisplatin in advanced cancer of the cervix: an update, *Sem Oncol* 18(1 suppl 3):11, 1991.

Ampil FL: Stage IVa carcinoma of the cervix, *Radiation Med* 8(5):184, 1990.

Barter JS et al: Diagnosis and treatment of pulmonary metastases from cervical carcinoma, *Gynecol Oncol* 38:347, 1990.

Bassan JS, Glaser MG: Bony metastasis in carcinoma of the uterine cervix, *Clin Radiol* 33:623, 1982.

Blythe JG et al: Bony metastases from carcinoma of the cervix, *Cancer* 36:475, 1975.

Burke TW et al: Clinical patterns of tumor recurrence after radical hysterectomy in stage Ib cervical carcinoma, *Obstet Gynecol* 69:382, 1987.

Christopherson WM, Parker JE: A critical study of cervical biopsies including serial sectioning, *Cancer* 14:213, 1961.

Coleman DL et al: Patterns of failure of bulky-barrel carcinomas of the cervix, *Am J Obstet Gynecol* 166:916, 1992.

Coleman RL et al: Radical hysterectomy for recurrent carcinoma of the uterine cervix after radiotherapy, *Gynecol Oncol* 55:29, 1994.

Delgato G, Goldson AL, Ashayeri E et al: Intraoperative radiation in the treatment of advanced cervical cancer, *Obstet Gynecol* 63:246, 1984.

El-Minawi MF, Perez-Mesa CM: Parametrial needle biopsy follow-up of cervical cancer, *Int J Obstet Gynecol* 12:1, 1974.

Flint A et al: Confirmation of metastasis by fine needle aspiration biopsy in patients with gynecologic malignancies, *Gynecol Oncol* 14:382, 1982.

Gallousis S: Isolated lung metastases from pelvic malignancies, *Gynecol Oncol* 7:206, 1979.

Hartenbach EM et al: Nonsurgical management strategies for the function complications of ileocolonic continent urinary reservoirs, *Gynecol Oncol* 59:358, 1995.

Hoskin PJ, Blake PR: Cis-platin, methotrexate and bleomycin (PMB) for carcinoma of the cervix: the influence of presentation and previous treatment upon response, *Int J Gynecol Cancer* 1:75, 1991.

Larson DM, Copeland LJ, Stringer CA, et al: Recurrent cervical carcinoma after radical hysterectomy, *Gynecol Oncol* 30:381, 1988.

Layfield LJ, Heaps JM, Berek JS: Fine-needle aspiration cytology accuracy with palpable gynecologic neoplasms, *Gynecol Oncol* 40:70, 1991.

Lele SB, Piver MS: Weekly cisplatin induction chemotherapy in the treatment of recurrent cervical carcinoma, *Gynecol Oncol* 33:6, 1989.

Lifshitz S, Railsback LD, Buchsbaum HJ: Intra-arterial pelvic infusion chemotherapy in advanced gynecologic cancer, *Obstet Gynecol* 52:476, 1978.

Lippman SM et al: 13-cis-retinoicretionic acid plus interferon α-2a: highly active systemic therapy for squamous cell carcinoma of the cervix, *J Natl Cancer Inst* 84:241, 1992.

Look KY et al: 5-Fluorouracil and low-dose leucovorin in the treatment of recurrent squamous cell carcinoma of the cervix, *Am J Clin Oncol* 15, 497, 1992.

Miyamoto T et al: Effectiveness of a sequential combination of bleomycin and mitomycin-C on an advanced cervical cancer, *Cancer* 41:403, 1978.

Monk BJ, Solh S, Johnson MT, Montz FJ: Radical hysterectomy after pelvic irradiation in patients with high rick cervical cancer or uterine sarcoma: morbidity and outcome, *Eur J Gynecol Oncol* XIV:506, 1993.

Montana GS, Martz KL, Hanks GE: Patterns and sites of failure in cervix cancer treated in the USA in 1978, *Int J Radiation* Oncology 20:87, 1991.

Morrow CP et al: Continuous pelvic arterial infusion with bleomycin for squamous carcinoma of the cervix recurrent after irradiation therapy, *Cancer Treat Rep* 61:1403, 1977.

Murphy WT, Schmitz A: The results of reirradiation of cancer of the cervix, *Radiology* 67:378, 1956.

Ng HT et al: The outcome of the patients with recurrent cervical carcinoma in terms of lymph node metastasis and treatment, *Gynecol Oncol* 26:355, 1987.

Omura GA: Current status of chemotherapy for cancer of the cervix, *Oncology* 6:27, 1992.

Park RC, Thigpen JT: Chemotherapy in advanced and recurrent cervical cancer, *Cancer Suppl* 71:1446, 1993.

Peeples WJ et al: The occurrence of metastasis outside the abdomen and retroperitoneal space in invasive carcinoma of the cervix, *Gynecol Oncol* 4:307, 1976.

Petrilli ES et al: Bleomycin pharmacology in relation to adverse effects and renal function in cervical cancer patients, *Gynecol Oncol* 14:350, 1982.

Piver MS, Lele SB, Malfetano JH: Cis-diamminedichloroplatinum II based combination chemotherapy for the control of extensive paraaortic lymph node metastasis in cervical cancer, *Gynecol Oncol* 26:71, 1987.

Potter ME, Alvarez RD, Gay GL et al: Optimal therapy of pelvic recurrence after radical hysterectomy for early stage cervical cancer, *Gynecol Oncol* 37:74, 1990.

Rettenmaier MA et al: Treatment of advanced and recurrent squamous carcinoma of the uterine cervix with constant intra-arterial infusion of cisplatin, *Cancer* 61:1301, 1988.

Rubin SC, Hoskins WJ, Lewis JL: Radical hysterectomy for recurrent cervical cancer following radiation therapy, *Gynecol Oncol* 27:316, 1987.

Russell AH, Tong DY, Figge DC et al: Adjuvant postoperative pelvic radiation for carcinoma of the uterine cervix: pattern of cancer recurrence in patients undergoing elective radiation following radical hysterectomy and pelvic lymphadenectomy, *Rad Oncol Biol Phys* 10:211, 1984.

Saphner T et al: Neurologic complications of cervical cancer: a review of 2261 cases, *Cancer* 64:1147, 1989.

Shield PW, Wright RG, Free K, Daunter B: The accuracy of cervicovaginal cytology in the detection of recurrent cervical carcinoma following radiotherapy, *Gynecol Oncol* 41:223, 1991.

Sommers GM et al: Outcome of recurrent cervical carcinoma following definitive irradiation, *Gynecol Oncol* 35:150, 1989.

Sorbe B, Frankendal B: Combination chemotherapy in advanced carcinoma of the cervix, *Cancer* 50:2028, 1982.

Stehman FB et al: Cis-platinum in advanced gynecologic malignancy, *Gynecol Oncol* 7:349, 1979.

Suit HD, Gallagher HS: Intact tumor cells in irradiated tissue, *Arch Pathol* 78:648, 1964.

Sutton GP et al: Phase II trial of ifosfamide and mesna in patients with advanced or recurrent squamous carcinoma of the cervix who had never received chemotherapy: a Gynecologic Oncology Group study, *Am J Obstet Gynecol* 168:805, 1993.

Terada K, Morley GW: Radical hysterectomy as surgical salvage therapy for gynecologic malignancy, *Obstet Gynecol* 70:913, 1987.

Thigpen T et al: Cis-platinum in the treatment of advanced or recurrent squamous cell carcinoma of the cervix, *Cancer* 48:899, 1981.

Thomas GM: Concurrent radiation and chemotherapy for carcinoma of the cervix recurrent after radical surgery, *Gynecol Oncol* 27:254, 1987.

Truelsen F: Injury of bones by roentgen treatment of the uterince cervix, *Acta Radiol* 23:581, 1942.

Van Herik M, Fricke RE: The results of radiation therapy for recurrent cancer of the cervix uteri, *AJR* 73:437, 1955.

Van Herik M et al: Late recurrence in carcinoma of the cervix, *Am J Obstet Gynecol* 108:1183, 1970.

Welander CE, Homesley HD, Barrett RJ: Combined interferon Alfa and doxorubicin in the treatment of advanced cervical cancer, *Am J Obstet Gynecol* 165:284, 1991.

Management of bilateral ureteral obstruction

Brin EN, Schiff M, Weiss RM: Palliative urinary diversion for pelvic malignancy, *J Urol* 113:619, 1975.

Carter J, Ramirez C, Waugh R et al: Percutaneous urinary diversion in gynecologic oncology, *Gynecol Oncol* 40:248, 1991.

Coddington CC, Thomas JR, Hoskins WJ: Percutaneous nephrostomy for ureteral obstruction in patients with gynecologic malignancy, *Gynecol Oncol* 18:339, 1984.

Delgato G: Urinary conduit diversion in advanced gynecologic malignancies, *Gynecol Oncol* 6:217, 1978.

Fisher HA et al. Nonoperative supravesical urinary diversion in obstetrics and gynecology, *Gynecol Oncol* 14:365, 1982.

Graham JB, Abab RS: Ureteral obstruction due to radiation, *Am J Obstet Gynecol* 99:409, 1967.

Pelvic recurrence after suboptimal surgery

Feuer GA, Fruchter R, Seruri E et al: Selection for percutaneous nephrostomy in gynecologic cancer patients, *Gynecol Oncol* 42:60, 1991.

Orr JW et al: Surgical treatment of women found to have invasive cervix cancer at the time of total hysterectomy, *Obstet Gynecol* 68:353, 1986.

Pelvic exenteration

Averette HE et al: Pelvic exenteration: a 15-year experience in a general metropolitan hospital, *Am J Obstet Gynecol* 150:179, 1984.

Barber HR: Relative prognostic significance of preoperative and operative findings in pelvic exenteration, *Surg Clin North Am* 49:431, 1969.

Barber HRK, Jones W: Lymphadenectomy in pelvic exenteration for recurrent cervix cancer, *JAMA* 215:1949, 1971.

Berman ML et al: Enteroperineal fistulae following pelvic exenteration: a 10-point program of management, *Gynecol Oncol* 4:368, 1976.

Bricker EM: Bladder substitution after pelvic evisceration, *Surg Clin North Am* 30:1511, 1950.

Bricker EM, Butcher HR, McAfee A: Results of pelvic exenteration, *AMA Arch Surg* 73:661, 1956.

Brunschwig A: What are the indications and results of pelvic exenteration? *JAMA* 194:274, 1965.

Brunschwig A, Pierce VK: Necropsy findings in patients with carcinoma of the cervix: implications for treatment, *Am J Obstet Gynecol* 56:1134, 1948.

Carlson JW et al: Rectus abdominis myocutaneous flap for primary vaginal reconstruction, *Gynecol Oncol* 51:323, 1993.

Creasman WT, Rutledge F: Is positive pelvic lymphadenectomy a contraindication to radical surgery in recurrent cervical carcinoma? *Gynecol Oncol* 2:282, 1974.

Hancock KC et al: Urinary conduits in gynecologic oncology, *Obstet Gynecol* 67:680, 1986.

Hatch KD et al: Low rectal resection and anastomosis at the time of pelvic exenteration, *Gynecol Oncol* 32:262, 1988.

Hoffman MS et al: Colorectal anastomosis on a gynecologic oncology service, *Gynecol Oncol* 55:60, 1994.

Ketcham AS et al: Pelvic exenteration for carcinoma of the uterine cervix: a 15-year experience, *Cancer* 26:513, 1970.

Krieger JS, Embree HK: Pelvic exenteration. *Cleve Clin Q* 36:1, 1969.

Lawhead RA: Pelvic exenteration for recurrent or persistent gynecologic malignancies: a 10-year review of the Memorial Sloan-Kettering Cancer Center Experience (1972-1981), *Gynecol Oncol* 33:279, 1989.

Lichtinger M et al: Small bowel complications after supravesical urinary diversion in pelvic exenteration, *Gynecol Oncol* 24:137, 1986.

Magrina JF: Types of pelvic exenterations: a reappraisal, *Gynecol Oncol* 37:363, 1990.

Matthews CM, Morris M, Burke TW et al: Pelvic exenteration in the elderly patient, *Proceedings of the Twenty-Second Annual Felix Rutledge Society Meeting,* 1991.

Miller B, Morris M, Rutledge FN et al: Aborted exenterative procedures for recurrent cervical cancer, *Proceedings of the Twenty-Second Annual Felix Rutledge Society Meeting,* 1991.

Morley GW, Lindenauer SM: Pelvic exenteration therapy for gynecologic malignancies: an analysis of 70 cases, *Cancer* 38:581, 1976.

Morley GW, Lindenauer SM, Young D: Vaginal reconstruction following pelvic exenteration, *Am J Obstet Gynecol* 116:996, 1973.

Ng C, Amis S: Radiology of continent urinary diversion, *Contemp Urorad* 29:557, 1991.

Orr JW et al: Urinary diversion in patients undergoing pelvic exenteration, *Am J Obstet Gynecol* 142:883, 1982.

Park TK, Choi DH, Kim SN et al: Role of induction chemotherapy in invasive cervical cancer, *Gynecol Oncol* 41:1007, 1991.

Penalver M et al: Gastrointestinal surgery in gynecologic oncology: evaluation of surgical techniques, *Gynecol Oncol* 28:74, 1987.

Roberts WS et al: Major morbidity after pelvic exenteration: a seven year experience, *Obstet Gynecol* 69 (4):617, April, 1987.

Rutledge FN, Burns BC Jr: Pelvic exenteration, *Am J Obstet Gynecol* 91:692, 1965.

Rutledge FN, McGuffee VB: Pelvic exenteration: prognostic significance of regional lymph node metastasis, *Gynecol Oncol* 26:374, 1987.

Rutledge FN et al: Pelvic exenteration: analysis of 296 patients, *Am J Obstet Gynecol* 129:881, 1977.

Shingleton HM et al: Clinical and histopathologic factors predicting recurrence and survival after pelvic exenteration for cancer of the cervix, *Obstet Gynecol* 73:1027, 1989.

Soper JT et al: Pelvic exenteration: factors associated with major surgical morbidity, *Gynecol Oncol* 35:93, 1989.

Stanhope CR et al: Urinary diversion with use of ileal and sigmoid conduit, *Am J Obstet Gynecol* 155:288, 1986.

Swan RW, Rutledge FN: Urinary conduit in pelvic cancer patients—a report of 16 years' experience, *Am J Obstet Gynecol* 119:6, 1974.

Symmonds RE, Pratt JH, Webb MJ: Exenteration operations: experience with 198 patients, *Am J Obstet Gynecol* 121:907, 1975.

Walton LA: The stress of radical pelvic surgery: a review, *Gynecol Oncol* 7:25, 1979.

Wheelers CR Jr: Incidence of fecal incontinence after coloproctostomy below five centimeters in the rectum, *Gynecol Oncol* 27:373, 1987.

Wheelers CR Jr: Recent advances in surgical reconstruction of the gynecologic caner patient, *Curr Opin Obstet Gynecol* 4:91, 1992.

Sarcoma, lymphoma, and melanoma of the cervix

Abdul-Karim RW et al: Sarcoma of the uterine cervix: clinicopathologic findings in three cases, *Gynecol Oncol* 26:103, 1987.

Akine Y et al: Carcinoma of the uterine cervix treated by irradiation alone: result of treatment at the National Cancer Center, Tokyo, *Acta Oncologica* 29:747, 1989.

Brand E et al: Rhabdomyosarcoma of the uterine cervix: sarcoma botryoides, *Cancer* 60:1552, 1987.

Kristiansen SB, Anderson R, Cohen DM: Case report: primary malignant melanoma of the cervix and review of the literature, *Gynecol Oncol* 47:398, 1992.

Montag RW, D'abaing G, Schlaerth JB: Embryonal rhabdomyosarcoma of the uterine corpus and cervix, *Gynecol Oncol* 25:171, 1986.

Mordel N et al: Malignant melanoma of the uterine cervix: case report and review of the literature, *Gynecol Oncol* 32:375, 1989.

Muntz GH et al: Stage IE primary malignant lymphomas of the uterine cervix, *Cancer* 68:2023, 1991.

Perren T et al: Case report: Lymphomas of the cervix and upper vagina: a report of five cases and a review of the literature, *Gynecol Oncol* 44:87, 1992.

Rotmensch J, Rosensheim NB, Woodruff JD: Cervical sarcoma: a review, *Obstet Gynecol Surv* 38:456, 1983.

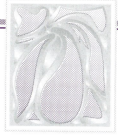

Endometrial Hyperplasia/Estrogen Therapy

Hyperplastic growth of the endometrium is somewhat analogous to dysplasia of the cervix. Undoubtedly, some of these lesions revert to normal spontaneously or with medical therapy, some persist as hyperplasia, and a few progress to endometrial adenocarcinoma. The diagnosis of endometrial hyperplasia can be made only on pathologic examination of the endometrium, and the pathologic literature has burdened us with a variety of terms and classifications. Unfortunately, there is no reliable, commonly used method of screening asymptomatic women for endometrial hyperplasia as there is for cervical dysplasia, so most patients with endometrial hyperplasia are diagnosed because they seek medical care for symptoms—usually abnormal uterine bleeding—and endometrial samples are subsequently obtained. Most endometrial hyperplasia is thought to result from persistent, prolonged estrogenic stimulation of the endometrium. The most common cause is a succession of anovulatory cycles, but hyperplasia may also result from excessive endogenously produced or exogenously administered estrogen (Figure 4-1). The association between unopposed estrogen and endometrial hyperstimulation is well recognized. The endometrial response to unopposed estrogen can be viewed as a spectrum of changes ranging from benign to malignant. This concept is supported by specimens from hysterectomies performed for endometrial adenocarcinoma, in which adjacent areas frequently show hyperplastic changes of varying degrees. The student is often confused by a discussion of hyperplasia because of the nomenclature. The terms *simple hyperplasia*, *glandular hyperplasia*, *cystic glandular hyperplasia*, and *endometrial hyperplasia* are synonymous. Adenomatous (complex) hyperplasia can occur with or without cytologic atypia, and this atypia may be severe enough to create difficulty in distinguishing the hyperplastic state from a well-differentiated adenocarcinoma. The process may be generalized throughout the endometrial cavity or localized to one or more areas. It may occur in any age group, and it is occasionally seen in teenage patients who have intermittent progesterone production and persistent estrogen stimulation without ovulation. In a similar manner, it is commonly observed during the menopause, when the process of ovulation is inconsistent. The next several paragraphs contain an initial discussion of the terminology most commonly used for endometrial hyperplasia in past literature followed by a newer, simplified classification that is more useful clinically.

PATHOLOGIC CRITERIA

The gross appearance of the endometrial cavity containing hyperplastic tissue is variable. In many instances the endometrium is markedly thickened or polypoid, with large quantities of tissue being obtained at the time of uterine curettage. The gross appearance of the endometrium can be confused with the very thick and succulent endometrium removed on days 26 to 28 of the normal secretory cycle. In other patients, particularly menopausal women, the uterine curettings are scant, and histologically only small foci of hyperplasia can be found. In general, endometrial hyperplasia is characterized by proliferation of both glands and stroma, resulting in the grossly thick, velvety, creamy yellow, often lobulated or pseudopolypoid appearance. In spite of the proliferation of both glands and stroma, focal crowding of the glands is apparent on histologic examination. The glands are tubular or slightly convoluted and vary considerably in size and shape. Occasionally, some of the glands may be

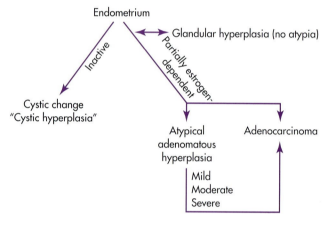

Figure 4-1 Histogenesis of endometrial carcinoma.

cystic and dilated. Secretory activity is either absent or focal and sporadic. Mitoses are present but oddly enough are not more numerous than in a proliferative endometrium. Nucleoli are prominent, and there is little or no budding of gland epithelium into the lumen.

Cystic ("Swiss Cheese") Hyperplasia

"Swiss cheese" hyperplasia is an outdated term that describes inactive endometrium with cystic change. Cystic change can be seen to a limited extent in virtually any endometrium. It is a prominent feature, however, in the endometrium of some menopausal women. Since the endometrium in these cases is not hyperplastic but thin and atrophic, the term is a misnomer. We believe that this term should be reserved exclusively for patients with inactive endometrium, and a preferable designation would be inactive endometrium with cystic change (Figure 4-2). Varying degrees of adenomatous hyperplasia may be seen concomitantly with these cystic changes, but the two histologic findings appear to be unrelated. In the opinion of most, no premalignant potential exists in the patient with pure inactive endometrium with cystic change.

Adenomatous Hyperplasia

The term *adenomatous hyperplasia* unfortunately remains in the jargon of the gynecologist and pathologist as a carry over from terminology used before 1984 when the International Society of Gynecologic Pathologists updated their classification of hyperplasia. The New classification can be found in Table 4-1, but some discussion

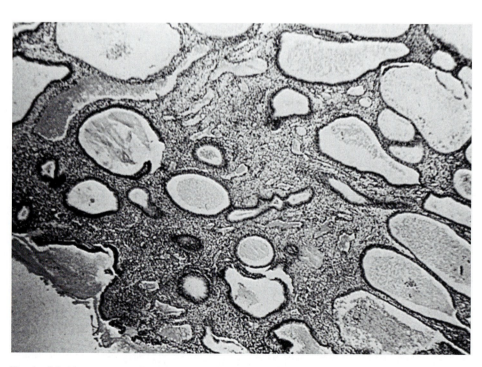

Figure 4-2 Photomicrograph of inactive endometrium with cystic change, sometimes called *cystic hyperplasia.*

of adenomatous hyperplasia is necessary in this period of transition. The term *adenomatous* suggests an emphasis on the number of glands and the subsequent crowding that occurs. Adenomatous hyperplasia (Figure 4-3) was viewed with much greater concern by gynecologists and pathologists. Mild degrees of adenomatous hyperplasia are sometimes called glandular hyperplasia. The distinction is histologic, made apparent because endometrial glands in adenomatous hyperplasia proliferate at the expense of the stroma. In those lesions labeled glandular hyperplasia, the crowding of glands is only focal, whereas in adenomatous hyperplasia crowding is prevalent. Indeed, the glands increase in number and complexity as the degree of hyperplasia increases, and conversely the intervening stroma diminishes in amount. The crowding of the glands may progress to a point where they are

"back to back" or separated from one another by only a very delicate band of fibrous stroma. The involvement of the endometrium may be focal or diffuse.

Atypical Adenomatous Hyperplasia

The term *atypical* refers to the cytologic atypia occurring in any hyperplasia (Figure 4-4). This atypia consists of nuclear enlargement, hyperchromasia, or irregularity in shape. These lesions have a great propensity for progression to adenocarcinoma and are often treated as if they were adenocarcinoma. Many pathologists and gynecologic oncologists further subdivide this category into mild, moderate, and severe atypical adenomatous hyperplasia. Severe atypical hyperplasia is characterized by anaplasia, or lessened differentiation of the glands particularly. The lining cells of the glands exhibit a pronounced variation in size, shape, cytoplasmic staining, and polarity. In a similar manner the nuclei are usually irregularly shaped and show marked variation in size and staining qualities. There is a generalized pallor of the cells, but this may not be uniform.

Severe atypical adenomatous hyperplasia has often been labeled *carcinoma in situ* of the endometrium, or stage 0 cancer of the endometrium. This relates to the concept held by most pathologists that adenocarcinoma of the endometrium begins as a focal change in the endometrial glandular epithelium. There is undoubtedly a stage that precedes endometrial stromal invasion, in which changes are limited to the endometrial glands. However, the gross appearance of the endometrium in carcinoma in situ is of little help, since it may be normal, thin, or focally polypoid.

Table 4-1 Classification of noninvasive endometrial proliferations

Histologic diagnosis	Cytologic atypia	Architectural pattern
Hyperplasia:		
Simple	Absent	Regular
Complex	Absent	Irregular; glands crowded back to back
Simple atypical	Present	Regular
Complex atypical	Present	Irregular; glands crowded back to back

Kurman RJ et al: *Cancer* 56:403, 1985.

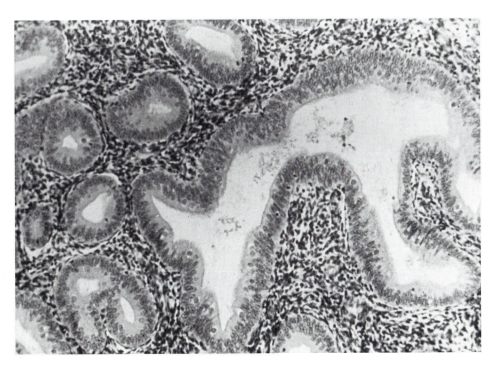

Figure 4-3 Photomicrograph of complex hyperplasia with one cystic gland.

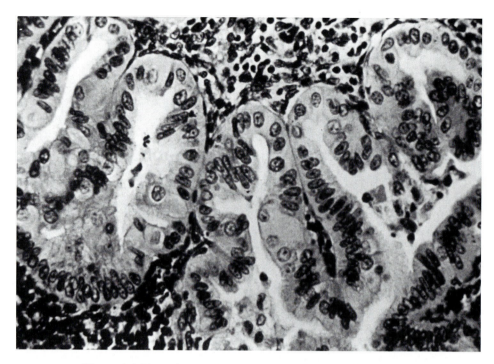

Figure 4-4 Photomicrograph of severe atypical complex hyperplasia.

Hertig based his diagnosis on the presence of glands composed of large eosinophilic cells with abundant cytoplasm. The nuclei tend to be pale with small chromatin granules and slightly irregular, folded, or scalloped nuclear membranes. Cytologic anaplasia is present, but there is no stromal invasion. It is doubtful whether the term *carcinoma in situ* of the endometrium is helpful, since there is no clear dividing line between severe forms of atypical adenomatous hyperplasia and this lesion described by Hertig. Our preference is to use the term *severe atypical adenomatous hyperplasia* rather than *carcinoma in situ*.

The classification of endometrial hyperplasia has been amply discussed over the years because of the need for a uniform terminology to describe the behavior of its various forms. Keeping these differences in terminology in mind is essential, not only in evaluating the various studies in the literature, but also in communicating with gynecologists and other pathologists. The clinician is faced with seemingly endless variations in terminology that almost preclude a rational approach to management. In 1984, the International Society of Gynecological Pathologists presented a classification (Table 4-1) that primarily takes into account cytological abnormalities. Endometrial hyperplasia that shows no evidence of cytological atypia is classified as simple or complex hyperplasia, depending on the extent of glandular complexity and crowding, whereas hyperplasia displaying cytological atypia, regardless of the architectural pattern, is classified as atypical hyperplasia. Thus there are four possible patterns of endometrial hyperplasia: simple without atypia, complex without atypia, simple with

Table 4-2   Comparison of follow-up of patients with simple and complex hyperplasia and simple and complex atypical hyperplasia (170 patients)

Type of hyperplasia	Patients N	Regressed N (%)	Persisted N (%)	Progressed to carcinoma N (%)
Simple	93	74 (80)	18 (19)	1 (1)
Complex	29	23 (79)	5 (17)	1 (3)
Simple atypical	13	9 (69)	3 (23)	1 (8)
Complex atypical	35	20 (57)	5 (14)	10 (29)

Kurman RJ et al: *Cancer* 56:403, 1985.

atypia (the least common pattern), complex with atypia (i.e., atypical hyperplasia). In order of increasing severity, these cases can be classified as simple hyperplasia, complex hyperplasia, and atypical hyperplasia. Simple and complex hyperplasias are much more likely to be reversible with progestational therapy than is atypical hyperplasia, which is also a significantly greater risk factor for concurrent or subsequent endometrial adenocarcinoma. This classification was supported by the work of Kurman and Norris (Table 4-2).

CLINICAL PROFILE

The symptom usually associated with the progression of endometrial hyperplasia is irregular, occasionally profuse uterine bleeding. This is often accompanied by lower abdominal cramps, which are caused by the accumulation of blood in the endometrial cavity and the expulsion of this blood and blood clots. In the young teenage patient this is usually associated with anovulatory cycles, as it is in the middle-aged perimenopausal patient. Endometrial hyperplasia has also been seen in association with granulosa cell tumors, ovarian thecomas, Stein-Leventhal syndrome (polycystic ovarian syndrome), and adrenocortical hyperplasia. The typical history of this group of patients reveals an interruption in cyclic menses, usually with skips and delays of menstrual flow or with prolonged periods of amenorrhea. This entire syndrome can also occur as a result of constant administration of exogenous estrogenic substances.

The significance of atypical endometrial cells detected by cervical cytology has been a subject of great interest to cytologists and gynecologists. It is now well established that the abnormal desquamation of the endometrium, reflected by the presence of atypical endometrial cells detected by routine cervical cytology, is associated with endometrial hyperplasia, adenocarcinoma, and other endometrial lesions. Cherkis studied 177 women with Papanicolaou smear findings of atypical endometrial cells. Adenocarcinoma was observed in 20% of the cases. Endometrial hyperplasia was present in 11% of the cases. Endometrial polyps were diagnosed in 10% of the cases. In view of these observations, a complete endometrial evaluation is indicated even in the asymptomatic patient who is discovered to have atypical endometrial cells detected by cervical cytology.

PREMALIGNANT POTENTIAL

It is generally agreed that patients with atypical hyperplasia are more likely to develop carcinoma than those with benign lesions of the endometrium, although the potential is difficult to quantify. Much of the confusion in past literature regarding the malignant potential of endometrial hyperplasia has been a result of inconsistent application of pathological terms, especially the term *adenomatous*. Some authors included the finding of cellular atypicality within the term *adenomatous* and many authors have not. Risk of invasive cancer for patients with atypical hyperplasia generally is considered to be 5% to 25%. The process appears to be relatively slow, and the progression from hyperplasia to carcinoma may take 5 years or more. In an interesting study done in 1970, Chamlian and Taylor found that, of 97 young women with endometrial hyperplasia, 24 (25%) had polycystic ovarian syndromes similar to the so-called Stein-Leventhal syndrome. In 14 of these women, the lesion progressed to adenocarcinoma 1 to 14 years after the initial diagnosis of endometrial hyperplasia, even though 41% of the patients underwent hysterectomy at some interval after diagnosis was made.

Atypical hyperplasia in the older post menopausal

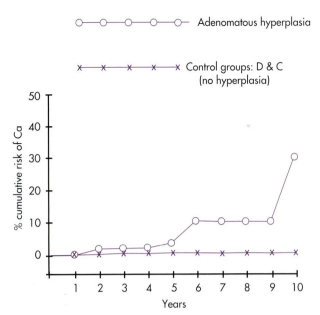

Figure 4-5 Ten-year follow-up study of two groups of patients, one with endometrial hyperplasia and the other without documented (documented by D&C) endometrial hyperplasia, showing markedly increased cumulative risk for cancer in the former. (From Gusberg SB, Frickll HC: *Corscaden's gynecologic cancer,* Baltimore, 1978, Williams & Wilkins.)

patient appears to have a higher rate of progression to adenocarcinoma. In 1947 Gusberg morphologically defined "adenomatous hyperplasia" and suggested that it is a precursor of endometrial carcinoma. Later, Gusberg and Kaplan did prospective follow-up studies on 191 patients with "adenomatous hyperplasia" diagnosed from 1934 to 1954. Of the 90 treated immediately by hysterectomy, 20% were found to have coexisting carcinoma, and 13% had borderline lesions. This left 101 patients to be followed. In this group, 8 patients (7.9%) went on to develop endometrial cancer (mean follow-up, 5.3 years). In the control group of 202 patients with postmenopausal bleeding but no hyperplasia or carcinoma on initial curettage, only 1 went on to develop endometrial carcinoma. Gusberg and Kaplan concluded that the cumulative risk for a patient with adenomatous hyperplasia followed for 9 to 10 years is significantly higher than the risk for a woman without hyperplasia (Figure 4-5). Adenocarcinoma of the endometrium is considered rare during the childbearing years. When it does occur, a significant number of the cases are associated with the polycystic ovarian syndrome and anovulatory cycles. In a study by Jackson and Dockerty of 43 patients with Stein-Leventhal syndrome, 16 (37.2%) had carcinoma of the endometrium.

In the 1980s, some leading gynecologic pathologists (e.g., Richart, Kurman, and Ferenczy) have challenged the continuum concept. They conclude that there appear to be two separate and biologically unrelated diseases of the endometrium—hyperplasia and neoplasia—and the important feature distinguishing the processes from one another is cytologic atypia. Hyperplastic lesions have been viewed as forming a continuum of morphologic severity, and the relatively common coexistence of hyperplasia and carcinoma in the same endometrium has reinforced the continuum concept. However, observations of cytologic changes in these endometrial proliferations have led to a reinterpretation of the traditional data. The continuum concept has been challenged. It now appears that cytologic atypia is the only important morphologic feature distinguishing endometrial lesions with invasive potential from benign ones.

Kurman followed 170 patients with all grades of endometrial hyperplasia without a hysterectomy being performed for at least 1 year and with no irradiation therapy administered. One third of the patients with each type of hyperplasia (nonatypical and atypical) were asymptomatic after the diagnostic curettage and required no additional treatment. Only 2% of the patients with nonatypical endometrial hyperplasia and 23% of the women with atypical endometrial hyperplasia progressed to carcinoma (p = 0.001). The two cases of nonatypical hyperplasia that progressed underwent a change to atypical hyperplasia before developing into carcinoma.

Endometrial glandular proliferations with marked nuclear atypia of the lining cells are corpus carcinoma precursors. The lesions show enlargement, rounding, and pleomorphism of the nuclei; high mean-maximal nuclear diameter, often aneuploid DNA content; and macronuclei. Ferenczy has suggested that these lesions with cytologic atypia are best referred to as endometrial intraepithelial neoplasia (EIN) and nonatypical lesions as endometrial hyperplasia (EH). Both may be under the influence of estrogen, but the EIN lesions develop from cells that are cancer-initiated (Figure 4-6). Obviously, both types could exist in the same endometrium. The value of such classification lies in the potential for directed therapy: conservative for EH lesions and aggressive for EIN lesions.

We adopted the classification of the International Society of Gynecological Pathologists and have thus dropped the term *adenomatous* from our working jargon. Simple hyperplasia and complex hyperplasia, not considered as potentially malignant lesions, are treated conservatively. Only patients with atypical hyperplasia are treated as potential candidates for progression to frank endometrial carcinoma. Adequate sampling of the endometrial cavity and review by a skilled gynecological pathologist is essential in making this distinction.

If atypia is not mentioned in the pathology report, the implication is that none is present. The presence of cytologic atypia is the most important predictor of malignant potential and resistance to medical therapy. Endometrial hyperplasia can be difficult to determine histologically and is frequently over diagnosed; in a review of 100 consultation cases, Winkler found that 69%

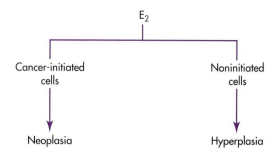

Figure 4-6 In the same endometrium, estradiol (E$_2$), a potent promoter of endometrial epithelial growth, may stimulate "carcinoma-initiated" cells to develop into neoplasia, and "non-initiated" cells may become hyperplastic under the hormone's influence. (From Ferenczy A, Gelfand MM, Tzipris F: *Ann Pathol* 3:189, 1983.)

were eventually down graded. The most common conditions confused with endometrial hyperplasia are endometrial polyps, endometrial metaplasias, menstrual patterns, and artifactual problems. Endometrial polyps may show hyperplastic glandular patterns, but may be distinguished by their polyp point configuration with an epithelial lining and a stalk containing thickened blood vessels. In menstrual patterns, stromal break down leads to closer approximation of endometrial glands, but this is not true glandular crowding.

Simple hyperplasia is characterized by a slight increase in the gland-to-stroma ratio, with mild degrees of glandular crowding. Glandular crowding is more pronounced in complex hyperplasia, but stromal still intervenes. Atypical hyperplasia is characterized by significant glandular crowding, but with some intervening stroma persisting. The nuclei of glandular epithelial cells are larger and rounder than normal, with variability in size. The pattern of well oriented oval nuclei is no longer present, with loss of polarity of the nuclei. The nuclei may appear "clear" owing to the margination of the chromatin under the nuclear membrane and prominent nucleoli also seen.

Distinguishing between atypical hyperplasia and endometrial carcinoma can be difficult, particularly in small endometrial samples. While myometrial invasion is conclusive evidence of carcinoma, curettings seldom contain myometrial fragments invaded by tumor. Many papers have endeavored to provide criteria to distinguish the atypical hyperplasia from carcinoma, but the main distinction is stromal invasion by the neoplastic glands. Although the concept of the endometrial carcinoma in situ has been proposed, this term is not widely recognized.

MANAGEMENT

The most important considerations in the management of endometrial hyperplasia are the age of the patient and the histologic pattern of the hyperplastic process. Treatment of a teenage patient with glandular hyperplasia will

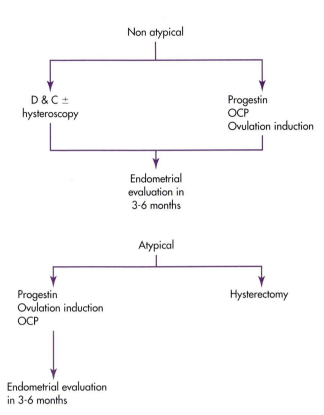

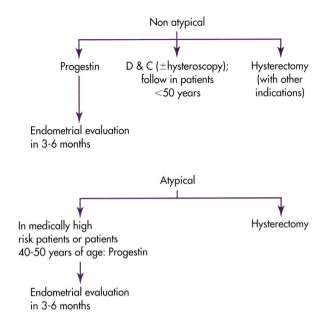

Figure 4-7 Management of patients with nonatypical endometrial hyperplasia who are 40 years of age or younger.

Figure 4-8 Management of patients with endometrial hyperplasia who are 40 years of age or older.

always be conservative, whereas the postmenopausal patient with atypical hyperplasia should, in most instances, be treated by hysterectomy and bilateral salpingo-oophorectomy. It should be kept in mind that various hyperplastic patterns may be found in nonmalignant endometrium of patients with concomitant endometrial carcinoma. Therefore, careful sampling of the endometrial cavity is a prerequisite to consideration for conservative therapy. In almost every series of hysterectomies for atypical endometrial hyperplasia, there have been a significant number of patients with concomitant unrecognized invasive adenocarcinomas. The problem of sufficient sampling of the endometrium, even with D&C, is important and should be kept in mind at all times when the patient is advised on therapy. As stated above, the presence of atypical cells and glands form the basis of a recommendation for aggressive therapy in patients with hyperplasia (Figure 4-7). Our preference for therapy has been as follows:

1. *Teenage girl.* This patient should be treated with estrogen-progestin artificial cycles for at least 6 months. Three months after completion of this treatment period, the endometrial cavity should be resampled. If benign endometrium is found on resampling, the patient should be observed for evidence of regular menses and patterns of ovulation. In the absence of ovulation the patient should be given periodic doses of medroxyprogesterone

(Provera), 10 mg orally each day for 10 days, to oppose the estrogen stimulation of her endometrium. This periodic use of progestin should continue until the patient has established an ovulatory pattern or is ready for ovulation induction and childbearing.

2. *Childbearing-age woman.* This patient should be treated with estrogen-progestin artificial cycles for 3 months. This period of therapy should be immediately followed by careful sampling of the endometrium to ensure reversion to a benign pattern. The patient should then be treated with clomiphene or menotropins (Pergonal) to induce ovulation. (Figure 4-7) If the patient is not interested in childbearing at that time, the continued use of estrogen-progestin artificial cycles is recommended.

3. *Perimenopausal woman.* This patient should be treated by hysterectomy or moderate doses of progestin alone. The decision for hysterectomy depends on the severity of the hyperplasia, the desire for sterilization, the presence of coexisting symptoms such as severe uterine bleeding, and/or the suspicion of an estrogen-secreting ovarian neoplasm. In general, our tendency is to recommend hysterectomy for patients with moderate to severe atypical hyperplasia and to use a trial of progestin for patients with lesser lesions and no concomitant pathologic findings. Our practice is to administer Provera, 20 mg PO daily for 10 days (days 16 to 25 in cycling women) repeated every 30 days for 6 months, or Depo-Provera, 200 mg IM every 2 months for three doses (Figure 4-8). The

endometrial cavity should be sampled by endometrial biopsy every 3 months. Patients will experience irregular bleeding and should be prepared for this to minimize anxiety.

4. *Postmenopausal woman.* This patient should undergo hysterectomy unless this is strongly contraindicated. A true postmenopausal woman (last menses 2 years or more ago) with atypical endometrial hyperplasia is often found to have coexisting foci of invasive adenocarcinoma or concomitant estrogen secreting ovarian neoplasms. Progestin therapy should be reserved for patients with severe medical problems that make them very poor operative candidates.

Progesterone and synthetic progestins both have produced reversion of benign and atypical hyperplasia to an atrophic pattern. This reversion also may be effected by induction of ovulation in women desirous of pregnancy. Some authors advocate immediate commencement of ovulation induction in patients desirous of pregnancy and believe that this maneuver is sufficient therapy for the endometrial hyperplasia as well. Our preference has been to continue the medical curettage (estrogen-progestin artificial cycles) for a period of up to 3 months before ovulation induction. Our preference for estrogen-progestin artificial cycles rather than progestin alone is based on ease of administration. The use of progestin alone results in irregular bleeding, which is often upsetting to the patient who is fearful of cancer. We found the estrogen-progestin cyclic therapy to be effective in reverting the endometrium in spite of the estrogen contained in this medication, and we are pleased with the smoothness of the cycles induced.

Progestins as the sole therapy eliminate in situ endometrial lesions in 62% of all cases, according to reports by Steiner et al. and Wilson and Kolstad. The incidence of invasive tumor in such patients treated with progestins is only 6%. Bonte et al. reported optimal responses with serum levels of 90 ng of medroxyprogesterone acetate (MPA) when treating both in situ and invasive endometrial cancer with progestins. MPA appears to partly inhibit hypothalamic and hypophyseal activities, especially luteinizing hormone production and, to a lesser extent, follicle-stimulating hormone production. Interestingly, estradiol and estrone serum levels are only slightly affected by MPA administration. At the cellular level, progestins appear to inhibit estrogen-induced RNA synthesis and thus exert their antimitotic action. Such progestin activity can be visualized partly by means of autoradiography with tagged thymidine. The cytoplasmic and nuclear receptors of estradiol and progestin, 17 β-estradiol and 20-α-dihydroprogestin dehydrogenase, would be the primary points of impact in both normal and malignant endometrium. The end result or the local effect of progestin on neoplastic endometrial tissue is apparently differentiation, maturation, secretion,

epithelial metaplasia, and atrophy. Gal reported success using megestrol acetate continuously (40 mg daily) in controlling endometrial hyperplasia in a group of women with high-risk factors for surgery. Similar results are possible using as little as 20 mg per day.

ESTROGENS AND ENDOMETRIAL NEOPLASIA

One of the factors that has prompted a returning and increasing interest in endometrial hyperplasia and endometrial cancer has been the role of ovarian hormones, notably estrogen, in this disease. The basis for considering estrogen as an etiologic factor is probably that hyperplasia of the endometrium is frequently associated with carcinoma, and the association of prolonged estrogen therapy and unopposed endogenous estrogens with endometrial hyperplasia has been widely recognized. The association is more suspect in the postmenopausal age group, in which 75% of cancer of the endometrium is found. In this age group, estrogen from any source can stimulate the endometrium unopposed by the action of progestin. In all likelihood, hyperplasia, excluding severe atypical hyperplasia, is not intimately related to carcinoma during the reproductive period, but the same entity encountered in the postmenopausal woman is strongly suggestive of cancer.

The role of estrogen and its possible relationship to endometrial cancer are receiving increased attention in both the scientific and the lay press (Table 4-3). Experiments of nature have provided us with information that implicate estrogen as a possible contributing factor to the development of endometrial cancer. It has been known for years that endometrial cancer can occur in patients with hormone-secreting tumors, particularly of the ovary. Many studies have been done on this since it was first

Table 4-3 Characteristics associated with incidence of endometrial cancer

Characteristic	Effect on incidence
Delayed menopause ("bloody menopause")	↑
Hypertension	↑
Diabetes	↑
Obesity	↑
High socioeconomic status	↑
Urban residence	↑
Positive family history	↑
Polycystic ovarian syndrome	↑
Exogenous estrogen in menopause	↑
Estrogen-secreting tumor	↑
Childbearing	↓
Delayed menarche	↓

reported by Novak and Yui in 1936 in the American literature. Gusberg and Kardon noted the highest correlation between endometrial cancer and the so-called feminizing ovarian tumors. They reported on 115 patients, 21% of whom were found to have corpus cancer and 43% of whom were found to have suspected cancer precursors such as endometrial hyperplasia and carcinoma in situ. They were nevertheless unable to draw any solid conclusions about the possible carcinogenic role of estrogen in humans. Norris and Taylor evaluated 203 patients with granulosa-theca cell tumors at the Armed Forces Institute of Pathology. They reported that only 9% of these patients had adenocarcinoma of the uterus but did not mention endometrial cancer precursors. Mansell and Hertig reviewed 80 feminizing tumors treated at the Free Hospital in Boston between 1905 and 1953. Only 11 patients had adenocarcinoma; however, 60% of the endometria did have changes suggestive of estrogen stimulation. McDonald et al. approached the situation from another viewpoint. Between 1905 and 1975, there were 44 patients with functional ovarian tumors and endometrial cancer at the Mayo Clinic. Unfortunately, the authors do not mention how many other functional ovarian tumors or adenocarcinomas of the endometrium they noted during that time interval. They also saw 28 patients with polycystic ovarian disease and endometrial cancer. They then compared these patients with 523 adenocarcinoma patients who were seen from 1952 to 1962. The 72 patients with endometrial cancer associated with functional tumors or polycystic ovaries had a predominance of stage I, grade I lesions, less myometrial involvement, and better survival rates compared with the other 523 adenocarcinoma patients. Some authors qualified the stromal tumors with the word *feminizing*, but others have not used this designation. It is well known that granulosa cell tumors can produce androgens, although to a smaller degree than those tumors that might produce estrogen.

Another situation in which endogenous estrogen might contribute to the development of endometrial cancer can be found in patients with polycystic ovary syndrome. The incidence of endometrial cancer has been reported to be as high as 25% in patients with Stein-Leventhal syndrome, although in actuality this number is probably considerably smaller. If the unopposed estrogen can be alleviated in this syndrome by wedge resection or clomiphene citrate, the estrogen-stimulated endometrium and its possible premalignant changes can be reversed. Kistner has reported that progestins can cause a regression of hyperplasia and carcinoma in situ of the endometrium in such patients.

Patients with ovarian dysgenesis (Turner syndrome) have also been reported to be at high risk for endometrial cancer because of the long-term supplemental unopposed estrogen that was given to these individuals beginning at an early age. Although several case reports have appeared in the literature, fewer than 50 patients have been reported to date.

It is also well known that estrone, which makes up the largest amount of estrogen produced in the postmenopausal woman, is a result of peripheral conversion of androstenedione. There appears to be a greater conversion of androstenedione to estrone in endometrial cancer patients than in healthy postmenopausal women. There is also increased estrone production in the woman who is postmenopausal, older, and obese. The cause of the increased production of estrone is unknown but one factor that is commonly involved relates to the increased conversion of precursors to estrone in large deposits of adipose tissue often found in these patients.

In view of the relative frequency with which the uterus is stimulated by estrogen, either naturally or synthetically through the use of hormone therapy, and the relative rarity of carcinoma of the endometrium, it is obvious that hyperestrogenism as the sole etiologic explanation for endometrial cancer is unsatisfactory. We must also accept the hypothesis of the presence of a properly sensitive substrate that overreacts to estrogen simulation. The available data from humans suggest that in predisposed individuals (those in whom a cancer-initiating factor has influenced the endometrium) the unopposed action of estrogen substances for considerable periods will result in endometrial adenomatous hyperplasia, anaplasia, carcinoma in situ, and eventually carcinoma.

The postmenopausal ovary continues to secrete substantial amounts of testosterone and androstenedione but virtually no estrogen. Increasing evidence supports the concept that after menopause most of the estrogens are derived from peripheral conversion of androgens of adrenal origin, with only a small contribution by the ovary. The origin of plasma sex hormones in postmenopausal women was further studied by determining plasma levels under basal conditions, after ACTH stimulation and dexamethasone suppression and after HCG stimulation. The findings indicate that the adrenal cortex is the almost unique source of plasma estradiol, estrone, progesterone, and 17-OH-progesterone and the most important source of plasma dehydro-3-epiandrosterone. The postmenopausal ovary appears to be responsible for about 50% of plasma testosterone and 30% of androstenediones, and HCG stimulation with 5000 IU daily for 3 days hardly influences steroid secretion by postmenopausal ovaries. Removal of the ovaries frequently fails to alter the quantity of estrogen produced in postmenopausal women. Even more interesting is the continuous presence of a small but definite amount of estrogen even after complete hypophysectomy in oophorectomized women.

Marrett et al. reported incidence rates for invasive cancer of the uterine corpus according to stage of disease (localized, nonlocalized) based on cases reported to the Connecticut Tumor Registry between 1960 and 1975. The 1960 to 1964 and 1965 to 1969 rates were very similar for both disease stages. However, in 1970 to 1975 the incidence of localized corpus cancer was 26% higher than in either of the previously studied periods. Women aged 50 to 59 years experienced the largest increase in localized disease, although all other age groups over 50 years also had higher rates in the most recent period of diagnosis. No increases were evident in women under 50 years. In addition, the frequency of the diagnosis of carcinoma in situ of the endometrium increased gradually over the 16-year period, and mortality from corpus cancer declined slightly. Over the same period there was an increase in the hysterectomy rate in Connecticut, and when the corpus cancer rate was adjusted for this variable, the rate increased another 5% to 15%. Factors associated with an increased risk of endometrial cancer (e.g., overweight, nulliparity, late menopause, diabetes mellitus, hypertension, Stein-Leventhal syndrome, cancer of other sites, pelvic irradiation, and administration of estrogens) were reviewed, and no evidence could be found that the prevalence of any of these, apart from estrogen use, has increased. Estrogens have been used for replacement therapy since the 1930s; by 1958, 1.6 million prescriptions were being filled nationally per year. This figure changed little between 1958 and 1965 but had doubled by 1966. This new higher level of use was maintained until 1971, after which time it began to increase. The increase in incidence of endometrial cancer that began in 1970 would lead to an estimated latency period of 4 to 8 years between initiation of drug exposure and diagnosis of cancer. Marrett et al. correctly concluded that the recent increase in the incidence of localized invasive endometrial cancer in women 50 years and over in Connecticut is likely to be at least partially caused by the increasing use of estrogen therapy. The fact that neither mortality from corpus cancer nor nonlocalized

disease incidence has increased in Connecticut since 1960 suggests that estrogen therapy may be predominantly associated with tumors that can be readily diagnosed at an early stage. Conversely, several countries (e.g., Norway and Czechoslovakia) have reported increased endometrial cancer rates in the absence of frequent use of exogenous estrogen in their populations.

In 1941 Greene described a strain of rabbits that developed "toxemia of pregnancy" and liver damage, whereupon such animals became infertile and developed endometrial hyperplasia and subsequent carcinoma of the endometrium, depending on the so-called hyperestrogenism. This was an excellent model of the infertile woman.

Cancer of the endometrium has not been produced experimentally in subhuman primates, but studies to date have suffered from the clear species variation of endometrial response to hormonal stimulation and the lack of appropriate genetic substrate in these animals, as well as the relatively short duration of most experiments of this type in this relatively long-lived animal. Although the development of adenocarcinoma of the endometrium in laboratory animals has been limited to the rabbit, guinea pig, and mouse, Scott and Wharton did produce "adenomatous hyperplasia" with diethylstilbestrol in monkeys.

In the past 25 years, numerous retrospective studies have correlated the use of exogenous estrogens in the postmenopausal woman with the increasing incidence of endometrial carcinoma (Table 4-4). Smith et al. from the University of Washington identified 317 women, aged 48 years or older, from two hospitals where they had been diagnosed as having adenocarcinoma of the endometrium between 1960 and 1972. A retrospective review of the hospital's records showed that for 152 (48%) of these women, exogenous estrogen therapy had been prescribed.

Table 4-4 Exogenous estrogen exposure and endometrial carcinoma

Year	Reference	Overall risk ratio	Characteristics of controls
1967	Dunn and Bradbury	1.1	Postmenopausal bleeding
1968	Pacheco and Kempers	0.5	Postmenopausal bleeding
1975	Smith et al.	4.5	Other gynecologic cancers; matched for age and site of diagnosis
1975	Ziel and Finkle	7.6	Matched for age, residence, and duration of health care in Kaiser system; intact uterus
1976	Mack et al.	8.0	Matched for residence, age, and marital status; intact uterus
1977	Gray et al.	3.1	Hysterectomy for benign condition in same time span; matched for age, parity, and weight
1977	McDonald et al.	4.9	Matched for age, residence, and duration of medical care; intact uterus
1978	Wigle et al.	2.2	Nongynecologic cancer
1978	Hoogerland et al.	2.2	Other gynecologic cancers; matched for age and site of diagnosis; intact uterus
1978	Horwitz and Feinstein	1.7	Dilation and curettage or hysterectomy for conditions other than endometrial carcinoma
1979	Antunes et al.	6.0	Matched for hospital, race, age, and date of admission; intact uterus
1979	Hammond et al.	3.8	Hypoestrogenic

Of the 317 patients without endometrial carcinoma but with other gynecologic cancers who were selected as a control group, only 54 (17%) had had exogenous estrogen prescribed previously. Appropriate statistical calculations revealed a 4.5-fold increased risk of developing endometrial cancer for the women exposed to estrogen in the retrospective study. Subsequent data from these same investigators revealed that the women developing endometrial carcinoma on exogenous estrogen therapy were phenotypically different from the typical obese, diabetic, hypertensive women usually associated with this neoplasm. Indeed, most of the women developing endometrial adenocarcinoma on exogenous estrogen therapy were much more normal in appearance with nonstriking medical histories for diabetes, hypertension, and obesity.

Ziel and Finkle from the Kaiser-Permanente Medical Center in Los Angeles published a retrospective review of their patients treated between July 1970 and December 1974. During that time period, 94 cases of endometrial carcinoma were discovered. The records of 54 (57%) of these patients showed them to have received prior therapy with conjugated estrogens. Selection of 108 women as controls (2 for each case) was based on comparable age, area of residence, and duration of health-plan membership. Only 29 (27%) of these women had been treated with conjugated estrogens. The risk ratio (RR) in this study was calculated to be 7.6.

The next report on this subject was published in June 1976 by Mack et al. and was conducted in a retirement community south of Los Angeles where 63 women were diagnosed between 1971 and 1975 as having endometrial carcinoma. As determined from medical records, patient interviews, or pharmacy prescription records, 56 (89%) of the patients were found to have taken some form of estrogen. These investigators selected four controls for each case. The control patients were residents of the community matched with the endometrial cancer patients for the time of entry into the community, age, and marital status. Of the group of 252 controls, 126 (50%) were found to have taken some form of estrogen, for a computed RR of 8.

Subsequently, a number of articles in the literature have evaluated the use of exogenous estrogen in patients with endometrial cancer. The study of McDonald et al. evaluating this relationship in Olmstead County (Rochester, Minnesota) noted 145 endometrial cancer patients over the period studied. They were compared with 417 controls. Whereas 27% of the endometrial cancer patients took estrogen, 28% of the controls took estrogen. The RR for all exogenous estrogen was 0.9; however, it increased to 2.3 if the drug was taken for longer than 6 months. If only conjugated estrogens were considered, regardless of duration, the RR was 2. It is of interest that only 16 patients out of the 145 took conjugated estrogens for longer than 6 months. The authors noted that the incidence of endometrial cancer in Olmstead County had actually decreased over the last three decades, even though estrogen use had increased from 5% to 21% during the time studied. When they evaluated their data in the manner that the previous three authors had, their RR became 2 as analyzed by Ziel and Finkle, 2.3 as analyzed by Smith et al., and 0.9 as analyzed by Mack et al.

Gray et al. evaluated their private practice experience with 205 endometrial cancer patients between 1947 and 1976, as compared with 205 controls who had hysterectomy for benign disease. Twenty-six percent of the cancer patients took estrogen, as compared with only 15% of the controls. The RR for conjugated estrogens was 3.1, but for all estrogen it was 2.1. The RR increased with years of use but was only significant above the 10-year interval. The authors stated that the actual number of cancers caused by exogenous estrogen is quite small. Only 31 of the 205 cancers could be attributed to estrogen use, even if all excess risk from estrogen leads to cancer.

Shapiro reported a case-control study of the risk of adenocarcinoma of the endometrium in relation to conjugated estrogens use. He found that 31% of 425 women with endometrial cancer and 15% of 792 controls reported having used conjugated estrogens; the RR estimate was 3.5. They also found that among women who had used estrogen for at least 1 year and then discontinued it, the risk of endometrial cancer remained significantly elevated, even after estrogen-free intervals of more than 10 years.

Hoover et al., in evaluating cancer of the uterine corpus after hormonal treatment for breast cancer, noted a slight increase in women who received estrogen after mastectomy. It was noted that in patients who did not receive estrogen there was a 40% greater incidence of uterine cancer than would be expected. Other studies have shown an increased RR for endometrial cancer in patients with breast cancer, since multiple primary cancers can occur in the same patient.

A study by Antunes et al. evaluated endometrial cancer patients between 1973 and 1977 in six hospitals in Baltimore. A total of 451 endometrial cancer patients were identified and compared with 888 controls. It was noted that if the controls were from the gynecologic service, the RR for estrogen use was 2.1; however, if the controls were from the nongynecologic services, the RR was 6. When the dosage, type of estrogen, and duration of use were considered, appropriate data were available on only 75% of the cancer patients and less than 50% of the controls. No pathologic data were presented, even though the authors stated that no overestimation of the material was made. The authors believe that the difference between the two groups of patients cannot be explained because a faster diagnosis was made in the estrogen versus the nonestrogen patient, yet only 30% of the cancer patients and 26% of the control patients were evaluated for this parameter.

In December 1975 the Obstetric Advisory Committee

of the FDA reviewed these reports and concluded that "the studies provided strong evidence that postmenopausal estrogen therapy increases the risk of endometrial cancer." On the basis of this conclusion, the FDA has developed a revised package insert for use by patients and physicians that will include a clear warning of the increased risk of endometrial cancer and a "clarification" of the indications for the use of estrogen in the menopausal or postmenopausal period.

Several additional retrospective studies have been done in a manner similar to those just cited, and similar conclusions were reached in most instances. Before the FDA position on this matter is accepted without question, a critical assessment of the reported data is necessary. All these studies have one feature in common: the use of retrospective case-control methodology. Women who had a diagnosis of endometrial carcinoma were selected as "cases" for comparison. Only then was the information gathered about prior exposure to exogenous estrogen use. Since calculation of an RR depends entirely on the different rates of estrogen exposure between the two groups, the choice of patients in the control group can obviously predetermine the results of such a study. The controls should be identical to the "cases" in every way except for the occurrence of the disease and the exposure to the ideologic factor or factors. The selection of the "controls" can introduce a so-called detection bias. Each of the studies done to date has been subjected to statistical criticisms based on the retrospective methodology. What is needed, of course, is a prospective study, but the execution of such a study would be difficult, and possibly unethical. Applying different rules about the inclusion of patients as cases but not as controls is unacceptable. For example, a prospective comparative study is being started to evaluate the possible carcinogenicity of estrogens. The two groups of women, all with intact uteri, would be selected and then allocated to treatment or no treatment on a random basis. With the passage of time, some women in each group would undergo hysterectomy for a number of reasons. These women would have to be taken into account in the evaluation of the final results of the study. In some of the studies cited above, the patients who underwent hysterectomy were specifically excluded from the control group. This and many other factors illustrate the potential pitfalls in the development of the case-control methodology.

Horowitz and Feinstein have questioned the studies that have shown a large RR between endometrial cancer and exogenous estrogen. They noted a bias in the selection of controls. They evaluated their cancer patients using two sets of controls. With the conventional controls similar to the other studies, 29% of the cancer patients had taken estrogen versus 3% of the controls, for an odds ratio of 11.98. The alternative set of controls, patients who had D&C or hysterectomy, were used to equalize the forces of diagnostic surveillance that might create major detected bias. In this group of patients an odds ratio of only 1.7 was present.

In addition, several reports in the literature have suggested no difference in estrogen use between endometrial cancer patients and controls. In 1967 Dunn and Bradbury noted that 28.6% of 56 patients with endometrial cancer took estrogen versus 27.5% of 83 control patients. The controls were those women who had postmenopausal bleeding but with atrophic endometrium on D&C. Pacheco and Kempers looked at a group of patients who had postmenopausal bleeding. Only 71 of 401 patients (18%) had an endometrial malignancy. Ninety-three (23%) of the patients took estrogen. Only 10% of those patients who had postmenopausal bleeding and took estrogen had cancer, whereas 18% of the patients who had postmenopausal bleeding not caused by cancer took estrogen. A study from Finland evaluated 317 endometrial cancer patients followed between 1970 and 1976 compared with 304 controls. Of the cancer patients, only 9% took estrogen, whereas 19% of the controls took estrogen.

ESTROGEN-PROGESTIN THERAPY

A great body of indirect evidence suggests that estrogen (endogenous and exogenous) can be an etiologic agent in the pathogenesis of endometrial adenocarcinoma. Similar evidence exists that any risk associated with exogenous estrogen use can be abrogated by simultaneous progestin use. A convincing study was reported by Sturdee et al. In the study vacuum endometrial curettage was performed on 348 women who had received various regimens of estrogen for an average of 97 months for menopausal symptoms. Cyclical unopposed oral estrogen treatment (98 cases) was associated with a 12% incidence of endometrial hyperplasia, but among the 102 women taking regimens including 10 to 13 days of progesterone there was zero incidence of hyperplasia. Among women treated with subcutaneous estrogen implants and monthly 5-day courses of oral progestin (50 patients), there was a 28% incidence of hyperplasia, including one case of adenocarcinoma. Regular withdrawal bleeding during treatment was associated with a lower incidence of endometrial hyperplasia (6%) than unscheduled breakthrough bleeding (18%), but the one patient with carcinoma had experienced regular bleeding only.

In contrast to several retrospective studies reporting an increased risk of endometrial cancer from estrogen use, Gambrell reported that the number of such cancers at Wilford Hall United States Air Force Medical Center has steadily declined, despite continued estrogen-progestin use. During the 5 years of the Wilford Hall prospective study there was a steady decline in the number of women using estrogens only and a steady increase in the use of the progestin challenge test to identify those postmenopausal women at greatest risk for endometrial cancer. The

Table 4-5   Incidence of endometrial cancer at Wilford Hall USAF Medical Center, 1975-1979, by therapy group

	Patient-years of observation	Patients with cancer	Incidence (per 100,000)
Estrogen-progestin users	7063	5	70.8
Estrogen users	2302	10	434.4
Estrogen vaginal cream users	1318	1	75.9
Progestin or androgen users	761	0	—
Untreated women	2477	6	242.2
TOTAL	13,921	22	158.0

Modified from Gambrell RD: *J Reprod Med* 27:531, 1982.

progestin challenge test was administered by giving a trial of progestin, either 5 mg norethindrone acetate (Norlutate) 10 mg or medroxyprogesterone acetate (Provera), for 10 days to each postmenopausal woman with an intact uterus. This included estrogen-treated climacteric women, as well as those with menopausal symptoms and asymptomatic postmenopausal women undergoing an annual evaluation. If withdrawal bleeding resulted from the progestin challenge, the progestin was continued for 10 days each month as long as withdrawal bleeding followed.

There has been considerable concern regarding the appropriate dosage of progestin needed to induce endometrial regression. Whitehead determined that the minimum daily progestin dose over 12 days for complete endometrial regression is 10 mg of medroxyprogesterone acetate, 0.7 mg for norethindrone, 75 mcg for levonorgestrel, 300 mg of micronized oral progesterone, and 10-20 mg of dehydrogesterone. These data are derived by endometrial sampling and transmission electron microscopy of ultrastructural elements.

Adenocarcinoma of the endometrium was diagnosed in 22 patients during 13,921 patient-years of observation, for an incidence of 158/100,000 women per year. The lowest incidence was observed in the largest group, the estrogen-progestin users, with an incidence of 70.8/100,000 women (Table 4-5).

Thus, progestational agents can negate the carcinogenic effect of estrogen on the endometrium. It has been demonstrated that 12 to 14 days of progestational therapy each month can eliminate hyperplasia, a probable precursor of endometrial cancer. It should be noted that progestational therapy theoretically can increase the risk of breast cancer and cardiovascular disease. Mitotic activity in the breast epithelium reaches a peak in the luteal phase of the menstrual cycle, suggesting that progesterone, when acting in conjunction with the luteal

phase estradiol peak, may serve as a breast cancer promoter. Yet, most clinical studies have failed to show convincing evidence of increased breast cancer in patients who take estrogen replacement therapy with or without progestin.

Literature on oral contraceptives suggests that the risk of arteriosclerotic disease is clearly related to the progestational component of the pill. Some progestational agents have the opposite effect of estrogens on HDL- and LDL-cholesterol. However, Barnes studied 35 women receiving conjugated estrogens or depo-medroxyprogesterone and found that similar effects resulted in plasma lipids. Cholesterol and low-density lipoprotein (LDL) decreased with both drugs. The high-density lipoprotein (HDL) was not significantly altered by either. This and other studies suggest that at least the progestin medroxyprogesterone when used with conjugate estrogens does not increase incidence of arteriosclerotic disease.

Silverberg and Makowski, as well as others, have described the development of endometrial carcinoma in patients taking oral contraceptive agents. In virtually every instance the agents used were sequential, and progestin was administered with the estrogen only in the last 7 days of each cycle. During the first 14 days of the cycle, the patient received large doses of synthetic estrogen alone. Whether sequential agents somehow predispose their recipients to endometrial cancer or whether those women who are predisposed to develop this tumor are protected **against** it by the use of a combined oral contraceptive **agent remains** to be determined. The sequential type of oral contraceptive has been voluntarily withdrawn from the market by the pharmaceutical companies producing it, so this question may remain moot. Currently available combination preparations, however, are associated with a 50% reduction in the incidence of endometrial carcinoma compared with the incidence in nonusers. The ability of progestins to reduce the incidence of estrogen-induced atypical endometrial hyperplasia probably explains this benefit for combination oral contraceptive users.

Yen and Rigg have demonstrated that the use of vaginal estrogen cream is associated with considerable systemic absorption, and potentially the same effects are possible as with oral administration. The absorption of estrogen from the vagina is often erratic, and as the vaginal epithelium thickens, absorption rates change. One can usually achieve a more constant level of absorption by using the oral or intramuscular route.

ESTROGENS AND BREAST CANCER

At present there is no conclusive evidence that there is an increased risk of breast carcinoma in postmenopausal women taking estrogen. In one study 735 women were followed for an average of 15 years after they began taking estrogens. Overall, 21 cases of breast carcinoma were found: 18 were expected. Hoover et al. reported on 1891 menopausal women treated with conjugated estrogens. The women were followed for an average of 12 years. In the treated group, 49 cases of breast carcinoma were observed: 39 were expected on the basis of the incidence in the general population. This difference was not statistically significant. The study's findings indicate that menopausal estrogen use does not protect against breast cancer, but neither does it appear to increase the risk of breast cancer markedly. However, with breast carcinoma, as with endometrial carcinoma, the possible association of estrogen use with increased risk remains and requires constant evaluation.

A much-publicized article by Bergkvist in 1989 examined the risk of breast cancer after noncontraceptive treatment with estrogen. A relative increase in risk was noted for some subsets utilizing synthetic estrogen, but no increase in risk was found with use of conjugated estrogens. Bergkvist published another article studying the prognosis after breast cancer diagnosis in women exposed to estrogen and estrogen-progestin replacement therapy. This second article looked directly at the outcome for patients who developed breast cancer as current or recent users of replacement therapy. It is of interest that the relative survival rate was significantly higher by about 10 percentage points at 8 years in patients who had received estrogen treatment—corresponding to an approximately 40% reduction in excess mortality. This more favorable course, which could be confirmed only in patients age 50 years or more at diagnosis, was most pronounced in recent users, that is, in women whose treatment was ongoing or had been discontinued within 1 year prior to diagnosis.

Gambrell et al. reported on prospective studies at Wilford Hall that failed to demonstrate that estrogen replacement therapy increased the risk of breast cancer. Their data suggested that estrogens may even provide some protection against mammary malignancy, particularly when combined with a progestin. Of the 5563 postmenopausal women followed for 24,559 patient-years of observation, 43 were found to have breast malignancy, an overall incidence of 174.8/100,000 women per year. There were 7 breast cancers among the estrogen-progestin users, an incidence of 95.6/100,000, and 15 breast cancers in the group taking estrogens only, an annual incidence of 137.3/100,000. The difference in incidence between the estrogen-progestin users and the estrogen users was significantly smaller than that between them and the untreated women (500/100,000; $p < 0.01$). Although the incidence of breast cancer in the estrogen users was less than in untreated women, the difference was not statistically significant but did indicate a trend ($p < 0.08$).

In a well-designed, 10-year double-blind study by Nachtigall et al. there were four breast cancers in the 84 placebo users and none in the 84 estrogen-progestin users; this finding was statistically significant ($p > 0.05$). An estrogen-window hypothesis has been proposed: breast cancer risk is thus related to the duration of unopposed estrogen exposure during the reproductive years of a woman's life. It may be that progestin-treated postmenopausal women have a lower risk of breast cancer just as they are protected against endometrial cancer; however, more clinical experience with postmenopausal progestin therapy is needed before any firm recommendations can be made for hysterectomized women. Hammond et al. observed 4 cases of mammary malignancy among 301 estrogen users followed for 5 or more years and 4 in the 309 untreated controls; his findings were not statistically significant. At this time we must conclude that estrogens do not significantly increase the risk except possibly with prolonged use (>10 years), and progestins may actually provide additional protection against breast cancer.

A 1995 report from Colditz on the Nurses' Health Study represents sixteen years of follow-up from 1976-1992. During that period, 1,935 cases of breast cancer were identified among more than 69,000 postmenopausal women. The analysis revealed that women who had used estrogen in the past (even for ten or more years) were not at increased risk of breast cancer. However, the relative risk for current users was 1.46 (Confidence Interval 1.22-1.74) for ten or more years of use. By virtue of the large numbers in the Nurses' Health Study and the careful analyses by the investigators, reports from this study must be given great credibility. The sixteen year follow-up report is disturbing because of the increased use in current users. However, estrogen users may be examined more frequently; detection bias is a great concern. It is noteworthy that current users had a 14% higher prevalence of mammography compared to never-users. This and other differences found in the study make the finding of an increased relative risk in long-term current users indefinite and not completely free of all confounding variables. The size of the statistical risk is not outside the range of influence by biases. This same study material was used to calculate a 40% to 50% reduction in the ischemic heart disease among this same group.

In another study of 1,686 and 2,077 controls done in the Eastern United States and reported by Kaufman, the relative risk for current use was 1.1 (C.I. 0.7-1.6). With a duration of use of 15 or more years, the relative risk was 0.9 (C.I. 0.4-1.9). Another study by Palmer, found no evidence for increased risk in either current or recent users or in users for up to 15 years. These latter two case-control studies failed to support the conclusion of the Nurses' Health Study that current users are at increased risk. In addition and importantly, these studies have consistently failed to demonstrate a link between increased risk and the duration of estrogen use.

Stanford reported in 1995 on a study of middle-aged women (ages 50-64), including 537 patients with primary breast cancer diagnosed between January 1, 1988 and June 30, 1990 who were ascertained through the Seattle-Puget Sound Surveillance, epidemiology, and End Results cancer registry and 492 randomly selected control women without a history of breast cancer. Menopausal hormones of some type had been used by 57.6% of breast cancer cases and 61.0% of comparison women. The women who had ever taken combined estrogen-progestin HRT, representing 21.5% of cases and 21.3% of controls, were not at increased risk of breast cancer (relative odds [RO] = 0.9). Compared with nonusers of menopausal hormones, those who used estrogen-progestin HRT for 8 or more years had, if anything, a reduced risk of breast cancer (RO = 0.4).

On the whole, the use of estrogen with progestin (HRT) does not appear to be associated with an increased risk of breast cancer in middle-aged women.

A meta-analysis is an increasingly popular statistical method by which many studies are combined and undergo vigorous analysis. Simply put, the purpose of a meta-analysis is to gain the statistical power that is lacking in individual studies. The term *"meta-analysis"* was coined in 1976 to indicate the reanalysis of data to answer new questions. The method was first used in social science, and then in the 1980s, in medicine. An Australian meta-analysis by Armstrong et al. of 23 studies of estrogen use and breast cancer concluded "unequivocally" that estrogen use did not alter the risk of breast cancer. In another meta-analysis by Dupont and Page, the authors concluded that "considerable and consistent" evidence existed that a daily dose of 0.625 mg conjugated estrogens taken for several years does not appreciably increase the risk of breast cancer. They found no evidence of an association between the duration of treatment and the risk of breast cancer at this dosage. On the other hand, the data suggested that a daily dose of 1.25 mg conjugated estrogens and higher may increase the risk in patients with a history of benign breast disease. A third analysis by Steinberg from the Center for Disease Control was conducted using what the authors called a "dose-response curve" for duration of use. The curve for each study analyzed was calculated by plotting breast cancer risk against duration of estrogen use. The combined dose-response slope represented the average change in risk associated with estrogen use over time. The analysis concluded that duration of estrogen use was associated with an increased risk of breast cancer, regardless of whether menopause was natural or surgical. No increase in risk was noted in the first 5 years of use, but after 15 years of use, the risk was increased by 30%. The effect was present irrespective of other risk factors, such as family history, parity, or history of benign breast disease. The effect of estrogen therapy on risk of breast cancer was enhanced in women with a positive family history of breast cancer.

A fourth meta-analysis reported by Sillero-Arenas in 1992 concluded that estrogen is associated with a very small, but statistically significant, increased relative risk of breast cancer, and that the increased risk is higher among current users. Confining their analysis to a dose of 0.625 mg conjugated estrogens; however, the Spanish epidemiologists conducting this study could not detect a statistically significant increased risk. Indeed, this meta-analysis concluded that an estrogen use of 0.625 mg conjugated estrogens is safe.

A fifth meta-analysis from the epidemiologists associated with the Nurses' Health Study concluded (based on 25 case-control and 6 cohort studies) that there is no increased risk of breast cancer in ever users of estrogen. Current use was associated with an increased risk (which was lost 2 years after using estrogen), and there was a slight increase with more than 10 years of use (there was no linear trend with increasing duration of use). The statistical power of this meta-analysis was in the ever use category, giving strength to its negative conclusion. This meta-analysis could not detect a link between risk of breast cancer and dosage. A possible effect of higher doses continues to be a concern since three of the meta-analyses indicated an increased risk with a daily dose of conjugated estrogens greater than 0.625 mg (or its equivalent).

It is interesting to note that all of the studies that have examined the mortality rates of women who were taking estrogen at the time of breast cancer diagnosis have documented improved survival rates. This undoubtedly reflects earlier diagnosis in users because the greater survival rate in current users is associated with a lower frequency of late stage disease. There is also evidence to suggest that estrogen users develop better differentiated tumors, and that surveillance/detection bias is not the only explanation for better survival. The risks associated with use of ERT for endometrial neoplasia were discussed earlier in this chapter.

BENEFITS OF ESTROGEN REPLACEMENT THERAPY

Estrogen replacement therapy (ERT) is usually beneficial for women experiencing involuntary hot flashes and sweating, as well as symptoms attributable to atrophy of the vagina or the urethra and to bladder trigone. Vasomotor symptoms, including hot flashes and sweating, are distinct and are troublesome to between 20% and 60% of postmenopausal women. Double-blind studies have established that estrogen therapy is beneficial in treating these symptoms. Emotional problems associated with these symptoms are best treated with estrogen and supportive therapy and, if necessary, with other drugs. Menopausal symptoms respond to low doses of estrogen (i.e., 0.625 mg conjugated estrogens). Among other manifestations (Table 4-6), estrogen deficiency results in a gradual reduction and eventual loss of the confined

Table 4-6 Estrogen target organs

Urogenital: ovary, uterus, fallopian tubes, vagina, bladder, urethra
Breast
Skin
Central nervous system: pituitary gland, hypothalamus, spinal cord
Gastrointestinal system: colon, pancreas, liver
Adrenal glands
Heart arteries
Bone

Table 4-7 The effect of estrogen treatment on cardiovascular morbidity in menopausal women (prospective studies)

Author	Year	Relative risk
Bush et al.	1983	0.4
Bush et al.	1987	0.3
Wilson et al.	1985	1.3-32*
Stampfer et al.	1985	0.3
Coldiz et al.	1987	0.42

*Smokers

epithelial layer of the vagina. Although not as marked, similar changes occur in the urethra and bladder epithelium as well. The results are increasing dryness in the vagina and, when deficiency is severe, vaginal irritation, pruritus vulvae, and urethritis.

Cardiovascular Disease

Cardiovascular morbidity, i.e., coronary heart disease and stroke, constitutes the most frequent cause of death among women in the United States. It accounts for about 650,000 deaths in the United States annually. The incidence of death caused by coronary heart disease in women is four times that which occurs as a result of any other disease, including malignancies of the female reproductive organs. With advancing age, the frequency and prevalence of cardiovascular risk factors also rise. High cholesterol levels are present in 40% of women over the age of fifty. High diastolic blood pressure is observed in 60% of women over the age of 65. The increased occurrence of risk factors is reflected in the increased frequency of cardiovascular disease in older women. The frequency of cardiovascular disease is low during the period of fertility, but as menopause approaches, it rises to three to six cases per thousand women, and at 70-75 years, it reaches fifty cases per thousand women. Aging is not a disease in itself, but it shows a high correlation with morbidity. The possible effects of estrogen and progestin on the incidence of cardiovascular disease in women is the subject of ongoing research and controversy with the majority of recent prospective studies supporting the beneficial effects of ERT. Most of the cohort studies prove that ERT effectively diminishes the risk of cardiovascular disease in 50-60 year old women (Table 4-7).

Blood cholesterol level is the main risk factor for cardiovascular disease in postmenopausal women. A high positive correlation has been found between levels of low-density lipoprotein (LDL) and coronary morbidity. Conversely, the level of high-density lipoprotein (HDL$_2$) shows a high negative correlation with the probability of coronary disease and with the extent of damage to the coronary vessels. Matthews has shown the beneficial effects of ERT on low and high-density lipoprotein levels.

In a prospective study, he showed clearly a corresponding rise in high-density lipoproteins and a decrease in low-density lipoproteins in ERT treated post menopausal patients. The association of increased HDL and decreased LDL levels with reduced risk of cardiovascular disease is well documented for both males and females.

In most of the epidemiological studies, the use of progestins was uncommon. Unfortunately, most progestins, although often recommended to reduce or eliminate the risk of endometrial cancer due to unopposed estrogen tend to lower HDL cholesterol and raise LDL cholesterol. One can devise regimens in which some estrogen benefit on lipids remains, but it is apparently attenuated to some extent by the addition of most progestins. Low doses of medroxyprogesterone acetate appear to maintain protection for the uterus without impairing benefits of estrogens on lipids.

Lobo reported on the impact of different dosages of medroxyprogesterone acetate (MPA) on metabolism and hemostasis in postmenopausal women treated with conjugated estrogens. In his prospective, double blind, study, 525 women were randomized to five treatment regimens at 26 sites in the United States and Europe. All participants received 0.625 mg of conjugated estrogens daily for up to 13 cycles; four groups also received MPA, either 2.5 or 5.0 mg/day continuously or 5.0 or 10.0 mg/day for the last 14 days of each cycle. Effects on lipid and carbohydrate metabolism and coagulation were evaluated.

All of the treatment groups experienced increases in high-density lipoprotein-cholesterol (HDL-C), the HDL$_2$-C subfraction and apolipoprotein A-1 compared to baseline; however, at each time point, the increases from baseline in the conjugated estrogens-only group were significantly greater than those for the conjugated estrogens-MPA groups. Additionally, all treatment groups had significant decreases in low-density lipoprotein-cholesterol (LDL-C) and apolipoprotein B. Decreases from baseline in total cholesterol (TC) levels were significantly greater than those in the conjugated estrogens-only group. HDL$_3$-C levels increased significantly from baseline in the conjugated estrogens-only group but not in the other treatment groups. Triglyceride levels increased significantly in all groups. The mean increase in the MPA-treated groups was less than that in the conjugated estrogens-only treatment group. Although MPA modified some of the effects of conjugated estrogens on lipid metabolism, the direction of changes in lipid parameters was unaltered.

With respect to carbohydrate metabolism, all treatment groups experienced fasting glucose levels, which were marginally lower than baseline. A slight decrease from baseline in fasting insulin levels was observed in all groups at all time points. After administration of oral glucose, blood glucose values at 30 minutes were significantly lower than baseline in the estrogens-only group but not with the other groups. The area under the curve for glucose increased from baseline in the MPA-treated groups; however, these changes were not significantly different than those observed in the estrogens-only group. Compared to baseline, insulin responses after oral glucose administration were significantly decreased in all groups.

The investigators also examined the effect of conjugated estrogens on prothrombin time, partial thromboplastin time, factor VII, factor X, antithrombin III activity, and plasminogen activity and concluded that, "No major changes of clinical significance occurred in hemostatic levels." The investigators reported that for each treatment group the majority of values for each parameter were within the normal ranges. Plasminogen activity increased significantly (p < 0.001) from baseline in all groups. With regard to the plasminogen activity, the authors suggest that, "The small decreases in antithrombin III . . . remained in the normal range and are most probably well counterbalanced by significant increases in plasminogen activity." The investigators reported no significant difference between the estrogens-only and estrogens plus MPA treated groups with regard to factor X, antithrombin III, or plasminogen values.

Additional data on the conjugated estrogens regimen was reported in the results of the Postmenopausal Estrogen/Progestin Intervention (PEPI) trial. In this 3-year, randomized, double-blind, placebo-controlled trial, the investigators evaluated differences in selected heart disease risk factors among 875 postmenopausal women who received placebo, conjugated estrogens, or one of three conjugated estrogens/progestin regimens. One of the regimens utilized in this study was identical to that present in conjugated estrogens.

The investigators reported that after 3 years of therapy, women taking the conjugated estrogens regimen experienced significant increases in HDL-C levels as compared to placebo. However, the increases were significantly less than that experienced by women taking conjugated estrogens alone. As compared to placebo, LDL-C values were significantly decreased in women taking the conjugated estrogens, with no significant difference between

groups. Total cholesterol levels decreased significantly among women taking the conjugated estrogens regimen as compared to placebo. Significant increases in serum triglyceride levels occurred in all treatment arms as compared to placebo. There were no significant changes in blood pressure, fasting insulin levels or 2-hour insulin levels among treatment groups. Treatment groups had significant increases in 2-hour glucose levels and significant decreases in fasting glucose levels compared with placebo. In pair wise comparisons, women in the placebo group had greater increases in fibrinogen than women in the active treatment groups, with no significant differences between active treatment groups. Among their findings, the investigators concluded that, ". . . oral estrogen taken alone or with MPA . . . is associated with improved lipoprotein and lower fibrinogen levels compared with placebo and . . . the magnitude of these differences is likely to be clinically significant."

Unlike the effect of oral contraceptives in younger women, estrogen replacement therapy (ERT) among postmenopausal women does not raise blood pressure. In a study of women aged 52 to 87 years living in a Southern California retirement community, Pfeffer observed the effect of estrogen use on blood pressure for at least a 5-month period in comparison with a carefully matched group of women who did not receive estrogen. No difference in blood pressure was seen between the two groups. Similar results were reported by Wren, who noted a significant fall in blood pressure when piperazine estrone sulfate was administered to 150 postmenopausal women.

In postmenopausal women treated with usual estrogen replacement doses, a doubling of the incidence of coronary heart disease has been observed in at least one study (Gordon), although the total mortality is not changed. This increase is in the occurrence of angina pectoris. The incidence of myocardial infarctions is not enhanced. On the other hand, Ross et al. reported a decrease in the death rate from ischemic heart disease in patients receiving conjugated estrogens when compared with matched controls.

Bain found that estrogen users aged 30 to 50 years who had bilateral oophorectomy showed a 0.4 relative risk of myocardial infarction. In the Lipid Research Clinics Program involving almost 2300 women aged 40 to 69 years observed for an average 5.6 years, Bush noted that the relative risk for estrogen users as compared with nonusers was 0.37. In short, probably because of its beneficial effect on lipids and blood pressure, as well as possibly on other factors, ERT has been associated with less overall morbidity and mortality from coronary and total cardiovascular disease. Also, estrogen in doses used for replacement therapy has not been associated with an enhanced incidence of stroke or thrombophlebitis.

At least 8 case-control studies and 7 cohort studies (Table 4-7) have examined the relationship between estrogen use and cardiovascular disease. Most studies have shown powerful protection against heart disease, reduction being about 50% in several large studies. The mechanism involved is unclear. Most attention has centered on the favorable changes induced in serum lipids by estrogens, but a protective effect against atherosclerosis independent of lipid changes has been demonstrated in animals. In the largest study of the effect of estrogen replacement therapy on cardiovascular disease, powerful protection was evident after controlling for the effects of cigarette smoking, hypertension, diabetes, high cholesterol levels, obesity, and a parental history of myocardial infarction. Hence, a strong family history of coronary artery disease may be a therapeutic indication for estrogen replacement therapy.

Findings from the epidemiological studies are not completely consistent. However, predominant evidence strongly suggests that women undergoing postmenopausal estrogen therapy ERT are at decreased risk for coronary heart disease (CHD). The consistency of the findings is more apparent in the better designed and analyzed studies. In the Nurses' Health Study reported by Stampfer, an attempt was made to determine whether the apparent benefits of estrogen could be explained by more frequent contact with the medical care system. One analysis included only subjects with a recent physician visit and the results were virtually unchanged, suggesting that this explanation was untenable. The second analysis included higher risk woman characterized by hypertension, diabetes, current cigarette smoking, high cholesterol, and obesity. If the estrogen effect is merely a marker of good health, one should expect little or no benefits in low risk women. However, the relative risk for estrogen use in these women was 0.5. Current users of estrogen appear to enjoy greater protection than past users. More protection is seen from estrogen among nonsmokers or light smokers but in even heavy smokers there appears to be a beneficial effect. Despite the fact that there are many gaps in our current knowledge, the preponderance of evidence from epidemiologic studies strongly supports the view that postmenopausal estrogen therapy can substantially reduce the risk of CHD.

Osteoporosis

Two anatomical areas are of interest in the bone remodeling process. The first is the axial skeleton, composed primarily of trabecular bone. The second is the appendicular skeleton, composed primarily of cortical bone. The remodeling cycle is the same in both types of bone. However, because of the greater surface area, approximately 40% of trabecular bone, as opposed to 10% of the cortical bone is in "turn over" each year. The osteoclast is responsible for the resorption of old bone, which results in the formation of a resorption cavity. Osteoblasts are then attracted to the cavity where they secrete osteoid, which is primarily type I collagen. The collagen is mineralized mainly with calcium, producing new bone with an appropriate mechanical strength. Under normal circumstances, the amount of bone removed is replaced with fresh bone; however, this process can become uncoupled if osteoclasts remove more bone than can normally be replaced by osteoblasts, resulting in net loss of bone mass. In menopausal women, accelerated bone loss is associated with high bone turn over rate and increased osteoclast activity. It is thought that estrogen inhibits osteoclast activity and increases proliferation of osteoblasts as well as collagen production.

Estrogen's beneficial effects in preventing or treating postmenopausal osteoporosis are becoming better recognized. At the same time there is growing recognition that osteoporosis is a major public health problem in the United States. The disease may account for as many as 1 to 2 million fractures each year, including about 350,000 hip injuries, 85% of which are sustained by women. Approximately 10% of patients with hip fractures die of surgical complications within 6 months of fracture. Approximately 25% of all white women over the age of 60 have spinal compression fractures resulting from osteoporosis. The risk of hip fracture is 20% by the age of 90, and hip fractures are about 2.5 times more common in women than in men. An increased rate of loss of both cortical and cancellous bone is associated with the menopause. In a follow-up study of 82 postmenopausal women 5 to 10 years after their first examination, Meema et al. concluded that (1) menopausal women as a group lost bone, and the beginning of this loss is less related to age than to loss of ovarian function; (2) the rate of loss was not significantly correlated with age; and (3) the bone loss was prevented by estrogen administration (i.e., 0.625 mg of conjugated estrogens). A similar beneficial effect of estrogen administration was shown by Lindsay et al. (Figure 4-9) in a short-term double-blind study of changes in metacarpal bone in oophorectomized women given an average daily dose of 25 mg of mestranol.

Nachtigall et al. conducted a 10-year double-blind prospective study to evaluate the effects of estrogen replacement therapy. They took a sample population of 84 pairs of randomly chosen postmenopausal patients who were matched for age and diagnosis. Half the patients received conjugated estrogens and cyclic progesterone while the other half received placebo. The estrogen-treated patients whose therapy was started within 3 years of menopause showed improvement or no increase in osteoporosis. The control patients demonstrated an increase in osteoporosis. A subsequent report by the same authors showed that there was no statistically significant difference in the incidence of thrombophlebitis, myocardial infarction, or uterine cancer in the two groups. Indeed, there was a lower incidence of breast cancer in the treated group. Estrogen-treated patients did show a higher incidence of cholelithiasis. The low number of cases precludes drawing any real conclusions from the data on diseases of low frequency. The study does exclude a high incidence of complications from estrogens.

In another crossover study comparing the effects of estrogen-progestin therapy with those of placebo, bone mineral content increased during the 3 years of combination hormone therapy but continued to decrease in the placebo-treated group (Figure 4-10). When placebo was given to some of the estrogen-progestin group, bone density decreased, whereas the placebo-treated women

had an increase in bone mineral content after being given estrogen-progestin therapy. Other factors are also important in preventing osteoporosis: at least adequate dietary (and possibly supplementary) calcium, exercise, and possibly vitamin D.

Estrogen Replacement Therapy (ERT) for Endometrial and Breast Cancer Survivors
ERT for the endometrial cancer survivor

Although estrogen administration has not been shown to have adverse effects on patients who have been treated for endometrial cancer, many physicians continue to be reluctant to administer this medication to these women. Presumably an occult and quiescent focus of metastatic disease could be exacerbated by the administration of exogenous estrogen. The potential detriments and the magnitude of the patient's discomfort if not taking exogenous estrogen has to be weighed against the relative risks involved. Obviously, women with low-grade tumors and lesions with minimal myometrial invasion are better candidates, since they are more likely to be disease free, especially if 2 or more years have elapsed since initial diagnosis and therapy.

Historically, hormone replacement is contraindicated for the patient who has had treatment for adenocarcinoma of the uterus. However, no data in the literature substantiate the detrimental effects of estrogen in these patients. It is not unusual to see a significant number of patients with appreciable postmenopausal symptoms after treatment for adenocarcinoma. Since the mid-1970s, we have treated individual patients with estrogen as necessary.

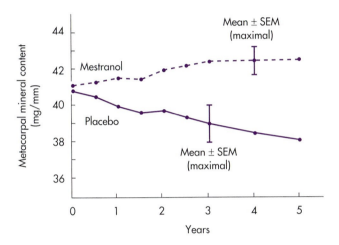

Figure 4-9 Mean metacarpal mineral content during 5-year follow-up of group observed from 3 years after bilateral oophorectomy (zero time). (From Lindsay R et al: *Lancet* 1:1038, 1976.)

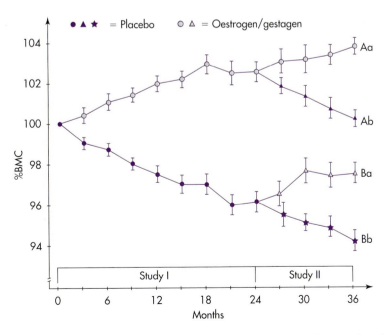

Figure 4-10 Bone mineral content as function of time and treatment in 94 (study I) and 72 (study II) women soon after menopause. (From Christensen C et al: *Lancet* 1:459, 1981.)

From 1975 to 1980, 221 patients with stage I adenocarcinoma of the endometrium were treated at the Duke University Medical Center. Forty seven patients were given posttreatment estrogen and were compared with 174 patients who did not receive estrogen. Multiple prognostic factors were evaluated between the two groups. The only significant variant was a larger number of estrogen-treated women with positive progesterone receptors compared with the non-estrogen-treated patients (no difference in estrogen receptors). Follow-up was available on only 42 patients. Of the 42 estrogen-treated patients, 1 (2%) had recurrence compared with 26 of 174 (15%) of non-estrogen-treated women (p < 0.05). A history of adenocarcinoma of the endometrium does not appear to be an absolute contraindication to estrogen replacement therapy.

In 1989, Lee and his associates reported a similar study. Their report described 144 patients with clinical stage I endometrial adenocarcinoma treated over an 11-year period at two military hospitals. Following staging, 44 selected patients were placed on oral estrogen replacement for a median duration of 64 months. In the estrogen user group, there were no recurrent endometrial cancers and no intercurrent deaths. Of the 99 non-estrogen users, there were 8 recurrences (8%) and 8 intercurrent deaths. Patients on estrogen replacement did have low risk factors for recurrence, namely, low tumor grade (grades 1 and 2), less than one half myometrial invasion, and no metastasis to lymph nodes or other organs. These authors also concluded that postoperative estrogen replacement therapy was safe in selected low-risk patients.

An additional retrospective study was done within the Division of Gynecologic Oncology at Irvine. Patients were treated at UCI Medical Center and Long Beach Memorial Women's Hospital between the years 1982 and 1993. All patients with advanced disease (stage III or IV), histology other than adenocarcinoma, or multiple primaries were excluded. An analysis of 132 patients with stage I or II adenocarcinoma of the endometrium was made; 65 (49%) of the patients received HRT some time after diagnosis and therapy, while 67 similar patients did not receive HRT or ERT and served as controls. The control patients were treated during the same period by the same physicians but were not interested in replacement therapy following initial treatment for their endometrial neoplasia. Sixty-one of the 65 patients receiving HRT took 0.3-1.25 mg (82% received 0.625 mg) of conjugated estrogens, three received only vaginal estrogen cream, and one patient used an estrogen patch. All patients also received medroxyprogesterone 2.5 mg by mouth daily.

A comparison of the HRT group to the control group was made with regard to several parameters. The mean age of diagnosis in the control group was significantly higher at 68.6 years (range 36 to 92) as compared to the HRT group with a mean age of 62.3 years (range 27-76). The mean parity was not significantly different with 2.2 and 2.4 respectively for the HRT and control groups. The mean duration of follow-up in the two groups was 58.2 and 31.1 months with the HRT group having the longer follow-up. One explanation for this observed difference is that the use of HRT following treatment became more popular in the later years of the period studied. Follow-up ranged from 2 to 11 months in the HRT group and 2 to 90 months in the control group. Greater than 95% of the HRT group was followed for at least 12 months and 77% had been followed for 24 months or more. This was considered important since 80% of the recurrences occurred within 24 months of treatment. The mean duration of HRT was 36.3 months with a range of 2 to 127 months. The interval of treatment to initiation of HRT ranged from 0 to 162 months with a mean interval of 21.3 months. The mean time to recurrence was nearly identical in both groups, 27.5 months in the HRT group versus 28.2 months in the control group. In the HRT group there was only one death, which was secondary to intercurrent disease and there were no deaths from the disease, and no patients alive with disease at the time of this study. By contrast, in the control group, there were a total of three deaths (4.5%), all of which were secondary to intercurrent disease.

Our data reveals no trend toward increased recurrence rates or poor outcomes in patients receiving HRT following therapy for early stage endometrial carcinoma. These preliminary results support the previous studies which indicate that estrogen replacement therapy appears safe, especially in selected patients.

Prospective randomized studies of this very important question are necessary. In the interim, physicians and patients must make their own individual decisions. Physicians should counsel patients carefully and document such counseling. In these authors' experience, patients are grateful for the relief, which is almost instantaneous; and observing their comfort is gratifying for the physician.

Two major questions emerge. The first is whether it would be prudent to have a treatment-free hiatus between therapy and the commencement of replacement therapy to reduce the likelihood that a patient with a metastatic focus might receive replacement therapy. The second is whether a progestin should be used in combination with the estrogen to abrogate any stimulatory effect on such an occult metastatic focus. We have concluded that the use of progestin with estrogen in these patients is reasonable and prudent. Medroxyprogesterone acetate has been suggested in a dose ranging from 2.5 mg to 10 mg daily. The most effective dose is unknown. Easier patient compliance and the adverse effect on the lipid profile of higher doses make the use of low to moderate daily doses of progestin more attractive. To that end, we recommend that the patient receive conjugated estrogens 0.625 mg and medroxyprogesterone acetate 2.5 mg daily in a continuous regimen. There are some inconsistencies in current practice. Many physicians feel more comfortable prescribing this regimen only to patients in the so-called "low-risk" categories of endometrial carcinoma. These low-risk categories include well-differentiated lesions with a low probability of recurrence. However, it is these well-differentiated lesions that are the potentially most sensitive to the hormone manipulative therapy, as demonstrated by the studies of the use of progestins for recurrent endometrial carcinoma. In point of fact, patients with grade 3 lesions are most likely to have a recurrence. On the contrary, this grade of lesion is unlikely to respond to either exogenous estrogen or progesterone. However, many clinicians continue to be hesitant to prescribe hormone replacement therapy for this latter group of patients. In summary, there seems to be no consistent line of reasoning separating good candidates from poor candidates for this regimen.

The other question, concerning an appropriate interval between initial therapy and commencement of hormone replacement therapy, is likewise convoluted. It is true that 80% to 90% of all recurrences occur in the first 2 years following initial therapy for endometrial carcinoma. If the suspected adverse effect of estrogen indeed exists, waiting 2 years to commence hormone replacement therapy would narrow the risk group by 80% to 90%. However, 2 years can be very lengthy for a symptomatic patient. Severe vaginal dryness can lead to serious and permanent marital difficulties. Loss of a positive effect on osteoporosis and the onset of ischemic heart disease may not be recovered. Discomfort, including insomnia and hot flashes, may persist relentlessly. If the physician feels that waiting 2 years is necessary, that physician must have come to the conclusion that there is substantive evidence that exogenous estrogen may adversely affect outcome for these patients. It therefore seems illogical that the physician would now be willing (2 years later) to subject the remaining 10% to 20% of patients to that increased risk. If there is an increased risk, it continues for 5 to 10 years for some percentage of patients. The question is whether estrogen therapy is truly contraindicated and whether it definitely affects survival negatively in these patients. Also, does the benefit to the patient outweigh the potential risk? These are the issues about which the physician must come to a decision.

In 1993, the American College of Obstetricians and Gynecologists released the following statement: "In women with a history of endometrial cancer, estrogens could be used for the same indications as for any other woman, except that the selection of appropriate candidates should be based on prognostic indicators and the risk the patient is willing to assume." In the absence of

good prospective studies, this statement appropriately leaves the issue with the patient and physician.

ERT for the breast cancer survivor.

The 'standard of practice' has been to prohibit breast cancer survivors from using hormone replacement therapy (HRT). However, in the last two decades there has been ever increasing evidence that postmenopausal estrogen replacement therapy (ERT) protects against osteoporosis and ischemic heart disease. This author believes firmly that a reappraisal of the 'standard of practice' is essential and long over due. The search for a prospective randomized study addressing this critical issue has been difficult and, to date, fruitless. The practitioner must now utilize indirect evidence in helping patients make a decision on this very important aspect of health and wellness for breast cancer survivors.

In 1989, Wile and DiSaia suggested that in the absence of a prospective study of ERT in breast cancer survivors, one could analyze situations in which these patients were inadvertently exposed to high levels of estrogen at times when they may have been harboring breast cancer cells. These situations were defined as pregnancy coincident with breast cancer, pregnancy subsequent to breast cancer, breast cancer in previous and current users of oral contraceptives (OCs), and breast cancer in postmenopausal women receiving ERT. Currently, approximately 185,000 cases of breast cancer occur in the United States annually. As 67% of these patients will survive this devastating disease to experience old age, we must address the advisability of HRT in this setting.

Approximately 10% to 20% of breast cancers occur in women aged 15 through 44, and between 0.5% and 4% may be diagnosed surrounding pregnancy and/or lactation. It has been established that the average breast cancer lies occultly in the breast some 5 to 8 years prior to diagnosis. This current knowledge of tumor growth rates suggests that cancers diagnosed up to 7 years after a delivery may have coexisted with a pregnancy.

Holleb, Farrow, and others have conclusively established that when pregnant patients with breast cancer are compared with non pregnant breast cancer patients of similar age and stage of disease, pregnancy does not confer a worse prognosis.

Women of reproductive age may choose to become pregnant after breast cancer treatment. Since the incidence of breast cancer in women of reproductive age is increasing, the number of pregnancies occurring after breast cancer treatment will probably increase. Many physicians have recommended against subsequent pregnancies, fearful that it might activate dormant cancer cells. However, pregnancy after breast cancer treatment does not appear to adversely affect survival. Mignot reported that survival of women who conceived even within six months after breast cancer treatment was not different from that of controls. Indeed, breast cancer patients who subsequently become pregnant seem to survive longer than comparable patients who do not become pregnant, even after eliminating biases for women with poor prognoses who are advised not to conceive and for women who are unlikely to become pregnant owing to recurrences.

Again, given the long natural history of this neoplasm, it is certain that a large number of patients subsequently diagnosed with breast cancer used OCs during the genesis and progression of their malignant disease process. The Rosner study was of particular interest, since 347 patients with primary breast cancer aged 50 years and under were analyzed. Among 112 OC users and 235 non users, no significant differences were found in the disease free survival, metastatic period, or overall survival. Users for less than 2 years had a similar survival to those whose OC use was of longer duration. Recent OC users (within 1 year of diagnosis) had a similar survival to that of those who stopped use more than one year prior to diagnosis. No significant differences were noted in survival between patients who began use 10 years or more before diagnosis and those beginning more recently. In summary, their data showed no adverse effect of OC use on the outcome of breast cancer, regardless of the duration of use or latency period.

Noncontraceptive estrogens where first marketed in the United States in 1942. Since then, these medications have been used extensively as ERT to relieve menopausal symptoms and, most recently, to prevent or retard the development of osteoporosis and ischemic heart disease in older women.

Bergkvist compared 261 women who developed breast cancer in a population-based cohort of estrogen-treated women with 6,617 breast cancer patients who had no recorded estrogen treatment. Complete follow-up was achieved during a period up to 9 years. The relative survival rate was significantly higher, by about 10 percentage points at 8 years, in patients who had received estrogen treatment—corresponding to an approximately 40% reduction in excess mortality. The times from the use of estrogen to diagnosis and the total duration of estrogen medication were unrelated to survival when the effect of recent use was taken into account in a multivariant analysis. A similar study by Strickland and colleagues demonstrated the same improved survival in patients in whom breast cancer was diagnosed while taking estrogen replacement therapy. This strongly argues against the so-called "fuel on the fire" theory proposed by those who prohibit ERT for breast cancer survivors.

An argument frequently used against the use of estrogen products in breast cancer survivors is that tamoxifen, "an antiestrogen," is effective treatment for patients with ER-positive breast cancer metastases. Indeed, tamoxifen is now used as adjuvant therapy in women with ER-positive breast cancers, regardless of

nodal or menopausal status. There is a 20% reduction in mortality associated with tamoxifen therapy among breast cancer patients who are 50 years of age or older. Approximately 50% of new breast cancers diagnosed in the United States are ER-positive. The question is whether tamoxifen is truly an "antiestrogen." This author believes that tamoxifen is really just a weak estrogen. Recent studies have shown that tamoxifen reduces the total cholesterol by an average of 10% to 12% and the low-density lipoprotein cholesterol by 20%. In premenopausal patients, standard dose of tamoxifen leads to a dramatic increase in the serum estradiol levels. Analogous to ERT, tamoxifen therapy appears to reduce the loss of bone mineral content. Indeed most of the biologic actions of tamoxifen are similar to those of a weak estrogen.

One need not postulate that tamoxifen is an "antiestrogen" to explain its positive therapeutic effect in breast cancer patients. Tamoxifen is a biologically active substance with activity in the nucleus and the cytoplasm that could explain its antitumor properties. Tamoxifen inhibits secretion by breast cancer cells of transforming growth factor alpha and epidermal growth factor while stimulating production of transforming growth factor-beta. Both transforming growth factor alpha and epidermal growth factor promote breast cancer. Transforming growth factor-beta inhibits growth of many epithelial cell lines, including estrogen receptor negative breast cancer cells. Additional antiproliferative effects of tamoxifen may relate to its inhibition of protein kinase C, its binding to calmodulin, and its ability to decrease insulin-like growth factor I. Therefore, the therapeutic effects of tamoxifen in breast cancer patients may be a function of biologic activities unrelated to its proclivity for the estrogen receptor.

In 1993, DiSaia et al. reported on their experience with 77 breast cancer survivors who had accepted HRT after breast cancer therapy. Patients were followed for a period of up to 15 years. The median age at diagnosis was 50 years. The median interval between diagnosis and the beginning of HRT was 23.8 months, with 37 patients starting within 24 months. The median duration of therapy was 27 months; all but 13 had taken progestin with estrogen. Most patients received HRT as conjugated estrogens. Approximately 40% of the patients received tamoxifen as well as HRT during some period of the treatment course. No differences were noted clinically (symptoms or physical findings) among the patients receiving tamoxifen in addition to HRT versus patients receiving only HRT. Seven women had breast cancer recurrence after starting HRT (average interval from diagnosis to relapse was 45.3 months). Of these patients, five were still taking HRT at the time of recurrence, whereas two had stopped HRT before recurrence was diagnosed. Of the 77 patients started on HRT, 71 had no evidence of disease at the time of their report. Three were alive with disease and three had died, one of complications of chemotherapy and two of progressive disease. Among the 70 patients with no evidence of recurrence only three have stopped taking HRT. The authors felt that their experience with this group of 77 patients did not support the "fuel on the fire" theory.

A more complete analysis of these situations is found in a review article by DiSaia. In fact, no prospective randomized study has ever tested the therapeutic impact of HRT on breast cancer survivors. Indirect evidence, outlined above, suggests that endogenous and exogenous estrogen has not influenced the outcome of patients treated for breast cancer. On the other hand, multiple reports have affirmed the beneficial effects of HRT in preventing ischemic heart disease and osteoporosis as well as improving the quality of life. When breast cancer survivors present and request information on HRT for relief of menopausal symptoms, and the other positive effects of which they are becoming increasingly aware, they deserve a comprehensive explanation. Because freedom from recurrent breast cancer can never be guaranteed, some women will develop recurrences coincident with any new hormone exposure; patients must understand this possibility. In our current climate of medical litigation, there is understandable reluctance to offer exogenous estrogen to women with a history of breast cancer; patient and physician education will be necessary to change these patterns. The possibility of developing a new lesion in the remaining breast tissue must be considered. A small number of studies have pointed to a slightly increased risk of developing breast cancer in specific subgroups of patients using ERT. In every incidence, the incidence of risk was minimal and/or of borderline significance. The patient must understand that everything we do in medical practice involves a risk/benefit analysis. This author feels that the proven benefits far outweigh the potential risk. However, the patient must be properly informed, so that she can make her own decisions regarding this important therapeutic tool. We must consider abandoning the practice of universally prohibiting the use of HRT in breast cancer survivors.

HOW TO USE ESTROGENS

In each instance, before estrogen therapy is begun, a thorough evaluation of the woman, including a complete history and physical examination with appropriate laboratory studies, should be done to discern any factors that may put the individual at an increased adverse risk. Any history of abnormal bleeding requires a histologic evaluation of the endometrium before initiation of estrogen therapy, and many authors have recommended that an endometrial evaluation be done even in the asymptomatic patient. Our feeling is that this is unnecessary in the patient with a normal pelvic examination and a history of an uneventful menopause. However, a

Table 4-8   Comparative physiologic doses of common estrogen preparations

Estrogen	Dose (mg)
Ethinyl estradiol	0.02
Diethylstilbestrol	0.25
Conjugated estrogens	0.625
Estrone	1.25

progestin challenge test of 10 mg of medroxyprogesterone or a similar drug for 5 days, as recommended by Gambrell et al., may be prudent before beginning therapy in such patients. Patients without a withdrawal bleed need not be sampled.

It is recommended that patients be started on 0.625 mg of conjugated estrogens or the equivalent (Table 4-8). The exception to this guideline is young women who have been surgically castrated, who must be started at a higher dose (1.25 mg/day) to adequately relieve symptoms. Doses should be increased only with the occurrence of very severe and intolerable symptoms. In each case, before estrogen therapy is instituted, the benefits and risks of this therapy should be weighed for the patient and discussed thoroughly. Some authorities recommend cyclic progestin therapy (the first or last 12 days of each monthly cycle) in addition to the exogenous estrogen to prevent excessive endometrial proliferation. There is considerable merit in this recommendation if the patient and physician will accept periodic menses even late in the postmenopausal period. In an attempt to avoid bleeding, still other authorities recommend giving both estrogen and progestin daily, either continuously or on weekdays only, with no medication on Saturdays and Sundays (Figure 4-11). These more recent regimens appear safe in large clinical studies.

The lowest dose of medroxyprogesterone that prevents endometrial hyperplasia is not known. The clinical studies reported in the literature reflect the use of 10 mg, and we have maintained that dose as optimum. Many patients cannot tolerate that dose, and a reduction is necessary for compliance.

In oligomenorrheic perimenopausal women, 10 mg of medroxyprogesterone should be administered daily for 10 days at intervals of 6 to 12 weeks. More frequent administration (every 6 weeks) will help reduce heavy or prolonged withdrawal bleeding. Many elderly patients are annoyed with the inconvenience of periodic vaginal bleeding, but reduction of estrogen doses below 0.625 mg of conjugated estrogens or its equivalent in an attempt to avoid cyclic bleeding may remove the beneficial effect of the estrogen therapy.

Brenner suggested two other regimens that may be helpful in decreasing the number of bleeding episodes that

Hormone replacement therapy

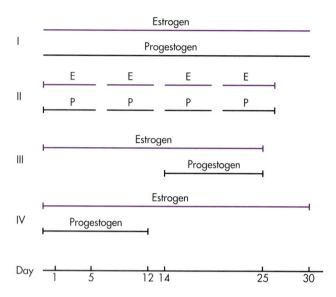

Figure 4-11 Suggested regimens for hormone replacement therapy.

Blood pressure*
Breast examination
Pelvic examination
Endometrial sampling if there is abnormal bleeding

*Monitoring is of questionable value.

are annoying to many patients. In the first, the estrogen-gestagen combination is used daily. Alternatively, he recommended a 5-day regimen of estrogen-gestagen with a drug holiday over the weekend. These regimens have been associated with a minimal amount of bleeding for patients who comply for 6 months or more. Further

studies are necessary to assure that these regimens are equally beneficial (see Figure 4-11).

In situations in which estrogen is contraindicated (e.g., endometrial carcinoma) menopausal symptoms may be somewhat relieved by daily ingestion of progestins such as megestrol acetate (Megace, 20 mg daily) or medroxy-progesterone (Provera, 10 to 20 mg daily). Although vasomotor symptoms are consistently relieved with the use of progestins, patients may complain of vaginal dryness and increased appetite with weight gain. Patients receiving exogenous estrogen therapy should be examined every 12 months for changes in uterine size, excessive breast stimulation, and elevated blood pressure (Table 4-9). Any patient who has any uterine bleeding in the postmenopausal period should be suspected of having endometrial carcinoma until adequate endometrial sampling has proved otherwise.

BIBLIOGRAPHY

Pathologic criteria

Bhagavan BS et al: Comparison of estrogen-induced hyperplasia to endometrial carcinoma, *Obstet Gynecol* 64:12, 1984.

Ferenczy A, Bergeron C: Endometrial hyperplasia. In Lowe D, Fox H, eds., *Advances in gynecological pathology*, London, England: Churchill Livingstone; 207, 1992.

Fox H, Buckley CH: The endometrial hyperplasias and their relationship to endometrial neoplasia, *Histopathology* 6:493, 1982.

Hertig AT, Sommerd SC: Genesis of endometrial carcinoma: study of prior biopsy, *Cancer* 2:946, 1949.

Ingram JM Jr, Novak E: Endometrial carcinoma associated with feminizing ovarian tumors, *Am J Obstet Gynecol* 61:774, 1951.

Kurman RJ, Norris HJ: Evaluation of criteria for distinguishing atypical endometrial hyperplasia from well-differentiated carcinoma, *Cancer* 49:2547, 1982.

Kurman RJ, Norris HJ: Endometrial hyperplasia and metaplasia. In Kurman RJ, editor: *Blaustein's pathology of the female genital tract*, New York, 1987, Springer Verlag.

Silverberg SG: Hyperplasia and carcinoma of the endometrium, *Semin Diagn Pathol* 5:135, 1988.

Sturdee DW et al: Relations between bleeding pattern, endometrial histology, and oestrogen treatment in menopausal women, *Br Med J* 1:1575, 1978.

Winkler B, Alvarez S, Richart RM et al: Pitfalls in the diagnosis of endometrial neoplasia, *Obstet Gynecol* 64:185, 1984.

Clinical profile

Chamlian DL, Taylor HB: Endometrial hyperplasia in young women, *Obstet Gynecol* 36:659, 1970.

Cherkis RC, Patten SF, Dickinson JC et al: Significance of atypical endometrial cells detected by cervical cytology, *Obstet Gynecol* 69 (5):786, 1987.

Emge LA: Endometrial cancer and feminizing tumors of the ovary, *Obstet Gynecol* 1:511, 1953.

Fechner RE, Kaufman RH: Endometrial adenocarcinoma in Stein-Leventhal syndrome, *Cancer* 34:444, 1974.

Gallup DG, Stock RJ: Adenocarcinoma of the endometrium in women 40 years of age or younger, *Obstet Gynecol* 64:417, 1984.

Lyon FA, Frisch MJ: Endometrial abnormalities occurring in young women on long-term sequential oral contraception, *Obstet Gynecol* 47:639, 1976.

Merriam JC Jr et al: Experimental production of endometrial cancer in the rabbit, *Obstet Gynecol* 16:253, 1960.

Pettersson B, Bergstrom R, Johansson EDB: Serum estrogens and androgens in women with endometrial carcinoma, *Gynecol Oncol* 25:223, 1986.

Sirota DK, Marinoff SC: Endometrial carcinoma in Turner's syndrome following prolonged treatment with diethylstilbestrol, *Mt Sinai J Med* 42:586, 1975.

Weiss NS, Szekely DR, Austin DF: Increasing incidence of endometrial cancer in the United States, *N Engl J Med* 294:1259, 1976.

Wood GP, Boronow RC: Endometrial adenocarcinoma and the polycystic ovary syndrome, *Am J Obstet Gynecol* 124:140, 1976.

Premalignant potential

Creasman WT: Estrogen replacement therapy: is previously treated cancer a contraindication? *Obstet Gynecol* 77 (2):308, 1991.

Ferenczy A, Gelfand MM, Tzipris F: The cytodynamics of endometrial hyperplasia and carcinoma: a review, *Ann Pathol* 3:189, 1983.

Gusberg SB: Precursors of corpus carcinoma, estrogens, and adenomatous hyperplasia, *Am J Obstet Gynecol* 54:905, 1947.

Gusberg SB, Moore DB, Martin F: Precursors of corpus cancer. II. A clinical and pathological study of adenomatous hyperplasia, *Am J Obstet Gynecol* 68:1472, 1954.

Gusberg SB, Hall RE: Precursors of corpus cancer. III. The appearance of cancer of the endometrium in estrogenically-conditioned patients, *Obstet Gynecol* 17:397, 1961.

Gusberg SB, Kaplan AL: Precursors of corpus cancer, *Am J Obstet Gynecol* 87:662, 1963.

Jackson RL, Dockerty MB: The Stein-Leventhal syndrome analysis of 43 cases with special reference to association with endometrial carcinoma, *Am J Obstet Gynecol* 73:161, 1957.

Kraus FT: High-risk and premalignant lesions of the endometrium, *Am J Surg Path* 9 (3):31, 1985.

Kurman RJ, Kalminski PF, Norris HJ: The behavior of endometrial hyperplasia: a long term study of "untreated" hyperplasia in 170 patients, *Cancer* 56:403, 1985.

Welch WR, Scully RE: Precancerous lesions of the endometrium, *Hum Pathol* 8:503, 1977.

Management

Bonte J et al: Hormonoprophylaxis and hormonotherapy in the treatment of endometrial adenocarcinoma by means of medroxyprogesterone acetate, *Gynecol Oncol* 6:60, 1978.

Bullock JL, Massey FM, Gambrell RD Jr: Use of medroxyprogesterone acetate to prevent menopausal symptoms, *Obstet Gynecol* 46:165, 1975.

Chu J, Schweid AI, Weiss NS: Survival among women with endometrial cancer: a comparison of estrogen users and nonusers, *Am J Obstet Gynecol* 143:569, 1982.

Gal D, Edman CD, Vellios F et al: Long-term effect of megestrol acetate in the treatment of endometrial hyperplasia, *Am J Obstet Gynecol* 146:316, 1983.

Rigg LA, Hermann H, Yen SS: Absorption of estrogens from vaginal creams, *N Engl J Med* 298:195, 1978.

Steiner GJ, Kistner RW, Craig JM: Histological effects of progestin on hyperplasia and carcinoma in situ of the endometrium—further observations, *Metabolism* 14:356, 1965.

Varma TR: Effect of long-term therapy with estrogen and progesterone on the endometrium of postmenopausal women, *Acta Obstet Gynecol Scand* 64:41, 1985.

Wilson PA, Kolstad P: *Hormonal treatment of preinvasive and invasive carcinoma of the corpus uteri in endometrial cancer*, London, 1973, William Heinemann Medical Books.

Estrogens and endometrial neoplasia

Aitken JM et al: Osteoporosis after oophorectomy for nonmalignant disease in premenopausal women, *Br Med J* 2:325, 1973.

Anderson JJ, Ferguson DJP, Raab GH: Cell turnover in the "resting" human breast: influence of parity, contraceptive pill, age and laterality, *Br J Cancer* 46:376, 1982.

Antunes CMF, et al: Endometrial cancer and estrogen use: report of a large case-control study, *N Engl J Med* 300:9, 1979.

Baker DP: Estrogen replacement therapy in patients with a previous diagnosis of endometrial carcinoma, *Comprehensive Therapy* 16(1):28, 1990.

Boston Collaborative Drug Surveillance Program, Boston University Medical Center: Surgical confirmed gall-bladder disease, venous thromboembolism, and breast tumors in relation to postmenopausal estrogen therapy, *N Engl J Med* 290:15, 1974.

Bryant GW: Admin of estrogens to patients with a previous diagnosis of endometrial adenocarcinoma, *Southern Med J* 83(6):725, 1990 (letter).

Chapman JA et al: Estrogen replacement in surgical stage I and II endometrial cancer survivors, *Am J Obstet Gynecol* 175:1195, 1996.

Christiansen C, Christiansen MS, Transbol I: Bone mass in postmenopausal women after withdrawal of oestrogen/progestogen replacement therapy, *Lancet* 1:459, 1981.

Creasman WT et al: Estrogen replacement therapy in the patient treated for endometrial cancer, *Cancer* 67:326, 1986.

Fremont-Smith M et al: Cancer of the endometrium and prolonged estrogen therapy, *JAMA* 131:805, 1946.

Gambrell RD Jr: Preventing endometrial cancer with progestins, *Contemp Obstet Gynecol* 17:133, 1981.

Gordon GE, Greenberg BG: Exogenous estrogen and endometrial cancer and invited review, *Postgrad Med* 59:67, 1976.

Gray LA, Christopherson WM, Hoover RN: Estrogens and endometrial carcinoma, *Obstet Gynecol* 49:385, 1977.

Greene HSN: Uterine adenomata in the rabbit: susceptibility as a function of constitutional factors, *J Exp Med* 73:273, 1941.

Gusberg SB, Kardon P: Proliferative endometrial response to thecal granulosa cell tumors, *Am J Obstet Gynecol* 3:633, 1971.

Henderson BE, Ross RK, Paganini-Hill A: Estrogen use and cardiovascular disease, *J Reprod Med* 30:814, 1985.

Hoogerlan DL et al: Estrogen use—risk of endometrial carcinoma, *Gynecol Oncol* 64:451, 1978.

Hoover R et al: Menopausal estrogens and breast cancer, *N Engl J Med* 295:401, 1976.

Horowitz RI, Feinstein AR: Alternative analytic methods for case-control studies of estrogens and endometrial cancer, *N Engl J Med* 299:1089, 1978.

Horowitz RI, Feinstein AR: Susceptibility bias and the estrogen-endometrial cancer controversy (meeting abstract), *Clin Res* 27:222A, 1979.

Kay CR: Progestogens and arterial disease: evidence from the Royal College of General Practitioners' study, *Am J Obstet Gynecol* 142:762, 1982.

Killacke MA, Halkes TB, Pierce VK: Endometrial endocarcinoma in breast cancer patients receiving anti-estrogens, *Cancer Threat Rep* 69:237, 1985.

Kistner RW: Histological effects of progestins on hyperplasia and carcinoma in situ of the endometrium, *Cancer* 12:1106, 1959.

Lee RB, Burke TW, Park RC: Estrogen replacement therapy following treatment for stage I endometrial carcinoma, *Gynecol Oncol*, 36-189, 1990.

Lyon FA: The development of adenocarcinoma of the endometrium in young women receiving long-term sequential oral contraception, *Am J Obstet Gynecol* 123:299, 1975.

MacDonald PC, Siiteri PK: The relationship between the extraglandular production of estrone and the occurrence of endometrial neoplasia, *Gynecol Oncol* 2:259, 1974.

Mack TM et al: Estrogens and endometrial cancer in a retirement community, *N Engl J Med* 294:1262, 1976.

Mansell H, Hertig AT: Granulosa-theca cell tumor and endometrial carcinoma: a study of their relationship and survey of 80 cases, *Obstet Gynecol* 6:385, 1955.

Marrett LD et al: Recent trends in the incidence and mortality of cancer of the uterine corpus in Connecticut, *Gynecol Oncol* 6:183, 1978.

McDonald TW et al: Exogenous estrogen and endometrial carcinoma: case control and incidence study, *Am J Obstet Gynecol* 49:385, 1977.

Nachtigall LE et al: Estrogen replacement therapy. I. A 10-year prospective study in the relationship to osteroporosis, *Obstet Gynecol* 53:277, 1979.

Norris HJ, Taylor HB: Prognosis of granulosa-theca tumors of the ovary, *Cancer* 21:255, 1968.

Pacheco JC, Kempers RD: Etiology of postmenopausal bleeding, *Obstet Gynecol* 32:40, 1968.

Riggs BL et al: Short and long-term effects of estrogen and synthetic anabolic hormone in postmenopausal osteoporosis, *J Clin Invest* 51:1659, 1972.

Rosenwaks Z et al: Endometrial pathology and estrogens, *Obstet Gynecol* 53:403, 1979.

Scott RB, Wharton LR Jr: The effects of excessive amounts of diethylstilbestrol on experimental endometriosis in monkeys, *Am J Obstet Gynecol* 69:573, 1955.

Shapiro S, Kelly JP, Rosenberg L: Risk of localized and widespread endometrial cancer in relation to recent and discontinued use of conjugated estrogens, *N Engl J Med* 313:968, 1985.

Silverberg SQ, Makowski EL: Endometrial carcinoma in young women taking oral contraceptives, *Obstet Gynecol* 46-503, 1975.

Smith DC et al: Estrogens and endometrial cancer in a retirement community, *N Engl J Med* 293:1164, 1975.

Weiss NS, Sayretz TA: Incidence of endometrial cancer in relation to the use of oral contraceptives, *N Engl J Med* 302:551, 1980.

Wigle DT, Grace M, Smith ESO: Estrogen use and cancer of the uterine corpus in Alberta, *Can Med Assoc J* 118:1276, 1978.

Woodruff DJ, Pickar JH: Incidence of endometrial hyperplasia in postmenopausal women taking conjugated estrogens (Premarin) with medroxyprogesterones or conjugated estrogens alone, *Am J Obstet Gynecol* 170:1213, 1994.

Ziel HK, Finkle WD: Increased risk of endometrial carcinoma among users of conjugated estrogens, *N Engl J Med* 293:1167, 1975.

Estrogen-progestin therapy

American College of Obstetricians and Gynecologists, Committee on Gynecologic Practice. Estrogen replacement therapy and endometrial cancer. ACOG Committee Opinion #80. Washington, DC: The American College of Obstetricians and Gynecologists, 1990.

Archer DF et al: Bleeding patterns in postmenopausal women taking continuous combined or sequential regimens of conjugated estrogens with medroxyprogesterone acetate, *Am J Obstet Gynecol* 83:686, 1994.

Armstrong BK et al: Oestrogen therapy after the menopause—boon or bane? *Med J Aust* 148:213, 1988.

Bain C et al: Use of postmenopausal hormones and risk of myocardial infarction, *Circulation* 64:42, 1981.

Jensen J, Riis BJ, Strom V et al: Continuous oestrogen-progestogen treatment and serum lipoproteins in postmenopausal women, *Br J Obstet Gynaecol* 94:130, 1987.

PEPI trial writing group. Effects of estrogen or estrogen/progestin regimens on heart disease risk factors in postmenopausal women, *JAMA* 273:199, 1995.

Prough SG, Aksel S, Wiebe RH et al: Continuous estrogen/progestin therapy in menopause, *Am J Obstet Gynecol* 157(6)1449, 1987.

Sherwin BB, Gelfand MM: A prospective one-year study of estrogen and progestin in postmenopausal women: effects on clinical symptoms and lipoprotein lipids, *Obstet Gynecol* 73(5-1):759, 1989.

Weinstein L: Efficacy of a continuous estrogen-progestin regimen in the postmenopausal patient, *Obstet Gynecol* 69(6)929, 1987.

Whitehead MI et al: The effects of cyclical oestrogen and sequential oestrogen progestogen therapy on the endometrium of postmenopausal women, *Acta Obstet Gynecol Scand Suppl* 65:91, 1977.

Whitehead MI, Siddle N, Lane G et al: The pharmacology of progestogens. In Mishell DR, editor: *Menopause: physiology and pharmacology,* St. Louis, 1987, Mosby.

Estrogens and breast cancer

Bergkvist L, Adami HO, Persson I et al: Prognosis after breast cancer diagnosis in women exposed to estrogen and estrogen-progestogen replacement therapy, *Am J Epidemiol* 130:221, 1989.

Bergkvist L, Adami HO, Persson I et al: The risk of breast cancer after estrogen and estrogen-progestin replacement, *N Engl J Med* 5:293, 1989.

Bonnier P et al: Clinical and biologic prognostic factors in breast cancer diagnosed during postmenopausal hormone replacement therapy, *Obstet Gynecol* 85:11, 1995.

Colditz GA, Walter BS, Willett C et al: Menopause and the risk of coronary heart disease in women, *N Engl J Med* 316:1105, 1987.

Colditz GA et al: Type of postmenopausal hormone use and risk of breast cancer: 12 year follow-up from the Nurses' Health Study, *Cancer Causes Control* 3:433, 1992.

Colditz GA et al: Hormone replacement therapy and risk of breast cancer: results from epidemiologic studies, *Am J Obstet Gynecol* 168:173, 1993.

Colditz GA et al: The use of estrogens and progestins and the risk of breast cancer in postmenopausal women, *New Eng J Med* 332:1589, 1995.

Cooper Dr. Butterfield J: Pregnancy subsequent to mastectomy for cancer of the breast, *Ann Surg* 171:429, 1970.

DiSaia PJ: Hormone replacement therapy in patients with breast cancer: a reappraisal, *Cancer* 71:1490, 1993.

DiSaia PJ et al: Hormone replace therapy in breast cancer (letter), *Lancet* 232-342, 1993.

Dupont WD Page DL: Menopausal estrogen replacement therapy and breast cancer: *Arch Intern Med* 151:67, 1991.

Gambrell RD Jr: Role of hormones in the etiology and prevention of endometrial and breast cancer, *Acta Obstet Gynecol Scand Suppl* 106:37, 1982.

Holleb AI, Farrow JH: The relation of carcinoma of the breast and pregnancy in 283 patients, *Surg Gynecol Obstet* 115:65,1962.

Hoover R, Gray LA Sr, Cole P et al: Menopausal estrogens and breast cancer, *N Engl J Med* 295:401, 1976.

Kaufman DW et al: Estrogen replacement therapy and the risk of breast cancer: results from the case-control surveillance study, *Am J Epidemiol* 134:1375, 1991.

Korenman SG: The endrocrinology of breast cancer, *Cancer* 46:874, 1980.

Mignot L, Morvan F, Berdah J et al: Pregnancy after breast cancer: results of a case study, *Presse Med* 15:1961, 1986.

Nachtigall LE et al: Estrogen replacement therapy. II. A prospective study in the relationship to carcinoma and cardiovascular and metabolic problems, *Obstet Gynecol* 54:74, 1979.

Palmer JR et al: Breast cancer risk after estrogen replacement therapy: results from the Toronto Breast cancer study, *Am J epidemiol* 134:1386, 1991.

Persson I et al: Combined oestrogen-progestogen replacement and breast cancer risk, *Lancet* 340:1044, 1992.

Rosner D, Lane W: Oral contraceptives use has no adverse effect on the prognosis of breast cancer, *Cancer* 57:591, 1986.

Sillero-Arenas M et al: Menopausal hormone treatment and breast cancer: a meta-analysis, *Obstet Gynecol* 79:286, 1992.

Stanford JL et al: Combined estrogen and progestin hormone replacement therapy in relation to risk of breast cancer in middle-aged women, *JAMA* 274 (2):137, 1995.

Steinberg KK et al: A meta-analysis pf the effect of estrogen replacement therapy on the risk of breast cancer, *JAMA* 265:1985, 1991.

Strickland DM et al: The relationship between breast cancer survival and prior postmenopausal estrogen use, *Obstet Gynecol* 80:400, 1992.

Wile AG, DiSaia PJ: Hormones and breast cancer, *Am J Surg* 157:438, 1989.

Benefits of estrogen replacement therapy

Bain C et al: Use of postmenopausal hormones and risk of myocardial infarction, *Circulation* 64:42m 1981.

Barnes RB, Roy S, Lobo RA: Comparison of lipid and androgen levels after conjugated estrogens or depomedroxyprogesterone acetate treatment in postmenopausal women, *Obstet Gynecol* 66:216, 1985.

Bass KM: Plasma lipoproteins as predictors of cardiovascular death in women, *Arch Intern Med* 153:2209, 1993.

Bush TL, Barrett-Conner E, Cowan LD et al: Cardiovascular mortality and non-contraceptive use of estrogen in women: results from the Lipid Research Clinics Program Follow-up Study, Circulation 75:1102, 1987.

Bush TL, Cowan LD, Barrett-Conner E et al: Estrogen use and all-cause mortality: preliminary results from the Lipid Research Clinics Program Follow-up Study, *JAMA* 249-903, 1983.

Christiansen C. Lindsay R: Estrogens, bone loss and preservation, *Osteoporosis Int* 1:7, 1990.

Corson SL: Impact of estrogen replacement therapy on cardiovascular risk, *J Reprod Med* 34:729, 1989.

Erenus M et al: Comparison of the impact of oral vs. transdermal estrogen on serum lipoproteins, *Fertil Steril* 61:300, 1994.

Gambrell RD, Teran AZ: Changes in lipids and lipoproteins with long-term estrogen deficiency and hormone replacement therapy, *Am J Obstet Gynecol* 165:307, 1991.

Gambrell RD Jr: The menopause: benefits and risks of estrogen-progestogen replacement therapy, *Fertil Steril* 37:457, 1982.

Gordon GS, Picchi J, Roof BS: Antifracture efficacy of long-term estrogens for osteoporosis, *Trans Assoc Am Physicians* 86:326, 1973.

Gordon T et al: Menopause and coronary heart disease, *Ann Intern Med* 89:157, 1978.

Hammond CB et al: Effects of long-term estrogen replacement therapy, I: metabolic effects, *Am J Obstet Gynecol* 133-525, 1979.

Hunt K, Vessey M, McPherson K: Mortality in a cohort of long-term users of hormone replacement therapy: an updated analysis, *Br J Obstet Gynaecol* 97:1080, 1990.

Knopp RH: The effect of postmenopausal estrogen therapy on the incidence of arteriosclerotic vascular disease, *Obstet Gynecol* 72(5):23S, 1988.

La Rosa JC: The varying effects of progestins on lipid levels and cardiovascular disease, *Am J Obstet Gynecol* 158(6-2):1621, 1988.

La Rosa JC: Estrogen: risk vs. benefit for the prevention of coronary artery disease, *Coron Artery Dis* 4:588, 1993.

Lindsay R et al: Long-term prevention of post-menopausal osteoporosis by oestrogen: evidence for an increased bone mass after delayed onset of oestrogen treatment, *Lancet* 1:1038, 1976.

Lobo RA: Estrogen and cardiovascular disease, *N Y Acad Sci* 592:286, 1990.

Lobo RA et al: Metabolic impact of adding medroxyprogesterone acetate to conjugated estrogens therapy in postmenopausal women, *Obstet Gynecol* 84(6)987-995, 1994.

Lufkin EG et al: Treatment of postmenopausal osteoporosis with transdermal estrogen, *Ann Intern Med* 117:1, 1992.

Matthews KA, Meilahn E, Kuller LH et al: Menopause and risk factors for coronary heart disease, *N Eng J Med* 321:641, 1989.

Meema S, Bunker ML, Meema HE: Preventive effect of estrogen on postmenopausal bone loss: a follow-up study, *Arch Intern Med* 135:1436, 1975.

Mendoza S et al: Postmenopausal cyclic estrogen-progestin therapy lowers lipoprotein (a), *J Lab Clin Med* 123:837, 1994.

Pfeffer RI, van den Noort S: Estrogen use and stroke in postmenopausal women, *Am J Epidemiol* 103:445, 1976.

Ross RK et al: Menopausal oestrogen therapy and protection from death from ischemic heart disease, *Lancet* 1:858, 1981.

Ross RK, Paganini-Hill A, Mack TM et al: Cardiovascular benefits of estrogen replacement therapy, *Am J Obstet Gynecol* 160:1301, 1989.

Selby PL, Peacock M: The effect of transdermal oestrogen on bone, calcium-regulating hormones and liver in postmenopausal women, *Clin Endocrin* 25:543, 1986.

Stampfer MJ, Colditz GW: Estrogen replacement therapy and coronary heart disease: a quantitative assessment of the epidemiologic evidence, *Prev Med* 20:47, 1991.

Stampfer MJ, Colditz GW, Willett WC et al: Menopause and heart disease: a review, *Ann N Y Acad Sci* 592:193, 1990.

Stampfer MJ, Colditz GA, Willett WC et al: A prospective study of postmenopausal estrogen therapy and cardiovasculat diseases: a ten-year follow-up from the Nurses' Health Study, *N Eng. J Med* 325:756, 1991.

Stampfer MJ, Sacks F, Salvini S et al: A prospective study of cholesterol, apolipoproteins, and the risk of myocardial infarction, *N Eng J Med* 325:373, 1991.

Stampfer MJ, Willett, WC, Colditz Gw et al: A prospective study of postmenopausal estrogen therapy and coronary heart disease, *N Eng J Med* 313:1044, 1985.

Sullivan JM, Zwaag RV, Lemp GF et al: Postmenopausal estrogen use and coronary atherosclerosis, *Ann Intern Med* 108:358, 1988.

Whitehead MI: Effects of hormone replacement therapy on cardiovascular disease: an interview, *Am J Obstet Gynecol* 69(6):929, 1987.

Wilson PWF, Garrison R, Castelli WP: Postmenopausal estrogen use, cigarette smoking, and cardiovascular morbidity in women over 50, *N Engl J Med* 313:1038,1985.

How to use estrogens

Adami HO, Bergstrom R, Holmberg L et al: The effect of female sex hormones on cancer survival, *JAMA* 263(16):2189, 1990.

Gambrell RD, Massey FM, Castaneda TA et al: Use of the progestogen challenge test to reduce the risk of endometrial cancer, *Obstet Gynecol* 55(6):732, 1980.

Henderson BE, Paganini-Hill A, Ross RK: Decreased mortality in users of estrogen replacement therapy, *Arch Intern Med* 151:75, 1991.

Henderson BE, Ross RK, Lobo RA et al: Reevaluating the role of progestogen therapy after the menopause, *Fertil Steril* 49(5):9S, 1988.

Mishell DR, Shoupe D, Moyer DL et al: Postmenopausal hormone replacement with a combination estrogen-progestin regimen for five days per week, *J Reprod Med* 36(5):351, 1991.

Steinberg KK, Thacker SB, Smith J et al: A meta-analysis of the effect of estrogen replacement therapy on the risk of breast cancer, *JAMA* 265(15):1985, 1991.

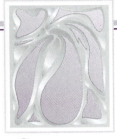

Adenocarcinoma of the Uterus

Cancer of the uterine corpus is the most common malignancy seen in the female pelvis today. It is estimated by the American Cancer Society that approximately 35,000 women will develop uterine cancer this year in the United States, making it the fourth most common cancer in women. The increased incidence of carcinoma of the endometrium has been apparent only during the last several years. In reviewing the predicted incidence for the 1970s, the American Cancer Society noted a 1½-fold increase in the number of patients with endometrial cancer; however there has been a decline in incidence during the late 1980s. Over the last several years, the incidence has remained fairly constant. During the period of increased incidence, predicted deaths from this malignancy actually decreased slightly. More recently, deaths from uterine cancer have increased. In 1990, the American Cancer Society estimated 4000 deaths from this cancer increasing to 6000 in 1996. The increased use of estrogen has been implicated in the apparent increased incidence during the 1970s and early 1980s; however, Norway and Czechoslovakia report a 50% to 60% increase in endometrial cancer, despite the fact that estrogens are rarely prescribed or are not generally available there. Regardless of the reason for the increased number of women with corpus cancer, this malignancy has become an important factor in the care of the female patient.

EPIDEMIOLOGY

Endometrial adenocarcinoma occurs during the reproductive and menopausal years. The median age for adenocarcinoma of the uterine corpus is 61 years, with the largest number of patients noted between the ages of 50 and 59 years. Approximately 5% of women will have adenocarcinoma before the age of 40, and 20% to 25% will be diagnosed before the menopause.

There are increasing data that note the use of combination oral contraceptives (OC) decreases the risk of developing endometrial cancer. The Centers for Disease Control (CDC) evaluated endometrial cancer cases of all women ages 20 to 54 years from eight population-based cancer registries and compared them with controls selected at random from the same centers. A comparison of the first 187 cases with 1320 controls showed that women who used OCs at some time had an 0.5 RR of developing endometrial cancer compared with women who had never used OCs. This protection occurred in women who used OCs for at least 12 months, and protection continued for at least 10 years after OC use. Protection was most notable for nulliparous women. These investigators estimate that about 2000 cases of endometrial cancer are prevented each year in the United States by past or current OC use. Cigarette smoking apparently decreases the risk of developing endometrial cancer. In a population-based case control study of women ages 40 to 60 years, Lawrence et al. found a significant decline in relative risk of endometrial carcinoma with increased smoking ($p < 0.05$). The RR decreased by about 30% when one pack of cigarettes was smoked per day, and another 30% when more than one pack was smoked per day. The effects of smoking did not appear to vary with menstrual status or exogenous estrogen. There was a fourfold increase in smoking-related odds ratio with body weight: the greatest reduction in risk by smoking was in the heaviest women. On the other hand, the estimated risk increased 12-fold in overweight women who were nonsmokers and whose primary source of estrogen was peripheral conversion of androgen to estrogen. Although smoking apparently reduces risk of developing early-stage endometrial cancer, this advantage is strongly outweighed by the increased risk of lung cancer and other major health hazards associated with cigarette smoking.

Multiple risk factors for endometrial cancer have been identified, and MacMahon divides these into three categories: variants of normal anatomy or physiology, frank abnormality or disease, and exposure to external carcinogens. Obesity, nulliparity, and late menopause are all variants of normal anatomy or physiology classically associated with endometrial carcinoma.

These three factors are evaluated in regard to the possible risk of developing endometrial cancer (Table 5-1). If a patient is nulliparous and obese and reaches menopause at age 52 or later, she appears to have a 5-fold increase in the risk of endometrial cancer over the patient who does not satisfy these criteria (Table 5-2). The type of obesity in patients with endometrial cancer has been evaluated. In a study from the University of South Florida, it was noted that women with endometrial cancer had greater waist-hip circumference ratios, abdomen to thigh skin and suprailiac to thigh skin ratios than matched control women. As these ratios increased, the relative risk of endometrial cancer increased. The researchers concluded that upper-body fat localization is a significant risk factor for endometrial cancer. In a large multicenter case-controlled study of 403 endometrial cases and 297 controls, Swanson and associates confirmed and amplified these findings. Women whose weight exceed 78 kg had a 2.3 times risk of those weighing less than 58 K. For women weighing greater than 96K, the RR increased to 4.3. Upper body obesity (waist to height ratio) was a risk factor independent of body weight. Patients in the highest quartile of both weight and waist to thigh circumference had a risk of 5.8 times. The amount of body fat has been associated with decreased circulating levels of both progesterone and sex hormone binding proteins. There was a strong inverse association between sitting height

Table 5-1   Endometrial cancer risk factors

	Risk factors	Risk
Obesity	Overweight	
	21-50 lb	3×
	>50 lb	10×
Nulliparity	Compared with	
	1 child	2×
	5 or more children	3×
Late menopause	Age	
	>52 yr	2.4×

Table 5-2   Multiple risk factors

Risk		
Nulliparous Top 15% in weight Menopause at 52 yr	5 × more than	Parous Lower two thirds in weight Menopause at <49 yr

and risk of endometrial cancer. This may be related to serum hormone-bound globulin (SHBG), which appears to be depressed in women with endometrial cancer. The level of SHGB is progressively depressed with increasing upper-body fat localization. With lower SHGB, there is a higher endogenous production of non-protein-bound estradiol. Since endometrial cancer is related to obesity, dietary habits appear to be important. Data suggest that the levels of estriol, total estrogens, and prolactin were lower and those of SHBG were higher in postmenopausal women who were vegetarians. Levi evaluated in a case-control study of dietary factors in 274 endometrial cancer patients and 572 controls from two areas in Switzerland and northern Italy. Extensive dietary history was obtained. Their data confirmed the relationship between obesity and endometrial cancer. Dietary related, they noted an increased association with total energy intake. After correcting for total energy intake, a risk was present with the frequency of consumption of most types of meats, eggs, beans, added fats, and sugar. Conversely, significant protection was noted with an elevated intake of most vegetables, fresh fruits, whole grain bread, and pasta. This reflected a low risk with increase intake of ascorbic acid and beta-carotene. Of dietary interest is that the intake of olive oil seemed beneficial in Switzerland but resembled other added fats in the Italian women. It has been previously noted that the amount and type of dietary fat influences estrogen metabolism as estrogen reabsorption from the bowel seems to be increased by diets rich in beef or fats.

Diabetes mellitus and hypertension are frequently

associated with endometrial cancer. Kaplan and Cole report a relative risk of 2.8 associated with a history of diabetes after controlling for age, body weight, and socioeconomic status. High blood pressure is prevalent in the elderly, obese patient but does not appear to be a significant factor by itself, even though 25% of endometrial cancer patients have hypertension or arteriosclerotic heart disease. As extensively detailed in Chapter 4, the relationship to unopposed estrogen and endometrial cancer is well documented. Fortunately, the addition of a progestin appears to be protective. Although the risk of unopposed estrogen is present, women on estrogen who develop endometrial cancer appear to have very favorable prognostic factors. Several, but not all studies, suggest that risk factors such as multiparity and obesity are lower in the estrogen users. Stage of disease and histologic grade appear to be lower in estrogen users. When corrected for stage and grade, estrogen users still have less myometrial invasion than non-estrogen users. The poor prognostic subtypes such as clear cell carcinoma and adenosquamous cancer appear less frequently in estrogen users. As a result, survival of estrogen-related endometrial cancer is much better than nonestrogen cancers. In fact, some studies note just as good, if not better, survival in estrogen users than in nonestrogen, non-endometrial cancers.

Incidence and survival is higher in whites compared to black women. Reasons for these differences are unexplained. An analysis of the GOG data base evaluated this factor in 600 white and 91 black women with clinical stage I or II endometrial cancer. A larger number of the African-American women were diagnosed after age 70, had a higher proportion of papillary serous and clear cell histologic types, and had more advanced disease, grade, vascular space involvement, depth of invasion and lymph node metastases than the whites women. Survival (5 year) for whites was 77% and for blacks 60%. Survival difference remained even in high risk groups such as grade 3 tumors (59% vs 37% respectively). The unadjusted hazard rate was 2.0, which was statistically significant. When adjusted for age, cell type, and extent of disease, the RR dropped to 1.2. The adjust risk rate suggests race is not a significant factor; nevertheless, race does denote an increase risk for poor prognostic factors, which clinically may be very important.

Tamoxifen is being used in an increasing amount in women with breast cancer. In addition, a study of the prophylactic use of tamoxifen in women without breast cancer has begun. Several cases of endometrial cancer have been reported in women on tamoxifen. It has not yet been determined if this relationship placed women on tamoxifen at higher risk for adenocarcinoma. It is hoped that several ongoing studies will answer this question. Tamoxifen, although an "antiestrogen," is known to have estrogenic properties. Women on tamoxifen also appear to have some protection from osteoporosis and against heart disease (decreased LDH and cholesterol), much like women on estrogen replacement therapy.

During the recent past, there has been a considerable amount of lay as well as professional publicity in regard to the possible association of tamoxifen with endometrial cancer. Tamoxifen was first introduced in the clinical trials in the early 1970s and approved in 1978 by the FDA for treatment of advanced breast carcinoma in the postmenopausal woman. Tremendous experience with this drug has been observed. It is estimated that over 3 million women in the United States have taken tamoxifen for almost 6 million women years of use. It is suggested that each year about 80,000 women in the United States will begin taking tamoxifen because of a diagnosis of breast cancer and will probably continue it for at least 5 years. With the prophylactic study now being performed, not only in the United States but overseas, this number will likely increase. The efficacy of tamoxifen has proved successful particularly in the postmenopausal patient and is usually considered the drug of choice in this group of women. Those patients with disease spread outside of the breast also appear to benefit substantially from its use. One of its major benefits has been the fact that in women taking tamoxifen there has been a substantial decrease in the incidence of a second cancer in the opposite breast compared to like women who were taking a placebo. In those patients in whom the drug may have been given prophylactically, recurrence has been markedly reduced compared to those not on the drug. Initial studies suggest the drug should be taken for 2 years and recently this has been extended to 5 years. Ongoing studies are evaluating its use for up to 10 years. Therefore there is no question that this drug, which has a relatively low toxicity rate, has proven to be extremely beneficial to women with breast cancer.

In 1985, Killackey reported three breast cancer patients on tamoxifen who subsequently developed endometrial cancer. During the last 10 years, approximately 250 endometrial cancer patients have been reported worldwide in breast cancer patients taking tamoxifen. In many instances, the literature is made up of case reports; however, several "series" have recently been reported. The one that has received the most notoriety is that of the prospective, randomized study of the National Surgical Adjuvant Breast and Bowel Project (NSABP). This study analyzed 2843 patients with node-negative estrogen-receptor positive invasive breast cancer randomly assigned to receive a placebo or 20 mg/day of tamoxifen. An additional 1220 tamoxifen-treated patients were registered and given the drug. The average time on the study was 8 years for the randomly assigned patients and 5 years for the registered patients. Of the 1419 patients randomly assigned to tamoxifen, 15 developed uterine cancer, of which two were sarcomas. One patient randomized to receive tamoxifen did take the drug and developed endometrial cancer 78 months after randomization. In the placebo group, two developed endometrial cancer; however, both were receiving tamoxifen at the time of their uterine malignancy. One patient developed a breast recurrence and was placed on tamoxifen and the other was given tamoxifen after colon cancer. Two of the endometrial cancer patients had been on tamoxifen for only 5 and 8 months, respectively, before their uterine diagnosis was made. There were five patients in the tamoxifen group who developed endometrial cancer after they had been off the drug for 7 to 73 months. In the registered patients who received tamoxifen, eight uterine tumors (7 endometrial) were subsequently diagnosed. Three of these patients had been on tamoxifen for less than a year (2, 2, and 9 months). The authors determined the average annual hazard rate per 1000 women of endometrial cancer in their patient population. This was 0.2/1000 in the placebo group, and 1.6/1000 for the randomized tamoxifen treated patients. In the registered patients receiving tamoxifen, the average annual hazard rate was 1.4/1000, similar to the randomized tamoxifen treated group. The hazard rate of endometrial cancer in the placebo was low when compared to the SEER data, as well as previous NSABP randomized tamoxifen-placebo studies. The latter data would suggest that the average annual hazard rate is 0.7/1000. This data based on very limited number of patients with endometrial cancer while on tamoxifen suggest that there may be a relative risk of 2.3 developing endometrial cancer while on tamoxifen. This does not take into account the well-known fact that women who develop breast cancer are at an increased risk for developing endometrial cancer irrespective of subsequent treatment. The relative risk of 1.72 to over 3 has been reported. The risk benefit of the prevention of recurrences and new breast cancer in comparison to new endometrial cancers were evaluated in the NSABP study. The benefits suggest that 121.3 fewer breast-related events per 1000 women treated with tamoxifen were seen compared to 6.3 endometrial cancers per 1000 women. Therefore the benefit from tamoxifen is apparent.

Initially, it was suggested that rate of tamoxifen-associated endometrial cancers might be equal to those associated with unopposed estrogen replacement therapy. Since tamoxifen is a weak estrogen, similar characteristics of the endometrial cancer were also implied; i.e., well differentiated superficially invasive cancers. Magriples, reporting a retrospective study, identified 15 women who had breast cancer, were on tamoxifen, and developed uterine cancers compared to 38 other breast cancer patients who developed uterine cancer but were not receiving tamoxifen. Tamoxifen was given at 40 mg/day for 3-10 years (mean 4.2 years). These investigators noted that 67% of the tamoxifen treated patients had high grade tumor compared to 24% in the untreated group. Five of the 15 patients died of endometrial cancer, compared to one in the untreated group. They suggested that tamoxifen-associated endometrial cancers carried a poor

prognosis. Barakat reviewed five studies, including Magriples, the NSABP, their own data from Memorial Sloan Kettering Hospital, and two studies from overseas. A total of 103 patients were evaluated in regard to histology, grade of tumor, FIGO staging, and deaths from uterine cancer. He did not find an increase in poor prognostic histology, tumor differentiation, or stage compared to what would be expected in a similar group of non tamoxifen uterine cancer patients. A recent evaluation by Jordan using the SEER data, as well as tamoxifen-associated endometrial cancer in the literature, reported similar findings.

It has been suggested by some individuals, based on extremely limited number of patients, that all women on tamoxifen should have the endometrium evaluated at regular intervals; i.e., yearly. The rationale for this recommendation suggests that uterine cancer is related to the tamoxifen. During the last 10 years, only 250 endometrial cancer patients have been reported in the literature worldwide. During that same time interval, it has been estimated that there have been approximately 350,000 uterine cancers in the United States alone. With over three million women in the United States having taken tamoxifen and only 250 women worldwide reported with tamoxifen-associated endometrial cancer, cost effectiveness of yearly endometrial evaluation does not appear warranted. Certainly, all women, irrespective of whether or not they are on tamoxifen, should have yearly gynecological examinations. The endometrium should be evaluated if the patient is symptomatic. Currently, we do not recommend endometrial sampling nor ultrasound evaluation of the endometrium just because an individual is on tamoxifen. The prophylactic tamoxifen study is evaluating yearly screening and that data will be most helpful in regard to determining optimal management of these patients.

DIAGNOSIS

The cost of screening for adenocarcinoma and its precursors in the total population would be prohibitive. Women on hormonal replacement therapy (estrogen and progesterone) do not need endometrial biopsy prior to institution of therapy or during replacement therapy unless abnormal bleeding occurs. Monthly withdrawal bleeding after progestin is not considered abnormal bleeding. On the other hand, breakthrough bleeding should be evaluated. The use of continuous estrogen alone increases the risk of adenocarcinoma. Estrogen plus progesterone appears to decrease the risk of adenocarcinoma and therefore is the preferred treatment. In asymptomatic high-risk patients, periodic screening may be advisable. Postmenopausal women with uterine bleeding must be evaluated for endometrial cancer, although only 20% of these patients will have a genital malignancy. As the patient's age increases after the menopause, there is a progressively increasing probability that her uterine bleeding is caused by endometrial cancer. Feldman found that age was the greatest independent risk factor associated with endometrial cancer or complex hyperplasia. In a women age 70 or over, the OR was 9.1. If complex hyperplasia was placed in the control group, the OR increased to 16. When a women was over 70 years old, her chance of having cancer when vaginal bleeding was present was about 50%. If she was also nulliparous and had diabetes, the risk was 87%. A perimenopausal patient who may have abnormal uterine bleeding indicative of endometrial cancer may not be evaluated because the patient or her physician interpret her new bleeding pattern as resulting from "menopause." During this time in a woman's life, the menstrual periods should become lighter and lighter and further and further apart. Any other bleeding pattern should be evaluated with carcinoma of the endometrium in mind.

A high index of suspicion must be maintained if the diagnosis of endometrial cancer is to be made in the young patient. Prolonged and heavy menstrual periods and intermenstrual spotting may indicate cancer, and endometrial sampling is advised. Most young patients who develop endometrial cancer are obese, in many instances, massively overweight, often with anovulatory menstrual cycles. Sequential oral contraceptives, which were also incriminated in young patients with endometrial cancer, should no longer be of concern, since these agents are no longer commercially available.

Historically, the fractional D&C has been the definitive diagnostic procedure used in ruling out endometrial cancer. In the 1920s, Kelly advocated the use of what amounts to an outpatient curettage to obtain adequate endometrial tissue for diagnostic study. Today most advocate the routine use of the endometrial biopsy as an office procedure to make a definitive diagnosis and spare the patient hospitalization and an anesthetic. Several studies have indicated that the accuracy of the endometrial biopsy in detecting endometrial cancer is approximately 90%. Hofmeister noted that 17% of the endometrial carcinomas diagnosed by routine office biopsy occurred in asymptomatic perimenopausal women. Unfortunately, in his study, in which the endometrial biopsy was used, several patients may have been missed, because not all of these individuals had a subsequent D&C. Other procedures have been developed to be used on an outpatient basis not only for diagnosis but also for screening. Those techniques using endometrial cytology to make the diagnosis of endometrial cancer have been less successful than those in which tissue itself is evaluated.

Cytologic detection of endometrial cancer by routine cervical Pap smear has generally been poor in comparison with the efficacy of the Pap smear in diagnosing early cervical disease. Several studies in the literature indicate that only one third to one half of the patients with adenocarcinoma of the endometrium have abnormal Pap smears on routine cervical screening. The main reason for the poor detection with the cervical Pap smear is that cells are not removed directly from the lesion as they are on the cervix. When a cytologic preparation is obtained directly from the endometrial cavity, malignant cells are present in higher numbers than those found if routine cervical or vaginal smears are obtained. Techniques that obtain only a cytologic preparation are generally inadequate if used alone.

Several commercial apparatuses are available for sampling the endometrial cavity on an outpatient basis. Devices that remove tissue for histologic evaluation have generally been good if tissue is obtained from the endometrial cavity. Stovall evaluated 40 known endometrial cancer patients with the Pipelle instrument. Ninety percent of the women were postmenopausal. Only in one patient was cancer not identified with the Pipelle. This patient had a prior D&C that revealed a grade I lesion. The Pipelle diagnosis was atypical adenomatous hyperplasia and the hysterectomy specimen revealed a focus of adenocarcinoma in situ. The pathologist noted that the obtainable tissue was acceptable for analysis in 100% of patients. Discomfort was recorded as mild in 80% and only 2 (5%) reported severe pain. In past years, we have used curettes such as the Duncan or Kevorkian successfully; however, in recent years, these have been replaced by the thin disposable suction type curette because they are as successful as the reusable instruments but appear to be less painful for the patient. In the symptomatic patient in whom inadequate tissue (or no tissue at all) is obtained for pathologic evaluation, a D&C must be considered.

The use of multiple diagnostic techniques to increase the capability of outpatient diagnosis appears to be most helpful. The use of cytologic and histologic methods will increase the detection rate of patients with endometrial cancer. If diagnosis of endometrial cancer can be made on an outpatient basis, the patient can avoid hospitalization and a minor surgical procedure. Any cytologic or histologic abnormality short of invasive cancer mandates a formal fractional curettage to rule out a small focus of invasive disease. All patients with persistent symptoms despite normal biopsy should submit to fractional curettage as well.

Hysterography and hysteroscopy have both been suggested as adjuvants in making the diagnosis of endometrial cancer and in establishing the extent of disease. Details seen with hysterography correlate well with surgical findings. Information that can be obtained includes tumor volume, tumor origin, extent of disease within the uterine cavity, shape of the cavity, and cervical involvement. Today hysterography is used infrequently, if at all, as a diagnostic procedure. Hysteroscopy has been used more frequently in the evaluation of patients with abnormal uterine bleeding and has the advantage of being done on an outpatient basis. Since many patients with endometrial cancer can be diagnosed with office biopsy, that is our preferred first diagnostic step. If the biopsy is negative and further evaluation is needed, we proceed to hysteroscopy. With its use, surgeons can direct biopsies of focal lesions that might be missed by D&C. Hysteroscopy can be used to evaluate the endocervical canal.

Ultrasound (U/S) has been suggested as a diagnostic tool in evaluating women with irregular bleeding, particularly the postmenopausal patient. (Figure 5-1, *A-C*)

The endometrial stripe as seen with the transvaginal U/S appears indicative of endometrial thickness. Several studies suggest that if a thin endometrial stripe is present a histologic diagnosis is not necessary, because atrophic endometrium would be present. Varner evaluated 80 postmenopausal women: 65 were asymptomatic with 38 on no hormones and 27 on hormones. There were 60 patients with U/S measured endometrial thickness of ≤4 mm and all on histologic evaluation noted atrophy or low

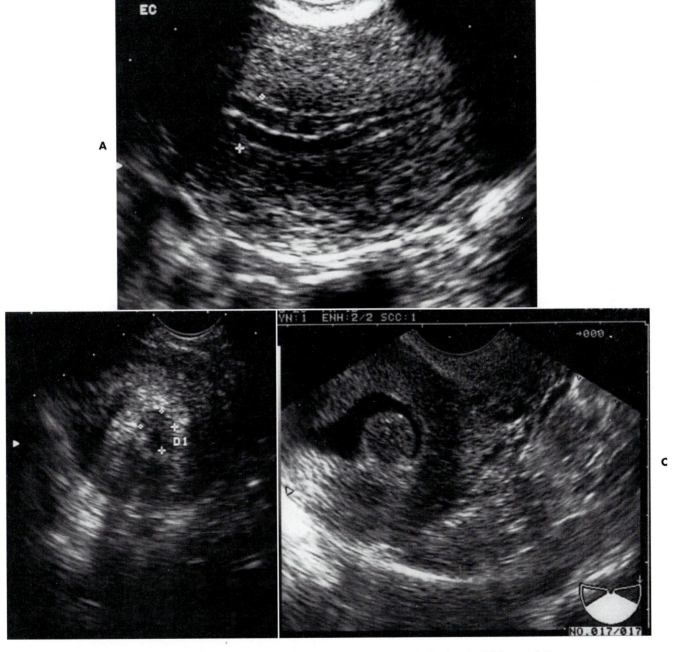

Figure 5-1 A, Ultrasound of the uterus showing the "triple line" indicating the thickness of the endometrium. **B,** Ultrasound of the uterus showing a "thickened endometrium" of >10 mm. **C,** Saline instillation of the endometrial cavity notes a well-defined submucous fibroid and not thickened endometrium.

estrogen stimulation. In women with measured endometrial thickness of 5-8 mm, the type of endometrium, including cancer, could not be distinguished. Unfortunately, for evaluation only two patients had cancer. Granberg evaluated 205 women with postmenopausal bleeding, 30 postmenopausal asymptomatic women, and 30 postmenopausal patients with known endometrial cancer. In the latter 60 patients, the endometrial thickness was 3.2 (mean) vs 17.7 respectively. In the 205 group, 18 were found to have endometrial cancer. No cancers were present in the endometrium that had an endometrial thickness of ≤8 mm. There was considerable overlapping of endometrial thickness by all histologic groups. The authors noted that if a 5 mm cut off was used, no false-negative findings were present. With this measurement, the positive predictive value was 87%, specificity 96%, and sensitivity of 100% for identifying endometrial abnormalities. Bourne, in evaluating 183 selected postmenopausal women of which 34 were asymptomatic and 12 had endometrial cancer, found an overlap of endometrial thickness between women with and without cancer. Other studies have suggested similar findings. It has been suggested that if U/S could save a large number of endometrial biopsies, there would be a large cost savings with less discomfort to the patient. As previously noted, significant pain with the newer disposable endometrial biopsy techniques affects only a small number of patients; and a certain number of patients, because of considerable endometrial thickness, will require endometrial sampling anyway. To date, cost effectiveness has not been demonstrated. Unfortunately, endometrial cancer has been identified when the endometrial thickness is less than 5 mm. Although studies may evaluate several hundred patients, most do not have many cancer patients included. To date, there is no general agreement of the cut off measurement at which endometrial sampling is not necessary. We prefer to sample the endometrium in symptomatic postmenopausal patients as the first diagnostic technique. If histology is "negative," the patient is followed. A D&C is done only if the patient continues to be symptomatic after the negative biopsy.

The U/S has also been evaluated as a means for determining depth of myometrial invasion. Gordon studied 15 known endometrial cancer patients with U/S and MRI. U/S was judged to be more accurate (less than or greater) than MRI; MRI was better in 3, both equally accurate in 4, and neither accurate in 3. It has been suggested by some that U/S can accurately predict myometrial invasion in about 75% of cases. Although knowing the depth of invasion preoperatively would be important information to the clinician, currently the data from studies as noted above would appear to be too premature or too costly to use routinely. We prefer to evaluate depth of myometrial invasion intraoperatively either with gross examination or frozen section.

The reliability of U/S in determining endometrial thickness in the postmenopausal patient does not appear to be applicable to women taking tamoxifen. In all studies, endometrial thickness in the tamoxifen patient is considerably thicker than the non-tamoxifen patient. Histologic evaluation revealed atrophic endometrium in a large number of these tamoxifen patients. Because of this discordance, Lahti evaluated 103 asymptomatic postmenopausal patients (51 on tamoxifen and 52 controls) with U/S, hysteroscopy and endometrial histology. In the tamoxifen group, 84% had endometrial thickness on U/S of ≥5 mm vs 19% in the non-tamoxifen group (51% vs 8% >10 mm respectively). Hysteroscopy findings noted 28% of uterine mucosa was atrophic vs 87% in non-tamoxifen controls. Histopathology noted atrophic endometrium in 60% of tamoxifen vs 79% in controls. The biggest difference between the two groups was 18% polyps in the tamoxifen group vs 0% in the control group. This latter finding appears to be frequently seen in the tamoxifen patient. So-called megapolyps measuring up to 12 cm in size have been described. Other uterine pathology has been attributed to tamoxifen and include increased uterine volume, lower impedance to blood flow in uterine arteries, endometriosis, focal periglandular condensation of stromal cells, and epithelium metaplasia.

Table 5-3 FIGO classification of endometrial carcinoma

Stage		
	Ia G123	Tumor limited to endometrium
	Ib G123	Invasion of less than half of the myometrium
	Ic G123	Invasin of more than half of the myometrium
	IIa G123	Endocervical glandular involvement only
	IIb G123	Cervical stromal invasion
	IIIa G123	Tumor invades serosa and/or adnexae and/or positive peritoneal cytology
	IIIb G123	Vaginal metastases
	IIIc G123	Metastases to pelvic and/or para-aortic lymph nodes
	IVa G123	Tumor invasion of bladder and/or bowel mucosa
	IVb	Distant metastases, including intra-abdominal and/or inguinal lymph node

Histopathology: Degree of differentiation
Cases of carcinoma of the corpus should be grouped according to the degree of differentiation of the adenocarcinoma as follows:
G1 = 5% or less of a nonsquamous or nonmorular solid growth pattern
G2 = 6% to 50% of a nonsquamous or nonmorular solid growth pattern
G3 = more than 50% of a nonsquamous or nonmorular solid growth pattern

Approved by FIGO, October 1988, Rio de Janeiro.

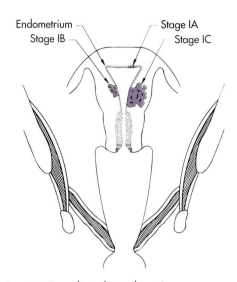

Stage IA: Tumor limited to endometrium
Stage IB: Invasion to less than one-half the myometrium
Stage IC: Invasion to more than one-half the myometrium

Stage I

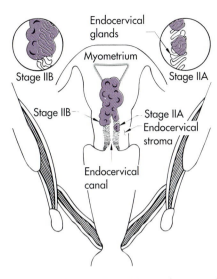

Stage IIA: Endocervical glandular involvement only
Stage IIB: Cervical stroma invasion

Stage II

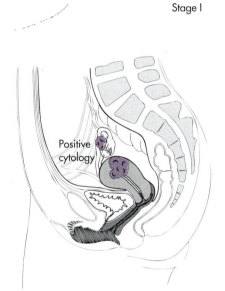

Stage IIIa

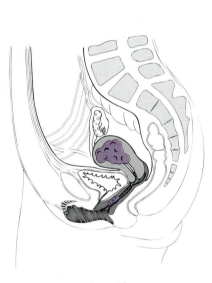

Stage IIIb

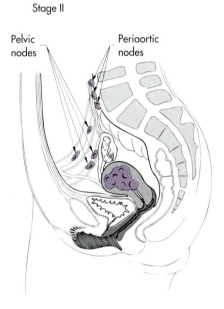

Stage IIIc

FIGO staging for endometrial cancer.

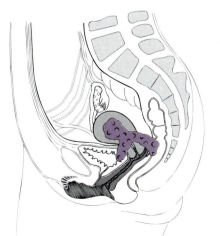

Stage IVa

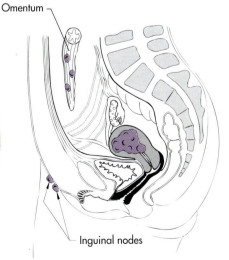

Stage IVb

Table 5-4   Distribution of endometrial carcinoma by stage (surgical)

Stage	Patients
I	4370 (73%)
II	723 (12%)
III	739 (12%)
IV	179 (3%)

From Pettersson F, editor: Annual report on the results of treatment in gynecological cancer, vol. 22, Stockholm, 1994, International Federation of Gynecology and Obstetrics.

PROGNOSTIC FACTORS IN ENDOMETRIAL ADENOCARCINOMA

Histologic type (pathology)
Histologic differentiation
Stage of disease
Myometrial invasion
Peritoneal cytology
Lymph node metastasis
Adnexal metastasis

Data now suggests that the markedly thickened endometrium (up to 40 mm) in tamoxifen patients is not thickened endometrium but proximal myometrium. Goldstein suggested endometrial saline infusion may help delineate the true endometrium from the underlying myometrium. With this technique, he was able to identify large polypoid lesions and other sonolucent cystic spaces that were initially thought to represent thickened endometrium.

After a tissue diagnosis of endometrial malignancy is established, the patient should have a thorough diagnostic evaluation before the institution of therapy. Before 1988, endometrial cancer was clinically staged. Because of the considerable discrepancy between clinical and actual stage, FIGO has now adopted a surgical pathological staging classification (Table 5-3; see Figure 5-1). Approximately 75% of patients with endometrial cancer present with stage 1 disease (Table 5-4). Routine hematologic studies and clotting profiles are obtained on all patients. Presurgical metastatic evaluation should include a chest film, intravenous urogram, and metabolic profiles. Sigmoidoscopy and barium enemas have been reserved for patients who demonstrate palpable disease outside the uterus or have recognizable symptoms of bowel disease. Brain, liver, and bone scans have been used only in patients who are suspected of having extant disease.

PROGNOSTIC FACTORS

Pretreatment evaluation of patients with malignant neoplasms, coupled with clinical pathologic experience, should allow the physician to individualize therapy for the best results. Multiple factors have been identified for endometrial carcinoma that appear to have significant predictive value for these women (see box top right). FIGO, in developing the recent classification for endometrial cancer, has taken into consideration two factors in the substage category within stage I (see Table 5-3). Essentially all reports in the literature agree that differentiation (grade) of tumor and depth of invasion are important prognostic considerations. The patient's clinical profile as it concerns prognosis has been evaluated. Several studies indicate that the age of the patient can be directly related to prognosis, in that younger women do much better than older women. This is probably because younger women tend to have more well-differentiated cancer than older women, and when corrected for grade, age does not appear to be an important prognostic factor. Bokhman suggests there are two pathogenic types of endometrial cancer. The first type arises in women with obesity, hyperlipidemia, and signs of hyperestrogenism, such as anovulatory uterine bleeding, infertility, late onset of menopause, and hyperplasia of the stroma of the ovaries and endometrium. The second pathogenic type of disease arises in women who have none of these disease states or in whom the disease states are not clearly defined. Bokhman's data suggest that patients with the first pathogenic type mainly have a well-differentiated or moderately differentiated tumor, superficial invasion of the myometrium, high sensitivity to progestins, and a favorable prognosis (85% 5-year survival in his material). The group of patients who fall into the second pathogenic group tend to have poorly differentiated tumors, deep myometrial invasion, a high frequency of metastatic disease in the lymph nodes, decreased sensitivity to progestin, and a poor prognosis (58% 5-year survival rate). Unfortunately, Bokhman does not provide a stage breakdown for the two pathogenic groups, although more than 70% of all of his patients had stage I disease. It is assumed from his description that a larger number of patients with the second pathogenic type had more advanced disease, and this may account for the poor prognosis. However, the etiologic role of hyperestrogenism suggested by this study is intriguing, particularly in view of the large number of patients with well-differentiated cancer, superficial invasion, and excellent prognosis in which exogenous estrogen association has been identified. Kauppila, Gornroos, and Nieminen, using only body weight as the determination, noted that in patients with stage I carcinoma of the endometrium the best 5-year survival rate occurred in the heaviest patients (greater than 75 kg), and again this seemed to be related to the fact that heavier patients had fewer anaplastic lesions than did lighter patients.

Pathology

Carcinoma of the endometrium may start as a focal discrete lesion, as in an endometrial polyp. It also may be diffuse in several different areas, in some situations involving the entire endometrial suface. Adenocarcinoma, the most common histologic type, is usually preceded by a predisposing lesion (atypical endometrial hyperplasia). Only those hyperplasias with cellular atypia are considered to be precursors of adenocarcinoma of the endometrium. As tumor volume increases, spread within the endometrium and/or myometrium takes place. As this process continues, dissemination to distant organs can take place. It is recognized that there are multiple prognostic factors in endometrial cancer (see subsequent section), including histological types and the grade of the cancer. A clinically enlarged uterus may be caused by increasing tumor volume, but this should not be used as the only gauge for significant local disease. Obviously, many patients can have enlarged uteri because of factors other than adenocarcinoma.

Adenocarcinoma is the most common histological subtype that may originate in the endometrium (Table 5-5). It is characterized by the presence of glands in an abnormal relationship to each other, with the hallmark of very little, if any, intervening stroma between the glands. There can be variations in the size of the glands, and infolding is common. The cells are usually enlarged, as are the nuclei, along with nuclear chromatin clumping and nucleolar enlargement. Mitosis may be frequent. Differentiation of adenocarcinoma (mild, moderate, severe—or grades 1-3) is important prognostically and is incorporated into the FIGO surgical staging. Most studies suggest approximately 60% to 65% of all adenocarcinomas are of this subtype.

For almost a century, it has been recognized that a squamous component may be associated with an adenocarcinoma of the endometrium. This occurs in about 25% of patients. For many years, patients with a squamous component were further stratified indicative of whether or not the squamous component appeared benign or malignant; the former designated adenocarcinoma (AA) and the latter adenosquamous carcinoma (AS). It was suggested that AA indicated a very good prognosis and those with AS had a poor survival. More recently, this distinction has been questioned in regards to its prognostic importance. Zaino, in reporting data from the GOG, suggests that the notation of squamous component per se irrespective of differentiation does not affect survival. Patients with clinical stage I and II cancers were evaluated and 456 with typical adenocarcinoma (AC) were identified as well as 175 with squamous differentiation (AC+SQ). The latter were subdivided into 99 with AA and 69 as AS. Multiple known prognostic factors were compared to differentiation of glandular and squamous component of the tumor. Age, depth of myometrial invasion, architectural, nuclear and combined grade were

Table 5-5   Endometrial carcinoma subtypes

Type	Number
Adenocarcinoma	589 (59.6%)
Adenocanthoma	215 (21.7%)
Adenosquamous carcinoma	68 (6.9%)
Clear cell carcinoma	56 (5.7%)
Papillary adenocarcinoma	46 (4.7%)
Secretory carcinoma	15 (1.5%)

Modified from Christopherson WM et al: *Am J Clin Pathol* 77:534, 1982.

similar for AC and AC+SQ, although patients with AA were better differentiated and had less myometrial invasion than AS. Both glandular and squamous differentiation correlated with frequency of pelvic and para-aortic node metastasis. Nodal metastasis when stratified for grade and depth of invasion was similar in AC and AC+SQ patients. The differentiation of squamous component is closely correlated with the differentiation of the glandular element and the latter is a better predictor of outcome. It would, therefore, appear that the previous designation of AA and AS has no added predictive properties than differentiation of glandular component and probably should be dropped as a diagnostic term. The authors suggest the term *squamous differentiation* should be used instead with differentiation of the glandular component noted as the important prognostic factor. Subsequently, Abeler and Kjorstad reviewed 255 cases and have made the same recommendations.

There has been an increasing emphasis on the importance of the histologic subtype of papillary adenocarcinoma. This subtype represents 1%-10% of all adenocarcinomas. Some authors have termed this *papillary serous adenocarcinoma*. Papillary carcinomas of the endometrium have been known for many years (Christopherson et al. credited Cullen with an illustration of this entity in 1900). Uterine papillary serous carcinoma (UPSC) is recognized as a distinct, highly aggressive carcinoma of the uterus. Of the two types of endometrial cancer (Type I with features of hyperestrogenism and Type II which are unassociated with hyperestrogen) UPSC falls in to the latter. These patients tend to be elderly, not obese, parous, have high grade tumor with extensive extrauterine disease and poor survival. Hendrickson, in the early 1980s, noted that in over 250 endometrial cancers, only 10% had histologic features of UPSC but these accounted for 50% of all treatment failures. The histopathology resembles a high grade serous carcinoma of the ovary that has a propensity for vascular/lymphatic vascular space involvement (LVSI). Well formed papillae are present lined by neoplastic cells with grade III cytology (Figure 5-2). Differentiation between papillary architecture and syncytial metaplasia with benign endometrial alterations must be made as the

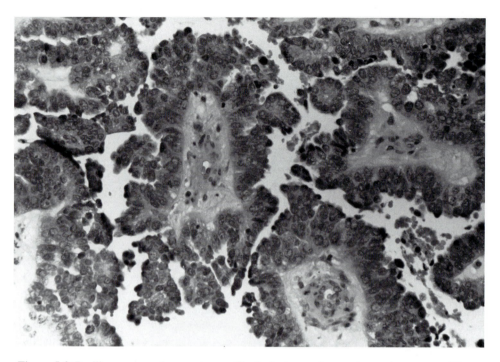

Figure 5-2 Papillary serous adenocarcinoma. Similarity to ovarian carcinoma is apparent. (Courtesy Dr. Gregory Spiegel.)

papillary architecture alone does not designate UPSC. The uterus grossly may appear normal but can have extensive myometrial invasion. Most UPSC tumors are aneuploid and have a high S-phase.

Subsequently, many small reports of this entity have appeared in the literature. One of the largest series has been reported by Goff and associates. They identified 50 patients with UPSC, 33 with pure UPSC, and 17 admixed with other histologies. Indicative of poor prognostic factors, 36 (72%) had extrauterine disease. Lymph node metastasis was found in 36% with no myometrial invasion, 50% with less than one half invasion, and 40% with outer one half invasion. Patients with LVSI have 85% incidence of extrauterine disease; however, 58% without LVSI had extrauterine disease. Grade and depth of invasion were not significant predictors of extant disease. Of particular significance was the fact that 14 (28%) of patients had disease limited to the endometrium, yet 36% had lymph node metastasis, 43% had intraperitoneal disease, and 50% with positive peritoneal cytology, essentially equal to the findings in patients with outer one half muscle invasion. In this study, the only significant prediction of extrauterine disease was LVSI. Even if disease is limited to a polyp, 30%-50% will have extrauterine disease.

With such a poor survival, adjuvant therapy has been applied in hopes of improving survival. Radiation therapy to the pelvis has been unsuccessful because most recurrences are outside the pelvis. Interestingly, Parkash and Carcangiu reported on 6 patients treated with radiation therapy for cervical carcinoma who developed

UPSC 10 years or more later (mean 16 years). This represented 7.5% of all the UPSC diagnosed at Yale during that time frame. Although others have also noted this relationship, prior radiation therapy does not appear to be an appreciable contributing factor. Several investigators using systemic therapy for ovarian cancer (since histologically the two entities are similar) have not noted similar benefits in UPSC as in ovarian cancer. MD Anderson treated 20 patients with UPSC using PAC. This included patients with measurable disease (advanced and recurrent disease) as well as adjuvant therapy. Only 2 of 11 with measurable disease had an objective response. Six patients had no extrauterine disease at the time of surgery and survival was better in this group, although no data was given. The 5-year survival for all patients was 23%. In contrast, Rosenberg and associates treated 10 clinical stage I UPSC cancers and 21 clinical stage I grade 3 patients with intense therapy of radical hysterectomy, bilateral pelvic lymphadenectomy, adjuvant pelvic radiation, and four courses of cisplatin and epirubicin. None of the UPSC died or relapsed during a median follow-up of 32 months compared with 16 of 30 (53%) historically controlled patients who were treated less intensely (P = 0.021). All of the intensely treated patients did not receive all planned treatment; in fact, only 53% completed the prescribed protocol. Three patients with UPSC did not receive radiation therapy, suggesting that the chemotherapy may be the most important aspect of the adjuvant therapy. This compared to 11/17 (64%) of historical controls that were treated with radiation and died of their disease. Hopefully, optimal adjuvant therapy

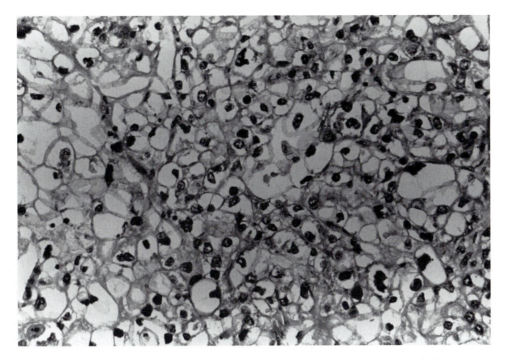

Figure 5-3 Clear cell carcinoma of the endometrium. Clear cell component is quite evident. (Courtesy Dr. Gregory Spiegel.)

for this aggressive subtype of endometrial cancer will be identified in the near future.

Clear cell carcinomas (Figure 5-3) are also infrequent in number but have distinct histologic criteria. Clear cell tumors are characterized by large polyhedral epithelial cells that may be admixed with typical non-clear cell adenocarcinomas. Some authorities accept the meso-nephritic-type hobnail cells as part of this pattern, whereas others believe that this histologic type should be excluded from the clear cell category. Silverberg and DeGiorgi, as well as Kurman and Scully, suggested a worse prognosis for clear cell adenocarcinoma than for pure adenocarcinoma. This was confirmed in studies by Christopherson et al. Even in stage I disease, only 44% of patients with clear cell carcinomas survive 5 years. Neither the FIGO classification nor nuclear grade correlate with survival. Photopulos et al. in a review of their material noted that their patients with this entity were older and tended to have a worse prognosis. They did note that patients with stage I clear cell carcinomas had a 5-year survival similar to that of patients with stage I pure adenocarcinoma of the endometrium.

So-called secretory adenocarcinoma (Figure 5-4) is an uncommon type of endometrial cancer. It usually represents well-differentiated carcinoma with progestational changes. It is difficult to differentiate it from secretory endometrium. Survival is good and comparable to that associated in the pure adenocarcinoma. Although it is an interesting histologic variant, the separation of the entity as it relates to treatment and survival is probably not warranted.

Histologic Differentiation

The degree of histologic differentiation of endometrial cancer has long been accepted as one of the most sensitive indicators of prognosis (Figure 5-5). The *Annual Report on the Results of Treatment in Gynecologic Cancer* has evaluated survival in regards to grade in patients with clinical stage I adenocarcinoma of the endometrium (Table 5-6). As the tumor loses its differentiation, the chance of survival decreases. In their review of 244 patients with stage I disease, Genest et al. noted that patients with grade 1 had a 5-year survival of 96%. This dropped to 79% and 70% for grades 2 and 3, respectively. In the GOG pilot study that surgically evaluated 222 clinical stage I endometrial cancers, only 42% were grade 1, and recurrences were only 4% compared with 15% and 41% in grades 2 and 3, respectively. Grade of tumor also correlates with other factors of prognosis. Table 5-7 shows the relationship between differentiation of the tumor and depth of myometrial invasion as reported by Creasman from the GOG study of 621 clinical stage I cancers. As the tumor becomes less differentiated, the chances of deep myometrial involvement increase. One should remember, however, that exceptions can occur: patients with a well-differentiated lesion can have deep myometrial invasion, whereas patients with a poorly differentiated malignancy might have only endometrial or superficial myometrial involvement.

Stage of Disease

The pretreatment staging of patients with malignant neoplasia is designed to have prognostic value by

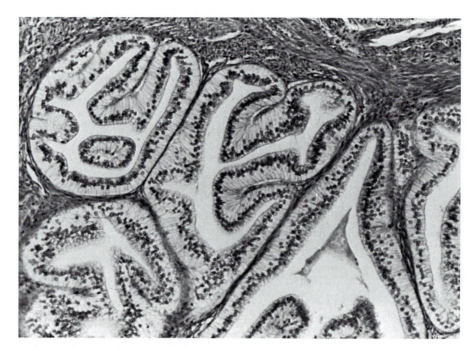

Figure 5-4 High-power view of well-differentiated secretory carcinoma invading inner one third of the myometrium. (Courtesy Dr. William M Christopherson, Louisville, Kentucky.)

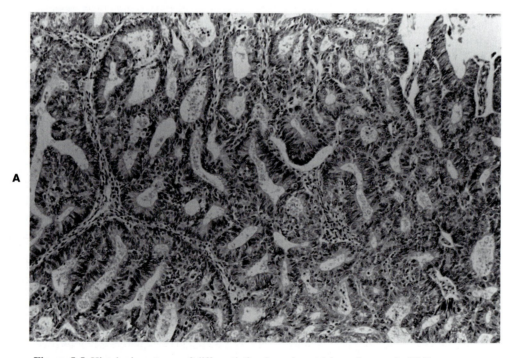

Figure 5-5 Histologic patterns of differentiation in endometrial carcinoma. **A,** Well-differentiated (G1).

Continued.

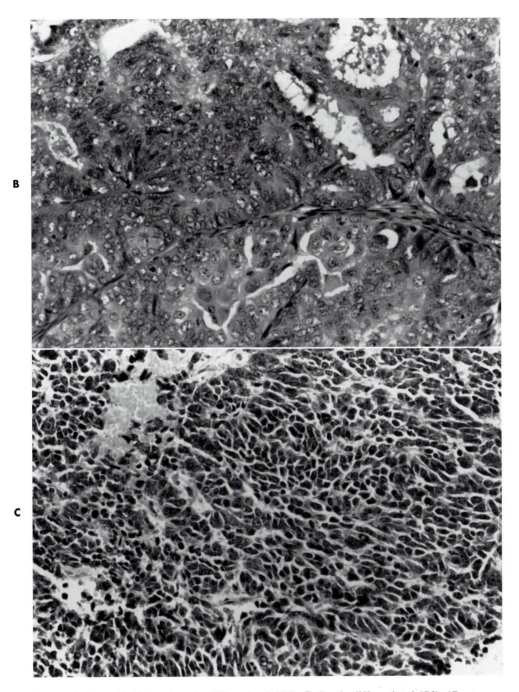

Figure 5-5, cont'd. B, Moderately differentiated (G2). **C,** Poorly differentiated (G3). (Courtesy Dr. Gregory Spiegel.)

determining the size and extent of tumor. The survival rate in regard to stage of disease has been consistent, and Table 5-8 shows the 5-year survival rate reported by FIGO. Prognosis for women with cervical involvement (stage II) is much worse than prognosis for earlier lesions. Previous endocervical curettage was used to determine whether or not the patient was stage II. Many false positives may occur through the use of this technique. The new surgical staging adopted by FIGO uses the uterine specimen as the final determination of endocervical involvement. A pretreatment endocervical curettage may guide therapy.

Location of the tumor within the endometrial cavity could be significant, since tumors low in the cavity can be expected to involve the cervix earlier than fundal lesions. It is shown in data from 621 stage I patients reported from the GOG that those with disease of the lower uterine segment have a higher incidence of pelvic lymph node metastases (16%) than those with only fundal disease (8%). There is a similar pattern of occurrence of perioaortic nodal metastases: a 16% incidence from disease of the lower uterine segment and a 4% incidence when only fundal disease is present.

Table 5-6 Relationship between tumor differentiation and 5-year survival rate—stage I (surgical)

Grade	Survival (N = 4370)
1	94%
2	88%
3	79%

From Pettersson F, editor: *Annual report on the results of treatment in gynecological cancer,* vol. 22, Stockholm, 1994, International Federation of Gynecology and Obstetrics.

Table 5-7 Correlation of differentiation and myometrial invasion in stage I cancer

Myometrial invasion	Grade		
	1	2	3
None	24%	11%	11%
Superficial	53%	45%	35%
Mid	12%	24%	16%
Deep	10%	20%	42%

Modified from Creasman WT et al: *Cancer* 60:2035, 1987.

Table 5-8 Five-year survival in endometrial cancer

Stage	Patients	Survival
I	8603	86%
II	1650	66%
III	1181	44%
IV	399	16%

From Pettersson F, editor: *Annual report on the results of treatment in gynecological cancer,* vol. 22, Stockholm, 1994, International Federation of Gynecology and Obstetrics.

It appears that the extent of disease within the endocervix is also of importance. Surwit et al. noted that in patients with stromal invasion of the cervix the survival rate was much lower at 3 years (47%) than in patients in whom involvement was limited to the endocervical glands or in whom no stroma was present in the endocervical curettage specimen (74%). The MD Anderson group, however, found no difference in survival of patients with stage II disease when gross cervical involvement was compared with occult disease. They also noted that stromal involvement made no survival difference in patients with occult disease. It should be noted that all these patients had preoperative radiation, and these results may not be a true representation of the disease process. In a GOG review of clinical stage II cancers that

Table 5-9 Relationship between depth of myometrial invasion and recurrence in patients with stage I endometrial carcinoma

Myometrial invasion	Recurrences
Endometrium only	7/92 (8%)
Superficial myometrium	10/80 (13%)
Medium myometrium	2/17 (12%)
Deep myometrium	15/33 (46%)

Modified from DiSaia PJ et al: *Am J Obstet Gynecol* 151:1009, 1985.

Table 5-10 Relationship between depth of myometrial invasion and 5-year survival rate (stage I)

Myometrial invasion	Survival rate
<1/3	2656/3224 (82.4%)
1/3-1/2	760/974 (78.0%)
>1/2	764/1144 (66.8%)

From Pettersson F, editor: *Annual report on the results of treatment in gynecological cancer,* vol. 22, Stockholm, 1994, International Federation of Gynecology and Obstetrics.

were surgically staged, over three fourths patients did not have disease involving cervix or had extant disease. Those patients with disease limited to the endocervical glandular tissue had a smaller number with extrauterine disease (39%) compared to those with cervical stromal invasion (50%). Once corrected for true surgical stage II disease, recurrence was similar for stage IIa and b cancers.

Myometrial Invasion

The degree of myometrial invasion is a consistent indicator of tumor virulence. DiSaia et al. noted that recurrences were directly related to depth of myometrial invasion in patients with stage I cancer treated primarily with surgery (Table 5-9). The Annual Report of FIGO demonstrated a decrease in the survival rate as myometrial penetration increased (Table 5-10). Lutz et al. determined that the depth of myometrial penetration was not as important as the proximity of the invading tumor to the uterine serosa. Patients whose tumors invaded to within 5 mm of the serosa had a 65% 5-year survival rate, whereas patients whose tumors were more than 10 mm from the serosa had a 97% survival rate.

The depth of myometrial invasion is associated with the other prognostic factors, such as the grade of the tumor. As noted by DiSaia et al., the survival rate for patients with poorly differentiated lesions and deep myometrial invasion is poor in contrast to that of patients who have well-differentiated lesions but no myometrial invasion. This suggests that virulence of the tumor may vary considerably, and as a result, therapy should depend on the individual prognostic factors.

Peritoneal Cytology

The importance of cytologic evaluation of peritoneal fluids, or washings, has been recognized as a prognostic and staging factor in pelvic malignancies. Creasman and Rutledge reported positive washings in 12% of patients with corpus cancer, although many of the patients with positive washings did have gross metastatic diseaseoutside the uterus. When 167 patients with clinical stage I carcinoma of the endometrium treated primarily by surgery had cytologic testings of peritoneal washings, 26 (15.5%) had malignant cells identified. Recurrences developed in 10 of these 26 patients (38%), compared with 14 of 141 (9.9%) patients with negative cytologic testing. Of the 26 patients with positive cytologic results, 13 (50%) had disease outside the uterus at the time of operation, and 7 (54%) have died of disease. Malignant cells were found in the peritoneal washings of 13 patients, but there was no disease outside the uterus; 6 (46%) patients have died of disseminated intra-abdominal carcinomatosis. In the GOG study of 621 patients, 76 (12%) had malignant cells, identified by cytologic examination of peritoneal washings. Of these patients, 25% had positive pelvic nodes, compared with 7% of patients in whom no malignant cells were found in peritoneal cytologic specimens (p < 0.0001). It is true that peritoneal cytology, to a certain degree, mimics other known prognostic factors; that is, if peritoneal cytologic specimens are positive, other known poor prognostic factors may also be identified.

Recurrences were evaluated according to known prognostic factors and whether malignant cells were present in peritoneal cytologic specimens. If malignant cells are not present in peritoneal cytologic specimens, the influence of known prognostic factors remains intact. However, when malignant cells are present in peritoneal fluid, this tends to neutralize the good prognostic factors, and cytologic findings become a predominantly important consideration.

Yazigi's study suggested that peritoneal cytology was not of prognostic significance. This study represented a patient population of two decades earlier in which the peritoneal cytology was not reviewed (in contrast to the pathology). In the original study, many patients were rejected because the original pathology could not be confirmed. Konski also noted no difference in survival regardless of the cytological findings; however, a significant number of those patients were treated with radiation therapy, which could have affected survival. More recently, Sutton, using multivariant analysis, noted that positive peritoneal cytology remained a significant prognostic factor. In a recent report from the GOG, 25 of 86 (29%) with positive cytology had regional or distant re-

currence, compared with 64/611 (10.4%) if cytology was negative. In a retrospective study from the MD Anderson Hospital, 28/567 (5%) had positive peritoneal cytology. Positive cytology was associated with significantly reduced progression-free interval (PFI). In a multivariant analysis of 477 cases, cytology was significantly associated with survival and PFI. Grimshaw noted 24/381 patients with positive cytology who had a significantly worse survival rate than those with negative cytology. When only patients with surgical stage I were compared, those with negative cytology had a better prognosis, but the difference was not statistically significant.

The role of peritoneal cytology and its implication in prognosis of endometrial cancer continues to be debated. Those studies which noted no or minimal effect were usually smaller in number than those noted with prognostic significance. Milosevic and colleagues, reviewed 17 studies. In 3820 patients, the prevalence of positive cytology was 11%. The three largest studies totalling over 1700 patients (Haroung, Turner and Morrow) using multivariate analysis noted malignant cytology was independently significantly associated with either recurrence or reduced survival. Pooled odds ratio for the entire series was 4.7 (CI 3.5-6.3) for disease recurrence. All studies note the highest correlation of malignant cytology with extrauterine disease. It does appear that, using multivariate analysis, the presence of malignant cytology is an important prognostic factor even when disease is limited to the uterus. Optimal therapy has not been determined to date. The use of intraperitoneal P-32 in patients with malignant cytologic specimens appears to be therapeutically efficacious, in that patients so treated did much better than patients with positive cytologic specimens but no intraperitoneal therapy (nonrandomized evaluation). Soper has reported an update of the Duke experience utilizing P-32 in patients with malignant peritoneal cytology. Sixty-five patients with positive washings were treated, of whom 53 were clinical stage I. Disease-free survival beyond 24 months was 89% for clinical stage I patients and 94% for surgical stage I patients. Significant acute and chronic complications were unusual unless combined with external irradiation. This therapy is identical to that used for ovarian cancer described in Chapter 11.

Once the peritoneal cavity is opened, an assessment of the amount of peritoneal fluid in the pelvis is made. If none is present, 100 to 125 ml of normal saline solution is injected into the pelvis. This can be done easily with a bulb syringe. The saline solution is admixed in the pelvis, withdrawn with the syringe, and sent for cytologic evaluation. Peritoneal cytology is obtained in all patients undergoing surgery for endometrial cancer.

Lymph Node Metastasis

A total abdominal hysterectomy and bilateral salpingo-oophorectomy have been the hallmarks of therapy for

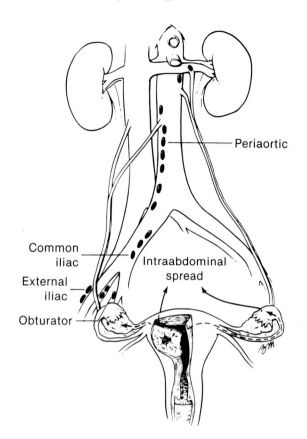

Periaortic

Common iliac

External iliac

Obturator

Intraabdominal spread

Figure 5-6 Spread pattern of endometrial cancer with particular emphasis on potential lymph node spread. Pelvic and peri-aortic nodes are at risk, even in stage I disease.

endometrial cancer. As a result, the significant incidence of lymph node metastases has been somewhat disregarded (Figure 5-6). Although contributions to the early and recent literature indicate that a significant number of women with endometrial cancer, even stage I, will develop lymph node disease, these potential metastatic sites have not been routinely included in the treatment plan. In 1973, Morrow et al. reviewed the recent literature and noted that in a collected series of 369 patients with stage I carcinoma of the endometrium, 39 had metastasis to the pelvic lymph node area. In 1976, Creasman et al. reported on an additional 140 patients, 16 of whom had positive pelvic nodes. These figures have been updated as additional cases have been reported in this study (Table 5-11). In this relatively large group of patients with clinical stage I carcinoma of the endometrium, almost 10% had metastases to the pelvic lymph node area. In the study by Morrow et al., only 31% of those patients with stage I disease and positive pelvic nodes survived 5 years, and most of these had been treated with postoperative radiation. Potish et al. have reported survival of patients with microscopic evidence of lymph node metastases who were treated with irradiation therapy as part of the primary treatment. Patients with surgically confirmed lymphatic spread had a survival of 67% at 5 years. Patients with surgically confirmed periaortic spread, with

Table 5-11 Incidence of pelvic node metastases

	Positive nodes/patients
Stage I	81/843 (9.6%)

From Boronow (1984) and Creasman (1987).

and without pelvic node involvement, had a 5-year survival of 47% and 43%, respectively. In the study by Creasman et al., 102 of the patients also had the periaortic fat pad removed for histologic evaluation, and it was found that 10 of these patients (9.8%) had metastasis to the periaortic area.

Boronow et al., in updating the GOG pilot study, noted that 23 of 222 (10.4%) stage I patients had pelvic node metastases. Of 156 patients in whom periaortic nodes were microscopically evaluated, 16 (10.2%) had metastases to this area. DiSaia, in reporting the long-term follow-up of these patients, noted a recurrence in 21 of 199 patients (10.5%) who had negative pelvic nodes, compared with recurrence in 13 of 23 patients (56%) whose pelvic nodes contained metastases. Recurrence with negative periaortic nodes was 15 of 140 patients (11%) versus recurrence in 10 of 17 patients (59%) when periaortic nodes were positive. Creasman, in reporting that GOG data on 621 patients with stage I disease, found that 58 (9%) have positive nodes in the pelvis and 34 have positive nodes in the periaortic area. Of these patients 11% had metastases to either pelvic nodes or periaortic nodes, or both.

The occurrence of lymph node metastases in patients with stage II carcinoma of the endometrium is considerably higher than occurrence in patients with stage I disease. Morrow et al. identified 85 patients in whom the pelvic lymph nodes were evaluated, and 31 (36.5%) had disease in the pelvic nodes. In the GOG study, 148 patients with clinical stage II cancers were surgically evaluated, 66 had cervical involvement. Three (17%) of the patients with only endocervical glandular involvement had pelvic node metastases compared to 35% of those with cervical stromal involvement. None of those with glandular involvement only had aortic node metastases compared with 23% of those with stromal invasion. In patients with stromal involvement, 46% had nodal metastases.

Adnexal Metastases

It is well recognized that endometrial cancer can, and frequently does, metastasize to the adnexa. Approximately 10% of patients with clinical stage I adenocarcinoma of the endometrium are found to have occult metastasis in the ovary at the time of surgery. In an analysis of 222 patients with clinical stage I carcinoma of the endometrium studied for surgical-pathologic evaluation, 16 (7%) were found to have metastasis in the adnexa.

This finding correlated with many, but not all, of the other prognostic factors. Spread to the adnexa did not seem to be related to the size of the uterus. The grade of the disease did not appear prognostically important in regard to this, in that 6% of patients with grade 1 tumors had adnexal disease compared with only 10% if poorly differentiated carcinoma was present. The depth of invasion, however, did appear to be significant, in that only 4% of patients with only the endometrium involved had adnexal spread, compared with 24% who had adnexal metastases if deep muscle was involved. If tumor was limited to the fundus of the uterus, only 5% of patients had disease in the adnexa; however, if the lower uterine segment or the endocervix was involved, one third had spread to the adnexa. Definite correlation was present in regard to adnexal metastasis and metastasis to both the pelvic and periaortic lymph node areas. When metastasis was present in the adnexa, 60% of patients had malignant cells present in the peritoneal cytology, compared with only 11% if the adnexa were not involved. Recurrences appeared in only 14% of these individuals who did not have metastasis to the adnexa, compared with recurrences in 38% of patients with adnexal metastasis. In the 621 patients reported from the GOG, 34/621 (5%) of patients had metastases to the adnexa. The new surgical staging classifies patients with adnexal metastases as IIIa.

Molecular Indices

Although many recognized prognostic factors such as grade of tumor with its subsequent effect (deep myometrial invasion and metastatic potential) can be said to be dependent on its molecular capabilities, this section deals with the more recent molecular biologic characteristics that have been identified with newer technology. Morphologic interpretations and subjectivity of traditional histopathologic features has led to development of rapid, more precise quantitative measures to assess cellular characteristics. Flow cytometry has been used in ploidy analysis (cellular nuclear DNA content) and to measure the proliferative fraction of tumor cells (S-phase). Single cells are obtained from fresh frozen or archival paraffin-embedded tissues through a mechanical disaggregation, enzymatic digestion or a combination thereof. DNA histograms reflect the cell cycle phase. G0 and G1 cells contain diploid nuclear DNA content. A small number of cells enter the S-phase and begin DNA replication (S-phase fraction). DNA ploidy can be denoted as the DNA index (DI) which is the numerical ratio of the DNA content of G0/G1 abnormal (tumor) peak to the DNA content of the G0/G1 peak of normal control population. A diploid tumor has a DI range of 0.95 to 1.05 and a tetraploid tumor has a DI range of 1.9 to 2.1. Peaks outside of these ranges are defined as aneuploid. Many studies have suggested that DNA content and S-phase fraction have prognostic significance. Univariant analysis have shown DNA ploidy as well as other long recognized

factors, i.e., grade to be important prognostically; however, on multivariate analysis, variations of independent prognostic significance has been reported. Podratz noted in paraffin embedded curettage specimens that recurrences and cancer-related deaths correlated with nondiploid pattern, S-phase fraction ≥9% and proliferative index ≥14%, the latter being the most independent prognostic factor. Proliferative index is the percent of S-phase plus percent of G2/metaphase, which is the fraction of tumor cell in an active proliferative phase. They did not correlate molecular status with other prognostic factors. Sorbe evaluated S-phase fraction on fresh-frozen tissue. On paraffin-embedded, tissue nuclear grade was evaluated and was the most significant and independent prognostic factor. On fresh frozen tissue, nuclear grade lost most of its prognostic value. The grade of tumor and S-phase fraction were independent and highly significant prognostic factors. These investigators used an S-phase fraction less than 10%. The DNA index was not significant. In 30% of cases it was impossible to assess either ploidy level or S-phase fraction. Von Minckwitz noted, in 161 endometrial cancer patients in which fresh frozen tissue was used, that aneuploid tumor and high S-phase fraction were more common in advanced stages. Positive receptor status correlated with diploid and low S-phase fraction. Prognosis correlated with diploid and S-phase status, and in multivariate analysis were both predictors of survival more than grade and estrogen receptor status in stage I disease. S-phase fraction cut off was set at 5%. Thornton, on the other hand, in evaluating 257 women with endometrial cancer with ploidy and proliferative indices found that they were related to stage, grade, and survival but not independent predictors of survival.

Other authors have evaluated DNA ploidy with other prognostic factors. Baak suggested the prognostic value of the ECPI-1 score (myometrial invasion, DNA ploidy and mean shortest nuclear axis) in stage I endometrial cancer patients. This score, which is mathematically derived, was found on multivariant analysis to be of most significance in regards to survival. Ambros and Kurman also noted in stage I cancer that the combination of DNA ploidy and vascular invasion associated change and myometrial invasion are the strongest prognostic factors.

Pisani evaluated several molecular biologic characteristics in regard to prognosis. This included HER-2/neu and p53 gene overexpression, DNA ploidy, and S-phase fraction evaluation on archival material from 128 patients with endometrial cancer. On multivariate analysis, p53 overexpression was the strongest independent factor to predict prognosis, although stage was also significant.

Although status of molecular biologic indices appear to be important in regard to prognosis, most studies are relatively small in number and use different techniques and cut off for S-phase significance. Whether the assay is done on paraffin or fresh frozen tissue also appears to affect results. Obviously, the necessity for standardization is needed before applicability and conclusions can be reached.

Other Factors

Capillary-like space (CLS) involvement

Hanson et al reported on 111 patients with stage I endometrium cancer and found CLS involvement in 16. This was most frequently found in patients with poorly differentiated tumors with deep invasion. These patients had a 44% recurrence rate, compared with 2% if CLS was not involved. This was an independent significant prognostic factor. In the GOG study of 621 patients, it was shown that 93 (15%) had CLS involvement. The incidences of pelvic and para-aortic node metastases were 27% and 19%, respectively. This compares with a 7% occurrence of pelvic node metastases and a 3% occurrence of para-aortic node metastasis when there is no CLS involvement.

Tumor size

Schink et al evaluated tumor size in 91 stage I patients. The incidence of lymph node metastases in patients with tumor size <2 cm was only 5.7%. If tumor was >2 cm in diameter, there were nodal metastases of 21% and up to 40% if the entire endometrium was involved. Patients with <2 cm lesions and less than one half myometrial invasion had no nodal metastasis. Using multivariant analysis, the authors showed that tumor size was an independent significant prognostic factor.

Hormonal receptors

Using multivariant analysis to analyze hormonal receptor status, Creasman et al. noted that in stage I and stage II cancers progesterone receptor-positive status was a highly significant independently prognostic factor in endometrial cancer. Without putting progesterone receptor status in the model and evaluating estrogen receptor in its stead, estrogen receptor-positive status was an independent prognostic factor but not to the degree of progesterone receptor-positive status.

Correlation of Multiple Prognostic Factors

At the completion of the original GOG study (Creasman, 1976; Boronow, 1984; DiSaia, 1985) of 222 stage I endometrial cancer patients who were surgically staged, results were reported and prognostic factors correlated. A subsequent study by the entire GOG of 621 patients with stage I endometrial cancer who were treated primarily with TAH, BSO, peritoneal cytology, and pelvic and periaortic selected lymphadenectomy has been reported. Data include size of the uterus, histology, grade, and depth of uterine muscle invasion, and this information is similar to that in preliminary reports as well as others. Only 25% of these patients had poorly differentiated cancers; and 22% had deep muscle invasion. Fifty-eight (9%) patients

had pelvic node metastases; 34 (6%) had metastases to the periaortic region. The size of the uterus, grade of tumor, and depth of muscle invasion correlated well with nodal metastasis (Tables 5-12 to 5-14). Of these patients, 35 (5%) had adnexal metastasis unappreciated before exploratory laparotomy. The chance of having disease in the adnexa increased as depth of invasion increased and when the lower uterine segment or endocervix was involved. As expected, there was a greater propensity for lymph node metastasis when disease was present in the lower uterine segment or in the cervix compared with the propensity among patients with disease limited to the fundus of the uterus. Seventy-six patients (12%) had malignant cells present in cytologic evaluation. Many of these prognostic factors interdigitated in that good prognostic factors occurred together, although it was not unusual to have several poor prognostic factors present in the same patient. When lymph node metastasis was evaluated relative to the six substages of clinical stage I disease, lymph node metastasis became more prevalent with increasing grade of tumor and increasing uterine size (Table 5-15).

Table 5-12 Clinical stage versus positive pelvic and aortic nodes

Stage	Pelvic	Aortic
Ia (N=346)	23 (7%)	11 (3%)
Ib (N=275)	35 (13%)	23 (8%)

Modified from Creasman WT et al: *Cancer* 60:2035, 1987.

Table 5-13 Grade versus positive pelvic and aortic nodes

Grade	Pelvic	Aortic
G1 (N = 180)	5 (3%)	3 (2%)
G2 (N = 288)	25 (9%)	14 (5%)
G3 (N = 153)	28 (18%)	17 (11%)

Modified from Creasman WT et al: *Cancer* 60:2035, 1987.

Table 5-14 Maximal invasion and node metastasis

Maximal invasion	Pelvic	Aortic
Endometrium only (N = 87)	1 (1%)	1 (1%)
Superficial muscle (N = 279)	15 (5%)	8 (3%)
Intermediate muscle (N = 116)	7 (6%)	1 (1%)
Deep muscle (N = 139)	35 (25%)	24 (17%)

Modified from Creasman WT et al: *Cancer* 60:2035, 1987.

Table 5-15   Clinical stage and grade versus pelvic and aortic node metastasis

Stage	Pelvic	Aortic
IaG1 (N = 101)	2 (2%)	0 (0%)
IaG2 (N = 169)	13 (8%)	6 (4%)
IaG3 (N = 76)	8 (11%)	5 (7%)
IbG1 (N = 79)	3 (4%)	3 (4%)
IbG2 (N = 119)	12 (10%)	8 (7%)
IbG3 (N = 77)	20 (26%)	12 (16%)

Modified from Creasman WT et al: *Cancer* 60:2035, 1987.

The patients in the GOG pilot study have been followed for 37 to 72 months after surgery; and since most recurrences appear within the first 2 years after therapy, it can be assumed that the majority of recurrences in this group of patients have already been identified. Sixty-eight (31%) patients were treated with surgery only, and an additional 97 (44%) received preoperative radium. All of the latter had surgery during the same hospitalization as their radium application. In at least one of the participating institutions, all patients at the beginning of the study received preoperative radium but with decreasing frequency as time elapsed: at the completion of the study it was unusual to place preoperative radium. Patients treated with surgery alone had a 9% recurrence; those treated with surgery plus radium had an 8% recurrence. Only 25% of the patients were thought to have disease significant enough (high risk) to require external irradiation as an individual determination. Patients treated with external irradiation had a 35% (20/57) recurrence. Since radiation therapy was given for patients who were thought to be at high risk, it appeared that the designation of high and low risk as determined by recurrence could be adequately determined. Only 25% of the patients in the study were determined to be at high risk, necessitating external irradiation. On the other hand, it was believed that 75% were not in need of radiation therapy, indicating a rather marked change in protocol as practiced by many institutions. When sites of recurrence were analyzed, only 2 (1%) patients had an isolated vault recurrence—1 patient having been treated with surgery only and the other with surgery plus radium. It appears from this study that the vaginal vault is not at high risk for recurrence, and the role of radium in endometrial cancer must therefore be questioned. An additional 5 patients had recurrence identified in the pelvis only. Of 37 recurrences, 27 (73%) were at distant sites outside the treatment field. It appears that local control with therapy was excellent, but in the future attention must be directed toward control of distant metastasis.

Recurrences correlated well with other prognostic factors such as grade, depth of invasion, location of tumor within the uterus, adnexal disease, peritoneal cytology, and lymph node metastasis. When recurrences were evaluated to determine if disease was intrauterine or extrauterine (adnexal disease, positive peritoneal cytology, lymph node metastasis, or intraperitoneal disease) irrespective of other prognostic factors, only 7% of those with intrauterine disease developed recurrences, compared with 43% if extrauterine disease was present at the time of surgery.

Risk factors in 895 patients with clinical stage I and II have recently been reported by the GOG. There were 789 stage I and 136 stage II patients evaluated. In some instances all prognostic factors were not available for analysis in all patients. In multivariant analysis, those patients with disease limited to the uterus were at increased risk for recurrence if there were deep myometrial invasion, vascular space involvement, or positive washings.

TREATMENT

Treatment for carcinoma of the uterus, particularly stage I, has evolved considerably over the last decade. This disease entity actually has a very long history of treatment development for the last century (see previous editions for a brief treatment history). With the more general acceptance of surgical staging for this disease, preoperative radiation has lost favor as standard therapy. Surgical staging allows a more complete identification of the true stage of disease. From surgical staging studies, it has been learned that about one fourth of clinical stage I patients have disease outside of the uterus and many clincial stage II patients do not have disease involving the cervix.

More recently, a considerable amount of data has been collected to evaluate vaginal recurrence and survival rate with surgery alone or combined therapy when mainly preoperative radium and surgery was used. Data have also been evaluated in regard to the grade of the tumor (Table 5-16) and, in some instances, the depth of myometrial involvement (Table 5-17). In patients who had preoperative or postoperative radiation, there appeared to be a lower incidence of vaginal vault recurrences, although there does not appear to be much difference in the grades 1 and 2 lesions. Vaginal vault recurrence did not appear to affect survival. The survival rate was similar in those treated by surgery only to that of those treated by radiation plus surgery, particularly in the grades 1 and 2 lesions. Patients with poorly differentiated adenocarcinoma treated with combined therapy had a slightly better survival rate, although most studies showed no statistical difference between these patients and those treated only with surgery.

The role of preoperative radiation in patients with endometrial carcinoma has been addressed by several authors. In a study from Germany, de Waal and Lochmuller compared patients with stage I or II carcinoma of the endometrium treated with preoperative intracavitary

Table 5-16 Survival rate in stage I carcinoma of the endometrium with regard to grade and treatment

	Survival	
Grade	Surgery only	Combined therapy
1	1295/1375 (94%)	2284/2389 (96%)
2	488/510 (96%)	1490/1721 (87%)
3	100/135 (74%)	398/498 (80%)

From Pettersson F, editor: *Annual report on the results of treatment in gynecological cancer,* vol. 21, Stockholm, 1991, International Federation of Gynecology and Obstetrics.

Table 5-17 Recurrences in stage I carcinoma of the endometrium with regard to depth of invasion and treatment

	Recurrence	
Residual	Surgery ± radium	Surgery and external radiation
Endometrium only	6/88 (7%)	0/4 (0%)
Inner and mid 1/3	3/68 (4%)	9/29 (31%)
Outer 1/3	3/9 (33%)	11/24 (46%)

Modified from DiSaia P et al: *Am J Obstet Gynecol* 151:1009, 1985

radiotherapy with those who received primary operation without radiotherapy. There was no difference in the 5-year survival rate or in the incidence of vaginal, pelvic sidewall, and distant metastases. The authors believed that preoperative radiotherapy did not appear to be of benefit in the management of patients with this malignancy. Patterson et al., in Rochester, New York, attempted to individualize treatment of a group of patients depending on grade of the tumor and the depth of myometrial invasion. In patients with grade 1 or 2 tumors, primary total abdominal hysterectomy and bilateral salpingo-oophorectomy were performed. If less than one third myometrial invasion was present in grade 1 or 2 tumors, no further treatment was carried out. There were 112 patients in this group. The authors' intent was to postoperatively radiate the pelvis in patients with less than one third myometrial involvement and grade 3 tumors, but they had no patients who fell into this category. In their 21 grade 1 or 2 patients who had greater than one third myometrial involvement, external irradiation to the whole pelvis was given irrespective of the grade. There were only 7 patients with grade 3 tumors noted at the time of D&C, and they received whole-pelvic irradiation preoperatively. Pre- or postoperative radium insertions were not a part of their planned treatment. The 5-year

survival rate was 96%, with 93% of their patients free of recurrence at that time. It was their belief that irradiation therapy could be individually applied, and in fact only 20% of their patients required this therapy.

In the only prospective randomized study done to date that evaluates the role of external pelvic radiation and radium versus radium alone in addition to surgery in stage I carcinoma of the endometrium, Onsrud, Kolstad, and Normann noted no difference in survival rate between the two groups of patients. Patients who received pelvic radiation had a 5-year survival rate of 88%, whereas those who did not receive external radiation had a 90% survival rate. When recurrence and survival were evaluated in regard to histologic grade and myometrial involvement, no difference was noted. In patients who received external radiation, there was less recurrence in the pelvis, but a larger number of patients had distant recurrences. Those who did not receive external radiation had a higher number of recurrences locally in the pelvis.

Most authorities, even those who are advocates of preoperative radiation, agree that in stage I, grade 1 lesions the procedure of choice is total abdominal hysterectomy and bilateral salpingo-oophorectomy alone. If extensive disease is present in the uterus or if metastasis outside the uterus is noted, appropriate radiation, progestins, and/or chemotherapy are given. There is no agreement on treatment of patients with grade 2 or 3 disease, as noted by the various modalities advocated in the literature. Some authors prefer preoperative radium either by Heyman packing plus vaginal ovoid or by tandem and ovoids if the uterus is small. A total abdominal hysterectomy with bilateral salpingo-oophorectomy is done 6 weeks later. Underwood et al. have recommended that the hysterectomy be done immediately after the radium is removed. If deep myometrial or distant disease is present, external radiation (4000 to 5000 cGy to the appropriate areas) is given. Underwood et al. have shown that depth of myometrial invasion is best determined by measuring the tumor-free area from serosa inward. If there is less than 5 mm of tumor-free area, they advocate external radiation (4000 to 5000 cGy to the whole pelvis) during the postoperative period because these patients will have a high risk for developing recurrence. If there is greater than 10 mm of tumor-free area, surgery alone appears adequate. Treatment of patients with 5 to 10 mm of tumor-free area is unresolved at the present time, although recurrence appears to take place more often than it does in disease with greater than 10 mm of tumor-free area.

Bond reported on 1703 stages Ia and Ib adenocarcinoma patients treated with or without vaginal irradiation after hysterectomy. There were fewer vaginal recurrences in those who received postoperative vaginal therapy (0% versus 3.4% in noninvasive lesions, and 4.3% versus 8.3% in invasive tumors). The vagina was the first site of recurrence in only 3.4% of cases, whereas 4 times as many patients developed pelvic or metastatic disease. Bond felt that postoperative vaginal irradiation was of value to a small percentage of patients but that it did not influence survival rate or the incidence of pelvic or metastatic disease in any histologic group and therefore does not recommend it as a routine measure. Chen, in a small study of 32 stage I patients with deep myometrial or grade 3 lesions, noted that 18 had no extrauterine disease. None of the 18 received postoperative radiation and all survived for more than 5 years. Of the 15 with extrauterine disease, all received postoperative therapy, but only 4 survived. It is his impression that for patients with surgically determined stage I disease, even with poor prognostic factors, surgery alone may be adequate therapy.

Elliott and colleagues from Australia reported on 811 clinical stage I and 116 clinical stage II endometrial cancers treated over a 25-year time interval. They have suggested that whole vaginal radiation postoperatively decreased isolated vaginal recurrence. Forty isolated vaginal recurrences (4.3%) were detected. Unfortunately over the years, multiple treatments were used, e.g., simple and radical hysterectomy, vault or whole vaginal radiation, as well as external radiation in various combinations. In low-risk patients (clinical stage I, grade 1 and 2 tumors confined to inner one third myometrium) vault recurrence was 2.5%, 2.5%, and 0% in patients treated with surgery alone, plus vault or whole vaginal radiation respectively. The low-risk group represented 53% of all patients. In multivariant analysis only total vaginal irradiation was independently protective. Almost 9% of patients treated with the total vaginal radiation had complications attributable to the radiation (see recommended treatment section).

The effectiveness of postoperative external radiation for nodal metastases has received increased attention with the increasing popularity of surgical staging. Patients with metastases to both para-aortic and pelvic nodes have received external irradiation to the affected area. Potish et al. used para-aortic radiation to treat 48 patients who had clincial or pathological evidence of metastases to this area. In the surgically confirmed patients, the authors noted a 67% 5-year survival if pelvic nodes alone were involved, 47% if para-aortic alone had metastases, and 43% if both areas were affected. Overall survival for the entire group was 52%; and 88% of the recurrences were outside of the treatment field. Morbidity appeared acceptable. Other authors, including those responsible for the follow-up of the GOG staging studies, have shown similar results. Some patients with metastases to lymph nodes have had long disease-free intervals with surgery only, but most investigators today would probably advocate postoperative radiation therapy in patients with metastases to the lymph nodes.

Therapy after surgical staging particularly in patients with disease limited to the uterus has not been evaluated in a prospective randomized study. Historically patients with deep invasion or poorly differentiated tumors received pelvic radiation as they were high risk and radiation therapy would decrease recurrence, although the data was lacking to substantiate that thesis. The GOG is currently evaluating surgery plus radiation therapy vs. surgery alone in moderate-risk patients. The GOG surgical-pathologic study suggests that when disease is limited to the uterus, except for those with grade 3 and greater than one third myometrial invasion, radiation therapy did not offer a benefit vs surgery alone. Kedar and associates retrospectively evaluated 262 surgically staged endometrial cancers. Multiple risk factors were evaluated. Tumor grade, myometrial invasion, presence of vascular invasion, cervical involvement, FIGO stage, and patient age were all independent prognostic factors. In patients with 0-1 risk factor, radiation therapy did not affect recurrence or survival. These patients had a 97% 5-year survival. Unfortunately, most patients with three or four risk factors do very poorly even with radiation therapy. One wonders if adjuvant therapy has any effect on survival as only a 17% 5-year survival was appreciated, even with 5 of 6 patients receiving radiation therapy. In the risk group 2 (2 risk factors), 24/28 received pelvic radiation with a suggestion of improved survival although statistical significance was not reached.

In the group-wide GOG study, 6% of patients with clinical stage I disease were noted to have intraperitoneal disease. Chen and Spiegel suggest that omental biopsies as a routine procedure should be accomplished as part of the operative procedure. In 84 patients with clinical stage I cancers, 7 (8.3%) had omental metastasis and 5 were identified only microscopically. Omental metastasis was identified with other risk factors, most notably papillary serous carcinoma. Particularly in high risk patients, omental biopsies appear to be warranted. Several studies note the role of vaginal hysterectomy in highly selected patients with endometrial cancer. These are usually in obese and high risk surgical patients. Survival rates are comparable to the abdominal approach. Lellé identified 60 patients from two institutions over almost 30 years who were treated with vaginal hysterectomy. The 5-year survival was over 90%. Two thirds of patients had grade 1 tumors and 41% had no myometrial invasion. In fact, a significant number of patients who were being operated on for hyperplasia or cancer was not diagnosed preoperation. These latter factors are the common theme in essentially all studies in which vaginal hysterectomy was the surgical therapy.

Suggested Treatment

When planning treatment, the physician must consider potential spread patterns (see Figure 5-6), but predictability of spread can be determined to a large degree by evaluation of prognostic factors. It is suggested that radiation therapy for adenocarcinoma of the endometrium should be used primarily in patients with poor prognostic factors or who may be inoperable. Therefore it would seem prudent to evaluate these factors and then apply radiation therapy selectively after surgery. Although the grade of the tumor can be determined before surgery, depth of myometrial invasion cannot be known until hysterectomy. Some patients with well-differentiated lesions can have deep myometrial involvement, and it appears that in this small group of patients the recurrence rate is higher and the survival rate lower than it is among patients with lesions of the same grade but limited invasion.

The data from the surgical-pathologic study correlating multiple prognostic factors reported earlier in this chapter suggest criteria that could be used to allow therapy to be planned selectively. From prognostic factors, such as grade of tumor, as predictors of extensive disease and recurrence (Table 5-18), it appears that in patients with grade 1, surgery can be limited to total abdominal hysterectomy, bilateral salpingo-oophorectomy, and peritoneal cytologic examination unless deep myometrial invasion is present. In many instances, an experienced oncologist can determine depth of invasion grossly with good correlation in the operating room. Reliability of frozen section with permanent evaluation of depth of invasion appears to be very good. Because of appreciable lymph node metastases in grades 2 and 3 disease, it is suggested that a pelvic and periaortic lymph node dissection be added to the surgical procedure described for grade 1 disease. It should be understood that lymphadenectomy in grade 2 adenocarcinoma is controversial. Further data are needed to determine its exact role in this group of patients. Adjunctive therapy, if needed, can then be planned, depending mainly on whether surgical-pathologic findings indicate intrauterine or extrauterine disease. If disease is intrauterine only, patients with grade 1 or 2 disease had 7/150 (4%) recurrence, and those with grade 3 and superficial disease had 2/14 (14%) recurrence, all of the latter at distant sites. It appears that surgery alone would be adequate treatment for these patients. In patients with grade 3 disease and significant muscle involvement, 4/10 (40%) recurrences were identified, with 3 of the 4 at distant sites. In these patients, one could probably justify postoperative external irradiation to the pelvis and consider adjunctive progestins or

chemotherapy. Unfortunately, patients responsive to progestins appear to need positive hormone receptors, and grade 3 tumors tend to be low in detectable receptors. Although doxorubicin (Adriamycin) has been considered the treatment of choice in recurrent adenocarcinomas, the complete response rate is only about 10%, and its role, if any, as an adjunct is yet to be defined (Figure 5-7).

When there is extrauterine disease (metastases to the adnexa and lymph nodes, intraperitoneally, or malignant cells in peritoneal cytologic specimens), the recurrence rate is high. Forty-eight of our patients had extrauterine disease, and 21 (43%) have had recurrences, 18 at distant sites. The necessity of developing adjunctive modalities to manage these metastases is apparent. It appears, however, that when disease is present in the pelvic or periaortic lymph nodes, postoperative irradiation therapy to these areas can be reasonably effective, since 40% of patients with nodal disease are tumor free at the time of analysis.

The hysterectomy should be extrafascial, and removal of the upper vagina does not appear to decrease vault recurrences (Figure 5-8). Peritoneal cytologic specimens should be obtained immediately after opening of the peritonal cavity (see description of the technique on p. 148). If ascites is present, appropriate samples of fluid should be sent for cytologic evaluation. When lymphadenectomy is done, the retroperitoneal spaces in the pelvis are opened in routine fashion. The vessels are outlined, and the lymph node-bearing tissue along the external iliacs from the bifurcation to the inguinal ligament is removed. The obturator fossa anterior to the obturator nerve is cleaned of lymphoid tissue. Lymph nodes along the common iliacs are also removed. No attempts to dissect behind or between the major vessels are made. The periaortic nodes are approached by retracting the small intestine into the upper abdomen and incising the peritoneum over the upper common iliac artery and lower aorta. The main vessels are outlined, and the ureter is retracted laterally. The tissue overlying the vena cava and the aorta is removed en bloc, beginning at the bifurcation of the aorta and extending caudad. The upper limit of the dissection (unless enlarged nodes are noted above this area) is usually the second and third portion of the duodenum as it crosses the main vessels retroperitoneally. Hemostasis can usually be accomplished with hemoclips. Using this technique, one should have a total of 20 to 30 lymph nodes available for histologic evaluation.

Patients with stage II carcinoma of the endometrium, because of extension of disease into the endocervix, will have a greater propensity for lymph node metastasis. Therapy should encompass likely metastatic sites and can be performed in several fashions. Primary surgery in the form of radical hysterectomy and pelvic lymphadenectomy has been acceptable therapy in the past, but it appears that simple hysterectomy, bilateral salpingo-

Table 5-18 Grade and risk factors in stage I cancer (clinical)

Grade	Lymph node metastasis	Deep muscle invasion	Recurrence
1	2%	4%	4%
2	11%	15%	15%
3	27%	39%	42%

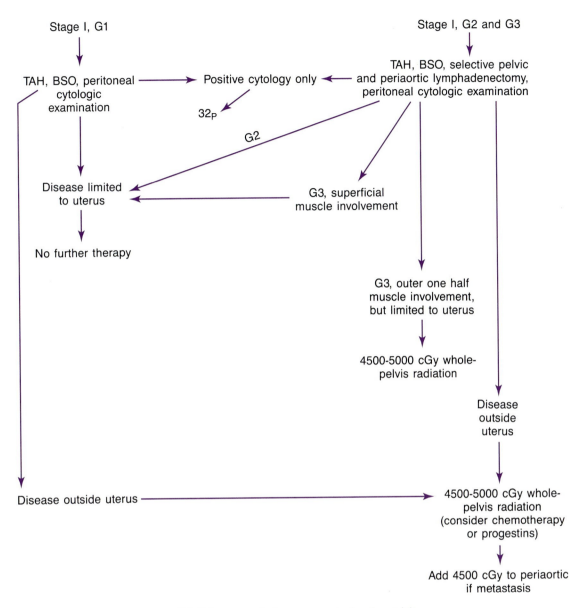

Figure 5-7 Primary surgical management of endometrial cancer.

oophorectomy, and pelvic and para-aortic lymphadenectomy would be adequate surgery today. Postoperative radiation therapy can be planned, depending on surgical pathological findings. If disease is limited to the uterus, postoperative radiation may not be necessary (Table 5-19). Others prefer to use external radiation in a dose of 4000 to 5000 cGy to the whole pelvis with at least one radium application before simple hysterectomy and bilateral salpingo-oophorectomy, which are usually performed 6 weeks after radiation therapy has been completed.

The role of adjunctive chemotherapy in addition to surgery and irradiation therapy has been addressed by the GOG in patients with high-risk stage I and occult stage II endometrial cancers. One hundred eighty-one patients were treated with TAH and BSO, peritoneal cytology, and selective pelvic and periaortic lymphadenopathy, followed by external irradiation (pelvic, with or without periaortic) and were then randomized to receive doxorubicin 60 mg/m^2 every 3 weeks for 8 doses. Patients participating in the doxorubicin arm of the protocol had a higher incidence of metastases to pelvic nodes (20% versus 10%) than those in the nondoxorubicin arm; otherwise, the risk factors were equal between the two groups. There were 22 of 92 (23%) recurrences in the doxorubicin arm versus 23 of 89 (26%) recurrences in the nondoxorubicin arm. Of those patients with recurrence, those who received doxorubicin had a greater chance of metastases to the abdomen than those who did not receive it (40% versus 17%). However, distant metastases occurred more frequently without the use of doxorubicin than with it (56% versus 18%).

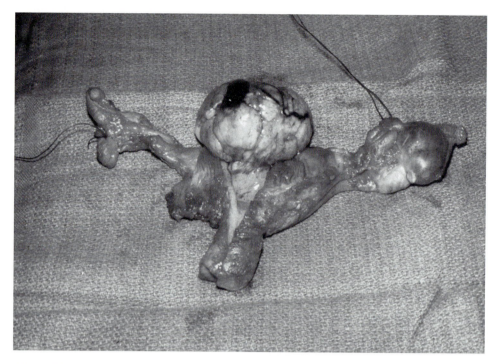

Figure 5-8 Total abdominal hysterectomy (TAH) and bilateral salpingo-oophorectomy (BSO) showing large polypoid adenocarcinoma of the endometrium with deep myometrial invasion.

Table 5-19 Recurrences in stage I and II patients surgically staged treated with surgery alone or surgery plus radiation (vault implant and/or external)

	Surgery only	Combined therapy
Negative risk factors	13/200 (6.5%)	17/190 (8.9%)
Positive risk factors*	31/78 (39.7%)	76/118 (64.4%)

Based on data from Morrow CP et al: *Gynecol Oncol* 40:55, 1991.
*Positive risk factors include disease outside uterus (adnexa, lymph nodes, intraperitoneal, positive cytology), isthmus/cervix involvement, and capillary space involvement.

Patients with occult stage II disease are managed surgically, as are those with stage I, grades 2 and 3 disease. It is well recognized that patients with endocervical involvement have a higher risk for extrauterine disease than those who have disease limited to the fundus. Some patients with endocervical involvement, however, do not exhibit other poor prognostic factors. Data from the surgical-pathologic study might suggest that if only endocervical disease is found, patients do well with surgery alone. It appears, however, that once the surgery has been done, postoperative irradiation therapy can be given if necessary, and studies have indicated that given in this sequence it is just as effective as if given preoperatively. To proceed with surgery initially would have an added benefit of making absolutely sure that, in fact, there was disease in the endocervix. It is not uncommon to designate a patient as having a stage II lesion on the basis of a fractional curettage because tumor cells are present, even though the cells may be "floaters." Onsrud et al., from the Norwegian Radium Hospital, have addressed this problem, and in a retrospective review they verified that only 96 of 174 cases (56%) originally recorded as stage II endometrial cancer in fact were stage II. Patients who were "overdiagnosed" had a survival rate similar to that of patients with stage I disease. It is interesting that in patients who truly had stage II disease, on histologic evaluation of the uterine specimen in a prospective clinical study, survial was not improved with the use of postoperative external irradiation over that of patients who had no external irradiation. A recent evaluation of 140 patients with clinical stage II cancers noted that only 35 (24%) in fact had surgical stage II disease. Knowing exact extent of disease appears to have a major impact not only on adjuvant therapy but also survival (prognosis).

There is no question that surgical staging can more accurately identify true extent of disease than clinical estimates. In clinical stage I disease, about one fourth of patients will have disease outside of the uterus and in patients thought to have stage II disease as many as 75% will have either less than stage II or extant disease. Implications in regard to therapy are great—not only in preventing unnecessary treatment but in directing more appropriate therapy, i.e., to known nodal disease. The question of possible increased morbidity has been

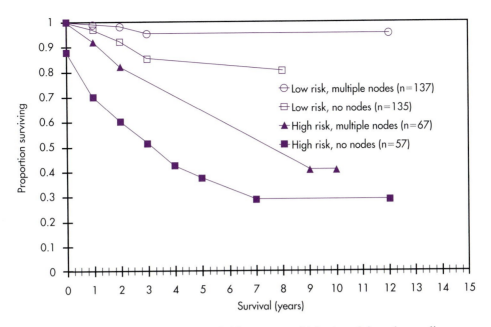

Figure 5-9 Survival by nodes sampled and risk groups: multiple-site pelvic node sampling vs no nodes. Low-risk group, $P = 0.026$; high-risk group, $P = 0.0006$. (Used with permission, Kilgore LC et al: *Gynecol Oncol* 56:29, 1995.)

addressed. It is suggested that there may be a significant increased complication rate with more extensive surgical staging. Moore and Larson have addressed morbidity from lymphadenectomy and noted no increased complications compared to the non-lymphadenectomy patients.

The question that has been asked since surgical staging has been proposed is whether or not survival may be affected. The implications of knowing true extent of disease suggests that certainly in individual situations survival may be affected. Kilgore and his colleagues at Alabama have published data that suggests not only is lymphadenectomy therapeutic but survival appears to be improved. They evaluated 649 patients with endometrial cancers, 212 had multiple-site pelvic node sampling, 205 had limited-site pelvic-node sampling, and in 208 nodes were not removed. Patients undergoing multiple-site lymphadenectomy had a significantly better survival than those patients not undergoing lymphadenectomy (p = 0.0002). Low-risk patients (disease confined to the uterus) with lymphadenectomy had better survival than those without lymphadenectomy (p = 0.026). High risk patients (disease in cervix, adnexa, uterine serosa, or washings) who underwent lymphadenectomy also had a better survival than those without lymphadenectomy (p = 0.0006) (Figure 5-9). Even when subsets were evaluated, the therapeutic benefits of the lymphadenectomy were apparent. Patients in both low and high risk categories who had lymphadenectomies and no post op radiation had a better survival than similar patients without lymphadenectomy but who received radiation therapy (Figure 5-10). Certainly, the therapeutic benefit of the lymphadenectomy is apparent. They also noted that

the extent of the lymphadenectomy was related to the number of metastatic lymph nodes identified.

Chuang noted that retroperitoneal recurrence in endometrial cancer was related to status of lymphadenectomy at time of primary surgery. If nodes were positive at primary surgery, retroperitoneal recurrence was not unusual while no recurrences were noted in retroperitoneum if both pelvic and para-aortic nodes were negative at initial surgery. In multivariant analysis, only presence of retroperitoneal nodal metastasis was significant for survival analysis.

Advanced disease presents an additional dilemma. With disease outside the uterus, therapy becomes limited with results less favorable. Behbakht evaluated prognostic factors in 137 patients with advanced disease (stage III and IV). Multivariant analysis noted age, parametrial involvement and abdominal metastasis as significant prognostic indicators. They also noted an increased frequency of advanced stage with papillary serous histology. Unfortunately, multiple therapies were used and conclusions concerning treatment cannot be made. Kadar and associates evaluated 58 patients with surgical stage III and IV disease. Extra pelvic peritoneal metastasis and positive peritoneal cytology affected survival. If either of these factors were present, a 2-year survival was only 25% compared to 83% if not present. Postoperative therapy varied but it did not appear to have any affect on survival.

Several chemotherapy combinations have been used in recurrent or advanced endometrial cancer. The GOG, in a randomized trial, compared doxorubicin with or without cisplatin. The combination experienced a 66% objective

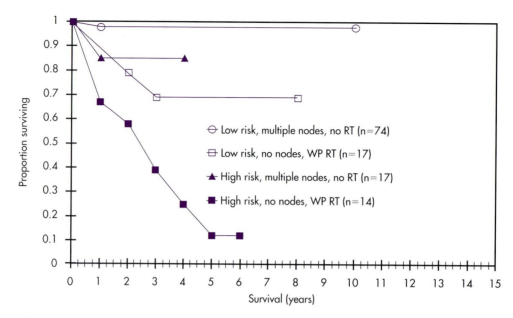

Figure 5-10 Survival comparisons of multiple-site pelvic node sampling to whole pelvic radiation therapy: multiple nodes without RT vs no nodes plus whole pelvic RT. Low risk, *P* = 0.003; high risk, *P* = 0.041. (Used with permission, Kilgore LC et al: *Gynecol Oncol* 56:29, 1995.)

response vs 35% for the single agent with median progressive free interval of 6.2 and 3.9 months respectively. Median survival was equal and only 9 months. A phase II trail of methotrexate, vinblastine, doxorubicin, and cisplatin (MVAC) was used by the Mayo and North Central Cancer Treatment Group in a like group of patients. In 30 patients, objective regression was noted in 20, complete in 8 (27%). Overall median survival was 10 months with objective responders surviving a median of 11 months. Toxicity was severe with severe treatment-related deaths.

Treatment of patients with stage III or IV disease must be individualized; however, in most instances hormonal treatment or chemotherapy, or both, must be used in addition to surgery and radiation therapy.

RECURRENCE

Even though the number of deaths caused by endometrial carcinoma is lower than the number associated with malignancies of the cervix and the ovary, the mortality is still significant, particularly in view of the number of patients with carcinoma of the uterus seen initially with stage I disease. Some recurrences, especially those that occur in the vaginal vault, can be treated successfully with surgery, radiation therapy, or a combination of the two. Many patients do extremely well and are long-term survivors. Unfortunately, many of the recurrences are seen outside the confines of the upper vagina and therefore are not amenable to surgery or radiation therapy. Radiation therapy may be of limited value in other patients, particularly if it has been used as part of primary

therapy. Therefore, hormonal treatment or chemotherapy may be the treatment of choice in many patients with recurrent carcinoma of the endometrium.

Progestins have been evaluated as adjunctive therapy in hopes of preventing recurrences. Lewis et al., in a randomized study, treated endometrial patients postoperatively with medroxyprogesterone (MPA) or placebo. The 4-year survival was similar in the two groups. Kauppila et al., in reporting on more than 1100 patients who received adjunctive progestin therapy for 2 years after surgery and irradiation therapy, found that even in stage I low-grade tumors, recurrences did appear; and it was their belief that prophylactic progestins were not of benefit to these patients. In a prospective study of 363 stage I patients who received adjuvant medroxyprogesterone for 12 months, DePalo et al. compared recurrence and survival with that of 383 stage I patients who did not receive medroxyprogesterone postoperatively. There was no difference in survival between the two groups. In a British study in which 429 patients with stage I or II cancers were randomized between postoperative MPA or observation, no difference in survival was seen after 5 years.

Progestins have been used for more than 20 years, and the objective responsiveness of recurrent carcinoma of the endometrium to these hormones has been substantiated. Historically, approximately one third of all patients with recurrent carcinoma of the endometrium are said to respond to the hormone, although patients with well-differentiated tumors have a higher response rate than those with moderately or poorly differentiated lesions. The GOG reported on 420 patients with advanced or

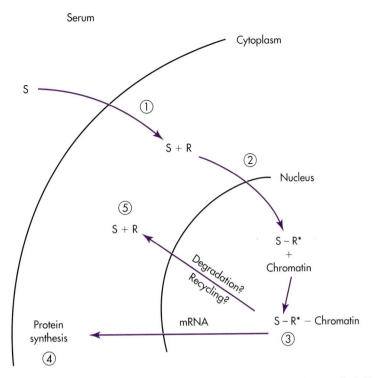

Figure 5-11 Simplified schema of steroid-receptor interactions in target tissue cell. *1,* Free steroid(s) diffuses across the cytoplasmic membrane and is bound by specific receptor(s). Recent studies with monoclonal antibody immunohistologic techniques indicate that estrogen receptor may be localized within nucleus. *2,* S-R complex is translocated into the nucleus and activated (*). *3,* Activated S-R complex interacts with chromatin and initiates mRNA transcription. *4,* mRNA initiates specific protein synthesis, producing hormonal effects. *5,* S-R complex is degraded and/or recycled. (From Soper JT, Christensen CW: *Clin Obstet Gynecol* 13:825, 1986.)

recurrent endometrial carcinoma treated with medroxyprogesterone acetate (MPA) 50 mg three times a day. Of the 219 patients with objective measurable disease, there were only 17 complete responders (8%) and 13 partial responders (6%). More than one half of the patients remained stable and one third progressed. Median survival was 10½ months. Grade 1 lesions responded more frequently than poorly differentiated carcinomas. The GOG evaluated, in randomized phase III trial, MPA at 1000 mg per day compared to 200 mg per day. In almost 300 patients, there was no difference in response rate or survival between the two groups.

More recently, considerable interest has been shown in the presence of specific estrogen-progesterone receptors in neoplastic human uterine tissue (Figure 5-11). These receptors are definitely present and vary from tumor to tumor. It has been shown that there is a greater number of both estrogen and progesterone receptors in well- differentiated lesions than in poorly differentiated ones (Table 5-20). In a small group of patients, it was noted that about one third of those with recurrent cancer had a positive receptor site analysis to both estrogen and progesterone. The receptor data may therefore correlate with clinical findings of responsiveness to progesterones in patients with recurrent cancer. Preliminary data suggest an excellent correlation (Table 5-21). Obviously, consider-

Table 5-20   Correlation of tumor differentiation with receptor content

Differentiation	E_2 and P_R positive
Well	28/40 (70%)
Moderate	21/38 (55%)
Poor	11/27 (41%)

From Creasman WT et al: *Am J Obstet Gynecol* 151:922, 1985.

able additional data are needed to verify these findings; however, the prospects are excellent. If direct correlation can be substantiated, the receptor site analysis can guide the types of progestin or chemotherapy given for recurrent endometrial cancer. If receptor site analysis is positive for both estrogen and progesterone, a patient's chances of responding to progestins are extremely good, even if she has a poorly differentiated lesion. On the other hand, if receptor site analysis is negative, the data suggest that the patient's response to progestins may be extremely low, making it more advisable to go directly to cytotoxic agents without wasting time on progestin therapy. Kauppila noted from five studies in the literature that 89% of progesterone receptor-positive tumors were hormonally

Table 5-21 Response to progestin therapy in regard to receptor content

Receptor content	Progestin response
Positive	44/55 (80%)
Negative	4/76 (5%)

Based on papers by Ehrlich, Benraad, Creasman, Martin, Kauppila, Pollow, Quinn.

responsive, compared to only 17% of progesterone receptor-negative tumors. The GOG noted that 4/10 (40%) of estrogen receptor-positive, progesterone receptor-positive tumors responded to progestins, compared to 5/41 (12%) of progesterone receptor-negative tumors.

Progestin therapy may be administered in several different ways. We prefer medroxyprogesterone (Depo-Provera), 400 mg IM at weekly intervals. Oral medroxyprogesterone (Provera) in the range of 150 mg/day and megestrol acetate (Megace), 160 mg/day, are other recommended progestins. Progestins are continued indefinitely if an objective response is obtained. If progression of disease is noted, progestins should be discontinued and chemotherapy considered.

With only modest response to progestins, other hormonal agents have been evaluated. Tamoxifen (TAM) has been shown to bind estrogen receptors and thereby block the access of the estrogen into the nucleus. It has also been suggested that TAM can increase the number of progesterone receptors in vivo. Combined results of several small studies noted a response rate of 22% (CR 8%) in 257 patients. These studies suggest that grade 1 lesions were more responsive than other grades of tumors. Progestins plus TAM have been evaluated in combination in recurrent carcinoma of the endometrium. Although TAM is theoretically attractive (it causes an increase in progesterone receptors for better progestin effect), studies of small groups of patients have not produced favorable results. The use of TAM is interesting, in view of the reports of endometrial cancer in patients taking TAM. This is in contrast to in vitro data that suggests that TAM does not stimulate, and in fact may inhibit, established endometrial cell line growth.

GnRH analogues have been evaluated in the treatment of endometrial cancer in a small number of patients. These analogues suppress gonadotropins with a reduction in estrogen but not cortisol levels. Gallagher treated 17 patients with recurrent endometrial cancer who had received previous progesterone therapy, with 6 (35%) having a response that continued for a median of 20 months. Further study is needed but it appears that GnRH analogues may have a direct inhibitory effect on cancer cells.

Because one third of the patients with recurrent carcinoma of the endometrium responded to progestins

and because hormone therapy is essentially nontoxic, evaluations of cytotoxic agents have not been pursued until recently. Initial data suggest that doxorubicin is an effective agent in the treatment of adenocarcinoma of the endometrium, with approximately a 35% response rate in patients not responding to progestins. In the report of the GOG experience, Thigpen noted that 16 of 43 (37%) patients with advanced or recurrent cancer experienced an objective response using doxorubicin alone. Unfortunately, response lasted only 7 months. The Eastern Oncology Group achieved only a 19% response rate in its doxorubicin trial; however, a dosage lower than the GOG dosage was used. When one evaluates the doxorubicin data, one notes that only about 10% of patients who received this drug had a complete response rate. Patients designated as giving a partial response had no greater survival rates than those who had no response to this cytotoxic agent. The role of doxorubicin as a single agent may be limited in this disease.

✓ Experience with cisplatin chemotherapy as a single agent has been reported by the MD Anderson Hospital group. Eleven of 26 patients (42%) had objective responses (10 partial responses and 1 complete response). Unfortunately, the mean duration of remission was 5 months, with the complete response lasting for 8 months. The same authors had previously reported their experience with doxorubicin and cyclophosphamide: 8 of 26 patients (30%) had partial responses for a mean duration of 4 months. Experience of the Gynecologic Oncology Group showed that only 1 of 23 patients treated with cisplatin responded; however, 20 of the 23 patients had been previously treated with other cytotoxic agents. Trope et al. noted a 36% response rate in 11 patients who were previously untreated with chemotherapy. In a subsequent study of 49 patients who had not been previously treated with a cytotoxic agent, 10 (20%), responded to cisplatin, and 2 (4%) were complete responders. Carboplatin, a cisplatin analog, has been evaluated in 48 patients with a 30% response, but only 2 (4%) complete responders.

Several other drugs have been used in phase II studies in this group of patients. These include ICRF 159 (Razoxane), piperazinedione, mAMSA (Amsacrine), mitoxantrone (Novantione), Dianhydrogalactitol, etoposide, methotrexate, and aminothiadiozole—all showed very little or no activity.

Several small nonrandomized reports in the literature suggest that multiple-agent chemotherapy can be effective in disseminated endometrial carcinoma. A large prospective randomized study was carried out by the GOG evaluating melphalan and 5-fluorouracil (5-FU) versus doxorubicin, 5-fluorouracil, and cyclophosphamide. Megestrol acetate was also used. Approximately one third of both groups achieved an objective response. The duration of the progression-free interval was essentially identical in the two groups, a median response rate of approximately 6 months. The median survival rate was

Table 5-22   Response to chemotherapy in regard to receptor content

	ER or PR negative	ER or PR positive
CR$^\times$ or PR$^+$ (4 mo)	7/10	1/5

Modified from Kauppila A et al: *Cancer* 46:2162, 1980.
$^\times$Complete response; $^+$partial response.

approximately 10 months in both groups, although complete responder median survival was 18.3 months and partial responder was 12.9 months. Toxicity from these regimens was appreciable. A similar study by the Eastern Oncology Group noted similar results.

In a prospective study by GOG, 336 patients who had advanced or recurrent adenocarcinoma were treated with doxorubicin, with or without cyclophosphamide. All these patients had failed to respond when given medroxy-progesterone acetate. Only 7 (5.4%) of those treated with doxorubicin had a complete response, but 18 (12.5%) who received doxorubicin plus cyclophosphamide were complete responders. Total response was 22% for doxorubicin and 30% for doxorubicin and cyclophosphamide. The median survival was 7 months for both groups, and there was no difference in survival between the two groups. Piver et al. treated 50 patients with melphalen, 5-fluorouracil, and medroxyprogesterone acetate, with or without tamoxifen, as first line chemotherapy. There was a 20% complete response rate and 48% total responses. The median progression-free survival was only 5 months for the whole group, but it was 24 months for the complete responders. Several small studies have evaluated cisplatin, cytoxan, and doxorubicin in phase II trials. In five studies with 127 evaluable patients, 63 (50%) responses were noted, and 24 (19%) were complete responders. The GOG is currently comparing doxorubicin to cisplatin and doxorubicin.

Obviously the ideal therapeutic agent for recurrent adenocarcinoma of the endometrium has not been found. Investigation in regard to new approaches, including role of recombinant hematopoietic colony stimulating factors, tumor necrosis factor, IL-2, and growth factors, may prove beneficial in the future.

Of interest is a report by Kauppila et al., who noted that patients with low estrogen or progesterone receptor values had a significantly greater response rate to combined cytotoxic therapy (doxorubicin, cyclophosphamide, 5-fluorouracil, and vincristine) than did patients with higher receptor values (Table 5-22). This observation must be confirmed, but the role of receptor analysis in recurrent adenocarcinoma of the endometrium may be extremely important in determining the best therapy for the individual patient.

It has been suggested by some that CA125 can be used to monitor therapy in patients with advanced or recurrent adenocarcinoma of the endometrium much as is done in ovarian cancer. Niloff and others have noted CA125 is elevated in as many as three fourths of these patients. Data is limited in regard to monitoring. Fanning and Piver did note in 21 women that clinical response, as well as subsequent relapse, correlated with CA125 levels on patients with advanced or recurrent disease. Monitoring with CA125 may be helpful.

Multiple Malignancies

Simultaneous or subsequent primary cancers involving the breast, ovary, and large intestines occur more frequently in endometrial cancer patients than might be expected. The reverse also appears true, in that women with breast or ovarian cancer have a higher than expected risk of developing subsequent primary cancers of the endometrium. As a result, the recommendation in a patient with one of these malignancies is to evaluate the other organ sites at the time of the diagnosis or during follow-up visits. Appropriate screening, such as mammography, should be emphasized.

Simultaneous malignancies of the ovary and endometrium are noted in about 8% of patients with carcinoma of the uterus, and twice that rate is noted in patients with ovarian carcinoma. Ovarian involvement in cases in which endometrial cancer is present has been reported in as high as 40% of autopsies and 15% of specimens obtained at the time of hysterectomy and bilateral salpingo-oophorectomy. In approximately one third of cases of endometroid carcinoma of the ovary, endometrial carcinoma has also been noted. When the simultaneous occurrence appears, the question arises whether these are simultaneous multiple malignancies or one is metastatic from the other. It appears that if metastasis is present, it is more common for it to go from the endometrium to the ovary than from the ovary to the endometrium. Metastasis to the ovary is suspected if the endometrial carcinoma involves significant myometrium, particularly with lymphatic or vascular channel invasion, or if the tumor is on the ovarian surface. If, on the other hand, the corpus carcinoma is small and limited to the endometrium or superficial myometrium, with associated atypical hyperplasia, and if the ovarian tumor is centrally located, then the tumors are probably independent of each other. Most common tumors are the endometroid type, but occasionally they can be of different histological types in the two organs. Most studies suggest that most of the synchronous ovarian and corpus carcinomas are independent primary tumors. The survival of patients with what is believed to be multiple primaries mimics the excellent prognosis of the individual cancer, suggesting that the two tumors are probably each stage I and not stage III. This has certainly been true when the simultaneous endometrial and ovarian carcinomas are of the endometroid type. In one study, the survival was 100% of the 16 patients reported. It appears that when such a situation is encountered (i.e., when there is no evidence of direct extension of either tumor), myometrial invasion is usually absent or superficial, there is no lymphatic or blood vessel invasion, there is atypical hyperplasia of the endometrium frequently associated with the cancer, both tumors are usually confined to the primary sites and have minimal spread, and tumor is predominantly within the ovary or the endometrium. Whether the histologic type is uniform or dissimilar, therapy should be appropriate for stage I disease, which in many instances may be treated adequately with surgery only (hysterectomy and bilateral salpingo-oophorectomy with appropriate surgical staging).

BIBLIOGRAPHY

Incidence and epidemiology

Antunes CMF et al: Endometrial cancer and estrogen use (report of a large case-control study), *N Engl J Med* 300:9, 1979.

Bokhman JV: Two pathogenetic types of endometrial carcinoma, *Gynecol Oncol* 15:10, 1983.

Caspi F, Perpinial S, Reif A: Incidence of malignancy in Jewish women with postmenopausal bleeding, *Isr J Med Sci* 13:299, 1977.

Center for Disease Control: Cancer in steroid hormone study: oral contraceptive use and the risk of endometrial cancer, *JAMA* 249:1600, 1983.

Cohen CJ, Deppe G: Endometrial carcinoma and oral contraceptive agents, *Obstet Gynecol* 49:390, 1977.

Dunn LJ, Bradbury JT: Endocrine factors in endometrial carcinoma, *Am J Obstet Gynecol* 97:465, 1967.

Gray LA, Christopherson WM, Hoover RN: Estrogens and endometrial carcinoma, *Obstet Gynecol* 49:385, 1977.

Greenblatt RB, Stoddard LB: The estrogen-cancer controversy, *J Am Geriatr Soc* 26:1, 1978.

Gusberg SB, Kardon P: Proliferative endometrial response to thecal granulosa cell tumors, *Am J Obstet Gynecol* 3:633, 1971.

Hoffman K, Nekhylndov L, Deligdisch L: Endometrial carcinoma in elderly women, *Gynecol Oncol* 58:198, 1995.

Hoover R et al: Cancer of the uterine corpus after hormonal treatment for breast cancer, *Lancet* 1:885, 1976.

Horwitz RL, Feinstein AF: Alternative analytic methods for case-control studies of estrogens and endometrial cancer, *N Engl J Med* 299:1090, 1978.

Husslein H, Brietenecker G, Tatra G: Premalignant and malignant uterine changes in immunosuppressed renal transplant recipients, *Acta Obstet Gynecol Scand* 57:73, 1978.

Kaplan DS, Cole P: Epidemiology of cancer of the endometrium, in press.

Kelley HW et al: Adenocarcinoma of the endometrium in women taking sequential oral contraceptives, *Obstet Gynecol* 47:200, 1972.

Lauritzen C: Oestrogens and endometrial cancer: a point of view, *Clin Obstet Gynecol* 4:145, 1977.

Lawrence C et al: Smoking, body weight, and early stage endometrial cancer, *Cancer* 59:1665, 1987.

Levi F, Franeschi S, Negri E, LaVecchia C: Dietary factors and the risk of endometrial cancer, *Cancer* 71:3775, 1993.

Mack TM et al: Estrogens and endometrial cancer in a retirement community, *N Engl J Med* 294:1262, 1976.

Mansell H, Hertig AT: Granulosa-theca cell tumor and endometrial carcinoma: a study of their relationship and survey of 80 cases, *Obstet Gynecol* 6:385, 1955.

Masubuchi K, Nemoto H: Epidemiologic studies on uterine cancer at Cancer Institute Hospital, Tokyo, Japan, *Cancer* 30:268, 1972.

McCarty KS Jr et al: Gonadal dysgenesis with adenocarcinoma of the endometrium: electron microscopic and steroid receptor analyses with a review of the literature, *Cancer* 42:510, 1978.

McDonald TW et al: Exogenous estrogen and endometrial carcinoma: case-control and incidence study, *Am J Obstet Gynecol* 127:572, 1977.

McDonald TW, Malkasian GD, Gaffey TA: Endometrial cancer associated with feminizing ovarian tumors and polycystic ovarian disease, *Obstet Gynecol* 94:654, 1977.

Novak E, Yui E: Relationship of endometrial hyperplasia to adenocarcinoma of the endometrium, *Am J Obstet Gynecol* 32:674, 1936.

Nyholm NCV, Neilsen AL, Norup P: Endometrial cancer in postmenopausal women with and without previous estrogen replacement treatment: Comparison of clinical and histopathological characteristics, *Gynecol Oncol* 49:229, 1993.

Ostor AG et al: Endometrial carcinoma in gonadal dysgenesis with and without estrogen therapy, *Gynecol Oncol* 6:316, 1978.

Pacheco JC, Kempers RD: Etiology of post-menopausal bleeding, *Obstet Gynecol* 32:40, 1968.

Rauramo L: Estrogen replacement therapy and endometrial carcinoma, *Front Horm Res* 5:117, 1978.

Schapira DV, Kumar NB, Lyman GH et al: Upper-body fat distribution and endometrial cancer risk, *JAMA* 266:1808, 1991.

Segaloff A: Steroids in carcinogenesis, *J Steroid Biochem* 6:171, 1975.

Silverberg E, Halleb A: Cancer statistics, 1971, *CA* 21:13, 1971.

Silverberg SG, Makowski EL: Endometrial carcinoma in young women taking oral contraceptives agents, *Obstet Gynecol* 46:503, 1975.

Smith DC et al: Association of exogenous estrogen and endometrial carcinoma, *N Engl J Med* 293:1164, 1975.

Steert H: Cancer of the endometrium in young women, *Surg Gynecol Obstet* 88:332, 1949.

Swanson CA, Potischman N, Wilbanks GD et al: Relationship of endometrial cancer risk to past and contemporary body size and body fat distribution, *Cancer Epid Biomarkers and Prev* 2:321, 1993.

Szekely DR, Weiss NS, Schweid A: Incidence of endometrial carcinoma in Kings County, Washington: a standardized histologic review, brief communication, *J Natl Ca Inst* 60:985, 1978.

Weiss NS: Noncontraceptive estrogens and abnormalities of endometrial proliferation, *Ann Intern Med* 88:410, 1978.

Wynder EL, Escher GC, Mantel N: An epidemiological investigation of cancer of the endometrium, *Cancer* 19:489, 1966.

Ziel HK, Finkle WD: Increased risk of endometrial carcinoma among users of conjugated estrogens, *N Engl J Med* 293:1167, 1975.

Pathology

Abeler UA and Kjorstad KE: Endometrial adenocarcinoma with squamous cell differentiation, *Cancer* 69:488, 1992.

Alberhasky RC, Connely PJ, Christopherson WN: Carcinoma of the endometrium. IV. Mixed adenosquamous carcinoma, *Am J Clin Pathol* 77:655, 1982.

Bokhman JV: Two pathogenic types of endometrial carcinoma, *Gynecol Oncol,* 15:10, 1983.

Chen JL, Trost DC, Wilkinson EJ: Endometrial papillary carcinoma: two clinical pathological types, *Int J Gynecol Pathol* 4:279, 1985.

Christopherson WN, Alberhasky RC, Connely PJ: Carcinoma of the endometrium. I. A clinicopathological study of clear cell carcinoma and secretory carcinoma, *Cancer* 49:1511, 1982.

Christopherson WN, Alberhasky RC, Connely PJ: Carcinoma of the endometrium. II. Papillary adenocarcinoma: a clinico-pathological study of 46 patients, *Am J Clin Pathol* 77:534, 1982.

Connely PJ, Alberhasky RC, Christopherson WN: Carcinoma of the endometrium. III. Analysis of 865 cases of adenocarcinoma and adenocanthoma, *Obstet Gynecol* 59:569, 1982.

Eifel P, Hendrickson M, Ross J et al: Simultaneous presentation of carcinoma involving the ovary and uterine corpus, *Cancer* 50:163, 1982.

Gordon J et al: Estrogen and endometrium carcinoma: an independent pathology review supporting original risk estimate, *N Engl J Med* 297:500, 1977.

Jeffrey JF, Krepart GV, Lotocki RJ: Papillary serous adenocarcinomas of the endometrium, *Obstet Gynecol* 67:670, 1986.

Johnsson JE, Norman O: Relation between prognosis in early carcinoma of the uterine body and hysterographically assessed localization and size of tumor, *Gynecol Oncol* 7:71, 1979.

Kurman RJ, Scully RE: Clear cell carcinoma of the endometrium: analysis of 21 cases, *Cancer* 37:872, 1976.

Mahle A: The morphological histology of adenocarcinoma of the body of the uterus in relationship to longevity, *Surg Gynecol Obstet* 36:385, 1923.

Ng ABP: Mixed carcinoma of the endometrium, *Am J Obstet Gynecol* 102:506, 1968.

Ng ABP, Reagan JW: Incidence and prognosis of endometrial carcinoma by histologic grade and extent, *Obstet Gynecol* 35:437, 1970.

Ng ABP et al: Mixed adenosquamous carcinoma of the endometrium, *Am J Clin Pathol* 59:765, 1973.

Photopulos GJ et al: Clear cell carcinoma of the endometrium, *Cancer* 43:1448, 1979.

Salazar OM et al: Adenosquamous carcinoma of the endometrium, *Cancer* 40:119, 1977.

Schwartz PE et al: Routine use of hysterography in endometrium carcinoma and postmenopausal bleeding, *Obstet Gynecol* 45:378, 1975.

Schwartz Z, Ohel G, Birkenfeld A et al: Second primary malignancy in endometria carcinoma patients, *Gynecol Oncol* 22:40, 1985.

Silverberg SG, Bolin MG, DeGiorgi LS: Adenoacanthoma and mixed adenosquamous carcinoma of the endometrium, *Cancer* 30:1307, 1972.

Silverberg SG, DeGiorgi LS: Clear cell carcinoma of the endometrium: clinical-pathological and ultra-structural findings, *Cancer* 31:1127, 1973.

Zaino RJ, Kurtman R, Herbald D et al: The significane of squamous differentiation, *Cancer* 68:2293, 1991.

Zaino RJ, Unger ER, Whitney C: Synchronous carcinomas of the uterine corpus and ovary, *Gynecol Oncol* 19:329, 1984.

Screening and diagnosis

Abate SD, Edwards CL, Vellias F: A comparative study of the endometrial jet-washing technique and endometrial biopsy, *Am J Clin Pathol* 58:118, 1972.

Anderson B: Diagnosis of endometrial cancer, *Clin Obstet Gynecol* 13:739, 1986.

Anderson B et al: Routine noninvasive hysterography in the evaluation and treatment of endometrial carcinoma, *Gynecol Oncol* 4:354, 1976.

Barakat RR: The effects of tamoxifen on the endometrium, *Oncol* 9:129, 1995.

Berezowsky J, Chalvardjian A, Murray D: Iatrogenic endometrial mega-polyps in women with breast carcinoma, *Obstet Gynecol* 84:727, 1994.

Bourne TH, Campbell S, Steer CV et al: Detection of endometrial cancer by transvaginal ultrasonography with color flow imaging and blood flow analysis, *Gynecol Oncol* 40:253, 1991.

Butler EB, Monahan PB, Warrell DW: Kuper brush in the diagnosis of endometrial lesions, *Lancet* 2:1390, 1971.

Cacciatore B, Lehtovirta P, Wahlstrom T et al: Preoperative sonographic evaluation of endometrial cancer, *Am J Obstet Gynecol* 160:133, 1989.

Chatfield WR, Bremner AD: Intrauterine sponge biopsy, *Obstet Gynecol* 39:323, 1972.

Cohen CJ, Gusberg SB: Screening for endometrial cancer, *Clin Obstet Gynecol* 18:27, 1975.

Cohen I, Rosen DJD, Shapria J et al: Endometrial changes with tamoxifen: comparison between tamoxifen-treated and nontreated asymptomatic postmenopausal breast cancer patients, *Gynecol Oncol* 52:185, 1994.

Creasman WT, Weed JC Jr: Screening techniques in endometrial cancer, *Cancer* 38:436, 1976.

Doering DL, Barnhill DR, Weiser EB et al: Intraoperative evaluation of depth of myometrial invasion in stage I endometrial carcinoma, *Obstet Gyencol* 74:930, 1989.

Feldman S, Cook EF, Harlow BL, Berkowitz RS: Predicting endometrial cancer among older women who present with abnormal vaginal bleeding, *Gynecol Oncol* 56:376, 1995.

Fisher B, Costantino JP, Redmond CK et al: Endometrial cancer in tamoxifen treated breast cancer patients: findings from the National Surgical Adjuvant Breast and Bowel Project (NSABP) B-14, *J Natl Cancer Inst* 86:527, 1994.

Goldstein SR: Unusual ultrasound appearance of the uterus in patients receiving tamoxifen, *Am J Obstet Gynecol* 170:447, 1994.

Gordon AN, Fleischer AC, Dudley BS et al: Preoperative assessment of myometrial invasion of endometrial adenocarcinoma by ultrasound and MRI, *Gynecol Oncol* 34:175, 1989.

Granberg S, Wikland M, Karlson B et al: Endometrial thickness as measured by endovaginal ultrasound for identifying endometrial abnormality, *Am J Obstet Gynecol* 164:47, 1991.

Hofmeister FJ: Endometrial biopsy: another look, *Am J Obstet Gynecol* 118:733, 1974.

Ismail SM: Pathology of endometrium treated with tamoxifen, *J Clin Path* 47:827, 1994.

Jordan VC, Assikis VJ: Endometrial carcinoma and tamoxifen: clearing up a controversy, *Clin Cancer Res* 1:467, 1995.

Kademian MT, Buehler DA, Wirtanen GW: Bipedal lymphangiography in malignancies of the uterine corpus, *AJR* 129:903, 1977.

Kedar RP, Bourne TH, Powles TJ et al: Effects of tamoxifen on uterus and ovaries of postmenopausal women in a randomized breast cancer prevention trial, *Lancet* 343:1318, 1994.

Killackey MA, Hakes TB, Pierce VK: Endometrial adenocarcinoma in breast cancer patients receiving anti-estrogen cancer treatment, Report 69:273, 1985.

Lahti E, Blanco G, Kauppila A et al: Endometrial changes in postmeno-pausal breast cancer patients receiving tamoxifen, *Obstet Gynecol* 81:660, 1993.

Magriples U, Naftolin F, Schwartz PE et al: High grade endometrial carcinoma in tamoxifen treated breast cancer patients, *J Clin Oncol* 11:485, 1993.

Milan AR et al: Endometrial cytology: using the Milan-Markley technique, *Obstet Gynecol* 48:111, 1976.

Nasri MH, Coast CJ: Correlation of ultrasound findings and endometrial histopathology in postmenopausal women, *Br J Obstet Gynaecol* 96:1333, 1989.

Ng ABP et al: Significance of endometrial cells in the detection of endometrial carcinoma and its precursors, *Acta Cytol* 18:356, 1974.

Stovall TG, Photopulos GJ, Poston WM et al: Pipelle endometrial sampling in patients with known endometrial carcinoma, *Obstet Gynecol* 77:954, 1991.

Varner RE, Sparks JM, Cameron CD et al: Transvaginal sonography of the endometrium in postmenopausal women, *Obstet Gynecol* 78:195, 1991.

Wolff JP et al: The value of hysterogram for the prognosis of endometrial cancer, *Gynecol Oncol* 3:103, 1975.

Prognostic factors

Ambros RA, Kurman RJ: Identification of patients with stage I uterine endometrial adenocarcinoma at high risk of recurrence by DNA ploidy myometrial invasion and vascular invasion, *Gynecol Oncol* 45:235, 1992.

Ayhan A, Turner R, Turner ZS et al: Correlation between clinical and histopathologic risk factors; i.e., lymph node metastasis in early endometrial cancer, *Int J Obstet Gynecol* 4:306, 1994.

Baak JPA, Snijders WP, Van Diest PJ et al: Confirmation of the prognostic value of the ECP1-1 score in FIGO stage I endometrial cancer patients with long follow up, *Int J. Gynecol Cancer* 5:112, 1995.

Benraad TJ et al: Do estrogen and progesterone receptors (E2R and PR) in metastasizing endometrial cancer predict the response to progestin therapy? *Acta Obstet Gynecol Scand* 59:155,1980.

Boronow RC et al: Surgical staging in endometrial cancer: clinical pathological findings of a prospective study, *Obstet Gynecol* 63:825, 1985.

Britton LC, Wilson TO, Gaffey TA et al: DNA ploidy in endometrial carcinoma: major objective prognostic factor, *Mayo Clin Proc* 65:643, 1990.

Cheon HK: Prognosis of endometrial carcinoma, *Obstet Gynecol* 34:680, 1969.

Cowles TA et al: Comparison of clinical and surgical staging in patients with endometrial cancer, *Obstet Gynecol* 66:413, 1985.

Creasman WT, DiSaia PJ, Blessing J: Prognostic significance of peritoneal cytology in patients with endometrial cancer and preliminary data concerning therapy with intraperitoneal radiopharmaceuticals, *Am J Obstet Gynecol* 141:921, 1981.

Creasman WT, McCarty KS Sr, McCarty KS Jr: Clinical correlation of estrogen, progesterone binding proteins in human endometrial adeno-carcinoma, Obstet Gyencol 55:363, 1980.

Creasman WT, Morrow CP, Bundy L: Surgical pathological spread patterns of endometrial cancer, *Cancer* 60:2035, 1987.

Creasman WT, Rutledge FN: The prognostic value of peritoneal cytology in gynecologic malignant disease, *Am J Obstet Gynecol* 110:773, 1971.

Creasman WT et al: Adenocarcinoma of the endometrium: its metastatic lymph node potential: a preliminary report, *Gynecol Oncol* 4:239, 1976.

Creasman WT et al: Influence of cytoplasmic steroid receptor content on prognosis of early stage endometrial carcinoma, *Am J Obstet Gynecol* 151:922, 1985.

De Muelenaere GFGO: Prognostic factors in endometrial carcinoma, *S Afr Med J* 49:1695, 1975.

DiSaia PJ et al: Risk factors in recurrent patterns in stage I endometrial carcinoma, *Am J Obstet Gynecol* 151:1009, 1985.

Ehrlich CE, Young PCM, Cleary RE: Cytoplasmic progesterone and estriol receptors in normal hyperplastic and carcinomas endometria: therapeutic implications, *Am J Obstet Gynecol* 141:539, 1981.

Genest P et al: Prognostic factors in early carcinoma of the endometrium, *Am J Clin Oncol (CCP)* 10:71, 1987.

Goff BA, Kato D, Schmidt RA et al: Uterine papillary serous carcinoma: patterns of metastatic spread, *Gynecol Oncol* 54:264, 1994.

Grimshaw RN, Tupper WC, Fraser RC et al: Prognostic value of peritoneal cytology in endometrial carcinoma, *Gynecol Oncol* 36:97, 1990.

Hanson NB et al: Prognostic significance of lymph-vascular space invasion in stage I endometrial cancer, *Cancer* 55:1753, 1985.

Haroung VR, Sutton EP, Clark SA et al: The importance of peritoneal cytology in endometrial carcinoma, *Obstet Gynecol* 72:394-8, 1988.

Hendrickson M et al: Adenocarcinoma of the endometrium: analysis of 256 cases of carcinoma limited to the uterine corpus, *Gynecol Oncol* 13:373, 1982.

Hendrickson MR, Longacre TA, Kempson RL: Uterine papillary serous carcinoma revisited, *Gynecol Oncol* 54:261, 1991.

Hendrickson MR, Ross J, Eifel PJ et al: Adenocarcinoma of the endometrium, *Gynecol Oncol* 13:373, 1982.

Javert CT: The spread of benign and malignant endometrium in the lymphatic system with a note on coexisting vascular involvement, *Am J Obstet Gynecol* 64:780, 1952.

Konski A, Poulter C, Keys H et al: Absence of prognostic significance, peritoneal dissemination and treatment advantage in endometrial cancer patients with postive peritoneal cytology, *Int J Radiat Oncol Biol Phys* 4:49, 1988.

Levenback C, Burke TW, Silva E et al: Uterine papillary serous carcinoma treated with PAC, *Gynecol Oncol* 46:317, 1992.

Lefevre H: Node dissection in cancer of the endometrium, *Surg Gynecol Obstet* 102:649, 1956.

Lurian JR, Rum Sey NK, Schink JC et al: Prognostic significance of positive peritoneal cytology in clinical stage I adenocarcinoma of the endometrium, *Obstet Gynecol* 74:175, 1989.

Lutz MH et al: Endometrial carcinoma: a new method of classification of therapeutic and prognostic significance, *Gynecol Oncol* 6:83, 1978.

MacMahon B: Risk factors for endometrial cancer, *Gynecol Oncol* 2:122, 1974.

Martin PM et al: Estriol and progesterone receptors in normal and neoplastic endometrium: correlations between receptors, histopathologic examination, and clinical response under progesterone therapy, *Int J Cancer* 23:321, 1979.

Milosevic MF, Dembo AD, Thomas GM: Clinical significant of malignant peritoneal cytology in stage I endometrial carcinoma, *Int J Gynecol Cancer* 2:225, 1992.

Morrow CP, Bundy BN, Kurman RJ et al: Relationship between surgical pathological risk factors and outcome in clinical stage I and II carcinoma of the endometrium, *Gynecol Oncol* 40:55, 1991. Nolan JF, Huen A: Prognosis in endometrial cancer, *Gynecol Oncol* 4:384, 1976.

Norris HJ, Taylor HG: Prognosis of granulosa thecal tumor of the ovary, *Cancer* 21:255, 1968.

Onsrud N et al: Endometrial carcinoma with cervical involvement (stage II): prognostic factors in value of combined radiological surgical treatment, *Gynecol Oncol* 13:76, 1982.

Parkash V, Carcangiu ML: Uterine papillary serous carcinoma after radiation therapy for carcinoma of the cervix, *Cancer* 69:496, 1992.

Pfister J, Kommess F, Sancrbrei V et al: Prognostic value of DNA ploidy and S-phase fraction in stage I endometrial carcinoma, *Gynecol Oncol* 58:149, 1995.

Pisani A, Barbuto DA, Chen D et al: HER-2/nen, p53, and DNA analysis as prognosticators for survival in endometrial carcinoma, *Obstet Gynecol* 85:729, 1995.

Plentyl AA, Friedman EA: *Lymphatic system of the female genitalia: the morphologic basis of oncologic diagnosis and therapy,* Philadelphia, 1971, WB Saunders.

Podratz KC, Wilson TO, Gaffey TA et al: DNA analysis facilitates the pretreatment identification of high-risk endometrial cancer patients, *Am J Obstet Gynecol* 168:1206, 1993.

Pollow K, Manz B, Grill JH: *Estrogen progesterone receptors in endometrial carcinoma.* In Jasonni VM, editor: *Steroids and endometrial cancer,* New York, Raven.

Potish RA et al: Paraaortic lymph node radiotherapy in the cancer of uterine corpus, *Obstet Gynecol* 65:251, 1985.

Quinn MA, Couchi M, Fortune V: Endometrial carcinoma: steroid receptors and response to medroxyprogesterone acetate, *Gynecol Oncol* 21:314, 1985.

Rosenberg P, Boeryd B, Simonsen E: A new aggressive treatment approach to high grade endometrial cancer of possible benefit to patients with stage I uterine papillary cancer, *Gynecol Oncol* 48:32, 1993.

Rutledge FN, Tan S, Fletcher G: Vaginal metastases from adenocarcinoma of the corpus uteri, *Am J Obstet Gynecol* 75:157, 1958. Sall S, Sonnenblick B, Stone ML: Factors affecting survival of patients with endometrial adenocarcinoma, *Am J Obstet Gynecol* 107:116, 1970.

Sandstrom RE, Welch WR, Green TH Jr: Adenocarcinoma of the endometrium in pregnancy, *Obstet Gynecol* 53(3 suppl):735, 1979.

Schink JC et al: Tumor size in endometrial cancer: a prospective factor for lymph node metastases, *Obstet Gynecol* 70:216, 1987.

Sorbe B, Risberg B, Thonthwaite J: Nuclear morphometry and DNA flow cytometry as prognostic methods for endometrial carcinoma, *Int J Gynecol Cancer* 4:94, 1994.

Surwit EA et al: Stage II carcinoma of the endometrium, *Int J Radiat Oncol Biol Phys* 5:323, 1979.

Sutton GP: The significance of positive peritoneal cytology in endometrial cancer, *Oncology* 4:21, 1990.

Tak WK et al: Myometrial invasion and hysterography in endometrial carcinoma, *Obstet Gynecol* 50:159, 1977.

Thornton JE, Ali S, O'Donovan P et al: Flow cytometric studies of ploidy and proliferative indices in the Yorkshire trail of adjuvant progestogen treatment of endometrial cancer, *Brit J Obstet Gynecol* 100:253, 1993.

Turner DA, Gershenon DM, Atkinson N et al: The prognostic significance of peritoneal cytology for stage I endometrial cancer, *Obstet Gynecol* 74:775, 1989.

Von Minckwitz G, Kuhn W, Kaufmann M et al: Prognostic importance of DNA ploidy and S- phase fraction in endometrial cancer, *Int J Gynecol Cancer* 4:250, 1994.

Yazigi R, Piver MS, Blumenson L: Malignant peritoneal cytology as prognostic indicator in stage I endometrial cancer, *Obstet Gynecol* 62:359, 1983.

Treatment

Arneson A: Clinical results and histological changes following irradiation treatment of cancer of the corpus uteri, *AJR* 36:461, 1936.

Badib AO et al: Radiotherapy in the treatment of sarcomas of the corpus uteri, *Cancer* 24:724, 1969.

Behbakht K, Jordan EL, Casey C et al: Prognostic indicators of survival in advanced endometrial cancer, *Gynecol Oncol* 55:363, 1994.

Bond WH: Early uterine body carcinoma: is postoperative vaginal irradiation any value? *Clin Radiol* 36:619, 1985.

Bruchner HW, Deppe G: Combination chemotherapy of advanced endometrial adenocarcinoma and Adriamycin, cyclophosphamide, 5-fluorouracil, and medroxyprogesterone acetate, *Obstet Gynecol* 50:105, 1977.

Carcangiu ML, Chambers JT: Uterine papillary serous carcinoma, *Gynecol Oncol* 47:298-305, 1992.

Chen SS: Operative treatment in stage I endometrial carcinoma with deep myometrial invasion and/or grade 3 tumor surgically limited to the corpus uteri: no recurrence with only primary surgery, *Cancer* 63:1843, 1989.

Cohen CJ, Deppe G, Bruchner HW: Treatment of advanced adenocarcinoma of the endometrium with melphalan, 5-flourouracil, and medroxyprogesterone acetate: a preliminary study, *Obstet Gynecol* 50:415, 1977.

Cohen CJ et al: Multidrug treatment of advanced and recurrent endometrial carcinoma: a Gynecologic Oncology Group study, *Obstet Gynecol* 63:719, 1984.

Corn BW, Lanciano RM, Greven KM et al: Impact of improved irradiation technique, age and lymph node sampling on the severe complication rate of surgically staged endometrial cancer patients: a multivariate analysis, *J Clinc Oncol* 12:510, 1994.

DePalo G et al: *Adjuvant treatment with medroxyprogesterone acetate in pathological stage I endometrial cancer with myometrial invasion.* In Volla, Racinet, Vrousos, editors: *Endometrial cancers, 5th Cancer Research Workshop,* Grenoble, 1985, p. 209, Korger, Basel.

Deppe G, Cohen CJ, Bruckner HW: Treatment of advanced endometrial carcinoma with cis-dichlorodiammine platinum (II) after intensive prior therapy, *Gynecol Oncol* 10:51, 1980. de Waal JC, Lochmuller H: Preoperative radium insertion in the management of carcinoma of the endeometrium, *Geburshilf Fraunheilkd* 42:394, 1982.

Elliott P, Green D, Coates M et al: The efficacy of postoperative vaginal irradiation in preventing vaginal recurrence in endometrial cancer, *Int J Gynecol Cancer* 4:84, 1994.

Fanning J, Piver MS: Serial CA125 levels during chemotherapy for metastatic or recurrent endometrial cancer, *Obstet Gynecol* 77:278, 1991.

Frick HC et al: Carcinoma of endometrium, *Am J Obstet Gynecol* 115:663, 1973.

Gallagher CJ, Oliver RTD, Oram DH et al: A new treatment for endometrial cancer with gonadotropin releasing hormonal analogue, *Brit J Obstet Gynecol* 98:1037, 1991.

Geisler HE: The use of megestrol acetate in the treatment of advanced malignant lesions of the endometrium, *Gynecol Oncol* 1:340, 1973.

Healy W, Brown R: Experience with surgical and radiation therapy in carcinoma of the corpus uteri, *Am J Obstet Gynecol* 38:1, 1939.

Hyeman J: The so-called Stockholm method and the results of treatment of uterine cancer with Radiumhemmet, *Acta Radiol* 16:129, 1935.

Javert C, Douglas R: Treatment of endometrial carcinoma, *AJR* 75:580, 1956.

Jones HW: Treatment of adenocarcinoma of the endometrium, *Obstet Gynecol Surv* 30:147, 1975.

Kadar N, Homesley HD and Malfetano JH: Prognostic factors in surgical stage III and IV carcinoma of the endometrium, *Obstet Gynecol* 84:983, 1994.

Kadar N, Malfetano JH, Homesley HD: Determinants of survival of surgically staged patients with endometrial carcinoma histologically confined to the uterus, *Obstet Gynecol* 80:655, 1992.

Kauppila A: Progestin therapy of endometrial, breast, and ovarian carcinoma, *Acta Obstet Gynecol Scand* 63:441, 1984.

Kauppila A, Gornroos N, Nieminen U: Clinical outcome in endometrial cancer, *Obstet Gynecol* 60:473, 1982.

Kauppila A et al: Treatment of advanced endometrial adenocarcinoma with combined cytotoxic therapy, *Cancer* 46:2162, 1980.

Kelly H: Radium therapy and cancer of the uterus, *Trans Am Gynecol Soc* 41:532, 1916.

Kelly RN, Baker WH: The effect of 17-alpha-hydroxyprogesterone caproate on metastatic endometrial cancer. In *Conference on Experiemental and Clinical Cancer Chemotherapy*, monograph 9, Bethesda, Md, 1960, National Cancer Institute.

Kennedy BJ: Progestins in the treatment of carcinoma of the endometrium, *Surg Gynecol Obstet* 127:103, 1968.

Kilgore LC, Patridge EE, Alvarez RD et al: Adenocarcinoma of the endometrium: survival comparison of patients with and without pelvic node sampling, *Gynecol Oncol* 56:26, 1995.

Kimmig R, Strowitzki T, Muller-Hocker J et al: Conservative treatment of endometrial cancer permitting subsequent triplet pregnancy, *Gynecol Oncol* 58:255, 1995.

Kistner RW: Histologic effects of progestin on hyperplasia and carcinoma in situ of the endometrium, *Cancer* 12:1106, 1959.

Kistner RW: The effects of progesteronal agents on hyperplasia and carcinoma in situ of the endometrium, *Int J Gynaecol Obstet* 8:561, 1970.

Kohorn EI: Gestagens and endometrial carcinoma, *Gynecol Oncol* 4:398, 1976.

Kottmeier H, Kolstad P, editors: *Annual report on the results of treatment of carcinoma of the uterus, vagina, and ovary*, vol 16, Stockholm, 1976, FIGO.

Larson DM, Johnson K, Olson FA: Pelvic and paraaortic lymphadenectomy for surgical staging of endometrial cancer: morbidity and mortality, *Obstet Gynecol* 79:998, 1992.

Lees D: An evaluation of treatment in carcinoma of the body of the uterus, *J Obstet Gynaecol Br Commonw* 76:615, 1969.

Lellé RJ, Morley GW, Peters WA: The role of vaginal hysterectomy in the treatment of endometrial carcinoma, *Int J Gynecol Cancer* 4:342, 1994.

Lewis B, Stallworthy JA, Cowdell R: Adenocarcinoma of the body of the uterus, *J Obstet Gynaecol Br Commonw* 77:343, 1970.

Lewis GC, Slack NH, Mortel R et al: Adjuvant progestogen therapy in primary definitive treatment of endometrial cancer, *Gynecol Oncol* 2:368, 1974.

Long JH, Langdon RM, Cha SS et al: Phase II trial of methotrexate, vinblastine, doxorubicin and cisplatin in advanced/recurrent endometrial carcinomas, *Gynecol Oncol* 58:240, 1995.

Macdonald RR, Thorogood J, Mason MK: A randomized trial of progestigens in the primary treatment of endometrial carcinoma, *Br J Obstet Gynaecol* 95:166, 1988.

Malkasian GD et al: Progestogen treatment of recurrent endometrial carcinoma, *Am J Obstet Gynecol* 110:15, 1971.

Mangioni C, DePalo G, DelVecchio M: Surgical pathologic staging in apparent stage I endometrial cancer, *Int J Gynecol Cancer* 3:373, 1993.

Monson RR, MacMahon B, Austin JH: Postoperative irradiation and carcinoma of the endometrium, *Cancer* 31:630, 1973.

Moore DH, Fowler WC, Walton LA et al: Morbidity of lymph node sampling in cancers of the uterine corpus and cervix, *Obstet Gynecol* 65:251, 1985.

Moore TO, Phillips PH, Nerenstone SR et al: Systemic treatment of advanced and recurrent endometrial carcinomas: current status and future direction, *J Clin Oncol* 9:1071, 1991.

Morrow CP et al: A randomized study of Adriamycin adjuvant chemotherapy for patients with high risk stage I and II (occult) endometrial carcinoma. Presented at the International Gynecologic Cancer Society, Amsterdam, October, 1987.

Morrow CP, DiSaia PJ, Townsend DE: Current management of endometrial carcinoma, *Obstet Gynecol* 42:399, 1973.

Niloff JM, Klug TL, Schaetzl E et al: Elevation of serum CA125 in carcinoma of fallopian tube, endometrium, and endocervix, *Am J Obstet Gynecol* 148:1057-8, l984.

Onsrud M, Kolstad P, Normann T: Postoperative external pelvic irradiation in carcinoma of the corpus stage I: a controlled clinical trial, *Gynecol Oncol* 4:222, 1976.

Orr JW, Holloway RW, Orr PF, Halimon JL: Surgical staging of uterine cancer: an analysis of perioperative morbidity, *Gynecol Oncol* 42:209, 1991.

Orr JW, Holloway RW, Orr PF et al: Surgical stating of uterine cancer, *Gynecol Oncol* 42:209, 1991.

Patterson E et al: Management of stage I carcinoma of the uterus, *Obstet Gynecol* 59:755, 1982.

Piver MS et al: Melphalan, 5-FU and medroxyprogesterone acetate in metastatic endometrial carcinoma, *Obstet Gynecol* 67:261, 1987.

Potish RA, Twiggs LB, Adcock LL et al: Paraaortic lymph node radiotherapy in cancer of the uterine corpus, *Obstet Gynecol* 65:251, 1985.

Rose PG, Cha SD, Tak WK et al: Radiation therapy for surgically proven para-aortic node metastasis in endometrial cancer, *Int J Radiat Oncol Biol Phys* 24:229, 1992.

Rozier JC, Underwood PB: Use of progestational agents in endometrial adenocarcinoma, *Obstet Gynecol* 44:60, 1974.

Rutledge FN: The role of radical hysterectomy in adenocarcinoma of the endometrium, *Gynecol Oncol* 2:331, 1974.

Salazar OM et al: The management of clinical stage I endometrial carcinoma, *Cancer* 41:1016, 1978.

Seski JC et al: Adriamycin and cyclophosphamide chemotherapy for disseminated endometrial cancer, *Obstet Gynecol* 58:88, 1981.

Seski JC: Cisplatin chemotherapy for disseminated endometrial cancer, *Obstet Gynecol* 59:225, 1982.

Soper JT et al: Intraperitoneal chromic phosphate P-32 suspension therapy in malignant peritoneal cytology and endometrial carcinoma, *Am J Obstet Gynecol* 153:191, 1985.

Thigpen JT: *Cis-platinum in the treatment of advanced or recurrent cervix and uterine cancer*. In Prestayka AW, Crooke ST, Carter SK, editors: *Cis-platin: current status and new developments*, New York, 1980, Academic Press.

Thigpen JT et al: Phase II trial of Adriamycin in treatment of advanced or recurrent endometrial carcinoma, *Cancer Treat Rep* 63:21, 1979.

Thigpen JT, Blessing JA, DiSaia, PJ et al: A randomized comparison of doxorubicin alone versus doxorubicin plus cyclophosphamide in the management of advanced or recurrent endometrial carcinoma, *J Clinc Oncol* 12:1408, 1994.

Thigpen T et al: Treatment of advanced early current endometrial cancer with medroxyprogesterone acetate, Society of Gynecologic Oncologists Abstract, February, 1985.

Thigpen T et al: A randomized comparison of Adriamycin with or without Cytoxan in the treatment of advanced recurrent adenocarcinoma, Abstract, ASGO, May, 1985.

Thigpen T, Blessing J, Homesley H et al: Phase III trial of doxorubin +/- cisplatin in advanced or recurrent endometrial carcinoma, *Proc Am Soc Clin Oncol* 12:26, 1993.

Trope C et al: A phase II study of cisplatin for recurrent corpus cancer, *Eur J Cancer* 16:1025, 1980.

Underwood PB et al: Carcinoma of the endometrium: radiation followed immediately by operation, *Am J Obstet Gynecol* 128:86, 1977.

Wharam MD, Phillips TL, Bagshawe MA: The role of radiation therapy in clinical stage I carcinoma of the endometrium, *AJR* 1:1081, 1976.

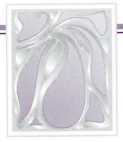

Sarcoma of the Uterus

CLASSIFICATION
CLINICAL PROFILE
LEIOMYOSARCOMA
MIXED MÜLLERIAN SARCOMA
ENDOMETRIAL STROMAL SARCOMA
Other Sarcomas
TREATMENT
Adjunctive Therapy
Recurrent Disease

**CLASSIFICATION OF UTERINE SARCOMAS
ENDORSED BY THE GYNECOLOGIC
ONCOLOGY GROUP**

Leiomyosarcomas
Endometrial stromal sarcomas
Mixed homologous müllerian sarcomas (carcinosar-
coma)
Mixed heterologous müllerian sarcomas (mixed meso-
dermal sarcoma)
Other uterine sarcomas

Sarcomas of the uterus are rare. This is fortunate because the prognosis is poor. The incidence of this tumor comprises only about 3% to 5% of all uterine tumors. These tumors arise primarily from two tissues: (1) endometrial sarcomas from the endometrial glands and stroma and (2) leiomyosarcomas from the uterine muscle itself. Other sarcomas, such as angiosarcoma and fibrosarcoma, arise in supporting tissues and are rare. As a result, the experience even in a large cancer referral institution is still limited. To a certain degree, this has led to a lack of unanimity with regard to certain criteria of diagnosis and definitive therapy.

CLASSIFICATION

In 1959 Ober suggested a classification of endometrial sarcomas to categorize these tumors by cell type and site of origin (Table 6-1). The tumors that are pure are composed of one cell type only, whereas those that are mixed are composed of more than one cell type. Homologous tumors contain tissue elements entirely indigenous to the uterus, whereas heterologous tumors are defined as those that contain tissue elements foreign to the uterus. Numerous modifications of this classification have

Table 6-1   Ober classification of uterine sarcomas

Homologous	Heterologous
Pure	
Stromal sarcoma (endolym- phatic stromal myosis)	Rhabdomyosarcoma
Leiomyosarcoma	Chondrosarcoma
Angiosarcoma	Osteosarcoma
Fibrosarcoma	Liposarcoma
Mixed	
Carcinosarcoma	Mixed müllerian tumors (mixed mesodermal tumor)

been made for various reasons. The Gynecologic Oncology Group (GOG) has accepted the histologic evaluation noted in the box above. This was done because the majority of sarcomas will fall into the four main histologic categories and data can be accumulated more rapidly so that definitive statements concerning diagnosis and therapy can be made.

CLINICAL PROFILE

The incidence of sarcoma of the uterus as reported in the literature is 1.7/100,000 women aged 20 years or more. Harlow reported on 1452 uterine sarcomas, of which 86% were either leiomyosarcoma or mixed mesodermal sarcoma. Both subtypes were more common in black women than in white women. The incidence of mixed mesodermal sarcoma was low through middle age, after which it rose sharply (Figure 6-1). The occurrence of uterine leiomyosarcoma, however, was most prevalent in middle-aged women and declined thereafter. The mean age of patients with a leiomyosarcoma (LMS) is the mid-fifties, 10 years younger than individuals with mixed mesodermal sarcoma (MMS) and endometrial stromal sarcoma (ESS). An abdominal mass or pain is a frequent complaint and finding. A rapidly enlarging uterus is a common entity. Particularly in the premenopausal patient, diagnosis of a myomatous uterus is commonly made preoperatively. In any rapidly enlarging uterus, especially in the postmenopausal patient, sarcomas must be considered (Figures 6-2 and 6-3). Menorrhagia or perimenopausal bleeding may occur in the younger patient. One must consider sarcomas when the patient initially has vaginal bleeding and a relatively large, friable polypoid mass extending through a dilated cervix into the vagina. This is particularly true in the postmenopausal patient. Associated clinical findings include obesity and hypertension in a third of the patients. A history of pelvic irradiation is noted in 5%-10% of patients with sarcoma. Meredith reported on a large series of women with histories of pelvic irradiation who later developed uterine cancers. The data reflected a tendency for patients previously irradiated for pelvic malignancy to have advanced-stage, extremely aggressive tumors compared with those previously irradiated for benign conditions.

In patients with these symptoms, a histologic evaluation is mandatory. If there is a tumor mass initially seen at the cervix, tissue is readily available for biopsy. A large polypoid mass may extend into the endometrial cavity, and the diagnosis can be readily based on either endometrial biopsy or curettage specimens (Figures 6-4 and 6-5). The diagnosis is more difficult to make preoperatively in patients with LMS because biopsy is difficult, and many lesions are incidentally found within a benign myoma. Some authors have reported that LMS may be present in the submucosa of the uterus in one third

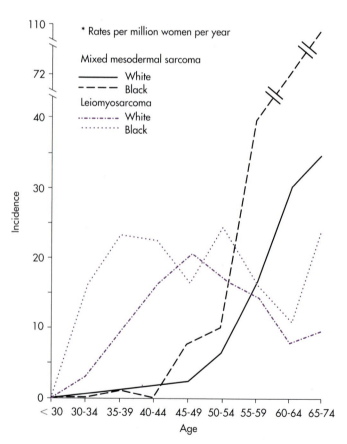

Figure 6-1 Incidence of uterine sarcoma among females by age, race, and histology: SEER areas, 1973-1981. (From Harlow BL, Weiss NS, Lofton S: *J Natl Ca Inst* 76(3):399, March 1986.)

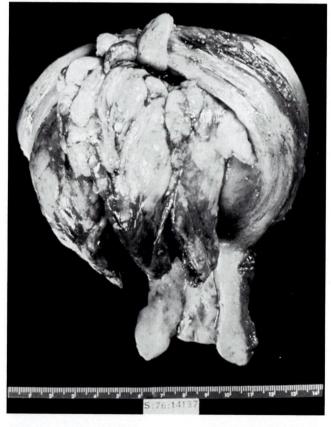

Figure 6-2 Large uterus with tumor filling the endometrial cavity. (Courtesy Department of Pathology, Duke University Medical Center.)

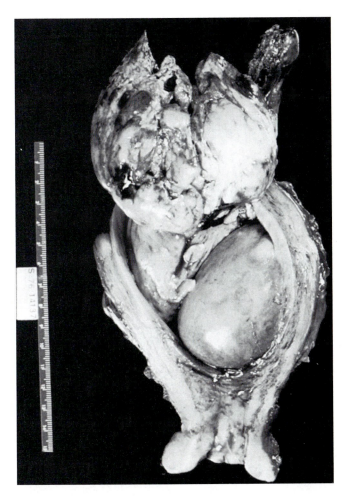

Figure 6-3 Same uterus as shown in Figure 6-2 with polypoid mass pulled out of the endometrial cavity. Significant myometrial involvement is apparent. Sarcoma extended to within 3 mm of the serosal surface. (Courtesy Department of Pathology, Duke University Medical Center.)

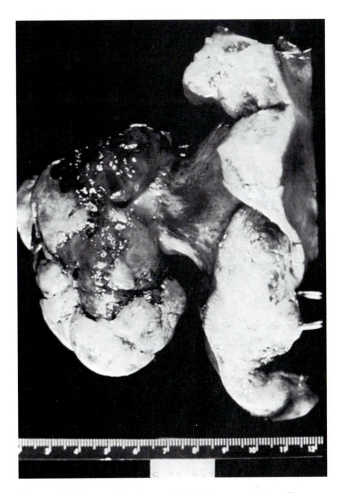

Figure 6-4 Large polyp that contains leiomyosarcoma. (Courtesy Department of Pathology, Duke University Medical Center.)

of patients; but even at that, biopsy is not easily accomplished. Although advanced disease accounts in part for the poor prognosis of sarcoma, an appreciable number of these patients have stage I disease (see corpus cancer staging in Table 5-3). As many as 50% of all sarcomas are stage I disease.

LEIOMYOSARCOMA

The older literature indicates that LMS is the most common sarcoma of the uterus; however, in an evaluation of recent data from the GOG, MMS represented about two thirds of all cases, whereas LMS was seen in only 16% of 447 patients. Other recent reports have also noted the preponderance of mixed mesodermal lesions. As indicated by its name, LMS may be associated with a myoma of the uterus, and the diagnosis may not be established until the hysterectomy specimen has been evaluated histologically.

There is considerable discussion about the histologic

criteria necessary for the diagnosis of LMS. The categories of cellular leiomyoma and bizarre leiomyoma add to the confusion of this entity but are considered to be benign. These two entities are distinguished from a true LMS mainly by the mitotic count of the tumor. Although cellular myoma and bizarre leiomyoma may appear at first sight to be malignant, in histologic evaluation they contain less than 5 mitoses per 10 high-power field (HPF), and with only surgery the prognosis is excellent. Taylor and Norris believed that mitotic count was extremely important in that if fewer than 10 mitoses per 10 HPF were identified, the lesion was benign regardless of the degree of cellular atypia. If more than 10 mitoses per 10 HPF were present, the prognosis was grave. More recently, Norris stated that tumors with fewer than 5 mitoses per 10 HPF rarely can metastasize. In a follow-up study from the Armed Force Institute of Pathology, O'Connor and Norris evaluated 73 smooth muscle tumors of the uterus with 5 to 9 mitotic figures per 10 HPF but lacking cytologic atypia (see box on p. 172). They concluded that the metastatic rate was too low to consider these as being sarcoma. Several of their patients were treated only with myomectomies with excellent results.

Figure 6-5 Whole-mount histologic section of tumor presented in Figure 6-4. Tumor was limited to the polyp. (Courtesy Department of Pathology, Duke University Medical Center.)

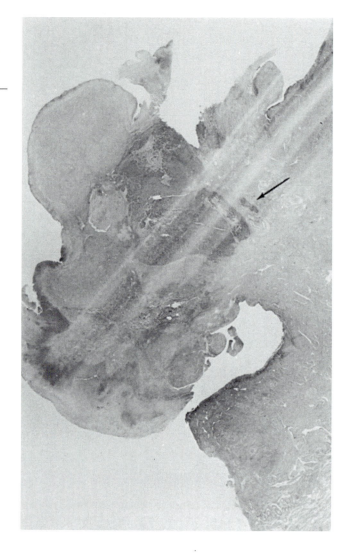

METASTATIC POTENTIAL OF SMOOTH-MUSCLE TUMORS OF THE UTERUS

Maximum MF/10 HPF	Atypia*	Diagnosis	Metastatic potential
1-4	Any degree	Leiomyoma	Very low
5-9	None	Leiomyoma with high mitotic activity	Very low
5-9	Grade 1*	Smooth-muscle tumor of uncertain malignant potential	Low
5-9	Grade 2 or 3*	Leiomyo-sarcoma	Moderate
10 or more	Grade 1*	Leiomyo-sarcoma	High
10 or more	Grade 2 or 3*	Leiomyo-sarcoma	Very high

O'Connor DM et al.: *Human Path* 21(2):226, 1990.
* Grade based on a scale of three.

They have suggested the following classification for smooth muscle tumors of the uterus:

1. If 1-4 mitoses per 10 HPF are present with any degree of atypia, metastatic potential is very low and the diagnosis should be leiomyoma.
2. If 5-9 mitoses per 10 HPF are present with no atypia, metastatic potential is very low and diagnosis is leiomyoma with high mitotic activity.
3. If 5-9 mitoses per 10 HPF are present with grade I atypia, metastatic potential is low and diagnosis is smooth-muscle tumor of uncertain malignant potential.
4. If 5-9 mistoses per 10 HPF are present with grade 2 or 3 atypia, metastatic potential is moderate and diagnosis is leiomyosarcoma.
5. In all other situations (>10 mitoses per 10 HPF, grade 1-3 atypias), the diagnosis is leiomyosarcoma.

Kempson and Bari believe that the mitotic count is important but state that prognosis is poor if more than 5 mitoses per 10 HPF are identified. Their experience with tumors containing 5 to 9 mitoses per 10 HPF indicates that the tumors usually behave aggressively and will metastasize. These authors believe that the degree of cellular atypism is of limited value by itself in determining the malignancy of smooth muscle tumors. In tumors with higher mitotic counts, there were usually a greater number of markedly atypical cells. This atypia was also seen in tumors with 5 to 9 mitoses per 10 HPF. Tumors with fewer than 5 mitoses per 10 HPF were thought to be benign regardless of the atypism of the cells. None of Kempson and Bari's patients with fewer than 5 mitoses per 10 HPF had disease outside the uterus, whereas distant disease was a common finding if more than 5 mitoses per 10 HPF were noted.

On the other hand, Silverberg believes that the mitotic count alone cannot be used as a strict histologic criterion because he had patients with fewer than 10 mitoses per 10 HPF who succumbed to their disease. He believes that the grade of the tumor, which reflects the cytologic atypia, is a better criterion than mitotic count alone. Essentially all investigators emphasized the gravity of the situation if intravascular invasion or disease outside the uterus is found. Silverberg believes that the single most important prognostic indicator is the menopausal status of the patient. Women who are premenopausal when the diagnosis is made tend to have a much better prognosis than those who are postmenopausal, even when criteria such as blood vessel invasion, growth pattern, grade, and mitotic counts are considered. LMSs occur in young patients and tend to be more localized when first diagnosed and probably exhibit a slower growth pattern than MMSs or ESSs.

Dinh and Woodruff studied 43 cases of uterine leiomyosarcoma followed 2 years or longer. The overall 5-year survival was 73%. Favorable prognostic features included the premenopausal status of the patient, the confinement of the tumor within a myoma, the low mitotic count (less than 4 mitotic figures in any one high-power field or fewer than 4 mitotic figures per 10 HPF), the absence of necrosis, and the presence of hyalinization in the adjacent tissue, suggesting confinement. Regardless of histopathologic features, the tumor that arises de novo in the myometrium has poorer prognosis than the lesion that develops in a leiomyoma. In a study of 70 LMS by Nordal, grading of the tumor was the most powerful predictor of survival. The 5-year survival was 83% for grade 1 and grade 2 tumors compared to 37% for grade 3 tumors for LMS and ESS. Chemotherapy for extrauterine disease did not appear to be effective.

Another 32 cases were reported by Vardi who found that the predominant symptoms were abnormal vaginal bleeding, pain or abdominal discomfort, or enlarged pelvic mass. Of the total group, 43.8% died of disease within the first 3 years after diagnosis. There was a 63.6% 5-year survival in women diagnosed while premenopausal, compared with 5.5% 5-year survival in postmenopausal women. Although almost all deaths and recurrences are during the 4 years after diagnosis, Gallup reported a recurrence 25 years after initial therapy.

Of the 477 sarcomas identified in the large clinical pathological evaluation of early-staged uterine sarcoma by the GOG, only 57 were LMS. Of these patients, 53 had lymph node status evaluated at the time of surgery, and metastases were noted in only 2 cases (4%). This compared to almost 18% lymph node metastases noted in mixed mesodermal tumors (MMT). Of the 57 patients, 36 (63%) experienced recurrence, with the vast majority of these at distant sites. Progression-free interval (PFI) was only 20.6 months for the LMS, considerably shorter than the interval for MMT. For all sarcomas, those that were well differentiated, limited to the endometrium, without vascular lymphatic space involvement, and with mitotic count less than 20 per 10 HPF had the best prognosis. Conversely, those with disease invading the cervix >5 cm in size or with extrauterine disease in the adnexae and lymph nodes had a significantly worse prognosis. With a 63% recurrence in LMS and only 4% lymph node metastases, many other factors obviously affect survival. Therapy used after surgery was not evaluated in this study.

Attempts have been made to correlate DNA analysis with prognosis in uterine sarcomas. Peters could not demonstrate prognosis with ploidy status or proliferative rate in patients with leiomyosarcomas. Wolfson evaluated DNA ploidy along with other prognostic factors in 62 patients. Using multivariate analysis, surgical stage was the most important prognostic factor although age and mitotic index also were important. Patients with diploid tumors had a median survival of 78.5 months compared to 35.1 months for aneuploid tumors (p = 0.07). Lennart also was unable to show DNA content and S phase fraction to be a significant factor.

MIXED MÜLLERIAN SARCOMA

A better term for mixed müllerian sarcomas may be *malignant mixed müllerian tumors*. This includes the homologous malignant mixed müllerian tumors and the heterologous malignant mixed müllerian tumors. Carcinoma and sarcoma must both be identified. Tumors should not be placed in the heterologous group unless there is definitive histologic evidence of tissue not normally found in the uterus, such as bone, cartilage, or skeletal muscle.

These tumors can be aggressive. They spread early to regional lymph nodes and adjacent tissue (Figure 6-6). In a study by DiSaia and associates from the MD Anderson Hospital, 101 patients were evaluated, and more than 60%

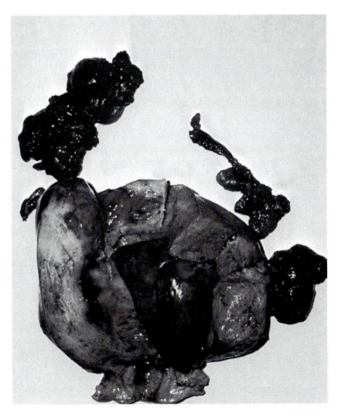

Figure 6-6 Uterine sarcoma with obviously enlarged lymph nodes, particularly on right side.

of these patients had disease outside the uterine corpus at the time the diagnosis was originally established. Microscopic invasion of blood vessels and lymphatic channels is frequent.

In a small pilot study from the GOG as reported by DiSaia, it was noted that in 28 patients with mixed müllerian sarcomas, stage I, 10 (35%) had metastasis to the pelvic lymph nodes. Four of these patients also had metastasis to the periaortic nodal area. In every instance of nodal involvement, the myometrial invasion was to the middle or outer one third of the uterine muscle. This phenomenon, of course, could be one of the explanations for poor prognosis, even in early-stage sarcomas. As a result, hematogenous spread, particularly to the lung and liver, is common. An appreciable number of patients may have a uterine polypoid growth pattern, which may be associated with myomas. Tumor hemorrhage and necrosis are common.

In the recent large study from the GOG of clinical stage I and II uterine sarcomas, the natural history of MMT, particularly in contrast to LMS, has been detailed. Unlike previous reports and the usual quoted data, the study found that MMT appears to have a considerable better prognosis than LMS. It had generally been accepted that LMS was more common and that the prognosis was better. In the 447 sarcomas, there were 165 homologous (HO) MMT, 134 heterogenous (HE) MMT, 57 LMS, and 91 others. Lymph node metastases were 15% for HO, 20% for HE, and only 4% for LMS. Recurrence rate was 41% for HO and 58% for HE (Table 6-2). The HO tumors had a progression-free interval (PFI) of 62.6 months, compared with 20.6 months for LMS and 22.7 months for HE. For both HE and HO, isolated pelvic recurrence was unusual (12% and 8%, respectively).

Another GOG study of 47 sarcoma patients followed for more than 5 years included 7 endometrial stromal sarcomas, 15 heterologous mixed müllerian tumors, 16 homologous mixed müllerian tumors, 7 leiomyosarcomas, and 2 unclassified tumors. Actual survival at 5 years was 73% with stage I, 80% with stage II, 10% with stage III, and 20% with surgical stage IV. Histologic type, when corrected for surgical stage, did not influence 5-year survival. Patients treated with preoperative or postoperative radiotherapy had a low incidence of local recurrence but were at risk for distant metastases.

If the heterologous elements present are rhabdomyoblasts or osteoblasts, the prognosis is poor according to Kempson and Bari. Their only survivors were patients whose tumors contained chondrosarcoma as the heterologous element. Patients with heterologous elements tended to have more advanced disease, both locally and distant, than those with homologous tumors. The survival rate was better in the homologous group but only when disease was limited superficially in the uterus.

In the most recent GOG study of 447 sarcomas, the types of heterologous elements did not seem to affect the frequency of lymph node metastases. Rhabdomyosarcoma was the most frequent type seen. The HE did have an adverse impact on survival, with a median PFI of only 22.7 months compared with 62.6 months with the HO type of MMT.

Peters reported a series of 103 patients with endometrial sarcomas, including 47 mixed homologous tumors, 32 mixed heterologous tumors, 21 pure homologous sarcomas (endometrial stromal sarcomas), and 3 pure heterologous sarcomas (rhabdomyosarcomas). Clinical characteristics were similar among the four groups. Twenty-nine percent of the patients with clinical stage I or II tumors had extrauterine disease discovered at surgery. Extent of the tumor at the time of surgery strongly correlated with outcome and only 2 patients with extrauterine disease were long-term survivors. Life table survival probability at 5 years was 58% with surgical stage I, 33% with surgical stage II, 13% with surgical stage III, 0% with surgical stage IV, and 5% in patients with recurrence. There was no difference in risk for treatment failure among pure endometrial stromal sarcoma, mixed homologous sarcoma, or mixed heterologous sarcoma. The strongest factor correlating with a poor outcome was deep myometrial invasion. An adverse trend was detected in patients with previous pelvic irradiation, with advancing age, and with increasing uterine size. Neither the presence of heterologous tumor elements nor cervical involvement was found to be a significant adverse prognostic factor.

ENDOMETRIAL STROMAL SARCOMA

The most common symptom of endometrial stromal sarcoma is irregular vaginal bleeding. Asymptomatic uterine enlargement and pelvic pain or mass are also common symptoms. The tumors are generally soft, fleshy, smooth, polypoid masses that may protrude into the endometrial cavity. The multiple-polyp form of the neoplasm has also been described, as has the characteristic yellow color of many of these lesions. Occasionally, the uterine wall is diffusely enlarged by tumor without the presence of an obvious tumor mass. Forty percent of the lesions extend beyond the uterus at the time of initial hysterectomy.

Table 6-2   Uterine sarcoma: Incidence of lymph node metastasis

	Positive nodes
MMT-HO	24/153 (16%)
MMT-HE	26/129 (20%)
LMS	2/53 (4%)

Modified from Major FJ, et al: Prognostic factors in uterine sarcoma: a Gynecological Oncology Group study, *Cancer* 71:1702-09, 1993.
MMT-HO, mixed mesodermal, homologous; MMT-HE, mixed mesodermal, heterologous; LMS, leiomyosarcoma.

Although individual reports suggested that ESSs has a better prognosis than other sarcomas, an analysis of the literature indicates that ESS is just as aggressive and the survival rate no better. Endometrial stromal tumors are usually considered in two groups: endolymphatic stromal myosis and ESS. The former is an infiltrating stromal lesion that usually follows an indolent course. Endolymphatic stromal myosis is usually considered a low-grade stromal sarcoma. The lesion can have an infiltrating growth pattern, and on cut surface tissue it can project out in a wormlike fashion. These wormlike projections may be found in the blood vessels of the broad ligament. Microscopically, there is little or no cellular atypia and there are few, if any, mitoses. Although metastasis can occur, the clinical course is usually indolent, and surgery only is usually adequate treatment. Endolymphatic stromal myosis may recur, but it does so after a long interval. On the other hand, ESSs infiltrate the myometrium to a greater degree and have a more aggressive course, with frequent metastasis and poor prognosis. Since these two lesions are similar, differentiation is important. Norris and Taylor separated the two tumors by the number of mitoses per 10 HPF. They believe that tumors with 10 or more mitoses per 10 HPF should be categorized as ESS and those with fewer mitoses should be categorized as endolymphatic stromal myosis. Kempson and Bari, in a review of their material, noted that 10 tumors contained more than 20 mitoses per 10 HPF, and 9 of the 10 patients died of disease. Seven patients had tumors that contained 5 or fewer mitoses per 10 HPF, and none have developed a recurrence. No tumors were seen with mitotic counts between 6 and 20 per 10 HPF. Pleomorphism was present in both groups of patients. Both tumors are composed of stromal cells with slight amounts of cytoplasm. They infiltrate and separate the muscle fibers of the uterus. Tumor is found frequently within lymphatic spaces.

A study of 24 "high grade" EESs at the Mayo Clinic found that prognosis was related to the extent of disease, size of primary tumor, and grade. Mitotic count was not a prognostic factor, nor was DNA pattern. Adjuvant radiation did not improve survival.

Other Sarcomas

Clement and Scully recently reported on 100 cases of müllerian adenosarcoma of the uterus. This is an unusual tumor with low malignant potential. Grossly the tumor is usually a polypoid mass that can fill the endometrial cavity. Involvement of the cervix and myometrium is less commonly seen. Histologic evaluation notes benign or atypical neoplastic glands with a sarcomatous stroma. In 78% of patients, the sarcomatous stroma was homologous. Stromal mitotic rate was 1-40 per 10 HPF. Extensive stromal fibrosis was common. Myometrial invasion was present in only 15, and deeply invasive in only 4. Recurrence became apparent in 23 patients, and in one third appeared 5 years after diagnosis. Recurrence was confined to the vagina, pelvis, or abdomen with two

exceptions. Of those with recurrence, only 11 died with tumor. Only the presence of myometrial invasion was associated with an increased risk of recurrence.

TREATMENT

Total abdominal hysterectomy and bilateral salpingo-oophorectomy have been considered the hallmark of therapy in uterine sarcomas. Some authorities have advocated the addition of bilateral pelvic lymphadenectomy, especially in the low-grade lesions, since local pelvic spread is common and the value of adjuvant therapy is in doubt or untested. It seems reasonable to assume that the 15%-20% of patients with disease that is apparently confined to the uterus have probably benefited from the lymph node dissection when positive specimens are subsequently identified. The use of radiation, either given preoperatively as intracavitary and/or external irradiation or given postoperatively with external irradiation and/or vaginal radium, has been advocated by many centers. Some authors, including radiotherapists, are now questioning the efficacy of adjunctive radiotherapy. True, there are patients who have received preoperative radiation and have no residual sarcoma present in the uterine specimen; however, the spread pattern and sites of recurrences detract from the possible benefits of radiation therapy.

When radiation therapy is given, 5000 to 6000 cGy to the pelvis has been advocated. Preoperative intracavitary radium is given in a dose of about 5000 mg-hr. Postoperative radium has been given to deliver 4000 cGy to the vaginal surface. If surgery is not anticipated, the amount of radiation, particularly in brachytherapy, has been increased. Perez et al. noted fewer central recurrences if the amount of external radiation was 5000 cGy or more, although the difference was not statistically significant.

Results of therapy, unless analyzed critically, may leave one with erroneous conclusions. Patients with LMS have a poorer survival rate than patients with MMT (Table 6-3). Some data suggest that patients treated with radiation therapy plus surgery have a better survival rate than those treated with surgery alone. Unfortunately, a randomized prospective study has not been done to

Table 6-3   Sarcoma type and survival

	Median survival (months)
MMT-HO	62.6
MMT-HE	22.7
LMS	20.6

Modified from Major FJ, et al: Prognostic factors in uterine sarcoma: a Gynecological Oncology Group study, *Cancer* 71:1702-09, 1993.
MMT-HO, mixed mesodermal, homologous; MMT-HE, mixed mesodermal, heterologous; LMS, leiomyosarcoma.

Table 6-4 Uterine sarcomas: survival rate in terms of stage, treatment, and pathology*

Stage	Cell type† (N)	5-year survival rate‡		
		S	S + R	R
I	MMS (63)	52%	48%	29%
	LMS (55)	58%	75%	33%
	ESS (24)	47%	88%	50%
II-IV	MMS (48)	5%	16%	0%
	LMS (33)	0%	13%	0%
	ESS (18)	0%	33%	0%

Modified from Salazar OM et al: *Cancer* 42:1152, 1978.
*Based on 142 patients with stage I disease (62% treated with S only, 30% treated with S + R, and 8% treated with R only) and 99 patients with stage II-IV disease (33% treated with S only, 46% treated with S + R, and 21% treated with R only).
†MMS, mixed mesodermal sarcoma; LMS, leiomyosarcoma; ESS, endometrial stromal sarcoma.
‡S, surgery; S + R, surgery + radiation; R, radiation.

Table 6-5 Uterine sarcoma: recurrence site

	MMT-HO N = 165	MMT-HE N = 134	LMS N = 57
Pelvic only	9%	12%	7%
Distant	33%	46%	56%
None	58%	42%	37%

Modified from Major FJ et al: Prognostic factors in uterine sarcoma: a Gynecological Oncology Group study, *Cancer* 71:1702-09, 1993.

answer this question. Collected data, however, allow some conclusions to be drawn. Salazar et al., presenting material and review of the literature of more than 900 patients, noted that in stage I disease there is no statistically significant difference between surgery alone and surgery plus irradiation in LMS, MMT, or ESS. This is true also of patients with more advanced disease. Patients who were treated with radiation therapy alone did considerably worse than those treated with surgery alone or surgery plus irradiation (Table 6-4).

What then is the possible role of radiation therapy in the management of uterine sarcomas? It appears that patients treated with radiation have a greater degree of local (pelvic) tumor control than patients treated with surgery only. This unfortunately was not reflected by an increased survival rate. In patients treated with radiation alone, the majority had recurrences, indicating that radiation therapy did not control these tumors.

Site and time of recurrence are important in our treatment consideration. In a pilot study, the GOG evaluated the surgical-pathologic spread patterns of sarcomas of the uterus. In patients with disease limited to the uterus, a significant number (16%) were found to have metastasis to the regional lymph nodes (see Table 6-2). As in endometrial cancer, survival was related to this factor, to the depth of myometrial invasion, and to whether the lower uterine segment or cervix was involved. It appears that patients with malignant cells in the peritoneal cytologic specimen also have an extremely poor prognosis and must be considered the same way as patients who have extant disease outside the uterus. Unfortunately, when recurrence appears, isolated pelvic occurrence is rare (Table 6-5). Since the main failure site is distant from the pelvis, the use of adjunctive local radiation is ineffective in increasing the overall survival rate.

We prefer to treat sarcomas primarily by surgery. A peritoneal cytologic specimen is obtained immediately after opening of the peritoneal cavity. A total abdominal hysterectomy and bilateral salpingo-oophorectomy are done if possible. Pelvic and periaortic lymphadenectomy is done as described in Chapter 5.

Adjunctive Therapy

Since there is such a poor survival rate with standard therapy, chemotherapy has been evaluated in an adjuvant setting. Several drugs have been found to be active agents when used singly in sarcomas. These include doxorubicin, dactinomycin, vincristine, cyclophosphamide, dimethyltriazeno imidazole carboxamide (DTIC), and methotrexate. Some studies suggest that doxorubicin is the best single agent for treatment of this group of tumors. Buchsbaum et al. used a combination of vincristine, dactinomycin, and cyclophosphamide (Cytoxan) (VAC) as prophylactic chemotherapy in 17 patients with stage I or II uterine sarcomas after their initial surgery. In the study, the intention was to give six courses of postoperative chemotherapy; however, only 10 of the 17 patients completed this therapy. Of the 10, 5 survived for 4 years or longer. The authors make the point that they have survivors with tumors containing more than 10 mitoses per 10 HPF. Using historic controls, they had no survivors with this number of mitoses and without chemotherapy. They suggested these results were better than their historic controls but are essentially equal to several studies in the literature in which surgery alone was used.

In a prospective randomized study by the GOG, doxorubicin was used as an adjunct in patients with stages I and II sarcomas in which all gross residual disease was removed. Radiation therapy could be used before randomization of the chemotherapy. Patients received either doxorubicin or no further therapy. In 156 evaluable patients no statistically significant difference in the progression-free interval or survivors was found in any category even after adjusting for maldistribution of cases. There was no benefit in this study using doxorubicin as an adjuvant therapy for treatment of uterine sarcomas. As previously noted, patients, even with early stage sarcoma, have recurrences and do so outside the treatment field (either surgical or radiation therapy); therefore it appears that the development of good systemic therapy is needed. Although studies are ongoing, to date it appears that proven adjuvant therapy is anecdotal at the best.

In summary, leiomyosarcomas, endometrial sarcomas, and mixed mesodermal tumors of the uterus should be considered separately. Key to a good prognosis is a careful staging procedure to ensure the absence of extrauterine disease. In addition, patients with mitotic counts of more than 20 mitoses per 10 HPF, with deep myometrial invasion, or with extensions of tumor beyond the confines of the uterus have been recommended for adjuvant chemotherapy protocols in the hope of improving outcome. It is not our practice to treat postoperatively patients with disease limited to the endometrium or superficial myometrium. Study continues, to determine the most appropriate drug combination for all uterine sarcomas. Adjuvant irradiation increases the rate of pelvic control but has not produced an increase in overall survival.

Recurrent Disease

Even in stage I disease, about one half the patients with uterine sarcoma will develop a recurrence, as will 90% of patients with stages II through IV disease. Therapy for recurrent disease is obviously needed. Several studies have been carried out evaluating different drug regimens in this group of patients. Hannigan reported on 39 patients with recurrent disease treated with doxorubicin, either alone or in combination with other chemotherapeutic agents. The median survival was 7.2 months, and no patient lived more than 32 months after the start of chemotherapy. The response rate was only 10.3%, and there were no complete responders. The GOG evaluated doxorubicin versus doxorubicin plus DTIC in a total of 240 patients with stages III, IV, and recurrent sarcomas of the uterus. There were 146 patients with measurable disease; no difference in response was noted between doxorubicin and doxorubicin plus DTIC. In the nonmeasureable category, the progression-free interval was similar between the two treatment arms. Patients with leiomyosarcomas had a significantly longer survival time than those with other cell types, but there was no advantage for either regimen. There was a trend favoring the combination in heterologous mixed mesodermal sarcomas, but the difference was not statistically significant and the survival rate was the same. The survival rate of the entire group was identical irrespective of the treatment given. Toxicity was appreciably increased with the addition of DTIC.

In another GOG protocol, doxorubicin with and without cyclophosphamide was evaluated in 104 patients with primary stage III, IV, or recurrent sarcoma of the uterus. The response rate was identical for both regimens; 19% (complete and partial). Median survival was essentially the same; 11.6 months for doxorubicin and 10.9 months for doxorubicin and cyclophosphamide.

Hannigan also reported on 74 patients with advanced and recurrent uterine sarcoma who were treated with a combination chemotherapy consisting of vincristine, dactinomycin, and cyclophosphamide. The probability of survival at 2 and 5 years was 23% and 15%, respectively. The response rate for patients with measurable disease was 28.9% (15.6% partial responses and 13.3% complete responses). The median duration of a complete response was 16 months, and that of a partial response was 5½ months. Some have suggested that the activity of this regimen can be increased by substituting doxorubicin for dactinomycin.

A phase II study using cisplatin in mixed mesodermal sarcoma, reported by Muss et al. (GOG), resulted in two complete and three partial responses in 28 evaluable patients. In 63 patients, cisplatin achieved a 19% response when used as first-line therapy which was similar to its effect as a second line therapy (18%) (GOG). Azizi et al. reported on 6 patients with metastatic uterine leiomyosarcoma treated with vincristine, doxorubicin, and DTIC. Complete remission was noted in 3 patients, and 1 partial response was recorded. One patient remained free of disease at 24 months. Lehrner et al. reported a complete response in a patient with metastatic (spinal cord, femur, and lung) ESS with surgery, radiation therapy, and chemotherapy using doxorubicin, vincristine, cyclophosphamide, and megestrol acetate. Piver reported on 20 patients treated with dimethlytriazeno-imidazole carboxamide (DTIC) and cis-diammine-dichloroplatinum II (DDP) given in two dosages (group 1, 1 mg/kg daily for 5 days and group 2, 20 mg/m$_2$ daily for 5 days). Of the 20 patients, 35% had an objective response. Of the 10 group 1 patients, 2 (20%) had an objective response (1 complete response, 1 partial) both as second-line chemotherapy. Of the group 2 patients, 5 (50%) have responded (3 complete, 2 partial) 1 as third-line and 4 as second-line chemotherapy.

The GOG has evaluated Ifosfamide and Mesna with and without cisplatin in patients with advanced, persistent or recurrent MMT in a Phase III study. This study of 188 patient (130 evaluable) has been completed but the results have not been reported to date. It is noted that in the 130 evaluable patients, there have been 38 (29%) CR and 24 (18%) PR. This response of over 50% is very encouraging. In an adjuvant setting, Ifosfamide, Mesna and cisplatin were used in stage I and II patients with MMT by the GOG. The study has been closed but again results are not available. Previous GOG studies found Etoposide to be ineffective in leiomyosarcoma but did note activity of doxorubicin, Ifosfamide-Mesna in this tumor type. The EORTC has evaluated advanced soft-tissue sarcoma in men and women in a Phase III study. Response rate, remission duration, and overall survival were similar in the three treatment arms (doxorubicin vs cyclophosphamide, vincristine, doxorubicin and dacarbenzine vs Ifosfamide and doxorubicin). Current on-going evaluation by the GOG is a Phase III study of accelerated hyperfractionated whole abdominal radiotherapy compared to Ifosfamide-Mesna and cisplatin in optimally debulked Stage I-IV carcinosarcoma of the uterus. Taxol in patients with advanced or recurrent uterine sarcoma is also being evaluated.

Van Rijswiyk studied the effects of chemotherapy on sarcomas. In a review of 28 studies, it was noted that in the adjuvant setting doxorubicin has not shown to prolong survival. Cisplatin and Ifosfamide have demonstrated activity, particularly in MMT. Combination of cisplatin and doxorubicin have resulted in 60%-70% response suggesting synergy between the two drugs in MMT. Resnik and the group at Yale treated 42 MMT patients with a combination of Etoposide, cisplatin and doxorubicin. In early staged disease (I and II), a 2-year survival of 92% was achieved. In advanced disease, 2-year survival was 33% (PFS was 20%). In four evaluable patients, 2CR and 2PR were observed.

In uterine endolymphatic stromal myosis, although found to have a good prognosis, many will recur even those with Stage I disease. It appears these tumors are hormone responsive and progestins have been used with good results.

BIBLIOGRAPHY

Clinical profile

Clement PB, Scully RE. Müllerian adenosarcoma of the uterus: a clinical pathological analysis of 100 cases with review of the literature, *Hum Pathol* 21:363, 1990.

Harlow BL, Weiss NS: The epidemiology of sarcomas of the uterus, *J Natl Ca Inst* 76:399, 1986.

Kempson RL, Bari W: Uterine sarcomas: classification, diagnosis, and prognosis, *Hum Pathol* 1:331, 1970.

Lennart K, Lennart B, Ulf S, Bernard T: Flow cytometric analysis of uterine sarcomas, *Gynecol Oncol* 55:339-42, 1994.

Major FJ, Blessing JA, Silverberg SG et al: Prognostic factors in early stage uterine sarcoma, *Int J Gynecol Pathol* 11:75-88, 1992.

Major FJ, Blessing JA, Silverberg SG et al: Prognostic factors in uterine sarcoma: a Gynecological Oncology Group study, *Cancer* 71:1702-09, 1993.

Meredith RF et al: An excess of uterine sarcomas after pelvic irradiation, *Cancer* 58:2003, 1986.

Nordal RN, Kjorstad KE, Stenweg AE, Tropé CE: Leimyosarcoma and endometrial stroma sarcoma of the uterus, *Int J Gynecol Cancer* 3:110-5, 1993.

Ober WB: Uterine sarcomas; histogenesis and taxonomy, *Ann NY Acad Sci* 75:568, 1959.

Peters WA, Howard DR, Anderson WA, Figge DC: Uterine smooth muscle tumor of uncertain malignant potential, *Obstet Gynecol* 83:1015-20, 1994.

Salazar OM et al: Uterine sarcomas; natural history, treatment and prognosis, *Cancer* 42:1152, 1978.

Schwartz Z et al: Uterine sarcoma in Israel: a study of 104 cases, *Gynecol Oncol* 20:354, 1985.

Wolfson AH, Wolfson DJ, Sittler SY et al: A multivariate analysis of clinicopathologic factors for predicting outcome in uterine sarcoma, *Gynecol Oncol* 52:56-62, 1994.

Leiomyosarcoma

Burns B, Curry RH, Bell MEA: Morphologic features of prognostic significance in uterine smooth muscle tumors; a review of 84 cases, *Am J Obstet Gynecol* 135:109, 1979.

Christopherson WM, Williamson EO, Gray LA: Leiomyosarcomas of the uterus, *Cancer* 29:1512, 1972.

Dinh TV, Woodruff JD: Leiomyosarcoma of the uterus, *Am J Obstet Gynecol* 144:817, 1982.

Gallup DG, Hobbs LH, Ross WB: Recurrence of uterine leiomyosarcoma 25 years after therapy, *Gynecol Oncol* 13:293, 1982.

O'Connor DM, Norris HJ: Mitotically active leiomyomas of the uterus, *Hum Pathol* 21:223, 1990.

Silverberg SG: Leiomyosarcoma of the uterus, *Obstet Gynecol* 38:613, 1971. Taylor HB, Norris HJ: Mesenchymal tumors of the uterus. IV. Diagnosis and prognosis of leiomyosarcomas, *Arch Pathol* 82:40, 1966.

Vardi JR, Tovel HM: Leiomyosarcoma of the uterus: clinico-pathologic study, *Obstet Gynecol* 56:428, 1980.

Mixed müllerian sarcoma

Baggish MS: Mesenchymal tumors of the uterus, *Clin Obstet Gynecol* 17:51, 1974.

DiSaia PJ, Catro JR, Rutledge FN: Mixed mesodermal sarcoma of the uterus, *AJR* 117:632, 1973.

DiSaia PJ et al: Endometrial sarcoma; lymphatic spread pattern, *Am J Obstet Gynecol* 130:104, 1978.

Marchese MJ et al: Uterine sarcomas: a clinico-pathologic study, 1965-1981, *Gynecol Oncol* 18:299, 1984.

Norris HF, Taylor HB: Mesenchymal tumors of the uterus. I. A clinical and pathological study of 53 endometrial stromal tumors, *Cancer* 19:755, 1966.

Peters WA, Kumar NB, Fleming WP: Prognostic features of sarcomas and mixed tumors of the endometrium, *Obstet Gynecol* 63:550, 1984.

Saksela E, Lampinen V, Procopé B: Malignant mesenchymal tumors of the uterine corpus, *Am J Obstet Gynecol* 120:452, 1974.

Endometrial stromal sarcoma

DeFusio PA, Gaffey TA, Malkasian GD et al: Endometrial stromal sarcomas: review of Mayo Clinic experience, 1945-1980, *Gynecol Oncol* 35:8, 1989.

Evans HL: Endometrial stromal sarcoma and poorly differentiated endometrial sarcoma, *Cancer* 50:2170, 1982.

Gilbert HA et al: The value of radiation therapy in uterine sarcoma, *Obstet Gynecol* 45:84, 1975.

Katz L et al: Endometrial stromal sarcoma: a clinico-pathologic study of 11 cases with determination of estrogen and progestin receptor levels in three tumors, *Gynecol Oncol* 26:87, 1987.

Lehrner LM, Miles PA, Enck RE: Complete remission of widely metastatic endometrial stromal sarcoma following combination chemotherapy, *Cancer* 43:1189, 1979.

Sutton GP, Blessing JA, Rosenoheim N et al: Phase II trial of Ifosfamide and Mesna in mixed mesodermal tumors of the uterus, *Am J Obstet Gynecol* 161:309, 1989.

Treatment

Azizi F et al: Remission of uterine leiomyosarcomas treated with vincristine, Adriamycin, and dimethyl-tri-zeno-imidazole carboxamide, *Am J Obstet Gynecol* 133:379, 1979.

Badib AO et al: Radiotherapy in the treatment of sarcomas of the corpus uteri, *Cancer* 2:724, 1969.

Buchsbaum HJ, Lifshitz S, Blythe JG: Prophylactic chemotherapy in stage I and II uterine sarcoma, *Gynecol Oncol* 8:346, 1979.

Grosh WW et al: Malignant mixed mesodermal tumors of the uterus and ovary treated with cisplatin-based combination chemotherapy, *Gynecol Oncol* 25:334, 1986.

Hannigan EV et al: Treatment of advanced sarcoma with vincristine, actinomycin D, and cyclophosphamide, *Gynceol Oncol* 15:224, 1983.

Hannigan EV et al: Treatment of advanced uterine sarcoma with Adriamycin, *Gynecol Oncol* 16:101, 1983.

Hannigan EV, Freedman RS, Rutledge FN: Adjuvant chemotherapy in early uterine sarcoma, *Gynecol Oncol* 15:56, 1983.

Kohorn EJ et al: Adjuvant therapy in mixed müllerian tumors of the uterus, *Gynecol Oncol* 23:212, 1986.

Muss HB et al: Treatment of recurrent or advanced uterine sarcoma: a randomized trial of doxorubicin versus doxorubicin and cyclophosphamide, *Cancer* 55:1648, 1985.

Omura GA, Blessing JA, Majors F et al: A randomized clinical trial of adjuvant Adriamycin in uterine sarcoma: a Gynecologic Oncology Group study, *J Clin Oncol* 3:1240, 1985.

Omura GA et al: A randomized study of Adriamycin with and without dimetyl triazenoimidazole carboxamide in advanced uterine sarcoma, *Cancer* 52:626, 1983.

Perez CA et al: Effects of irradiation on mixed müllerian tumors of the uterus, *Cancer* 43:1274, 1979.

Piver MS, Lele SB, Patsner B: Cis-diammine-dichloroplatinum plus dimethyl-triazenoimidazole-carboxamide as second- and third-line chemotherapy for sarcomas of the female pelvis, *Gynecol Oncol* 23:371, 1986.

Piver MS, Rutledge FN, Copeland L et al: Uterine endolymphatic stroma myosis: a collaborative study, *Obstet Gynecol* 64:173-8, 1984.

Resnik E, Chambers SK, Carcangiu ML et al: A phase II study of etoposide, cisplatin and doxorubicin chemotherapy in mixed müllerian tumors of the uterus, *Gynecol Oncol* 56:370-5, 1995.

Salazar OM et al: Uterine sarcomas; analysis of failures with special emphasis on the use of adjuvant radiation therapy, *Cancer* 42:1161, 1978.

Santos A, Tursz T, Mouridsen H et al: Doxorubicin versus Cyvadic versus doxorubicin plus ifosfamide in first line treatment of advanced soft tissue sarcoma, *J Clin Oncol* 13:1537-45, 1995.

Sorbe B: Radiotherapy and/or chemotherapy as adjuvant treatment of uterine sarcomas, *Gynecol Oncol* 20:281, 1985.

Thigpen JT, Blessing JA, Wilbanks GD: Cisplatin as second line chemotherapy in the treatment of advanced or recurrent leiomyosarcoma of the uterus, *Am J Clin Oncol* 9:18, 1986.

Thigpen JT et al: A phase II trial of cis-diamminedichlo-roplatinum (DDP) in treatment of advanced or recurrent mixed mesodermal sarcoma of the uterus, *Proc ASCO/AACR* 23:110, 1982.

Thigpen JT, Blessing JA, Beecham J et al: Phase II trial of cisplatin as first line chemotherapy in patients with advanced or recurrent uterine sarcoma, *J Clin Oncol* 9:1962-6, 1991.

Van Rijswijk REN, Tognon E, Burger CW et al: The effect of chemotherapy on the different components of advanced carcinosarcomas of the female genitalia tract, *Int J Gynecol Cancer* 4:52-60, 1994.

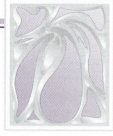

7

Gestational Trophoblastic Neoplasia

Gestational trophoblastic neoplasia has been known since antiquity. Hippocrates, four centuries before the birth of Christ, described the hydatidiform mole as dropsy of the uterus and attributed it to unhealthy water. In the thirteenth century, the tombstone of Countess Henneberg noted that at 40 years of age she had delivered 365 children: half were christened John and half were christened Elizabeth. William Smellie, in 1700, was the first to use the terms *hydatidid* and *mole*. In the early nineteenth century, Velpeau and Boivin recognized the hydatidiform mole as cystic dilation of the chorionic villi. In 1895 Felix Marchand demonstrated that the hydatidiform mole, and less commonly a normal pregnancy or abortion, preceded the development of choriocarcinoma. He described proliferation of the syncytium and the cytotrophoblast of the villi in molar pregnancies. In the early part of the twentieth century, Fels, Ehrhart, Roessler, and Zondek demonstrated that an excess of chorionic gonadotropic hormones could be identified in the urine of patients with hydatidiform moles.

Gestational trophoblastic neoplasia (GTN) is the term now commonly applied to choriocarcinoma and related tumors. It appears to be more appropriate because it is indicative of the spectrum of trophoblastic diseases (hydatidiform mole, invasive mole, and choriocarcinoma). Before the mid-1950s, the prognoses of these diseases, particularly the end stage (choriocarcinoma), were dismal. Even though Hertz in the late 1940s demonstrated that fetal tissues required a large amount of folic acid and could be inhibited by the antifolic compound methotrexate, it was not until 1956 that Li et al. reported the first complete and sustained remission in a patient with metastatic choriocarcinoma by using methotrexate. Since then, a considerable amount of knowledge and experience has been obtained, and GTN is recognized today as the most curable gynecologic malignancy. Several reasons are apparent for this change of events: (1) a sensitive marker is produced by the tumor—human chorionic gonadotropins (hCG)—and the amount of hormone present is directly related to the number of viable tumor cells; (2) this malignancy is extremely sensitive to various chemotherapeutic agents; (3) one can identify high-risk factors in this disease process and thereby individualize treatment; and (4) the aggressive use of multiple modalities is possible, such as single- and multiple-agent chemotherapy regimens, radiation, and surgery.

HYDATIDIFORM MOLE

In early studies, a considerable variation in the incidence of hydatidiform mole in different geographic regions was reported with the highest rates in certain areas of Asia. Many of those studies have been questioned because of the differences in the denominator used to calculate the rates. The most reliable studies suggest that the incidence of hydatidiform mole is slightly less than 1/1000 pregnancies in most of the world and possibly as high as 2/1000 in Japan. There may be some difference in ethnic groups in polysocial societies. In a study from Hawaii, the incidence was lower in white and native Hawaiians and highest in Filipino and Japanese populations. Whether this difference is genetic or cultural is unknown. In analyzing the effects of maternal age on the incidence of hydatidiform mole, the Duke group studied 2202 patients with hydatidiform moles and compared them with a contemporary control group that compared all types of pregnancy events. A significant increase in the incidence of mole was seen in women 15 years old or younger and 40 years of age or older. A significantly lower incidence was seen in women aged 20-29 years. The greatest relative risks were in women 50 years of age or older (RR=519). There appears to be no difference in parity among patients with molar pregnancies and patients with normal pregnancies. Age and parity do not appear to affect the clinical outcome of an individual with hydatidiform mole. Gestational age at the time of diagnosis of the hydatidiform mole does not appear to influence subsequent sequelae.

Nutritional factors may well have an effect on the incidence of hydatidiform mole. It has been suggested by Berkowitz et al. that a deficiency of animal fat and fat-soluble vitamin carotene may contribute to this disease. A prevalance of vitamin A deficiency corresponds to geographic locations where there is a high incidence of hydatidiform mole. Athough there are carotene-rich vegetables available in these countries, there is a lack of dietary fat for carotene absorption.

Patients with molar pregnancies have an increased risk of trophoblastic disease in later conceptions. It has been estimated that women with a previous mole have over ten times the risk of having another mole compared to women who have never had one. This risk increases if a women has more than one mole. Bagshawe noted the risk was 1/76 pregnancies for a second mole after the first one but increase to 1 in 6.5 pregnancies in women who already have had two moles. Sand reported that after two prior episodes of gestational trophoblastic disease, the risk of repeated disease is 28%. Goldstein et al. noted that 9 of 1339 patients (1 in 150) had at least two consecutive molar pregnancies. One patient had four moles. Other centers have reported incidences as high as 1 in 50 women. With recurrent molar pregnancies, there is an increased risk of malignant sequelae, although patients with consecutive molar pregnancies may have subsequent normal pregnancies. Berkowitz et al. noted that four of their patients with repeated moles later had full-term pregnancies. Lurain noted that 5 of 8 patients with consecutive moles had normal full-term pregnancies.

In a case-controlled study from Baltimore, factors found to be associated with gestational trophoblastic disease included professional occupation, history of prior spontaneous abortions, and the mean number of months from last pregnancy to the index pregnancy. Contraceptive history, irradiation, ABO blood groups, and smoking factors of the male partner were not relevant.

Symptoms

Essentially all patients with complete hydatidiform mole have delayed menses for varying periods, and most patients are considered to be pregnant. Vaginal bleeding occurs, usually during the first trimester. The bleeding may be a dark brown discharge or bright red in quantities sufficient to require blood transfusion. In one series this was present in 97% of complete moles. Nausea and vomiting are reported in almost one third of patients with hydatidiform mole, although Curry et al., in a report of patients with hydatidiform mole, noted only 14% of 347 patients with this symptom. This symptom, of course, can be confused with nausea and vomiting accompanying a normal pregnancy. Preeclampsia in the first trimester of pregnancy has been said to be almost pathognomonic of a hydatidiform mole, although this occurred in only 12% of the patients in the study by Curry et al. but was present in 27% of patients reported from Boston. Although proteinuria, hypertension, and hyperreflexia may be common, convulsions appear to be rare. Hyperthyroidism occurs rarely, but when present it can precipitate a medical emergency. Manifestations of hyperthyroidism that affect blood values can occur in as many as 10% of patients; however, clinical manifestations occurred in fewer than 1% of the patients of Curry et al., although it has been found to be as high as 7% in other reports. It appears the classic symptoms of a complete mole may be changing. The Boston group compared symptoms in their complete moles seen from 1988-1993 to those seen in 1965-1976. Vaginal bleeding was still the most common symptom but occurred in only 84% vs 97% in the earlier group. Excessive uterine size, preeclampsia, and hyperemesis were present in only 28%, 1.3%, and 8% respectively in the most recent group compared with 51%, 27%, and 26% respectively in the former group. Anemia was present in only 5% in current patients compared with 54% of the older group. The reason for these differences may be due to an earlier diagnosis (12 weeks vs 16 weeks) in the current group. The earlier diagnosis may be the results of using a more sensitive hCG determination and ultrasound earlier in the pregnancy. In only 75% of the current group who had an ultrasound was there a diagnosis of mole suggested. It may be more difficult to make the diagnosis in early pregnancy with the ultrasound. The incidence of persistent gestational trophoblastic tumor, however, is similar between the two groups. Hyperthyroidism and respiratory distress were not seen in any of the current group vs 7% and 2% in the former group.

Hyperthyroidism in molar pregnancy is caused by the

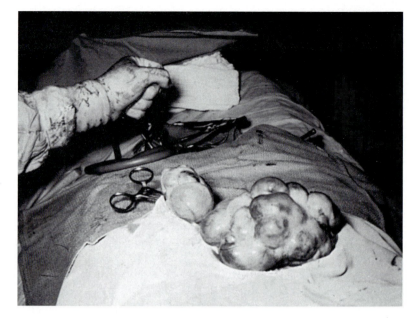

Figure 7-1 Thecal luteal cysts that are markedly enlarged. Cysts are caused by increased hCG production from molar pregnancy. Thecal luteal cysts will resolve spontaneously as hCG titer drops.

production of a thyrotropin-like compound by the molar tissue. There appears to be a central pathophysiologic role for the hCG molecule in the acceleration of thyroid function that occurs in patients with hydatidiform mole and GTN. This is mainly a result of the correlation between hCG level and endogenous thyroid function and of hCG having intrinsic thyroid-stimulating activity. With elevated levels of hCG, there is a binding of the hCG molecule by the TSH receptor site, resulting in hyperfunction of the thyroid gland. Clinical manifestations of hyperthyroidism disappear once the molar pregnancy is treated. Antithyroid therapy may be indicated for a short period. The most significant symptom of complete mole is acute respiratory distress thought to be due, at least in part, to trophoblastic pulmonary embolization. Other factors, such as changes associated with toxemia, hyperthyroidism, and other conditions, may be contributing.

Classically, a patient with a hydatidiform mole is said to have a uterine size excessive for gestational age, and this is found in about 50% of patients with moles; however, approximately one third of patients have uteri smaller than expected for gestational age. In the recent Boston study, excessive uterine size was present in 28%, equal to dates in 58%, and less than dates in 14% of patients. Thecal luteal cysts of the ovary may be large and are caused by the excessive hCG produced by the molar pregnancy (Figure 7-1). About 15% of patients with intact molar pregnancies have enlarged thecal luteal cysts. Patients with associated thecal luteal cysts appear to have a higher incidence of developing malignant sequelae of trophoblastic disease. The combination of enlarged ovaries with uteri large for gestational age results in an extremely high risk for malignant sequelae of trophoblastic disease and required subsequent therapy (57%). It should be emphasized that the symptoms elicited in this section are seen mainly in patients with complete moles.

Patients with partial moles do not usually exhibit excessive uterine size, thecal luteal cysts, toxemia, hyperthyroidism, or respiratory problems. In most patients with partial mole, the clinical diagnosis is missed or incomplete abortion. The necessity for thorough histopathological evaluation of missed or incomplete abortion material is self-evident.

Diagnosis

In many patients the first evidence to suggest the presence of a hydatidiform mole is the passage of vesicular tissue (Figure 7-2). Several techniques are available to substantiate diagnosis when pathologic material is not available for analysis. A quantitative pregnancy test of greater than 1,000,000 IU/L, an enlarged uterus, and vaginal bleeding suggest a diagnosis of hydatidiform mole. A single hCG determination, however, is not diagnostic. Occasionally, a single high hCG titer may be seen with a normal single or multiple pregnancy; this should not be used as the determining factor in making a diagnosis of hydatidiform mole. Conversely, a "normal" hCG titer for an anticipated gestational age can be seen with a mole.

Although several prepathologically diagnostic techniques have historically been used to identify a mole (amniography, uterine arteriography), today ultrasound has become the test of choice (Figure 7-3). In a molar pregnancy, the characteristic ultrasound notes multiple echoes, which are formed by the interface between the molar villi and the surrounding tissue without the normal gestational sac or fetus present. In rare instances a fetus may coexist with a mole (Figures 7-4 and 7-5). The group at Yale has proposed the combined use of ultrasound and hCG to determine if a hydatidiform mole is present. In 36 patients with moles, when ultrasound was used alone, 15 (42%) did not have a definite diagnosis on first examination. When hCG titer (threshold of 82,350 mlU/ml) was

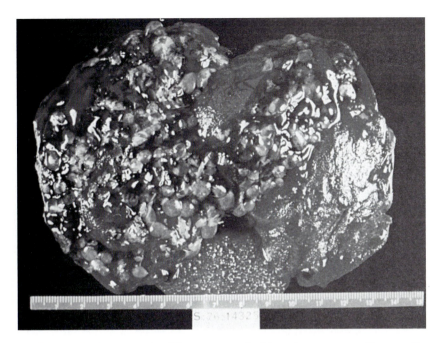

Figure 7-2 Typical enlarged cystic villi are apparent in this molar pregnancy. (Courtesy Department of Pathology, Duke University Medical Center.)

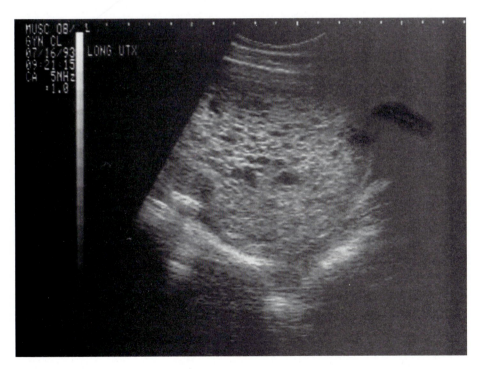

Figure 7-3 Ultrasound of a molar pregnancy. Multiple cystic spaces are noted in the enlarged uterus.

combined with ultrasound, 32 patients (89%) were correctly identified as having hydatidiform moles.

Complete and partial moles

The classic (complete) mole is well recognized histologically by the presence of trophoblastic proliferation and hydropic degeneration and the absence of vasculature. No fetus, cord, or amniotic fluid is identified. A normal karyotype (46 XX) is present in 90% of complete moles. There is fertilization of "an empty egg" by a single sperm carrying 23 chromosomes. This haploid set of chromosomes reduplicates to give a 46 karyotype. The usual 46 XX is a result of the doubling of the paternal set of chromosomes. Rarely, an empty egg may be fertilized by

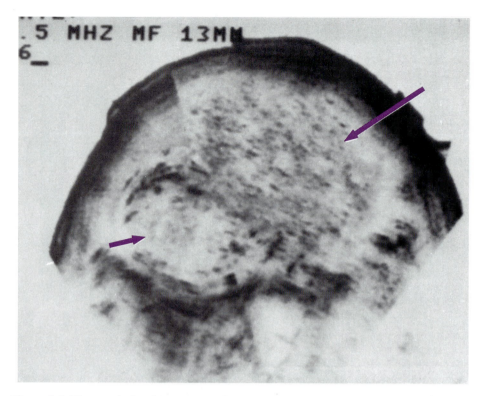

Figure 7-4 Ultrasound of molar pregnancy *(large arrow)* coexistent with fetus *(small arrow)*. (Courtesy Dr. Julius Butler, Minneapolis, Minnesota.)

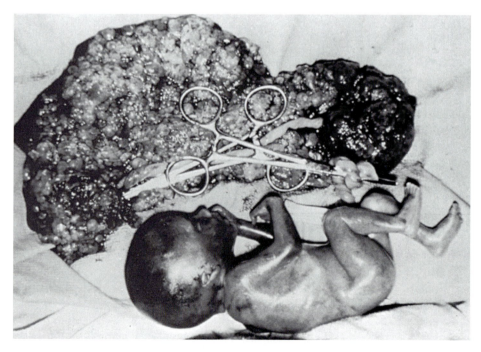

Figure 7-5 Molar pregnancy and fetus as noted on ultrasound in Figure 7-4. (Courtesy Dr. Julius Butler, Minneapolis, Minnesota.)

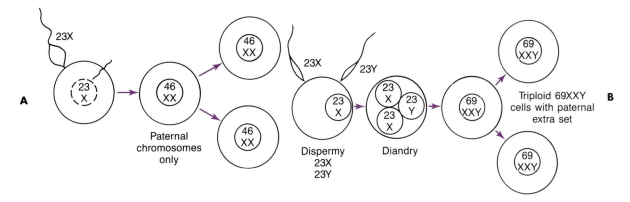

Figure 7-6 A, Paternal chromosomal origin of a complete classic mole (46XX). **B,** Triploid chromosomal origin of a partial mole (69 XXY-dispermy). (Reproduced with permission from Szulman AE, Surti U: The syndromes of partial and complete molar gestation, *Clin Obstet Gynecol* 27(1):177, 1984.)

two sperm, one carrying the X and the other the Y chromosome (Figure 7-6, *A*). About 6%-10% of complete moles have a 46 XY chromosomal pattern, again derived paternally.

In contrast, the partial hydatidiform mole consists of both placenta and fetus. There is usually marked swelling of the villi, but it is focal and slower in development. The focal trophoblastic hyperplasia usually affects the syncytial layer only. The fetus usually dies during the first trimester; rarely are living infants born in the second or third trimester. The fetus is usually growth retarded and shows signs of chromosomal abnormalities. Partial moles usually have a triploid karyotype. A normal egg is usually fertilized by dispermy, which can carry either sex chromosome, resulting in 69 chromosomes with a sex configuration of XXX, XXY, or XYY. The extra haploid set may also result from the failure of sperm meiosis during the first or second reduction division (see Figure 7-6, *B*).

At Charing Cross Hospital, in a 10-year period, 5989 patients with mole were registered, of whom 424 (7.1%) required chemotherapy. Partial mole had been diagnosed at the referring hospital in 857 (14.3%). Eleven patients were subsequently referred for treatment, yet only 5 were confirmed as partial moles. There are some clinical differences between complete and partial molar pregnancies. Patients with partial moles tend to be older, with longer gestational age, than individuals with complete moles. In patients with complete moles, it is not unusual to have large uteri relative to gestational ages; however, this is unusual in patients with partial moles. Preeclampsia occurs less frequently in patients with partial moles; when it does occur, it usually does so well into the second trimester. It is unusual to make the distinction between partial and complete mole preoperatively. The usual clinical diagnosis of a partial mole is missed abortion or incomplete abortion. The hCG titers are usually lower in patients with partial moles than in those with complete moles and tend to return to normal promptly. In a study

of 240 partial molar pregnancies from the New England Trophoblastic Disease Center, 16 (6.6%) developed metastatic disease. From nine published reports, 39 of 1125 (3.5%) patients with partial moles developed persistent disease and 7 (0.6%) developed metastatic disease. Metastatic trophoblastic disease has been reported after evaluation of partial mole, although this appears to be a rare occurrence. A partial mole is a pathologic diagnosis, and clinical diagnosis should not be relied upon without pathologic confirmation. Although the malignant sequela is apparently much less frequent after a partial mole than after a complete mole, hCG titers should be monitored after evacuation of all molar pregnancies.

Risk Factors

The size of the uterus at time of diagnosis has been considered for many years to be of significance in regard to malignant sequelae. It must be remembered that moles can occur in normal-size or small-for-date uteri. Curry et al. evaluated this in 347 patients with moles and noted that those with normal-size and large-for-date uteri had a 25% chance of developing GTN, compared with only 11% in patients with small-for-date uteri. Patients with enlarged ovaries, irrespective of uterine size, had a 49% chance of GTN appearing in the future. If patients had enlarged ovaries and large-for-date uteri, 57% developed GTN, compared with only 16% if the uteri and ovaries were not enlarged. Berkowtiz noted that patients with symptoms of marked trophoblastic growth (serum hCG >100,000 mIU/ml, excessive uterine size for dates, and prominent theca lutein cysts) are at high risk for persistent GTT. These patients had local invasion and metastasis in 31% and 8.8% respectively compared to 3.4% and 0.6% in those without symptoms of marked trophoblastic growth.

If time of evacuation was between 11 and 15 weeks, there was an increased incidence (29%) of malignant sequelae, compared with only 4% if less than 10 weeks and 19% if more than 16 weeks. The method of evacuation also appeared to be significant, in that 36% of those treated with hysterotomy developed GTN, compared with 19% and 20% if D&C or hysterectomy were used (Curry et al.). This probably reflects that the size of the uterus is an important prognostic factor—not the method of evaluation per se. With the increased use of suction curettage, even for uteri larger than 20 weeks in size, the role of hysterotomy is limited, if not eliminated. These data remind one that even if a hysterectomy is chosen for "evacuation," all patients must be followed in the same manner, as discussed later in this chapter.

Stone et al. noted that their patients who had passed moles and were taking oral contraceptives had a delayed rate of decline of hCG and a twofold increased risk of developing invasive sequelae. In a retrospective study Berkowitz et al. were unable to confirm these observations. Morrow et al., in a retrospective review of 149 patients with molar pregnancies, compared patients who received oral contraceptives with those who used non-hormonal contraceptives after evacuation. They concluded that there was no evidence that the use of estrogen-progesterone oral contraceptives before hCG remissions increased the risk of malignant sequelae following molar pregnancies. Ho Yuen and Burch followed 194 patients with moles. In 177 patients whose beta-hCG spontaneously returned to normal, they found no difference in the decline rate between those who used IUD, barrier, and other methods and those who used oral contraceptives. In the 17 patients who developed invasive disease, a greater proportion of women ingested more than 50 μg of estrogen than those in the group of 177 patients. These authors suggest that it may be the dose of estrogen rather than the oral contraceptive itself that influences the postmolar sequence. The GOG, in a prospective randomized study, evaluated 216 women of whom one half received oral contraceptives (OCs) and one half used barrier contraception following molar pregnancy. In this study there was neither an increased risk of postmolar disease nor a delay in time to normal titer when OCs were compared to the barrier method. This study should reassure physicians concerning the safety of OCs in the postmolar patient. It is our practice to start patients on OCs immediately following evacuation, unless there are other contraindications, while monitoring the serum hCG.

Evacuation

Several techniques have been used in the past to evacuate a molar pregnancy. These have included D&C (routine and suction), hysterotomy, hysterectomy, and various induction techniques. Before the use of suction curettage, hysterotomy was frequently used on uteri that were greater than 12 to 14 weeks in size. Suction curettage is now the method of choice for evacuation of a mole, and the role of hysterotomy is extremely limited unless major

hemorrhage is present. Suction curettage can be done even when the uterus is larger than 20 weeks in size. Blood loss has been moderate. We recommend that all patients with molar pregnancy have evacuation by suction D&E, with a laparotomy setup available for patients with large uteri. After a moderate amount of the tissue has been removed, administration of intravenous oxytocin (Pitocin) is begun. When the suction curettage has been completed and involution has begun, a sharp curettement is done, and this tissue is submitted separately for pathologic evaluation.

A primary hysterectomy may be selected as the method for evacuation if the patient is not desirous of future pregnancies. If at the time of hysterectomy thecal luetal cysts are encountered, the ovaries should be left in situ, because these will regress to normal as the hCG diminishes to a normal level. One must remember that even if hysterectomy is used as the method of evacuation, patients must be followed in the same manner as when other evacuation techniques are used.

Follow-up of Molar Pregnancy

Since hCG is produced by molar pregnancies and is a sensitive marker of trophoblastic cells present in the body, the patient who has had a mole evacuated must be followed very closely by this parameter. This can be done *only* with a sensitive bioassay or radioimmunoassay. Pregnancy tests using either biologic or immunologic materials may be inadequate, depending on their sensitivities. Patients *must* be followed with radioimmune assays for beta-hCG.

After evacuation the patient should have serial radioimmune beta-hCG determinations at 1-2 week intervals until there are two normal determinations. This would indicate a spontaneous remission and should occur in approximately 80% of patients with complete moles. The hCG titer should then be repeated bimonthly for at least 6-12 months. It is imperative that the patient use some type of contraception during this period, since a subsequent normal pregnancy cannot be differentiated from GTN by the hCG determination. Unless otherwise contraindicated, oral contraceptives may be used. Regular pelvic examinations should be done at 2-week intervals until the hCG titers return to normal levels. During this time, repeat examinations at 3-month intervals should be done (see box on p. 185). In the patient who has gone into spontaneous remission (negative titers, examinations, and chest films for 6-12 months) and who is desirous of further pregnancies, contraception can now be stopped. Some investigators now feel a normal titer for 6 months is sufficient, and subsequent pregnancies may occur after that time. Molar pregnancies occur in only about 1% of subsequent pregnancies, and many patients with histories of molar pregnancies have subsequently had normal gestations without difficulty. It appears that the pregnancy history following a mole is very similar to that of nonmole

---

MANAGEMENT OF HYDATIDIFORM MOLE

1. Beta-hCG determination every 1-2 weeks until negative two times
   a. Then bimonthly for 1 year
   b. Contraception for 6-12 months
2. Physical examination, including pelvic every 2 weeks until remission
   a. Then every 3 months for 1 year
3. Chest film initially
   a. Repeat only if hCG titer plateaus or rises
4. Chemotherapy started immediately if:
   a. hCG titer rises or plateaus during follow-up
   b. Metastases are detected at any time

---

patients in regard to term live births, first and second trimester abortions, anomalies, stillbirths, prematurity and primary cesarean section rate. Chemoprophylaxis, although rarely used today, appears to have no adverse effects on subsequent pregnancies. Subsequent pregnancy outcome appears similar irrespective of whether the mole is complete or partial.

Lurain et al. from the John I. Brewer Trophoblastic Disease Center have reported their experience with 738 patients with complete hydatidiform moles. In their study, 596 patients had spontaneous remission to normal of hCG titers, although only 390 (65%) had done so by 60 days. An additional 206 patients reached normal titers during the next 110 days. Of all of the patients, 142 (19%) were treated with chemotherapy because of rising or plateauing hCG titers. In addition, 125 patients had invasive moles, and 17 had choriocarcinomas. Only 15% of the 142 treated patients, or 3% of the total patients, had disease outside the uterus. These authors believe that the continued use of individual patient hCG regression patterns rather than deviations from a normal hCG regression curve (as suggested by Morrow and Kohorn) to make treatment decisions is in the patient's best interest. Morrow and Kohorn treated an increased number of patients (36% and 27%, respectively) using the regression curve, compared with studies in the literature using the individual patient's hCG regression pattern. It appears that the use of the hCG regression curve may result in more patients being treated than necessary, and it did not prevent metastatic disease in patients so treated. All the patients in the Lurain et al. study, by either spontaneous or therapeutic modalities, had remained in remission.

The time required for complete elimination of hCG from patients depends on the initial level of hCG, the amount of viable trophoblastic tissue remaining after evacuation, the excretion and serum half-life of hCG, and the sensitivity of the hCG test used. hCG is secreted by the kidneys at a fairly constant rate, and the serum half-life of hCG is 23.9 hours after intravenous injection of hCG and 37.2 hours after a normal-term delivery. Ho Yuen and Cannon followed 120 patients with moles with serial beta-hCG and found that the average time to reach undetectable levels was 73 days after evacuation, with half the patients having undetectable levels at 8 to 9 weeks after evacuation.

If the hCG titer plateaus or rises during the observation period, this is indicative of persistent or recurrent GTN, and the patient must be evaluated and started on chemotherapy; however, today the necessity of having a normal hCG at 60 days or a plateau of 2-3 weeks does not appear to be absolute as an indication for starting chemotherapy in postmolar patients. Any obvious metastases found on clinical examination or chest film also dictate the immediate use of chemotherapy.

Prophylactic Chemotherapy

Goldstein et al. suggested that dactinomycin can decrease the possibility of a patient with a hydatidiform mole developing subsequent malignancy. Kim et al. prospectively randomized 71 patients with complete moles into two groups: 39 patients who were treated with single courses of methotrexate and folinic acid, and 32 patients who were not treated. Of those treated, 10% developed persistent trophoblastic disease, compared with 31% of those who were not treated. In the treated group, disease was diagnosed later and required more courses of chemotherapy until complete remission than in the nontreated group. All 14 patients with persistent disease experienced complete remission with therapeutic chemotherapy. These authors concluded that although chemoprophylaxis reduced the incidence of persistent trophoblastic disease in patients at high risk, it increased tumor resistance and morbidity, and they felt that prophylactic chemotherapy was not indicated. Because 80% of the patients with molar pregnancy will go into a spontaneous remission and not require any therapy and because serial sensitive hCG determinations can identify the 20% who will develop malignant sequelae, it does not seem appropriate to treat all patients. The toxicity from prophylactic chemotherapy may be severe: deaths have been reported in some patients receiving this therapy.

GESTATIONAL TROPHOBLASTIC NEOPLASIA

The hydatidiform mole precedes malignant disease in approximately 50% of patients. There is an antecedent normal pregnancy in 25% of patients and an abortion or ectopic pregnancy in the other 25%. There may or may not be persistent uterine bleeding after the antecedent pregnancy. If the malignant GTN appears within a relatively short time after pregnancy, the index of suspicion is relatively high. Unfortunately, in many instances the preceding pregnancy occurred years before,

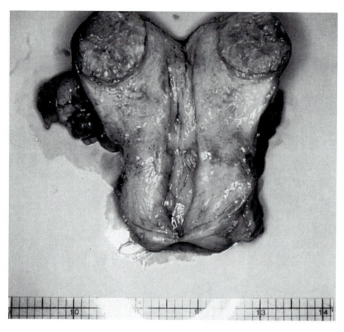

Figure 7-7 Choriocarcinoma present deep in myometrium. D&C would not identify residual disease.

and malignant GTN is usually not considered in the differential diagnosis. Essentially all types of symptoms have been described in patients with this disease. Lesions have been noted in the lower genital tract; and, unfortunately, many of these lesions when biopsied have been reported as "anaplastic malignant disease." Metastatic disease can be found in the gastrointestinal tract and genitourinary system, as well as in the liver, lung, and brain. Patients have had thoracotomies and craniotomies for diagnostic purposes, and only when the histologic evaluation suggested GTN were diagnostic hCG determinations obtained. Again, a high index of suspicion can prevent these invasive diagnostic procedures, which in most instances are unnecessary. A quantitative pregnancy test if positive is diagnostic but if negative it does not rule out disease. The serum beta-hCG determination is relatively fast, simple, inexpensive, and diagnostic.

In a patient with abnormal uterine bleeding a D&C may or may not be of benefit. If malignant trophoblastic disease is identified pathologically, this is, of course, helpful. Unfortunately, disease may be deep in the myometrium and unobtainable by curettage (Figure 7-7). In other instances, patients with GTN may have no localized disease in the uterus and have only metastatic disease.

Diagnosis and Evaluation

In 1973 Hammond et al. suggested a new categorization for GTN. To a certain degree, this has replaced the old terminology of chorioadenoma destruens and choriocarcinoma, since those designations tended to identify as

---

CLASSIFICATION OF GESTATIONAL TROPHOBLASTIC NEOPLASIA

I. Nonmetastic disease: no evidence of disease outside uterus
II. Metastatic disease: any disease outside uterus
   A. Good prognosis metastatic disease
      1. Short duration (last pregnancy <4 months)
      2. Low pretreatment hCG titer (<100,000 IU/24 hr or <40,000 mIU/ml)
      3. No metastasis to brain or liver
      4. No significant prior chemotherapy
   B. Poor prognosis metastatic disease
      1. Long duration (last pregnancy >4 months)
      2. High pretreatment hCG titer (>100,000 IU/24 hr or >40,000 mIU/ml)
      3. Brain or liver metastasis
      4. Significant prior chemotherapy
      5. Term pregnancy

---

separate and distinct entities what is truly a spectrum of disease. This new classification (see box above) treats GTN as a spectrum of neoplasia and allows identification of high-risk factors in this disease process. By so doing, one is able to individualize therapy and thereby treat a specific patient more appropriately.

There have been several suggested modifications or staging proposals. In 1976 Bagshawe suggested the use of a prognostic scoring system instead of a staging system.

Table 7-1   WHO scoring system

Prognostic factors	Score			
	0	**1**	**2**	**4**
Age	≤ 39	>39		
Antecedent pregnancy	HM	Abortion	Term	
Months from last pregnancy	4	4 to 6	7 to 12	12
hCG (IU/L)	10^3	10^3-10^4	10^4-10^5	10^5
ABO (female × male)		O × A	B	
		A × O	AB	
Largest tumor (cm)		3 to 5	5	
Site metastases		Spleen	GI	Brain
		Kidney	Liver	
Number of metastases		1 to 4	4 to 8	8
Prior chemotherapy			Single drug	2 or more drugs

≤ 4: low risk; 5-7: middle risk; ≥ 8: high risk.

The World Health Organization (WHO) adopted a modification of Bagshawe's scoring system (Table 7-1).

FIGO for many years staged this disease classically as an anatomic designation. Because of insufficient discrimination between low and high-risk subsets of patients, FIGO has added risk factors as substages to each stage. Risk factors include pre-therapy hCG levels >100,000 mIU/ml and duration of disease longer than 6 months. If no risk factors are present, patients are assigned to substage A, 1 risk factor to substage B, and 2 risk factors to substage C (Table 7-2). The WHO scoring system identified 9 factors with 29 variables (or scores), which makes it cumbersome. Most investigators have found that essentially all patients with scores less than 8 survived with mainly single-agent chemotherapy. In patients with scores greater than 8, the actual number does not necessarily predict whether patients will survive with multiple agent chemotherapy.

Soper and his colleagues at Duke have recently evaluated the three currently used staging classifications (FIGO, WHO, and clinical classification). They used a data base of 454 women treated at their institution. Multivariant Cox modeling identified prior therapy, type of antecedent pregnancy, number of metastatic sites and duration of disease as independent prognostic factors. All three staging systems identified high and low risk patients with statistically significant and equal efficiency. Survival of previously untreated patients with FIGO stage IIIb or higher was essentially equivalent. FIGO Stage I-IIIa correlated with nonmetastatic good prognosis metastatic disease categories. The FIGO system correlated the outcome and provides stratification of patients with pulmonary metastatic disease into prognostic groups.

When a diagnosis of GTN has been suggested or established, proper evaluation must be performed. The

Table 7-2   FIGO staging for trophoblastic tumors

Stage I	Disease confined to the uterus
Stage Ia	Disease confined to the uterus with no risk factors
Stage Ib	Disease confined to the uterus with one risk factor
Stage Ic	Disease confined to the uterus with two risk factors
Stage II	GTT extends outside the uterus but is limited to the genital structures (adnexa, vagina, broad ligament)
Stage IIa	GTT involving genital structures without risk factors
Stage IIb	GTT extends outside of the uterus but limited to genital structures with one risk factor
Stage IIc	GTT extends outside of the uterus but limited to the genital structures with two risk factors
Stage III	GTT extends to the lungs with or without known genital tract involvement
Stage IIIa	GTT extends to the lungs with or without genital tract involvement and with no risk factors
Stage IIIb	GTT extends to the lungs with or without genital tract involvement and with one risk factor
Stage IIIc	GTT extends to the lungs with or without genital tract involvement and has two risk factors
Stage IV	All other metastatic sites
Stage IVa	All other metastatic sites without risk factors
Stage IVb	All other metastatic sites with one risk factor
Stage IVc	All other metastatic sites with two risk factors

Risk factors affecting staging include the following: (1) hCG >100,000 mIU/ml; (2) duration of disease >6 months from termination of the antecedent pregnancy. The following factors should be considered and noted in reporting: (1) prior chemotherapy for known GTT; (2) placental site tumors should be reported separately; (3) histological verification of disease is not required.

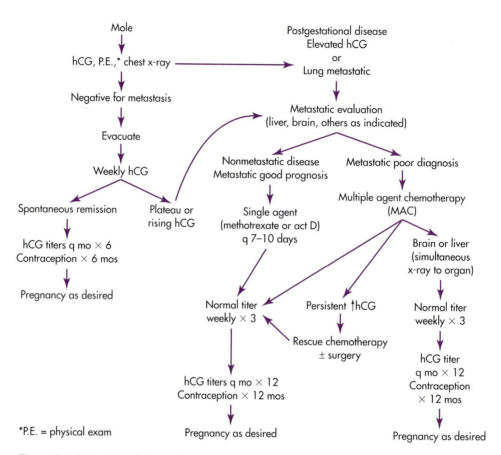

Figure 7-8 Evaluation of the molar pregnancy and the patient with gestational trophoblastic disease.

top box on p. 189 lists the minimum workup suggested for these patients. Identification of foci of disease should be established if at all possible. Since GTN can metastasize in the liver, lung, and brain, quite commonly these areas are evaluated in depth. In an evaluation of 324 women with gestational trophoblastic disease, investigators at Duke University evaluated whether all patients with GTD needed extensive investigation as has been practiced. They noted in the asymptomatic patient that the history and physical examination, quantitative hCG, and chest x-ray are 100% sensitive in identifying those who require further evaluation to diagnose metastatic gestational trophoblastic disease that has poor prognosis. Only patients with lung or vaginal metastases or obvious symptoms had evaluation for liver or brain metastases. With these criteria, patients with high-risk metastases were identified with 100% sensitivity and 63% specificity. This information certainly can result in cost saving to the patient. After these tests have been obtained, categorization of disease can be performed and specific therapy begun.

The treatment results of 395 patients with GTN from the Brewer Trophoblastic Disease Center (Lurain et al.)

were reported in 1982. Lurain et al. preferred to continue the traditional classification of invasive mole and choriocarcinoma but did subdivide each into nonmetastatic and metastatic disease. Since tissue is not always available in these patients, it appears that the continued use of a histologic classification can be burdensome and unworkable in some patients. Several authors suggested that the use of hCG makes the histologic diagnosis unnecessary (Figure 7-8).

Nonmetastatic Trophoblastic Disease

Nonmetastatic trophoblastic disease is the first part of the spectrum of GTN and the most common (see the top box on p. 189). By definition, disease is limited to the uterus, with this conclusion usually arrived at as an exclusion diagnosis, since metastasis cannot be identified. Particularly if subsequent fertility is desired, a pelvic arteriogram can be performed and disease identified within the uterus. This may be a guide, especially if chemotherapy is unsuccessful.

Patients with nonmetastatic trophoblastic disease can be treated with single-agent chemotherapy (see the bottom box on p. 191). For years methotrexate as primary

---

WORKUP OF GESTATIONAL TROPHOBLASTIC NEOPLASIA

History and physical examination
Chest film
Pretreatment hCG titer
Hematologic survey
Serum chemistries
CT of brain
Ultrasound of pelvis   } only if above denotes abnormality
Liver scan

SINGLE-AGENT CHEMOTHERAPY

1. Methotrexate 20-25 mg IM every day for 5 days
   (repeat every 7 days if possible)
2. Dactinomycin 10-12 µg/kg IV every day for 5 days
   (repeat every 7 days if possible)
3. Methotrexate 1 mg/kg IM on days 1, 3, 5, and 7
   Folinic acid 0.1 mg/kg IM on days 2, 4, 6, and 8
   (repeat every 7 days if possible)

---

therapy has been the treatment of choice at the Southeastern Regional Center for Trophoblastic Disease. If patients have abnormal liver function, methotrexate should not be used, since this agent is metabolized in the liver. Other investigators have used dactinomycin as primary therapy with equally good results. They believe that the toxicity from dactinomycin is less than that from methotrexate. Alternate chemotherapy with methotrexate and dactinomycin has been reported. This regimen has been used in the hope of decreasing chemotherapy toxicity.

Berkowitz et al., at the New England Trophoblastic Center, have used methotrexate with folinic acid rescue in 106 patients with GTN (89 nonmetastatic and 12 low-risk metastatic). Ninety-six (90%) patients achieved complete remission with this regimen, and 77 (80%) required only one course. Almost 95% of nonmetastatic patients obtained remission, compared with 59% who had low-risk metastatic disease. Resistance to methotrexate with folinic acid rescue was greater in patients with excessive hCG titers and disseminated disease. Toxicity was low, particularly in comparison with the standard methods of giving methotrexate. These investigators have updated their experience in 185 patients with gestational trophoblastic disease. Ninety percent of 163 patients with nonmetastatic disease and 68% of 22 patients with low-risk metastatic disease were placed into complete remission with methotrexate and folinic acid. More than 80% were placed into remission with only one course of chemotherapy. All patients with methotrexate resistance achieved remission with other agents. At Charing Cross, 347 of 348 (99.7%) low-risk patients treated with methotrexate and folinic acid survived; however 69 (20%) had to change treatment because of drug resistance and 23 (6%) additional patients needed to change treatment because of drug-induced toxicity. An analysis of the data from the Southeastern Trophoblastic Disease Center at Duke University indicated that resistance to methotrexate with folinic acid was greater than that noted in previous experience using standard methotrexate for nonmetastatic disease.

Although this difference was statistically significant, when one considers the increased number of patients receiving standard methotrexate who must be switched to another agent because of toxicity, this difference between the two regimens becomes less significant. Because of the lower toxicity and because all patients treated in this category were eventually put into remission, methotrexate with folinic acid rescue is considered as first-line therapy for nonmetastatic trophoblastic disease in the United States. Wong et al. noted that administration of methotrexate, alone or with folinic acid, resulted in comparable sustained biochemical remission rates; however, the patients receiving the latter treatment achieved remission earlier, but experienced a higher incidence of hepatic toxicity in contrast to other reports.

In the Far East, 5-fluorouracil has been used successfully as a single agent in gestational trophoblastic disease. Sung et al. have used large doses (25 to 30 mg/kg) of 5-fluorouracil administered by slow IV drip (over an 8-hour period) in 173 cases of invasive mole and 139 cases of choriocarcinoma. In 212 cases, 5-fluorouracil was used as initial therapy. There was an overall remission rate of 98.4% for invasive mole and 93% for choriocarcinoma. In 100 patients who developed resistance to 6-mercaptopurine or methotrexate, 5-fluorouracil was successful in 93.6% of patients with invasive mole and 71.7% of those with choriocarcinoma. The number of recurrences after successful 5-fluorouracil therapy was 3 (1.4%). Toxicity was minimal.

The GOG has evaluated other therapeutic regimens in nonmetastatic gestational trophoblastic disease. Actinomycin D 1.25 mg/m^2 was given as a single IV dose every 2 weeks. Of 31 patients who were treated, 29 (94%) achieved remission after an average of 4.4 (range of 2 to 15) courses of therapy. The two patients who failed to respond to pulse therapy were subsequently cured by alternative treatment. The frequency of toxicity was acceptable. The advantages of pulse Actinomycin D over other treatments include ease of administration, greater patient convenience, and improved cost effectiveness.

In another GOG study, 65 patients initially were given methotrexate 30 mg/m^2 weekly. On preliminary review of 27 patients, 21 had a complete response and toxicity was minimal (no grade III or IV). The six nonresponders received Actinomycin D and are in remission. In a

---

MANAGEMENT OF SINGLE-AGENT CHEMOTHERAPY

A. Chemotherapy as noted in the bottom box on p. 189
   1. Repeated at 7-10 days intervals depending on toxicity
   2. Contraception begun (oral if not contraindicated)
B. Drug continued as above until hCG titer is normal
C. Chemotherapy changed if:
   1. Titer rises (10% or more)
   2. Titer plateaus
   3. Evidence of new metastasis
D. Laboratory Values—chemotherapy not repeated unless:
   1. WBC >3000/cu mm
   2. Polys >1500/cu mm
   3. Platelets >100,000/cu mm
   4. BUN, SGOT, SGPT essentially normal
E. Other toxicity mandating postponement of chemotherapy
   1. Severe oral or gastrointestinal ulceration
   2. Febrile course (usually present only with leukopenia)
F. Remission defined as three consecutive normal weekly hCG titers

---

REMISSION AND FOLLOW-UP IN GESTATIONAL TROPHOBLASTIC NEOPLASIA

1. Three consecutive normal weekly hCG assays (1-3 courses after normal)
2. hCG titers every 2 weeks for 3 months
   Then monthly for 3 months
   Then every 2 months for 6 months
   Then every 6 months
3. Frequent pelvic examination
4. Contraception for at least 6 months

Table 7-3   Role of therapy in nonmetastatic gestational trophoblastic neoplasia

Therapy	Remission	
Chemotherapy only	106/122	
Chemotherapy + hysterectomy (2°)	9/9	
Chemotherapy + pelvic infusion	3/7	122/122
Chemotherapy + pelvic infusion + hysterectomy (3°)	4/7	
Chemotherapy + 1° hysterectomy	17/17	
TOTAL	139/139 (100%)	

Based on data from Hammond CB, Weed JC Jr, Currie JL: *Am J Obstet Gynecol* 136:844, 1980.

---

subsequent follow-up study, the GOG evaluated weekly methotrexate with 40 mg/m^2 escalating to a maximum of 50 mg/m^2 if major toxicity was not seen. In 46 of 62 patients (74%), complete response was achieved in nonmetastatic GTD. Fifteen of the 16 failures had complete response with subsequent chemotherapy. This higher dose is no more effective than lower-dose regimens (30 mg/m^2) and has similar toxicity.

Therapy should be repeated at 7-day intervals if at all possible. Criteria noted in the box above must be strictly adhered to so that toxicity will not become life threatening. Severe oral mucosal ulcerations can result from single-agent methotrexate and become so severe that oral intake is impossible. This type of toxicity would preclude frequently repeated courses. It has not been seen with the methotrexate-folinic acid regimen. The therapy should be continued until negative hCG titers are obtained. A remission is defined as three consecutive normal weekly hCG titers. However, if a patient's hCG titer rises or if there is a titer plateau after two courses of chemotherapy, an alternative drug should be tried. Evidence of new metastasis while the patient is being treated is also an indication for changing the chemotherapy. After the hCG titers return to normal levels, appropriate follow-up is mandatory. This is outlined in the box top right. It is important that some type of contraception be used for at least 6 months after remission. Unless otherwise contraindicated, oral contraceptives can be used. If a patient remains in remission for longer than 6 months and desires further childbearing, this can now be allowed. Experience indicates that patients successfully treated can expect normal reproduction in the future. There appears to be no increase in congenital anomalies. Subsequent fertility or fetal wastage is not chemotherapeutic-dose dependent, although the number of drugs given (three or greater) did appear to decrease conception rate in the Charing Cross data.

Treatment of nonmetastatic GTN has been 100% successful. A total of 139 patients with this disease so treated at the Southeastern Trophoblastic Center have entered into remission (Tables 7-3 and 7-4). Of 122 patients treated with chemotherapy, 106 have entered into remission. In 9 patients who failed to go into remission a hysterectomy was done, followed by remission. In an attempt to preserve fertility, 7 patients had pelvic infusion, and 3 were successful. The other 4 were treated successfully by tertiary hysterectomy (see Table 7-3). In patients who no longer desire fertility it has been suggested that a primary hysterectomy during the first course of chemotherapy can shorten the treatment period. In 17 patients so treated, remission was obtained in a shorter period and with fewer courses of chemotherapy

Table 7-4   Role of therapy in nonmetastatic gestational trophoblastic neoplasia

Therapy	Patients	Days hospitalized	Number of courses of chemotherapy
Chemotherapy + 1° hysterectomy	17	32.8	2.2
Chemotherapy only (cure)	106	50.8	4.0
Chemotherapy + 2° surgery	16	121.2	8.3

Based on data from Hammond CB, Weed JC Jr, Currie JL: *Am J Obstet Gynecol* 136:844, 1980.

Table 7-5   Fertility in nonmetastatic gestational trophoblastic neoplasia

Desired fertility	109/122 (89%)
Subsequent pregnancies (47 patients)	57
Normal infants	45 (2 sets of twins)
Spontaneous abortion	7
Therapeutic abortion	3
Mole	2

Based on data from Hammond CB, Weed JC Jr, Currie JL: *Am J Obstet Gynecol* 136:844, 1980.

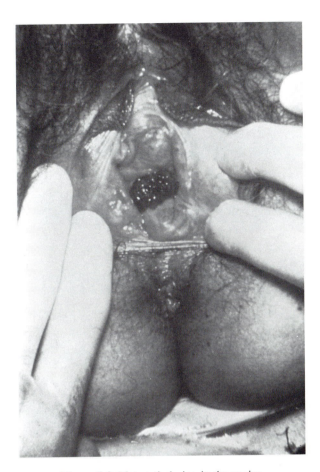

Figure 7-9 Metastatic lesion in the vagina.

(see Table 7-4). Patients who required secondary surgery in addition to chemotherapy were more difficult to place into remission, requiring more courses of chemotherapy and a considerably longer period of hospitalization. An attempt to preserve fertility was the reason for the delay in subsequent surgery. Of patients desiring fertility, 89% went into remission with preservation of the uterus (Table 7-5). Fifty-seven subsequent pregnancies in 47 patients occurred. There were two subsequent molar pregnancies. Bagshawe's group evaluated occurrence of pregnancy after cytotoxic chemotherapy (445 long-term survivors) and found that 97% of those who wished for a pregnancy (49% of all studied) conceived, and 86% had at least one live birth (all had received methotrexate). Of the 47 women whose combination chemotherapy included cyclophosphamide, 37 had live births. Those who received three or more drugs were less likely to have live births than those who received methotrexate alone or those who received methotrexate with only one other drug. There was not an excess of congenital malformations. It should be remembered that to substantiate remission, patients who have primary or secondary hysterectomy must be followed in exactly the same manner as those who are treated primarily with chemotherapy.

In summary, it appears that single-agent methotrexate or Actinomycin D is the treatment of choice for nonmetastatic GTD, at least in the western world. One should expect 100% survival, although second-line chemotherapy may be required in as many as one third of patients. All regimens suggested have been effective. The protocol followed should include consideration of cost effectiveness and convenience to the patient. Close monitoring is critical and protocols must be followed.

Good Prognosis Metastatic Trophoblastic Neoplasia

Patients with GTN who on evaluation are found to have metastatic disease are categorized as good prognosis when none of the following is present: (1) brain or liver metastasis; (2) urinary hCG titer greater than 100,000 IU/24 hr or serum beta-hCG titer greater than 40,000 mIU/ml; (3) previous chemotherapy; and (4) symptoms (antecedent pregnancy) longer than 4 months (Figures 7-9 and 7-10). This category is equivalent to FIGO stage IIIA with minor exceptions. It has been suggested by the Southeastern Trophoblastic Center that patients who had antecedent term pregnancies and developed GTN should be placed in the poor prognosis category. There is no general agreement in the literature concerning this item. In another publication, three fourths of the patients who

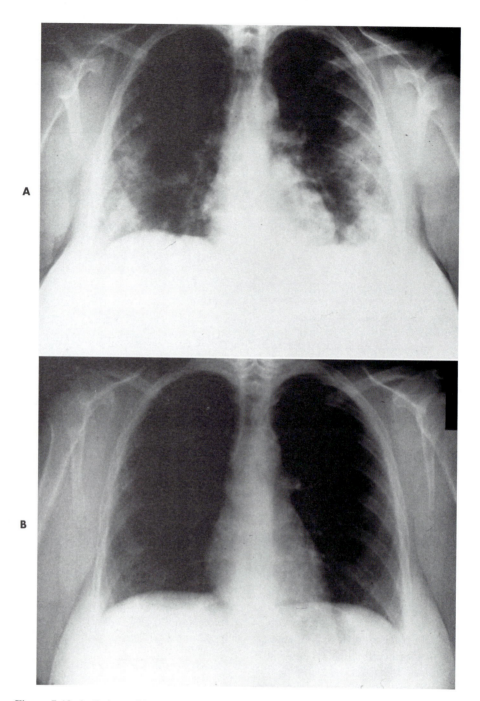

Figure 7-10 A, Patient with multiple pulmonary nodules from metastatic GTN. **B,** After complete clearance of metastatic pulmonary nodules with chemotherapy.

had an antecedent full-term pregnancy were categorized as poor prognosis using the above four criteria. The five patients who were categorized as having good prognosis disease following full-term pregnancy were succesfully treated with chemotherapy and/or surgery. The New England Trophoblastic Center reported on 15 patients with choriocarcinoma following term pregnancy. Five patients died; however, all had brain and other organ metastases at the time of diagnosis. Eight patients with nonmetastatic or good prognosis metastatic disease

achieved complete response. In addition, two patients with other poor prognostic factors were placed into remission. This issue remains unresolved.

Therapy for good prognosis metastatic GTN can be the same as that described for nonmetastatic disease (see bottom box on p. 189). Methotrexate is considered by many to be the drug of choice for patients with good prognosis metastatic trophoblastic neoplasia. They are treated with 20 to 25 mg intramuscularly every day for 5 days, and this course is repeated after a 7-day drug-free

Table 7-6   Modified Bagshawe chemotherapy

Day	Hour	Treatment
1	0600	Hydroxyurea 500 mg P.O.
	1200	Hydroxyurea 500 mg P.O.
	1800	Hydroxyurea 500 mg P.O.
	1900	Dactinomycin 200 µg IV
	2400	Hydroxyurea 500 mg P.O.
2	0700	Vincristine 1 mg/m^2 IV
	1900	Methotrexate 100 mg/m^2 IV
		Methotrexate 200 mg/m^2 infused over 12 hr
		Dactinomycin 200 µg IV
3	1900	Dactinomycin 200 µg IV
		Cyclophosphamide 500 mg/m^2 IV
		Folinic acid 14 mg IM
4	0100	Folinic acid 14 mg IM
	0700	Folinic acid 14 mg IM
	1300	Folinic acid 14 mg IM
	1900	Folinic acid 14 mg IM
		Dactinomycin 500 µg IV
5	0100	Folinic acid 14 mg IM
	1900	Dactinomycin 500 µg IV
6	No treatment	
7	No treatment	
8	1900	Cyclophosphamide 500 mg/m^2 IV
		Doxorubicin 30 mg/m^2 IV

Table 7-7   Role of therapy in good prognosis metastatic gestational trophoblastic neoplasia

Chemotherapy only	35/40	⎫ 40/40
Chemotherapy + hysterectomy (2°)	5/5	⎬
Chemotherapy + 1° hysterectomy	15/15	⎭
TOTAL	55/55 (100%)	

Based on data from Hammond CB, Weed JC Jr, Currie JL: *Am J Obstet Gynecol* 136:844, 1980.

interval if toxicity allows. Liver and kidney function, as well as the hemopoietic survey, must be evaluated, and therapy should not be instituted unless these values are adequate. When negative titers have been achieved, one additional course is routinely given. If resistance to methotrexate occurs, manifested by rising or plateauing titers or by the development of new metastasis, or if negative titers are not achieved by the fifth course of methotrexate, patients are switched to dactinomycin. If resistance to both drugs develops, the patients should then be started on a multiple-agent protocol such as methotrexate, dactinomycin, and chlorambucil (MAC) or the modified Bagshawe protocol (MBP) (Table 7-6). If there is no evidence of metastatic disease and titers are still elevated, a uterine site for the disease should be vigorously sought (such as identifying foci in the uterus by pelvic arteriography). In patients desiring further fertility, pelvic artery infusion may be considered. Hysterectomy may be performed if future fertility is not desired.

At the Southeastern Trophoblastic Center, 93 patients with good prognosis metastatic GTN have been treated (Table 7-7). Of the first 55 patients analyzed, there were 40 treated with chemotherapy only, and 35 were placed in remission. The other 5 had secondary hysterectomy, with clearing of their disease. An additional 15 patients had chemotherapy and hysterectomy performed primarily, all of whom were placed into remission. Patients who had

chemotherapy and primary hysterectomy went into remission in a shorter time and with fewer courses of chemotherapy than patients treated with chemotherapy alone or chemotherapy plus secondary surgery. When compared with the nonmetastatic GTN patients, more courses of chemotherapy were required in good prognosis metastatic GTN patients treated in a similar manner, with the exception of those who had chemotherapy plus secondary surgery. The efficacy of primary surgery is apparent, although this finding is probably related to extent of disease within the good prognosis metastatic GTN category.

The Boston group reported their experience with 48 patients with low-risk metastatic disease. All patients were treated with methotrexate alone or with folinic acid or dactinomycin initially. After the first course of chemotherapy, no further therapy was given as long as the hCG levels continued to fall. Twenty-five patients (51%) required a change to another chemotherapy regimen, with 7 (14%) receiving combination therapy. Mean number of courses was 3.4 in all patients but 4.5 in those with resistant disease. Fourteen patients (29%) underwent some type of surgical intervention, including hysterectomy (8), thoracotomy (2), adnexectomy (3), and uterine resection (1). The prognostic score (WHO) was not useful in predicting which patient required alternative single-agent or combination chemotherapy. All patients achieved sustained remission.

Poor Prognosis Metastatic Trophoblastic Neoplasia

Patients who have been categorized as having poor prognosis metastatic GTN (see box top left on p. 196) present the physician and the medical team with a major challenge. Many of these patients have been previously treated with chemotherapy and are resistant to that treatment while accumulating considerable toxicity and depleting bone marrow reserves. Multiple-agent chemotherapy is recommended in this disease, and a multiple-modality approach is necessary in many patients. These patients should be treated in centers that have special interest and expertise in this disease. Most patients require prolonged hospitalization for as long as several months.

POOR PROGNOSIS METASTATIC GESTATIONAL TROPHOBLASTIC NEOPLASIA

Brain or liver metastasis
Urinary hCG >100,000 IU/24 hr or serum beta-hCG
 >40,000 mIU/ml
Unsuccessful prior chemotherapy
Symptoms that have lasted longer than 4 months
Gestational trophoblastic neoplasia after term pregnancy (?)

TREATMENT OF POOR PROGNOSIS GESTATIONAL TROPHOBLASTIC NEOPLASIA

Methotrexate 15 mg IM every
 day for 5 days
Dactinomycin 10-12 μg/kg IV   } Every 12-14 days
 every day for 5 days
Chlorambucil 10 mg P.O. every
 day for 5 days
Brain or liver radiation therapy 2000-3000 cGy

Table 7-8   Role of therapy in poor prognosis metastatic gestational trophoblastic neoplasia

Therapy	Remission
Chemotherapy ± radiation therapy	20/23 (87%)
Chemotherapy + 1° surgery	17/29 (58%)
Chemotherapy + 2° surgery	5/11 (45%)
TOTAL	42/63 (66%)

16 patients died of disease
5 patients died of toxicity

Based on data from Hammond CB, Weed JC Jr, Currie JL: *Am J Obstet Gynecol* 136:844, 1980.

They will have life-threatening toxicity from therapy and in some instances require specialized care such as total parenteral nutrition and other life-support measures during periods of minimal host resistance.

Before 1969, at the Southeastern Trophoblastic Disease Center, patients with this disease were treated by single-agent therapy, and in the first seven patients so treated only one was placed into remission. Beginning in 1969, patients with poor prognosis GTN were started initially on triple chemotherapy, as outlined in the second box above. Triple chemotherapy (MAC) is repeated at 12 to 14 days, depending on the toxicity and using the parameters established for single-agent therapy (see box top left on p. 190). Cerebral or hepatic metastases are treated concurrently with 2000 to 3000 cGy (in 10 days) to the whole brain or liver. If the hCG titer rises or plateaus after two courses of MAC, the chemotherapy is changed.

Liver metastases appear to carry a worse prognosis than brain metastases. Liver metastases are usually associated with widespread metastases. In a review of the recent literature, it appeared that 21 of 56 (38%) with liver metastases achieved a complete remission, in contrast to 40 of 69 (58%) with brain metastases. Patients with brain metastases noted on initial evaluation tended to respond better than patients who developed brain lesions during therapy. Those with metastasis to multiple sites are at a significant risk for treatment failure. All investigators do not use radiation to the liver. Bakri noted chemotherapy alone with cisplatin, etoposide, and actinomycin D put 5 of 8 patients with liver metastasis into remission while none of 6 treated with MAC survived. It also appears that patients with a prognostic score greater than 8 are at high risk (see Table 7-1); however, this has not been universally noted. At the New England Trophoblastic Disease Center, 30 patients with high-risk scores were treated, and the mean score of those who died was similar to that of those who survived (11 for the former, 13 for the latter). Unfortunately, several of the items included in the WHO scoring system are of little or limited significance.

The Southeastern Trophoblastic Center reported on 63 patients with poor prognosis GTN. The remission rate for these patients is 66% (Table 7-8). Patients treated by chemotherapy with concurrent radiation therapy have the best prognosis: 87% went into remission. If primary or secondary surgery is needed, the prognosis worsens. In 67 patients primarily treated at Duke, survival was 79% compared to 63% survival in all 120 patients with this disease categorization. Failed initial therapy before referral supports the poor prognosis if this factor is present. These patients require longer hospitalization and more courses of chemotherapy to place them into remission than do patients with nonmetastatic or good prognosis metastatic disease.

Although the anticipated outcome for poor prognosis GTN is considerably less favorable than that for nonmetastatic and good prognosis metastatic disease, it has shown marked improvement over the years. As previously noted, of the first 7 patients treated with single-agent chemotherapy only one survived. During the 10 years from 1968 through 1978, 73% of the patients were placed into remission; however, during the next 3 years, 17 of 19 (90%) went into remission. This has been accomplished not only with the new chemotherapeutic regimens but also with the aggressive multiple-modality approach and conscientious support of these patients during their critical illness. In addition, deaths from toxicity have decreased considerably during this time.

Of the 63 patients with poor prognosis metastatic GTN, only 19 were able to preserve their reproductive capacity. Only four of these patients have had subsequent pregnancy, resulting in one spontaneous abortion and four normal deliveries.

Patients with high-risk disease, defined by Lurain et al. as (1) immediate pretreatment hCG titer more than 100,000 IU/L or time longer than 4 months from antecedent pregnancy, (2) brain or liver metastases, (3) antecedent term pregnancy (since 1975), and (4) prior unsuccessful chemotherapy treatment, were initially treated with methotrexate or dactinomycin before 1968. Since then, all individuals received MAC chemotherapy. Cerebral metastases were treated simultaneously with whole-organ irradiation therapy. The overall remission rate in 395 patients with GTN was 83% (329 patients). All patients with invasive mole, irrespective of whether their disease was nonmetastatic or metastatic, were in remission, but only 75 out of 100 (75%) patients with metastatic choriocarcinomas were in remission. In the analysis of treatment failures Lurain et al. noted three factors primarily responsible:

1. *Extensive disease.* Many patients had extensive disease present at the time of initial treatment: 11 of 48 (23%) were dead within 1 month of diagnosis. Of these 11 patients, 5 had such extensive disease at diagnosis that not even one full course of chemotherapy could be administered before death.

2. *Inadequate initial treatment.* In the analysis of treatment given before referral, 10 of 15 (67%) patients had not received optimal therapy. In comparison of patients monitored and treated at the Brewer Trophoblastic Disease Center with patients monitored (beta-hCG) at the Center but treated elsewhere, the cure rate was 94% vs 55%, respectively. Of patients transferred to the Center after treatment failures, 59% were cured, compared with 93% of patients treated totally at the Center. It was noted that only 9 of 24 (38%) patients with metastatic choriocarcinoma referred elsewhere after treatment were placed in remission. It is therefore extremely important that patients who fall into the high-risk category have proper consultation and referral to an institution with expertise in this disease, since the first treatment given to these patients will probably determine their outcome.

3. *Failure of presently used chemotherapy protocols in advanced disease.* Before MAC was used in high-risk patients, there was a 39% cure, compared with up to 90% remission with the multiple-agent regimens. Secondary chemotherapy yields very poor results. Lurain et al. have been unable to achieve a single complete remission with second-line chemotherapeutic agents.

Using the designation of high-risk metastatic gestational trophoblastic disease, Lurain and Brewer treated 46 patients primarily and 27 patients with recurrence with MAC. Adjuvant surgery and radiotherapy were used in selected patients. Overall cure rate was 63% (29) for primary treatment and 30% (8) for secondary treatment. Patients with primary diagnosis of invasive mole had a 100% remission rate compared with 59% with choriocarcinoma. Patients with metastases to the lung and vagina did better than those who had metastases to other sites (74% vs 44%). Those with term pregnancies did worse than those with hydatidiform mole or abortion (50% vs 75%). The greater the number of risk factors, the worse the remission rate.

The Boston group used a modified triple chemotherapy (MAC III: methotrexate with folinic acid, dactinomycin, and cyclophosphamide) in this group of patients and achieved a 67% (34/51) complete response. During the period 1980 to 1985, 18 of 20 patients (90%) were placed into complete remission. All 17 deaths that occurred in this high-risk group had mean prognostic scores (WHO) of 13. Patients with a score of 7 or less achieved complete remission.

Because of low remission rate of poor prognosis metastatic gestational trophoblastic disease (high prognostic index score) compared with nonmetastatic and metastatic good prognosis gestational trophoblastic disease, new drugs and regimens have been used as primary and secondary chemotherapy. The initial excellent reports of the MBP therapy (Bagshawe) or the modified Bagshawe (CHAMOMA) were enthusiastically received, and many investigators suggested CHAMOMA should be the first-line therapy in poor prognosis metastatic disease. Bagshawe reported 75% (32 patients) remission rate in high-risk trophoblastic disease using the CHAMOMA regimen. Wong et al. treated 50 patients (high risk and patients with resistant disease) with CHAMOMA. Forty-one (82%) achieved complete remission. Bagshawe, using the CHAMOMA VP regimen (CHAMOMA alternating with etoposide), reported that 83% (of 12 patients) are in remission. The GOG has recently completed a prospective randomized study comparing MAC with CHAMOMA in poor prognosis metastatic gestational trophoblastic disease. Twenty-two patients received MAC and 20 the modified CHAMOMA. There have been six deaths caused by disease in the CHAMOMA group and none in the MAC-treated patients. Five MAC failures were rescued by surgery and/or chemotherapy; only one of 8 CHAMOMA failures was rescued. Forty-four percent of CHAMOMA patients experienced life-threatening hematological toxicity, compared with only 9% of the MAC patients. MAC appears to be at least as effective as, and less toxic than, the modified Bagshawe (CHAMOMA) regimen.

Etoposide (VP16212) is an effective drug in treating patients with high risk or resistant disease. Wong et al. used oral etoposide to treat 60 patients who developed persistent or metastatic gestational trophoblastic disease.

EMA-CO CHEMOTHERAPY*

Course 1 (EMA)

Day 1   Etoposide, 100 mg/m², IV infusion in 200 ml
        of saline
        Dactinomycin, 0.5 mg, IV stat
        Methotrexate, 100 mg/m², IV stat
                    200 mg/m², IV infusion over
                    12 hours
Day 2   Etoposide, 100 mg/m², IV infusion, in
                    200 ml of saline over 30 minutes
        Dactinomycin, 0.5 mg, IV stat
        Folinic acid, 15 mg, IM or orally every
                    12 hours for 4 doses beginning 24 hours
                    after start of methotrexate

Course 2 (CO)

Day 8   Vincristine, 1.0 mg/m², IV stat
        Cyclophosphamide, 600 mg/m², IV infusion

*This regimen consists of two courses. Course 1 is given on days 1 and 2. Course 2 is given on day 8. These courses can usually be given on days 1 and 2, 8, 15 and 16, 22, etc., and the intervals should not be extended without cause.

Table 7-9   Recurrences in gestational trophoblastic neoplasia

Disease	Recurrences
Nonmetastatic	3/139 (2.1%)
Good prognosis metastatic	3/55 (5.4%)
Poor prognosis metastatic	13/63 (21%)

Based on data from Hammond CB, Weed JC Jr, Currie JL: *Am J Obstet Gynecol* 136:844, 1980.

Table 7-10   Results of treatment (Duke University)

Disease	Remission
Nonmetastatic	139/139 (100%)
Good prognosis metastatic	55/55 (100%)
Poor prognosis metastatic	42/63 (66%)
TOTAL	236/257 (92%)

Modified from Hammond CB, Weed JC Jr, Currie JL: *Am J Obstet Gynecol* 136:844, 1980.

Twelve had metastatic gestational trophoblastic disease. Fifty-nine patients achieved complete response. Three patients developed recurrence.

EMA-CO, a new combination that includes etoposide, dactinomycin, methotrexate with folinic acid, vincristine, and cyclophosphamide (see box above) has also received attention. Newlands treated 56 high-risk patients with 84% long-term survival. An update noted an 80% complete response and 82% survival in 76 high-risk patients who had received no prior chemotherapy. Toxicity was minimal. In 17 patients with prognostic scores greater than 15, Bolis reported a response rate of 86%. Schink and associates reported 83% complete response and 100% survival in 12 patients with high risk disease treated primarily at their institution. The two partial responses and one relapse were successively treated with cisplatin/etoposide with or without bleomycin. Reproductive function was preserved in 9 with 4 pregnancies in 3 patients (2 term, 1 preterm delivery and 1 mole complicated by osmolar trophoblastic tumor.)

Surwit suggests that increasing the dose of etoposide and adding cisplatin to the high-dose methotrexate may produce a better response in high-risk metastatic disease. Using this regimen, four high-risk patients have been placed in remission, one with the prognostic score of 17 who presented with both brain and liver metastases.

Recurrence

Recurrence for all categories of GTN is presented in Table 7-9. In patients with advanced initial disease, there is a greater chance of recurrence, as one would expect. Particularly in good and poor prognosis metastatic GTN, subsequent chemotherapy past the first normal titer is given as a precautionary measure in the hope of decreasing the chance of recurrence. It is of utmost importance that once a patient is placed into remission the follow-up protocol be adhered to strictly. With an aggressive multiple-modality approach developed through extensive experience, 100% of patients with nonmetastatic and good prognosis metastatic trophoblastic disease have been placed into remission. Only two thirds of the patients with poor prognosis metastatic disease have been placed into remission; however, this number has increased over the years: 90% of those treated during the past 3 years are in remission (Table 7-10). The fact that GTN is potentially curable in 100% of the cases must be attributed to the patience, expertise, and ingenuity of the physicians who have developed and who continually evaluate methods for making this the most curable of all gynecologic malignancies.

Surwit et al., using MBP, were able to obtain complete remission in 5 of 6 patients who developed resistance to MAC. In an update of the Duke experience, Weed et al. treated 18 patients with poor prognostic disease (16 with resistance after previous chemotherapy) with MBP. Of the 18, 10 (56%) are alive and have been free of disease for more than 12 months after a negative hCG titer. Jones, using a modified CHAMOMA in which the same drugs as in MBP are used in different sequence with additional vincristine, treated eight patients resistant to triple chemotherapy. All experienced initial response, with one patient in full remission and two alive with disease. Newlands and Bagshawe, using VP16-213 alone or in combination with methotrexate and vincristine or bleomycin, observed six responses and six improvements among 21 resistant patients. Of these patients, 12 are still in treatment, and 3 have died. Six patients are "complete response" at 2 to 22 months. Lurain et al. noted no complete remission or survivals in patients found resistant to first-line drugs. Surgery appears to play an important role in recurrent as well as primary disease. Among 28 women with recurrent disease treated at Duke, 14 underwent a hysterectomy and 10 (83%) survived. These patients were chosen for hysterectomy because there was no evidence of extrauterine disease. This compares to 32 patients treated with primary hysterectomy combined with chemotherapy, and all sustained remission. The Duke group also noted that 4 of 9 patients who had thoracotomy with pulmonary wedge resection of resistant choriocarcinoma survived. It should be noted that resection of pulmonary disease is unnecessary in the majority of patients. Tumor regression as noted on chest x-rays lags behind the hCG response. It may take several months for the disappearance of pulmonary nodules after completion of chemotherapy. Tomoda has proposed guidelines for resection of pulmonary nodules. In essence, solitary pulmonary nodule is present with elevated hCG and no other evidence of disease is present. Fourteen of 15 patients who satisfied these criteria survived after pulmonary resection compared to none of 4 who had other unfavorable clinical findings.

Placental Site Trophoblastic Tumor

This rare tumor has the potential for metastasis and death. Approximately 100 cases have been reported in the literature. It may be found after abortion, mole, or normal pregnancy. Bleeding, the most common symptom, can appear shortly after termination of pregnancy or years later. The bleeding is often accompanied by uterine enlargement and a pregnancy diagnosis is often entertained. A pregnancy test may be positive. Gross uterine findings may vary from a diffuse nodular enlargement of the myometrium, which is usually well circumscribed, to a large polypoid projection into the uterine cavity with involvement of the myometrium. Invasion may extend to the serosa or even with extension to the adnexae. Microscopically, it is difficult to differentiate from benign trophoblastic infiltration. It is characterized by mononuclear infiltration of the uterus and its blood vessels with occasional multinucleated giant cells. The predominant cell is intermediate trophoblast with large polyhedral cells and pleomorphic nuclei. Occasionally, syncytial trophoblast giant cells are present. Mitotic counts have not been a reliable prognostic factor. Placental site trophoblastic tumors must be distinguished from choriocarcinoma and occasionally can be interpreted as sarcomas. Histochemical stains for hPL are usually diffusely positive but only focally positive for hCG. The serum hCG, although elevated enough to give a positive pregnancy test, is often low, even with metastasis, and therefore it is a poor predictor of prognosis. Most of these tumors behave in a benign fashion, although they may act malignant with at least 20 deaths reported, indicating approximately a 15%-20% mortality rate. Metastases have been reported at various sites. Some patients may be cured with a D&C only but hysterectomy is considered optimal therapy and is usually adequate in most situations. Historically, metastatic placental site tumors have not responded to multiple agent chemotherapy; however, there are patients with metastasis to the lung that apparently have been cured with chemotherapy. In most instances, response to chemotherapy is short lived.

BIBLIOGRAPHY

Epidemiology and risk factors

Aziz MF, Kampono N, Moegni EN: Epidemiology of gestational trophoblastic disease at the Doctor Cipto Mangunkusumo Hospital, Jakarta, Indonesia, *Adv Exp Med Biol* 176:165, 1984.

Bagshawe KD: *Choriocarcinoma: the clinical biology of the trophoblast and its tumours*, London, 1969, Edward Arnold.

Bagshawe KD: Risks and prognostic factors in trophoblastic neoplasia, *Cancer* 38:1373, 1976.

Bandy LC, Clarke-Pearson LD, Hammond CB: Malignant potential of gestational trophoblastic disease at the extreme age of reproductive life, *Obstet Gynecol* 64:395, 1984.

Berkowitz RS, Goldstein DP, Bernstein MR: Choriocarcinoma following term pregnancy, *Gynecol Oncol* 17:32, 1984.

Brewer JI, Halpern B, Torok EE: *Gestational trophoblastic disease: selected clinical aspects and chorionic gonadotropin test methods.* In Hickey RG, editor: *Current problems in cancer*, Chicago, 1979, Year Book Medical.

DuBeshter B: High risk factors in metastatic GTD, *J Reprod Med* 36:9013, 1991.

Hertig AT, Sheldon WH: Hydatidiform mole—a pathological clinical correlation of 200 cases, *Am J Obstet Gynecol* 53:1, 1947.

Ho Yuen B, Burch P: Relationship of oral contraceptives and the intrauterine contraceptive devices to the regression of concentrations of the beta-subunit of human chorionic gonadotropins and invasive complications after molar pregnancy, *Am J Obstet Gynecol* 145:214, 1983.

Ho Yuen B, Cannon W: Molar pregnancy in British Columbia: estimated incidence and post evacuation regression pattern of the beta-subunit of human chorionic gonadotropins, *Am J Obstet Gynecol* 139:316, 1981.

Jones WB: Trophoblastic tumors—prognostic factors, *Cancer* 48:602, 1981.

Morrow CP et al: The influence of oral contraceptives on the postmolar human chorionic gonadotropin regression curve, *Am J Obstet Gynecol* 151:906, 1985.

Nisula BC, Taliadours GS: Thyroid function in gestational trophoblastic neoplasia: evidence that the thyrotrophic activity of chorionic gonadotropin mediates the thyrotoxicosis of choriocarcinoma, *Am J Obstet Gynecol* 138:77, 1980.

Sand PK, Hurain JR, Brewer JI: Repeat gestational trophoblastic disease, *Obstet Gynecol* 63:140, 1984.

Stone N et al: Relationship of oral contraception to development of trophoblastic tumor after evacuation of a hydatidiform mole, *Br J Obstet Gynaecol* 83:913, 1976.

World Health Organization Scientific Group: Gestational trophoblastic disease, *WHO Tech Rep Ser* 692:1, 1983.

Moles

Bagshawe KD, Lawler SD, Paradmas FJ et al: Gestational trophoblastic tumours following initial diagnosis of partial hydatidiform mole, *Lancet* 335:1074, 1990.

Berkowitz RS, Cramer DW, Bernstein MR: Risk factors for complete molar pregnancy from a case control study, *Am J Obstet Gynecol* 152:1016, 1985.

Berkowitz RS, Goldstein DP, Bernstein MR: Evolving concepts of molar pregnancy, *J Reprod Med* 36:40, 1991.

Berkowitz RS, Goldstein DP, Bernstein MR: Natural history of partial molar pregnancy, *Obstet Gynecol* 66:677, 1983.

Berkowitz RS, Goldstein DP, Bernstein MR: Reproductive experiences after complete and partial molar pregnancy and gestational trophoblastic tumors, *J Reprod Med* 36:3, 1991.

Berkowitz RS et al: Oral contraceptives and postmolar trophoblastic disease, *Obstet Gynecol* 58:474, 1981.

Curry SL et al: Hydatidiform mole: diagnosis, management, and long-term follow-up of 347 patients, *Obstet Gynecol* 45:1, 1975.

Curry SL, Schlaerth JB, Kohorn EI et al: Hormonal contraception and trophoblastic sequelae after hydatidiform mole, *Am J Obstet Gynecol* 160:805, 1989.

Goldstein DP, Berkowitz RS: Current management of complete and partial molar pregnancy, *J Reprod Med* 39 139-46, 1994.

Palmer JR: Advances in the epidemiology of gestational trophoblastic disease, *J Reprod Med* 39:155-62, 1994.

Rice LW, Berkowitz RS, Lage JM et al: Persistent gestational trophoblastic tumor after partial hydatidiform mole, *Gynecol Oncol* 36:358, 1990.

Soto-Wright V, Bernstein M, Goldstein DP et al: The changing clinical presentation of complete molar pregnancy, *Obstet Gynecol* 86:775-9, 1995.

Szulman AE, Surti U: The syndrome of hydatidiform mole. I. Cytogenetics and morphologic correlation, *Am J Obstet Gynecol* 131:665, 1978.

Szulman AE, Surti U: The syndrome of hydatidiform mole. II. Morphologic evaluation of the complete and partial mole, *Am J Obstet Gynecol* 132:20, 1978.

Szulman AE, Surti U: The clinical pathologic profile of the partial hydatidiform mole, *Obstet Gynecol* 59:597, 1982.

Vassilakos P, Riotton G, Kajii T: Hydatidiform mole: two entities—a morphologic and cytogenetic study with some clinical considerations, *Am J Obstet Gynecol* 127:167, 197.

Prophylactic chemotherapy

Goldstein DP: Five years' experience with the prevention of trophoblastic tumors by the prophylactic use of chemotherapy in patients with molar pregnancy, *Clin Obstet Gynecol* 13:945, 1970.

Kim DS et al: Effects of prophylactic chemotherapy for persistent trophoblastic disease in patients with complete hydatidiform mole, *Obstet Gynecol* 67:690, 1986.

Diagnosis

Bagshawe KD, Lawler SD, Paradmas FJ et al: Gestational trophoblastic tumours following initial diagnosis of partial hydatidiform mole, *Lancet* 335:1074, 1990.

Berkowitz RS, Goldstein DP, Bernstein MR: Evolving concepts of molar pregnancy, *J Reprod Med* 36:40, 1991.

Curry SL, Schlaerth JB, Kohorn EI et al: Hormonal contraception and trophoblastic sequelae after hydatidiform mole, *Am J Obstet Gynecol* 160:805, 1989.

Hunter V, Christensen RE, Olt G et al: Efficacy of the metastatic screening in the staging of gestational trophoblastic disease, *Cancer* 65:1647, 1990.

Rice LW, Berkowitz RS, Lage JM et al: Persistent gestational trophoblastic tumor after partial hydatidiform mole, *Gynecol Oncol* 36:358, 1990.

Romero R et al: New criteria for diagnosis of gestational trophoblastic disease, *Obstet Gynecol* 66:553, 1985.

Soper JT, Evans AC, Conaway MR et al: Evaluation of prognostic factors and staging in gestational trophoblastic tumor, *Obstet Gynecol* 84:969-73, 1994.

Treatment

Ayhan A, Ergeneli MH, Yuce K et al: Pregnancy after chemotherapy for gestational trophoblastic disease, *J Reprod Med* 35:522, 1990.

Azab MB, Pejovic M, Theorose C et al: Prognostic factors in gestational trophoblastic tumors: a multivariant analysis, *Cancer* 62:585, 1988.

Azab TC, Droz JP, Assouline A et al: Treatment of high risk gestational trophoblastic disease with chemotherapy combination containing cisplatin and etoposide, *Cancer* 64:1824, 1989.

Bagshawe KD: Treatment of trophoblastic tumors, *Ann Acad Med* 5:273, 1976.

Bagshawe KD: Treatment of high risk choriocarcinoma, *J Reprod Med* 29:813, 1984.

Bagshawe KD, Wilde CE: Infusion therapy for pelvic trophoblastic tumors, *J Obstet Gynaecol Br Commonw* 71:565, 1964.

Bagshawe KD, Dent J, Newlands ES et al: The role of low dose methotrexate and folic acid in gestational trophoblastic tumors (GII), *Br J Obstet Gynecol* 96:795, 1989.

Bakri YN, Subhi J, Amer M et al: Liver metastasis of gestational trophoblastic tumor, *Gynecol Onc* 48:110-3, 1993.

Berkowitz RS, Goldstein DP, Bernstein MR: Methotrexate with Citrovorum factor rescue as primary therapy for gestational trophoblastic disease, *Cancer* 50:2024, 1982.

Berkowitz RS, Goldstein DP, Bernstein MR: Ten-year experience with methotrexate and folinic acid as primary treatment for gestational trophoblastic disease, *Gynecol Oncol* 23:111, 1986.

Berkowitz RS, Goldstein DP, Bernstein MR: Methotrexate infusion and folinic acid in the primary therapy of non-metastatic gestational trophoblastic tumors, *Gynecol Oncol* 36:56, 1990.

Bolis G, Bonazzi C, Landoni F et al: EMA/CO regime in high risk GTT, *Gynecol Oncol* 31:439, 1988.

Brace KC: The role of irradiation in the treatment of metastatic trophoblastic disease, *Radiology* 91:539, 1968.

Curry S, Blessing J, DiSaia P et al: A prospective randomized comparison of MAC versus modified Bagshawe regimen in poor prognosis gestational trophoblastic disease, *Obstet Gynecol* 73:357, 1989.

DuBeshter B, Berkowitz RS, Goldstein DP: Metastatic gestational trophoblastic disease: experience at the New England Trophoblastic Disease Center, 1965-1985, *Obstet Gynecol* 69:390, 1987.

DuBeshter B, Berkowitz RS, Goldstein DP et al: Management of low risk metastatic gestational trophoblastic tumors, *J Reprod Med* 36:36, 1991.

Finkler NJ, Berkowitz RS, Driscoll SC et al: Clinical experience with placental site trophoblastic tumors at the New England Trophoblastic Disease Center, *Obstet Gynecol* 71:854, 1988.

Goldstein DP et al: Methotrexate with Citrovorum factor rescue for gestational trophoblastic neoplasms, *Obstet Gynecol* 53:93, 1978.

Hammond CB, Lewis JL Jr: *Gestational trophoblastic neoplasms.* In Schirra J, editor: *Davis' gynecology and obstetrics*, vol 1, New York, 1977, Harper & Row.

Hammond CB, Parker RT: Diagnosis and treatment of trophoblastic disease, *Obstet Gynecol* 35:132, 1970.

Hammond CB, Weed JC Jr, Currie JL: The role of operation in the current therapy of gestational trophoblastic disease, *Am J Obstet Gynecol* 135:844, 1980.

Hammond CB et al: Treatment of metastatic trophoblastic disease: good and poor prognosis, *Am J Obstet Gynecol* 115:4, 1973.

Hertz R, Lewis JL Jr, Lipsett MB: Five years' experience with chemotherapy of metastatic choriocarcinoma and related trophoblastic tumors in women, *Am J Obstet Gynecol* 82:631, 1961.

Homesley HD: Development of single-agent chemotherapy regimens for gestational trophoblastic disease, *J Reprod Med* 39:185-92, 1994.

Homesley HD, Blessing JA, Rettenmaier M et al: Weekly intramuscular methotrexate for nonmetastatic gestational trophoblastic disease, *Obstet Gynecol* 72:413, 1988.

Homesley HD, Blessing JA, Schlaerth J et al: Rapid escalation of weekly IM MTX for NMGTD, *Gynecol Oncol* 39:305, 1990.

Kurman RJ, Scully RE, Norris HJ: Trophoblastic pseudotumor of the uterus: an exaggerated form of "syncytial endometritis" simulating a malignant tumor, *Cancer* 38:1214, 1976.

Li M, Hertz R, Spencer DB: Effects of methotrexate therapy upon choriocarcinoma and chorioadenoma, *Proc Soc Exp Biol Med* 93:361, 1956.

Lurain JR, Brewer JI: Treatment of high risk gestational trophoblastic disease with MAC chemotherapy, *Obstet Gynecol* 65:830, 1985.

Lurain JR: High risk metastatic gestational trophoblastic tumors, *J Reprod Med* 39:217-22, 1994.

Lurain JR et al: Fatal gestational trophoblastic disease, an analysis of treatment failures, *Am J Obstet Gynecol* 144:391, 1982.

Lurain JR et al: Gestational trophoblastic disease: treatment results at the Brewer Trophoblastic Disease Center, *Obstet Gynecol* 60:354, 1982.

Maroulis GB et al: Arteriography and infusional chemotherapy in localized trophoblastic disease, *Obstet Gynecol* 45:397, 1975.

McDonald TW, Ruffolo EH: Modern management of gestational trophoblastic disease, *Obstet Gynecol* 38:167, 1983.

Newlands ES, Bagshawe KD, Begent RHJ et al: Development in chemotherapy for medium and high risk patients with GTT, *Br J Obstet Gynaecol* 93:63, 1986.

Newlands ES, Bagshawe KD, Begent RHJ et al: Results with the EMA/CO regime in high risk gestation trophoblastic tumors, *Br J Obstet Gynecol* 98:550, 1991.

Ross GT et al: Sequential use of methotrexate and actinomycin D in the treatment of metastatic choriocarcinoma and related trophoblastic diseases in women, *Am J Obstet Gynecol* 93:223, 1965.

Schink JC, Singh DK, Radmaker AW et al: EMA/CO for the treatment of metastatic, high risk gestational trophoblastic disease, *Obstet Gynecol* 80:817, 1992.

Scully RE, Young RH: Trophoblastic pseudotumor: a reappraisal, *Am J Surg Pathol* 5:75, 1981.

Smith EB et al: Treatment of non-metastatic gestational trophoblastic disease: results of methotrexate alone versus methotrexate-folinic acid, *Am J Obstet Gynecol* 144:88, 1982.

Soper T: Surgical therapy for gestational trophoblastic disease, *J Reprod Med* 39:168-74, 1994.

Sung AC, Wu FC, Wang YB: Reevaluation of 5-FU as a single agent for gestational malignant trophoblastic disease, *Adv Exp Med Biol* 176:355, 1984.

Surwit EA, Childey JM: High risk metastatic GTD, *J Reprod Med* 39:45, 1991.

Tomoda Y, Arii Y, Kaseki S et al: Surgical indications for resection in pulmonary metastasis of choriocarcinoma, *Cancer* 46:2723, 1980.

Twiggs LB, Hatch K, Petrilli ES: A chemotherapeutic trial of bactinomycin with pulse fashion scheduling in the treatment of nonmetastatic trophoblastic disease, *Gynecol Oncol* (abstracts), Feb, 1986.

Vaitukaitis JB, Braunstein GD, Ross GT: A radioimmunoassay which specifically measures human chorionic gonadotrophin in the presence of human luteinizing hormone, *Am J Obstet Gynecol* 113:751, 1972.

Weed JC Jr et al: Chemotherapy with the modified Bagshawe protocol for poor prognosis metastatic trophoblastic disease, *Obstet Gynecol* 59:377, 1982.

Wong LC, Choo YC, Ma HK: Methotrexate with Citrovorum rescue in gestational trophoblastic disease, *Am J Obstet Gynecol* 152:59, 1985.

Wong LC, Choo YC, Ma HK: Primary oral etoposide therapy in gestational trophoblastic disease: an update, *Cancer* 58:14, 198

Posttreatment pregnancy

Goldstein DP, Berkowtiz RS, Bernstein MR: Reproduction performance after molar pregnancy in gestational trophoblastic tumors, *Clin Obstet Gynecol* 27:221, 1984.

Miller JM Jr, Surwit EA, Hammond CB: Choriocarcinoma following term pregnancy, *Obstet Gynecol* 53:207, 1979.

Rustin GJ et al: Pregnancy after cytotoxic chemotherapy for gestational trophoblastic tumours, *Br Med J Clin Res* 288:103, 1984.

Placental site tumors

Finkler NJ, Berkowitz RS, Driscoll S et al: Clinical experience with placental site trophoblastic tumors at the New England Trophoblastic Disease Center, *Obstet Gynecol* 71:854-7, 1988.

Kurman RJ (ed) in *Blaustein's Pathology of the Female Genital Tract*, Springer-Verlag, New York, 1994, 1074-78.

Kuman RJ, Scully RE, Norris HJ: Trophoblastic pseudotumor of the uterus, *Cancer* 38, 1214-25, 1988.

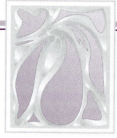

Invasive Cancer of the Vulva

In the 1994 FIGO annual report, cancer of the vulva has accounted for 5% of all female genital malignancies. During recent years, it appears that this incidence has been increasing. Green reported that in his experience carcinoma of the vulva accounted for 5% of all gynecologic malignancies seen from 1927 through 1961, but in the next 12 years it increased to 8%. He believed that this increase in incidence was a result of the continued rise in the average age of the female population in later years, causing an increase in the number at risk to develop the disease. Vulvar cancer, with the exception of the rare sarcomas, appears most frequently in women between 65 and 75 years old (Figure 8-1), and in some series almost half are 70 years of age or older. On the other hand, vulvar cancers can also appear in young patients; Rutledge et al. at the MD Anderson Hospital and Tumor Institute noted that about 15% of all vulvar cancers occur in women younger than 40 years. Many of these younger patients have microcarcinomas associated with diffuse intraepithelial neoplasia of the vulva skin.

Choo found 17 patients younger than 35 years of age with invasive carcinoma of the vulva. Of these, 8 had microinvasion. Many of the associated features seen in patients with vulvar cancer, such as diabetes, obesity, hypertension, and arteriosclerosis, may just reflect the increased incidence of these diseases as one gets older.

Over the years, the possible association of vulvar carcinoma and venereal or granulomatous lesions of the vulva has been noted. The incidence tends to be greater in the older literature and much less in more recent reports, probably reflecting to a certain degree a lower incidence of syphilis. The association of condyloma acuminatum with vulvar carcinoma is well known, but no cause-and-effect relationship has been confirmed as yet. The HPV virus is suspect in the etiology of squamous neoplasia of the vulva, as it is in similar lesions of the cervix.

INVASIVE SQUAMOUS CELL CARCINOMA
Histology

The overwhelming majority of all vulvar cancer is squamous in origin. The vulva is covered with skin, and any malignancy that appears elsewhere on the skin can occur in this region. Table 8-1 depicts the incidence of vulvar neoplasia from several collected studies in the literature. Our discussion will focus mainly on squamous cell carcinoma because of its preponderance, but as a generalization, the other lesions can also be treated similarly, except where noted.

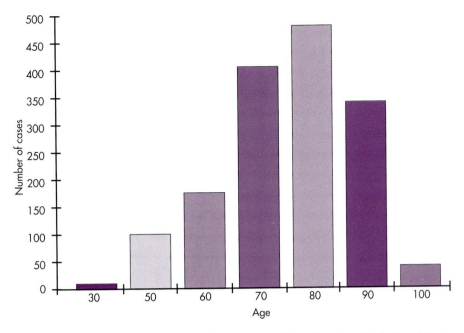

Figure 8-1 Invasive squamous epithelial cell carcinoma of the vulva. Age distribution. (From *Annual Report Gynecological Cancer FIGO*, vol. 22, 1994.)

Table 8-1 Incidence of vulvar neoplasms by histologic type*

Tumor type	Percent
Epidermoid	86.2
Melanoma	4.8
Sarcoma	2.2
Basal cell	1.4
Bartholin gland	
Squamous	0.4 ⎫ 1.2
Adenocarcinoma	0.6 ⎭
Adenocarcinoma	0.6
Undifferentiated	3.9

Modified from Plentl AA, Friedman EA: *Lymphatic system of the female genitalia*, Philadelphia, 1971, WB Saunders.
*Based on 1378 reported cases.

Clinical Profile

The development of squamous cell carcinoma of the vulva may be similar to the process that occurs on the cervix. However, no race or culture is spared, and gravidity and parity are not involved in the pathogenesis of this neoplasm. Actually, vulvar cancer is common in the poor and elderly in most parts of the world, and this has led to the hypothesis that inadequate personal hygiene and medical care are often contributing factors in this disease. In truth, the cause of cancer of the vulva is unknown—few data support the concept that these neoplasms often develop from vulvar dystrophies (Figure 8-2). In many cases the initial lesion appears to arise from

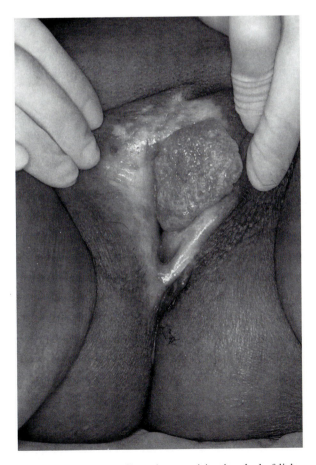

Figure 8-2 Squamous cell carcinoma arising in a bed of lichen sclerosis.

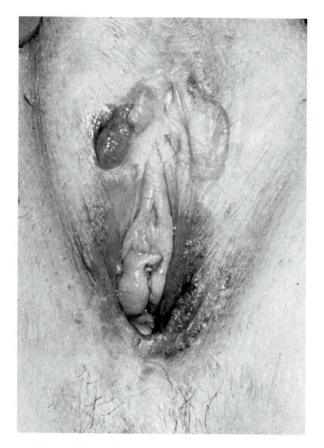

Figure 8-3 Small, well-localized lesion of the vulva.

Table 8-2	Signs and symptoms of vulvar cancer
Signs and symptoms	Percent
Pruritus	45.0
Mass	45.0
Pain	23.0
Bleeding	14.0
Ulceration	14.0
Dysuria	10.0
Discharge	8.0
Groin mass	2.5

Table 8-3   Indications for excisional biopsy of vulva nevi

Change in surface area of nevus
Change in elevation of a lesion—raised, thickened, or nodular
Change in color—especially brown to black
Change in surface—smooth to scaly or ulcerated
Change in sensation—itching or tingling

an area of intraepithelial neoplasia that subsequently develops into a small nodule that may break down and ulcerate (Figure 8-3). On other occasions, small, warty or cauliflower-like growths evolve, and these may be confused with condyloma acuminatum. Long-term pruritus or a lump or mass on the vulva is present in more than 50% of patients with invasive vulvar cancer (Table 8-2). In most reported series of carcinoma of the vulva there is (1) delay in treatment of the patient who has symptoms for 2 to 16 months before seeking medical attention; and/or (2) medical treatment of vulvar lesions for up to 12 months or longer without biopsy for definitive diagnosis or referral.

Fortunately, vulvar cancer is commonly indolent, extends slowly, and metastasizes fairly late. Hence we have a good opportunity for preventing the serious advanced stages of this disease through education of patients and physicians. Lawhead has proposed a technique for routine vulvar self-examination and urges that this practice be incorporated into every woman's preventive health care regimen. Biopsy *must* be done on all suspicious lesions of the vulva, including lumps, ulcers, or pigmented areas, even in the patient not complaining of burning or itching (Table 8-3). Our own group has looked at the clinical and histological features of vulvar carcinomas analyzed for HPV status. Of 21 invasive

carcinomas of the vulva analyzed, 10 were found to contain HPV 16 DNA. Others have confirmed this observation, suggesting that HPV-DNA associations with malignancy of the vulva are similar to those observed elsewhere in the genital tract. The correlation is not as strong as in VIN. Anderson among others noted a variable detection rate of HPV nucleic acids in vulvar cancer. Only 13% of the invasive lesions contained HPV when analyzed by in situ hybridization.

A rare variant of epidermoid carcinoma with distinct clinical and pathological features is known as verrucous carcinoma (Figure 8-4). Its lesions, which may involve the cervix and vagina as well as the vulva, present as a warty, fungating, ulcerated mass with a bulky, elevated appearance reminiscent of benign HPV lesions. Identification of this variant is important because the biologic behavior of the disease greatly influences therapy.

Distinction from ordinary condylomata is aided by the absence of fibrovascular cores within the proliferating papillary masses of tumor. Surgical excision is the foundation of therapy, with lymphadenectomy of questionable value except where nodes are obviously involved. Radiotherapy is contraindicated because of its ineffectiveness and reports indicate that it can be an instigator of more aggressive behavior by this tumor.

Location and Spread Pattern

Primary disease can appear anywhere on the vulva. Approximately 70% arise primarily on the labia. Disease more commonly occurs in the labium majora; however, it

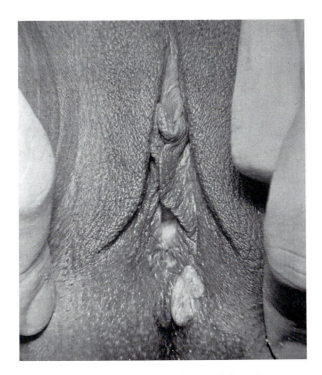

Figure 8-4 Verrucous carcinoma of the vulva.

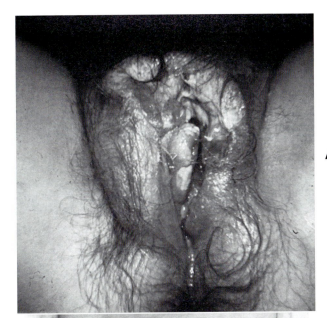

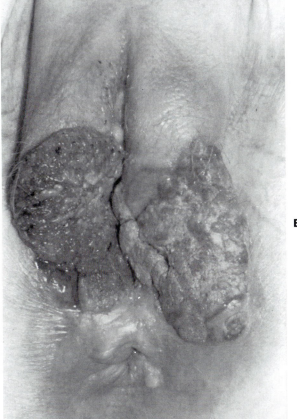

Figure 8-5 A, Large ulcerating squamous cell malignancy of the vulva with destruction of the clitoris and the urethra. **B,** Large exophytic squamous cell carcinoma of the vulva.

may appear on the labium minora, clitoris, and perineum. The disease is usually localized and well demarcated, although occasionally it can be so extensive that the primary location cannot be determined (Figure 8-5, *A* and *B*). Multifocal growth pattern in invasive squamous cell carcinoma of the vulva is uncommon, except for the so-called kissing lesions that can occur as isolated lesions, usually on the upper labia.

Fundamental to the understanding of therapy for invasive cancer of the vulva is thorough knowledge of the lymphatic drainage of this organ. In general, the four histologic types of invasive cancer behave similarly and use primarily the lymphatic route for initial metastases (Figure 8-6).

Lymphatic drainage of the external genitalia begins with minute papillae, and these are connected in turn to a multilayered meshwork of fine vessels. These fine vessels extend over the entire labium minora, the prepuce of the clitoris, the fourchette, and the vaginal mucosa up to the level of the hymenal ring (Figure 8-7). Drainage of these lymphatics extends toward the anterior portion of the labium minora, where they emerge into three or four collecting trunks whose course is toward the mons veneris, bypassing the clitoris. Vessels from the prepuce anastomose with these lymphatics. Similarly, vessels from the labium majora proceed anteriorly to the upper part of the vulva and mons veneris, there joining the vessels of the prepuce and labium minora. These lymphatic vessels abruptly change direction, turning laterally, and terminate in ipsilateral or contralateral femoral nodes. Drainage is usually limited initially to the

medial upper quadrant of the femoral node group. The nodes are located medial to the great saphenous vein above the cribriform fascia and in turn may drain secondarily through the cribriform fascia to the deep femoral group.

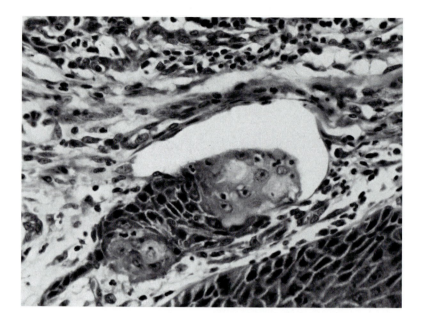

Figure 8-6 Photomicrograph of a tumor nodule invading a vulvar lymphatic.

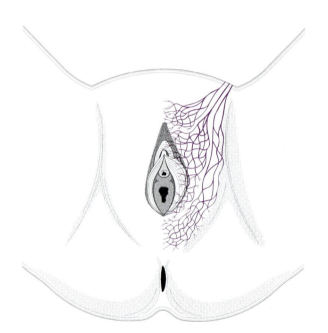

Figure 8-7 Lymphatic drainage of the external genitalia.

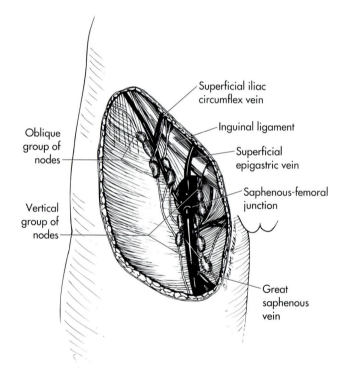

Figure 8-8 The superficial inguinal lymph nodes can be divided into the horizontal group and the perpendicular group.

The superficial inguinal lymph glands, located immediately beneath the integument and Camper fascia, are large and from eight to ten in number. Most authors agree that the superficial inguinal lymph glands are the primary nodal group for the vulva and can serve as the sentinel lymph nodes of the vulva (Figure 8-8). The deep femoral nodes, which are by classic teaching located beneath the cribriform fascia, are the secondary nodal recipients and are involved before drainage into the deep pelvic nodes occurs. The Cloquet node, the last node of the deep femoral group, is located just beneath the Poupart ligament. The multilayered meshwork of lymphatics on the vulva itself is always limited to an area medial to the

genitocrural fold (Figure 8-9). Lymphatic drainage of the vulva is a very progressive systematic mechanism, and therapy can be planned depending on where in the lymphatic chain tumor is present.

Borgno and colleagues examined 100 inguinal lymphadenectomy specimens at autopsy and demonstrated that the deep femoral nodes are always situated within the openings in the fascia at the fossa ovalis, and no lymph nodes are distal to the lower margin of the fossa ovalis,

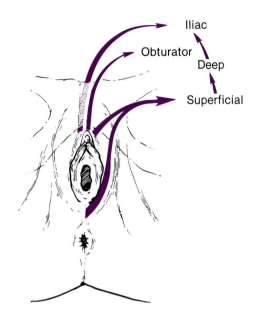

Figure 8-9 Lymphatic spread of vulvar malignancy. See text for details.

under the fascia cribrosa. The implication is that a carefully done deep femoral lymphadenectomy does not require removal of the fascia lata (cribriform fascia), since *no* lymph nodes were found between the femoral vein and artery lateral to the artery and distal to the lower margin of the fossa ovalis beneath the cribriform fascia. They also found that the node of Cloquet or Rosenmüller, which is the uppermost node among the deep femoral lymph nodes, was absent in 54% of the specimens dissected. Their observations have been confirmed by our own experience. When during surgery, traction is persistently applied to the lymphovascular/fat tissue above the cribriform fascia, all inguinal nodes can be removed. No

nodal tissue was found in our patients where the cribriform fascia and the fat beneath were submitted separately for pathological review.

Although lymphatics from the clitoris directly to the deep pelvic lymph nodes are described, their clinical significance appears to be minimal. It is unusual to find a case in which metastasis is present in the pelvic lymph nodes without metastatic disease in the inguinal lymph nodes, even when the clitoris is involved. Curry et al. noted 58 patients with clitoral involvement of 191 studied; none had positive deep pelvic nodes without involvement of inguinal nodes also. Similar results were observed by Ericksson in a study of 38 patients with carcinomas of the clitoris. Ericksson found also that the deep inguinal or femoral nodes were never positive in the absence of positive superficial inguinal nodes.

The incidence of positive inguinal and pelvic nodes varies considerably, as noted in Table 8-4. Unfortunately, most of these studies were unstaged, although, in general, the larger the tumor, the greater the propensity for inguinal and pelvic node metastases (Table 8-5). Morley noted a 20.7% incidence of lymph node involvement if there was a T1 lesion (less than 2 cm in diameter). In T2 lesions (greater than 2 cm but limited to the vulva), the incidence of lymph node involvement more than doubled to 44.8%. Malfetano reported the incidence of inguinal node metastases in patients with stages III and IV lesions to be 53% and 90%, respectively.

An exception to vulvar cancer is verrucous carcinoma of the vulva. This is a special and unusual variant of squamous cell carcinoma that is locally invasive but nonmetastasizing. Microscopically, a condyloma may be initially diagnosed. There is usually a uniform lack of malignant features histologically. Adequate material, including underlined stroma for pathologic evaluation, is

Table 8-4   Incidence of positive nodes

Series	Number of cases	Positive groin or pelvic nodes (%)	Positive pelvic nodes (%)
Taussig (1938)	65	46.2	7.7
Cherry and Glucksman (1955)	95	44.2	—
Green et al. (1958)	238	58.8	—
Stening and Elliot (1959)	50	40.0	12.0
Way (1960)	143	42.0	16.1
Macafee (1962)	82	40.2	—
Collins et al. (1963)	71	31.0	8.5
Rutledge, Smith, and Franklin (1970)	101	47.6	11.1
Faukbeudal (1973)	55	22.0	—
Morley (1976)	374	37.0	—
Krupp and Bahm (1978)	195	21.0	4.6
Curry, Wharton, and Rutledge (1980)	191	30.0	4.7
Simonsen (1984)	122	50.0	10.0
Sutton (1991)	150	24.0	—
Homesley (1992)	277	29.2	—

Table 8-5 Groin node metastasis for each tumor diameter

Tumor diameter (cm)	N	Positive groin nodes (%)
<1.0	61	18.0
1.1-2.0	129	19.4
2.1-3.0	175	31.4
3.1-4.0	81	54.3
4.1-5.0	48	39.6
>5.0	85	51.8
TOTAL	579	34.2

A GOG study: Homesley, HD: Gyn Oncol, 49:279, 1993.

necessary to differentiate verrucous carcinoma from the condyloma. The tumor may invade deeply into the underlying tissue, often requiring extensive surgery, and has a propensity to recur locally. Woodruff noted a lack of lymph node metastases in 27 patients (literature and his patients) who were treated with radical vulvectomy and inguinal lymphadenectomy. As a result, he advocates a more conservative approach, with wide excision and tumor-free margins as the therapeutic aim.

Staging

Many staging systems have been applied to invasive cancer of the vulva. In 1988 the current International Federation of Gynecology and Obstetrics (FIGO) staging system (Table 8-6), based on the TNM classification, was adopted for international use. The old system of clinical staging was unfortunately contingent on the ability of the clinician to assess node involvement by palpation. The new staging system is based on surgical findings.

There appears to be a large discrepancy between clinical and surgical-pathologic evaluation of lymph node status. This has been documented in a study by Iversen with 258 patients seen at the Norwegian Radium Hospital. Overdiagnosis (clinically suspicious but negative pathologically) was seen in 40 of 258 patients (15%). Of the 100 patients with metastasis to the inguinal lymph nodes, 36 did not have clinically suspicious nodes. Patients with "micrometastasis" (clinically nonsuspicious but microscopically positive nodes) had a significantly better survival rate than those with gross metastasis. As a result of these repeated findings, it was suggested that staging be based on surgical-pathologic evaluation instead of clinical basis alone. FIGO agreed, and a new staging has been in place since 1988. In 1995, FIGO instituted a subclassification of stage I (Table 8-6). The reader must remain aware that many reports in the literature used the old staging system, where data were compiled on cases treated before 1988, and must consider this when analyzing these publications.

Donaldson et al. thoroughly evaluated the prognostic parameters in 66 patients with squamous cell carcinomas of the vulva. The size of the lesion dictated incidence of lymph node metastasis (19% metastasis if lesion was less than 3 cm and 72% if greater than 3 cm). Likewise, grade of tumor correlated with nodal metastasis (one third of well-differentiated tumors had metastasis, compared with 75% of the poorly differentiated lesions). Of 38 patients, 11 (29%) had nodal involvement if invasion of the primary lesion was 5 mm or less, compared with 17 of 28 (61%) if invasion was greater than 5 mm. If tumor did not involve lymphatic or vascular spaces, only 2 of 33 (6%) had positive nodes, whereas 26 of 33 patients (79%) with lymphatic or vascular space involvement had metastasis to the regional lymph nodes. None of 25 patients with lesions invading less than 5 mm and without lymphatic or vascular space involvement had lymph node metastasis. Iversen et al., reporting on 117 patients with stage I cancer, noted the same prognostic factors, confirming earlier reports. From these data and from other reports by Boyce, Andersen, and Shimm, it appears that conservative therapy may be applied on an individual basis with minimal risk to patients.

Management

Since Way reported an improved survival rate in carcinoma of the vulva by using the en bloc dissection of radical vulvectomy plus inguinal and pelvic lymphadenectomy, this has become the mainstay of treatment in vulvar cancer. With this therapy, the corrected 5-year survival rate for stages I and II disease has been reported by many authors to be approximately 90%.

For many years a deep pelvic lymphadenectomy was routinely performed with the radical vulvectomy and inguinal lymphadenectomy irrespective of the size of the vulvar lesion or the presence or lack of disease in the inguinal lymph nodes. Most surgeons now limit the initial procedure to radical vulvectomy and bilateral inguinal lymphadenectomy and do not proceed with pelvic node therapy unless metastasis is demonstrated in the inguinal node area. If the presence of tumor is documented in the inguinal nodes, a pelvic lymphadenectomy is an option for therapy, on the involved side only. This philosophy is a result of the observation that the deep pelvic nodes are essentially never involved with metastatic disease when the more superficial inguinal nodes are uninvolved. A study by Curry et al. of the MD Anderson Hospital showed that in 191 patients only 9 (4.7%) had positive deep pelvic nodes, and all 9 patients also had metastatic disease in the groin nodes. There is a definitive increase in morbidity from pelvic node dissection in conjunction with inguinal node dissection; thus, there is a valid reluctance to perform pelvic lymphadenectomy unless necessary. In most patients the surgeons will elect to treat the pelvic nodes with radiation therapy rather than extend the operative procedure and incur the additional morbid-

Table 8-6   FIGO staging of invasive cancer of the vulva

Stage 0

Tis   Carcinoma in situ, intraepithelial carcinoma

Stage I

T1   N0   M0   Tumor confined to the vulva and/or perineum—2 cm or less in greatest dimension (no nodal metastasis)

                     Stage Ia   Lesions 2 cm or less in size confined to the vulva or perineum and with stromal invasion no greater than 1.0 mm* (no nodal metastasis)

                     Stage Ib   Lesions 2 cm or less in size confined to the vulva or perineum and with stromal invasion greater than 1.0 mm (no nodal metastasis)

Stage II

T2   N0   M0   Tumor confined to the vulva and/or perineum—more than 2 cm in greatest dimension (no nodal metastasis)

Stage III   Tumor any size with

T3   N0   M0   (1) Adjacent spread to the lower urethra and/or the vagina, or the anus, and/or

T3   N1   M0   (2) Unilateral regional lymph node metastasis

T1   N1   M0

T2   N1   M0

Stage IVa

T1   N2   M0   Tumor invades any of the following: Upper urethra, bladder, mucosa, rectal mucosa, pelvic bone, and/or bilateral regional node metastasis

T2   N2   M0

T3   N2   M0

T4   Any   N   M0

Stage IVb Any T Any N M1   Any distant metastasis including pelvic lymph nodes

*The depth of invasion is defined as the measurement of the tumor from the epithelial-stromal junction of the adjacent most superficial dermal papilla to the deepest point of invasion.

ity. The pelvic nodes are positive approximately 25% of the time when the inguinal nodes have documented metastatic disease. In turn, approximately 20% of the patients with positive pelvic nodes will survive 5 years or more. Thus if all patients with positive inguinal nodes underwent pelvic lymphadenectomy, the procedure would result in approximately a 5% salvage rate for that group of patients. This type of statistical reasoning has encouraged many individuals to use radiation therapy when the deep pelvic nodes are at risk, especially in the elderly or medically infirm patient. It is not known whether similar statistics are true for patients who receive radiation therapy to the deep nodes instead of lymphadenectomy.

Unilateral lesions (defined as 1 cm or more from the midline) presents another possible variation for therapy. Homesley presented the GOG experience with such lesions (Table 8-7) and confirmed the low incidence of contralateral node involvement, making ipsilateral inguinal lymphadenectomy a rational initial approach.

The Gynecologic Oncology Group (GOG) did a

Table 8-7   Unilateral lesions—percentage of positive groin nodes by tumor thickness

Tumor thickness (mm)	Ipsilateral positive only	Contralateral positive only	Bilateral positive	Total	N
≤2	6.8	0.0	0.0	6.8	59
3-5	20.4	1.9	2.8	25.0	108
6-10	28.8	3.8	11.3	43.8	80
≥11	36.7	6.7	6.7	50.0	30
TOTAL	21.7	2.5	5.1	29.2	277

A GOG study: Homesley HD: *Gyn Oncol* 49:279, 1993.

prospective randomized study in patients with vulvar carcinoma who had more than one positive groin node. Of 114 patients with surgical findings of more than one positive inguinal node, as additional therapy one group was treated with radiotherapy and the other group was treated with pelvic node dissection. In 1986, the GOG

(Homesley) reported that the former group had a 68% relative 2-year survival rate and the latter group had a 54% relative 2-year survival rate. The authors now prefer to recommend pelvic lymph node irradiation therapy (Figure 8-10) for patients with positive inguinal nodes.

Combined radiation therapy and surgery, as well as radiation alone and local surgery alone, have been applied to this disease. No adequate prospective studies comparing various therapies or combinations of such are available for analysis. The older literature notes superior results with radical vulvectomy and lymphadenectomy as compared with radiation therapy alone or surgery plus radiation therapy. It was also noted that patients who had vulvectomy alone did worse than patients in whom lymphadenectomy was also included.

Daly and Million advocated radical vulvectomy combined with elective node irradiation from stages I and II squamous cell carcinoma of the vulva. In a small number of patients, they found that this treatment combination was well tolerated with no node failures, no irradiation complications, no delay in healing of the surgical site, and an average hospitalization of 13 days. The dose to the inguinal nodes was between 5000 and 5500 cGy, and the midplane pelvic dose was between 4500 and 5000 cGy. Although this is an interesting approach, the small number of patients treated to date does not prove that elective node irradiation will eliminate subclinical node

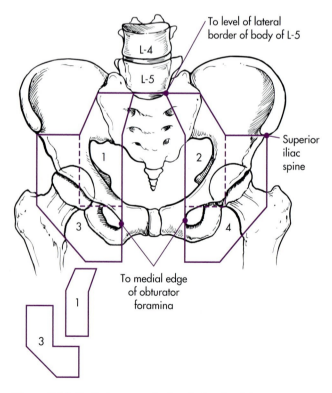

Figure 8-10 Radiation ports for inguinal and pelvic treatment. 1, 2 = anteroposterior pelvic and inguinal port; 3, 4 = anterior boost, or "wing." (From Prolog: *Gynecologic oncology and surgery,* ed 2, The American College of Obstetricians and Gynecologists, 1991, p 51.)

disease from vulvar carcinoma. Since the incidence of inguinal node involvement in stages I and II disease is about 20% to 40%, it will take a reasonably large series of patients followed for a significant time to establish the validity of Daly and Million's hypothesis.

Boronow also emphasized the possible role of irradiation therapy in vulvar vaginal cancers. His report dealt mostly with advanced disease involving vaginal mucous membrane, necessitating an exenterative procedure if a primary surgical approach was used. As an alternative, he recommends surgical extirpation of the lymph nodes with a combination of external and interstitial radiation for control of the central lesion. In a small, highly individualized series, this approach appeared promising. Similar reports by Fairey and Hacker substantiated this initial work by Boronow. Others suggested the use of radiation therapy concomitant with chemotherapy prior to surgery to provide optimum reduction in the size of the central lesion. Radiotherapy has not hitherto been widely used for vulvar cancer because of the technical difficulties associated with directing external beam to this area and the very sensitive moist vulvar skin and mucous membrane, which tolerate irradiation poorly. Low anterior and posterior fields must be used, resulting in intense exposure of the vulvar skin because the axis of the x-ray beam runs parallel (and often within) to the skin and mucous membrane. Vulvitis results, and interruption of therapy is often necessary because of patient discomfort. Similarly, radiation therapy to enlarged, obviously positive inguinal nodes becomes technically difficult, and removal of at least the enlarged nodes, with subsequent x-ray therapy to the area, has been our preference. Preoperative doses of 4500 to 5000 cGy to either groin or vulvar areas produce a hazardous situation for any subsequent surgical approach.

Russell reported on 25 women with locoregionally advanced squamous cancer of the vulva. Eighteen patients were previously untreated and all patients received external beam radiation and synchronous radio potentiating chemotherapy. Complete clinical response was obtained in 16 of 18 previously untreated patients and in 4 of 7 patients with recurrent disease.

It has been suggested that in selected stage IV carcinomas of the vulva, ultraradical surgery may be applicable. Cavanagh and Shepherd, in a review of their data and the literature, identified 53 patients since 1973 who were treated with exenteration and radical vulvectomy and were eligible for a 5-year follow-up. Most of the patients were young, and 47% were alive without recurrence. In their series Cavanagh and Shepherd found all survivors to have negative pelvic lymph nodes.

Technique of radical vulvectomy

We often employ a single arching skin incision parallel to and 2 cm below the inguinal ligament. An effort should be made to spare the fat pad on the mons pubis, especially if the cancer is located posteriorly. This facilitates closure of the vulvectomy defect and provides a fat cushion over the body of the pubic bone (Figure 8-11, *A*). The skin incision can be tailored (Figure 8-11, *B*) to remove a larger amount of skin in the inguinal region if large fixed lymph nodes are found. Another possibility is to limit the skin incision to the inguinal area, especially for small posterior lesions, and thereby preserve the bridge of skin between the inguinal and vulvar incisions ("3 incision technique" Figure 8-12). All tissue is removed from the inguinal and femoral lymph node bundles and immediately sent for

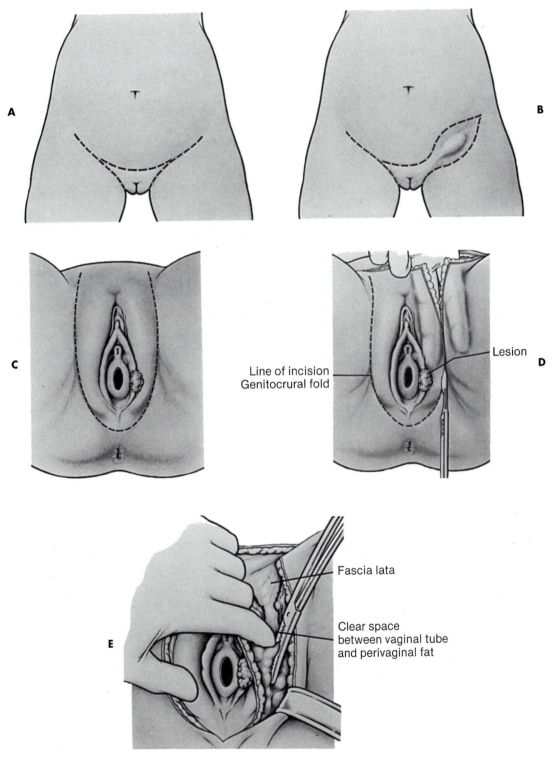

Figure 8-11 A, Groin incision for moderate size lesions. **B,** Groin incision for a patient with a matted left inguinal node. **C** and **D,** Vulvar incision along genitocrural fold. **E,** Clamping the perivaginal tissue.   *Continued.*

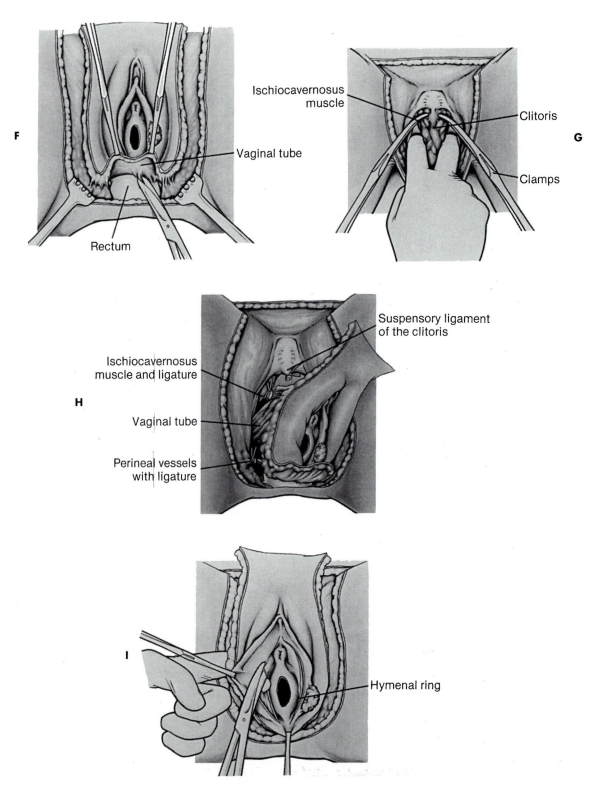

Figure 8-11, cont'd F, Vagina being separated from the rectum. **G,** Clamping the ischiocaverno-sus muscle and crura of the clitoris. **H,** Molulized specimen is prepared for excision. **I,** Exci-sion along the inner margin of the specimen.

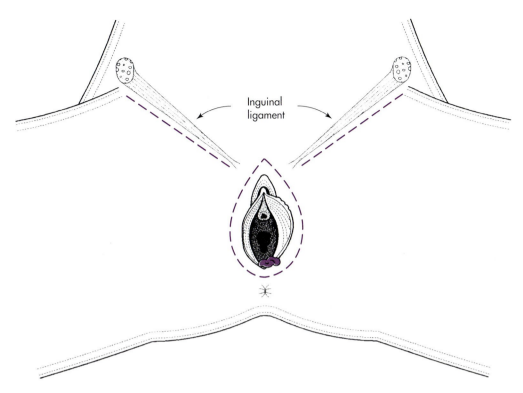

Figure 8-12 Three incision technique for vulvar cancer.

frozen section analysis. If metastatic disease is found, a retroperitoneal pelvic lymphadenectomy can be performed on the involved side as an alternative to the more widely utilized whole-pelvis radiation after surgery. This procedure is done through the same inguinal skin incision by incising the fascia of the anterior abdominal muscles 1 cm above the inguinal ligament. The pelvic parietal peritoneum is then dislocated by means of blunt dissection, and a standard lymphadenectomy is done. The sartorius muscle is removed from its insertion on the anterior iliac spine and sutured to the inguinal ligament to completely cover the femoral nerve, artery, and vein in the femoral triangle. Closed-system suction drains are then placed in the groin dissection and in the pelvic retroperitoneum, and the skin incision is closed by means of a running polyglycolic acid (PGA) suture. Attention is then turned toward the vulvectomy itself. The line of incision extends anteriorly from the previously developed inguinal incision, laterally to the genitocrural fold, and posteriorly midway between the anus and posterior fourchette (Figure 8-11, *C*). A bloodless space can be dissected between vulvar fat and the subcutaneous tissue of the thigh, using a finger dissection (Figure 8-11, *D*). Peon clamps are then serially placed on the perivaginal fat. The tissue is transected and ligated with 0 chromic catgut at the level of the fascia of the thigh (Figure 8-11, *E*). The posterior dissection is performed sharply (Figure 8-11, *F*). Special attention is directed toward the location of the anus and rectum. It is sometimes helpful for the operator to place a finger in the rectum to ascertain its location and

avoid damage during this part of the procedure. The clitoris is then isolated and its suspensory ligament clamped, divided, and suture-ligated at its inferior attachment to the pubic bone. It is often helpful at this point to attempt to isolate the ischiocavernosus muscle and divide this structure as laterally as possible (Figure 8-11, *G*). The pudendal artery and vein are ligated bilaterally (Figure 8-11, *H*). At this point of the procedure, only the vagina remains attached to the vulva. A decision about the amount of vagina to be removed should be relative to the location and size of cancer and based on a knowledge of the lymphatic drainage of the vulva. For small unilateral lesions, removal of a wide margin of contralateral vagina can be avoided (Figure 8-11, *I*). Every effort should be made to avoid resection of the urethra unless it is close to the cancer. If indicated, the distal 1 to 2 cm of this organ can be removed without damage to the functional sphincter. The perineal defect is closed primarily with mattress sutures of 0 PGA laterally and posteriorly. Tension on this closure can be prevented, if necessary, by sharp and blunt mobilization of the vaginal barrel and/or subcutaneous tissue of the thigh. The most anterior extent of the dissection is not sutured primarily; it is allowed to granulate secondarily. This prevents distortion of the urethra and alteration of the urinary stream.

Patients are given a broad-spectrum cephalosporin for 1 week after surgery. Bed rest is maintained for 2 to 3 days, and constipating agents are given for up to 1 week, depending on the degree of perianal dissection. Vigorous local cleansing of the perineal and groin incisions is continued until these incisions are completely healed.

Operative Morbidity and Mortality for Radical Vulvectomy and Bilateral Inguinal Lymphadenectomy

In the early series of Way, operative mortality approached 20%. In the last two decades, this has been reduced to 1% or 2%. Frequently this procedure is carried out in the ninth and tenth decades of life with surprising safety.

The complication encountered most frequently is wound breakdown, which occurs in well over 50% of patients in most series. This aspect of the morbidity is usually limited to skin loss at the margin of the groin incision. Podratz et al. at the Mayo Clinic noted impaired primary wound healing in 148 of 175 patients (85%) who were treated with radical vulvectomy and inguinal lymphadenectomy. Removing lesser amounts of skin and decreasing the undermining of the skin flaps have reduced the incidence of wound breakdown. Suction drainage has also added to this decreasing morbidity. Careful debridement and vigorous care to keep the wounds clean and dry almost always result in adequate healing.

Lymphedema of the lower extremities is another major problem, especially in patients who have had inguinal and deep pelvic node dissection (Figure 8-13). In the study reported by Podratz et al., varying degrees of lymphedema of the lower extremities occurred in 69% of their patients. The incidence of this debilitating long-term complication can be reduced by routine use of custom-made plastic support hose during the first postoperative year while collateral pathways of lymph drainage are being developed. Rutledge has for many years advised that post lymphadenectomy patients also receive low-dose prophylactic antibiotic therapy (similar to that used to prevent subacute bacterial endocarditis) to prevent streptococcal lymphangitis in the lower extremities, which dramatically increases the incidence of lymphedema. Established lymphedema can be kept under control in many patients with routine use of pneumatic-hose devices that have become widely available.

The development of a lymphocyst in the groin area is an infrequent occurrence, and it usually resolves spontaneously. The incidence can be reduced by careful ligation of all the lymph-bearing tissue during the groin dissection. Occasionally, intermittent aseptic aspiration of the fluid facilitates resolution of these collections.

The use of radiation therapy as apriori treatment (especially in patients with fixed inguinal nodes) can result in significant vulva edema. This is specially true when low fields are used to include vulvar disease. Figure 8-14 illustrates severe edema in a patient treated primarily with radiation therapy. Necrosis is seen at 5:00 o'clock,

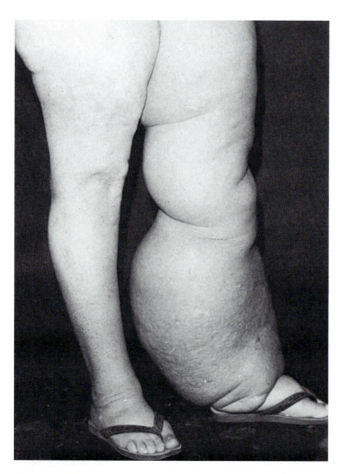

Figure 8-13 Marked lymphedema of left leg after inguinal and pelvic lymphadenectomy.

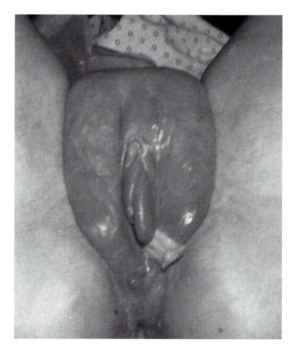

Figure 8-14 Severe edema of the vulva following radiation therapy with necrosis at the site of the primary lesion.

which is residual from the large lesion occupying that area prior to radiation.

Symptoms related to stress incontinence and the development of cystocele or rectocele are sometimes reported by these patients. These conditions are secondary to the loss of the support of the lower end of the vagina and subsequent enlargement of the introitus. The findings also may simply reflect the increased frequency of pelvic visceral prolapse among older women.

Removal of significant vulvar tissue, particularly the clitoris, can result in decreased sexual satisfaction. Loss of the subcutaneous tissue prevents mobility of the external genitalia, which can also hinder sexual pleasure. Although this has been a detriment in many patients, others state that orgasm is still obtainable after vulvectomy.

Survival Results

Survival in cancer of the vulva is, as with all other malignancies, directly related to the extent of disease at the time diagnosis is made and treatment is undertaken.

Because this malignancy is initially diagnosed in the elderly woman, many patients succumb to intercurrent disease while tumor free. In stages I and II disease, the corrected 5-year survival rate should approach 90%. A 75% corrected 5-year survival rate for all stages of vulvar cancer is not unusual. Hacker et al. reported a 5-year survival rate of 98% in stage I cancer and 90% stage II. Regardless of the stage, if negative lymphatic nodes were present, there was a 96% survival rate. This dropped to 66% if positive nodes were present. If only one inguinal node had metastasis, the survival rate was 94%, dropping to 80% if two positive nodes were involved. Similar results were noted from the Mayo Clinic data. If lymph nodes were negative, the 5-year survival rate was 90%. However, in their material the survival rate dropped precipitously if even one lymph node had metastasis (57%). Overall survival results by stage are found in Table 8-8 and Figure 8-15.

If, however, the lymph nodes are negative irrespective of stage, in many series more than 90% of these patients will survive 5 years (corrected survival), whereas only 40%-50% will survive if the lymph nodes are positive (Table 8-9). Curry et al. noted that, in patients with three or fewer unilateral groin nodes involved with metastasis, the 5-year survival rate was still good (17/25, or 68%); however, of five patients in whom more than three nodes were involved, none survived. None of the patients with three or fewer unilateral involved nodes had deep pelvic node metastases. Boyce and Shimm reported similar results, with prognosis worsening not only with an increase in the number of positive nodes but to a lesser extent in the presence of bilateral inguinal node involve-

Table 8-8   Survival by stage

Stage	Percent
I	91
II	81
III	48
IV	15

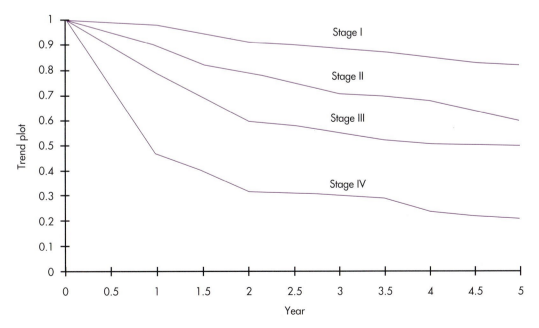

Figure 8-15 Invasive squamous epithelial cell carcinoma of the vulva. Actuarial survival by stage. (From *Annual Report Gynecological Cancer FIGO,* vol 22, 1994.)

Table 8-9   Survival rates for carcinoma of the vulva

Series	Status of nodes	Number of patients	Percent surviving	
			Positive	Negative
Way (1960)	Positive	45	42	
	Negative	36		77
Macafee (1962)	Positive	33	33	
	Negative	49		70
Collins et al. (1963)	Positive	19	21	
	Negative	32		69
Franklin and Rutledge (1971)	Positive	33	39	
	Negative	53		100
Morley (1976)	Positive	64	39	
	Negative	130		92
Krupp and Bahm (1978)	Positive	40	36	
	Negative	154		91
Green (1978)	Positive	46	33	
	Negative	61		87
Benedet et al. (1979)	Positive	34	53	
	Negative	86		81
Boyce (1985)	Positive	30	50	
	Negative	49		82
Shimm (1986)	Positive	33	52	
	Negative	65		77
Cavanagh et al. (1990)	Positive	77	39	
	Negative	126		85

Table 8-10   Survival rates for patients with positive pelvic nodes

Series	5-year survival rate (%)
Way (1957)	2/9 (22.2)
Green et al. (1958)	2/16 (12.5)
Way (1960)	3/8 (37.5)
Merrill and Ross (1961)	1/3 (33.3)
Collins et al. (1963)	1/6 (16.7)
Franklin and Rutledge (1971)	3/12 (25.0)
Morley (1976)	1/6 (16.7)
Curry, Wharton, and Rutledge (1980)	2/9 (22.2)
Boyce (1985)	0/6 (0)
Shimm (1986)	0/7 (0)
TOTAL	15/82 (18.3)

ment. Of the patients with more than four unilateral nodes, 50% had deep pelvic node metastasis, and if bilateral groin nodes were involved, 26% had positive pelvic nodes. In patients with positive pelvic nodes, the survival rate is poor. Collected series indicate that only one fifth of patients with deep pelvic node metastasis survived 5 years (Table 8-10).

Tolerance of the Elderly Patient to Therapy

As stated above, many cases of squamous cell carcinoma of the vulva occur in patients who are in the eighth, ninth, and tenth decades of life. Because the average life span of women has increased, gynecologic malignancies in true geriatric patients have become common. In fact, more than half of all cancers occur in elderly patients; the probability of developing cancer within a 5-year span climbs from 1 in 700 at the age of 25 to 1 in 14 by the age of 65. Cancer is the second leading cause of death in persons more than 65 years of age. Why there is an increase in incidence of cancer in this population has not been clearly established, although a number of factors may be involved. These include the possibility of decreased immunosurveillance, longer duration of carcinogenic exposure, and an increased susceptibility of aging cells to carcinogenesis.

In younger patients, the "clinical dictum" is to attempt to attribute all signs and symptoms of cancer to a single diagnosis. The opposite is true, however, for older patients in whom the clinical features probably are caused by multiple diagnoses because of common occurrences of concomitant medical illnesses. The pervasive notion that elderly patients are less tolerant of chemotherapy, surgery, and radiation therapy is generally untrue. The majority of older people who have few concomitant medical problems can tolerate all these modalities, especially surgery, quite well. Although elderly patients should not be categorically excluded from aggressive therapy because of their age, treatment may need modification to accommodate changes that occur with age. For example, it is clear that older patients who are treated with intensive chemotherapy have a much higher initial toxicity rate because of bone marrow suppression. Therefore doses should be initiated at a reduced level and then increased as tolerated to avoid difficulty. On the other hand, surgical therapy such as radical vulvectomy with bilateral inguinal lymphadenectomy is well tolerated by elderly patients, even those in their 90s. Undoubtedly, this is because body cavities are not violated. Much of the risk lies in the anesthesia required.

Recurrence

Recurrence may be local or distant, and more than 80% will occur in the first 2 years after therapy, demanding initial close follow-up. Surprisingly, over half the recurrences are local and near the site of the primary lesion. This is more common in patients with large primary tumors and/or metastatic disease in the lymph nodes revealed at initial surgery. A study from the MD Anderson Hospital suggests that local recurrences are commonly seen even when the margins are declared clear on the original operative specimen. On the other hand, the high incidence of local recurrences demands careful attention to adequate margins in the removal of the primary lesion. In many instances, local recurrences can be successfully treated by local excision and/or interstitial radiation. Patients with recurrent local disease in the lymph node area or distant disease are difficult to treat, and the salvage rate is poor. Simonsen reported a 40% salvage with local recurrence and an 8% survival at 5 years with regional metastases. Both groups were treated with a combination of surgery and irradiation therapy. Prempree had similar results using radiation alone. Disease limited to the introitus gave the best prognosis: 6 of 6 patients survived. As expected, extensive recurrences have the poorest prognosis, especially when bone metastases occur. Patients with distant recurrences have been treated at our institution with cisplatin based chemotherapy and a 30% overall response rate has been achieved. Responses are more likely outside the radiation field.

EARLY VULVAR CARCINOMA

In 1974, Wharton et al. described an entity they called microinvasive carcinoma of the vulva. These lesions were 2 cm or smaller in diameter and invaded the stroma to a depth of 5 mm or less. In 25 such patients none had positive lymph nodes, developed recurrence, or died as a result of vulvar cancer. These results imply that microinvasive carcinoma of the vulva is a definable stage, in that this group may be treated by conservative surgery. As a result of this article, several patients with stage I lesions

and limited stromal invasion were treated by radical vulvectomy only. Several of these patients subsequently developed recurrent or metastatic carcinoma and died of their disease. In 1975, Parker et al. at Duke University presented their evaluation of patients with early invasive epidermoid carcinoma of the vulva. They believed that the term *microinvasive* was not applicable to vulvar neoplasia. Of their patients, 60 had a stage I (TI) lesion of 2 cm or smaller. Fifty-eight of these patients had stromal invasion 5 mm or less in depth. Of the 58 patients, 3 (5%) had pelvic node metastases: 2 of these 3 showed invasion of vascular channels, and the third patient showed cellular anaplasia. The Duke study concluded that if a strict histologic evaluation of the excised vulvar lesion showed invasion of 5 mm or less, an absence of vascular or lymphatic channel invasion, and no anaplasia an operational approach less radical than radical vulvectomy, inguinal dissection, and/or pelvic lymphadenectomy could be used for selected patients. This would reduce the morbidity and not increase mortality.

Andersen constructed three different models of groups at low risk for metastasis in squamous cell carcinoma of the vulva region. He concluded that a definite, distinct profile of low-risk patients would require data from very large patient accruals and international collaboration.

There is at present no universally agreed-on definition for superficial invasion carcinoma of the vulva, although the term has been used by many authors. One of the problems of defining the lesion is determining its clinically important dimensions and how these dimensions should be measured. The measurements of the diameter of the lesion and the depth of invasion are the most commonly used. In studies that used the 5 mm depth of invasion parameter, 874 cases collected by Wilkinson with 5 mm or less depth of invasion revealed 107 patients (12.2%) with inguinal lymph node metastasis (Table 8-11). The depth of invasion by tumor acceptable as superficial invasion has been quite variable and is further confused by there being little agreement on how the measurement should be made. Although 5 mm depth of invasion was accepted by many authors, others utilize a 3 mm depth. In patients with tumors with 3 mm depth of invasion the frequency of lymph node metastasis is lower (Table 8-12). There remains considerable inconsistency regarding pathologists' methods of measuring depth of invasion. In most current publications a method is described that measures from the most superficial dermal-epidermal junction of the most superficial adjacent dermal papillae. Others have used a method that measures from the surface of the lesion. Although this latter method is simpler, it appears not to be as reflective of true invasion. The importance of vascular invasion adjacent to the vulva carcinoma in predicting lymph node metastasis, or prognosis, remains controversial. However, there are data that support the hypothesis that vascular space involvement by tumor at the site of the primary tumor is

Table 8-11 Superficially invasive vulvar carcinoma: frequency of lymph node metastasis with lesions 5 mm in depth or less

Author	Total cases	Number with lymphadenectomy	Node metastasis	% of total with node metastasis
Wharton et al.	25	10	0	0
Dean et al.	7	1	0	0
Parker et al.	58	37	3	5.2
DiPaolo et al.	12	11	4	33.3
Kunschner et al.	17	13	0	0
Kabulski and Frankman	23	23	5	21.7
Magrina et al.	96	71	9	9.4
DiSaia et al.	19	19	1	5.3
Barnes et al.	18	7	2	11.1
Iversen et al.	70	70	5	7.1*
Donaldson et al.	38	38	11	28.9
Fu et al.	13	12	2	15.4
Buscema et al.	58	40	6	10.3
Wilkinson et al.	30	27	2	6.7
Kneale et al.	92	61	6	6.5
Hoffman et al.	75	46	10	13.3
Sedlis et al.	187	187	33	18.0
Dvoretsky et al.	36	NR	6	16.7
Rowley et al.	22	22	2	9.0
Berman et al.	50	50	1	2.0
TOTAL	946	745	108	11.4

From Wilkinson EJ: *Clin Obstet Gynecol* 28 (1):188, March 1985.
NR, not reported.
*Inguinal or distant metastasis.

Table 8-12 Superficially invasive vulvar carcinoma: frequency of lymph node metastasis with lesions 3 mm in depth or less

Author	Total cases	Number with lymphadenectomy	Node metastasis	% of total with node metastasis
Jafari and Cartnick	6	6	1	16.6
Iversen et al.	48	48	2*	4.2
Chu et al.	26	13	0	0
Buscema et al.	19	19	1	5.3
Wilkinson et al.	29	25	2	6.8
Hoffman et al.	60	NR	2	3.3
Kneale et al.	68	NR	4	5.8
Dvoretsky et al.	28	NR	2	7.1
Rowley et al.	18	18	1	5.5
Berman et al.	31	31	1	3.2
TOTAL	333	160	16	4.8

NR, not reported.
*Groin recurrence.

associated with increased frequency of lymph node metastasis.

The International Society for the Study of Vulvar Disease (ISSVD) has proposed the following pathologic definition of microinvasive carcinoma of the vulva: a squamous carcinoma having a diameter of 2 cm or less, as measured in the fresh state, with a depth of invasion of 1 mm or less, measured from the epithelial-stromal junction of the most superficial adjacent dermal papilla to the deepest point of invasion. The presence of vascular space involvement by tumor would exclude the lesion from this definition. These lesions probably do not need

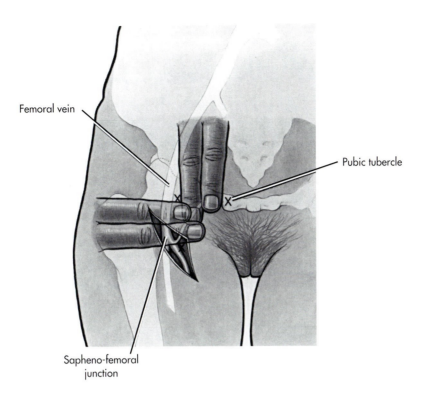

Femoral vein

Pubic tubercle

X

X

Sapheno-femoral
junction

Figure 8-16 Incision can be made as noted so that superficial inguinal nodes can be removed easily. (Modified from Cabanas RM: An approach to the treatment of penile carcinoma, *Cancer* 39:456, 1977.)

an inguinal lymphadenectomy of any type and are now classified as stage Ia. A review of the literature reveals only two cases of stage Ia with lymph node metastasis.

Donaldson reported a patient with 1.1 mm of stromal invasion with tumor in vascular spaces who was found to have metastatic tumor in two ipsilateral inguinal lymph nodes. There does not appear to be a definitive correlation between tumor differentiation and lymph node metastasis or survival. There may be an association between depth of tumor invasion and tumor differentiation, with deeply invasive tumors being more undifferentiated. More study of this issue is needed.

Podratz et al. reported a 5-year survival rate of 90% if the primary lesion was less than 1 cm, 89% if the lesion was 1 to 2 cm, and 83% if the lesion was 2 to 3 cm. They found that the 5- and 10-year survival rates of patients with stage I disease were independent of the extent of the surgical procedure, suggesting that more selectivity of the treatment is feasible without sacrifice of curability.

There continues to be a lack of unanimity concerning the proper surgical approach to the patient with an early invasive carcinoma of the vulva. Reports illustrating metastatic disease in inguinal lymph nodes conflict with other reports that suggest radical vulvectomy only. The morbidity produced by radical vulvectomy, both to body image and sexual function, makes this issue worthy of serious consideration. As a result, DiSaia, Creasman, and Rich proposed an alternate approach to this early disease

that attempts to preserve vulvar tissue without sacrificing curability when possible metastatic disease exists. This approach uses the inguinal nodes as sentinel nodes in the treatment planning when the central lesion is 1 cm or less in diameter and focal invasion is limited to 5 mm or less (see the description of metastatic lymph node spread pattern on pp. 204-208).

The patient is prepared for radical vulvectomy with a bilateral inguinal lymphadenectomy if the operative findings warrant a maximal surgical effort. An 8 cm incision is made parallel to the inguinal ligament two finger-breadths (4 cm) beneath the inguinal ligament and two finger breadths (4 cm) lateral to the pubic tubercle (Figure 8-16). This allows access to the inguinal lymph nodes of both the upper oblique and inferior vertical set. The incision is carried down through the Camper fascia, and at this point skin flaps are bluntly and sharply dissected superiorly and inferiorly, allowing access to the fat pad containing the superficial nodes. The sentinel nodes are located in the fatty layer of tissue above and beneath the Camper fascia, in part anterior to the cribriform plate and also protruding from beneath the fascia lata (Figure 8-17). The dissection should be carried superiorly to the inguinal ligament and inferiorly to a point approximately 2 cm proximal to the opening of the Hunter canal. The dissection should be carried laterally to the sartorius muscle and medially to the adductor longus muscle fascia (Figure 8-18). Blunt dissection with the

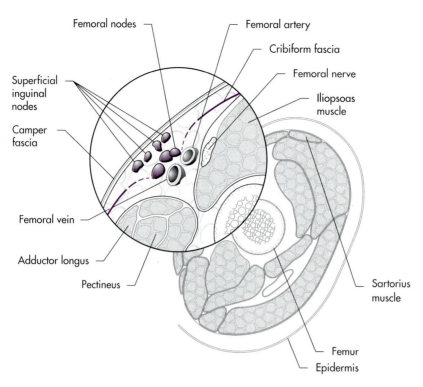

Figure 8-17 Many inguinal nodes are located between the Camper fascia and the cribriform fascia, as noted on cross section through femoral triangle. Additional nodes are clustered in the foramen ovalis, in part protruding from beneath the plane of the cribriform fascia. (Modified from Cabanas RM: An approach to the treatment of penile carcinoma, *Cancer* 39:456, 1977.)

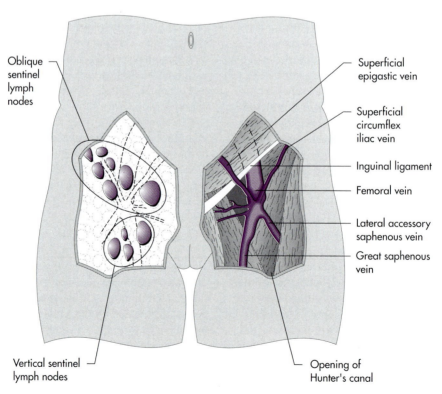

Figure 8-18 The right side demonstrates the two groups of lymph nodes making up the "sentinel" nodes. The left side notes the limits of the dissection with the cribriform fascia removed. The triangle that is dissected in a full inguinal lymphadenectomy is clearly identified on the patient's left side. The inguinal ligament forms the base of the triangle, and the opening of Hunter's canal becomes the apex. The triangle is bound laterally by the sartorius muscle and medially by the adductor muscles and fascia.

handle of the scalpel facilitates identification of the cribriform fascia, which is most easily identified just below the inguinal ligament or in the area of the saphenous opening. The cribriform fascia unites with the fascia lata and thus is contiguous with the fascia on the surface of the adductor longus and sartorius muscles; this may facilitate its identification. The portion of the fascia covering the femoral triangle is perforated by the saphenous vein, lymph nodes of the vertical set, and by numerous blood and lymphatic vessels, hence the name cribriform fascia. If the dissection is carried out properly, the adventitia of the femoral vessels should not be clearly seen except through the vessel openings mentioned above. As stated previously, Borgno demonstrated that the deep inguinal or femoral nodes are exposed in the fossa ovalis and other openings of the cribriform fascia, allowing access to all inguinal nodes with this technique. The result is that a dissection that utilizes the boundaries described above and at the same time is carried out to the level of the cribriform fascia with optimum traction on the lymphovascular/fat bundle of the inguinal area will produce a specimen that contains all of the inguinal/femoral nodes.

The excised nodes are immediately sent for frozen section analysis—the finding of positive nodes mandates a complete inguinal dissection, including removal of the cribriform fascia and fatty tissue beneath. If there is no metastatic disease, simple closure of the incision is done using a subcuticular suture of polyglycolic acid over two medium-sized suction drainage tubes.

A wide local excision of the vulvar skin is then performed, ensuring a margin of 2-3 cm of normal skin on all sides of the primary lesion. Adequate subcutaneous tissue should be taken down to the perineal fascia, especially beneath the primary lesion. It has been our practice to submit mucous membrane and skin margins as separate specimens.

After hemostasis is established, a decision must be made regarding primary closure of the defect vs intraposition of a split-thickness skin graft. When a split-thickness graft is used, the graft is usually taken from the medial aspect of the right thigh at 0.018-inch thickness. With an air-driven dermatome, this can be accomplished easily with minimal morbidity. The donor site is dressed, and an occlusive pressure dressing is applied. The skin graft is then sutured to the defect using 4-0 PGA suture and a pressure dressing in a manner previously described by Rutledge and Sinclair.

If metastatic disease is found in the inguinal nodes, a classic radical vulvectomy and inguinal lymphadenectomy must be done. The approach outlined here attempts to gain optimal curability and preserve optimal cosmesis and sexual function.

Berman reported the latest series of 50 patients utilizing this technique. Lesions up to 2 cm in diameter were accepted, whereas they were limited to 1 cm in the

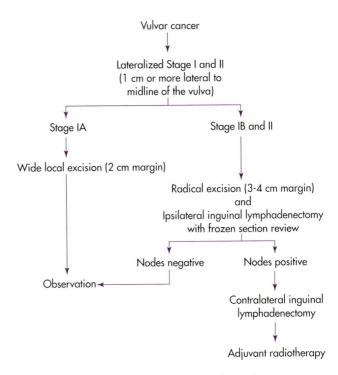

Figure 8-19 Algorithm for management of lateralized stage I or II vulvar cancer.

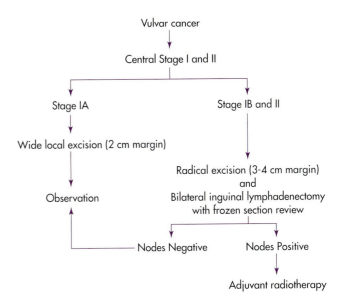

Figure 8-20 Algorithm for management of central stage I or II vulvar cancer.

first report by DiSaia. Depth of invasion was, as in the first report, limited to 5 mm. Only one of 50 patients had lymph node metastases, and that one died of her disease. Five local recurrences were noted in the other 49 patients, and these were successfully managed with reexcision of the vulvar lesion. The upper limits of size and depth of invasion acceptable for this approach is a judgment for the

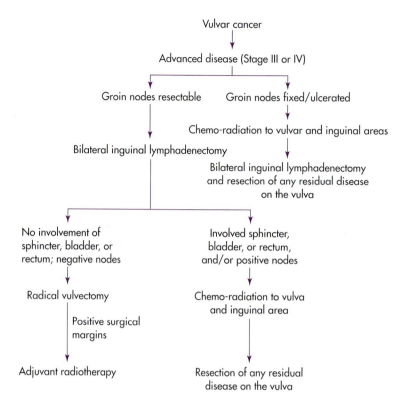

Figure 8-21 Algorithm for management of advanced (stage III or IV) vulvar cancer.

clinician; but the authors currently believe it should be limited to stage I lesions with 5 mm or less of invasion.

Stehman reported the GOG experience with 121 patients with stage I disease and invasion less than 5 mm treated as described by DiSaia. There were 19 recurrences, and unlike DiSaia and Berman there were 5 groin only recurrences and 7 deaths. In our experience with more than 100 patients, there has not been any groin recurrence or deaths. The difference is likely in the extent of the inguinal lymphadenectomy. Our practice is to remove all the nodes and fat in the area (illustrated in Figure 8-8) down to the cribriform fascia, including nodes that are partially under the fascia appearing at the holes in that fascia. Algorithms seen in Figures 8-19 to 8-21 are the author's suggestions for management.

PAGET'S DISEASE

Paget's disease of the vulva is rare. Even among vulvar neoplasias it is an unusual finding. It occurs in women in the seventh decade of life but can be seen in young patients, just as with squamous carcinoma of the vulva. Symptoms of pruritus and tenderness or the identification of a vulvar lesion is most frequently seen. These symptoms may be present for years before the patient seeks medical attention. The vulvar lesion may be localized to one labium or involve the entire vulvar epithelium. It is not unusual for the disease process to extend to the perirectal area, buttocks, inguinal area, or mons. Recently, extension into the vagina has been reported.

Clinical and Histologic Features

On examination, the vulvar lesions are usually hyperemic, sharply demarcated, and thickened, with foci of excoriation and induration. Often the vulvar skin is thick and smooth, leading to the impression of leukoplakia. It is not unusual for the hyperemic areas associated with a superficial white coating to give the impression of "cake-icing effect." This finding is classic and, if present, is almost pathognomonic for Paget's disease (Figures 8-22, *A* and *B*). Typically, areas of leukoplakia are mixed with patches of redness where excoriation has occurred because of intense pruritus. On palpation, the vulvar changes appear to be superficial. This maneuver is extremely important, for one must rule out an underlying adenocarcinoma, which is usually self-evident because of thickness or a mass-like effect under the epithelial changes. It is unusual not to appreciate an underlying adenocarcinoma clinically; however, one must take adequate biopsies of the lesion, relative to width as well as depth of tissue, to enable adequate histologic evaluation. The use of fine-needle aspiration biopsy to evaluate subcutaneous masses of the vulva, as well as other sites, should be encouraged as a rapid diagnostic technique. This procedure is associated with low morbidity and

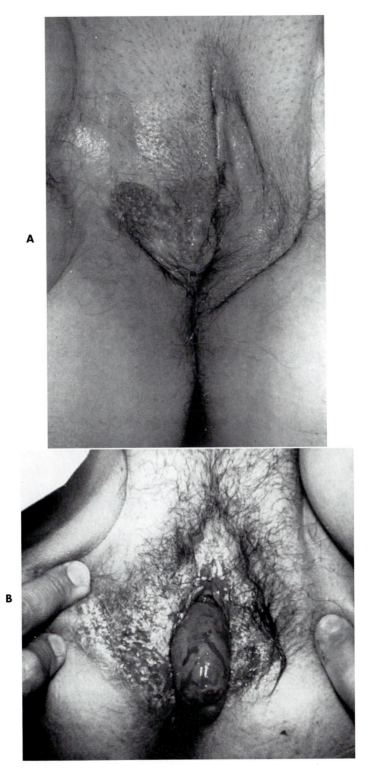

Figure 8-22 A, Paget's disease of the vulva involving the lower half of the right labium major. The white medial portion is characteristic of "cake-icing effect." The red lateral aspect is also commonly seen and termed "violaceous coloring." **B,** Paget's disease with uterine prolapse.

allows greater planning before undertaking major surgery. It is our practice to perform a needle aspiration of any thickness or mass that is palpated beneath the skin involved with Paget's disease. It appears that there are two separate lesions: intraepithelial extramammary Paget's disease and pagetoid changes within the skin associated with an underlying adenocarcinoma. Therapy for these two lesions is considerably different, and a definitive diagnosis is therefore imperative.

A thickened, often acanthotic epidermis is the typical histologic finding. Characteristic large cells with clear granular cytoplasm are found within the epidermis (Figure 8-23). Often a single layer of squamous cells separates the Paget cells from the epidermis, but neoplastic cells may be an immediate contact with the dermis. Intraepidermal formation of glands with true lumina may also be present. The hair follicles may also be involved with Paget cells. These cells contain intracytoplasmic mucin demonstrated by Mayer muci-carmine or Alcian blue. A mixed inflammatory infiltrate of variable intensity composed usually of lymphocytes and plasma cells is present in the upper dermis. Misdiagnosis of carcinoma in situ or melanoma has been made; however, adequate tissue for evaluation and a proper clinical description tends to eliminate this confusion. Sufficient tissue for histologic evaluation will readily identify an underlying adenocarcinoma.

Clinical Course and Management

If only intraepithelial Paget's disease is present, the clinical course may be prolonged and indolent. In a patient originally diagnosed with only intraepithelial Paget's disease, there can be recurrence, but it is usually seen as an intraepithelial lesion only, without an underlying adenocarcinoma. From a review of our material and the literature, we believe that when extramammary Paget's disease with an underlying adenocarcinoma is present, it is the result of simultaneous diagnoses or, more

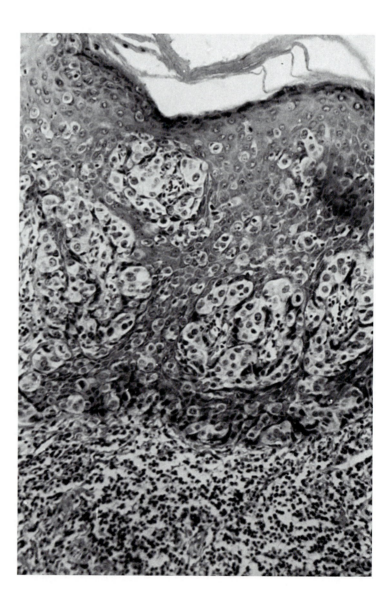

Figure 8-23 Histologic picture of Paget's disease of the vulva. Large cells with clear cytoplasm are apparent in epidermis. Note heavy lymphocytic infiltration in dermis.

likely, a secondary infiltration of the vulva skin by cells from a primary adenocarcinoma of underlying apocrine glands. It appears that we are dealing with two separate diseases and not a spectrum. The exclusively intraepithelial disease presentation, by far the more common one seen by the clinician, remains a local phenomenon even with recurrences. Paget's disease with an underlying adenocarcinoma can be aggressive, with metastasis to the regional lymph nodes, as well as distant spread.

The literature has been confusing with regard to the association of invasive carcinoma and concomitant intraepithelial Paget's disease. Invasive underlying adenocarcinomas have been reported in up to 20% of patients with histologically confirmed Pagetoid cells in the vulva skin. Our experience suggests a much lower incidence. Similarly, older studies suggest that up to 25% of patients have a concomitant carcinoma at another site, such as breast, colon, anus, or cervix. Here, too, our experience has not been in agreement, with only a rare patient having a simultaneous lesion.

Since Paget's disease without an underlying adenocarcinoma appears to be a true intraepithelial neoplasia, it can be treated as such. Wide local excision to include the entire lesion is usually sufficient. Even with apparent wide margins, it is not unusual to find Paget's disease extending to the edge of the surgical margin. Histologically, one may find neoplastic cells present in normal-appearing skin for a variable, but often considerable, distance beyond the seemingly sharp margin of the clinically evident lesion. It is difficult to avoid cutting across intraepithelial tumor, and therefore intraoperative examination of the surgical margins by cryostat frozen sectioning is imperative (Figure 8-24). It is our custom to incise the periphery of the operative specimen and immediately send identifiable strips of surgical margin for cryostat frozen sectioning. If the presence of tumor cells is reported, additional margins can then be excised. Recurrences are common when the surgical margins contain neoplastic cells. Unfortunately, recurrences are also not unusual with negative margins, leading some surgeons to abandon the use of frozen section surgical margins. These new lesions can be handled in the same manner as the primary disease: that is, by wide local excision. Our studies show that removal of full-thickness skin plus a microscopic amount of subcutaneous fat routinely results in an operative specimen that is 6 mm thick (Figure 8-25). Because the base of the hair follicles in vulva skin is at a depth of 4 mm, one need not be concerned about the possibility of leaving neoplastic cells that may have involved hair shafts. Lesions can be extensive in the primary and recurrent stages, and treatment should be given accordingly. The use of a skin graft to cover the removed tissue may be warranted and should be used freely. Recently, DiSaia reported on two patients who developed recurrent Paget's disease in the middle of a split thickness skin graft. A process labeled

"retrodissemination" was given as an explanation for this curious phenomenon whereby Pagetoid cells from peripheral occult sites of persistent disease are postulated to metastasize back into a skin graft site.

Besa reported good results when radiotherapy was used in conjunction with surgery or for patients for whom surgery was not possible. A dose of 50-55 Gy appeared to be adequate. Voight reported a dramatic response of extramammary Paget carcinoma in a man with chemotherapy utilizing carboplatin and 5-fluorouracil with folinic acid, suggesting another possible approach when surgery is not appropriate.

Patients in whom an underlying adenocarcinoma is identified in association with Paget's disease of the vulva should be treated in the same manner as patients with other invasive malignancies of the vulva. This usually includes radical vulvectomy and inguinal lymphadenectomy. If the lymph nodes have no evidence of metastatic disease, the prognosis is good; however, if metastases are present in the lymph nodes, the prognosis is guarded. No statement concerning the role of radiation therapy and

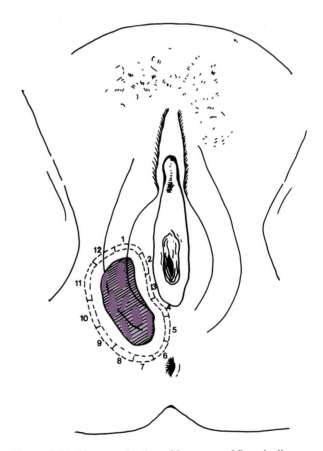

Figure 8-24 Diagram of vulva with an area of Paget's disease involving the right labium majus. The two parallel lines lateral to the lesion represent the surgical margin sent intraoperatively for frozen-section analysis. The margin is serially cut in a clockwise fashion, labeled, and analyzed. If any segment of the margin reveals Paget's disease, the resection is extended in that direction. (From *Bergen S et al: Gynecol Oncol* 33:151, 1989.)

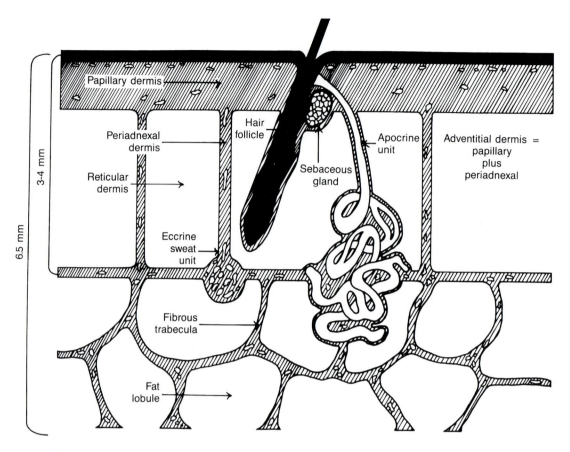

Figure 8-25 Schematic of vulvar skin anatomy showing the extension of skin appendages into the subdermal adipose tissue. (From Bergen S et al: *Gynecol Oncol* 33:151, 1989.)

chemotherapy in this disease can be made, since the experience has been limited and inconclusive.

MELANOMA

Melanoma of the vulva, although it is the second most common invasive cancer occurring in this area, is still rare. This malignancy probably arises from a lesion containing a junctional or a compound nevus. As a result, it is suggested by some authorities that all pigmented nevi on the vulva should be prophylactically excised. The box *(right)* defines the high-risk group and describes the characteristics of pigmented lesions of the vulva or any skin that determine the need for excisional biopsy.

The clinical characteristics are as elsewhere on the body; melanomas are usually pigmented, raised, and may be ulcerated (Figure 8-26). The median age of patients with these lesions is 65 in a series reported by Tasseron. Melanomas are often misdiagnosed as undifferentiated squamous cell cancers, especially when they are histologically amelanotic. Electron microscopy can be helpful when the diagnosis continues to be in doubt. The patient may have experienced pruritus, bleeding, or enlargement of a pigmented area. Most vulvar melanomas are located

---

INDIVIDUALS AT RISK FOR DEVELOPING MELANOMA ARE THOSE WHO HAVE ONE OR MORE OF THE FOLLOWING:

1. A family history of melanoma in blood relatives
2. Poor or no tanning ability, often with a history of sunburn in adolescence
3. Unusual moles with any of the following characteristics:
   Dark (blue-black) look
   Speckled or splotchy color pattern
   Jagged or fuzzy border
4. Recent change in size, shape, or color of a mole
5. Any mole larger than a dime

---

on the labia minora or clitoris. Prognosis is related to the size of the lesion and the depth of invasion. The Clark classification, commonly used for melanomas elsewhere on the skin, is of prognostic benefit for the vulva also. Clark's classification, which uses histologic levels, is outlined in Table 8-13. In 1970, Breslow recognized that survival was relative to the greatest thickness of the invasive portion of the melanoma by micrometer measure (Figure 8-27). The Breslow technique appeals to many because of its simplicity. Evidence exists that these lesions can metastasize to deep nodes in the absence of inguinal node involvement, although this has not been our experience. In 1975, Chung reported a third system of level of involvement of vulvar melanoma (Figure 8-28).

Although it has been suggested that all patients with melanoma of the vulva should be treated with radical vulvectomy and inguinal and pelvic lymphadenectomy, there has been a tendency of late to be more conservative. Radical local excision with a 2 cm margin for thin lesions (up to 7 mm) and 3-4 cm for thicker lesions appears to be adequate for most well circumscribed lesions. Since prognosis is directly related to depth of invasion, therapy can be tailored accordingly. If the disease is intraepithelial, cure should be very close to 100%. Even with level I or II melanoma (Clark classification), a wide local

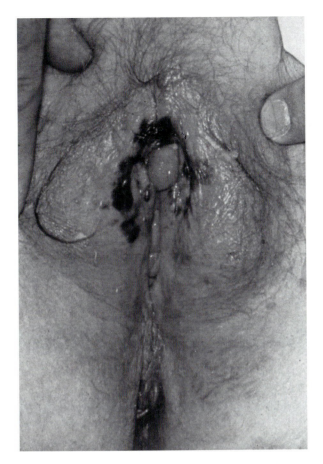

Figure 8-26 Melanoma of the vulva. Typical pigmented neoplasm is present.

Table 8-13   Clark's staging classification by levels

Level	Definition
I	In situ melanoma: all demonstrable tumor is above the basement membrane in the epidermis
II	Melanoma extends through the basement membrane into the papillary dermis
III	The tumor fills the papillary dermis and extends to the reticular dermis but does not invade it
IV	The tumor extends into the reticular dermis
V	The tumor extends into the subcutaneous fat

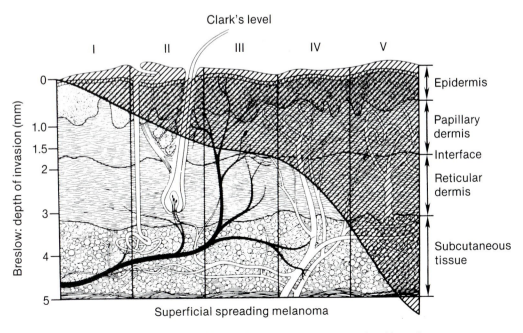

Figure 8-27 Comparison of Clark and Breslow classifications for skin melanomas.

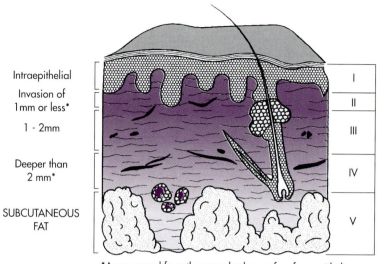

Intraepithelial

Invasion of
1mm or less*

1 - 2mm

Deeper than
2 mm*

SUBCUTANEOUS
FAT

I

II

III

IV

V

*As measured from the granular layer of surface epithelium

Figure 8-28 Chung system of reporting melanoma involvement.

Table 8-14   Correlation of melanoma thickness with patient survival

Thickness	8-year survival rates
<0.85 mm	100%
0.85-1.5 mm	99%
1.5-4 mm	66%
>4 mm	25% to 35%

From Jaramillo BA et al: *Obstet Gynecol* 66 (3):398, 1985; and Day CL et al: *N Engl J Med* 305:1155, 1981.

excision may be adequate treatment. As the melanoma extends deeper, the chance of lymph node metastasis increases, and the prognosis decreases considerably. Podratz reported that 10-year survival rates associated with Clark's level II, III, IV, and V tumors were 100%, 83%, 65%, and 23%, respectively. Histologic growth patterns also influence survival: 5-year survival rates for superficial spreading and nodular melanomas were 71% and 38%, respectively. Ten-year survival rates were 66% and 25%, respectively. Utilizing the Breslow method, Jaramillo, as well as Day, reported nearly 100% survival in patients with lesions less than 1.5 mm in thickness, 65% to 70% survival in patients with lesions 1.5 to 4 mm, and 25% to 35% survival with lesions greater than 4 mm (Table 8-14). Trimble reported on 80 patients treated at Memorial Sloan Kettering Cancer Center with a median follow-up of 193 months. By Chung level, 10-ten year survival for each grade was: I, 100%; II, 81%; III, 87%; IV, 11%; V, 33%. The role of the lymphadenectomy in this disease is probably more prognostic than therapeutic. If disease is limited to the vulva, regardless of its extent, and the lymph nodes are negative, the survival rate is good. It is rare that a patient with positive inguinal nodes has a long-term survival rate: virtually all patients with positive pelvic nodes eventually succumb to the disease.

SARCOMA

Sarcoma of the vulva is rare, and even in large referral institutions the experience is limited. Symptoms and findings are the same as those noted with squamous cell carcinoma. DiSaia et al., in a review of 12 patients, noted that this lesion occurred in a younger group of patients (mean age 38 years) than did other vulvar malignancies. The histologic grade of the sarcoma appears to be the most important factor in prognosis. If a patient has an undifferentiated rhabdomyosarcoma, prognosis is poor, since these lesions tend to grow and metastasize very rapidly. However, a well-differentiated leiomyosarcoma will be slow growing and develop late recurrences. Therapy generally would be radical vulvectomy and bilateral inguinal lymphadenectomy except in the low-grade lesions, in which nodal involvement is rare and wide local excision should be considered. Patients undergoing wide local excision are at risk of local recurrence and should be observed closely.

BARTHOLIN GLAND CARCINOMA

Adenocarcinoma of Bartholin gland is a rare lesion occurring only in about 1% of all vulvar malignancies (Figure 8-29). The peak incidence is in women in their mid-sixties, although it has been reported in a teenager. Because of its location, the tumor can be of considerable size before the patient is aware of symptoms. Dyspareunia may be one of the first symptoms, although the finding of a mass or ulcerative lesion may be the first indication to the patient of her disease. An enlargement in the Bartholin gland area in a postmenopausal woman should be considered a malignancy until proven otherwise. The lesion can have a tendency to spread into the ischiorectal fossa and can have a propensity for (1) lymphatic spread to the inguinal nodes via the common lymphatic spread for vulvar cancer and (2) for posterior spread to the pelvic nodes directly. Almost half of all carcinomas said to be of Bartholin gland origin are squamous cell carcinomas. In most instances, strict histologic criteria have not been followed. Every attempt should be made to differentiate between a true Bartholin gland cancer and a squamous cell carcinoma of the vulva arising in proximity to the Bartholin gland. Prognosis is good if lymph node metastasis is not present.

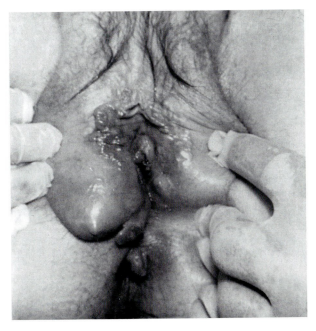

Figure 8-29 Adenocarcinoma of Bartholin gland with local skin metastasis.

Therapy includes radical vulvectomy with a large, wide, extensive dissection around the gland and inguinal lymphadenectomy. To have adequate margins, there may be a need to remove a considerable amount of vagina and, on occasion, part of the rectum. It appears that pelvic lymphadenectomy is not indicated unless the inguinal nodes are involved. A more conservative approach in early selected patients may be appropriate. The largest series is reported by Copeland, with 36 patients whose 5-year survival was 84%. Distribution of the tumors in FIGO stages included 9 stage I, 15 stage II, 10 stage III, and 2 stage IV. Cell types were squamous, 27; adenomatous, 6; adenoid cystic, 2; and adenosquamous, 1. Of 30 patients with lymph node dissections 14 (47%) had nodal metastasis, and 11 remain free of disease. Disease recurred in 9 patients (6 local recurrences, 2 distant, 1 local and distant), and 4 were treated successfully. Less impressive results were reported by Wheelock in a series of 10 patients.

Adenoid cystic carcinoma of the Bartholin gland is a rare entity manifested by frequent local recurrences and slowly progressive disease, including pulmonary metastasis, sometimes many years following initial therapy. Recommended primary treatment is wide local excision, obtaining clear margins, and an ipsilateral inguinal lymphadenectomy followed by careful monitoring. Recurrences are best treated with surgery.

BASAL CELL CARCINOMA

Basal cell carcinoma is usually small, occurs on the labia majora, and may have a central ulceration (Figure 8-30). The stromal infiltration is usually circumscribed and orderly and, as elsewhere in the body, has a slow and indolent growth rate and, rarely if ever, involves the lymphatics. Metastatic basal cell carcinoma of the vulva

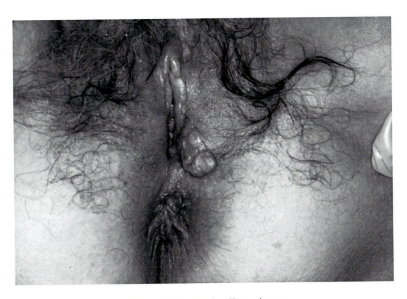

Figure 8-30 Basal cell carcinoma.

has been reported as a rare occurrence. For the most part, these lesions behave as elsewhere in the body, with local invasion as the rule. A typical lesion has a rolled, pearly border showing fine telangiectatic vessels on the surface and a central ulceration. The patient complains that the lesion itches slightly, bleeds a little, and then seems to heal. The process repeats itself as the lesion slowly increases in size. Local excision is adequate, with primary closure the usual rule. If a large lesion is present after local excision, a skin graft may be applied. Basal cell carcinoma must be differentiated pathologically from the so-called basosquamous cell carcinoma, which must be treated as one would treat a squamous cell carcinoma of the vulva.

BIBLIOGRAPHY

Invasive squamous cell carcinoma

Andersen WA et al: Vulvar squamous cell carcinoma and papillomaviruses: Two separate entities? *Am J Obstet Gynecol* 165:329, 1991.

Andreasson B, Nyboe J: Value of prognostic parameters in squamous cell carcinoma of the vulva, *Gynecol Oncol* 22:341, 1985.

Andrews SJ et al: Therapeutic implications of lymph nodal spread in lateral T_1 and T_2 squamous cell carcinoma of the vulva, *Gynecol Oncol* 55:41, 1994.

Berek JS, Heaps JM, Fu YS et al: Concurrent cisplatin and 5-fluorouracil chemotherapy and radiation therapy for advanced-stage squamous cell carcinoma of the vulva, *Gynecol Oncol* 42:197, 1991.

Binder SW, Huang I, Fu YS et al: Risk factors for the development of lymph node metastasis in vulvar squamous cell carcinoma, *Gynecol Oncol* 37:9, 1990.

Borgno G, Micheletti L, Barbero M: Topographic distribution of groin lymph nodes: a study of 50 female cadavers, *J Reprod Med* 35:1127, 1990.

Boronow RC: Therapeutic alternative to primary exenteration for advanced vulvo-vaginal cancer, *Gynecol Oncol* 1:233, 1973.

Boronow RC, Hickman BT, Reagan MT et al: Combined therapy as an alternative to exenteration for locally advanced vulvovaginal cancer. II. Results, complications and dosimetric and surgical considerations, *Am J Clin Oncol* 10:171, 1987.

Boyce J et al: Prognostic factors in carcinoma of the vulva, *Gynecol Oncol* 20:364, 1985.

Bryson SCP, Dembo AJ, Colgan TJ et al: Invasive squamous cell carcinoma of the vulva: defining low and high risk groups for recurrence, *Int J Gynecol Cancer* 1:25, 1991.

Carson LF, Twiggs LB, Okagaki T et al: Human papillomavirus DNA in adenosquamous carcinoma and squamous cell carcinoma of the vulva, *Obstet Gynecol* 72:63, 1988.

Cavanagh D, Shepherd JH: The place of pelvic exenteration in the primary management of advanced carcinoma of the vulva, *Gynecol Oncol* 13:318, 1982.

Cavanagh D, Fiorica JV, Hoffman MS et al: Invasive carcinoma of the vulva: changing trends in surgical management, *Am J Obstet Gynecol* 163:1007, 1990.

Crosby JH, Bryan AB, Gallup DG et al: Fine-needle aspiration of inguinal lymph nodes in gynecologic practice, *Obstet Gynecol* 73:281, 1989.

Curry SL, Wharton JT, Rutledge F: Positive lymph nodes in the vulvar squamous carcinoma, *Gynecol Oncol* 9:63, 1980.

Daly JW, Million RR: Radical vulvectomy combined with elective node irradiation for T^2N^0 squamous carcinoma of the vulva, *Cancer* 34:161, 1974.

Deppe G, Cohen CJ, Bruckner HW: Chemotherapy of squamous cell carcinoma of the vulva: a review, *Gynecol Oncol* 7:345, 1979.

Donaldson ES et al: Prognostic parameters in invasive vulvar cancer, *Gynecol Oncol* 11:184, 1981.

Ericksson E, Eldh J, Peterson LE: Surgical treatment of carcinoma of the clitoris, *Gynecol Oncol* 17:291, 1984.

Fairey RN et al: Radiation treatment of carcinoma of the vulva, 1950 to 1980, *Am J Obstet Gynecol* 151 (5):591, 1985.

Franklin EW III, Rutledge FN: Prognostic factors in epidermoid carcinoma of the vulva, *Obstet Gynecol* 37:892, 1971.

Franklin EW III, Rutledge FN: Epidemiology of epidermoid carcinoma of the vulva, *Obstet Gynecol* 39:165, 1972.

Green TH: Carcinoma of the vulva; a reassessment, *Obstet Gynecol* 52:462, 1978.

Grimshaw RN, Aswad SG, Monaghan JM: The role of anovulvectomy in locally advanced carcinoma of the vulva, *Int J Gynecol Cancer* 1:15, 1991.

Hacker NF et al: Management of regional lymph nodes and their prognostic influence in vulvar cancer, *Obstet Gynecol* 61:408, 1983.

Hacker NF et al: Preoperative radiation therapy for locally advanced vulvar cancer, *Cancer* 54 (10):2056, 1984.

Hoffman MS, Roberts WS, La Polla JP et al: Carcinoma of the vulva involving the perianal or anal skin, *Gynecol Oncol* 35:215, 1989.

Hoffman MS, Roberts WS, La Polla JP et al: Recent modifications in the treatment of invasive squamous cell carcinoma of the vulva, *Obstet Gynecol Surv* 44:227, 1989.

Homesley HD: Lymph node findings and outcome in squamous cell carcinoma of the vulva, *Cancer* 74:2399, 1994.

Homesley HD et al: Radiation therapy versus pelvic node resection for carcinoma of the vulva with positive groin nodes, *Obstet Gynecol* 68:733, 1986.

Homesley HD et al: Prognostic factors for groin node metastasis in squamous cell carcinoma of the vulva (a Gynecologic Oncology Group Study), *Gynecol Oncol* 49: 279, 1993.

Homesley HD, Bundy BN, Sedlis A et al: Assessment of current International Federation of Gynecology and Obstetrics staging of vulvar carcinoma relative to prognostic factors for survival (a Gynecologic Oncology Group study), *Am J Obstet Gynecol* 164(4):997, 1991.

Hopkins MP, Morley GW: Pelvic exenteration for the treatment of vulvar cancer, *Cancer* 70:2835, 1992.

Hopkins MP, Reid GC, Morley GW: The surgical management of recurrent squamous cell carcinoma of the vulva, *Obstet Gynecol* 75:1001, 1990.

Isaacs JH: Verrucous carcinoma of the female genital tract, *Gynecol Oncol* 4:259, 1976.

Iversen T: The value of groin palpation in epidermoid carcinoma of the vulva, *Gynecol Oncol* 12:291, 1981.

Japaze H, Dinh TV, Woodruff JD: Verrucous carcinoma of the vulva: study of 24 cases, *Obstet Gynecol* 60:462, 1982.

Kaufman RH, Woodruff JD: Historical background in developmental stages of the new nomenclature, *J Reprod Med* 17:133, 1976.

Krupp PJ, Bahm JW: Lymph gland metastases in invasive squamous cell cancer of the vulva, *Am J Obstet Gynecol* 130:943, 1978.

Kurzl R, Messerer D, Baltzer J et al: Comparative morphometric study on the depth of invasion in vulvar carcinoma, *Gynecol Oncol* 29:12, 1988.

Lawhead RA Jr: Vulvar self-examination, *Am J Obstet Gynecol* 158 (5):4, 1988.

Levin W, Goldberg G, Altaras M et al: The use of concomitant chemotherapy and radiotherapy prior to surgery in advanced stage carcinoma of the vulva, *Gynecol Oncol* 25:20, 1986.

Magrina JF et al: Stage I squamous cell cancer of the vulva, *Am J Obstet Gynecol* 134:453, 1979.

Malfetano J, Piver MS, Tsukada Y: Stage III and IV squamous cell of the vulva, *Gynecol Oncol* 23:192, 1986.

Malmström H, Janson H, Simonsen E et al: Prognostic factors in invasive squamous cell carcinoma of the vulva treated with surgery and irradiation, *Acta Oncol* 29:915, 1990.

Morley GW: Infiltrative carcinoma of the vulva: results of surgical treatment, *Am J Obstet Gynecol* 124:874, 1976.

Morley GW: Cancer of the vulva: a review, *Cancer* 48:597, 1981.

Morrow CP, Rutledge FN: Melanoma of the vulva, *Obstet Gynecol* 39:745, 1972.

Nuovo GJ et al: Correlation of histology and detection of human papillomavirus DNA in vulvar cancers, *Gynecol Oncol* 43:275, 1991.

Piura B et al: Recurrent squamous cell carcinoma of the vulva: a study of 73 cases, *Gynecol Oncol* 48:189, 1993.

Piver MS, Xynos FP: Pelvic lymphadenectomy in women with carcinoma of the clitoris, *Obstet Gynecol* 49:592, 1977.

Planner RS, Hobbs JB: Intraepithelial and invasive neoplasia of the vulva in association with human papillomavirus infection, *J Reprod Med* 33:503, 1988.

Podratz KC, Symmonds RE, Taylor WF: Carcinoma of the vulva: analysis of treatment failures, *Am J Obstet Gynecol* 143:340, 1982.

Prempree T, Amornmarn R: Radiation treatment of recurrent carcinoma of the vulva, *Cancer* 54 (9):1943, 1984.

Reid GC, DeLancey JO, Hopkins MP et al: Urinary incontinence following radical vulvectomy, *Obstet Gynecol* 75:852, 1990.

Remmenga S, Barnhill D, Nash J et al: Radical vulvectomy with partial rectal resection and temporary colostomy as primary therapy for selected patients with vulvar carcinoma, *Obstet Gynecol* 77:577, 1991.

Roberts WS, Hoffman MS, La Polla JP et al: Management of radionecrosis of vulva and distant vagina, *Am J Obstet Gynecol* 164:1235, 1991.

Rotmensch J, Rubin SJ, Sutton HG et al: Preoperative radiotherapy followed by radical vulvectomy with inguinal lymphadenectomy for advanced vulvar carcinomas, *Gynecol Oncol* 36:181, 1990.

Rusk D, Sutton GP, Look KY: Analysis of invasive squamous cell carcinoma of the vulva and VIN for the presence of human papilloma DNA, *Obstet Gynecol* 77:918, 1991.

Russell AH et al: Synchronous radiation and cytotoxic chemotherapy for locally advanced or recurrent squamous cancer of the vulva, *Gynecol Oncol* 47, 14, 1992.

Rutledge FN, Mitchell MF, Munsell MF et al: Prognostic indicators for invasive carcinoma of the vulva, *Gynecol Oncol* 42:239, 1991.

Sharma SK, Isaacs JH: Bone metastasis in vulvar carcinoma, *Gynecol Oncol* 20:156, 1985.

Shimm DS et al: Prognostic variables in the treatment of squamous cell carcinoma of the vulva, *Gynecol Oncol* 24:343, 1986.

Siller BS et al: T2/3 Vulva Cancer: A case-control study of triple incision versus *en bloc* radical vulvectomy and inguinal lymphadenectomy, *Gynecol Oncol* 57:335, 1995.

Simonsen E: Invasive squamous cell carcinoma of the vulva, *Ann Chir Gynaecol* 73:331, 1984.

Simonsen E: Treatment of recurrent squamous cell carcinoma of the vulva, *Acta Radiol Oncol* 23:345, 1984.

Sutton GP et al: Trends in the operative management of invasive squamous carcinoma of the vulva at Indiana University, 1974-1988, *Am J Obstet Gynecol* 164:1472, 1991.

Taussig FJ: A study of the lymph glands in cancer of the cervix and cancer of the vulva, *Am J Obstet Gynecol* 36:1319, 1958.

Thomas GM et al: Review; Changing Concepts in the management of vulvar cancer, *Gynecol Oncol* 42:9, 1991.

Way S: The surgery of vulvar carcinoma: an appraisal, *Clin Obstet Gynecol* 5:623, 1978.

Wharton JT, Gallager S, Rutledge FN: Microinvasive carcinoma of the vulva, *Am J Obstet Gynecol* 118:159, 1974.

Early vulvar carcinoma

Barnes AE et al: Microinvasive carcinoma of the vulva: a clinicopathologic evaluation, *Obstet Gynecol* 56:234, 1980.

Berman ML, Soper JT, Creasman WT et al: Conservative surgical management of superficially invasive stage I vulvar carcinoma, *Gynecol Oncol* 35:352, 1989.

Burger MPM et al: The importance of the groin node status for the survival of T1 and T2 vulval carcinoma patients, *Gynecol Oncol* 57:327, 1995.

Burke TW: Changing surgical approaches to vulvar cancer, *Curr Opin Obstet Gynecol* 4:86, 1992.

Burke TW, Stringer CA, Gershenson DM et al: Radical wide excision and selective inguinal node dissection for squamous cell carcinoma of the vulva, *Gynecol Oncol* 38:328, 1990.

Buscema J, Stern JL, Woodruff JD: Early invasive carcinoma of the vulva, *Am J Obstet Gynecol* 140:563, 1981.

Cabanas RM: An approach to the treatment of penile carcinoma, *Cancer* 39:456, 1977.

Choo YC: Invasive squamous carcinoma of the vulva in young patients, *Gynecol Oncol* 13:158, 1982.

Chu J et al: Stage I vulvar cancer: criteria for microinvasion, *Obstet Gynecol* 59:716, 1982.

Degefu S, O'Quinn AG, Dhurandhar HN: Paget's disease of the vulva and urogenital malignancies: a case report and review of the literature, *Gynecol Oncol* 25:347, 1986.

DiPaola GR, Gomez-Rueda N, Arrighi L: Relevance of microinvasion in carcinoma of the vulva, *Obstet Gynecol* 45:647, 1975.

DiSaia PJ, Creasman WT, Rich WM: An alternate approach to early cancer of the vulva, *Am J Obstet Gynecol* 133:825, 1979.

Dvoretsky P et al: The pathology of superficially invasive thin vulvar squamous cell carcinoma, *Int J Gynecol Pathol* 3:331, 1984.

Hacker NF et al: Superficially invasive vulvar cancer with nodal metastases, *Gynecol Oncol* 15:65, 1983.

Hoffman JS, Kumar NB, Morley GW: Microinvasive squamous carcinoma of the vulva: search for a definition, *Obstet Gynecol* 61:615, 1983.

Hughes RP: Early diagnosis and management of premalignant lesions and early invasive cancers of the vulva, *South Med J* 64:1490, 1971.

Iversen T, Aberler V, Aalders J: Individualized treatment of stage I carcinoma of the vulva, *Obstet Gynecol* 57:85, 1981.

Jafari K, Cartnick EN: Microinvasive squamous cell carcinoma of the vulva, *Am J Obstet Gynecol* 125:274, 1976.

Kneale B, Elliott P, Fortune D: Microinvasive carcinoma of the vulva. Proceedings of the International Society for the Study of Vulvar Disease, 7th World Congress, Lake Buena Vista, Florida, 1983, *J Reprod Med* 29(7):454, 1984.

Kunscher AI, Kanbour A, David B: Early vulvar carcinoma, *Am J Obstet Gynecol* 132:599, 1978.

Magrina JF: Microinvasive squamous cell cancer of the vulva. Paper presented to the Society of Gynecologic Oncologists, Scottsdale, Arizona, January, 1979.

Microinvasive cancer of the vulva; Report of the ISSVD Task Force. Proceedings of the International Society for the Study of Vulvar Disease, 6th World Congress, Cambridge, England, 1981, *J Reprod Med* 29:454, 1984.

Nakao CY et al: "Microinvasive" epidermoid carcinoma of the vulva with an unexpected natural history, *Am J Obstet Gynecol* 120:1123, 1974.

Parker RT et al: Operative management of early invasive epidermoid carcinoma of the vulva, *Am J Obstet Gynecol* 123:349, 1975.

Plentl AA, Friedman EA: *Lymphatic system of the female genitalia*, Philadelphia, 1971, WB Saunders.

Podczaski E, Sexton M, Kaminski P et al: Recurrent carcinoma of the vulva after conservative treatment of "microinvasive" disease, *Gynecol Oncol* 39:65, 1990.

Rastkar G et al: Early invasive and in situ warty carcinoma of the vulva: clinical, histologic, and electron microscopic study with particular reference to viral association, *Am J Obstet Gynecol* 143:814, 1982.

Rowley KC, Gallion HH, Donaldson ES et al: Prognostic factors in early vulvar cancer, *Gynecol Oncol* 31:43, 1988.

Sedlis A et al: Positive groin lymph nodes in vulvar cancer with superficial tumor penetration, Society of Gynecologic Oncology, Miami, Feb, 1984.

Sedlis A, Homesley H, Bundy BN et al: Positive groin lymph nodes in superficial squamous cell vulvar cancer: a Gynecologic Oncology Group study, *Am J Obstet Gynecol* 156:1159, 1987.

Stehman FB et al: Early stage I carcinoma of the vulva treated with ipsilateral superficial inguinal lymphadenectomy and modified radical hemivulvectomy: a prospective study of the Gynecologic Oncology Group, *Obstet Gynecol* 79:490, 1992.

Stehman FB et al: Groin dissection versus groin radiation in carcinoma of the vulva: a Gynecologic Oncology Group study, *Int J Radiat Oncol Biol Pty* 24:39, 1992.

Van der Velden J et al: A stage Ia vulvar carcinoma with an inguinal lymph node recurrence after local excision: a case report and literature review, *Int J Gynecol Cancer* 2:157, 1992.

Wilkinson EJ: Superficial invasive carcinoma of the vulva, *Clin Obstet Gynecol* 28(1):188, 1985.

Wilkinson EJ, Rico MJ, Pierson KK: Microinvasive carcinoma of the vulva, *Int J Gynecol Pathol* 1:29, 1982.

Paget's disease

Baehrendtz H et al: Paget's disease of the vulva: the Radiumhemmet series 1975-1990, *Int J Gynecol Cancer* 4:1, 1994.

Balducci L, Athar M, Smith GF et al: Metastatic extramammary Paget's disease: dramatic response to combined modality treatment, *J Surg Oncol* 38:38, 1988.

Bergen S, DiSaia PJ, Liao SY et al: Conservative management of extramammary Paget's disease of the vulva, *Gynecol Oncol* 33:151, 1989.

Besa P et al: Extramammary Paget's disease of the perineal skin: role of radiotherapy, *I J Rad Oncol* 24: 73, 1992.

Creasman WT, Gallager HS, Rutledge F: Paget's disease of the vulva, *Gynecol Oncol* 3:133, 1975.

Curtin JP, Rubin SC, Jones WB et al: Paget's disease of the vulva, *Gynecol Oncol* 39:374, 1990.

DiSaia PJ et al: A report of two cases of recurrent Paget's disease of the vulva in a split-thickness graft and its possible pathogenesis-labeled "retrodissemination," *Gynecol Oncol* 57:109, 1995.

Feuer GA, Shevchuk M, Calanog A: Vulvar Paget's disease: the need to exclude an invasive lesion, *Gynecol Oncol* 38:81, 1990.

Fine BA: Case Report: Minimally invasive Paget's disease of the vulva with extensive lymph node metastases, *Gynecol Oncol* 57:262, 1995.

Fishman DA et al: Extramammary Paget's disease of the vulva, *Gynecol Oncol* 56:266, 1995.

James LP: Aprocrine adenocarcinoma of the vulva with associated Paget's disease, *Acta Cytol* 28:178, 1984.

Stacy D, Burrell MO, Franklin EW: Extramammary Paget's disease of the vulva and anus: use of intraoperative frozen(-)section margins, *Am J Obstet Gynecol* 155:519, 1986.

Tasseron EWK et al: A clinicopathological study of 30 melanomas of the vulva, *Gynecol Oncol* 46:170, 1992.

Taylor PT, Stenwig JT, Klausen H: Paget's disease of the vulva: a report of 18 cases, *Gynecol Oncol* 3:46, 1975.

Voigt H, Bassermann R, Nathrath W: Cytoreductive combination chemotherapy for regionally advanced unresectable extramammary Paget carcinoma, *Cancer* 70:704, 1992.

Watring WG, Roberts JA, Lagasse LD et al: Treatment of recurrent Paget's disease of the vulva with topical bleomycin, *Cancer* 41:10, 1978.

Melanoma

Bailet JW, Figge DC, Tamimi HK et al: Malignant melanoma of the vulva: a case report of distal recurrence in a patient with a superficially invasive primary lesion, *Obstet Gynecol* 70:515, 1987.

Balch CM et al: Efficacy of 2 cm surgical margins for intermediate thickness melanomas (1 to 4 mm): Results of a multi-institutional randomized surgical trial, *Ann Surg* 218:262, 1993.

Blessing K, Kernohan NM, Miller ID et al: Malignant melanoma of the vulva: clinicopathological features, *Int J Gynecol Cancer* 1:81, 1991.

Bradgate MG, Rollason TP, McConkey CC et al: Malignant melanoma of the vulva: a clinicopathological study of 50 women, *Br J Obstet Gynaecol* 97:124, 1990.

Breslow A: Thickness, cross-sectional areas and depth of invasion in the prognosis of cutaneous melanoma, *Ann Surg* 172(5):902, 1970.

Chung AF, Woodruff JM, Lewis JL: Malignant melanoma of the vulva: a report of 44 cases, *Obstet Gynecol* 45:638, 1975.

Clark WH Jr et al: The histogenesis and biologic behaviour of primary human malignant melanomas of the skin, *Cancer Res* 29:705, 1969.

Jaramillo BA et al: Malignant melanoma of the vulva, *Obstet Gynecol* 66(3):398, 1985.

Look KY, Roth LM, Sutton GP: Vulvar melanoma reconsidered, *Cancer* 72:143, 1993.

Morris JM: A formula for selective lymphadenectomy, its application in cancer of the vulva, *Obstet Gynecol* 50:152, 1977.

Morrow CP, DiSaia PJ: Malignant melanoma of the female genitalia: a clinical analysis, *Obstet Gynecol Surv* 31:233, 1976.

Podratz KC et al: Melanoma of the vulva: an update, *Gynecol Oncol* 16:153, 1983.

Rose PG et al: Conservative therapy for melanoma of the vulva, *Am J Obstet Gynecol* 159:52, 1988.

Trimble EL, Lewis JL Jr, Williams LL et al: Radical local excision often sufficient for vulvar melanoma, Management of vulvar melanoma, *Gynecol Oncol* 45:254, 1992.

Veronesi U, Cascinelli N: Narrow excision (1 cm margin): a safe procedure for thin cutaneous melanoma, *Arch Surg* 126:438, 1991.

Sarcoma

Bakri YN et al: Case Report: vulvar sarcoma: a report of four cases, *Gynecol Oncol* 46:384, 1992.

DiSaia PJ, Rutledge FN, Smith JP: Sarcoma of the vulva, *Obstet Gynecol* 38:180, 1971.

Bartholin gland carcinoma

Copeland LJ et al: Adenoid cystic carcinoma of Bartholin gland, *Obstet Gynecol* 67(1):115, 1986.

Copeland LJ et al: Bartholin gland carcinoma, *Obstet Gynecol* 67 (6):794, 1986.

Ghamande SA et al: Case Report: mucinous adenocarcinomas of the vulva, *Gynecol Oncol* 57:117, 1995.

Lelle RJ, Davis KP, Roberts JA: Adenoid cystic carcinoma of the Bartholin's gland: the University of Michigan Experience, *Int J Gynecol Cancer* 3:000, 1993.

Leuchter RS et al: Primary carcinoma of the Bartholin gland: a report of 14 cases and review of the literature, *Obstet Gynecol* 60:361, 1982.

Wheelock JB et al: Primary carcinoma of the Bartholin gland: a report of ten cases, *Obstet Gynecol* 63 (6):820, 1984.

Yazigi R, Piver MS, Tsukada Y: Microinvasive carcinoma of the vulva, *Obstet Gynecol* 123:349, 1975.

Basal cell carcinoma

Winkelmann SE, Llorens AS: Case report: metastatic basal cell carcinoma of the vulva, *Gynecol Oncol* 38:138, 1990.

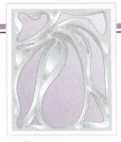

Invasive Cancer of the Vagina and Urethra

Table 9-1   Incidence of vaginal cancer

Series	Number of genital malignancies	Percent vaginal cancer
Smith (1955)	8199	1.5
Ries and Ludwig (1962)	14,785	2.1
Smith (1964)	6050	1.8
Wolff and Douyon (1964)	4665	1.8
Rutledge (1967)	5715	1.2
Palumbo et al. (1969)	2305	1.9
Daw (1971)	564	1.9
Gallup (1987)	not given	3.1
Manetta (1988)	2149	1.3
Eddy (1991)	2929	3.1

SQUAMOUS CANCER OF THE VAGINA
Clinical Profile

It is interesting that there is a greater frequency of malignant disease in the organs situated on either end of the vaginal canal than in the vagina itself. Indeed, one may say that primary cancer of the vagina is one of the rarest of the malignant processes in the human body (Table 9-1). The relative immunity of the vaginal tissues to malignant change is in sharp contrast to that of the uterine cervix. When primary cancer does occur in the vagina, it usually is in the upper half (Table 9-2) and it is generally epidermoid carcinoma. By convention, any malignant neoplasm involving both cervix and vagina that is histologically compatible with origin in either organ is classified as cervical cancer. The age incidence of this disease is between 35 and 90 years (Figure 9-1). If the lesion arises in the upper position of the vagina, extension

Table 9-2   Involvement of vagina

Series	Upper third	Middle third	Lower third
Livingstone (1950)	34	4	42
Bivens (1953)	22	3	14
Mobius (1956)	89	0	29
Arronet, Latour, and Tremblay (1960)	14	8	3
Whelton and Kottmeier (1962)	20	13	19
Blunt (1965)	13	15	10
Daw (1971)	24	14	13
Benedet (1983)	46	3	19
Manetta (1990)	22	8	16
Eddy (1991)	33	5	8
TOTAL	317 (56%)	73 (13%)	173 (31%)

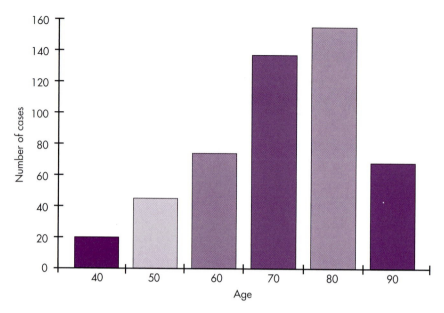

Figure 9-1 Carcinoma of the vagina. Distribution by age. (From *Annual Report Gynecological Cancer FIGO,* vol 22, 1994.)

occurs in much the same pattern as is seen in cervical carcinoma: metastasis to obturator, iliac, and hypogastric lymph nodes is the usual spread pattern. If the lesion is low in the vagina, extension is similar to that observed in carcinoma of the vulva: inguinal nodes are involved early and later extension is to the deep pelvic nodes.

Secondary carcinoma of the vagina is seen much more frequently than primary disease. Extensions of cervical cancer to the vagina probably account for the greatest number of so-called vaginal cancers. In addition, true secondary lesions from more remote foci are not infrequently seen. Examples are cancers of the endometrium, ovary, urethra or bladder, and rectum and malignant trophoblastic disease. Primary lesions are usually in the histologic classification of squamous cell carcinoma. Melanoma, sarcoma, and recently adenocarcinoma have also been described as primary vaginal cancers (Table 9-3). Interest in the possible relationship of DES intrauterine exposure to clear cell adenocarcinoma of the vagina has resulted in the reporting of significant numbers of cases of adenocarcinoma of the vagina in both exposed and unexposed individuals.

The cause of squamous cell carcinoma of the vagina is unknown. The predominance of lesions in the upper third and on the posterior wall of the vagina (Figure 9-2) has led to speculation that an accumulation of irritating or macerating substances pools in the posterior fornix and produces a chronic irritation leading to a malignant degeneration. Reports have been published about possible predisposing factors, such as use of a vaginal pessary, prolapse of the vaginal wall, syphilis, leukorrhea, and "leukoplakia," but none of these hypotheses has been

Table 9-3 Histologic distribution of primary vaginal cancer

Cell type	Percent
Squamous	85
Adenocarcinoma	6
Melanoma	3
Sarcoma	3
Misc	3

validated. In two reports by Manetta, the distribution of lesions (that is, posterior wall vs anterior and lateral) showed no definitive predominance for a posterior site.

It seems logical to assume that some of the factors that promote carcinoma of the cervix may be equally damaging to vaginal epithelium. This thought provokes the controversy as to the value of the Papanicolaou smear for screening patients after hysterectomy for benign disease. Bell reported 87 patients with primary cancer of the vagina, 31 of whom had undergone total hysterectomy for benign disease. Benedet found that 19 of his 97 patients had surgery for benign diseases. Peters reported that 38% (25/68) of his series were patients who had undergone prior hysterectomies for benign disease. Bleeding was the most common symptom in all these series and usually connoted relatively advanced disease. The Papanicolaou smear is effective in detecting vaginal cancer in an asymptomatic patient. The issue then becomes somewhat philosophic and must involve considerations of cost effectiveness. We suggest that smears be done every 2 or 3 years, even in patients who have had hysterectomies for benign disease. This recommendation is made with the assumption that the natural history of vaginal cancer is similar to that of squamous carcinoma of the cervix. This cost-effective recommendation is a compromise over the recommendation for annual screening of cervix cancer.

The signs and symptoms of invasive vaginal cancer are similar to those of cervical cancer. Vaginal discharge, often bloody, is the most frequent symptom in most series. Irregular or postmenopausal vaginal bleeding is the initial symptom in many patients with invasive lesions, and a gross lesion is obvious on speculum examination. Urinary symptoms are more common than with cervical cancer because neoplasms lower in the vagina are close to the vesicle neck with resulting compression of the bladder at an earlier stage of the disease. As the lesion spreads locally, it often involves the paracolpium, bladder, rectum, or vulva. The elasticity of the posterior vaginal fornix allows lesions in this area to become quite large, especially in sexually inactive elderly women. The decreased distensibility of the anterior vaginal wall, creating bladder symptoms, should favor early recognition and curability—however, the reverse is true, possibly because of early involvement of adjacent structures such as the bladder neck and urethra. The diagnosis of vaginal

cancer is usually delayed. Several general explanations have been offered for this observation. Many patients are elderly, sexually inactive, and unlikely to have periodic vaginal examinations. In addition, the lesions are rare, and physicians often fail to consider the possibility until the patient has symptoms of advanced disease.

Lymphatic Drainage of the Vagina

The lymphatic vasculature of the vagina begins as an extremely fine capillary meshwork in the mucosa and submucosa (Figure 9-3). In the deep layers of the submucosa and muscularis, there is a similar, parallel, but coarser network. Irregular anastomoses have been demonstrated between the two. Both systems drain into small trunks that combine at the lateral aspect of the vagina and form a number of collecting trunks. It is at this point that the efferent lymph drainage channels of the organ originate. The lymphatic trunks of the upper vagina drain into the most dorsal group of iliac nodes, usually

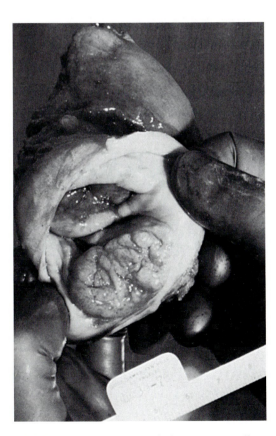

Figure 9-2 Lesion of posterior fornix in squamous cell carcinoma.

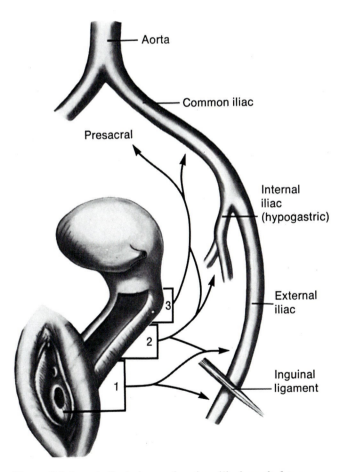

Figure 9-3 Lymphatic drainage of vagina: (1) channels from lower third drain into femoral and external iliac nodes; (2) channels from middle third drain into hypogastric nodes; (3) channels from upper third drain into common iliac, presacral, and hypogastric nodes. (Modified from Plentl AA, Friedman EA: *Lymphatic system of the female genitalia,* Philadelphia, 1971, WB Saunders.)

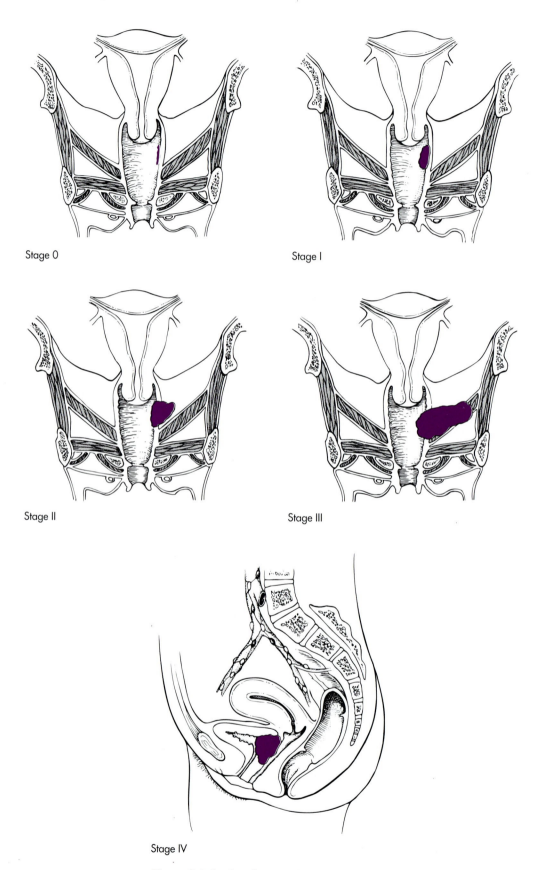

Stage 0

Stage I

Stage II

Stage III

Stage IV

Figure 9-4 Staging diagrams for vaginal cancer.

represented by the common iliac and hypogastric nodes. The distal, or lower, vagina is drained by a lymphatic network that anastomoses with that of the vestibule to end in the regional lymph nodes of the femoral triangle. The lymphatic system of the vagina is complex, and the simple patterns suggested here are not necessarily always accurate. The course and destination of lymphatic channels from specific regions of the vagina are not entirely consistent, and there is a great deal of crossover. All lymph nodes in the pelvis may at one time or another serve as primary sites or regional drainage nodes for vaginal lymph and its contents.

Staging (Figure 9-4)

Patients with invasive squamous cell carcinoma or other cancers of the vagina should be investigated for evidence of local or distant spread in a manner analogous to that of cervical cancer. All patients should have at least the following diagnostic studies in addition to a thorough history and physical examination: chest film, intravenous pyelogram (IVP), cystoscopy, and proctosigmoidoscopy. Optional, but often helpful, studies are lymphangiogram and barium enema. Barium enema is definitely indicated for patients suspected of having recent diverticulitis, since it may be important in planning radiation therapy. Staging according to the International Federation of Gynecology and Obstetrics is clinical and not surgical; a summary of the staging classification follows:

Stage 0   Carcinoma in situ, intraepithelial carcinoma
Stage I   Carcinoma is limited to the vaginal wall
Stage II   Carcinoma has involved the subvaginal tissue but has not extended onto the pelvic wall
Stage III   Carcinoma has extended onto the pelvic wall
Stage IV   Carcinoma has extended beyond the true pelvis or has involved the mucosa of the bladder or rectum; bullous edema or tumor bulge into the bladder or rectum is not acceptable evidence of invasion of these organs
Stage IVa   Spread of the growth to adjacent organs and/or direct extension beyond the true pelvis
Stage IVb   Spread to distant organs

Perez has suggested modification of stage II. Stage IIa lesions would involve the submucosal area of the vagina but not extend into the true paracolpium. Stage IIb lesions would significantly involve the paracolpium but not extend to the pelvic wall. Such classification would usually be an indirect measure of tumor bulk and may have relevance to prognosis and response. Involvement of the pubic symphysis will place a patient in the Stage III category.

Management

Cases of squamous cell carcinoma reported in the gynecologic literature have been treated primarily by radiotherapy. Treatment is tailored to the stage and extent of the disease. Large carcinomas of the vault or vaginal walls are treated initially with external irradiation. This shrinks the neoplasm so that local radiation therapy will be more effective. Cancers of the upper portion of the vagina in patients with intact uteri are treated with techniques similar to those used for carcinoma of the cervix. External irradiation in a dose of 4000 to 5000 cGy is given initially in bulky stage I and stage II cancers (Table 9-4). In some centers, on completion of external therapy, vaginal ovoids and an intrauterine tandem (Fletcher-Suit or similar applicators) are used to deliver a surface dose of 6000 cGy in 72 hours or 8000 cGy in two applications of 48 hours each separated by 2 weeks, depending on the initial thickness and regression of the lesion. An interstitial implant is considered by others to be judicious instead of, or in combination with, the intracavitary technique just described. If the uterus has been removed, local therapy must be individualized, and one should consider the following: (1) ovoids, (2) transvaginal cone, and (3) interstitial implant. Stage III and stage IV lesions anywhere in the vagina are treated initially with 5000 cGy external radiation during a period of 5 to 6 weeks. The deep nodes must of course be included in the treatment fields, since large tumors have a high incidence of regional lymphatic metastasis. After receiving 5000 cGy, the patient should be reevaluated for an additional 1000 to 2000 cGy external radiation to reduced fields. An

Table 9-4 Radiotherapy of vaginal cancer

Stage	External irradiation	Vaginal therapy
Stage 0	Surgical excision perferred for localized disease	7000 cGy surface dose
Stage I		
1-2 cm lesion	Omit	Interstitial irradiation, 6000-7000 cGy
Larger lesions	4000-5000 cGy whole pelvis	Interstitial implant delivering 3000-4000 cGy
Stage II	4000-5000 cGy whole pelvis	Same as above
Stage III	5000 cGy whole pelvis (optional 1000-2000 cGy through reduced fields)	Interstitial implant, 2000-3000 cGy (if tumor regression is satisfactory)
Stage IV (pelvis only)	Same as above	Same as above

interstitial implant in the residual disease is usually needed for large neoplasms. A large-volume implant is often best delivered using a Syed/Neblett applicator (Figure 9-5) and its accompanying perineal template (Figure 9-6) to achieve a comprehensive isodose distribution (Figure 9-7) to the paracolpium. Tumors involving the distal one third of the vagina frequently metastasize to the inguinal nodes, and these nodes are best treated by radical inguinal dissection before radiation therapy. Postoperative radiation can be delivered to the whole pelvis (and inguinal areas if necessary) following inguinal lymphadenectomy. Small carcinomas of the vagina may be treated with interstitial radiation therapy alone; a single or double plane or even a volume implant may be necessary, depending on the location of the cancer. In most instances a minimum of 6000 to 7000 cGy is delivered to the neoplasm in 5 to 7 days.

For patients who have lesions involving the upper half, especially the upper third, of the vagina after hysterec-

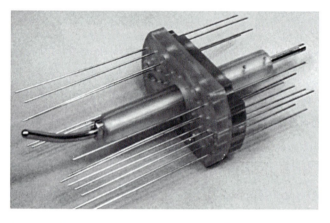

Figure 9-5 Interstitial-intracavitary implant (Syed/Neblett applicator).

tomy, serious consideration should be given to an "open implant." A laparotomy is done to remove loops of small bowel and other structures that may have adhered to the apex of the vagina after previous pelvic surgery. With the patient in stirrups, simultaneous access to the vagina and the perineum enables optimum guidance of needles for a volume implant during the laparotomy. The laparotomy also provides opportunity for the creation of an "omental carpet" (Figures 9-8 and 9-9) that can be brought into the pelvis to act as bolus between the implant and the viscera and also provide a new source of blood supply to the irradiated tissue at the vaginal cuff. We think this approach results in more effective dosimetry and diminishes complications for lesions involving the upper portion of the vagina after hysterectomy.

In general, the radiation therapy plan must reflect consideration of the depth of invasion of the lesion. Lesions with appreciable invasion of the paracolpium must be treated with whole-pelvis irradiation followed by an interstitial implant in the tumor bed. As stated earlier, some physicians prefer intracavitary vaginal applicators to deliver the local radiation. However, interstitial therapy should be strongly considered for most patients, since surface applicators deliver a poor depth dose to the submucosal tissue. An exception to the earlier recommendations may be valid in institutions where skilled personnel can give transvaginal external irradiation instead of interstitial irradiation to shallow residual lesions. Although one is often dealing with a radiosensitive neoplasm in a relatively radioresistant bed (the vagina), serious limitations may nonetheless exist. The proximity of relatively radiosensitive normal tissues, such as the bladder and rectum, provides a real challenge to the therapist, especially in the treatment of tumors located in the lower third of the vagina. Proper planning of radiation therapy and individualization of treatment plans are

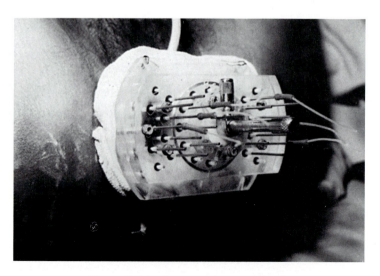

Figure 9-6 Implant procedure completed.

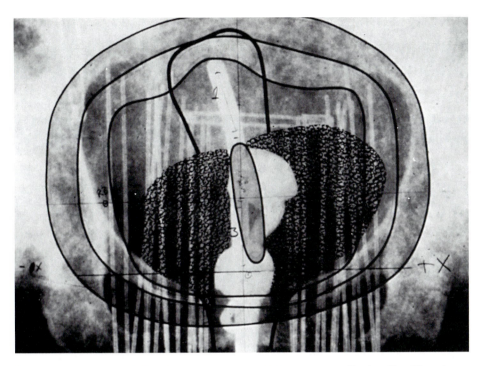

Figure 9-7 Computerized dose distribution plot overlaid on x-ray localization film. There is extensive involvement of parametria and paracolpium.

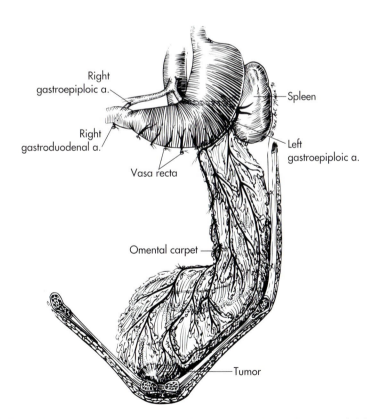

Figure 9-8 Development of omental carpet with transection of the right gastroepiploic artery and placement along the descending colon into the pelvis. (From DiSaia PJ et al: Malignant neoplasia of the upper vagina, *Endocurie/Hypertherm Oncol* 6:251, 1990.)

essential to minimize the more serious complications of acute and long-term radiation sequelae in these organs. The difficulty in applying radiation systems to vaginal cancer led some, like Wertheim and Brunschwig, to advocate radical surgery as primary therapy. However, the complications associated with these radical procedures, especially in older patients, have become a serious limiting factor to the surgical approach. Our belief is that in most instances radical surgery should be reserved for radiation failures. The incidence of complications follow-

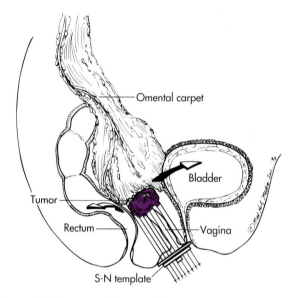

Figure 9-9 Placement of omental tissue around the apex of the vagina containing neoplasm after reflecting the bladder and the rectum. (From DiSaia PJ et al: Malignant neoplasia of the upper vagina, *Endocurie/Hypertherm Oncol* 6:251, 1990.)

ing irradiation therapy is relatively low. Serious complications occur in about 10% of patients and consist primarily of rectal stenosis, rectovaginal fistulae, and severe rectal bleeding requiring diversion. As many as 35% of patients experience cystitis or proctitis during or shortly after therapy but symptoms usually resolve spontaneously. A few patients have extensive vaginal necrosis that usually resolves with prolonged conservative management.

Survival Results

The number of patients who survive vaginal cancer has increased to a point where the pessimism detailed in the older literature can be abandoned (Figure 9-10). In a review of 104 patients Smith (1964) found 6.8% survivors among 29 patients with cancer of the lower third of the vagina, 25% in 48 patients with middle-third tumors, and 37% in 27 patients with upper-third lesions. In 1958 Merrill and Bender reported a 29% survival rate in 14 patients with upper-third lesions and an 11% rate in 9 patients with distal-third involvement. A more encouraging study by Rutledge in 1967 reported 3- and 5-year survival rates of 42% and 44%, respectively, for patients treated primarily with radiotherapy. Comparable survival results at 5 years were reported by Prempree et al. who used radiotherapy for stage I (83%), stage II (63%), stage III (40%), and stage IV (0%) lesions. Their absolute 5-year cure rate for all stages was 55.5%. A more encouraging report from the Rutledge service (MD Anderson Hospital) by Krepart et al. reveals considerable improvement, especially in early lesions (Table 9-5). This is confirmed by Eddy, who reported on 84 patients with primary vaginal carcinoma. Of these patients, 25 (29%)

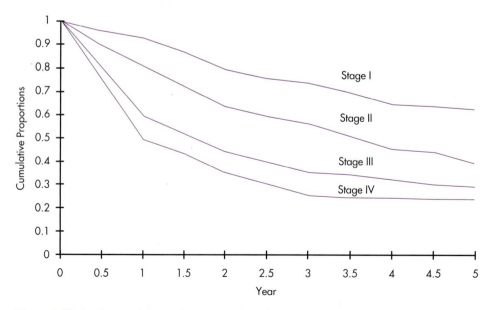

Figure 9-10 Carcinoma of the vagina. Actuarial survival by stage. Cumulative proportion surviving. (From *Annual Report Gynecologic Cancer FIGO*, vol 22, 1994.)

had prior total hysterectomies and an additional 3 patients (3%) had prior subtotal hysterectomies. There was a previous history of radiation therapy in 15% and/or invasive cervical cancer in 23% of the patients. Detection of cancer was accomplished by routine cytology in 19% of the cases, palpation of an asymptomatic mass in 12%, or palpation of a symptomatic mass in 9%. Seventy-five percent of the patients were treated with irradiation therapy (survival figures are shown in Table 9-5).

In 1982 Perez and Camel reported their long-term follow-up of patients treated with radiation therapy for invasive carcinoma of the vagina. The actuarial disease-free 5-year survival rate for stage I (39 patients) was 90%; stage IIa (39 patients), 58%; stage IIb (21 patients), 32%; stage III (12 patients), 40%; and stage IV (8 patients), 0%. Of 39 patients with stage I carcinoma, 37 (95%) showed no evidence of vaginal or pelvic recurrence. Most of them received interstitial or intracavitary therapy or both; the addition of external beam irradiation did not significantly increase survival or tumor control. In stage IIa (para-vaginal extension) 22 of 34 (64.7%) patients were controlled with a combination of brachytherapy and external beam irradiation; only 2 of 5 (40%) treated with brachytherapy alone exhibited tumor control in the pelvis. The incidence of complications was 9.7% for all stages.

In 1991 Reddy published similar results for stage I and stage II lesions of the vagina treated with curative radiotherapy and reported a 5-year survival of 78% for stage I and 71% for stage II patients. In addition, Stock (1995) reported local control rates of 72% for stage I and 62% for stage II disease (Table 9-6).

Recurrence

These neoplasms appear to behave like cervical or vulvar epidermoid cancer by first recurring locally. More than 80% of patients with recurrent disease have pelvic recurrence noted clinically, and most recurrences appear within 2 years of primary therapy. Distant sites of involvement occur later and much less frequently. Recurrent or persistent vaginal cancer requires ultraradical surgery of an exenterative type, and little has been written specifically on this subject. Krepart reported a 51% overall recurrence rate in a series on vaginal cancers, and 40% of the patients with recurrent or persistent disease responded (apparent cures) when radical surgical procedures were done. Therefore radiation therapy should be planned carefully, and the therapist should prepare for reevaluation of the patient during therapy for possible alterations in the treatment plan to give optimal results. Reuben reported on the grave prognoses of a series of patients who had recurrences of vaginal carcinoma. Of 33 patients with tumors that recurred, 30 died of disease. The average length of survival from recurrence was 8 months. Of the 33 patients, 18 had pelvic disease recurrence and 15 had extrapelvic disease recurrence. In the past, chemotherapy for recurrent squamous cell carcinoma of the vagina has been relatively ineffective, but cisplatin appears to be an effective agent when used in a manner similar to that used for recurrent cervical cancer.

Thigpen reported on 16 patients with squamous cell carcinoma of the vagina treated in a phase II study of cisplatin, 50 mg/m^2 intravenously every 3 weeks. The results were disappointing. There was only one responder, and this was a complete responder who had extrapelvic disease and who had received no prior therapy. Most of the patients with recurrence in previously irradiated fields showed no response; 5 of the remaining 15 patients had stable disease.

Special Problems

Brown et al. reported no new cases of in situ and/or invasive carcinoma of the vagina developing after radiation therapy for carcinoma in situ or early invasive carcinoma. Their report discouraged overt aggressive therapy for early-stage tumors because of the good prognosis for these lesions and the adverse effects of

Table 9-5   Vaginal cancer—comparison of survival

Authors	Number of cases	Stage and survival				
		I	II	III	IV	All stages
Krepart (1979)	14	65%	60%	35%	39%	51%
Nori et al. (1981)	36	71%	66%	33%	0%	42%
Perez (1982)	105	81%	42%	30%	9%	50%
Prempree (1982)	80	78%	57%	39%	0%	8%
Puthawala et al. (1983)	27	100%	75%	22%	0%	56%
Benedet et al. (1983)	75	71%	50%	15%	0%	45%
Reuben (1985)	68	79%	52%	54%	0%	49%
Gallup et al. (1987)	28	100%	50%	0%	25%	42.8%
Eddy (1991)	84	70%	45%	35%	28%	50%
Stock (1995)	100	67%	53%	0%	15%	46%

Table 9-6 1° Vaginal carcinoma local control and disease-free survival by stage

| FIGO stage | # | Five years | |
		Local control (%)	DFS (%)
I	23	72	67
II	58	62	53
III	9	0	0
IV	10	21	15

Stock RG et al: A 30 year experience in the management of primary carcinoma of the vagina: analysis of prognostic factors and treatment modalities, *Gyn Onc* 56:45, 1995.

high-dose irradiation on the pliability of the vagina and on sexual function. Lee and Symmonds reported the results in 66 patients treated previously with wide local excisions or partial vaginectomies and in patients with multicentric disease treated with total vaginectomies (7 patients). Only 1 patient had recurrent carcinoma of the vagina resulting in her death. Thus options for therapy exist, and treatment for each patient should be individualized: age, level of sexual activity, and patient preference are often deciding factors. In the young, sexually active patient with diffuse involvement of the vaginal epithelium, total or subtotal vaginectomy with split-thickness skin graft reconstruction of the vagina often allows for excellent long-term results.

When radiation therapy is chosen, patients who have carcinoma in situ and superficial stage I tumors can be treated with intracavitary insertion alone. For invasive carcinoma thicker than 0.5 cm and localized to one wall, the addition of an interstitial single-plane implant enhances the probability of tumor control without exposing all the mucosa to excessive doses.

Peters has described superficially invasive squamous cell carcinoma of the vagina as a lesion that invades less than 2.5 mm from the surface, is lacking involvement of lymph-vascular spaces, and is developed in a field of carcinoma in situ. His experience with six patients suggests that local therapy was sufficient, and no attempt was made to treat pelvic nodes either surgically or with irradiation. Our experience with a similar small group of patients has been the same, and we continue to favor surgical excision as treatment of choice for early focal lesions of the vagina. This experience, if confirmed by others, might allow for preservation of optimum sexual function in young patients who have these very early invasive squamous and adenocarcinoma lesions.

Perez and Camel reported on 15 patients with in situ carcinoma; 14 were controlled with interstitial or intracavitary therapy. Clement and Benedet reported a case of adenocarcinoma of the vagina in a 40-year-old woman with a negative history for intrauterine DES exposure.

The lesion was diagnosed 15 months after hysterectomy for in situ squamous cell carcinoma and in situ adenocarcinoma of the cervix. The lesion was successfully treated by wide local excision.

Pride and Buchler suggested that vaginal carcinoma may occur more frequently in patients who received pelvic irradiation 10 or more years before the appearance of the new lesion. Of patients previously treated for cervical cancer, those who had received radiation therapy (5 or more years previously) were more likely to develop vaginal cancer than those whose cervical cancers had been treated surgically, according to Murad et al. The occurrence of abnormal vaginal cytologic findings after radiation is common, and many have ignored these dysplastic lesions as if they were routine results of irradiation therapy. However, material from the MD Anderson Hospital suggests that 30% of these "dysplastic" or "intraepithelial" lesions will progress to invasive cancer if left untreated. In this report, 28 patients with dysplasia or carcinoma in situ of the vagina after previous pelvic radiation therapy were observed for progression, and 9 developed invasive carcinoma. The median length of time from diagnosis of the intraepithelial lesion to invasion was 33.7 months. Therefore treatment of these intraepithelial lesions by local excision, laser vaporization, or topical chemotherapy with 5-fluorouracil should be seriously considered.

Boronow emphasized the possible role of radiation therapy in vulvovaginal cancers. His report dealt mostly with advanced disease involving a great deal of vaginal mucous membrane, as well as the vulva, necessitating an exenterative type of procedure if a primary surgical approach was used. As an alternative, he recommended surgical extirpation of the inguinal lymph nodes with a combination of external and interstitial irradiation for control of the central lesion. His results were encouraging, showing a 5-year survival rate of 75%. In 1981 Philips et al. published a report of 16 patients with vulvovaginal carcinoma treated by pelvic exenteration. There was a 5-year cure rate of 44% overall and 50% in the four patients with only vaginal disease. We agree with Boronow's comments in the discussion of this report by Phillips et al. in which a plea is made for preferring treatment plans that preserve bladder and/or rectum. When the lower portion of the vagina and/or vulva is involved, surgical resection of the groin nodes should precede radiation therapy. In Boronow's report 4 of 9 patients with surgically proven positive groin nodes survived for 5 years.

In vaginal cancer of a hysterectomized patient, the geometry is usually unfavorable for local radiation therapy. In addition, the proximity of the bladder base and urethra makes the risks of a urinary-vaginal fistula appreciable (Figure 9-11). Therapy must be individualized, and radical surgery should be reserved for failures. The radiotherapist must be flexible, using combinations

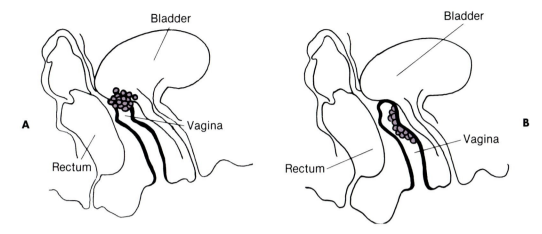

Figure 9-11 Diagrammatic representation of typical locations of vaginal cancer in previously hysterectomized patient illustrating proximity of bladder and urethra. **A,** Lesion at vaginal apex. **B,** Lesion at upper anterior vaginal wall. (Courtesy Dr. A Robert Kagan, Los Angeles, California.)

of external radiation with transvaginal and/or interstitial and/or intracavitary therapy as necessary. For large lesions involving the upper portion of the vagina, serious consideration should be given to using the "open implant" technique described previously.

Kanbour et al. reported on a 25-year experience with vaginal carcinoma at Magee Women's Hospital, where there were 51 cases of invasive disease and 23 cases of carcinoma in situ. Of the 23 cases of in situ carcinoma of the vagina, 16 (70%) were synchronous with or subsequent to cervical cancer; of the 51 cases with invasive disease, 14 (27%) had concurrent or antecedent cervical cancer. This striking high frequency of vaginal cancer in association with cervical neoplasia emphasizes the multicentric occurrence of carcinoma in the female lower genital tract.

RARE VAGINAL CANCERS
Adenocarcinoma/Clear Cell Adenocarcinoma

Before 1965, clear cell adenocarcinoma of the cervix in women under the age of 30 was reported only rarely, and vaginal clear cell adenocarcinoma was seemingly unknown (Figure 9-12). In April 1970, Herbst and Scully reported seven cases of primary vaginal adenocarcinoma in females between the ages of 15 and 22 years. These seven cases exceeded the number of cases in the world literature in adolescent females born before 1945. Because of this case clustering, an epidemiologic study of the patients and their families was initiated to identify associative factors. With the addition of another patient to the study, it was discovered that the mothers of seven of the eight patients with vaginal adenocarcinoma had been treated with diethylstilbestrol (DES), a nonsteroidal synthetic estrogen, in the first trimester of the relevant pregnancy. Since that time, additional cases of vaginal and cervical adenocarcinoma have been reported in patients whose mothers ingested nonsteroidal estrogen during pregnancy. DES and related drugs were used to support high-risk pregnancy and reduce fetal wastage in the mid-1940s and 1950s, but their use then declined. As of 1992, 594 cases of vaginal and cervical (approximately 40% involve the cervix) adenocarcinoma have been accessioned by the registry established by Herbst and colleagues. Among the cases in which a maternal history was obtainable, the proportion that were positive for medication with DES or chemically related estrogens was two out of three. Similarly, one of ten histories has been positive for an unknown medication prescribed for a high-risk pregnancy; one of four has been negative. In six of the cases, progestins had been administered and in another three cases, a steroidal estrogen had been administered.

The youngest patient was 7 years of age at the time of diagnosis, and the oldest patient was 42 years old, with a peak frequency at the age of 19 years for patients with a history of DES exposure (Figure 9-13). The risk of development of these carcinomas in the DES-exposed female through the age of 24 years has been estimated to be 0.14 to 1.4 per 1000. About 68% of the individuals with clear cell adenocarcinoma of the cervix had a history of hormone exposure, and 86% of those with primary vaginal tumors. The incidence of cervical and vaginal lesions combined has decreased markedly since the peak of 31 cases reported in 1975.

A careful study has been done of cases in which details were available concerning the administration of DES to the mothers of afflicted daughters. A wide variation existed in both dose and duration of DES treatment. In some cases the total dose was far less than 500 mg; in other instances it exceeded 15,000 mg. In one case the dose was 1.5 mg daily; in others the dose was more than

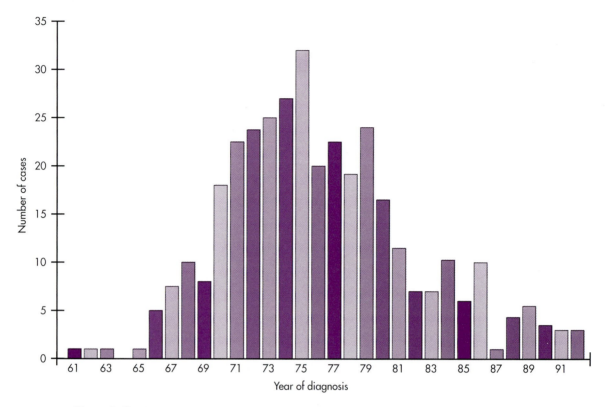

Figure 9-12 Histogram of number of cases by year of diagnosis (n = 361). (From Mittendorf R, Herbst AL: Diethylstilbestrol: an update. In DeVita VT Jr, editor: *Cancer Prevention*, Philadelphia, 1992, Lippincott.)

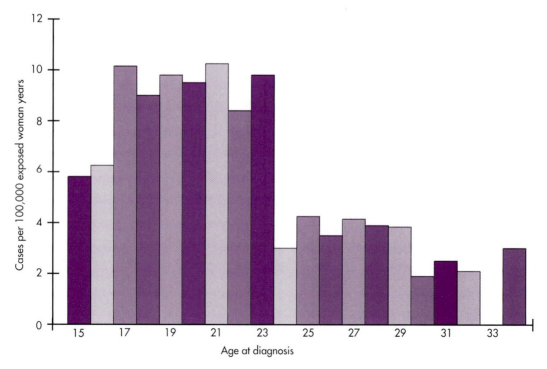

Figure 9-13 Histogram of age incidence of CCA for DES-daughters. (From Mittendorf R, Herbst AL: Diethylstilbestrol: an update. In DeVita VT Jr, editor: *Cancer Prevention*, Philadelphia, 1992, Lippincott.)

200 mg daily. It has not been possible to correlate the dose or the duration of treatment with the incidence or pattern of cancer in the cases studied. However, in all cases with accurate treatment dates the drug was begun before the eighteenth week of pregnancy. There was a lower risk for cancer among women whose mothers began diethylstilbestrol after the twelfth week of pregnancy. It is not known how many exposed females are in the United States, but estimates place this population at 0.5 to 2 million. Ninety percent of the cases have occurred in patients 14 years of age or older.

Data do not substantiate that DES intrauterine exposure is a carcinogenic event. A large body of evidence, however, suggests that such an exposure may be teratogenic with increased adenosis and other uterine anomalies. The elevated rate of prior spontaneous abortion and a history of vaginal bleeding during pregnancy among the mothers whose daughters developed clear cell adenocarcinoma raise the possibility that an inherited genetic predisposing factor may have a role in some of these cases. A higher frequency of birth weight less than 5½ pounds in the cancer cases compared with the DESAD (National Collaborative Diethylstilbestrol Adenosis Project) controls may also suggest maternal complications as predisposing factors in cancer development or an inherent disadvantage of premature babies to resist subsequent carcinogenic factors such as viral infection. In addition, analyses of month of birth show a prevalence of fall births in the cancer cases, whether compared with births of the DESAD controls or with the birth-month distribution expected from the United States census figures. Patients born in the fall were conceived primarily in the winter months, during the prevalence of influenza virus. Viruses have been associated with some cancers, and animal studies suggest immunologic deficiency after diethylstilbestrol exposure in rodents. Thus a viral role in clear cell adenocarcinoma is suggested but these data at this time do not permit more than speculation in regard to a potential role. It is also possible that these observed differences, and even that of DES exposure, are artifactual and not indicative of any influence on the development of clear cell adenocarcinoma. One important possibility is that the susceptibility bias itself, which incidentally resulted in the use of the drug for the problem pregnancy, is a prime source of the observed effect in the case-controlled studies. With the decreasing incidence apparent in recent years, many of these questions may go unanswered.

Oral contraceptive use was analyzed in 339 cases. The survival rate of current users was somewhat higher than that of nonusers: 90% vs 80%. Further evaluation of the data, however, showed a higher proportion of stage I cases among the current users (73% vs 35%), and this finding could account for their improved survival. Also, 39% of oral contraceptive users had their tumors detected at routine screening examinations in comparison to 14% of nonusers. Thus medical surveillance appears to have led to the detection of a higher proportion of low-stage tumors in oral contraceptive users, resulting in improved survival.

Patients 15 years of age and younger appeared to have more aggressive carcinomas than those 19 years of age and older. Abnormal bleeding was the initial symptom in most of the patients, but 20% were asymptomatic, and carcinomas were discovered on routine pelvic examinations. Cytologic testing has proved useful, but a false negative rate of up to 20% has been reported, probably because of the heavy polymorphonuclear infiltration seen with these lesions. The carcinomas may occur anywhere on the vagina or cervix, but most have been in the upper part of the vagina, particularly on the anterior wall (Figure 9-14). Adenosis (the presence of glandular epithelium or its mucinous products in the vagina) has been found accompanying vaginal clear cell adenocarcinoma in virtually all cases. Adenosis is benign tissue, but it may be the nonneoplastic precursor of the clear cell adenocarcinoma in some cases, although direct transitions from adenosis to cancer have not been identified. The same observations apply to cervical eversion (ectropion, "congenital erosion") and clear cell adenocarcinoma of the cervix. Both vaginal adenosis and cervical eversion are very common in DES-exposed females, in contrast to the rare carcinomas. Therefore these lesions are benign, with minimal, if any, potential for transformation into adenocarcinoma. Both surgery and radiation have been effective in treating these tumors (Table 9-7), although many patients have been followed for fewer than 5 years. The optimal therapy for clear cell carcinoma of the cervix and vagina has not been established. Incidence of lymph node metastases is fairly high, with approximately 16% in stage I and 30% or more in stage II. The neoplasm tends to remain superficial, suggesting the possibility that this disease can be treated locally, especially if the lesion is small. It has been reported that a few very small lesions have been treated by local excision and/or local interstitial irradiation alone with good results and subsequent pregnancies.

The Registry for Research on Hormonal Transplacental Carcinogenesis has reported a study examining the effectiveness of various forms of therapy for early-stage vaginal clear cell adenocarcinomas. Of 219 stage I vaginal clear cell adenocarcinomas, 20% received local therapy and 80% underwent conventional therapy. Actuarial survival rates at 5 and 10 years for patients managed with local therapy (92% and 88%) and conventional therapy are equivalent. This study indicates that for certain early cancers local therapy, which can conserve reproductive function, is an effective mode. Another recent study showed that pregnancy does not appear to affect the prognosis or behavior of clear cell adenocarcinoma. However, one instance of pelvic node metastases has been reported in a patient with less than 3 mm of

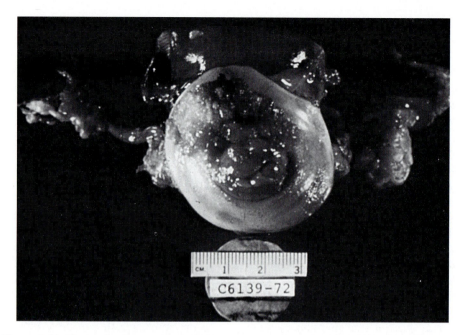

Figure 9-14 Clear cell adenocarcinoma (radical hysterectomy and upper gavinectomy specimen). Note involvement of cervix and anterior wall of upper vagina.

Table 9-7 **Suggested management of clear cell adenocarcinoma of the cervix and vagina**

Stage	Surgery	Radiation
Cervix		
Ib	Radical hysterectomy with clear vaginal margins and bilateral pelvic lymphadenectomy	5000 cGy WP* in patients with positive pelvic nodes
IIa	Radical hysterectomy with bilateral pelvic lymphadenectomy and upper vaginectomy	5000 cGy WP in patients with positive pelvic nodes
IIb	Consider exenteration for radiation failures	5000 cGy WP tandem and ovoids
IIIa and b	Consider exenteration for radiation failures	6000 cGy WP tandem and ovoids
IV	Individualize	
Vagina		
I (upper one third of vagina)	Radical hysterectomy with bilateral pelvic lymphadenectomy and upper vaginectomy	5000 cGy WP in patients with positive pelvic nodes
I (lower two thirds of vagina)	Radical hysterectomy with bilateral pelvic lymphadenectomy and total vaginectomy with vaginal reconstruction	5000 cGy WP vaginal application or interstitial implant
II	Consider exenteration for radiation failures	5000 cGy WP interstitial implant
III	Consider exenteration for radiation failures	6000 cGy WP interstitial implant
IV	Individualize	

*WP, Whole pelvis.

invasion. If the growth is confined to the cervix or upper vagina, or both, radical hysterectomy with upper vaginectomy and pelvic lymphadenectomy with retention of the ovaries is the recommended therapy. In young patients, avoidance of pelvic radiation is desirable in view of the increased risks of long-term morbidity (radiation-induced carcinogenesis and progressive vasculitis) in patients surviving many decades after full-dose pelvic irradiation and the possible decrease of optimal vaginal function. More extensive tumors and lesions involving the lower two thirds of the vagina are more suitable for radiation, which would include the pelvic nodes and parametrial tissues. Although some experienced surgeons have used radical hysterectomy with total vaginectomy and split-thickness skin graft vaginal reconstruction in this group of patients, we are dissatisfied with the surgical margins (especially on the bladder) of this procedure and have followed the radiation therapy techniques of Wharton et al. from the MD Anderson Hospital in Houston, Texas. At our institutions, radical pelvic surgery (exenteration) is reserved for radiation failures in patients with central persistence of the neoplasm and involvement of the lower two thirds of the vagina. In 1979 Herbst et al. reported a discouraging 37% recurrence rate among 22 patients treated by conventional irradiation, but 21 of these 22 patients had large vaginal adenocarcinomas and probably would not have been good surgical candidates for vaginectomy.

Because of the wide differences in treatment from one institution to another, the comparative efficacy of the various approaches is difficult to evaluate. Transvaginal local excision of stage I vaginal adenocarcinoma, which is associated with higher recurrence rates than are transabdominal approaches, appears to be an inferior treatment. Some institutions have attempted treatment with radiation transvaginal cone and/or implant, especially for small vaginal tumors following local excision. The identification of the risk of pelvic lymph node spread, even in cases of small stage I tumors, led to the recommendation that retroperitoneal node dissection should be carried out before the local treatment. Currently Herbst's registry files contain data on 76 individuals who have had varying combinations of local treatment; 7 have subsequently borne children. These cases must be individualized, and the patient must accept the increased risk of recurrence.

Survival is stage related, and the follow-up of many of the cases is still too short for calculating a meaningful 5-year survival rate or for comparing the efficiency of various modes of therapy at this time. However, follow-up of 588 patients for periods up to 15 years yielded an actuarial 5-year survival rate of 80% (Table 9-8). Survival percentages are highly correlated with tumor stage. The following percentages were found for patients at these stages: stage I, 91%; stage II vaginal, 82%; stage IIa cervical, 80%; stage IIb cervical, 56%; stage III, 37%. The overall survival rate of 80% is somewhat better than the 65% crude survival rate reported for squamous cell carcinoma of the cervix and much higher than the 35%-45% overall survival rate reported for squamous cell carcinoma of the vagina. The better prognosis might be the result of early detection, since it is occurring mainly in young patients exposed to DES.

Recurrences of Clear Cell Adenocarcinoma

Two cases of recurrence were observed 7 years after apparently successful treatment; this emphasizes the importance of prolonged follow-up of these patients. It appears that a higher proportion of clear cell adenocarcinomas metastasize to the lungs and supraclavicular area than of squamous cell carcinomas of the vagina and cervix.

Table 9-8   Five- and ten-year survival rates for 588 patients with clear cell adenocarcinoma of the vagina and cervix by stage

Stage	5-year survival (%)	10-year survival (%)
I	91	85
IIa	80	67
IIb	56	47
II (vagina)	82	67
III	37	25
IV	0	0

Herbst AL: Neoplastic diseases of the vagina. In Mishell Dr Jr et al., (eds): *Comprehensive Gynecology*, ed. 3, St. Louis: Mosby-Year Book, 1997.

In a study by Herbst et al. in 1979, 346 patients were analyzed for frequency, site, and treatment of recurrent disease. Twenty of the 346 were never free of disease after initial therapy, and 19 had died at the time of the report. Fifty-eight patients had recurrences; most of these were diagnosed within 3 years after primary tumor treatment. Sixty percent had recurrence in the pelvis, almost half of these being in the vagina. Twenty-one patients (36%) had recurrence in the lungs, and 12 (20%) had recurrence in the supraclavicular lymph nodes. Surgery and radiation have been effective in the control of pelvic recurrences in some cases. The results of chemotherapy have generally been disappointing. Isolated responses to individual cytotoxic agents have been noted, but there are no documented objective responses with the use of progestational agents. In most cases no response was observed. Objective responses (greater than 50% reduction of tumor size for longer than 3 months) were observed in 8 out of 34 cases in which chemotherapy regimens were analyzed. Two patients who received doxorubicin (Adriamycin) had objective remissions, but in one of these an alkylating agent was also given. Two patients who received combination chemotherapy (5-FU, methotrexate, vincristine, cyclophosphamide [Cytoxan], and prednisolone; and 5-FU, dactinomycin, and cyclophosphamide) also had objective remissions. No total remissions were observed. There were no responses in 9 cases in which a progestational agent alone was used.

In a 1983 report by Herbst from the Registry for Research on Hormonal Transplacental Carcinogenesis, follow-up data of 409 patients for periods up to 15 years were published. In this study 55 patients had an initial recurrence in the pelvis (60% of the total group with recurrence) up to 7 years after initial therapy. This emphasizes the importance of prolonged follow-up. Of the 58 patients with recurrences, 12 survived 3 or more years after treatment of their first recurrence. A second recurrence was observed in 17 of the patients, and 12 of them died within 1 year of the diagnosis. However, 3 patients had survived more than 2 years after treatment of their second recurrence.

Primary adenocarcinoma of the vagina can occur, in both premenopausal and postmenopausal women, unrelated to intrauterine DES exposure. Some cases that were thought to have arisen in association with vaginal adenosis or from foci of endometriosis generally resembled endocervical or endometrial carcinomas. Because of their content of clear cells, others were considered to be of mesonephric origin. A few exceptional cases may have arisen from Gartner duct remnants and thus may have truly been mesonephric in origin. These have been recognized and reported more frequently in the last two decades because of the DES disclosures. Therapy for these adenocarcinomas is presently analogous to that for their squamous counterpart.

Vaginal metastases from adenocarcinoma of other pelvic and abdominal organs are not uncommon. Lesions of cervical and endometrial origin are most common. Ovary, tube, colon, and rectum, as well as renal cell neoplasms, can also be present with vaginal metastasis.

Malignant Melanoma

Malignant melanoma of the vagina is rare and comprises less than 0.5% of all vaginal malignancies and 0.4% to 0.8% of all malignant melanomas in the female. The main presenting symptoms are vaginal bleeding, vaginal discharge, and the feeling of a mass. The tumors are predominantly located in the lower third of the vagina, commonly on the anterior wall. It is primarily a disease of postmenopausal women. Lesions may be single or multiple, pigmented or nonpigmented, arising from melanocytes present in the epithelium of the vagina (Figure 9-15).

Multiple therapies have been attempted during the past several decades, and surgery remains the treatment of choice. The surgical approach must be tailored to the location of the lesions. Neoplasms that involve the lower third of the vagina are usually treated in a manner similar to that used for vulvar melanoma, with radical vulvectomy, partial vaginectomy, and inguinal and deep node dissection. Neoplasms that involve the upper two thirds of the vagina require some form of exenteration for optimal results. Radiation therapy in general has not proven effective, and the results of chemotherapy have been equally disappointing; thus the radical surgical approach remains the primary therapy where applicable. Survival figures for this group of lesions are difficult to determine because of the infrequent occurrence of this disease. However, it appears that the survival rate is poor if any nodes are positive. The value of adjuvant chemotherapy in such instances has been disappointing to date. Patients with negative nodes who have disease involving the upper two thirds of the vagina and are treated by exenteration have about a 50% probability of surviving 5 years or more. The overall survival rate for vaginal melanoma is

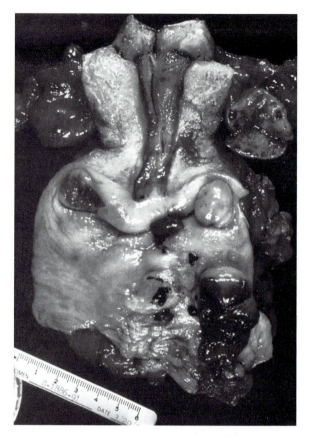

Figure 9-15 An exenteration specimen showing an open uterus, tubes, and ovaries with multifocal melanotic lesions of the vagina in a patient who underwent vaginectomy with her exenteration.

about 15%. Many patients have advanced disease at the time of diagnosis. Treatment must be based on the extent of the disease, location, patient tolerance, and depth of invasion. More and more emphasis is placed on the depth of invasion. Superficial lesions (Clark levels I and II) can be managed with less than exenterative-type surgery, whereas more deeply invasive tumors must be managed with extended radical surgery with some expectation of a favorable outcome, as reported by Van Nostrand. Survival appears to be more favorable with depths of invasion of less than 2 mm.

The dissection of lymph nodes that are clinically negative for melanoma of the vagina, urethra, and vulva continues to be controversial. For levels I and II lesions, there appears to be little value in lymphadenectomy if nodes are clinically negative. Patients with levels IV and V lesions with positive nodes rarely survive, but local control may be achieved with lymphadenectomy. Our practice is to perform an elective lymph node dissection for levels III to V lesions. Although the Clark and Breslow classifications were organized for skin lesions, we have found them very helpful in prognosticating mucosal tumors as well.

Recurrences occur primarily in the pelvis and lung.

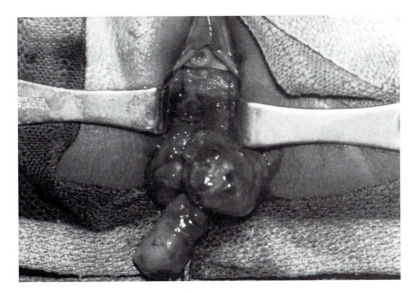

Figure 9-16 Sarcoma botryoides (rhabdomyosarcoma) in a 3-year-old child.

The interval to recurrence varies, but it is usually less than 1 year. Survival from point of recurrence averages 8 months.

Sarcoma

Spindle cell sarcomas of the vagina, such as leiomyosarcoma and fibrosarcoma, have rarely been reported. Tavassoli and Norris reported on 60 smooth muscle tumors of the vagina. Only five neoplasms recurred, and these were all greater than 3 cm, with more than five mitotic figures per 10 HPF. Local excision was the treatment of choice when the tumor was well differentiated and well circumscribed and the margins were not infiltrated. In general, these lesions behave in a manner similar to that of their corresponding cell types on the vulva in that the well-differentiated lesions have a much better prognosis than the pleomorphic types, which tend to have poor prognosis regardless of therapy. The vagina, like the vulva, has a rich lymphatic and vascular network, possibly contributing to the early dissemination of these neoplasms (especially the pleomorphic types). In general, hematogenous dissemination occurs surprisingly late in the course of the disease, so that the importance of local therapy is underlined. However, after local excision of a circumscribed lesion and postoperative local radiation therapy, the value of pelvic radiation therapy is unclear. In most instances where it has been successfully applied, the lesions were well differentiated and well circumscribed, suggesting that surgery itself was curative.

An unusual and tragic lesion that predominately afflicts children is sarcoma botryoides (Figure 9-16). These lesions are usually multicentric and tend to arise in the anterior wall at the apex of the vagina. Whereas these lesions were formerly treated by exenterative procedures, in recent years equal success has been obtained with less radical surgery and adjuvant chemotherapy, with or without radiotherapy. Piver et al. and Hilgers have both reported on this approach, and unpublished information suggests that it is equally effective when compared with exenterative surgery for local control.

There is a tendency for this tumor to originate higher in the genital tract in older patients. In all patients, the tumor may be multifocal but this is rare and should not be taken as a basis for extensive surgery. The tendency for genitourinary rhabdomyosarcoma to spread to regional lymph nodes is well established. The Intergroup Rhabdomyosarcoma Study reported a 26% incidence of known lymph node metastasis. The pelvis is the most common site for primary recurrences.

A combination of vincristine, dactinomycin, and cyclophosphamide appears to be very effective in this disease and results in a marked reduction in tumor size when the drug combination is used as initial therapy, permitting more conservative surgery. Although there is continued use of external irradiation therapy in many centers, its role in managing sarcoma botryoides of the female genital tract remains unclear. Small lesions appear to be adequately treated with chemotherapy and surgery. Also, in a report by Flamant a combination of chemotherapy and radiation therapy without surgery has been reported as curative of localized vaginal lesions.

Endodermal Sinus Tumor

This rare carcinoma occurring in the vaginas of infants is most likely of germ cell origin. Norris uses the terms *mesonephroma* or *mesonephric carcinoma* because of an alternative theory of their origin. The disease usually occurs in infants under the age of 2, and survivals have been poor, with fewer than 25% of patients alive at 2 years. Lesions most often occur on the posterior vaginal wall or fornices. Combination therapy (surgery and chemotherapy) appears appropriate. Patients who have vaginal endodermal sinus tumors usually are seen because of vaginal bleeding or discharge and have polypoid or sessile tumors. In the majority of cases the differential diagnosis of endodermal sinus tumor is that of embryonal rhabdomyosarcoma (sarcoma botryoides). This is the most common vaginal tumor of children and almost always develops in patients under 5 years of age: the average age at the time of diagnosis is 3 years. The characteristic grape-like appearance of the sarcoma botryoides differs from that of the usual endodermal sinus tumor. In addition, the edematous and cellular areas that are composed of immature skeletal muscle cells characteristic of embryonal rhabdomyosarcoma bear no resemblance to the histology of endodermal sinus tumor.

After a review of the world's literature, Young reported on 32 patients with endodermal sinus tumors. At the time of the report, 18 had died of their disease despite radical surgical therapy. In addition to the review, Young reported on six patients who were treated by surgery and who then received vincristine, dactinomycin, and cyclophosphamide. Two of the six patients also received radiation therapy. All were alive and free of disease from 2 to 9 years after surgery. Similar results with the same combination have been reported by Copeland. Thus it appears that chemotherapy, with or without radiation therapy, following conservative surgical excision can be effective in controlling this neoplasm.

URETHRAL CANCER

Primary carcinoma of the female urethra is a rare neoplasm with a relatively poor prognosis, except when disease is limited to the anterior or distal urethra. The incidence is 1 in 1500 female cancer admissions and accounts for less than 0.1% of all female genital malignancies. Because of the rarity of the disease, only a few reports with significant numbers of treated patients have been published. The Cancer Committee of FIGO has not yet proposed a stage grouping for carcinoma of the urethra.

The majority of urethral lesions are squamous growths originating from the mucosa and, less commonly, adenocarcinomas originating from the paraurethral ducts. Sarcomas and melanomas have rarely been described.

Lesions of the distal third of the urethra are elongated growths palpable through the anterior vaginal wall or exophytic neoplasms obscuring the urethral orifice. Because they can be confused with urethral carbuncle, urethral polyp, or mucosal ectropion, biopsy should be done to confirm diagnosis.

Unlike its role in vulvar cancer, the role of radiotherapy for this lesion is substantial. The proximal half of the urethra must be preserved to ensure urinary continence. This often leads to local failure when a surgical approach is chosen as the sole modality. Interstitial irradiation to the central lesion has thus gained wide acceptance for this site. Our recommendation has been to dissect the inguinal lymph nodes as both a diagnostic and a therapeutic procedure. Discovery of lymph node metastases should be followed by pelvic and local irradiation. Pelvic lymphadenectomy is usually omitted, even with positive inguinal nodes, since whole-pelvis irradiation should follow as soon as the groin incisions have healed. In our experience, radiation therapy alone has been less successful in controlling groin metastases, leading to the difficult problem of a fungating necrotic lesion eroding through the skin of the groin in a previously irradiated area. No instances of local groin failure have resulted from removal of the inguinal node metastases with subsequent radiation therapy. Lesions of the distal urethra appear to have a better prognosis than those of the upper lumen. The poor results in carcinoma of the upper urethra appear to be caused by early lymphatic dissemination to inaccessible pelvic and periaortic nodes.

Weghaupt reported on 62 patients with primary carcinoma of the female urethra treated with combined radiation therapy. Treatment was strictly individualized, but an administered tumor dose of 5500 to 7000 cGy was always attempted. Forty-two patients (67.7%) had tumors of the anterior urethra, and in 20 women (32.3%) the posterior urethra was involved. In 19 patients (30.6%) the clinical diagnosis of lymph node involvement was made. The overall 5-year survival was 64.5%. Patients with anterior urethral carcinoma had a higher 5-year survival (71.4%) than patients with posterior carcinoma (50%). These are the most favorable results reported in the literature and probably reflect sophisticated use of radiation therapy techniques.

BIBLIOGRAPHY

Squamous cancer of the vagina

Andersen ES: Primary carcinoma of the vagina: a study of 29 cases, *Gynecol Oncol* 33:317, 1989.

Ball HG, Berman ML: Management of primary vaginal carcinoma, *Gynecol Oncol* 14:154, 1982.

Barclay DL: Carcinoma of the vagina after hysterectomy for severe dysplasia or carcinoma in situ of the cervix, *Gynecol Oncol* 8:1, 1979.

Bell J et al: Vaginal cancer after hysterectomy for benign disease: value of cytologic screening, *Obstet Gynecol* 64:699, 1984.

Benedet JL et al: Primary invasive carcinoma of the vagina, *Obstet Gynecol* 62:715, 1983.

Blunt VAW: Primary carcinoma of the vagina, *Aust NZ J Obstet Gynecol* 5:29, 1965.

Boronow RC: Therapeutic alternative to primary exenteration for advanced vulvovaginal cancer, *Gynecol Oncol* 1:233, 1973.

Brinton LA, Nasca PC, Mallin K et al: Case-control study of in situ and invasive carcinoma of the vagina, *Gynecol Oncol* 38:49, 1990.

Brown AR, Fletcher GH, Rutledge FN: Irradiation of in situ and invasive squamous cell carcinoma of the vagina, *Cancer* 28:1278, 1971.

Burger MPM et al: The importance of the groin node status for the survival of T1 and T2 vulval carcinoma patients, *Gynecol Oncol* 57:327, 1995.

Chu AM, Beechinor R: Survival and recurrence in the radiation treatment of carcinoma of the vagina, *Gynecol Oncol* 19:298, 1984.

Davis KP, Stanhope CR, Garton GR et al: Invasive vaginal carcinoma: analysis of early-stage disease, *Gynecol Oncol 42:131, 1991.*

Daw E: Primary carcinoma of the vagina, J Obstet Gynaecol Br Commonw 78:853, 1971.

DiDomenico A: Primary vaginal squamous cell carcinoma in the young patient, Gynecol Oncol 35:181, 1989.

DiSaia PJ, Syed AMN, Puthawala AA: Malignant neoplasia of the upper vagina, *Endocrine/Hypertherm Oncol* 6:251, 1990.

Eddy GL, Singh KP, Gansler TS: Superficially invasive carcinoma of the vagina following treatment for cervical cancer: a report of six cases, *Gynecol Oncol* 36:376, 1990.

Eddy GL, Marks RD Jr, Miller MC III et al: Primary invasive vaginal carcinoma, *Am J Obstet Gynecol* 165 (2):292, 1991.

Fine BA et al: The curative potential of radiation therapy in the treatment of primary vaginal carcinoma, *Am J Clin Oncol* 19(1):39, 1996.

Frick HC et al: Primary carcinoma of the vagina, *Am J Obstet Gynecol* 101:695, 1968.

Gallup DG et al: Invasive squamous cell carcinoma of the vagina: a 14 year study, *Obstet Gynecol* 69 (5):782, 1987.

Gray L et al: In situ and early invasive carcinoma of the vagina, *Obstet Gynecol* 34:226, 1969.

Herbst AL, Green TH, Ulfelder H: Primary carcinoma of vagina, *Am J Obstet Gynecol* 106:210, 1970.

Hintz BL et al: Radiation tolerance of the vaginal mucosa, *Int J Radiat Oncol Biol Phys* 6:711, 1980.

Hoffman MS et al: Upper vaginectomy for in situ and occult, superficially invasive carcinoma of the vagina, *Am J Obstet Gynecol* 166:30, 1992.

Houghton CRS, Iverson T: Squamous cell carcinoma of the vagina: a clinical study of the location of the tumor, *Gynecol Oncol* 13:365, 1982.

Johnston GA, Kotz J, Boutselis JG: Primary invasive carcinoma of the vagina, *Surg Gynecol Obstet* 156:34, 1983.

Joseph RE et al: Small cell neuroendocrine carcinoma of the vagina, *Cancer* 70:784, 1992.

Kanbour AI, Klionsky B, Murphy AI: Carcinoma of the vagina following cervical cancer, *Cancer* 34:1838, 1974.

Krepart G et al: Invasive squamous cell carcinoma of the vagina. Paper presented at Felix Rutledge Society, Houston, Texas, 1975.

Kucera H, Vavra N: Radiation management of primary carcinoma of the vagina: clinical and histopathological variables associated with survival, *Gynecol Oncol* 40:12, 1991.

Kucera H et al: Radiotherapy of primary carcinoma of the vagina: management and results of different therapy schemes, *Gynecol Oncol* 21:87, 1985.

Lee RA, Symmonds RE: Recurrent carcinoma in situ of the vagina in patients previously treated for in situ carcinoma of the cervix, *Obstet Gynecol* 48:61, 1976.

Manetta A, Gutrecht EL, Berman ML et al: Primary invasive carcinoma of the vagina, *Obstet Gynecol* 76:639, 1990.

Manetta A, Pinto JL, Larson JE et al: Primary invasive carcinoma of the vagina, *Obstet Gynecol* 72:77, 1988.

Murad TM et al: The pathologic behavior of primary vaginal carcinoma and its relationship to cervical cancer, *Cancer* 35:787, 1975.

Nanavati PJ et al: High-dose-rate brachytherapy in primary stage I and II vaginal cancer, *Gynecol Oncol* 51:67, 1993.

Nori D, Hilaris BS, Shu F: Radiation therapy of primary vaginal carcinoma, *Int J Radiat Oncol Biol Phys* 70:20, 1981.

Nori D et al: Radiation therapy of primary vaginal carcinoma, *Int J Radiat Oncol Biol Phys* 9:1471, 1983.

Palumbo L et al: Primary carcinoma of the vagina, *South Med J* 62:1048, 1969.

Perez CA, Arneson AN, Galakatos A: Treatment of carcinoma of the vagina, *Cancer* 31:36, 1973.

Perez CA, Camel HM: Long-term follow-up in radiation therapy of carcinoma of the vagina, *Cancer* 49:1308, 1982.

Peters WA, Kumar NB, Morley GW: Carcinoma of the vagina: factors influencing treatment of outcome, *Cancer* 55:892, 1985.

Peters WA, Kumar NB, Morley GW: Microinvasive carcinoma of the vagina: a distinct clinical entity? *Am J Obstet Gynecol* 153:505, 1985.

Phillips B, Buchsbaum HJ, Lifshitz S: Pelvic exenteration for vulvovaginal carcinoma, *Am J Obstet Gynecol* 141:1038, 1981.

Prempree T: Role of radiation therapy in the management of primary carcinoma of the vagina, *Acta Radiol Oncol* 21:195, 1982. Prempree T et al: Radiation management of primary carcinoma of the vagina, *Cancer* 40:109, 1977.

Pride GL, Buchler DA: Carcinoma of vagina 10 or more years following pelvic irradiation therapy, *Am J Obstet Gynecol* 127:513, 1977.

Pride GL et al: Primary invasive squamous carcinoma of the vagina, *Obstet Gynecol* 53:218, 1979.

Puthawala A et al: Integrated external and interstitial radiation therapy for primary carcinoma of the vagina, *Obstet Gynecol* 62:367, 1983.

Reddy S et al: Radiation therapy in primary carcinoma of the vagina, *Gynecol Oncol* 26:19, 1987.

Reddy S et al: Results of radiotherapeutic management of primary carcinoma of the vagina, *Int J Rad Oncol Biol Phys* 21:1041, 1991.

Reuben SC, Young J, Mikuta JJ: Squamous carcinoma of the vagina: treatment, complications, and long-term follow-up, *Gynecol Oncol* 20:346, 1985.

Ries J, Ludwig H: Zur Therapie des primaren Karzinoms der Vagina, *Strahlentherapie* 118:92, 1962.

Rutledge FN: Cancer of the vagina, *Am J Obstet Gynecol* 97:635, 1967.

Smith FR: Clinical management of cancer of the vagina, *Ann NY Acad Sci* 114:1012, 1964.

Spirtos NM, Doshi BP, Kapp DS et al: Radiation therapy for primary squamous cell carcinoma of the vagina: Stanford University experience, *Gynecol Oncol* 35:20, 1989.

Stock RG, Chen AS, Seski J: A 30-year experience in the management of primary carcinoma of the vagina: analysis of prognostic factors and treatment modalities, *Gynecol Oncol* 56:45, 1995.

Thigpen JT et al: A phase II trial of cisplatin in advanced recurrent cancer of the vagina: a GOG study, *Gynecol Oncol* 23:101, 1986.

Urbanski K et al: Primary invasive vaginal carcinoma treated with radiotherapy: analysis of prognostic factors, *Gynecol Oncol* 60:16, 1996.

Usherwood MM: Management of vaginal carcinoma after hysterectomy, *Am J Obstet Gynecol* 122:352, 1975.

Whelton JA, Kottmeier HL: Primary carcinoma of the vagina, *Acta Obstet Gynecol Scand* 41:22, 1962.

Adenocarcinoma/clear cell adenocarcinoma

Bornstein J, Kaufman RH, Adam E et al: Human papillomavirus associated with vaginal intraepithelial neoplasia in women exposed to Diethylstilbestrol in utero, *Obstet Gynecol* 70:75, 1987.

Clement PB, Benedet JL: Adenocarcinoma in situ of the vagina, *Cancer* 43:2479, 1979.

Demars LR et al: Case Report: Primary non-clear cell adenocarcinomas of the vagina in older DES-Exposed women, *Gynecol Oncol* 58:389, 1995.

Greenberg ER et al: Breast cancer in mothers given Diethylstilbestrol in pregnancy, *N Engl J Med* 311:1393, 1984.

Greenwald P et al: Vaginal cancer after maternal treatment with synthetic estrogens, *N Engl J Med* 285:390, 1971.

Hanselaar AGJM, Van Leusen NDM, De Wilde PCM et al: Clear cell adenocarcinoma of the vagina and cervix, *Cancer* 67 (7):1971, 1991.

Haskel S, Chen SS, Spiegel G: Vaginal endometrioid adenocarcinoma arising in vaginal endometriosis: a case report and literature review, *Gynecol Oncol* 34:232, 1989.

Herbst A, Anderson D: Clear cell adenocarcinoma of the vagina and cervix secondary to intrauterine exposure to Diethylstilbestrol, *Sem Surg Oncol* 6 (6):343, 1990.

Herbst AL: *DES (Diethylstilbestrol) program follow-up of mother and offspring*, 1987 Newsletter, University of Chicago, 1987.

Herbst AL et al: Epidemiologic aspects and factors related to survival in 384 registry cases of clear cell adenocarcinoma of the vagina and cervix, *Am J Obstet Gynecol* 135:876, 1979.

Herbst AL et al: Clear cell adenocarcinoma of the genital tract in young females: registry report, *N Engl J Med* 287:1259, 1972.

Herbst AL, Scully RE: Adenocarcinoma of the vagina in adolescence: a report of seven cases, including six clear cell carcinomas (so-called mesonephromas), *Cancer* 25:745, 1970.

Herbst AL et al: Risk factors of the development of Diethylstilbestrol-associated clear cell adenocarcinoma, *Am J Obstet Gynecol* 154:814, 1986.

Hormio M, Soloheimo AM: Clear cell adenocarcinoma of the female genital tract, *Acta Obstet Gynecol Scand* 49:259, 1970.

Manetta A, Gutrecht EL, Berman ML et al: Primary invasive carcinoma of the vagina, *Obstet Gynecol* 76:639, 1990.

Mittendorf R, Herbst Al: Diethylstilbestrol: an update. In DeVita VT, Jr: *Cancer Prevention*, JB Lippincott Company, Pennsylvania, 1992.

Rosenfeld PA, Lowe BA: Solitary metastasis of renal adenocarcinoma to the vagina: a case report, *J Reprod Med* 35:295, 1990.

Rutledge F: Cancer of the vagina, *Am J Obstet Gynecol* 97:635, 1967.

Senekjian EK, Frey K, Herbst AL: Pelvic exenteration in clear cell adenocarcinoma of the vagina and cervix, *Gynecol Oncol* 34:413, 1989.

Senekjian EK et al: Clear cell adenocarcinoma (CCA) of the vagina and cervix in association with pregnancy, *Gynecol Oncol* 24:207, 1986.

Senekjian EK, Frey KW, Anderson D et al: Local therapy in stage I clear cell adenocarcinoma of the vagina, *Cancer* 60:1319, 1987.

Melanoma

Borazjani G, Prem KA, Okagaki T et al: Primary malignant melanoma of the vagina: a clinicopathological analysis of 10 cases, *Gynecol Oncol* 37:264, 1990.

Breslow A: Thickness, cross-sectional areas, and depth of invasion in the prognosis of cutaneous melanoma, *Ann Surg* 172(5):902, 1970.

Breslow A: Tumor thickness, level of invasion, and node dissection in stage I cutaneous melanoma, *Am J Surg* 182:572, 1975.

ClarkWH Jr et al: The histogenesis and biologic behavior of primary human malignant melanomas of the skin, *Cancer Res* 29:705, 1969.

Geisler JP et al: Pelvic exenteration for malignant melanomas of the vagina or urethra with over 3 mm of invasion, *Gynecol Oncol* 59:338, 1995.

Liu L, Hou Y, Li J et al: Primary malignant melanoma of the vagina: a report of seven cases, *Obstet Gynecol* 70:569, 1987.

Morrow CP, DiSaia PJ: Malignant melanoma of the female genitalia: a clinical analysis, *Obstet Gynecol Surv* 31:233, 1976.

Reid GC, Schmidt RW, Roberts JA et al: Primary melanoma of the vagina: a clinicopathologic analysis, *Obstet Gynecol* 74:190, 1989.

Van Nostrand KM et al: Primary vaginal melanoma: improved survival with radical pelvic surgery, *Gynecol Oncol* 55:234, 1994.

Sarcoma

Copeland LJ et al: Sarcoma botryoides of the female genital tract, *Gynecol Oncol* 66:262, 1985.

Flamant F et al: Embryonal rhabdomyosarcoma of the vagina in children, *Eur J Cancer* 15:527, 1979.

Curtin JP et al: Soft-tissue sarcoma of the vagina and vulva: a clinicopathologic study, *Obstet & Gynecol* 86(2):269, 1995.

Hilgers R: Pelvic exenteration for vaginal embryonal and rhabdomyosarcoma, *Gynecol Oncol* 45:175, 1975.

Ingemanson C, Alfredsson J: Recurrent fibromyoma of the vagina, *Acta Obstet Gynecol Scand* 49:271, 1970.

Kaufman RH, Gardner HL: Tumors of the vulva and vagina: benign mesodermal tumors, *Clin Obstet Gynecol* 8:953, 1965.

La Vecchia C, Draper J, Franceshi S: Childhood nonovarian female genital tract cancer in Britain, *Cancer* 54:188, 1984.

Mahesh Kumar AP et al: Combined therapy to prevent complete pelvic exenteration for rhabdomyosarcoma of the vagina or uterus, *Cancer* 37:118, 1976.

Mitchell M, Talerman A, Sholl JS et al: Pseudosarcoma botryoides in pregnancy: report of a case with ultrastructural observations, *Obstet Gynecol* 70:522, 1987.

Ngan HYS, Fisher C, Blake P, Shepherd JH: Vaginal sarcoma: the Royal Marsden experience, *Int J Gynecol Cancer* 4:337, 1994.

Norris HJ, Bagley GP, Taylor HB: Carcinoma of the infant vagina: a distinctive tumor, *Arch Pathol* 90:473, 1970.

O'Connell MEA et al: Intravaginal iridium-192 in the management of embryonal rhabdomyosarcoma, *Clin Oncol* 3:236, 1991.

Ortega JA: A therapeutic approach to childhood pelvic rhabdomyosarcoma without pelvic exenteration, *J Pediatr* 94:205, 1979.

Piver MS et al: Combined radical surgery, radiation therapy and chemotherapy in infants with vulvovaginal embryonal and rhabdomyosarcoma, *Obstet Gynecol* 45:522, 1973.

Rutledge FN, Sullivan M: Sarcoma botryoides, *Ann NY Acad Sci* 142:694, 1967.

Rywlin AM, Simmons RJ, Robinson MJ: Leiomyoma of vagina recurrent in pregnancy: a case with apparent hormone dependency, *South Med J* 62:1449, 1969.

Schram M: Leiomyosarcoma of the vagina: report of a case and review of the literature, *Obstet Gynecol* 12:195, 1958.

Tavassoli FA, Norris HJ: Smooth muscle tumors of the vagina, *Obstet Gynecol* 53:689, 1979.

Endodermal sinus tumor

Aartsen EJ, Delemarre JFM, Gerretsen G, Endodermal sinus tumor of the vagina: radiation therapy and progeny, *Obstet Gynecol* 81:893, 1993.

Allyn DL, Silverberg SG, Salzberg AM: Endodermal sinus tumor of the vagina, *Cancer* 27:1231, 1971.

Andersen WA et al: Endodermal sinus tumor of the vagina, *Cancer* 56:1025, 1985.

Copeland LJ et al: Endodermal sinus tumor of the vagina and cervix, *Cancer* 55:2558, 1985.

Young RH, Scully RE: Endodermal sinus tumor of the vagina: a report of nine cases in review of the literature, *Gynecol Oncol* 18:380, 1984.

Urethral cancer

Bolduan JP, Farah RN: Primary urethral neoplasms: review of 30 cases, *J Urol* 25:198, 1981.

Delclos L, Wharton JT, Fletcher GH et al: The role of brachytherapy in the treatment of primary carcinoma of the vagina and female urethra. In George FW, editor: *Modern interstitial and intracavitary radiation management*, vol 6, New York, 1981, Masson.

Dodson MK et al: Female urethral adenocarcinoma: evidence for more than one tissue of origin? *Gynecol Oncol* 59:352, 1995.

Fagan GE, Hertig AT: Carcinoma of the female urethra, *Obstet Gynecol* 6:1, 1955.

Geisler JP et al: Pelvic exenteration for malignant melanomas of the vagina or urethra with over 3 mm of invasion, *Gynecol Oncol* 59:338, 1995.

Mayer R, Fowler JE, Clayton M: Localized urethral cancer in women, *Cancer* 60:1548, 1987.

Meis JM, Ayala AG, Johnson DE: Adenocarcinoma of the urethra in women: a clinicopathologic study, *Cancer* 60:1038, 1987.

Roberts TW, Melicow MM: Pathology and natural history of urethral tumors in females: a review of 65 cases, *Urology* 10:583, 1977.

Taggart CG, Cortro JR, Rutledge FN: Carcinoma of the female urethra, *AJR* 114:145, 1972.

Weghaupt K, Gerstner GJ, Kucera H: Radiation therapy for primary carcinoma of the female urethra: a survey over 25 years, *Gynecol Oncol* 17:58, 1984.

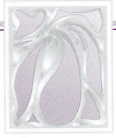

CHAPTER

10

The Adnexal Mass and Early Ovarian Cancer

ADNEXAL MASS

Anatomically, the adnexa consist of the fallopian tubes, broad ligament, ovaries, and structures within the broad ligament that were formed from embryologic rests. The differential diagnosis in management of the adnexal mass is complex because of the scope of the disorders that it encompasses and the numerous therapies that may be appropriate (Table 10-1). It is the risk of malignancy that propels the system, as well as the fundamental concept that early diagnosis and treatment in cancer are related to lessened mortality and morbidity. An adnexal mass often involves ovarian substance because of the propensity of the ovary for neoplasia. Fewer neoplasms occur in the fallopian tube, although that structure may commonly be involved in an inflammatory process that manifests as an adnexal mass. It is estimated that 5%-10% of women in the United States will undergo a surgical procedure for a suspected ovarian neoplasm during their life time, and 13%-21% of these women will be found to have an ovarian malignancy. The overwhelming majority of adnexal masses are benign, and it is important to determine preoperatively whether a patient is at a high risk for ovarian malignancy to minimize the number of operative procedures performed that are self-limiting processes. To determine whether an adnexal mass requires surgery and what the appropriate preparation and intervention should be, the preoperative evaluation should be a complete history and physical examination, as well as liberal use of transvaginal ultrasonography and a CA 125 determination. Management then depends on a combination of many predictive factors, including the age and the menopausal status of the patient, the size of the mass, ultrasonographic features, the presence or absence of symptoms, the CA 125 level, and unilaterality vs bilaterality. Age is probably the most important factor for determining the potential for malignancy.

The differential diagnosis of an adnexal mass varies considerably with the age of the patient. In premenarchal and postmenopausal women, an adnexal mass should be considered highly abnormal and must be immediately investigated. In premenarchal patients, most neoplasms are germ cell in origin and require immediate surgical exploration (Table 10-2). Stromal, germ cell, and epithelial tumors are all seen in postmenopausal women. Any enlargement of the ovary is abnormal in this older age group and should be considered malignant until proved

Table 10-1   Differential diagnosis of adnexal mass

Organ	Cystic	Solid

Ovary	Functional cyst
	Neoplastic cyst
	   Benign
	   Malignant
	Endometriosis
		Neoplasm
		   Benign
		   Malignant

Fallopian tube	Tuboovarian abscess Hydrosalpinx Parovarian cyst	Tuboovarian abscess Ectopic pregnancy Neoplasm
Uterus	Intrauterine pregnancy in a bicornate uterus	Pedunculated or interligamentous myoma
Bowel	Sigmoid or cecum distended with gas and/or feces	Diverticulitis Ileitis Appendicitis Colonic cancer
Miscellaneous	Distended bladder Pelvic kidney Urachal cyst	Abdominal wall hematoma or abscess Retroperitoneal neoplasm

Table 10-2   Frequency distribution of adnexal masses in childhood

Mass	Age of patient at diagnosis (0-20 yr) No.	%
Nonneoplastic	335	64
Simple or follicular cyst	117	23
Corpus luteum cyst	143	28
Other*	75	14
Neoplastic	186	36
Benign	144	28
Malignant	42	8
Germ cell	17	3
Stromal	9	2
Epithelial	14	3
Gonadoblastoma	2	1
TOTAL	521	

*Endometrioma, polycystic ovary syndrome, pelvic inflammatory disease, ectopic pregnancy.
Modified from Van Winter, Simmons, and Podratz, *Am J Obstet Gynecol* 170:1780, 1994.

otherwise. Many clinicians believe that any palpable ovary in a postmenopausal patient suggests malignancy and requires further study and probably laparotomy.

In the menstruating patient (reproductive-age period), the differential diagnosis is varied; both benign and malignant tumors of multiple organs can occur. Occasionally, extragenital lesions, which are often quite large and cystic, are found on pelvic examination; exploratory laparotomy is indicated because of the size alone. These extragenital lesions include peritoneal cysts, omental cysts, retroperitoneal lesions, and diseases of the gastrointestinal tract (cecum, appendix, sigmoid, and even small bowel, any of which can fall into the pelvis and become adherent). If one suspects gastrointestinal origin of the mass, appropriate radiographic studies usually help in the definitive diagnosis.

The adnexal mass is usually secondary to disease of one of the genital organs in the reproductive-age patient. Detection of pelvic abnormalities is more frequent in women of reproductive age because these patients have relatively frequent periodic screening for cancer detection and contraceptive counseling. Although most pelvic masses occur in this age range, fortunately the majority are histologically benign. Detection of an adnexal mass is greatly facilitated by a rectovaginal examination (see Figure 3-14), which allows more complete access to the cul-de-sac as well as the more superficial areas of the pelvic basin. This approach permits deeper penetration of the examining fingers. The author recommends a rectovaginal examination as the primary method for examining the pelvis.

Differential Diagnosis

Adnexal mass of gynecologic origin

This category includes disorders of the uterus, fallopian tubes, ovaries, and their adjacent structures. The process that creates the mass can be congenital, functional, neoplastic, or inflammatory.

Uterine masses. Pregnancy should always be kept in mind as a cause of uterine enlargement. Most physicians are familiar with the unreliability of a menstrual history and any patient in the reproductive-age period with a pelvic mass should first have pregnancy ruled out. This can be done by any of a variety of pregnancy tests or by detection of a fetus with ultrasound.

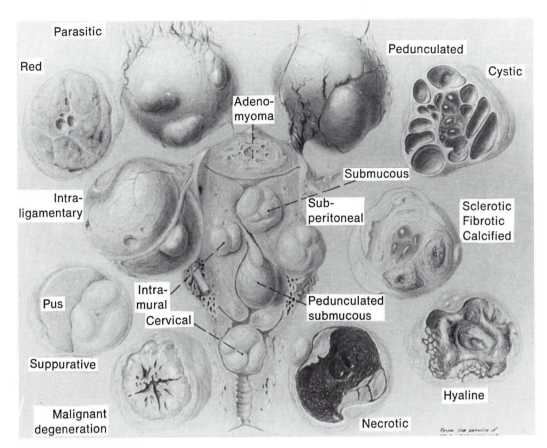

Figure 10-1 Myomas can initially be seen in multiple sizes and states of growth, disease, and degeneration. (Courtesy Dr. Erle Henriksen, Los Angeles, California.)

Myomas of the uterus are the most common uterine neoplasms (Figure 10-1). They are usually discrete, relatively round tumors that are quite firm to palpation and may be single or multiple. Myomas may be located within the myometrium (intramural), just beneath the endometrial lining (submucous), or on the surface of the uterus (serous). Frequently a myoma may be found in the broad ligament attached to the lower uterine segment by a rather thin pedicle. This will often confuse and lead the examiner to believe that the mass originates in the ovary or tube. In the United States, myomas are found in at least 10% of white women and 30%-40% of black women over the age of 35. In the postmenopausal age group, it is said that the incidence increases to 30% in white women and 50% in black women. Fortunately these neoplasms usually shrink after menopause, especially in patients not receiving high doses of exogenous estrogen stimulation. It appears that most of these benign neoplasms are somewhat estrogen dependent. Growth is commonly seen during pregnancy, probably secondary to elevated hormone levels. Degeneration, infarction, and infection can occur in these lesions, and these complications are all associated with considerable lower-abdominal pain. Sarcomatous elements, associated with myomas less than 0.1% of the time, are most often recognized postoperatively. Symptoms of associated sarcomatous elements

may include a rapidly enlarging pelvic mass, often accompanied by pain and tenderness. The mean age at diagnosis for these lesions is 50-55, with a range of 25-85 years of age.

It should be remembered that an enlargement of the uterus in the postmenopausal patient is rarely caused by fibroids, particularly if the enlargement develops in a short time ("rapid" growth). The use of HRT in and of itself is not an explanation for such an enlargement The most probable diagnosis is a malignancy, and physicians must prepare to do an appropriate surgical procedure even if the D&C is negative.

Other conditions that can cause enlargement of the uterus are adenomyosis and endometrial carcinoma or sarcoma. Endometrial carcinoma can enlarge the uterus to as much as four times normal size. The diagnosis of endometrial carcinoma is of course made by D&C of the endometrial cavity or other appropriate endometrial sampling.

Ovarian masses

Functional cysts. Among the most frequently found masses involving the adnexa are the nonneoplastic cysts related to the process of ovulation that are sometimes referred to as functional cysts. They are by far the most common clinically detectable enlargements of the ovary

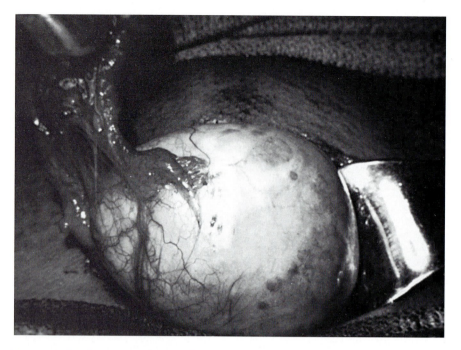

Figure 10-2 Follicular cyst (8 cm). Fimbrial adhesions from fallopian tube are also noted.

occurring during the reproductive years. They are of great significance primarily because they cannot be readily distinguished from true neoplasms on clinical grounds alone. Among the nonneoplastic cysts and hyperplasias of the ovary are:

1. Functional cysts, both follicular and corpus luteum types
2. Theca lutein cysts
3. Pregnancy luteoma
4. Sclerocystic ovaries
5. Endometriotic cysts

If ovulation does not occur, a clear fluid-filled follicular cyst (Figure 10-2) lined by granulosa cells may result that can reach sizes as large as 10 cm in diameter. These cysts usually resolve spontaneously within a few days to 2 weeks but can persist longer. When ovulation occurs, a corpus luteum is formed that may become abnormally enlarged through internal hemorrhage or cyst formation. Such cysts are often associated with variable delays in the onset of menses and confusion regarding the possibility of an ectopic pregnancy. Pregnancy testing has greatly facilitated this differential diagnosis.

Theca lutein cysts result from overstimulation of the ovary by human chorionic gonadotropin (hCG) and on histologic examination are characterized by extensive luteinization of the stroma surrounding the follicle. Although the occurrence of theca lutein cysts is not common in a normal pregnancy, they are often associated with hydatidiform moles and choriocarcinoma. Gross examination of the ovary containing theca luetin cysts shows a structure almost completely replaced by lobulated thin-wall cysts that vary in size and are smooth and yellow.

ADNEXAL MASS: INDICATIONS FOR SURGERY

1. Ovarian cystic structure >5 cm that has been followed 6-8 weeks without regression
2. Any solid ovarian lesion
3. Any ovarian lesion with papillary vegetation on the cyst wall
4. Any adnexal mass greater than 10 cm in diameter
5. Ascites
6. Palpable adnexal mass in a premenarchal or postmenopausal patient
7. Torsion or rupture suspected

Corpus luteum, follicular, and theca lutein cysts are benign and represent an exaggerated physiologic response of the ovary. In most instances, they involute over time, but they do present a problem requiring a differential diagnosis. Further discussion of the management of the suspected functional cyst is included later in this chapter.

Ovarian neoplasms. Although it is not unrealistic to consider every ovarian neoplasm or ovarian mass potentially malignant, in truth only 20% of all ovarian neoplasms are pathologically malignant. Only occasionally is it possible to differentiate benign from malignant tumors on the basis of history and physical examination (see box above). In most instances the diagnosis can be made only after both gross and microscopic examination of the mass. The ovary is composed of tissue derived from coelomic epithelium, germ cells, and mesenchyme, and clinically, ovarian neoplasms can be divided into solid and cystic types.

By far the most common benign cystic neoplasms of the ovary are serous and mucinous cystadenomas and cystic teratomas (dermoids). Cystadenomas may vary from 5-20 cm in size and are thin-walled, ovoid, and unilocular. The fluid contained within the neoplasms is usually yellow tinged and thin to viscous in quality. Benign cystic teratomas are usually no larger than 10 cm and can be identified grossly by the presence of sebaceous material or hair noted on sectioning the neoplasm.

Malignant cystic neoplasms are usually of the serous or mucinous cystadenocarcinoma variety. In the absence of definite solid areas, these lesions may be difficult to distinguish from their benign counterparts. Papillary surface excrescences, areas of necrosis, and internal papillations are very suggestive of malignancy. However, in the absence of obvious implants elsewhere in the peritoneal cavity, histologic review of the material is necessary to establish the diagnosis.

Benign solid tumors of the ovary are usually of connective tissue origin (fibromas, thecomas, or Brenner tumors). They vary in size from very small nodules found on the surface of the ovary to very large neoplasms weighing several thousand grams. On physical examination, these neoplasms are usually quite firm, slightly irregular in contour, and mobile. Meigs syndrome is an uncommon clinical entity in which a benign ovarian fibroma is seen with ascites and hydrothorax.

The malignant solid neoplasms of the ovary are most commonly adenocarcinomas arising in the ovary or metastatic from other sites. The firm masses noted on pelvic examination often appear to be associated with undifferentiated adenocarcinomas that have a poor prognosis. This clinical impression should be tempered by the knowledge that patients with inflammatory processes (e.g., chronic pelvic inflammatory disease) can demonstrate the firmest of palpable masses. In addition, elevated serum levels of several estrogens and androgens have been found in patients with solid ovarian neoplasms; fortunately these neoplasms (arrhenoblastoma, gynandroblastoma, and hilar cell tumor) are either benign or of low malignant potential.

Most neoplasms of the ovary are asymptomatic unless they have been subject to rupture or torsion. Widespread intraperitoneal dissemination can occur in ovarian carcinoma and be totally asymptomatic until ascites causes an initial symptom of abdominal distention. On the other hand, any adnexal enlargement may cause menstrual abnormalities and a sensation of pelvic pressure from distortion of the bladder and rectum.

A true neoplasm of the ovary (e.g., serous and mucinous cystadenomas and benign cystic teratomas) do not resolve spontaneously. Whether these benign lesions are precursors of malignancies is as yet an unanswered question. Intraepithelial neoplasia has been reported in otherwise benign serous cystadenomas, and in early-stage invasive epithelial cancer several authors have described the presence of transitional changes from normal epithelium to intraepithelial neoplasia to invasive cancer. Some have argued that if benign epithelial adenomas give rise to invasive cancers, it follows that surgical removal of these lesions should reduce the incidence of ovarian cancers. However, the reported increase in the incidence of surgical procedures for ovarian cysts in the past two decades has not affected the incidence of invasive ovarian cancer.

Endometriosis. Endometriosis is a condition in which implants of normal-appearing endometrial glands and stroma are found outside their normal location in the uterine cavity. The most common sites for endometriosis are the ovaries, the supporting ligaments of the uterus, and the peritoneum of the cul-de-sac and bladder. The occurrence of endometriosis is most common in women 35-45 years of age and is more common in white and nulliparous women. When the ovary is involved, that structure may become enlarged and cystic as a collection of dark, chocolate-colored fluid accumulates within an ovarian cyst. These cysts rarely exceed a diameter of 12 cm, but they are often indistinguishable from ovarian neoplasms. Nodularity of the uterosacral ligaments and other structures within the cul-de-sac may be helpful in the differential diagnosis. Pelvic pain is by far the most usual symptom of endometriosis. Although physical activity and sexual intercourse usually increase the discomfort, the amount of endometriosis present does not seem to correlate with the intensity of the symptoms. For some, pain produced from small peritoneal implants appears to be incapacitating.

Tubal masses

Neoplasms arising from the fallopian tube are rare. More commonly, adnexal masses secondary to tubal disease are inflammatory or represent an ectopic pregnancy. Distinction between tubal and ovarian masses on the basis of examination alone is often quite difficult.

In the acute phase of salpingitis, the fallopian tube is distended by grossly purulent material. This infection may be secondary to gonorrhea or other organisms, including anaerobes. As the salpingitis process progresses, the adjacent ovary may become involved, creating a so-called tubo-ovarian abscess. Although this acute process may resolve, the patient is often subject to reinfection. As a result of repeated chronic infectious processes, the tubal ostia may close or firmly adhere to the adjacent ovary, and the fallopian tube will fill with a clear fluid. As the structure distends, it creates a mass that can easily be mistaken for an ovarian cyst. Although the symptoms of acute pelvic inflammatory disease are distinct (pelvic pain, fever, increased vaginal discharge, and abnormal uterine bleeding), the symptoms of chronic pelvic infection may be subtle. Even the traditional elevation of the erythrocyte sedimentation rate and/or leukocyte count may be absent in as many as 30% of

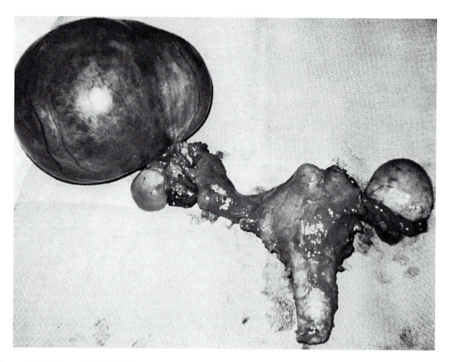

Figure 10-3 Large fluid-filled right parovarian cyst (specimen from total abdominal hysterectomy and bilateral salpingo-oophorectomy).

patients with chronic pelvic inflammatory disease and adnexal masses.

A cystic mass in the adnexal region may be neither ovarian nor tubal in origin but caused instead by remnants of embryologic structures. The parovarium, located within the portion of the broad ligament containing the fallopian tube, consists of vestigial remnants of the wolffian duct. Parovarian cysts are found as distal remnants of the wolffian duct system (Figure 10-3). They are characteristically located between the fallopian tube and the ovary and, when large, are often found with the fallopian tube stretched over the top of the cyst. These parovarian cysts are most commonly unilocular and filled with clear yellow fluid.

Approximately 98% of ectopic pregnancies are tubal. Unfortunately, a pelvic mass can be found on examination in fewer than half the cases of tubal pregnancy, and urinary pregnancy tests may be negative. Rupture usually occurs when the distended fallopian tube reaches a diameter of 4 cm. Tubal pregnancy may be difficult to distinguish from pelvic inflammatory disease, torsion of the adnexa, or bleeding corpus luteum cysts, since all produce pain and/or abnormal bleeding. Culdocentesis may be helpful in ruling out a hemoperitoneum or pelvic inflammatory disease.

Carcinoma of the fallopian tube is rare and accounts for less than 0.5% of all female genital tract malignancies. Indeed, most of these neoplasms are discovered by serendipity, a preoperative diagnosis of ovarian neoplasm being most common. Grossly, the fallopian tube is usually enlarged, smooth walled, and sausage shaped. Occasionally, patients present with the symptom of several weeks of profuse watery vaginal discharge, the so called "Hydrops tubal profluens."

Pelvic masses of nongynecologic origin

Bowel. By far the most common entity of the gastrointestinal tract that initially appears to be an adnexal mass is fecal material in the sigmoid colon and/or cecum, which may on initial pelvic examination be palpated as a soft, mobile, tubular mass. Patients should be reexamined after appropriate cleansing enemas to confirm or rule out this possibility.

Inflammatory disorders of the large and small intestine can also be detected on pelvic examination. Diarrhea, nausea and vomiting, anorexia, or passage of blood or mucus per rectum should suggest these gastrointestinal tract disorders. Patients with diverticulitis, even with abscess formation, sometimes exhibit remarkably minor symptoms initially. Careful questioning to detect subtle changes in gastrointestinal symptoms is often rewarding. Periappendiceal abscesses may be formed as a result of rupture of the appendix and present as pelvic masses. Unfortunately, they vary in location, although they are generally found on the right side of the pelvis and are usually fixed and firm and tender to palpation. Diverticulitis is a more common disorder with increasing age. Although it is usually located in the sigmoid colon, the mass may be midline or right-sided. Occasionally, inflammation of the ileum (regional ileitis) may present as

---

DIAGNOSTIC EVALUATION OF THE PATIENT WITH AN ADNEXAL MASS

Complete physical examination
Sounding of uterus (after ruling out pregnancy)
CT scan with contrast or intravenous pyelogram
Colonoscopy and/or barium enema, if symptomatic
Pelvic untrasound (optional to rule out pregnancy)
Laparoscopy, laparotomy

Table 10-3   Pelvic findings in benign and malignant ovarian tumors

Clinical findings	Benign	Malignant
Unilateral	+++	+
Bilateral	+	+++
Cystic	+++	+
Solid	+	+++
Mobile	+++	++
Fixed	+	+++
Irregular	+	+++
Smooth	+++	+
Ascites	+	+++
Cul-de-sac nodules	−	+++
Rapid growth rate	−	+++

a right adnexal mass as the loops of thickened and inflamed ileum become fixed in the pelvis.

Gastrointestinal malignancy is suggested by the presence of blood in the stool, anemia, and alterations in bowel habits. Occurrence of neoplasms of the large intestine is particularly common with increasing age, and 60%-70% occur on the left side within the reach of the palpating finger or flexible sigmoid scope. On the other hand, carcinoma of the cecum often presents as a right-sided adnexal mass, and on examination, induration and irregularity may be found in the involved area. Appropriate roentgenographic and endoscopic studies are helpful in establishing these diagnoses (see box above).

Miscellaneous

Pelvic examination should always be performed under optimal circumstances. The patient's bladder should be empty. Many patients with 10 cm midline masses thought to be ovarian neoplasms have been admitted to university hospitals. These masses disappeared with catheterization of their bladders. Whenever possible, the rectum and rectosigmoid should also be empty when a pelvic examination is done. This avoids the problem of fecal material being misdiagnosed as an adnexal mass.

The rare pelvic kidney should always be kept in mind as a possible cause of a pelvic mass. Tragic reports of excision of such a mass in a patient with one kidney are found in the literature. A preoperative intravenous pyelogram (IVP) or CT scan with contrast in a patient with a large pelvic mass can help make this diagnosis.

Retroperitoneal disorders may also be palpated on pelvic examination. Retroperitoneal sarcomas, lymphomas, and teratomas of the sacrococcygeal areas are commonly noted on rectovaginal examination and misdiagnosed as an adnexal mass.

Management

Pelvic examination remains the most widely used method of identifying an ovarian mass in its earliest stages, although incidental discovery of a pelvic mass when imaging the pelvis (CT-scan, ultrasound, or MRI) for other reasons is a growing method of identification. Knowledge of the size, shape, contour, and general

location within the pelvis helps the physician arrive at the most likely diagnosis. Benign tumors are commonly smooth walled, cystic, mobile, unilateral, and smaller than 8 cm (7 cm is the exact diameter of a new tennis ball). Malignant tumors are usually solid or semisolid, bilateral, irregular, fixed, and associated with nodules in the cul-de-sac. Ascites is usually found with malignant neoplasms (Table 10-3). Koonings showed that women with bilateral neoplasms had a 2.6-fold greater risk of malignancy than women with unilateral neoplasms.

Certain studies may precede surgical exploration. Roentgenologic examination of the abdomen may reveal the outline of a pelvic mass, and the finding of "teeth" indicates a benign teratoma. However, all calcifications are not "teeth," and psammoma bodies in serous adenocarcinoma of the ovary are other commonly found radiopaque entities also noted on roentgenologic examination. IVP is useful in the management of a pelvic mass because ureteral displacement and distortion of the bladder contour may be used to judge the size of the mass. In addition, kidney position and function can also be evaluated. Ureteral obstruction or displacement should be noted before laparotomy, particularly when retroperitoneal dissection is anticipated to remove tumor bulk. Transvaginal sonography, CT scan, and/or MRI scans occasionally are necessary to further define the nature of the mass.

Specific diagnostic assays (e.g., tumor markers) for ovarian cancer are also available. Some germ cell neoplasms produce hCG, LDH or alpha-fetoprotein (AFP), but most early-staged ovarian neoplasms are not associated with reliable tumor markers. Although serum CA-125 levels appear to be elevated in many serous cystadenocarcinomas, overall it is positive and roughly 50% of stage I lesions.

Contrast studies of the gastrointestinal tract should be used liberally, especially when there is suspicion that the

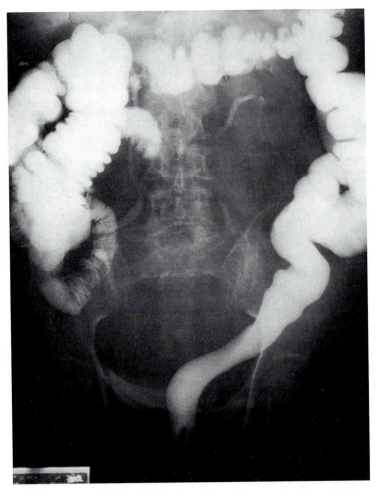

Figure 10-4 Barium enema film in a patient with large mucinous cystadenoma of right ovary.

mass is gastrointestinal in origin (Figure 10-4). Ultrasonography has not been as diagnostically helpful as expected, except to exclude intrauterine or extrauterine pregnancy. Although ultrasound can be helpful in detecting solid-fluid interfaces and distinguishing between solid and cystic masses, these determinations do not help in the eventual management of the patient and therefore seem redundant when a distinct mass has been palpated. Occasionally, ultrasound can be helpful in confirming the suspicion of an adnexal mass in an obese or uncooperative patient. Its routine use for all adnexal masses is discouraged.

Diagnostic laparoscopy may be helpful in distinguishing a uterine myoma from an ovarian neoplasm. Laparoscopy is helpful in any situation where the source of a pelvic mass is uncertain, and locating the source determines whether treatment is to be surgical or nonsurgical. This is especially true with smaller masses (7 cm or smaller) in patients of reproductive age, in whom expectant therapy should be seriously considered.

Deciding which patient needs surgical exploration can best be done by considering the characteristics of the adnexal mass. Any mass larger than 10 cm in diameter should be surgically explored. Ninety-five percent of ovarian cysts smaller than 5 cm in diameter are nonneoplastic. In addition, functional cysts are seldom larger than 7 cm in diameter and are usually unilateral and freely mobile. Patients usually are not taking oral contraceptive drugs. A physician can presume that during the reproductive years an adnexal mass as described above is a functional or hyperplastic change of the ovary rather than a true neoplasm. The transitory existence of functional cysts is of prime importance in distinguishing them from true neoplasms. Tradition and clinical experience have shown that functional cysts usually persist for only a few days to a few weeks, and reexamination during a later phase of the menstrual cycle has been a reliable procedure in confirming this diagnosis. Many gynecologists prescribe oral contraceptives to accelerate the involution of the functional cyst on the presumption that these cysts are gonadotropin-dependent. The unconfirmed theory is that the inhibitory effect of the contraceptive steroids on the release of pituitary gonadotropins should shorten the life span of these cysts, hastening their identification as

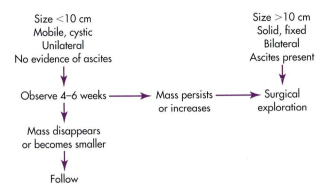

Figure 10-5 Management of premenopausal women with an adnexal mass.

Table 10-4   Benign ovarian tumors

I. Nonneoplastic tumors
   A. Germinal inclusion cyst
   B. Follicle cyst
   C. Corpus luteum cyst
   D. Pregnancy luteoma
   E. Theca lutein cysts
   F. Sclerocystic ovaries
   G. Endometrioma
II. Neoplastic tumors derived from coelomic epithelium
   A. Cystic tumors
      1. Serous cystoma
      2. Mucinous cystoma
      3. Mixed forms
   B. Tumors with stromal overgrowth
      1. Fibroma, adenofibroma
      2. Brenner tumor
III. Tumors derived from germ cells
   A. Dermoid (benign cystic teratoma)

functional or nonneoplastic lesions. Failure of the enlargement to regress during one menstrual cycle (4 to 6 weeks) mandates operative intervention (Figure 10-5). A careful study by Spanos was conducted on 286 patients who had adnexal cysts. Combination oral contraceptives were prescribed, and the women were reexamined in 6 weeks. In 72% of the women, the masses disappeared during the observation period. Of the 81 patients whose masses persisted, none were found to have a functional cyst at laparotomy. The fact that five of the removed tumors were malignant underscores the importance of avoiding unnecessary delay in the operative investigation of these patients. It also has made the authors slow to recommend operative laparoscopy for removal of such masses. In the premenarchal or postmenopausal period any ovarian enlargement should result in surgical intervention.

BENIGN OVARIAN TUMORS (Table 10-4)

The differentiation between benign and malignant ovarian enlargements is often the exclusive decision of the pathologist, but a short discussion of these lesions is pertinent even in a textbook of oncology. Although functional ovarian cysts are usually asymptomatic, they can on occasion be accompanied by a minor degree of lower abdominal discomfort, pelvic pain, or dyspareunia. In addition, rupture of one of these fluid-filled structures can result in additional peritoneal irritation and possibly an accompanying hemoperitoneum; however, this is rarely serious. More intense lower abdominal discomfort will result when these ovarian tumors undergo torsion or infarction. Similar to functional cysts of the ovary, benign ovarian neoplasms do not produce any symptoms that readily differentiate them from malignant tumors or from various other pelvic diseases. Although these tumors are more prone to twist, resulting in infarction, malignant neoplasms may have the same fate. Indeed, one of the most unfortunate features of benign ovarian neoplasms is that they are indistinguishable clinically from their

malignant counterparts. Although it is not known whether malignant ovarian tumors arise de novo or develop from benign tumors, there is strong inferential evidence that at least some benign tumors will become malignant. All too often, the first symptom of cancer in an ovarian tumor is increasing abdominal distention, although benign ovarian neoplasms may become apparent because of increasing abdominal girth, and indeed the "giant tumors" of the ovary are often benign mucinous cystadenomas. True functional cysts of the ovary will regress in a 4- to 6-week follow-up period of observation. All persistent adnexal enlargements must be considered malignant until proven otherwise.

Laparoscopically Managed Benign Cysts

The operative approach for presumptively benign ovarian cyst has been the laparotomy. Advances in ultrasonography have provided an opportunity to predict benign masses preoperatively. With the use of specific ultrasound criteria, benign masses can be predicted with a high degree of certainty especially in premenopausal women. Careful patient selection is critical for the appropriate use of laparoscopy for removal of adnexal masses. Patient age, the clinical exam, and ultrasound findings provide important information that help determine the appropriate operative approach. Laparoscopy should be used cautiously in the presence of any mass with clinical or ultrasonographic characteristics suspicious for malignancy. It is also contraindicated for management of an adnexal mass in the presence of an elevated serum CA-125 value in a postmenopausal woman.

Ultrasonographic examination of the pelvis, particularly transvaginal, is a reliable and consistent method for evaluation of the size and the consistency of a pelvic mass. Masses that are cystic, unilocular, less than 10 cm, unilateral and have regular borders are likely to be benign. The presence of irregular borders, papillations, solitary thick septa, ascites, or matted bowel should raise concern about the possibility of malignancy. Using strict ultrasonographic criteria, physicians accurately predict benign masses in over 95% of patients. Functional cysts, hemorrhagic cysts, dermoids, and endometriomas will often have characteristic appearances on ultrasound. Functional cysts are usually unilocular and have regular, thin borders. In premenopausal women, the majority of fairly cystic masses less than 7 cm will resolve spontaneously within 6-8 weeks. Hemorrhagic cysts contain interior echoes that can vary in intensity from low to high levels and can be focal or diffuse. The ultrasound appearance of these cysts usually changes over time, and most regress spontaneously. Cysts that appear to be functional or hemorrhagic on ultrasound that persist should be removed to rule out neoplasia.

Dermoids have a variable appearance on ultrasound. They may appear as a cystic mass that contain foci of echogenic material in a nondependent distribution or a highly echogenic area suggesting bone or teeth. Endometriomas usually have regular but slightly thickened borders. They often will contain low level and diffused internal echoes, although fresh hemorrhage may appear more highly echogenic. These masses that meet strict ultrasonic criteria for benign lesions may be considered for a laparoscopic approach. If any suspicious ultrasound findings are seen, operative laparoscopy is less appropriate, and laparotomy should be seriously considered.

CA-125, a tumor associated antigen has been studied to determine its value in preoperative differentiation of benign and malignant pelvic masses. In patients less than 50 years of age, an elevated CA-125 level is associated with a malignant mass less than 25% of time. If the patient is over 50, an elevated CA-125 level is associated with a malignant mass 80% of the time. A more detailed discussion of CA 125, is contained in Chapter 11. Of note for this discussion is the fact that only 50% of patients with stage I epithelial cancer of the ovary will have an elevated CA-125 level.

All patients scheduled for operative laparoscopy with an adnexal mass should also consent for possible laparotomy; the surgeon should be prepared to proceed with staging laparotomy without delay if malignancy is uncovered. All patients are operated on under general anesthesia in the laparoscopy stirrups. A Foley catheter is inserted into the bladder to avoid injury to that structure secondary to overdistention during prolonged cases. A 10-mm laparoscope provides a wide field of vision and excellent light. The initial inspection of the peritoneal cavity is done before attaching the video camera because the eyepiece gives a clearer assessment of the fine details and color differentiation than most video systems.

Cell washings are obtained from the pelvis and upper abdomen and saved for proper staging if a malignancy is found. Any lesions or suspicious areas are sampled and sent for frozen section. If obvious carcinoma, ascites, or a positive frozen section is found, the surgeon should proceed with immediate staging laparotomy through a midline incision. If a decision is made to proceed with operative laparoscopy, the video camera is attached, allowing the assistant and a nurse to participate in the procedure. Laproscopic fenestration of the mass and biopsy provide the most accurate method of diagnosing malignancy. A large window should be cut in the wall of the cyst; its size should vary with the size of the cyst but it is usually about 2 cm smaller than the cyst to a maximum of 4-5 cm. The cavity of the cyst is carefully inspected, usually while being irrigated with Ringer's solution. Bleeding points from the biopsy site are controlled with hemostatic coagulation, utilizing one of the energy sources available to the surgeon. Biopsy specimens are submitted to the laboratory for immediate tissue diagnosis.

Nezhat reported his experience with 1209 patients with adnexal masses who were managed laparoscopically. Of 1011 cases with surgical management, ovarian cancer was discovered intraoperatively in four. The management of a cystic mass included aspiration of fluid, which was sent for cytological examination, followed by opening of the cyst and inspecting the wall for any irregular thickening. Frozen-section biopsy specimens were obtained if the surgeon thought any surfaces were suspicious. An ovarian cystectomy-oophorectomy was then performed, and tissue was sent for permanent-histological examination. The Nezhat study suggests that experienced surgeons using intraoperative histological sampling may safely evaluate adnexal masses laparoscopically.

Hasson reported another series of 102 women with ovarian cysts who were managed laparoscopically. Eighty three of the women were treated with laparoscopic fenestration and biopsied, with or without coagulation or removal of the cyst lining. Only one of 56 functional, simple or paraovarian cysts recurred during the study. Two of the 18 ovarian endometriomas treated with fenestration and coagulation or removal of the lining recurred, whereas eight of nine such lesions recurred when treated with fenestration alone. There were no surgical complications.

Serous Cystadenoma

Serous cystadenomas are more common than the mucinous type of tumor but as a rule they do not attain the very large size characteristic of their mucinous counterparts. Grossly, the characteristic feature of the tumor is papillary projections on the surface, which at times are so numerous that a cauliflower pattern is produced. Although most of the inner wall of the cyst may be smooth (Figure 10-6), it may also contain a large number of these papillae.

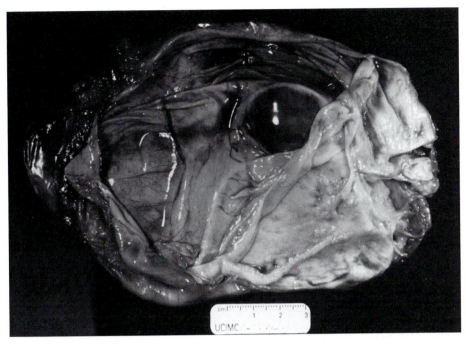

Figure 10-6 Gross photograph of an opened serous cyst adenoma that contains 500 cc of clear straw-colored fluid. Note the papillary projections on the inner surface especially on the right.

Microscopically, the epithelium is usually of the low columnar type, and at times cilia are present. Particularly characteristic of this type of cyst is the frequent finding of small cancerous granules, the so-called psammoma bodies, which are an end product of degeneration of the papillary implants. Aure et al. suggests that these psammoma bodies are indicative of a functional immunologic response. Associated fibrosis may lead to the so-called cystadenofibroma, which represents a similar lesion found in the breast.

Mucinous Cystadenoma

Mucinous cystadenomas (Figure 10-7) may become huge. Several have been reported to weigh 100 to 200 pounds. Grossly, they are round or ovoid masses with smooth capsules that are usually translucent or bluish-whitish gray. The interior is divided by a number of discrete septa into loculi containing generally a clear, viscid fluid. Papillae are rarely noted. However, microscopically the lining epithelium is of a rather tall, pale-staining secretory type with nuclei at the basal pole; the presence of goblet cells is common. The cells will be found to be rich in mucin if suitable stains are obtained. It is believed that this type of cyst usually arises from simple metaplasia of the germinal epithelium. It may arise occasionally from a teratoma in which all the other elements have been blotted out. It rarely occurs from a Brenner tumor in which there has been mucinous transformation of the epithelium.

Bilaterality may be found in as many as 10% of patients with serous cystadenomas, in contrast with mucinous cystadenomas, where there is essentially no significant incidence of bilaterality. This information is helpful when the surgeon needs to make a judgment about surgical inspection of the opposite ovary in a young woman desirous of further childbearing. If the other ovary is of normal size, shape, and configuration, surgical evaluation is not needed.

Pseudomyxoma Peritonei (Figure 10-8)

Of major concern are mucinous cysts that perforate and initiate intra-abdominal transformation of the peritoneal mesothelium to a mucin-secreting epithelium. This altered peritoneal mesothelium continues to secrete mucus, according to Woodruff and Novak, with gradual accumulation in the peritoneal cavity of huge amounts of gelatinous material, constituting the so-called pseudomyxoma peritonei. Evacuation of this material at operation is almost invariably followed by reaccumulation because of the impossibility of altering the secretion of the mucinous mesothelium.

Among 13 cases of pseudomyxoma, Shanks noted that 10 cases originated in benign ovarian tumors, 2 cases originated in malignant ovarian tumors, and 1 arose from an appendiceal mucocele. Of 7 survivors, 2 had recurrences: 1 after 14 years and 1 after 6 years.

Treatment remains primarily surgical, and because of the recurrent nature of the lesion, it may be repetitive. Intraperitoneal alkylating agents have been used with some success; however, according to Limber at al., the use of x-ray therapy, radioactive materials, and mucolytic

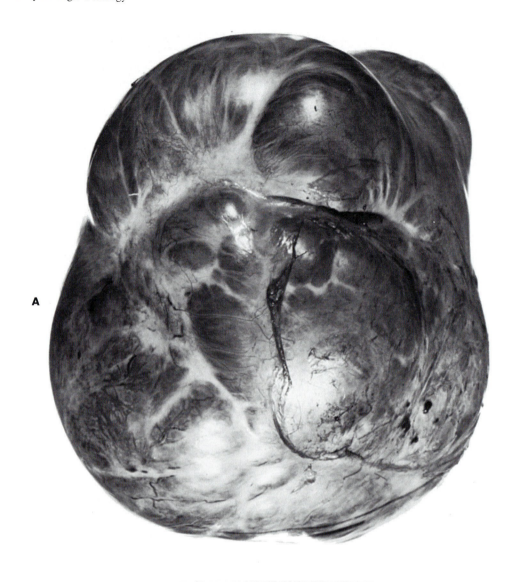

Figure 10-7 Mucinous cystadenoma. **A,** Gross appearance.   *Continued.*

agents has been disappointing. Long et al. reported a 45% 5-year and a 40% 10-year survival rate. In 1990, Mann reported his experience with nine patients. He concluded that chemotherapy, including the use of cisplatin was not effective, and long-term nutritional support provided a good quality of survival for select patients.

Brenner Tumor

Brenner tumor (Figure 10-9), a rather uncommon type of ovarian neoplasm, is grossly identical to a fibroma. Microscopically, one finds a markedly hyperplastic fibromatous matrix interspersed with nests of epithelioid cells. The epithelioid cells under high magnification show a "coffee bean" pattern caused by the longitudinal grooving of the nuclei. The cell nests show a frequent tendency toward central cystic degeneration, producing a superficial resemblance to a follicle. Although it was originally believed that Brenner tumors arise from simple Walthard cell rests, it has been conclusively demonstrated that Brenner tumors can arise from diverse sources, including the surface epithelium, rete ovarii, and ovarian stroma itself. It was originally stressed that Brenner tumors were uniformly benign, but in the last several decades there have been scattered reports of a number of malignant Brenner tumors. Brenner tumors are generally thought to be endocrinologically inert, but in recent years several cases have been associated with postmenopausal endometrial hyperplasia, and a frequent estrogen effect has been attributed to this neoplasm. Even more recently, a characteristic Brenner tumor has been associated with virilism.

Benign lesions are managed by simple excision.

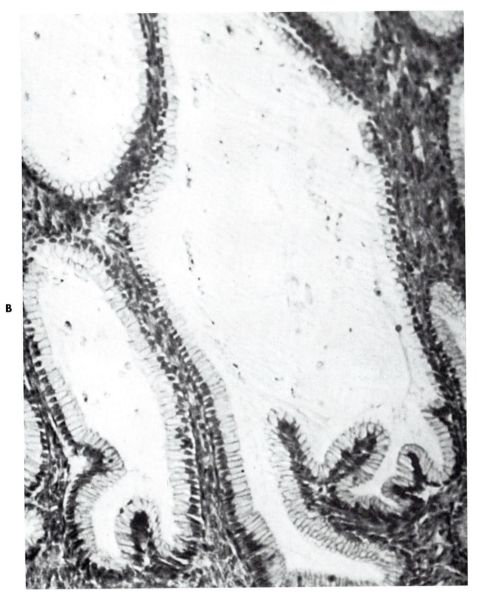

Figure 10-7, cont'd Mucinous cystadenoma. **B,** Histologic section showing tall epithelial lining with pale-staining nuclei at basal pole.

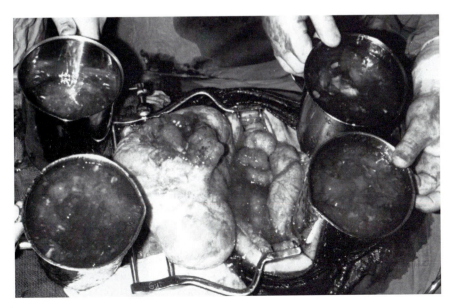

Figure 10-8 Laparotomy of patient with pseudomyxoma. Note the large amount of mucinous material.

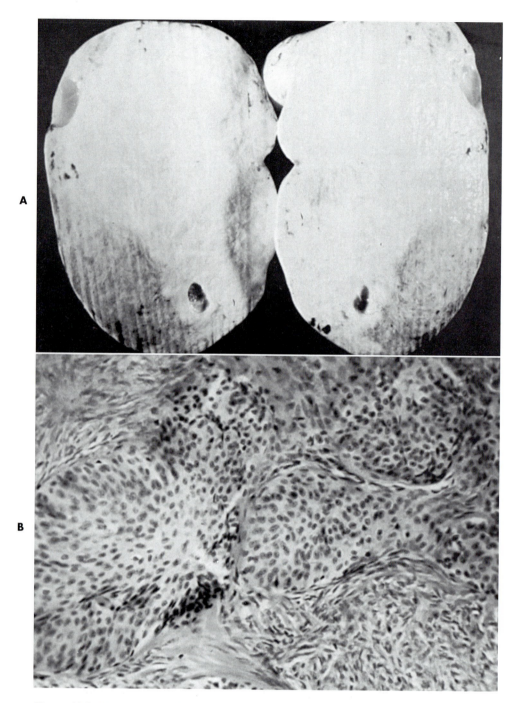

Figure 10-9 Brenner tumor. **A,** Gross appearance—solid, firm, white cut surface. **B,** Histologic section—hyperplastic fibromatous matrix interspersed with nests of epitheloid cells.

Treatment of malignant Brenner tumors is unsettled, and various forms of chemotherapy have been used with little reported successes.

Dermoid Cyst (Benign Cystic Teratoma)

Dermoid cysts are rarely large, often bilateral (15% to 25%), and occur with disproportionate frequency in younger patients. Grossly, there is a rather thick, opaque, whitish wall, and on opening the cyst one frequently finds hair, bone, cartilage, and a large amount of greasy fluid, which rapidly becomes sebaceous on cooling. Microscopically one may find all types of mature ectoderm, mesoderm, and such endodermal elements as gastrointestinal mucosa. Stratified squamous epithelium, hair follicles, sebaceous and pseudoriferous glands, cartilage, neural and respiratory elements, and indeed all elements normally seen in fetal life may be present. When malignant degeneration occurs in these benign cystic teratomas, it is usually of a squamous type: it has been reported in 1% to 3% of these tumors. These neoplasms

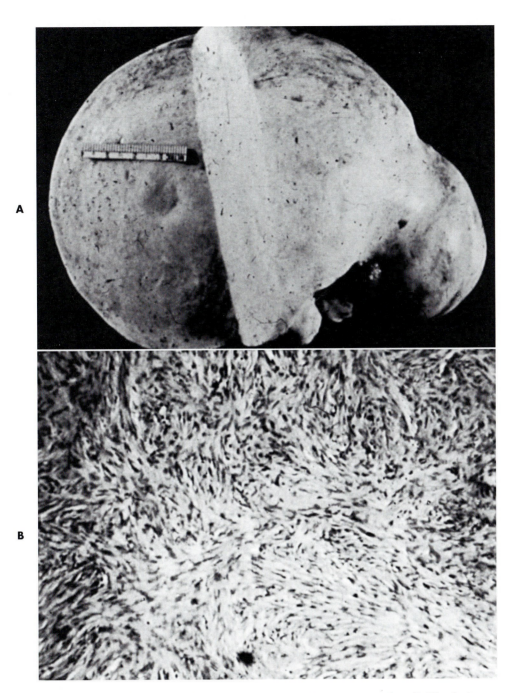

Figure 10-10 Ovarian fibroma. **A,** Gross appearance—white, firm cut surface. **B,** Histologic section—whorls of fibromatous matrix.

are thought to arise from early ova that have been triggered by some type of parthenogenetic process.

Management of these lesions in a patient desirous of further childbearing is cystectomy. Care must be taken to remove the entire capsule of the neoplasm to avoid recurrence. In most instances, a significant portion of normal ovary can be preserved and reconstituted. Some controversy exists relating to the necessity for creating a bivalve in the opposite ovary because of the high incidence of bilaterality with these lesions. In our experience, bilaterality is rare when the opposite ovary is normal in appearance; therefore, we do not recommend the procedure in these circumstances. Care should be taken to prevent spillage of the contents of the dermoid cyst because this material can cause a chemical peritonitis.

Fibroma

The occurrence of fibromas (Figure 10-10) is not at all infrequent. Sometimes they are first noted as very small nodules on the ovarian cortex. In other instances they can be extremely large, filling the entire pelvis and lower abdomen. The tumors are characterized by their firmness and resemblance to myomas, and they are frequently misdiagnosed as such. The cut surface has a homogeneous grayish-white and firm appearance, although areas of cystic degeneration are common in larger tumors. Microscopically one finds stellate or spindle-shaped cells arranged in fusiform fashion. The cells are uniformly well differentiated, with nothing to suggest malignancy. Hyalinization is frequent, particularly in the larger tumors, and if fat stains are done, admixtures of theca cells may be seen. Meigs syndrome is characterized by ascites, hydrothorax, and an ovarian tumor that was originally believed to be specifically a fibroma; however, many other types of ovarian tumors are now known to be associated with this syndrome, such as Brenner tumors and Krukenberg tumors. The cause of Meigs syndrome is not completely understood, but it seems that the hydrothorax occurs via certain lymphatics through the diaphragm. Following removal of the ovarian neoplasm, there is a prompt resolution of both abdominal and pleural fluid.

Adnexal Masses in Childhood

In a study by Ehren et al., 63 children and adolescents with benign or malignant ovarian tumors were reported. Abdominal pain was the most common complaint; 22% had torsion. The most common sign on initial examination was a palpable abdominal mass (45 of 54 patients). Benign teratoma was the final diagnosis in 41 (65%) of the patients, and 29 had calcification apparent on abdominal x-ray film. All patients younger than 12 years with ovarian neoplasms had germ cell lesions, although an epithelial tumor has been reported in a 4-year-old patient. Two patients experienced precocious puberty and, interestingly, both had embryonal carcinoma. In this 63-patient study, appendicitis was the most usual misdiagnosis. Twenty-one percent had malignant tumors. Breen and Maxson noted that 35% of ovarian tumors in children were malignant.

Van Winter reported on 521 adnexal masses in infancy, childhood, and adolescence: 92% were benign, including 335 nonneoplastic and 144 of 186 (77%) neoplastic lesions. The frequency of ovarian malignancies correlated inversely with patient age. Germ cell, stromal, and epithelial malignancies accounted for 40%, 21%, and 33%, respectively, of the 42 cancers. Nonconformance between preoperative and postoperative diagnoses were noted in 94 cases. The most common preoperative diagnosis necessitating reassignment was acute appendicitis. During the last decade of his study, ultrasonography and computed tomography did not miss a single malignancy. The majority of these patients presented with a pain or a mass (Table 10-5). The histology found in these lesions is presented in Table 10-2.

PALPABLE OR ENLARGED POSTMENOPAUSAL OVARY (Figure 10-11)

During the postmenopausal years, when the ovary becomes smaller and quiescent after cessation of menses, the presence of a palpable ovary must alert the physician to the possibility of an underlying malignancy. Physiologic enlargement and functional cysts should not be present in postmenopausal ovaries. The postmenopausal

Table 10-5 Symptoms at initial presentation of 521 adnexal masses in children

Symptom	Patients (no.)
Pain*	271
Mass†	151
Menstrual irregularity‡	71
Dysmenorrhea	50
Amenorrhea, primary	12
Amenorrhea, secondary	35
Increased abdominal girth	34
Urinary complaints§	16
Hirsutism	13
Premature sexual development	6

*Mass was secondarily discovered in 150 of these patients.
†Without accompanying pain.
‡Metrorrhagia, menorrhagia, oligomenorrhea.
§Frequency, dysuria, suprapubic pressure.
From Van Winter, Simmons and Podratz, *Am J Obstet Gynecol* 170:1780, 1994.

Postmenopausal palpable ovary syndrome
The PMPO syndrome

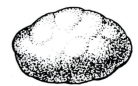

Normal ovary
Premenopause
3.5 × 2 × 1.5 cm

Early menopause
(1-2 years)
2 × 1.5 × 0.5 cm

Late menopause
(2-5 years)
1.5 × 0.75 × 0.5 cm

Figure 10-11 Comparison of ovary size during progressive periods of a woman's life. (From Barber HRK, Graber EA; The PMPO syndrome [post-menopausal palpable ovary syndrome], *Obstet Gynecol Surv* 28:357, 1973. Copyright © 1973 The Williams & Wilkins Co, Baltimore.)

gonad atrophies to a size of 1.5 × 1 × 0.5 cm on the average, and at that size it should not be palpable on pelvic examination. The possibility of malignancy must therefore be carefully assessed when an ovary is palpable in a postmenopausal woman. Goswamy et al. studied ovaries from 2221 postmenopausal women with regard to ovarian volumes (Figure 10-12). They noted that there were three ranges of volume and that volume appeared to be increased in obese and multiparous women.

When laparotomy is done, the approach should be made with the assumption that the patient may have an early ovarian carcinoma. Cytologic washings and careful exploration of the abdomen should be done, as in any patient being staged for ovarian cancer. A vertical abdominal incision is strongly recommended; this would allow careful assessment of the subdiaphragmatic surfaces. In our experience, only 10% of patients with a palpable postmenopausal ovary who are subjected to oophorectomy are found to have a malignant ovarian neoplasm. By far the most common finding is a benign ovarian lesion such as fibroma or Brenner tumor (Figure 10-13). This has led us to reevaluate our former practice of recommending laparotomy in most of these patients.

Goldstein reported on 42 postmenopausal women with simple adnexal cysts. He included only patients available for follow-up who had cysts ≤5 cm in maximum diameter that were unilocular and without ascites. Of these patients, 26 underwent prompt surgical exploration. All exhibited benign histopathology. In 16 patients, serial sonographics surveillance was performed every 3 to 6 months. Two of these patients had exploratory laparotomy at 6 and 9 months of observation; the first operation, for increasing size and septation, demonstrated a cystadenofibroma, and

the second operation, for increasing pain, demonstrated a degenerating myoma. The remaining 14 patients were followed from 10 to 73 months without any change in the size or character of their cysts. Goldstein concluded that small, unilocular postmenopausal cysts had a low incidence of malignant disease and that serial ultrasound follow-up, without surgical intervention, should have a major role in clinical management of such patients. Others, such as Parker, have suggested that these low-risk postmenopausal cysts should be managed with operative laparoscopy.

Miller reported on 20 postmenopausal patients who underwent surgical exploration to evaluate an asymptomatic palpable ovary. Thirteen patients (65%) were found to have an ovarian neoplastic process. Three of the neoplasms were malignant or of borderline malignant potential, resulting in overall malignancy rate of 15% for the postmenopausal palpable ovary syndrome. This is consistent with our experience and that of Flynt and Gallup who reported on 11 patients, none of which had a malignant ovarian neoplasm. The majority of neoplasms in this group of patients is benign. However, the actual number of postmenopausal women who have been followed and subsequently reported in the literature is extremely small (Table 10-6). Lerner accurately predicted a benign outcome in 247/248 patients studied. He used color-flow Doppler analysis in improving the accuracy of ultrasonic characterization of ovarian masses. However, this technique has not been as accurate when used by others.

A diagnosis of ovarian cancer should be suspected when a postmenopausal woman presents with a pelvic mass. The presence of ascites, which can be detected clinically or by ultrasound markedly increases the probability of a diagnosis of malignancy. In addition, CA 125, although nonspecific in the premenopausal patient population, is very sensitive in the postmenopausal patient when used in combination with a clinical impression and an abnormal ultrasound. CT-scan, which is more sensitive than the ultrasound, is often not necessary. Early surgical intervention is a key component in the treatment of these patients, and extensive diagnostic testing should be discouraged.

SCAN-DETECTED MASSES

With the increased utilization of computed tomography, MRI scans, and ultrasound, an increasing number of "pelvic masses" are being identified. It is not unusual today for a patient to come to the office with a scan in hand. In many instances, no mass is felt on pelvic examination. This causes a management dilemma, particularly in the postmenopausal woman. Experience has dictated that a pelvic mass in the postmenopausal woman needs surgical evaluation, but the decision to operate should be relative to identification of the mass on pelvic

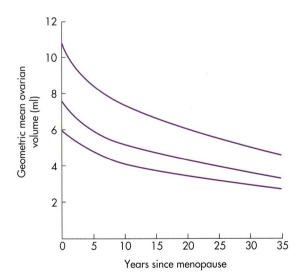

Figure 10-12 The 95th centiles for high, medium, and low expected ovarian volumes (geometric means) based on data from 2221 postmenopausal women. (From Goswamy RK et al: *Br J Obstet Gynaecol* 98:795, 1988.)

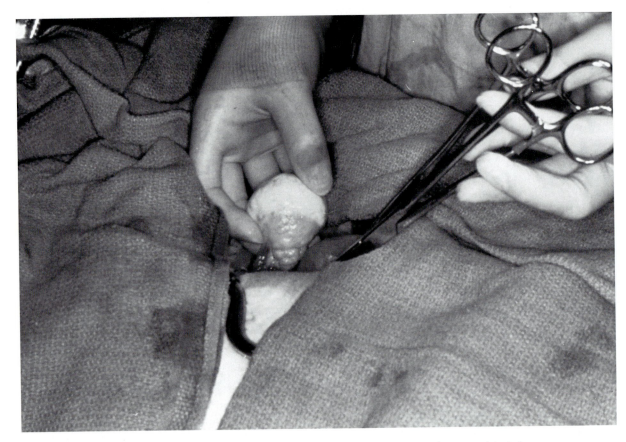

Figure 10-13 A 5 cm adenofibroma found in surgery in a postmenopausal woman detected preoperatively and diagnosed by ultrasonography as a solid mass.

Table 10-6 Small postmenopausal adnexal mass studies

Series	N	Inclusion criteria	N operative	% CA
Hall (1986)	13	Simple cyst	13	8
Goldstein (1989)	42	Unilateral cyst <5 cm	28	0
Andolf (1989)	58	<5 cm, simple	29	0
	11	<5 cm, multicystic, echoes	10	10
	33	>5 cm, simple	27	10
	50	>5 cm, multicystic, echoes	45	30
Wolf (1991)	22	<5 cm, simple	1	0

Modified from Curtin JP: Management of the adnexal mass, *Gynecol Oncol* 55:S42, 1994.

examination. In many instances when surgery has been performed for scan-detected masses, no malignancies have been identified, even when the scans indicated that the masses were "solid." Hydrosalpinx and old follicular cysts have often been found. On other occasions, the mass is a fluid-filled pocket of adhesions in a patient with a history of previous pelvic surgery. Obviously, these situations must be individualized, and a false-positive rate for "pelvic masses" identified only by imaging must be accepted.

BORDERLINE MALIGNANT EPITHELIAL OVARIAN NEOPLASMS

In the last three decades, clear evidence has been presented that there is a group of epithelial ovarian tumors with histologic and biologic features intermediate to those of clearly benign and those of frankly malignant ovarian neoplasms. These borderline malignancies, which account for approximately 15% of all epithelial ovarian cancers, were often referred to as proliferative cystadenomas. These lesions tend to occur more frequently in the younger population than the obviously malignant epithelial ovarian carcinomas that are seen more frequently in the older patient population (Figure 10-14). There is a 10-year survival rate of approximately 95% for stage I lesions in these borderline neoplasms. However, symptomatic recurrence and death may occur as many as 20 years after therapy in a few patients, and these neoplasms are correctly labeled as being of low malignant potential.

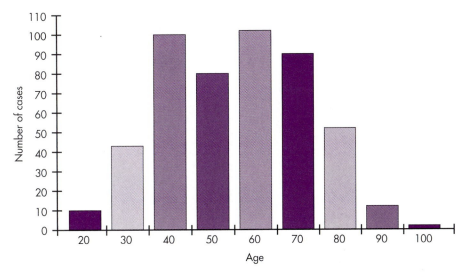

Figure 10-14 Epithelial borderline tumors of the ovary. Age distribution. (From *Annual Report Gynecological Cancer FIGO*, vol 22, 1994.)

Borderline serous epithelial tumors (Figure 10-15) definitely occupy an intermediate position between the benign serous cystadenomas and the frankly malignant serous cystadenocarcinomas in their histologic features and prognostic aspects. Grossly, the borderline serous tumors are similar to the previously described benign serous cystadenomas, which have papillary projections, but the borderline tumors possibly show an increased incidence of bilaterality. In addition, the papillary component is usually more abundant in the borderline lesions than in the perfectly benign serous cystadenoma. Survival in these lesions differs significantly from their obviously malignant counterpart (Figure 10-16).

The histologic criteria characterizing the borderline tumors can be summarized as follows:

Stratification of the epithelial lining of the papillae

Formation of microscopic papillary projections or tufts arising from the epithelial lining of the papillae

Epithelial pleomorphism Atypicality Mitotic activity

No stromal invasion present

According to Janovski and Paramananthon, at least two of these features must be present for the tumor to qualify as borderline. Although borderline serous epithelial tumors of the ovary are well established and were accepted by the International Federation of Gynecology and Obstetrics in 1964, they remain a controversial issue. Although there is no doubt that there exists a group of low-grade malignant tumors among the serous cystadenocarcinomas of the ovary, it is doubtful whether qualifying terms such as *borderline* are always appropriate. Unfortunately, terms like *borderline* may create a false sense of security among some physicians. These patients should be observed as closely as any patient with ovarian cancer.

In 1973, Hart and Norris reported a series of borderline

mucinous tumors confined to either or both ovaries at the time of diagnosis, with a corrected 10-year actuarial survival rate of 96%. Whereas the origin of the serous tumors from germinal epithelium is generally accepted, the histogenesis of mucinous tumors is more problematic. Grossly, these neoplasms do not differ significantly from their benign counterparts. They are multilocular, cystic, frequently voluminous masses with smooth outer surfaces. The inner lining, also similar to that of benign mucinous cystadenomas, is generally smooth, although papillary structures and solid thickening of the capsule have been observed in about 25% to 50% of lesions reported. Microscopically, in contrast to that of the benign mucinous cystadenoma, the epithelial lining of the borderline tumor is characterized by stratification of two to three layers. In the benign tumors, the cells show no atypism or pleomorphism, but the epithelium of the borderline lesions does demonstrate atypism, with irregular, hyperchromatic nuclei and enlarged nuclei. Mitotic figures are also seen.

For treatment of borderline lesions, the physician should strive to completely extirpate the tumor. If disease is unilateral, a salpingo-oophorectomy or a carefully performed ovarian cystectomy is appropriate, on condition that a thorough evaluation of the other ovary (biopsy if necessary), a peritoneal cytologic examination, and a partial omentectomy are done. Julian and Woodruff evaluated 65 patients who had low-grade papillary serous carcinoma of the ovary and found that 100% of the 50 patients who had unilateral adnexectomy and 90% of the 10 patients who had complete operation were alive at 5 years. Lim-Tan reported on 35 patients with ovarian serous borderline tumors treated by unilateral cystectomy or bilateral cystectomy. Tumor persisted or recurred only in the ovary that had been subjected to cystectomy in 2

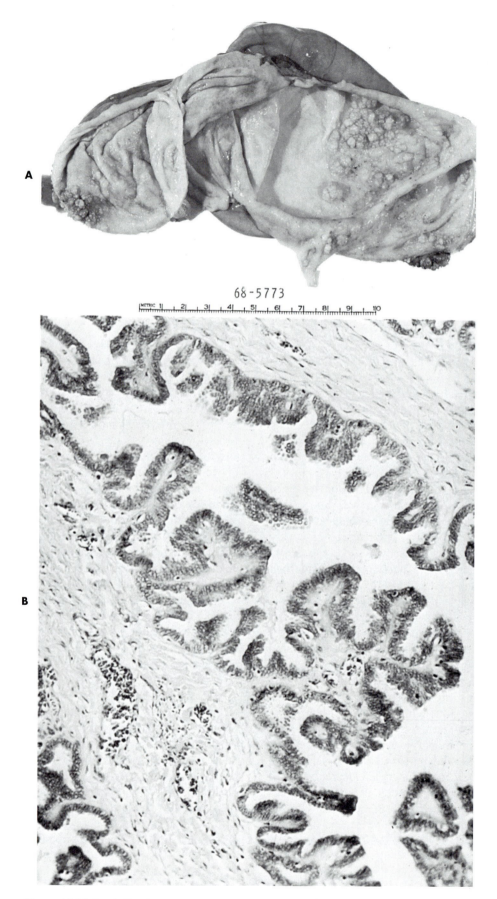

Figure 10-15 Borderline serous carcinoma. **A,** Gross appearance. **B,** Histologic section showing stratification of epithelial lining in papillary projections.

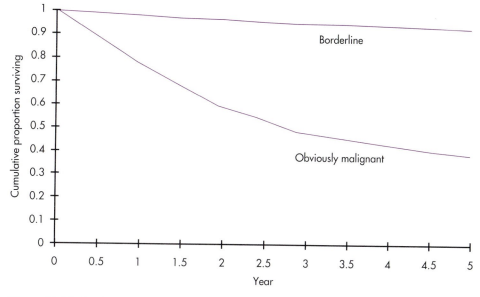

Figure 10-16 Carcinoma of the ovary. All stages. Cumulative proportion surviving by borderline tumors compared with obviously malignant cases. (From *Annual Report Gynecological Cancer FIGO,* vol 22, 1994.)

(6%) of the 33 patients, with stage I tumors in both the ipsilateral and contralateral ovary in one patient (3%) and only in the contralateral ovary in the other patient (3%). All the patients were alive without evidence of disease 3 to 18 years after initial operation, with the average follow-up of 7.5 years. Scattered reports of similar smaller series suggest that these lesions may be managed with ovarian cystectomy alone in patients desirous of further childbearing where acceptance of a small risk is appropriate.

If there is bilateral ovarian involvement, especially when papillary projections are found on the external surface of the tumor, or if peritoneal spread is noted, a more radical surgical approach, such as total abdominal hysterectomy with bilateral salpingo-oophorectomy and radical excision of involved pelvic peritoneum, is advocated. Peritoneal cytology, partial omentectomy, and selected pelvic and periaortic lymphadenectomy should also be done in these patients with more advanced disease. Advanced (stage III) borderline lesions can occur with metastases to lymph nodes. Survival even of these advanced lesions is appreciable.

Appropriate treatment for stage I borderline neoplasms of the ovary, other than surgical resection, remains uncertain. Kolstad et al. randomized patients with stage I borderline lesions into two groups, one treated by pelvic radiotherapy and the other by pelvic radiotherapy and intraperitoneal radioactive colloidal gold. The actuarial survival rates were 92.5% and 87.2%, respectively; several patients died of complications of the gold therapy. In these instances, therapy seemingly resulted in a significant lowering of survival compared with three other series. Use of intraperitoneal chromic phosphate alone, without pelvic radiotherapy, is usually associated with

fewer intra-abdominal complications and may be more appropriate therapy.

Creasman reported on 55 patients with stage I borderline or low-malignant-potential lesions of the ovary. He concluded that surgical removal of the disease was as efficacious for adequate therapy as was postoperative pelvic irradiation or adjunctive chemotherapy. Both Gershenson and Bell have reported on patients with ovarian serous borderline tumors with peritoneal implants. Gershenson had a 95% disease-free survival rate at 5 years and a 91% disease-free survival rate at 10 years. On the other hand, Bell reported 13% of patients died of tumor and one patient was alive with widespread progressive tumor. Death from tumor was 4% at 5 years and 23% at 10 years. Drescher studied the significance of DNA content and nuclear morphology in these lesions. Their results suggest that measurement of DNA ploidy and nuclear morphology using image analysis can provide important prognostic information in patients with borderline ovarian tumors. Work such as this is important because some of these lesions progress in an aggressive manner, leading the clinician to consider chemotherapy. It would be comfortable to have a mechanism for distinguishing lesions that are biologically aggressive from lesions that persist in a state of equilibrium, posing no threat to the patients' health and welfare.

Trimble reported an excellent review of epithelial ovarian tumors of low malignant potential in 1994. For serous and mucinous tumors of low malignant potential (LMP), the mean age at diagnosis falls close to 40 years of age, approximately two decades earlier than the mean age at diagnosis for invasive epithelial ovarian cancer. In a meta-analysis of 12 case-controlled studies conducted in the United States, Harris found a mean age of 44 for women with tumors of LMP compared with a mean age of 52.9 for women with invasive ovarian carcinoma. The meta-analysis conducted by the Collaborative Ovarian Cancer Group found protective factors against the development of tumors of LMP to be pregnancy, breast feeding, and use of oral contraceptives. A history of infertility increased the risk of tumors of LMP (odds ratio 1.9), and the use of infertility drugs further increased the risk of developing a tumor of LMP, above that of women with no history of infertility (odds ratio 4.0).

Kurman and Trimble reviewed survival in 22 studies of serous tumors of LMP, excluding those patients with invasive peritoneal implants. For 538 patients with stage I disease, survival was 99%, with a mean follow-up of 7 years. Even in the series for 415 patients with stage II and stage III disease, survival was 92% with the mean follow up of 7 years. In reviewing the causes of death in this series, 3 patients died of radiation-associated complications, 9 died from chemotherapy-associated complications, 8 died from bowel obstruction, and 8 died from invasive carcinoma; 18 patients were reported as "dying of disease" without additional information. In short, more patients seemed "to die with disease than of disease." In addition, more patients died of treatment-related complications than died of bowel obstruction from progressive disease.

PROPER IDENTIFICATION OF AN EARLY OVARIAN NEOPLASM

The combined 5-year survival rates quoted for stages I and II epithelial cancer of the ovary vary from 50%-70% and from 40%-50%, respectively. These survival rates are disappointing in view of the presumptive removal of all tumor at the time of surgery.

To date there have been several prospective studies evaluating metastasis to the diaphragm in women with presumed stage I or stage II ovarian carcinoma (Table 10-7). In each instance, the surgeon doing the initial procedure believed that the lesion was confined to the ovary and/or pelvis. The incidence of such unsuspected metastases was 15.7% in the collective series (11.3% for stage I and 23.0% for stage II).

Knapp and Friedman, Delgado et al., and Musumeci et al., evaluated prospectively aortic node metastasis in patients with stages I or II ovarian carcinoma. Collectively they found that 10.3% of stage I and 10.0% of stage II patients had aortic node disease. Knapp and Friedman found that the omentum was a site of microscopic metastasis in 4.7% of the patients with stages I and II ovarian epithelial cancer. Keettel et al. were among the first to report that in the absence of clinical ascites, a significant number of patients with localized ovarian cancer have free-floating intraperitoneal cancer cells, demonstrated by cytologic washings. In their report, 36% of the stage I patients had malignant cells in the cytologic washings. The report and three other studies were collated

Table 10-7 Incidence of subclinical metastases in stages I and II ovarian carcinoma

Series	Diaphragm (%)	Aortic nodes (%)	Malignant cytologic washings (%)
Knapp and Friedman	—	12.5	—
Rosenoff et al.	43.7	—	—
Delgado et al.	0.0	20.0	—
Spinelli et al.	23.0	—	—
Musumeci et al.	—	7.0	—
Keettel et al.	—	—	36.0
Creasman et al.	—	—	10.0
Morton, Moore, and Chang	—	—	50.0
Piver, Barlow, and Lele	3.2	0.0	25.8
TOTAL	15.7	10.3	29.8
Stage I	11.3	10.3	32.9
Stage II	23.0	10.0	12.5

Modified from Piver MS, Barlow JJ, Lele SB: *Obstet Gynecol* 52:100, 1978.

by Piver et al. for a total of 87 women with presumed stages I or II ovarian carcinoma. A total of 29.8% of these patients were found to have free-floating cancer cells in the pelvis or paracolonic spaces. Therefore, many of the failures in the stages I and II categories were undoubtedly patients with occult dissemination not realized at the time of the initial surgical procedure. (For recommendations on the optimal surgical procedure at initial laparotomy, see the section on Diagnostic Techniques and Staging in Chapter 11.)

MANAGEMENT OF EARLY OVARIAN CANCER IN YOUNG WOMEN

Traditionally, operative treatment has been the mainstay of management in ovarian carcinoma. The technical aspects of the initial laparotomy have a greater bearing on outcome than many subsequent therapeutic decisions. Hysterectomy with bilateral salpingo-oophorectomy continues to be the most cogent therapy for ovarian carcinoma. The opposite ovary is removed because of the frequency of bilateral synchronous tumors and the possibility of occult metastases, which in the normal-appearing opposite ovary have varied from 6%-43%, depending on the report and stage of the disease. Because the uterine serosa and endometrium are often sites of occult metastasis and because the prevalence of synchronous endometrial carcinoma is relatively high, hysterectomy is also indicated. Occasionally, however, unilateral oophorectomy has been done in young, childless women, and the tumors subsequently were found to be malignant. Not to proceed with further therapy is a calculated risk, the justification for which exists in statements made, summarized below, by many authoritative gynecologists.

REQUIREMENTS FOR CONSERVATIVE MANAGEMENT IN EPITHELIAL OVARIAN CANCER

1. Stage Ia
2. Well differentiated
3. Young woman of low parity
4. Otherwise normal pelvis
5. Encapsulated and free of adhesions
6. No invasion of capsule, lymphatics, or mesovarium
7. Peritoneal washings negative
8. Adequate evaluation of opposite ovary and omental biopsy negative
9. Close follow-up probable
10. Excision of residual ovary after completion of childbearing

Modified from DiSaia PJ, Townsend DE, Morrow CP: *Obstet Gynecol Surv* 29:581, 1994. Copyright © 1974 by The Williams & Wilkins Co.

Table 10-8   Recurrence rate in patients with low malignant potential lesions with conservative surgery

Author	Incidence of recurrence (%)	
Casey et al.	0/7	(0)
Chambers et al.	2/20	(20)
Lim-Tan et al.	4/35	(11)
Manchul et al.	0/15	(0)
Rice et al.	0/32	(0)
Sawada et al.	1/5	(20)
Tazelaar et al.	3/20	(15)
Trope et al.	0/14	(0)
TOTAL	10/148	(7)

Modified from Trimble EL: Management of Low Malignant Potential Ovarian Tumors, *Gynecol Oncol* 55:S52, 1994.

For the young, nulliparous woman with a stage Ia tumor, the safety of more conservative operations to preserve childbearing is uncertain. Munnell reviewed 127 cases of ovarian cancer treated by operation that included bilateral salpingo-oophorectomy and 38 cases in which conservative therapy was used. Excluding the uncommon carcinomas in the series, the 5-year survival figures for the 28 patients treated conservatively and for the 105 patients treated more radically is 75%. In patients with mucinous tumors, 78% who had complete operation (23 patients) and 100% who had conservative operation (8 patients) survived 5 years. Similarly, Parker et al. found no difference in the 5-year survival rate regardless of whether patients were treated by hysterectomy and bilateral salpingo-oophorectomy or by unilateral salpingo-oophorectomy alone.

The requirements for conservative management of stage Ia ovarian cancer are listed in the box above. Unilateral salpingo-oophorectomy may be the definitive treatment for a young woman of low parity found to have a well-differentiated serous, mucinous, endometrioid, or mesonephric carcinoma of the ovary. The tumor must be unilateral, well encapsulated, free of adhesions, and not associated with ascites or evidence of extragonadal spread. Peritoneal washings for cytology should be taken from the pelvis and upper abdomen, and the opposite ovary should be evaluated for disease. If the opposite ovary is of normal size, shape, and configuration, surgical evaluation is not routinely done. The incidence of microscopic metastases in the opposite ovary has been calculated by Munnell and others to be approximately 12%. The periaortic and pelvic wall nodes must be carefully palpated and sampled, and an adequate sample of the omentum must be taken for biopsy. In our experience, it is rare for grade I ovarian lesions to metastasize to pelvic or periaortic nodes. However, any grossly abnormal nodal tissue must be suspect for being a focus of a rare metastatic lesion. In addition, the preserved pelvic organs should be reasonably normal, since there is little to be gained by retaining the opposite ovary in a patient who is not fertile. With the finding of carcinoma in any of these areas, conservative surgery must be abandoned. After the patient has completed childbearing, some consideration should be given to the removal of the other ovary to eliminate the risk of another ovarian malignancy. Because the incidence of epithelial cancer of the ovary increases when a woman reaches the sixth decade and because a patient with a history of such a lesion harbors the unfortunate milieu that could promote another epithelium lesion, it is only logical to remove the vestigial ovarian tissue after childbearing.

The key issue in patients treated conservatively for stage Ia epithelial tumors of the ovary is the histology. Mucinous and endometrioid lesions fare better than serous lesions, the grade I and borderline lesions being the most easily treated conservatively. Serous lesions are said to be 7 times more frequently bilateral than mucinous carcinomas.

Conservative therapy, designed by preservation of some ovarian tissue, appears to be safe, although no prospective trials have compared conservative surgery to bilateral salpingo-oophorectomy. Trimble collected eight series (Table 10-8). In a study of this data, there were only 10 recurrences in 148 patients for an incidence of 6.8%. In our own experience, we have observed the development of papillary serous carcinoma in a contralateral ovary 5 years after conservative therapy in the form of unilateral salpingo-oophorectomy that was performed on a 29-year-old patient.

The role of adjuvant therapy, whether radiotherapy or chemotherapy, in tumors of LMP has not yet been established. Several prospective, randomized studies of adjuvant therapy in patients with invasive ovarian

Table 10-9 Dysgerminoma: stage I

	Cases	Treatment	Recurrence rate	5-year survival rate
Radiumhemmet	22	UO + radiation therapy	18%	95%
AFIP	46	UO	22%	91%
AFIP	21	TAH, BSO	10%	90%

UO, Unilateral oophorectomy; *TAH, BSO,* total abdominal hysterectomy and bilateral salpingo-oophorectomy; *AFIP,* Armed Forces Institute of Pathology.

carcinoma have included patients with tumors of LMP. In one trial, conducted by the GOG, 55 patients with stage I disease were randomized to no further therapy, pelvic radiation therapy, or oral Melphalan for 18 months. They noted one recurrence, on the radiation therapy arm, and concluded that the total abdominal hysterectomy with bilateral salpingo-oophorectomy was adequate treatment for patients with stage I disease.

In a recent study of 33 women from the Mayo Clinic, ages 16 to 29, who had stage Ia ovarian cancer, it was shown that unilateral salpingo-oophorectomy or just resection of the ovary resulted in no recurrences in a period of follow-up from 3 to 10 years. These results are encouraging, but they are not the final answer, since many low-grade lesions are prone to late recurrence. Some centers are now studying the role of ovarian cystectomy alone for low-grade stage I epithelial neoplasms. Others have permitted stage I, grade 2 and 3 lesions, and stage Ic neoplasms to undergo ovarian tissue-sparing surgery followed by chemotherapy in an attempt to preserve fertility. These investigations await further observation and confirmation as to long-term safety. Chemotherapy administered following such ovarian tissue-sparing procedures is likely to destroy the remaining ova, especially in patients over 30 years of age.

Colombo reported data on 99 patients below age 40 with stage I ovarian cancer. Conservative surgery was performed in 56 of the patients (36 stage Ia, 1 stage Ib, and 19 stage Ic). Relapses occurred in 3 stage Ia (grades 1, 2, and 3) patients. One recurrence was in the residual ovary and the patient was rescued by surgery; the other two patients relapsed at distant sites and died as a result of their tumors. Seventeen patients who desired to become pregnant did so, for a total of 25 conceptions. Colombo suggested a platinum based regimen to lower the recurrence rate even further. A GOG study reported no difference in survival for patients with stages Ic or II or poorly differentiated stages Ia and Ib cancer randomized to receive either Melphalan or intraperitoneal ^{32}P. The same report showed no advantage to adjuvant treatment with Melphalan for patients with stages Ia or Ib, well or moderately differentiated tumor.

Only one trial testing cis-platinum as adjuvant treatment of early disease has been published. In this study, 347 patients with epithelial ovarian cancer without residual tumor following primary surgery were randomized to adjuvant intraperitoneal ^{32}P therapy or six courses of cisplatin. Disease free survival and overall survival were similar in the two arms even after adjustment for prognostic variable. Bolis reported two multicenter clinical trials in Italy. After surgical staging and stratification by center, eligible patients were randomized according to a computer generated list. In the first study, 92 patients with stage Ia or Ib, grade 2 or 3 tumors were randomly assigned to receive either cisplatin for six cycles or no further treatment. With a median follow-up of 69 months, 5-year disease free survival was 83% for the platinum group and 64% for the observation group. However, no difference in the overall survival could be detected. Indeed, the patients who relapsed in the no treatment arm appeared to be salvageable with chemotherapy begun at the time of reoccurrence.

The management of dysgerminoma is frequently singled out as an example for conservative surgery. Table 10-9 shows the statistics in patients treated in various manners. The exquisite radiosensitivity and chemosensitivity of dysgerminoma allows one to be somewhat liberal in its management. Although the recurrence rate is approximately 20% in stage I, the overall survival rate is almost 95% because of the exceptional response to radical radiation therapy or chemotherapy. It is interesting to note that the incidence of recurrence is approximately the same despite the initial treatment. The treatment of recurrences results in approximately a 75% 5-year salvage rate. In the last decade, many centers have chosen to use multi-agent chemotherapy rather than irradiation for advanced or recurrent dysgerminoma. Preferred regimens are similar to those used for other malignant germ cell tumors of the ovary (see Chapter 12).

SPILL OF TUMOR

The subject of tumor spill has been quite controversial in gynecologic oncology for some time. It is logical to assume that implantation and germination of cancer cells are conceivable and probable when a malignant cyst ruptures at the time of surgery. The question remains only to prove that this is so.

The early studies of Munnell did not support the theoretic possibility that rupture of a malignant ovarian

Table 10-10   Tumor-free survival in stage I ovarian cancer

Series	Neoplasm ruptured	Neoplasm unruptured
Purola and Nieminen (1968)	18/30 (60%)	83/100 (83%)
Williams, Symmonds, and Litwak (1973)	3/7 (43%)	57/58 (98%)
Parker, Parker, and Wilbanks (1970)	16/27 (59%)	12/20 (60%)
Dembo et al. (1989)	98/119 (82%)	168/199 (84%)
Sevelda et al. (1989)	23/30 (76%)	23/30 (76%)

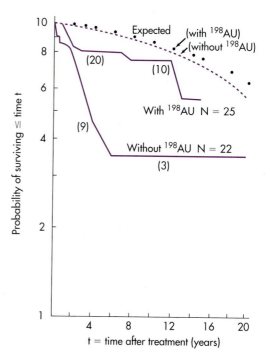

Figure 10-17 Probability of survival in stage I epithelial ovarian cancer with rupture of neoplasm at surgical removal, with and without intraperitoneal radioactive colloidal gold therapy. (From Decker DG, Webb MJ, Holbrook MA: *Am J Obstet Gynecol* 115:751, 1973.)

tumor would enhance dissemination. He studied 99 patients with stages I or II ovarian cancer and had an overall 5-year survival rate of 71%. In his retrospective study, 27 of the patients had had spill at the time of surgery. Of these patients, 22 (81%) survived 5 years. Of these 27 patients, postoperative irradiation was administered to 21, and there was a 66% 5-year survival rate in this group of 21. Six of the patients did not receive x-ray therapy, and all six survived 5 years. It appears from this very limited retrospective study that spill eruption does not endanger the patient's prognosis and that if this does occur, postoperative irradiation is not necessarily indicated. Since the number of patients studied here is small, it is necessary to carefully study the histology in the 6 patients who did not receive x-ray therapy. One might find that these were highly differentiated lesions, maybe of borderline quality. There is, in addition, an obvious bias interjected here in that the patients with more malignant lesions probably received radiation therapy. There have been very few studies with enough patients to shed further light on this subject (Table 10-10). However, a report by Decker et al. of the Mayo Clinic, involving some 223 stage I cases of ovarian epithelial cancer, revealed that rupture during surgery did seem to lower the survival curve (Figure 10-17). Another study by Grogan from Harvard analyzed 124 patients with ovarian cancer. Rupture of an ovarian tumor cyst during surgery occurred in 16 of 124 patients. For our purposes, however, only 9 patients should be considered, because only these patients had stage I lesions. Of these 9 patients, 6 survived 5 years or more, 1 died of a massive myocardial infarction, and the other 2 succumbed to their malignancies. The 6 patients who survived had well-differentiated grade I histologic patterns. Both patients who died of tumor had poorly differentiated histologic pictures. They had received radiation therapy following hysterectomy and bilateral salpingo-oophorectomy but the radiation therapy was delivered in very moderate dosages of 2500 to 3000 cGy on a 200 kv machine. This is far below optimal

radiation therapy. Parket et al. and Dembo et al. could find no difference in survival between patients with stage I cancers whose ovaries were ruptured at the time of surgery and those in whom rupture did not occur. Many of these retrospective studies have no information regarding the status of peritoneal cytology prior to manipulation of the neoplasm. Indeed, it is the patient with a negative peritoneal cytology that suffers spill who is of concern. Sevelda reported on 60 stage I patients with negative peritoneal washings at the beginning of the primary laparotomy. In 30 patients, rupture occurred, and in the other 30 the tumor could be removed with the capsule intact. After an average follow-up of 75 months, the probability of survival was 76% in both groups. However, all but 10 of the patients received whole-abdomen radiation postoperatively, which obscures a conclusion as to the true meaning of spill.

Sainz reported on 79 patients with stage I invasive epithelial ovarian cancer treated at the Massachusetts General Hospital. Of these 79 patients, 36 had stage Ia tumors, 20 stage Ic secondary to intraoperative rupture (Ic-rupture), and 17 stage Ic secondary to capsule invasion, serosal disease, or positive ascites/ washings. There were four recurrences and subsequent deaths among the 20 women with stage Ic-ruptured tumors (20%), compared to only one (3%) of the 36 women with stage Ia. The median follow-up time for the two groups was 97 and 78 months, respectively; overall survival was

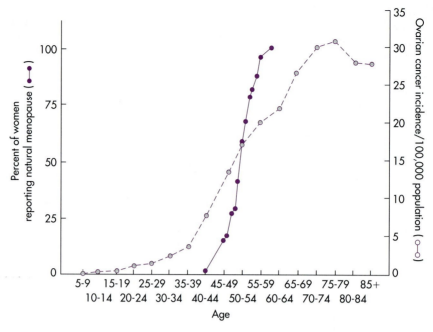

Figure 10-18 Incidence of ovarian cancer and onset of natural menopause vs age.

97 and 73 months. There were two recurrences (12%), one death (6%) among the 17 women with stage Ic disease and no rupture. Survival experience of this last group was not significantly different to that of the Ic-rupture group. Sainz concluded that intraoperative rupture of malignant epithelial ovarian neoplasms may worsen the prognosis of patients with stage I ovarian epithelial cancer. In the same year (1994), Sjövall reported on 247 patients with stage I disease who were at risk of spill. There was no difference in survival in patients whose tumors had intact capsules and the patients in whom rupture occurred during surgery—78% and 85%, respectively. On the other hand, a significant difference in survival was found between patients in whom rupture occurred before surgery and those with intraoperative rupture—59% and 85%, respectively. Their conclusion was that manipulation during surgery that results in puncture or rupture does not have a negative influence on the outcome for patients. However, rupture occurring at some interval prior to surgery may lead to seeding in the peritoneal cavity.

The issue is difficult to resolve because one is very prone to treat more vigorously patients who have spill at the time of surgery, and this may equalize the survival rates in the groups of patients. In the era when whole-abdomen irradiation with pelvic boost was the only therapy that could be offered these patients, some hesitation in instituting postoperative therapy appeared to be justified. However, we now have comparatively less morbid chemotherapeutic regimens that can be adequately used postoperatively. A reasonable and seemingly adequate recommendation in these instances is a course of chemotherapy administered in the form of a platinum-based regimen for six cycles and then a "second-look" procedure to verify the absence of disease within the pelvic and abdominal cavities. Others have recommended the use of intraperitoneal colloidal isotopes such as ^{32}P. No prospective study comparing these seemingly valid approaches has been reported. If rupture does occur, lavage of the peritoneal cavity with sterile water is recommended to cause lysis of the cells, and this may be helpful. The peritoneal surfaces will absorb the water, so care should be taken to prevent delays in retrieving the fluid.

PROPHYLACTIC OOPHORECTOMY

The early diagnosis of ovarian carcinoma is as difficult and infrequent now as in the past. Although survival figures for this disease may be recently improving to a slight degree, the prognosis is still very grave. One is therefore led to at least consider the impact of prophylactic oophorectomy on women, especially women undergoing pelvic surgery for benign disease when childbearing is completed and preservation of ovarian tissue is not essential.

At some time during their lives, 1%-2% of all women develop ovarian carcinoma. The risk increases after the age of 40 with a peak incidence between 55 and 60 years of age, closely paralleling the peak incidence of menopause in Western countries (Figure 10-18). One is tempted to speculate that the gonadotropin changes or other factors associated with menopause might at times function as a promoting agent in the carcinogenic process. However, no scientific data are available in this regard.

The function of the ovary lies (1) in its role of ova production for procreation and (2) as the primary site of estrogen production. After the need for ova has passed in a woman's life, only estrogen production remains as an essential function. The adverse effects of oophorectomy on several metabolic parameters are well known; understanding of the endocrinology, sexuality, and psychology of the postmenopausal patient (natural or surgical) has increased considerably during the past decade, and good methods of adequate substitution for the loss of ovarian function are now available.

In 1981 Grundsell reported on a series of 352 women with ovarian carcinoma and studied the incidence of previous pelvic surgeries performed on these patients. Twenty-one (6%) had undergone previous pelvic surgery, and 16 (4.6%) of these patients had surgery at some time after the age of 40. Others (Table 10-11) have reported similar results (Bloom, Gibbs, Grogan, Kofler, and Terz). McKenzie, Christ, and Paloucek reported that as many as 3.6% of women who have pelvic surgery with preservation of ovarian tissue will need subsequent surgery for benign lesions of the ovary (Table 10-12), further influencing the argument for prophylactic oophorectomy.

Averette et al. found that 18.2% of patients reported previous hysterectomy with ovarian conservation in a recent national survey of 12,316 ovarian cancer cases. Of these, hysterectomies were abdominal in 7.2%, vaginal in 4.2%, and unspecified in another 6.8%. A subsequent analysis, Boike et al. found that 57.4% of hysterectomies were performed after the age of 40. Thus a potential 1286 ovarian cancer cases could have been prevented if prophylactical oophorectomy had been practiced in women undergoing hysterectomy at the age of 40 or older. Assuming an annual incidence of 24,000 new ovarian cases and that 5%-14% of these cases had previous hysterectomies with conserved ovaries, it is estimated that at least 1000 cases could have been prevented if prophylactic oophorectomy were diligently practiced over the age of 40.

We are obviously influenced by the frequent task of caring for patients with advanced ovarian carcinoma. The occurrence of this disease in patients who had previous pelvic surgery and in whom the ovaries could have been

removed is certainly frustrating. Randall has shown that unilateral oophorectomy does not influence the subsequent incidence of ovarian carcinoma.

All patients in whom prophylactic oophorectomy is under consideration should be thoroughly informed about the possible adverse effects as well as the advantages. The patient must make the decision without undue pressure from her physician. All thoughts of further childbearing must be settled. Open discussion should be encouraged, especially in areas of body image, libido, and other psychosexual concerns. With this as background, we feel that prophylactic oophorectomy should be offered to all perimenopausal patients (40 to 50 years of age) undergoing pelvic surgery.

Table 10-11   Ovarian carcinoma/preserved ovaries

Author	Year	Pevious pelvic surgery (%)	
		All ages	>40 yr
Bloom	1962	10.6	
Grogan	1967	8.2	
Terz	1967	8.8	3.8
Gibbs	1971	11.8	
Kofler	1972	8.1	8.1
Grundsell	1980	6.0	4.6

Table 10-12   Ovarian carcinoma/preserved ovaries

Author	Year	Previous pelvic surgery (%)	
		All ages	>40 yr
Bloom	1962	10.6	
Grogan	1967	8.2	
Terz	1967	8.8	3.8
Gibbs	1971	11.8	
Kofler	1972	8.1	8.1
Grundsell	1980	6.0	4.6
Averette	1994	18.2	10.1

BIBLIOGRAPHY

Adnexal mass

Borne TH et al: Color blood flow imaging aids ovarian cancer diagnosis, *Today in Medicine/Obstet Gynecol*, April to June 1993.

Cohen I et al: Ovarian tumors in postmenopausal breast cancer patients treated with Tamoxifen, *Gynecol Oncol* 60:54, 1996.

Curtin JP: Management of the adnexal mass, *Gynecol Oncol* 55:S42, 1994.

Fathalla MF: Factors in the causation and incidence of ovarian cancer, *Obstet Gynecol Surv* 27:751, 1972.

Graham JB, Graham RM: Ovarian cancer and asbestosis, *Environ Res* 1:115, 1967.

Grundsell H et al: Some aspects of prophylactic oophorectomy and ovarian carcinoma, *Ann Chir Gynaecol* 70:36, 1981.

Harvald B, Hauge M: Heredity of cancer elucidated by a study of unselected twins, *JAMA* 186:749, 1963.

Hasson HM: Laparoscopic management of ovarian cysts, *J Reprod Med* 35:863, 1990.

Henderson WJ et al: Talc and carcinoma of the ovary and cervix, *J Obstet Gynaecol Br Common* 78:6, 1971.

Kawai M et al: Transvaginal Doppler ultrasound with color flow imaging in the diagnosis of ovarian cancer, *Am Coll Obstet Gynec* 79:163, 1992.

Lee RA, Symmonds RE: Presacral tumors in the female: clinical presentation, surgical management, and results, *Obstet Gynecol* 71:216, 1988.

Nezhat F et al: Four ovarian cancers diagnosed during laparoscopic management of 1011 women with adnexal masses, *Am J Obstet Gynecol* 167:790, 1992.

Plaxe SC et al: Ovarian intraepithelial neoplasia demonstrated in patients with stage I ovarian carcinoma, *Gynecol Oncol* 38:367, 1992.

Puls LE et al: Transition from benign to malignant epithelium in mucinous and serous ovarian cystadenocarcinoma, *Gynecol Oncol* 47:53, 1992.

Randall CL, Hall DW, Armenia CS: Pathology in the preserved ovary after unilateral oophorectomy, *Am J Obstet Gynecol* 84:1233, 1962.

Spiert H: The role of ionizing radiations in the causation of ovarian tumors, *Cancer* 5:478, 1952.

Weiner Z et al: Differentiating malignant from benign ovarian tumors with transvaginal color flow imaging, *Am Coll Obstet Gynec* 79:159, 1992.

Ovarian tumors

Andolf E, Jorgensen C: Simple adnexal cysts diagnosed by ultrasound in postmenopausal women, *J Clin Ultrasound*, 16:301, 1988.

Andolf E, Jorgensen C: Cystic lesions in elderly women, diagnosed by ultrasound, *Br J Obstet Gynecol* 96:1076, 1989.

Arey LB: Origin and form of Brenner tumor, *Am J Obstet Gynecol* 81:743, 1961.

Asadourian LA, Taylor HB: Dysgerminoma: an analysis of 105 cases, *Obstet Gynecol* 33:370, 1969.

Aure JC, Hoeg K, Kolstadt P: Psammoma bodies in serous carcinoma of the ovary, *Am J Obstet Gynecol* 109:113, 1971.

Aure JC, Hoeg K, Kolstadt P: Radioactive colloidal gold in the treatment of ovarian carcinoma, *Acta Radiol* 10:399, 1971.

Bergman F: Carcinoma of the ovary: a clinicopathological study of 86 autopsied cases with special reference to mode of spread, *Acta Obstet Gynecol Scand* 45:211, 1966.

Bourne T, Campbell S, Steer C: A possible new screening technique for ovarian cancer, *Br Med J* 299:1367, 1989.

Caspi E, Schreyer P, Bukovsky J: Ovarian lutein cysts in pregnancy, *Obstet Gynecol* 42:388, 1972.

Christ JE, Lotze EC: The residual ovary syndrome, *Obstet Gynecol* 46:551, 1975.

Cianfrani T: Neoplasms in apparently normal ovaries, *Am J Obstet Gynecol* 41:211, 1973.

Creasman WT, Rutledge F: The prognostic value of peritoneal cytology in gynecologic malignant disease, *Am J Obstet Gynecol* 120:773, 1971.

Creasman WT et al: Stage I borderline ovarian tumors, *Obstet Gynecol* 59:93, 1982.

Decker DG, Webb MJ, Holbrook MA: Radiogold treatment of epithelial cancer of ovary: late results, *Am J Obstet Gynecol* 115:751, 1973.

Delgado G et al: Para-aortic lymphadenectomy in gynecologic malignancies confined to the pelvis, *Obstet Gynecol* 50:418, 1977.

Dembo AJ et al: Prognostic factors in patients with stage I epithelial ovarian cancer, *Obstet Gynecol* 75(2):263, 1990.

de Neef JC, Hollenbeck ZJR: The fate of ovaries preserved at the time of hysterectomy, *Am J Obstet Gynecol* 96:1088, 1966.

DiSaia PJ et al: Individualized treatment of ovarian cancers, *Am J Obstet Gynecol* 128:619, 1977.

Dockerty MB, Masson JC: Ovarian fibromas: a clinical and pathologic study of 283 cases, *Am J Obstet Gynecol* 47:741, 1944.

Eriksson L, Kjellgren O, von Schoultz B: Functional cyst or ovarian cancer: histopathological findings during 1 year of surgery, *Gynecol Obstet Invest* 19:155, 1985.

Finn CB et al: Is stage I epithelial ovarian cancer overtreated both surgically and systematically? Results of a five-year cancer registry review, *Br J Obstet Gynecol* 99:54, 1992.

Finn CB et al: Can we predict a high risk group in stage I epithelial ovarian cancer? *Int J Gynecol Cancer* 3:226, 1993.

Graham J, Burstein P, Graham R: Prognostic significance of pleural effusion in ovarian cancer, *Am J Obstet Gynecol* 106:312, 1970.

Graham JB, Graham RM, Schueller EF: Preclinical detection of ovarian cancer, *Cancer* 17:1414, 1964.

Granberg S, Norstrom A, Wikland M: Tumors in the lower pelvis as imaged by vaginal sonography, *Gynecol Oncol* 37:224, 1990.

Grogan RH: Accidental rupture of malignant ovarian cysts during surgical removal, *Obstet Gynecol* 30:716, 1967.

Grogan RH: Reappraisal of residual ovaries, *Am J Obstet Gynecol* 97:124, 1967.

Hart WR, Norris HJ: Borderline and malignant mucinous tumors of the ovary: histologic criteria and clinical behavior, *Cancer* 31:1031, 1973.

Hester LL, White L: Radioactive colloidal chromic phosphate in the treatment of ovarian malignancies, *Am J Obstet Gynecol* 103:911, 1969.

Higgins RV, van Nagell JR, Donaldson ES: Transvaginal sonography as a screening method for ovarian cancer, *Gynecol Oncol* 34:402, 1989.

Julian CG, Woodruff JD: The biologic behavior of the low-grade papillary serous carcinoma of the ovary, *Obstet Gynecol* 40:860, 1973.

Keettel WC, Pixley EE, Buchsbaum HJ: Experience with peritoneal cytology in the management of gynecologic malignancies, *Am J Obstet Gynecol* 120:174, 1974.

Knapp RC, Friedman EA: Aortic lymph node metastases in early ovarian cancer, *Am J Obstet Gynecol* 119:1013, 1974.

Kolstadt P et al: Individualized treatment of ovarian cancer, *Am J Obstet Gynecol* 128:619, 1977.

Koonings PP et al: Bilateral ovarian neoplasms and the risk of malignancy, *Am J Obstet Gynecol* 162:167, 1990.

Kurjak A et al: Transvaginal colour Doppler assessment of pelvic circulation, *Acta Obstet Gynecol Scand* 68:131, 1989.

Kurman RJ, Craig JM: Endometrioid carcinoma of the ovary, *Cancer* 29:1653, 1972.

Limber GK, King RE, Silverberg SG: Pseudomyxoma peritonei: a report of ten cases, *Ann Surg* 128:587, 1973.

Long RT, Spratt JS, Dowling E: Pseudomyxoma peritonei: new concepts in management with a report of 17 patients, *Ann Surg* 117:162, 1969.

Maiman M, Seltzer V, Boyce J: Laparoscopic excision of ovarian neoplasms subsequently found to be malignant, *Obstet Gynecol* 77(4):563, 1991.

Malkasian GD Jr, Dockerty MB, Symmonds RE: Benign cystic teratomas, *Obstet Gynecol* 29:719, 1967.

Malmström H, Simonsen E, Westberg R: A phase II study of intraperitoneal carboplatin as adjuvant treatment in early-stage ovarian cancer patients, *Gynecol Oncol* 52:20, 1994.

Mann WG et al: The management of pseudomyxoma peritonei, *Cancer* 66:1636, 1990.

McGowan L, Stein DB, Miller W: Cul-de-sac aspiration for diagnostic cytologic study, *Am J Obstet Gynecol* 96:413, 1966.

McKenzie LL: On discussion of the frequency of oophorectomy at the time of hysterectomy, *Am J Obstet Gynecol* 100:724, 1968.

Meigs JV, Cass JW: Fibroma of the ovary with ascites and hydrothorax with a report of 7 cases, *Am J Obstet Gynecol* 33:249, 1937.

Munnell EW: Is conservative therapy ever justified in stage IA cancer of the ovary? *Am J Obstet Gynecol* 103:641, 1969.

O'Hanlan KA: Case Report Resection of a 303.2-pound ovarian tumor, *Gynecol Oncol* 54:365, 1994.

Pezner RD: Limited epithelial carcinoma of the ovary treated with curative intent by the intraperitoneal instillation of radiocolloids, *Cancer* 42:2563, 1978.

Piver MS, Barlow JJ, Lele SB: Incidence of subclinical metastasis in stage I and II ovarian carcinoma, *Obstet Gynecol* 52:100, 1978.

Piver MS et al: Intraperitoneal chromic phosphate in peritoneoscopically confirmed stage I ovarian adenocarcinoma, *Am J Obstet Gynecol* 144:836, 1982.

Piver MS et al: Five year survival for stage Ic or stage I grade 3 epithelial ovarian cancer treated with cisplatin based chemotherapy, *Gynecol Oncol* 46:357, 1992.

Purola E, Nieminen V: Does rupture of cystic carcinoma during operation influence the prognosis? *Ann Chir Gynaecol Fenn* 57:615, 1968.

Rubin SC: Platinum-based chemotherapy of high-risk stage I epithelial ovarian cancer following comprehensive surgical staging, *Obstet & Gynecol* 82:143, 1993.

Samanth KK, Black WC: Benign ovarian stromal tumors associated with free peritoneal fluid, *Am J Obstet Gynecol* 107:538, 1970.

Sevelda P, Dittrich C, Salzer H: Prognostic value of the rupture of the capsule in stage I epithelial ovarian carcinoma, *Gynecol Oncol* 35:321, 1989.

Shanks HGI: Pseudomyxoma peritonei, *J Obstet Gynaecol Br Common* 68:212, 1961.

Spanos WJ: Preoperative hormonal therapy of cystic adnexal masses, *Am J Obstet Gynecol* 116:551, 1973.

Spanos WJ et al: Complications in the use of intra-abdominal ^{32}P for ovarian carcinoma, *Gynecol Oncol* 45:243, 1992.

Taylor KJW, Conway DI, Hull MGR: Ultrasound and Doppler flow studies of the ovarian and uterine arteries, *Br J Obstet Gynaecol* 92:240, 1985.

Vergote IB et al: Analysis of prognostic factors in stage I epithelial ovarian carcinoma: importance of degree of differentiation and deoxyribonucleic acid ploidy in predicting relapse, *Am J Obstet Gynecol* 169:40, 1993.

Webb MJ et al: Factors influencing survival in stage I ovarian cancer, *Am J Obstet Gynecol* 116:222, 1973.

Williams TJ, Dockerty MB: Status of the contralateral ovary in encapsulated low grade malignant tumors of the ovary, *Surgery* 143:763, 1976.

Wolf SI, Gosnik BB, Feldsman MR: Prevalence of simple adnexal cysts in postmenopausal women, *Radiology* 180:65, 1991.

Woodruff JD, Julian CG: Histologic grading and morphologic changes of significance in the treatment of semi-malignant and malignant ovarian tumors, *Proc Natl Cancer Conf* 6:346, 1970.

Yoonessi M, Murray RA: Brenner tumors of the ovary, *Obstet Gynecol* 54:90, 1979.

Childhood adnexal masses

Blom PG, Torkildsen EM: Ovarian cystadenocarcinoma in a 4-year-old girl: report of a case and review of the literature, *Gynecol Oncol* 13:242, 1982.

Breen JL, Maxson WS: Ovarian tumors in children and adolescents, *Clin Obstet Gynecol* 20:607, 1977.

Carlson DH, Griscom NT: Ovarian cysts in the newborn, *AJR* 116:664, 1972.

Deprest J et al: Case report: ovarian borderline mucinous tumor in a premenarchal girl: review on ovarian epithelial cancer in young girls, *Gynecol Oncol* 45:219, 1992.

Ehren IM, Mahour GH, Isaacs H: Benign and malignant ovarian tumors in children and adolescents, *Am J Surg* 147:339, 1984.

Haefner HK, Roberts JA, Schmidt RW: The university experience of clinical and pathological findings of ovarian neoplasms in children and adolescents, *Adolesc Pediatr Gynecol* 5:182, 1992.

Norris HG, Jensen RD: Relative frequency of ovarian neoplasms in children and adolescents, *Cancer* 30:713, 1972.

Schwöbel MG, Stauffer UG: Surgical treatment of ovarian tumors in childhood, *Prog Pediatr Surg* 26:112, 1991.

Smith JP, Rutledge RN, Sutow WW: Malignant gynecologic tumors in children; current approaches to treatment, *Am J Obstet Gynecol* 116:261, 1973.

Van Winter JT, Simmons PS, Podratz KC: Surgically treated adnexal masses in infancy, childhood, and adolescence, *Am J Obstet Gynecol* 170:1780, 1994.

Postmenopausal adnexal cysts

Andolf E, Jorgensen C: Simple adnexal cysts diagnosed by ultrasound in postmenopausal women, *J Clin Ultrasound* 16:301, 1988.

Barber HR, Graber EA: The PMPO syndrome (postmenopausal palpable ovary syndrome), *Obstet Gynecol* 38(6):921, 1971.

Creasman WT, Soper JT: The undiagnosed adnexal mass after the menopause, *Clin Obstet Gynecol* 29(2):446, 1986.

Flynt JR, Gallup DG: The postmenopausal ovary syndrome: a fourteen year review, *Milit Med* 146(10):686, 1981.

Goldstein SR: Ultrasound for the postmenopausal patient, *Female Patient* 15:61, 1990.

Goldstein SR et al: The postmenopausal cystic adnexal mass: the potential role of ultrasound in conservative management, *Obstet Gynecol* 72(1):8, 1989.

Goswamy RK et al: Ovarian size in postmenopausal women, *Br J Obstet Gynaecol* 95(8):795, 1988.

Hall DA, McCarthy KA: The significance of the postmenopausal simple adnexal cyst, *J Ultrasound Med* 5(9):503, 1986.

Lerner JP et al: Transvaginal ultrasonographic characterization of ovarian masses with a improved, weighted scoring system, *Am J Obstet Gynecol* 170:81, 1994.

Luxman D et al: The postmenopausal adnexal mass: correlation between ultrasonic and pathology finding, *Obstet Gynecol* 77:726, 1991.

Miller RC et al: The postmenopausal palpable ovary syndrome: a retrospective review with histopathologic correlates, *J Reprod Med* 36:568, 1991.

Parker WH, Berek JS: Management of selected cystic adnexal masses in postmenopausal women by operative laparoscopy: a pilot study, *Am J Obstet Gynecol* 163:1574, 1990.

Rulin MC, Preston AL: Adnexal masses in postmenopausal women, *Obstet Gynecol* 70(4):578, 1987.

Snider DD et al: Evaluation of surgical staging in stage I low malignant potential ovarian tumors, *Gynecol Oncol* 40:129, 1991.

Westhoff C et al: CA 125 levels in menopausal women, *Obstet Gynecol* 76:428, 1990.

Borderline lesions (low malignant potential)

Bell DA, Weinstock MA, Scully RE: Peritoneal implants of ovarian serous borderline tumors: histologic features and prognosis, *Cancer* 62:2212, 1988.

Casey AC et al: Epithelial ovarian tumors of borderline malignancy: long term follow-up, *Gynecol Oncol* 50:316, 1993.

Chambers JT et al: Borderline ovarian tumors, *Am J Ob/Gyn* 159:1088, 1988.

Creasman WT et al: Stage I borderline ovarian tumors, *Obstet Gynecol* 59:93, 1982.

Drescher W et al: Prognostic significance of DNA content and nuclear morphology in borderline ovarian tumors, *Gynecol Oncol* 48:242, 1993.

Fort MG et al: Evidence for the efficacy of adjuvant therapy in epithelial ovarian tumors of low malignant potential, *Gynecol Oncol* 32:269, 1989.

Gershenson DM, Silva EG: Serous ovarian tumors of low malignant potential with peritoneal implants, *Cancer* 65:578, 1990.

Harris R, Whittemore AS, Itnyre J, and the Collaborative Ovarian Cancer Group. Characteristics relating to ovarian cancer risk: collaborative analysis of 12 US Case-control studies. III. Epithelial tumors of low malignant potential in white women, *Am J Epidemiol* 136:1204, 1992.

Janovski NA, Paramananthon TL: *Ovarian Tumors,* Stuttgart, 1973. Georg Thieme Verlag.

Kurman RJ, Trimble CL: The behavior of serous tumors of low malignant potential: are they ever malignant? *Int J Gynecol Pathol* 12:120, 1993.

Lim-Tan SK et al: Ovarian cystectomy for serous borderline tumors: a follow-up study of 35 cases, *Obstet Gynecol* 72:775, 1988.

Manchul LA et al: Borderline epithelial ovarian tumors: a review of 81 cases with an assessment of the impact of treatment, *Int J Radiat Oncol Biol Phys* 22:867, 1992.

Rice LW et al: Epithelial ovarian tumors of borderline malignancy, *Gynecol Oncol* 39:195, 1990.

Sawada M et al: Stage I epithelial ovarian tumors of low malignant potential, *Jpn J Clin Oncol* 21:30, 1991.

Shiraki M et al: Case Report: Ovarian serous borderline epithelial tumors with multiple retroperitoneal nodal involvement: metastasis or malignant transformation of epithelial glandular inclusions? *Gynecol Oncol* 46:255, 1992.

Tazelaar HD et al: Conservative treatment of borderline ovarian tumors, *Obstet Gynecol* 66:417, 1985.

Trimble CL, Trimble EI: Management of epithelial ovarian tumors of low malignant potential, *Gynecol Oncol* 55: S52, 1994.

Trope et al: Are borderline tumors of the ovary over treated both surgically and systematically? A review of four prospective randomized trials, including 253 patients with borderline tumors, *Gyncol Oncol* 51:236, 1993.

Proper identification of an early ovarian neoplasm

Bolis G et al: Multicenter controlled trial in patients with epithelial ovarian cancer Stage I, *Proc Int Gynecol Cancer Soc* 157 (abstract), 1989.

Colombo N et al: Controversial issues in the management of early epithelial ovarian cancer: conservative surgery and role of adjuvant therapy, *Gynecol Oncol* 55:S47, 1994.

Einhorn N et al: Prospective evaluation of serum CA 125 levels for early detection of ovarian cancer, *Obstet Gynecol* 80:14, 1992.

Trimbos JB et al: Watch and wait after careful surgical treatment and staging in well-differentiated early ovarian cancer, *Cancer* 67(3):597, 1991.

Spill of tumor

Sainz de la Cuesta R et al: Prognostic importance of intraoperative rupture of malignant ovarian epithelial neoplasms, *Obset Gynecol* 84:1, 1994.

Sjöval K, Nilsson B, Einhorn N: Different types of rupture of the tumor capsule and the impact on survival in early ovarian carcinoma, *Int J Gynecol Cancer* 4:333, 1994.

Prophylactic oophorectomy

Averette HE, Nguyen HN: The role of prophylactic oophorectomy in cancer prevention, *Gynecol Oncol* 55:S38, 1994.

Boike G et al: National survey of ovarian carcinoma. Women with prior hysterectomy: a failure of prevention? *Gynecol Oncol* 49(1):112, 1993.

Kemp GM, Hsiu JG, Andrews MC: Case Report: Papillary peritoneal carcinomatosis after prophylactic oophorectomy, *Gynecol Oncol* 47:395, 1992.

Kerlikowske K, Brown JS, Grady DG: Should women with familial ovarian cancer undergo prophylactic oophorectomy? *Obstet Gynecol* 80:700, 1992.

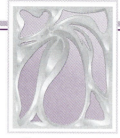

Epithelial Ovarian Cancer

Malignant neoplasms of the ovary present an increasing challenge to the physician. They are the cause of more deaths than any other female genital tract cancer. About 26,500 new cases are diagnosed each year in the United States, and about 14,500 deaths occur annually as a result of this disease (Figure 11-1). It accounts for 5% of all cancers among women. In the United States, deaths from this cause occur at a rate of one every 45 minutes, and one in every 56 women will develop this disease. The gynecologic oncologist is frustrated by the paucity of knowledge of the etiologic factors in ovarian cancer and by the failure to achieve a significant reduction in mortality from these neoplasms over the past six decades.

CLASSIFICATION

The student of ovarian pathology is often confused by the prodigious variation in histologic structure and biologic behavior. Currently the most popular and practical scheme of classification is based on the histogenesis of the normal ovary, shown in the box on p. 283. The early development of the ovary may be divided into four major stages. During the first stage, undifferentiated germ cells (primordial germ cells) become segregated and migrate from their sites of origin to settle in the genital ridges, which are bilateral thickenings of coelomic epithelium. The second stage occurs after arrival of the germ cells in the genital ridges and consists of proliferation of the coelomic epithelium and the underlying mesenchyme. During the third stage, the ovary becomes divided into a peripheral cortex and a central medulla. The fourth stage is characterized by the development of the cortex and the involution of the medulla. The histogenetic classification categorizes ovarian neoplasms with regard to their derivation from coelomic epithelium, germ cells, and mesenchyme.

The majority (85% to 90%) of malignant ovarian tumors seen in the United States are epithelial. They can be further grouped into histological types as follows:

Serous cystadenocarcinoma, 42%

Mucinous cystadenocarcinoma, 12%

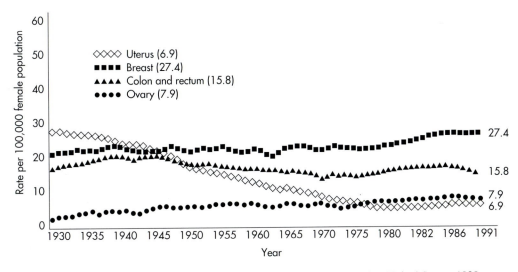

Figure 11-1 Age-adjusted cancer death rates for selected sites in females, United States, 1920-1991. (Modified from *Cancer facts and figures,* New York, 1991, American Cancer Society, Inc.)

HISTOGENETIC CLASSIFICATION OF OVARIAN NEOPLASMS

I. Neoplasms derived from coelomic epithelium
   A. Serous tumor
   B. Mucinous tumor
   C. Endometrioid tumor
   D. Mesonephroid (clear cell) tumor
   E. Brenner tumor Undifferentiated carcinoma
   F. Carcinosarcoma and mixed mesodermal tumor

II. Neoplasms derived from germ cells
   A. Teratoma
      1. Mature teratoma
         a. Solid adult teratoma
         b. Dermoid cyst
         c. Struma ovarii
         d. Malignant neoplasms secondarily arising from mature cystic teratoma
      2. Immature teratoma (partially differentiated teratoma)
   B. Dysgerminoma
   C. Embryonal carcinoma
   D. Endodermal sinus tumor
   E. Choriocarcinoma
   F. Gonadoblastoma

III. Neoplasms derived from specialized gonadal stroma
   A. Granulosa-theca cell tumors
      1. Graulosa tumor
      2. Thecoma
   B. Sertoli-Leydig tumors
      1. Arrhenoblastoma
      2. Sertoli tumor
   C. Gynandroblastoma
   D. Lipid cell tumors

IV. Neoplasms derived from nonspecific mesenchyme
   A. Fibroma, hemangioma, leiomyoma, lipoma
   B. Lymphoma
   C. Sarcoma

V. Neoplasms metastatic to the ovary
   A. Gastrointestinal tract (Krukenberg)
   B. Breast
   C. Endometrium
   D. Lymphoma

Endometrioid carcinoma, 15%
Undifferentiated carcinoma, 17%
Clear cell carcinoma, 6%
There seems to be limited prognostic significance to the histological type of malignant epithelial ovarian cancer independent of clinical stage, extent of residual disease, and histologic grade. Histologic grade is an important independent prognostic factor in patients with epithelial tumors of the ovary (Figure 11-2). This is certainly true for patients who have early stage disease, and considerable evidence suggests that it is also true of patients who have advanced disease. The distribution of histological types is approximately similar to those institutions reported by FIGO (Figure 11-3).

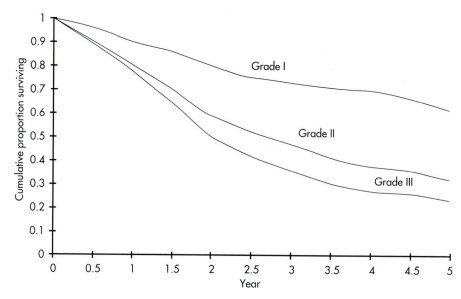

Figure 11-2 Serous cystadenocarcinoma of the ovary. Cumulative proportion surviving by degree of differentiation. (From *Annual Report Gynecological Cancer* FIGO, vol 22, 1994)

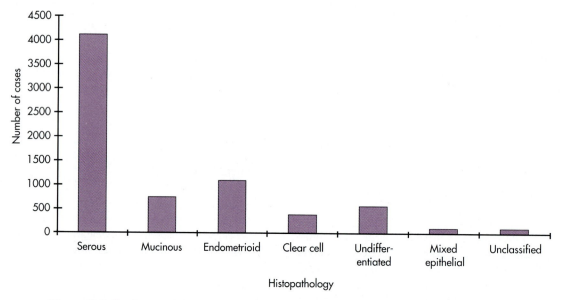

Figure 11-3 Carcinoma of the ovary. Histopathology of obviously malignant cases. Distribution by age. (From *Annual Report Gynecological Cancer* FIGO, vol. 22, 1994)

INCIDENCE, EPIDEMIOLOGY, AND ETIOLOGY (Figure 11-4)

Approximately 23% of gynecologic cancers are of ovarian origin, but 47% of all deaths from cancer of the female genital tract occur in women who have gynecologic cancer of ovarian origin. Cancer of the ovaries is the fourth most frequently occurring fatal cancer in women in the United States. It ranks high as a cause of female deaths in Canada, New Zealand, Israel, and countries of northern Europe. Approximately 12 of every 1000 women in the United States older than 40 years will develop ovarian cancer (Table 11-1), but only 2 or 3 of the 12 will be cured. The remainder will have repeated bouts of intestinal obstruction as the tumor spreads over the surface of the bowel, develop inanition and malnutrition, and literally starve to death.

Malignant neoplasms of the ovaries occur at all ages, including infancy and childhood (Figure 11-5). Throughout childhood and adolescence, US death rates for neoplasms of the ovary are exceeded only by those for

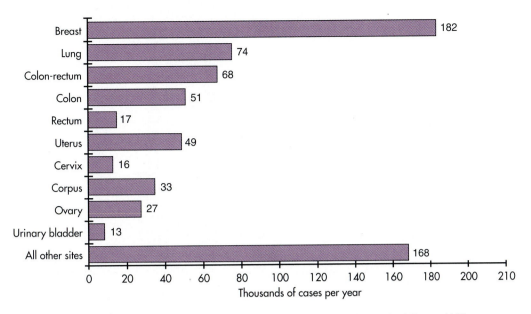

Figure 11-4 Estimated incidence of cancer of leading sites in females, United States, 1995. (From *Cancer facts and figures,* New York, 1995, American Cancer Society, Inc.)

Table 11-1   Percent probability at birth of ever developing cancer, United States (1995)

	Female	
All sites	39.26	(1 in 3)
Breast	12.30	(1 in 8)
Cervix	1.1	(1 in 91)
Corpus	2.2	(1 in 45)
Lung	5.17	(1 in 19)
Ovary	1.8	(1 in 56)
Colon-rectum	5.92	(1 in 17)

From American Cancer Society: Cancer Facts and Figures 1995.

leukemia, lymphomas, and neoplasms of the central nervous system, kidney, connective tissue, and bone. Overall death rates for neoplasms of the ovary are greater in nonwhite Americans younger than 39 years; after age 40, however, death rates for white women are significantly higher. The major histologic types occur in distinctive age ranges (Table 11-2). Malignant germ cell tumors are most commonly seen in females younger than 20 years, whereas epithelial cancers of the ovary are primarily seen in women older than 50 years. Beginning with the 40-44 year age group, which has a rate of 15.7 cases per 100,000, the incidence rates increase dramatically with age. The rate more than doubles after age 50, to about 35 cases per 100,000. Highest incidence rates are found in the 65-85 year age group, where the peak rate of 54 cases per 100,000 is found in the 75-79 year age group. The largest number of ovarian cancer patients is found in the 60-64 year age group. More than one third of the cases

occur in patients 65 years or older. Elderly women are more likely than younger women to be in advanced stages of ovarian cancer at initial diagnosis, and 5-year relative survival rates for elderly women are almost one half the rate observed in women younger than 65 years of age. Studies of the Connecticut Tumor Registry suggest that the age-adjusted rate of all ages has remained about the same over the last 30 years (Table 11-3).

Familial Ovarian Cancer

Several reports describe families in which girls and women of the same or succeeding generations develop similar neoplasms of the ovaries. Most of these neoplasms were serous carcinomas, but other types were also observed. Cancers of the breasts, colon, and other sites were also found more commonly in female members of these afflicted families. Investigators at the National Cancer Institute have studied four families in which women of two or three generations have developed papillary-serous adenocarcinomas at ages past 35. Koch studied cancer incidence in relatives of 197 patients with ovarian cancer and relatives of age-matched controls. The number of relatives with ovarian cancer was significantly higher in the cases than in the controls, with a limited relative risk of 2.61. However, only 9 of the 197 ovarian cancer cases studied (4.6%) presented with a positive history for a first-order relative with ovarian cancer. Ovarian epithelial cancer is currently affecting 2 in every 70 women in the United States. Preliminary data suggest that having a single first-order relative with history of ovarian cancer increases the risk to close to 5%. Rare families exist in which the risk is much greater (as high as 50%). Several familial ovarian cancer registries have been established throughout the United States to track this

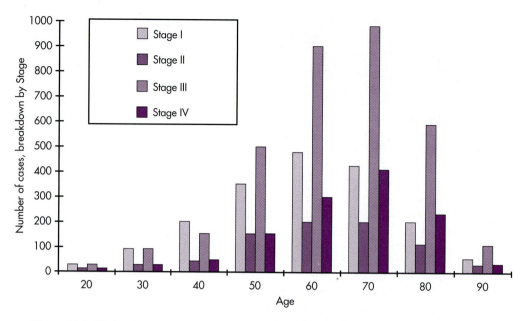

Figure 11-5 Obviously malignant ovarian epithelial tumors. Age distribution by stage. (From *Annual Report Gynecological Cancer* FIGO, vol 22, 1994.)

Table 11-2   Primary ovarian neoplasms related to age

Type	Up to 20 yr	20-50 yr	Over 50 yr
Coelomic epithelium	29%	71%	81%
Germ cell	59%	14%	6%
Specialized gonadal stroma	8%	5%	4%
Nonspecific mesenchyme	4%	10%	9%

Table 11-3   Lifetime probability of ovarian cancer by age in women with one relative with ovarian cancer

Age (year)	Lifetime probability of ovarian cancer (%)	Lifetime probability of ovarian cancer with one relative (%)
30	1.6	5
35	1.6	5
40	1.6	4.8
45	1.5	4.5
50	1.4	4.4
55	1.3	4.1
60	1.2	3.6

From Kerlikowske K, Brown JS, Grady DG: *Ob/Gyn* 80:700, 1992.

phenomenon. The lifetime risk for ovarian cancer in the population as a whole is approximately 1.4%; with one first-degree relative, it is 5%; with two or more first-degree relatives, it rises to 7%. Among the latter group, there is a 3% chance of having hereditary ovarian cancer syndrome; in those families, the lifetime risk of ovarian cancer is at least 40%.

Firm guidelines for prophylactic oophorectomy have not been established. The majority of patients who develop ovarian epithelial cancer have no family history of such. Franceschi et al. reported eight families with multiple occurrences of epithelial ovarian cancer (22 cases). There was a high proportion of serous and undifferentiated carcinoma, bilateral ovarian involvement, multiple primary cancers, and unfavorable prognosis. Piver reported two families; in one family the patient's two sisters, her first cousin, and her first cousin's daughter all had adenocarcinoma of the ovary. In such families genetic counseling should be considered, as well as prophylactic oophorectomy. In addition, the dysgenetic gonads of sex chromatin-negative individuals, most of

whom are phenotypic females, are prone to develop a distinctive, usually benign neoplasm called gonadoblastoma.

Three different hereditary syndromes of cancer have been identified. The first is a site-specific familial ovarian cancer syndrome in which women are at high risk for the development of ovarian carcinoma only. A woman may be at risk if her mother or sister has ovarian carcinoma. The second is a breast-ovarian cancer syndrome. Women in families with this syndrome have an increased incidence of breast and ovarian carcinomas, alone or in combination. These women may have a 50% risk of ovarian carcinoma if their mothers or sisters had breast and/or ovarian carcinoma. This syndrome has been associated with the BRCA-1 gene. In addition, there is evidence for a second breast/ovarian cancer gene, BRCA-2. The third type is the cancer family syndrome in which both males and females are at increased risk of acquiring colon cancer, and to a lesser extent other cancers, including gastric carcinoma, thyroid carcinoma, and sarcoma. Most of the colon cancers are in the proximal colon and not easily diagnosed by a limited rectosigmoid evaluation. Women in these families are at increased risk for carcinoma of the ovary, endometrium, and breast. All three syndromes have a pattern of early-onset cancer and vertical transmission consistent with autosomal dominant inheritance.

Because of the autosomal dominant pattern of inheritance seen in these syndromes, a 50% risk can be predicted in all offspring and siblings of inflicted individuals. Many advise consideration of prophylactic oophorectomy of female offspring in these families as soon as childbearing is completed. Most of the cancers have been detected in women between 35 and 45 years of age; thus, if oophorectomy is not performed, biannual ultrasonographic and pelvic examinations should be considered beginning at 25 years of age. Unfortunately, neither this method of surveillance nor prophylactic oophorectomy has resulted in complete safety. Several high-risk women have had intra-abdominal carcinomatosis, histologically indistinguishable from ovarian carcinoma, several years after prophylactic oophorectomy. The occurrence of these cancers is consistent with the hypothesis that at least some ovarian carcinomas are multicentric neoplasms arising from the embryonic mesothelium or coelomic epithelium from which the peritoneum and germinal epithelium of the ovary arise. Therefore, oophorectomy may not completely eliminate the individual's risk of ovarian carcinoma.

It is important to distinguish women in families with hereditary ovarian cancer syndromes from those who have family members with ovarian cancer. A medical history is the primary method for identifying women from families with hereditary ovarian cancer syndromes. A complete history should include establishing a woman's family history of ovarian cancer, breast cancer, endometrial cancer, and non-polyposis colorectal cancer; determining the age of occurrence of these cancers in the family members; and verifying the diagnoses with autopsy or pathology reports. Women suspected of having a hereditary ovarian cancer syndrome should have a family pedigree constructed by a physician or a genetic counselor competent in determining the presence of an autosomal dominant inheritance pattern. The authors feel that these patients should be maintained on oral contraceptive therapy until such time that they desire childbearing. Patients less than 35 years of age with a history of hereditary ovarian cancer syndrome should be monitored with a pelvic exam, pelvic ultrasound, and CA-125 determination every 6 months. At the age of 35, these patients should be encouraged to consider the prophylactic removal of the ovaries.

As with other prevalent epithelial cancers, epidemiologic evidence strongly suggests that environmental

Table 11-4 Incidence and death rate of ovarian cancer for various countries

	Incidence per 100,000	Death rate per 100,000
Sweden	14.9	12.9
Norway	14.2	9.5
USA (white)	13.3	7.3
Israel	12.7	
German Democratic Republic	11.8	
West Germany	11.5	11.0
United Kingdom	11.1	9.1
Switzerland	10.6	
Finland	7.9	
Brazil	6.1	
India	4.6	
Japan	2.7	2.1
Netherlands		12.1

From Heintz AP et al: Epidemiology and etiology of ovarian cancer, *Obstet Gynecol* 66:127, 1985.

factors are major etiologic determinants in cancer of the human ovary. The highest rates are recorded in highly industrial countries (Table 11-4), which suggests that physical or chemical products of industry are major causes of epithelial neoplasms. A notable exception is highly industrialized Japan, where rates for malignant neoplasms of the ovary have been among the lowest recorded in the world. Interestingly, one observes a higher rate of ovarian cancer in Japanese immigrants in the United States and their offspring, eventually approaching that of Anglo-Saxon whites by the second and third generation. This suggests strongly that the causative carcinogens are probably in the immediate environment, such as food, personal customs, and other influences that change gradually during the cultural transition. To date there are no clues as to which dietary items or other environmental contacts might be specifically carcinogenic for the ovary.

Whittemore and others have shown that the odds for invasive epithelial ovarian cancer vary with the number of term pregnancies each woman experiences. This observation coincided with the data illustrating a reduction in the disease incidence with the use of oral contraceptives (see Table 11-4). The hypothesis that oral contraceptive use reduces the risk of epithelial ovarian cancer was suggested by Casagrande et al. in 1979. In 1982 Rosenberg et al. reported a case-control study of women younger than 60 years. Combination oral contraceptives were used by 26% of the cancer patients and 35% of the controls. The relative risk estimate for combination oral contraceptive use was 0.6 (Table 11-5). The reduction in risk appears to persist for as long as 10 years after use has ceased and to be greater for longer durations of use but these results were not statistically significant. Their findings were not explained by parity or by differences in other identified potential confounding factors. Their conclusion was that the use of combination oral contraceptives protects against epithelial ovarian cancer. This theory of "incessant ovulation" suggests that the epithelial lining of the ovary may be sensitive to the constant trauma of ovulation, which in turn can act as a promoting factor in the carcinogenic process. Further observation and study of this interesting hypothesis are necessary. Gross determined the effect of oral contraceptive use on the cumulative incidence of epithelial ovarian cancer from ages 20-40, 20-50, and 20-55. The women were categorized into four groups: positive family history, negative family history, parous, and nulliparous. The cancer and steroid hormone study data was used in all four groups. The cumulative number of epithelial ovarian cancer cases estimated to occur per 100,000 oral contraceptive (OC) users compared to never users decreased with increasing duration of OC use. Their results suggest that 5 years of use by nulliparous women can reduce their ovarian cancer risk to the level seen in parous women who never use OCs, and that 10 years of OC use by women with a positive family history can reduce their risk to a level below that of women whose family history is negative and who never use OCs. Based on this data, the recommendation is strongly made that patients with family history of ovarian cancer seriously consider utilizing OCs when pregnancy is not being sought.

Two different studies suggest that prolonged use of fertility drugs such as Clomid may increase the risk of borderline and invasive ovarian neoplasms. Rossing examined the risk of ovarian tumors in a cohort of 3,837 women evaluated for infertility between 1974 and 1985 in Seattle, Washington. Computer linkage with a population based tumor registry was used to identify women whose tumors were diagnosed before January 1st, 1992. There were 11 invasive or borderline malignant ovarian tumors, compared with an expected number of 4.4. Nine of the women in whom ovarian tumor developed had taken Clomid; the adjusted relative risk among these women, as compared with that of infertile women who had not taken this drug was 2.3. Five of the nine women had taken the drug during 12 or more monthly cycles. Further investigations are underway to clarify this association. The concept is appealing when one considers the reduction in incidence noted with the use of OCs and parity.

McGowan, on the basis of a study of 197 women with ovarian cancer, estimated that nulligravidas were 2.45 times more likely to develop malignant ovarian tumors and 2.9 times more likely to develop ovarian carcinoma of low potential malignancy than were women who had been pregnant three or more times (Table 11-6). The risk of ovarian cancer in their series was reduced to 1.27 among women who had been pregnant at least once. In Gerow's series, women with ovarian cancer demonstrated a marked decrease in the number of live births. Several studies have confirmed this observation. One possible interpretation could be that the endocrinologic status of pregnancy protects against ovarian cancer and that the lack of this protection places infertile women at higher risk for ovarian cancer. A second explanation could be that

---

Table 11-5 How oral contraceptive use affects the risk of ovarian cancer

Duration of oral contraceptive use	Number of women who developed ovarian cancer	Controls	Relative risk
Never	242	1,532	1
3-6 months	26	280	.6
7-11 months	14	134	.7
1-2 years	65	602	.7
3-4 years	40	397	.6
5-9 years	39	594	.4
≥10 years	13	328	.2

From Centers for Disease Control and Steroid Hormone Study: The reduction in risk of ovarian cancer associated with oral contraceptive use, *NEJM* 316:650, 1987.

Table 11-6 Odds ratio for invasive epithelial ovarian cancer according to parity

Number of term pregnancies	Cases	Percentage	Population studies		Odds ratio
			Controls	Percentage	
0	322	24	765	14	1
1	164	12	605	11	.6
2	376	28	1515	27	.53
3	265	19	1259	22	.48
4	135	10	774	14	.36
5	56	4	345	6	.33
≥6	45	3	346	6	.29

Adapted from Whittemore AS et al: *Am J Epidemiol* 136:1184, 1992.

infertility in ovarian cancer is the result of the same abnormal gonadal status. This theory would explain why infertile women are more at risk than never-married and never-pregnant women.

Parazzini et al. studied the influence of various menstrual factors on the risk of epithelial ovarian cancer. They reported that the risk rose with later age at menopause and with early menarche. Confirmation of this work is not yet at hand. Studies of dietary fat have been inconclusive, and other dietary factors are not at present considered well established.

Still others have suggested that ovarian cancer may be initiated by a chemical carcinogen via the vagina, uterus, and fallopian tubes, and the substances promoting cancer may even be the steroid-rich antral fluid from ruptured follicles. For years Woodruff et al. suggested this hypothesis of migration of chemical carcinogens from the vagina to the pelvic peritoneum. There is ample clinical evidence of the migration of chemical substances from the vagina to the peritoneal cavity and ovaries. Venter demonstrated with the use of radionuclides that upward migration is possible. Certainly many different chemical substances are regularly used in the vulvovaginal areas, and some of these could be implicated in carcinogenesis.

Cramer et al. reported on the opportunities for genital exposure to talc in 215 white females with epithelial ovarian cancer and in 215 controls from the general population matched by age, race, and residence. Ninety-two (42.8%) women in the case group regularly used talc as a dusting powder on the perineum or on sanitary napkins, compared with 61 (28.4%) of the controls. This provides some support for an association between talc and ovarian cancer hypothesized because of the similarity of ovarian cancer to mesotheliomas and the chemical relationship of talc to asbestos, a known cause of mesotheliomas. The authors also investigated opportunities for potential talc exposure after pelvic surgery from rubber products such as condoms and diaphragms. No significant differences were noted between cases and controls and these exposures, although the intensity of talc exposure from these sources was likely to be affected by variables not assessed in the study.

No epidemiologic or experimental evidence exists to incriminate viruses in the development of neoplasms of the human ovary. Attempts to isolate viruses from cultures of human ovarian cancer cells have been unsuccessful to date. Because of its gonadotropic properties, mumps virus is an obvious candidate among known viruses for oncogenic activity in the ovary. Case-control studies have revealed a possible negative association with mumps parotitis but these historic accounts were not supported by skin tests or serologic evidence of reactivity to mumps virus. Menczer et al. reported on 84 ovarian cancer patients and 84 controls with nonmalignant conditions matched by age and ethnic origin who were interviewed with regard to clinical mumps history, and their sera were tested for mumps complement-fixing antibodies. Ovarian cancer patients differed from the controls in the response to past mumps infection in two reports: (1) they appeared to be more likely to have developed subclinical mumps, as evidenced by the lower rate of clinical mumps history, despite serologic evidence of similar infection rates among those with positive and those with negative clinical mumps history, and (2) they tended to have lower persistent mumps complement-fixing antibody titers. Menczer et al. interpreted these results as possibly indicating that an immunologic incompetence enables development of ovarian cancer, possibly through a direct etiologic role of mumps virus. At present, however, the evidence for mumps virus as an etiologic agent in ovarian cancer remains speculative.

Knowledge of the etiologic mechanisms involved in cancer of the ovary is limited to fragments of information. The multi-institution therapy programs offer an ideal population of women for case-control studies. Each patient should be questioned for a history of preexisting gynecologic abnormalities, documented by clinical or laboratory data where possible, and for information about exposure to environmental carcinogens. There are many programs of this nature.

SIGNS, SYMPTOMS, AND ATTEMPTS AT EARLY DETECTION (SCREENING)

Although diverse ovarian tumors generally manifest in a similar manner, the diagnosis of early ovarian cancer is more a matter of chance than a triumph of the scientific method. As enlargement occurs (Figure 11-6), there is progressive compression of the surrounding pelvic structures, producing vague abdominal discomfort, dyspepsia, urinary frequency, and "pelvic pressure" (Table 11-7). The insidious onset of ovarian cancer needs no elaboration. As the neoplasm reaches a diameter of 15 cm, it begins to rise out of the pelvis and may account for abdominal enlargement. It is time, however, to change the generally accepted notion that there are no early symptoms of ovarian cancer. Symptoms often include vague abdominal discomfort, dyspepsia, and other mild digestive disturbances, which may be present for several months before the diagnosis. Such complaints are usually not recognized as anything more than "middle-age indigestion." A high index of suspicion is warranted in all women between the ages of 40 and 69 who have persistent gastrointestinal symptoms that cannot be diagnosed. Unfortunately, the majority of such nonspecific complaints are often functional in origin, causing the internist or family physician to dismiss the possibility of ovarian cancer. Indeed, it is only when the patient has gross enlargement of the abdomen marking the occurrence of ascites and extension of the neoplastic process to the abdominal cavity (Figure 11-7) that she receives appropriate diagnostic evaluation.

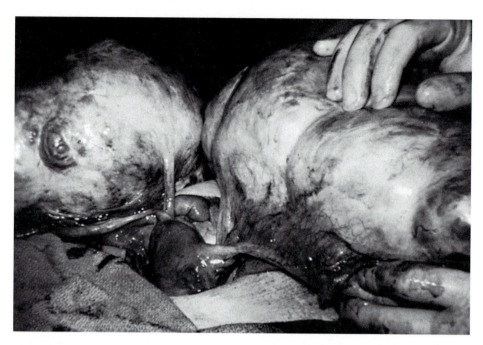

Figure 11-6 Large bilateral ovarian neoplasms: low-grade mucinous adenocarcinoma.

Table 11-7 Most frequent presenting symptoms of ovarian cancer

Symptom	Relative frequency
Abdominal swelling	XXXX
Abdominal pain	XXX
Dyspepsia	XX
Urinary frequency	XX
Weight change	X

Table 11-8 Surgical findings

	Benign	Malignant
Surface papilla	Rare	Very common
Intracystic papilla	Uncommon	Very common
Solid areas	Rare	Very common
Bilaterality	Rare	Common
Adhesions	Uncommon	Common
Ascites (100 ml)	Rare	Common
Necrosis	Rare	Common
Peritoneal implants	Rare	Common
Capsule intact	Common	Infrequent
Totally cystic	Common	Rare

Methods for early diagnosis have been investigated in limited studies employing cul-de-sac aspiration for peritoneal cytologic assessment and frequent pelvic examinations. All these endeavors have failed to show a significant impact on early diagnosis of this disease. These ovarian neoplasms grow quickly and painlessly. Any persistent ovarian enlargement should be an immediate indication for exploratory laparotomy. The diagnosis rests with the pathologist. The size of the tumor does not indicate the severity of disease. Indeed, some of the largest neoplasms are benign histologically. In addition, many large adnexal masses may be of nonovarian etiology. Frequently encountered nonovarian causes of apparent adnexal masses are diverticulitis, tubo-ovarian abscess, carcinoma of the cecum or sigmoid, pelvic kidney, and uterine or intraligamentous myomas. At the time of surgery, it may be difficult to discern the malignant potential of a particular ovarian neoplasm (Table 11-8). There is sufficient overlap of morphologic criteria to cause considerable confusion. Again, the diagnosis rests with the histologic examination of the specimen.

Immunologic diagnosis of subclinical ovarian cancer by means of identification of specific tumor-associated antigens in the serum has yet to materialize. Several tumor-associated antigens, including CA-125, have been identified and purified. Unfortunately, their detection within the serum in the presence of minimal neoplastic tissue has not been possible. A search for other antigens that might be clinically more useful in early diagnosis is under way.

It has been suggested that every women should have a periodic pelvic examination, pelvic ultrasonographic examination, and a CA-125 test to make sure she does not harbor an occult ovarian cancer. Enthusiasm for early detection of ovarian cancer is laudable. However, it has been calculated that 10,000 routine pelvic examinations

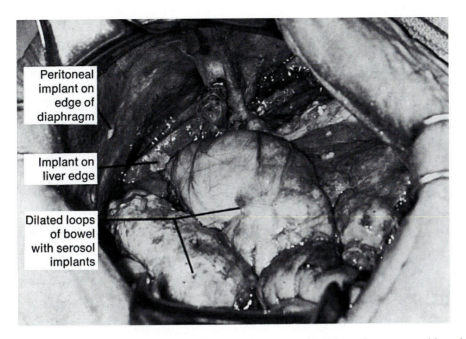

Peritoneal
implant on
edge of
diaphragm

Implant on
liver edge

Dilated loops
of bowel
with serosol
implants

Figure 11-7 Findings at laparotomy in patient with stage III epithelial ovarian cancer and bowel obstruction. Note wide distribution of surface implants.

Table 11-9   Non-malignant conditions that may elevate CA 125 concentrations

Gynecologic	Nongynecologic
Acute pelvic inflammatory disease	Active hepatitis
Adenomyosis	Acute pancreatitis
Benign ovarian neoplasm	Chronic liver disease
Endometriosis	Cirrhosis
Functional ovarian cyst	Colitis
Meig's syndrome	Congestive heart failure
Menstruation	Diabetes (poorly controlled)
Ovarian hyperstimulation	Diverticulitis
Unexplained infertility	Mesothelioma
Uterine myomata	Nonmalignant ascites
	Pericarditis
	Pneumonia
	Polyarteritis nodosa
	Postoperative period
	Renal disease
	Rodent exposure (HAMA)
	Systemic lupus erythematosus

would be required to pick up one early ovarian cancer in an asymptomatic patient population. As already noted, the use of CA-125 as a screening technique has not been rewarding especially in premenopausal women. Many conditions of a benign nature, as well as most GI malignancies, may elevate the CA-125 (Table 11-9). The value of ultrasonography in the screening for early ovarian carcinoma has received much attention. Her-

rmann analyzed data on 312 operated patients regarding initial ultrasound readings (Table 11-10) and found a predictive value for cancer of 73%. Campbell and his co-workers report early detection of five primary ovarian cancers in approximately 5000 women screened by abdominal ultrasound (Table 11-11). Although transvaginal ultrasound may increase the accuracy of noting adnexal enlargements, it undoubtedly also increases costs, especially in terms of the follow-up of patients noted to have enlargement. To date, no one has demonstrated that any screening technique significantly affects mortality, even if one screens high risk patients (Table 11-12). More recent advances in ultrasound technology, especially transvaginal color Doppler ultrasound, provide evaluation of vascular flow, the increase of which may indicate malignancy, as well as additional information on the malignant potential of adnexal masses. This may be very helpful in reducing the number of unnecessary laparotomies for such masses but further investigation is needed.

One strategy to improve the effectiveness of ovarian cancer screening would be to target populations at increased risk of the development of the disease, such as individuals with a positive family history of ovarian cancer. Bourne et al. reported the results of such a strategy in screening patients with Transvaginal Sonography (TVS) in combination with color flow Doppler imaging and morphologic assessment. In screening 1601 patients, 57% required repeat TVS to confirm the presence of a mass. Six ovarian cancers were diagnosed (2 stage I, 3 low malignant potential tumors, and 1 stage III). Karlan et al. reported screening 597 patients with a family history of cancer utilizing CA-125, TVS and color flow Doppler

Table 11-10 Overall accuracy of sonographic diagnosis compared with pathologic findings in 312 operated patients

Surgical/histological findings	N	No mass found (N = 54)	Benign (N = 200)	Malignant (N = 58)
			Sonographic findings	
			Mass found (N = 258)	
Normal pelvis	39	32	7	0
Nonneoplastic disease	24	11	13	0
Endometrial malignancy with normal ovaries	8	2	3	3
Benign tumors (ovary and uterus or uterus)	191	7	170	14
Ovarian tumors or borderline malignancy	4	0	1	3
Ovarian cancers	46	2	6	38

Predictive value for cancer 38/52, 73%
Predictive value for benign 177/185, 95%

From Herrmann UJ et al: Sonography and ovarian cancer, *Obstet Gynecol* 69:777, 1987.

Table 11-11   Uncontrolled trials of ovarian cancer screening

| | | | **General population volunteers** | |
| | | | **Ovarian cancer** | |
Report	Country	Participants	Stage I	Total
Einhorn et al., 1992	Sweden	5550	2	6
Campbell et al., 1990	UK	5479	5	9
Jacobs et al., 1993	UK	21,959	3	11
DePriest et al., 1993	US	3220	2	3
TOTAL	All	36,208	12	29

Table 11-12   Uncontrolled trials of ovarian cancer screening

| | | | **Volunteers with positive family history** | |
| | | | **Ovarian cancer** | |
Report	Location	Participants	Stage I	Total
Bourne et al., 1993	UK	1601	5	6
Karlan et al., 1993	Los Angeles	597	1	1
Schwartz et al., 1991	Connecticut	>200	—	—
Muto et al., 1993	Boston	386	—	—
Crade, 1993	Long Beach	389	—	—

imaging. Initially, 115 patients had an abnormal TVS, and 68 had an abnormal CA 125 level. After repeat TVS, because of abnormal findings from color flow Doppler imaging, 19 patients underwent surgery. At the time of the report, one LMP tumor had been diagnosed.

Another strategy to improve sensitivity and specificity in screening for ovarian cancer involves the use of multiple serum tumor markers. Because less than 50% of patients with stage I ovarian cancer will have an elevated CA 125, the addition of other markers in screening strategy could potentially improve sensitivity. Studies addressing this concept have to date not been fruitful. The National Institute of Health consensus developing conference on ovarian cancer screening in 1994 published the following conclusions:

1. There is no evidence available yet that the current screening modalities of CA 125 and transvaginal ultrasonography (TVS) can be effectively used for widespread screening to reduce mortality from ovarian cancer nor that their use will result in decreased rather than increased morbidity and mortality. Routine screening has resulted in unnecessary surgery with potential risks. Clearly, it is important to identify and validate effective screening modalities. Currently available technology for screening should be employed in the context of clinical trials to determine the efficacy of these modalities and their effect on ovarian cancer mortality. In addition, research must be continued to identify additional markers and imaging techniques that will be useful. If a woman has one first-degree relative with ovarian cancer (making her life time risk of developing the disease 5%) but no clinical trials are available to her, she may feel that despite the absence of prospective data, this is sufficient risk for her to be screened. This alternative and opportunity should be available to the woman and her physician.

2. If a woman is undergoing pelvic surgery, removal of the ovaries at that time would almost fully eliminate her risk of ovarian cancer (although there remains a minimal risk of peritoneal carcinomatosis). If the woman is premenopausal, discussion of estrogen replacement therapy is important prior to removal of the ovaries, since for some younger women, if estrogen replacement is not utilized, the risk of premature menopause and the potential for cardiovascular disease and osteoporosis may outweigh the risk of ovarian conservation and the potential for ovarian cancer.

DIAGNOSTIC TECHNIQUES AND STAGING (Figure 11-8)

Routine pelvic examinations detect only 1 ovarian cancer in 10,000 asymptomatic women. However, pelvic examination remains the most practical means of detecting early disease. Pain is usually a late complication, seen with early disease only when associated with a complication such as torsion, rupture, or infection. Any ovary palpated in a patient 3 or more years after menopause should raise a high index of suspicion of an early ovarian neoplasm. These patients should be considered for immediate laparoscopy and/or laparotomy when there is a high suspicion of malignancy on ultrasound, e.g., solid mass, >5 cm and/or intra cystic papillations.

Routine laboratory tests are not of great value in the diagnosis of ovarian tumors. The major value of labora-

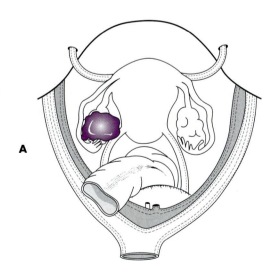

One ovary, capsule intact; no tumor on ovarian surface.

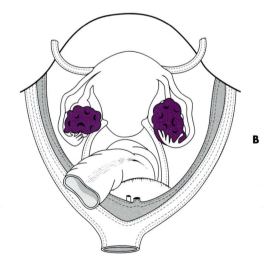

Both ovaries, capsule intact; no tumor on ovarian surface.

Figure 11-8 Ovarian epithelial carcinoma. **A,** Stage Ia. **B,** Stage Ib.   *Continued.*

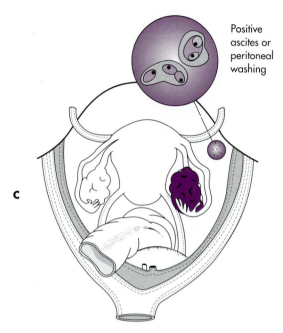

Positive ascites or peritoneal washing

C

One or both ovaries with capsule ruptured or tumor on ovarian surface; malignant cells in ascites or peritoneal washings.

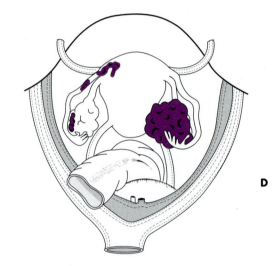

D

Extension and/or implants on uterus and/or tubes; adnexae.

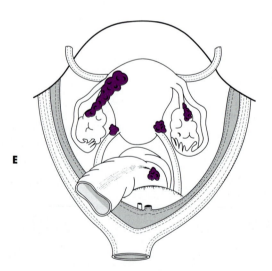

E

Extension and/or implants to other pelvic tissues; pelvic wall, broad ligament, adjacent peritoneum, mesovarium.

Figure 11-8, cont'd. Ovarian epithelial carcinoma. **C,** Stage Ic. **D,** Stage IIa. **E,** Stage IIb.

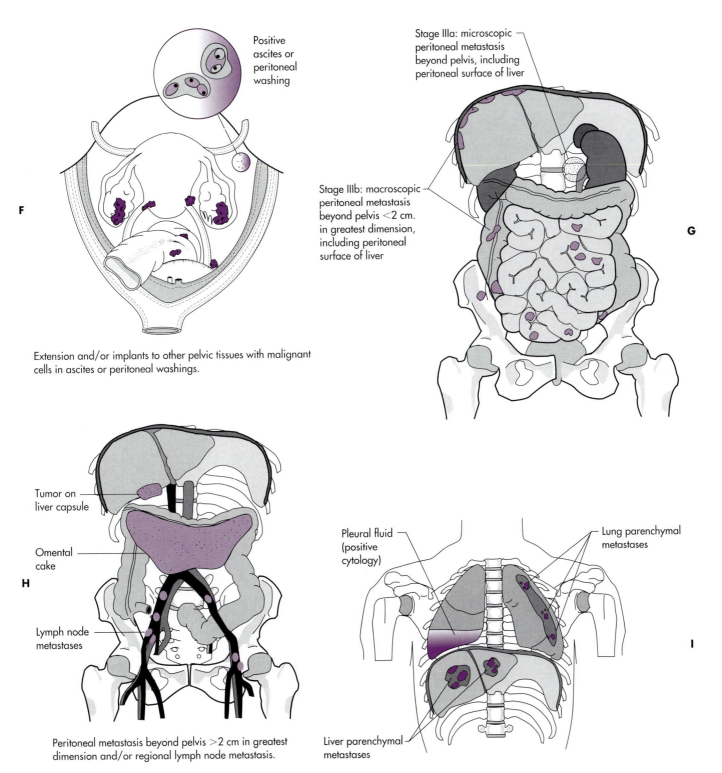

Figure 11-8, cont'd. Ovarian epithelial carcinoma. **F,** Stage IIc. **G,** Stages IIIa and IIIb. **H,** Stage IIIc. **I,** Stage IV.

Table 11-13   Carcinoma of the ovary: staging classification using the FIGO nomenclature

Stage	Description
Stage I	Growth limited to the ovaries
Stage Ia	Growth limited to one ovary; no ascites present containing malignant cells; no tumor on the external surfaces; capsule intact
Stage Ib	Growth limited to both ovaries; no ascites present containing malignant cells; no tumor on the external surfaces; capsules intact
Stage Ic*	Tumor stage Ia or stage Ib but with tumor on the surface of one or both ovaries; or with capsule ruptured; or with ascites present containing malignant cells or with positive peritoneal washings
Stage II	Growth involving one or both ovaries with pelvic extension
Stage IIa	Extension and/or metastases to the uterus and/or tubes
Stage IIb	Extension to other pelvic tissues
Stage IIc*	Tumor stage IIa or stage IIb but with tumor on the surface of one of both ovaries; or with capsule(s) ruptured; or with ascites present containing malignant cells or with positive peritoneal washings
Stage III	Tumor involving one or both ovaries with peritoneal implants outside the pelvis and/or positive retroperitoneal or inguinal nodes; superficial liver metastasis equals stage III; tumor is limited to the true pelvis but with histologically verified malignant extension to small bowel or omentum
Stage IIIa	Tumor grossly limited to the true pelvis with negative nodes with histologically confirmed microscopic seeding of abdominal peritoneal surfaces
Stage IIIb	Tumor of one or both ovaries; histologically confirmed implants of abdominal peritoneal surfaces, none exceeding 2 cm in diameter; nodes negative
Stage IIIc	Abdominal implants 2 cm in diameter and/or positive retroperitoneal or inguinal nodes
Stage IV	Growth involving one or both ovaries with distant metastasis; if pleural effusion is present, there must be positive cytologic test results to allot a case to stage IV; parenchymal liver metastasis equals stage IV

As published in *Am J Obstet Gynecol* 156:263, 1987.
*In order to evaluate the impact on prognosis of the different criteria for alloting cases to stage Ic or IIc, it would be of value to know if rupture of the capsule was (1) spontaneous or (2) caused by the surgeon and if the source of the malignant cells detected was (1) peritoneal washings or (2) ascites.

COMPLETE WORKUP FOR OVARIAN CANCER

Careful history
Physical examination
Pelvic examination and Pap smear
Proctosigmoidoscopy, where indicated
CBC and urinalysis
Blood chemistries, including CA-125
Chest film
IVP }
Barium enema } or CT scan with contrast
Pelvic ultrasound

---

tory tests is in ruling out other pelvic disorders (shown in the box above). Pelvic ultrasound or abdominal roentgenograms may reveal calcifications consistent with myomas or tooth-like calcifications consistent with benign teratomas. Intravenous pyelogram is often helpful in ruling out disease in adjacent pelvic structures. A barium enema is probably advisable with any pelvic mass and in a postmenopausal woman, but the need for a CT scan can be individualized. A similar comment can be made for proctosigmoidoscopy, which is particularly valuable in patients who have lower intestinal symptoms. The outcome in ovarian cancer relies so heavily on early diagnosis that procrastination with numerous diagnostic procedures is somewhat hazardous. Laparotomy is the ultimate test as to the nature of the disorder. Paracentesis for the purpose of obtaining a cell block and cytologic smear of the peritoneal fluid appears unnecessary and is, at times, dangerous. If one is dealing with a self-contained malignant cyst, such a procedure can result in a spillage of malignant cells into the peritoneal cavity. In addition, regardless of whether the fluid contains neoplastic cells, laparotomy is still necessary to remove the large benign neoplasm or to define the extent of the malignant process. In addition, up to 50% of ascitic fluid samples from patients with true ovarian malignancies will be negative for malignant cells on cell block analysis. Diagnostic paracentesis in a patient with ascites and a pelvic-abdominal mass is therefore both unnecessary and dangerous.

The staging of ovarian cancer is surgical (Table 11-13) and based on the operative findings at the commencement of the procedure. A longitudinal midline incision is recommended to facilitate removal of the neoplasm and to permit adequate visualization of the entire abdominal cavity, including the under surface of the diaphragm.

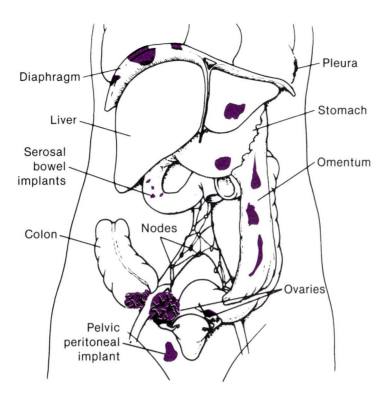

Figure 11-9 Spread pattern for epithelial cancer of the ovary. (From DiSaia PJ: *Hosp Pract* 22(4), April 5, 1987.)

Ovarian cancer is classically a serosal spreading disease (Figure 11-9), and thus all peritoneal surfaces must be carefully inspected, especially when disease is thought to be limited to the pelvis. Although lymphatic spread to retroperitoneal nodes is common in ovarian cancer, the disease most often spreads intraperitoneally: free-floating cells shed from the primary tumor are capable of implanting on any peritoneal surface. Any peritoneal fluid found when the peritoneal cavity is opened should be aspirated and submitted for cytologic examination. In the absence of peritoneal fluid, four washings should be taken by lavaging the peritoneal surfaces: the under surface of the diaphragm as the first specimen (Figure 11-10), lateral to the ascending and descending colon as the second and third specimens, and the pelvic peritoneal surfaces as the fourth specimen. These specimens are obtained by lavaging these areas with 50-75 ml of saline solution and retrieving the fluid for cell block analysis. Care should be taken to visualize and palpate all peritoneal surfaces, including the underside of the diaphragm, the surface of the liver, and the small and large bowel mesentery. Fiber optic light sources are particularly helpful in properlyvisualizing the peritoneal surfaces of the upper abdomen through a vertical lower abdominal incision. The omentum should be scrutinized and any suspicious areas removed by excision or biopsy. If the disease is apparently limited to the pelvis, it is judicious to excise the most dependent portion of the omentum or any portion of the

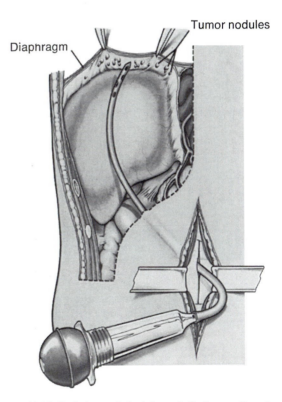

Figure 11-10 Technique of obtaining subdiaphragmatic cytologic washings at laparotomy. Saline lavage of space between diaphragm and dome of liver is easily accomplished; fluid pockets collecting in the lateral recesses are aspirated with bulb syringe.

omentum adherent to pelvic structures. Often microscopic disease will be present in the omentum but not obvious grossly. Data from one institution suggest that routine omentectomy may be of benefit in improving survival, but additional data are needed to validate this suggestion. Recommended surgical therapy is presented in sequence in the box below. If the disease is limited to the pelvis, great care should be taken to avoid rupture of the neoplasm during its removal. All roughened or suspicious surfaces in the peritoneal cavity should be removed as biopsy specimens. This includes adhesions, which should be excised not incised, since they often contain microscopic disease. Several studies are under way to investigate the efficacy of "blind" peritoneal biopsies and routine retroperitoneal node dissections in the proper staging of early epithelial cancer of the ovary (Table 11-14). These studies are preliminary, and a firm recommendation cannot be made until results of these studies are conclusive. It is not our practice to routinely perform biopsies on normal-appearing peritoneum or diaphragmatic surfaces. Any abnormal-appearing surface is always regarded as suspicious, and biopsies are readily performed. Proper staging is the key to an accurate prognosis (Table 11-15).

THERAPEUTIC OPTIONS FOR PRIMARY TREATMENT

Borderline Malignant Epithelial Neoplasms

In the last three decades clear evidence has shown the existence of epithelial ovarian tumors whose histologic and biologic features are between those of clearly benign and frankly malignant ovarian neoplasms. These borderline malignancies, which account for approximately 15% of all epithelial ovarian cancers, are often referred to as proliferative cystadenomas and are more completely discussed in Chapter 10. As compared to obviously malignant epithelial neoplasms of the ovary, epithelial

---

SURGICAL THERAPY IN OVARIAN CANCER

1. Peritoneal cytologic examination
2. Determination of extent of disease
   a. Pelvis
   b. Peritoneal surfaces
   c. Diaphragms
   d. Omentum
   e. Lymph nodes
3. Removal of all tumor possible (total abdominal hysterectomy and bilateral salpingo-oophorectomy) plus node sampling and omentectomy

---

Table 11-15   Carcinoma of the ovary. Obviously malignant cases. All histopathological classes. 5-year actuarial survival by stage.

Stage	Number	5-year survival (%)
Ia	845	83.5
Ib	188	79.3
Ic	606	73.1
IIa	140	64.6
IIb	272	54.2
IIc	336	61.3
IIIa	171	51.7
IIIb	366	29.2
IIIc	1903	17.7
IV	1291	14.3
TOTAL	6118*	

From annual report on the results of treatment in gynecological cancer, *FIGO*, Vol 22, 1994.
*Includes cases with specified stage.

Table 11-14   Aortic lymph node metastases in epithelial ovarian cancer

Series	Stage I Positive lymphangiography	Stage I Positive biopsy	Stage II Positive lymphangiography	Stage II Positive biopsy	Stage III-IV Positive lymphangiography	Stage III-IV Positive biopsy	Total Positive lymphangiography
Hanks and Bagshawe (1969)	2/9	—	2/6	—	4/7	—	8/22
Parker et al. (1974)	3/13	—	2/29	—	12/27	—	17/69
Knapp and Friedman (1974)	—	5/26	—	—	—	—	—
Delgado et al. (1977)	1/5	—	1/5	—	—	3/5	2/10
Buchsbaum et al. (1989)*	—	4/95	—	8/41	—	7/46	—
Burghardt (1991)	—	1/20	—	4/7	—	51/78	—
TOTAL		10/141		12/48		61/129	

*All patients had optimal carcinoma with metastatic lesions less than 3 cm.

borderline tumors tend to afflict a younger population (Figure 10-14). A 10-year survival rate of approximately 95% has been obtained in these borderline neoplasms (Figure 10-16). However, symptomatic recurrence and death may develop as many as 20 years after therapy in a few patients. These neoplasms can correctly be labeled as being of low malignant potential. On the basis of their almost benign behavior, many gynecologists advocate conservative therapy, especially in patients who are desirous of further childbearing and have stage Ia disease (Chapter 10).

The following can be said about ovarian tumors of low malignant potential, or so-called borderline malignancies:

1. Patients have a high survival rate.
2. Even lesions that behave in a malignant fashion usually have a typical indolent course.
3. There is occasional spontaneous regression of peritoneal implants.
4. Only a small percentage of cases are fatal.
5. The diagnosis must be based on examination of the original ovarian tumor without considering whether it has spread.
6. Extensive sectioning of the neoplasm is necessary to rule out truly invasive characteristics.

Serous lesions appear to be more common than mucinous lesions, but both have similar natural histories. The majority of patients with borderline serous tumors have stage I tumors—70%-85% in most series. About 30% of patients have extraovarian tumor at the time of diagnosis, with equal numbers in stages II and III. Stage IV borderline tumors of low malignant potential have been described, but they are rare. Most tumor-related deaths occur in patients with stage II or III neoplasms, but there are several important differences from true adenocarcinoma of the ovary. First, more than 50% of patients with extra-ovarian tumors survive, even though resection is incomplete. Second, patients who ultimately die of tumor do so many years after initial diagnosis. The protracted clinical course of these tumors makes prolonged follow-up an essential component of any scientific investigation. The long survival and the apparent cure of patients with advanced-stage proliferating serous tumors is puzzling and had led to speculation that some patients have multifocal proliferations of coelomic epithelium involving one or both ovaries and extraovarian sites, including some unusual ones, such as sites within pelvic and abdominal lymph nodes. Both clinical and pathologic evidence is available to support the hypothesis that extraovarian tumor, in at least some of these patients, represents multifocal proliferation rather than an implantation or metastasis.

Appropriate treatment for patients with serous or mucinous tumors of low malignant potential remains to be determined (Chapter 10). The standard surgical therapy is total abdominal hysterectomy and bilateral salpingo-oophorectomy. Genadry believes that adjuvant therapy is unwarranted regardless of clinical stage, since any extraovarian neoplasm should be viewed as multifocal and in situ, rather than metastatic. This issue obviously requires additional study that includes careful evaluation in grading of extraovarian tumor deposits, as well as ovarian neoplasms, and correlation of their appearances with outcome.

According to both Julian and Woodruff and Malloy et al., recurrent lesions may develop after latent intervals as long as 20-50 years. After long follow-up, as many as 25% of the patients studied succumbed to their tumors. Recurrences are usually histologically similar to the primary tumors, suggesting that the cells of borderline tumors probably do not undergo progressive anaplasia with the passage of time. Occasionally, lymph node metastases develop but hematogenous metastases and extension outside the peritoneal cavity are uncommon, although subcutaneous metastases have been rarely reported.

The treatment of stage III disease remains unsettled. Many clinicians believe that neither radiation therapy nor chemotherapy is effective against these slow-dividing cell populations. No prospective or well-controlled studies have been done on advanced disease, although scattered reports of response to various chemotherapeutic agents have been recorded. Fort reported on the experience from Memorial Sloan Kettering Cancer Center with low-malignant-potential epithelial ovarian tumors treated with chemotherapy. Twenty-nine patients with stage I, 5 patients with stage II, 11 patients with stage III, and 1 patient with stage IV were studied. Nineteen patients had residual disease following surgery. All 19 received adjuvant chemotherapy, radiation therapy, or a combination. Twelve patients with residual disease were found to be free of disease at second assessment surgery following adjunctive therapy. This review indicates that adjunctive therapy can eradicate residual disease in some patients with epithelial ovarian tumors of low malignant potential. This has not been the experience of most. The authors have found surgical excision of disease the most effective therapy and have utilized repeated explorations, reserving chemotherapy for patients who develop ascites, change histology or demonstrate very rapid growth (Figure 11-11).

Treatment of Malignant Epithelial Neoplasms

The most common epithelial cancers of the ovary are histologically categorized as serous, mucinous, endometrioid, and clear cell (mesonephroid) types (Figures 11-12 to 11-15). Although there has been some controversy in the past, it is now apparent that these different histologic varieties behave similarly, stage for stage and grade for grade. Some types, such as the mucinous and endometrioid varieties, are more commonly found in lower stages, with more well-differentiated lesions accounting for the confusion in the earlier literature. Prognosis, survival, and therapy for these various forms of epithelial cancer are hereafter considered collectively.

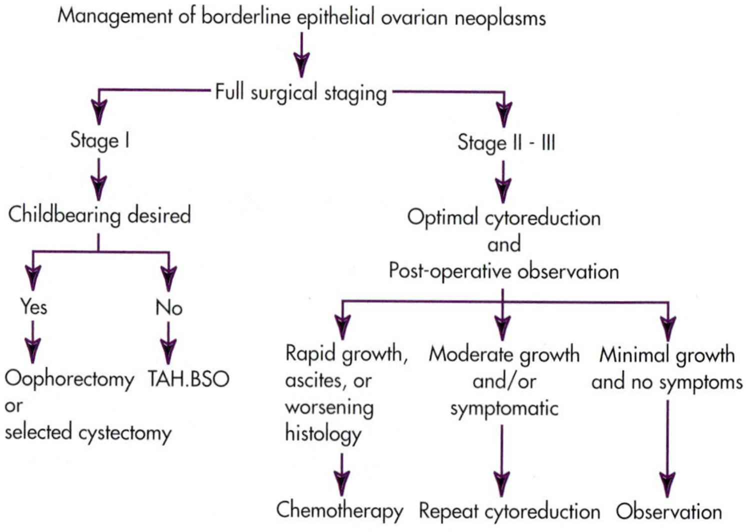

Management of borderline epithelial ovarian neoplasms

Full surgical staging

Stage I → Stage II - III

Figure 11-11 Algorithm for the management of borderline epithelial ovarian neoplasms.

Stage I → Childbearing desired → Yes / No

Yes → Oophorectomy or selected cystectomy

No → TAH.BSO

Stage II - III → Optimal cytoreduction and Post-operative observation

Rapid growth, ascites, or worsening histology → Chemotherapy

Moderate growth and/or symptomatic → Repeat cytoreduction

Minimal growth and no symptoms → Observation

One theory of ovarian epithelial cancer growth suggests that the disease initially grows locally, invading the capsule and mesovarium, and then invades adjacent organs by contiguous growth and lymphatic spread. When the malignancy reaches the external surface of the capsule, cells may exfoliate into the peritoneal cavity, where they are free to circulate and later implant. Local and regional lymphatic metastasis may occur involving the uterus, fallopian tubes, and pelvic lymph nodes. Involvement of the periaortic lymph nodes by way of the infundibulopelvic ligament is also common.

Woodruff suggested another mechanism of disease spread that may be operational in epithelial ovarian cancer. He suggests that the entire coelomic epithelium can give rise to this lesion under the influence of carcinogenic agents that may gain access to the peritoneal cavity from the vagina through the fallopian tubes. Indeed, the lesion could then originate in a multifocal distribution, "like a measles rash," over large portions of the coelomic epithelium. This theory would explain the common observation of advanced stage disease in a patient who was carefully examined in a short time previously and was apparently free of disease with no palpable pelvic mass.

Probably the most important variable influencing the prognosis in each case of ovarian cancer is the stage or extent of disease. A staging system has been devised that allows a comparison of treatment results among different institutions.

Although staging does not mandate treatment, discussing treatment by stage is often helpful. Survival depends on the stage of the lesion, the grade of differentiation of the lesion, gross findings at surgery (see box above), the amount of residual tumor remaining after surgery, and the additional treatment after surgery. The 5-year survival figures from the International Federation of Gynecology and Obstetrics (FIGO) 1994 report (Figure 11-16) are:

GUIDELINES FOR STAGING IN EPITHELIAL OVARIAN CANCER

- 4 peritoneal washings (diaphragm, right and left abdomen, pelvis)
- Careful inspection and palpation of all peritoneal surfaces
- Biopsy or smear from undersurface of right hemidiaphragm
- Biopsy of all suspicious lesions
- Infracolic omentectomy
- Biopsy or resection of any adhesions
- Random biopsy or normal peritoneum of bladder reflection cul-de-sac, right and left paracolic recesses, and both pelvic side walls (in the absence of obvious implants)
- Selected lymphadenectomy of pelvic and para-aortic nodes
- TAH, BSO, and excision of all masses where prudent

Stage Ia	84%
Stage Ib	79%
Stage Ic	73%
Stage IIa	65%
Stage IIb	54%
Stage IIc	61%
Stage IIIa	52%
Stage IIIb	29%
Stage IIIc	18%
Stage IV	14%

The overall 5-year survival rate was 31%. There is improved survival for all stages in patients with well-differentiated lesions, in those with all or most of the tumor removed at surgery, and in those who received postoperative irradiation and/or chemotherapy.

Text continued on p. 302.

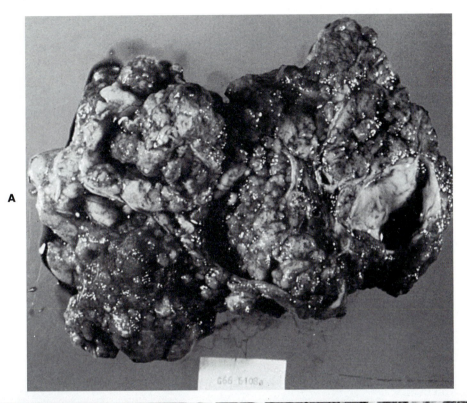

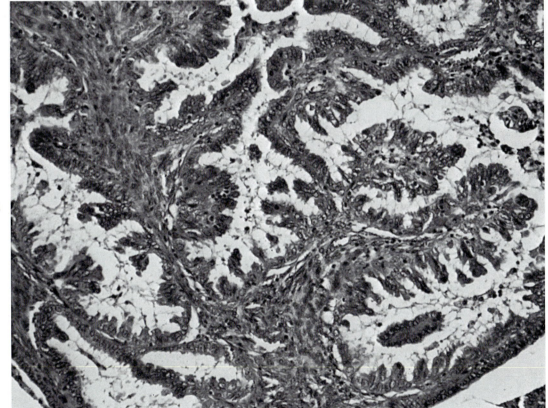

Figure 11-12 Papillary serous adenocarcinoma of ovary. **A,** Gross appearance with soft, friable proliferating papillae. **B,** Histologic appearance with prominent fibrous stalks and non-mucin-producing epithelial cells.

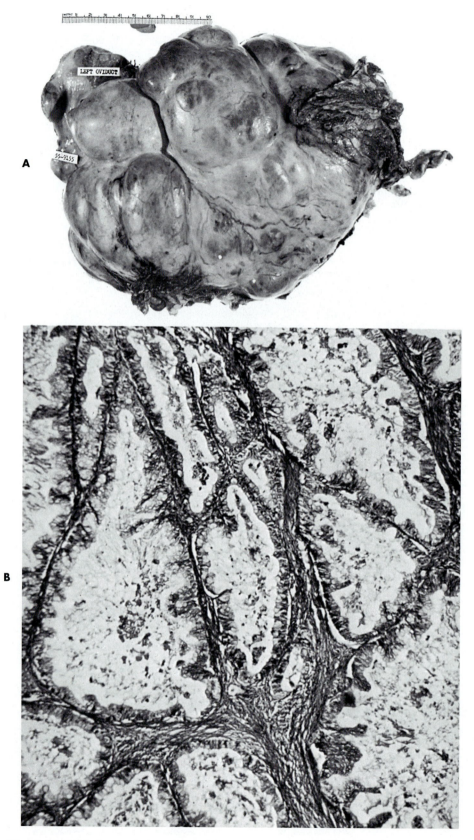

Figure 11-13 Mucinous adenocarcinoma of ovary. **A,** Gross appearance. **B,** Microscopic appearance. Note tall, columnar, mucin-producing cells.

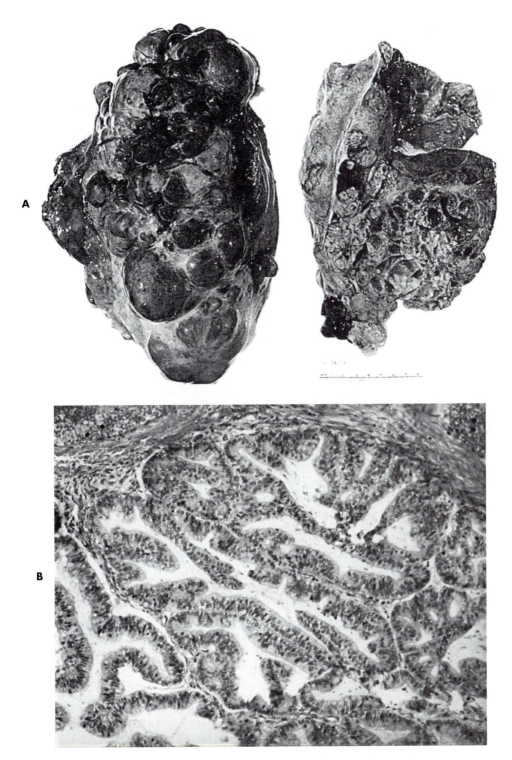

Figure 11-14 Endometroid adenocarcinoma of ovary. **A,** Gross cystic and solid appearance.
B, Histologic appearance with columnar and pseudostratified epithelial cells showing prominent
elongated hyperchromatic nuclei.

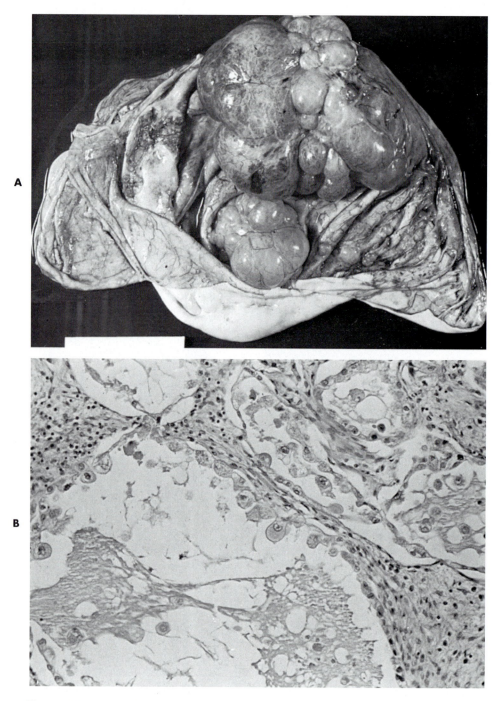

Figure 11-15 Clear cell adenocarcinoma ovary. **A,** Gross solid and cystic appearance. **B,** Microscopic view showing hobnail or peg cells.

Stages Ia, Ib, and Ic

Total abdominal hysterectomy and bilateral salpingo-oophorectomy with careful surgical staging is undoubtedly the best therapy for stage I lesions (Table 11-16). At many institutions, omentectomy is also done for stage I lesions, especially if adjunctive therapy is planned in the form of intraperitoneal instillation of radioactive colloidal phosphorus. In addition to being an organ that may harbor microscopic disease in patients with apparent stage I lesions, the omentum is an organ to which radioactive colloidal substances such as ^{32}P have a great affinity, and thus its removal theoretically allows a greater amount of radioactive substance to be available for distribution over the visceral and parietal peritoneal surfaces of the abdomen. The value of omentectomy in and of itself as a therapeutic modality for stage I disease has yet to be conclusively established.

Recent evidence suggests that pelvic and periaortic nodes may be involved 10%-20% of the time in apparent stage I disease, and the value of lymphadenectomy as a

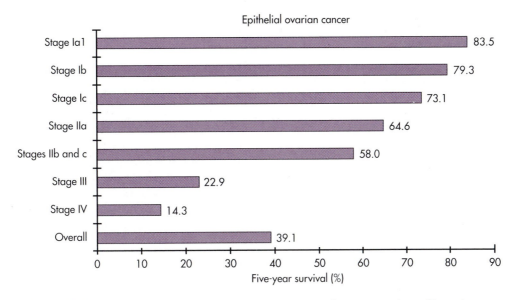

Figure 11-16 Multicentered data on the treatment of 7509 ovarian cancer patients. (From *Annual report on the results of treatment in gynecological cancer,* FIGO, vol 22, 1994).

Table 11-16 Stage I ovarian cancer (Mayo Clinic)

Extent grossly	Survival
Intracystic papillations	90%
Extracystic excrescences	68%
Ruptured cyst	56%
Adherent cyst	51%

Based on data from Webb MJ et al: *Am J Obstet Gynecol* 116:222, 1973.

diagnostic and therapeutic procedure is now under study. Burghardt reported on 23 patients with stage I epithelial cancers of the ovary, all of whom had complete pelvic lymphadenectomies. Seven patients (30%) were found to have lymph node involvement. Buchsbaum reported a lower incidence of positive pelvic nodes from the large GOG study (0.0% for apparent stage I, 19.5% for apparent stage II, and 11.1% for apparent stage III). However, the GOG study included only patients with metastatic lesions less than 3 cm in diameter. Burghardt et al. reported on a series of patients with all sizes of lesions upon whom complete pelvic and periaortic lymphadenectomies had been done, and the involvement of pelvic nodes was much higher (15% for stage I, 57% for stage II, and 64% for stage III). Creasman et al. reported four patients with ovarian cancer who, after chemotherapy or combined immunochemotherapy, were found to have retroperitoneal disease at the time of a second-look exploratory laparotomy, even though there was no evidence of intra-abdominal residual cancer. Ovarian cancer can metastasize to pelvic and periaortic lymph nodes, and

therefore these areas must be evaluated to assess appropriately the true extent of disease in patients with ovarian cancer.

Some institutions prefer chemotherapy as postoperative therapy with stage Ib and Ic lesions and with undifferentiated histology. In the more recent era, this adjuvant therapy is usually a platinum analog alone or in combination with an alkylating agent and/or TAXOL. In the management of low-grade (grade 1) lesions, the physician must weigh the possible benefits of adjuvant chemotherapy vs the risks. The authors have discontinued recommending chemotherapy for patients with stage Ia, grade I lesion.

Patients with stage I, grade 3 lesions present a difficult problem. The incidence of recurrence in this group approaches 50% in some series. Traditionally these patients were treated with single-agent chemotherapy, but in recent years many have been given multiple-agent therapy because of the very impressive preliminary data suggesting that multiple drugs are more effective than single agents. It is our belief that this group of patients should receive adjuvant multiple-agent chemotherapy despite the fact that no clear data exists showing superior results as compared to single agent therapy. Philosophically, it is difficult to withhold the apparent best therapy from a group of patients who may have the best situation for a chemotherapy "cure"; in addition, this group is usually youthful and better able to tolerate vigorous adjuvant therapy than older patients.

The most appropriate adjuvant therapy for patients with stage I lesions in whom total abdominal hysterectomy and bilateral salpingo-oophorectomy have been done is a subject of considerable controversy. Some have advocated no further therapy, whereas others insist on a period of chemotherapy or intraperitoneal instillation of radioactive colloid. Still others suggest whole abdominal irradiation with or without chemotherapy. We favor platinum-based multi-agent therapy for this group of high-risk patients. The only prospective study available that addresses this subject is found in data of the Gynecologic Oncology Group (Table 11-17).

The study by the Gynecologic Oncology Group (GOG) and the Ovarian Cancer Study Group (OCSG) has been reported in which patients with stages Ia and Ib, grade 1 or 2 disease, were randomized between those who received melphalan (0.2 mg/m^2/daily PO for 5 days) for 12 cycles and those who received no further therapy. The 5-year survival in both arms of the study was excellent (>90%). Considering the toxicity, the expense, the inconvenience, and the risk of second malignancy associated with alkylating agent therapy, defining those patients who require no additional therapy will be important should these data be confirmed. A second GOG-OCSG trial included all patients who had stage Ic disease with no microscopic residua, patients who had stages Ia and Ib disease with ruptured capsule, patients who had stages Ia and Ib, grade 3 lesions, and patients who had stage II disease when there was no evidence of macroscopic residua. These patients were randomized to receive melphalan or 15 mCi of intraperitoneal colloidal ^{32}P. Survival and disease-free survival were similar in both arms of the study (approximately 80%; see Table 11-17). The frequency of severe side effects was low in both treatment arms. However, ^{32}P was associated with fewer side effects than melphalan, and only 25% of patients treated with ^{32}P experienced any type of toxicity. Because of the ease, convenience to patients, minimal toxicity, and cost currently suggested, intraperitoneal ^{32}P should be seriously considered as a standard for further investigations.

In the young woman with stage Ia disease who is desirous of further childbearing, unilateral salpingo-oophorectomy may be associated with minimal increased risk of recurrence, provided a careful staging procedure is performed and due consideration is given to grade and apparent self-containment of the neoplasm.

Stages IIa, IIb, and IIc

In many institutions, the treatment of choice for stages IIa and IIb disease is total abdominal hysterectomy and bilateral salpingo-oophorectomy, omentectomy, and instillation of ^{32}P. Other centers prefer abdominal and pelvic irradiation as postoperative therapy. Still other institutions have had reasonable success with a combination of pelvic irradiation and systemic chemotherapy. A fourth more commonly used treatment plan is to follow surgery with chemotherapy, usually with platinum-based combination therapy and then consider a second-look procedure if the patient is clinically free of disease at completion of therapy. As in stage I disease, the value of omentectomy remains inconclusive. However, most authorities agree that in all stages, omentectomy serves as a valuable diagnostic tool. Here, as in stage I disease, the variety of treatment plans is a reflection of retrospective studies that report acceptable survival rates following a number of therapy approaches. One issue appears to be clear: the entire abdomen should be considered at risk, and the treatment plan should include some form of therapy for at least all peritoneal surfaces. Even at very large institutions only a few cases of stage I and stage II disease are seen, making prospective randomized studies difficult. Fortunately, these problems are currently being studied by cooperative groups, and Table 11-17 describes the result of one such study. Careful surgical staging is essential to successful treatment planning.

Stage III

In stage III, as in other stages, every effort should be made to remove the uterus with both adnexa. In addition, every effort should be made short of major bowel surgery to remove the bulk of the tumor, including the large omental cakes. Retrospective studies have suggested strongly that the survival rate in patients with stage III disease related to the residual tumor after surgery, such that patients with minimal residual appear to have better prognoses with adjunctive therapy (Table 11-18). Adjunctive therapy in

---

Table 11-17 Adjuvant therapy in stage I and stage II epithelial ovarian cancer (GOG study)

Regimen	Number of patients	5-yr survival (%)
Stage Ia or Ib, grade 1 and 2		
No therapy	38	91
Melphalan (1.0 mg/kg)	43	98
Stage I "high risk"* or stage II		
Melphalan (1.0 mg/kg)	68	81
Intraperitoneal ^{32}P (15 mc)	73	78

From Young RC et al: *N Engl J Med* 322:1021, 1990.
*Stage Ia or Ib with capsule ruptured or surface involvement, stage Ic.

Table 11-18 Relationship of residual tumor size and median survival (months)

Author	Number of patients	Optimal (<2 cm)	Suboptimal (>2 cm)
Griffiths et al.	102	28	11
Wharton et al.	104	27	15
Hacker et al.	47	22	6
Sutton et al.	56	39	22

the form of abdominal and pelvic irradiation is used in many centers but has found less and less favor in recent years. Unless the residual masses are no larger than 2 cm at any focus in the abdomen, irradiation is not likely to be effective. Thus, patients with bulky residual disease should be treated with chemotherapy. Most centers now prefer multiple-agent platinum-based chemotherapy for this group of patients because of the excellent response rates reported in the literature (see Combination chemotherapy on pp. 317-322). It should be pointed out, however, that comparative long-term survival rates for multiple-agent and single-agent chemotherapy are yet to be reported.

The duration of treatment using multiple-agent therapy is usually 6-12 months or until maximal doses of certain dose-limited drugs, such as doxorubicin (Adriamycin) and cisplatin, have been reached. If the patient survives this period and has no clinical evidence of disease, a second-look procedure is often considered.

Reported evidence suggests that even in the optimal group (patients with residua no greater than 1-2 cm in diameter at any site), the survival and response rates with chemotherapy are equivalent to that of abdominal and pelvic irradiation (Figure 11-17). The long-term morbidity of radiation therapy is much greater, and this factor has considerably influenced postoperative therapy for stage III disease such that most centers prescribe multi-agent chemotherapy. As yet, there are no convincing studies reported of patients who were randomized between those who received radiotherapy and those who received multiple-agent chemotherapy. Initial prospective studies by several groups randomized patients between those who received single-agent chemotherapy and those who received multiple-drug regimens, and most concluded

(with regard to tumor response) that polychemotherapy had significant advantage over single-agent regimens. This issue is important since the morbidity of polychemotherapy is considerably greater than that of the single-agent alkylating-agent regimen.

Stage IV

The ideal management of stage IV disease is to remove as much cancer as possible and to administer chemotherapy after surgery. The overall survival for this group of patients is similar to that of stage III (Figure 11-18).

Maximal Surgical Effort

It has been axiomatic among many gynecologic oncologists that it is judicious to excise as much tumor as possible when disseminated disease is encountered at the time of primary operation for ovarian cancer. Although it was known that significant palliation may be achieved by reduction of a heavy tumor burden, until recently there had been little firm evidence that the usual "debulking" procedures directly improve survival. Munnell reported a 28% 5-year survival rate among patients who had undergone a "maximal surgical effort" as compared with a 9% 5-year survival rate among patients who had had partial resection and a 3% 5-year survival rate among patients who had had biopsy only. In Munnell's 14 survivors the "maximal surgical effort" consisted of hysterectomy, bilateral salpingo-oophorectomy, and omentectomy.

Aure et al. demonstrated significant improvement in survival among stage III patients only if all gross tumor had been removed (Figure 11-19). Similar results were recently obtained by Griffiths, who used a multiple linear regression equation with survival as the dependent variable to control simultaneously for the multiple

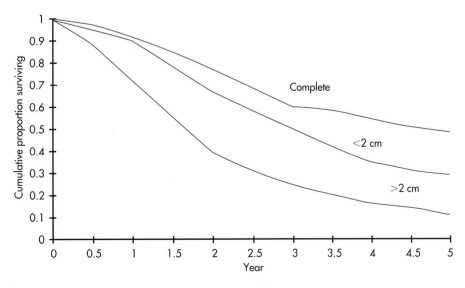

Figure 11-17 Carcinoma of the ovary stage IIIc class Ic. Actuarial survival by completeness of surgery. Cumulative proportion surviving. (From *Annual Report Gynecological Cancer* FIGO, vol 22, 1994.)

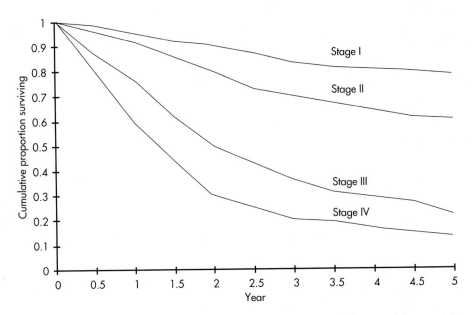

Figure 11-18 Obviously malignant cases of ovarian carcinoma. Cumulative proportion surviving by stage. (From *Annual Report Gynecological Cancer* FIGO, vol 22, 1994.)

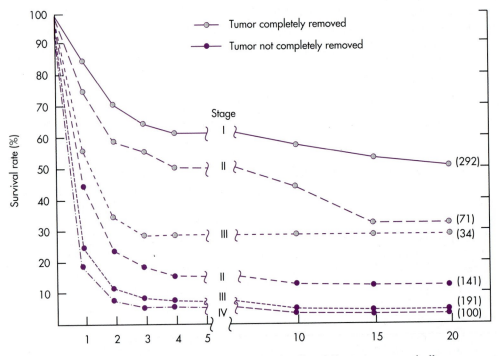

Figure 11-19 Survival rates stage for stage in patients in whom all tumor was surgically removed vs patients in whom all tumor was not completely removed. (From Aure JC, Hoeg K, Kolstad P: *Obstet Gynecol* 37:1, 1971.)

therapeutic and biologic factors that contribute to the ultimate outcome in the individual patient. The most important factors proved to be histologic grade of the tumor and size of the largest residual mass after primary surgery. The operation itself contributed nothing to survival unless it effected the reduction in the size of the largest residual tumor mass below the limit of 1.6 cm.

The so-called debulking procedure has gained considerable attention in the management of ovarian cancer. The concept is simply to diminish the residual tumor burden to a point where adjuvant therapy will be optimally effective. All forms of adjuvant therapy are most effective when a minimal tumor burden exists. This is particularly true of ovarian carcinoma, which is one of the solid

Table 11-19 The effect of cytoreductive surgery on residual disease as found by second-assessment surgery

Author	% negative second look		
	No residual	Optimal residual	Suboptimal residual
Barnhill (1984)	67	61	14
Cain (1986)	76	50	28
Smirz (1985)	75	—	25
Webb (1982)	95	36	20
Podratz (1983)	82	44	33
Curry (1981)	79	45	22
Dauplat (1983)	100	100	40
Hoskins (1989)	75	45	25
MEAN	81	52	23

tumors more sensitive to chemotherapy. A careful and persistent surgeon can often remove large tumor masses that on first impression appear to be unresectable. Using the clear retroperitoneal spaces, one can usually identify the infundibulopelvic ligament and ureter and then isolate the vessels of the infundibulopelvic ligament and the blood supply of the ovary. Once these vessels have been ligated and transected, retrograde removal of large ovarian masses is easier and safer. The ureter must be kept under direct vision throughout the dissection so that probability of traumatizing this pelvic structure is minimized. A clear space usually exists on the transverse colon whereby large omental cakes of ovarian carcinoma can be removed after the right and left gastroepiploic vessels have been ligated. Removal of large ovarian masses and omental involvement often reduces the tumor burden by 80%-90%. The theoretic value of debulking procedures lies in the obvious reduction of cell numbers and the advantage this affords to adjuvant therapy. This is especially relevant in bulky solid tumors such as ovarian cancer, where removal of large numbers of cells in the resting phase (G_0) can propel the residual cells into the more vulnerable proliferating pool. Several careful retrospective studies have repeatedly demonstrated improved survival rate in patients who can be surgically brought to a status of minimal tumor burden (Table 11-19). A recent report of the very large experience of the MD Anderson Hospital and Tumor Institute illustrated a significantly improved salvage rate in patients with stage II and stage III epithelial cancers of the ovary when initial surgery was followed by no gross residual tumor or no single residual tumor mass exceeding 1 cm in diameter. This report reflects a 70% 2-year survival rate in stage III patients in whom no gross disease remained and a 50% survival rate when residual nodules were limited to 1 cm in diameter. This compares favorably with the usually

quoted overall survival rates. GOG has attempted to better define primary cytoreductive surgery with a detailed analysis of the results of surgery in patients with advanced disease. Their initial study compared survival in the stage III patients who were found at surgery to have abdominal disease of ≤1 cm to patients found to have disease >1 cm but were surgically cytoreduced to ≤1 cm. If surgery was the only important factor, survival should have been equivalent in both groups. This was not the case. Patients found to have small volume disease survived longer than patients cytoreduced to small volume disease at surgery. In a second study, GOG investigators evaluated the effect of the diameter of the largest residual disease on survival in patients with suboptimal cytoreduction. They demonstrated that cytoreduction so that the largest residual mass to ≤2 cm resulted in a significant survival benefit, but that all residual diameters >2 cm had equivalent survival (Figure 11-20). Therefore unless the patient can be cytoreduced to ≤2 cm, residual diameter did not influence survival. In evaluating optimally and suboptimally cytoreduced patients, these GOG investigators showed that three distinct groups emerged: microscopic residual, residual disease of ≤2 cm, and residual disease of >2 cm (Figure 11-21). It is clear from these studies, that patients with microscopic disease have a 4-year survival of about 60%, while patients with gross disease ≤2 cm have a 4-year survival of 35%. On the other hand, patients who cannot be cytoreduced to ≤2 cm have a 4-year survival of less than 20%. Most striking, however, is the failure of cytoreductive surgery to have any effect on survival unless the largest diameter of residual disease is ≤2 cm.

The effect of maximal cytoreductive surgery can be seen in the percentage of negative second looks (Table 11-19). Even though cytoreductive surgery seems to have therapeutic value, controversy continues. The primary unresolved issue is whether the poor prognosis associated with bulky disease is caused by the presence of increased tumor burden (in which case cytoreductive surgery would be of potential benefit) or associated with differences in tumor biology or a decreased sensitivity to chemotherapeutic regimens. If the latter possibilities are indeed the case, cytoreductive surgery is not likely to have a major impact on survival. The implication is thus that those patients who have disease that can be cytoreduced are a select group with good prognoses on the basis of factors independent of the cytoreductive surgery. It is not clear how many patients with bulky disease can actually successfully undergo cytoreduction of tumor masses smaller than 2 cm and in how many patients such aggressive surgery is medically contraindicated. Furthermore, if chemotherapy is delayed because of complications of cytoreductive surgery, this may have a deleterious effect on long-term survival. Finally, the most appropriate time to do cytoreductive surgery has not been determined: before any chemotherapy, after 1 to 3 cycles of induction chemotherapy, or after completion of a full 6 to 12 month

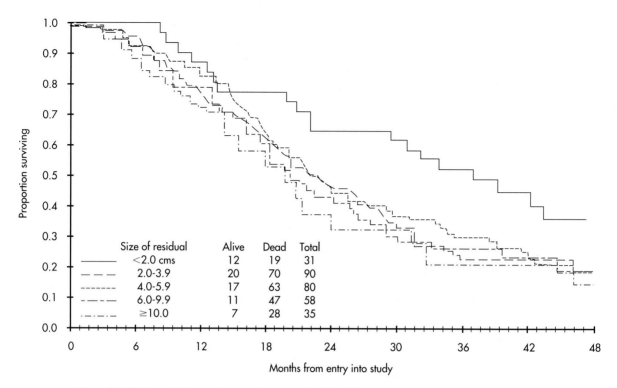

Figure 11-20 Survival by maximum diameter of residual disease. (From Hoskins WJ et al: *Am J Obstet Gynecol* 170:974, 1994.)

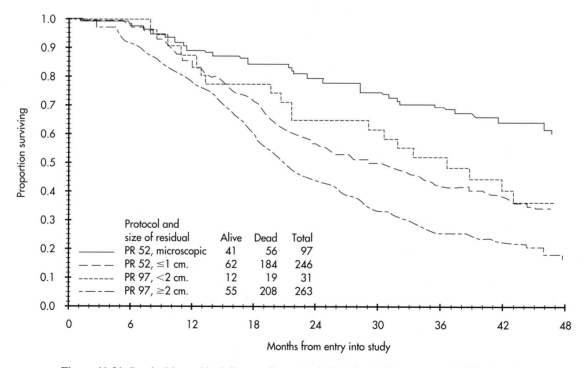

Figure 11-21 Survival by residual disease, Gynecologic Oncology Group protocols (PR) 52 and 97. (From Hoskins WJ et al: *Am J Obstet Gynecol* 170:974, 1994.)

induction course of chemotherapy. The percentage of patients with advanced ovarian cancer who can effectively undergo cytoreductive surgery seems to range from 43%-87%, depending on the report reviewed. This difference may reflect the individual skills of the surgeons but it more likely represents different referral patterns and other selection factors. None of the studies reported to date proves that debulking surgery is a therapeutically important maneuver, instead of just a prognostic variable. The answer to this question will require a prospective randomized trial. Although this or similar trials may change subsequent recommendations, it currently seems appropriate to recommend that patients who are diagnosed as having advanced ovarian cancer should undergo resection of all masses when this is technically feasible. However, because the complications of cytoreductive surgery can be high, aggressive surgery that requires multiple bowel resections or lower urinary tract diversion should be restricted to carefully controlled clinical trials.

The enthusiasm for the debulking of ovarian cancer has led to many techniques for achieving that end. Some clinicians have advocated the use of an ultrasound surgical aspirator. Others suggested electrosurgical debulking with an argon beam coagulator. Still others suggest that the resection of the diaphragmatic peritoneum or muscle may have a role in cytoreductive surgery. The impact of all of these techniques on patient survival is somewhat unclear. One must be cautious about techniques that are executed successfully only in the hands of the enthusiastic and await confirming reports.

The literature on secondary cytoreductive surgery in the treatment of advanced epithelial ovarian cancer is fairly evenly divided between those who believe it is of benefit and those who do not. All the studies are hampered at present by relatively small numbers, and many of the patients were not treated with what can be considered optimal first-line therapy. Two of the better reports are by Hoskins and by Morris. Hoskins and his colleagues at Memorial Sloan-Kettering retrospectively reviewed 67 patients who were found to have a positive second-look laparotomy. Between 1978 and 1986, 50 of their patients were actually candidates for secondary cytoreduction. Of these, 16 had all gross and macroscopic disease resected. No information is given regarding the type of surgery required or the morbidity incurred but the 5-year survival for this group of patients with no macroscopic residual disease was 51%. This was not statistically different from the survival of another 17 patients found to have macroscopic disease only at the time of second-look. Patients with any gross residual disease following secondary cytoreductive surgery did very poorly. On the other hand, Morris, at the MD Anderson Hospital, retrospectively reviewed 30 patients who underwent very radical secondary cytoreduction for clinical evidence of recurrent disease. Optimum debulking, which the authors define as tumor nodules less than 2 cm in diameter, was

achieved in 51% of the patients, but no significant survival advantage was seen for these patients.

Pecorelli reported an experience of the European Gynecological Oncology Group whereby eligible patients with residual lesions of >1 cm after primary surgery were given three cycles of cyclophosphamide and cisplatin and then randomized between conventional debulking surgery vs no surgery followed by continued cyclophosphamide and cisplatin chemotherapy. The study end points were progression free and overall survival. Three hundred and nineteen patients were randomized. An analysis of 278 patients was presented at the Society for Gynecologic Oncology in San Francisco, in February, 1995. Intervention surgery was performed on 140 patients and no further surgery was performed on 138 patients. At the time of intervention surgery, 65% of the patients had tumor lesions of >1 cm. In 45% of these patients, the disease could be reduced to lesions of >1 cm. No significant morbidity was noted from the surgical procedures. Both progression free and overall survival were significantly longer for the surgery group. The 2-year survival for the surgery group was 56% as opposed to 46% for the no surgery group. The median survival rates were 26 and 20 months respectively. In a multivariate analysis, surgery was an independent diagnostic factor. Overall, the benefit of surgery after being adjusted for all prognostic factors was risk reduction of 33%. Patients randomized to the intervention debulking surgery had a significantly longer progression free and overall survival. Patients who undergo extensive surgery are at increased risk for wound disruption; therefore, mass closure techniques for abdominal wall closure should be utilized (Figure 11-22).

Role of Radiation Therapy

Radiation therapy techniques include intraperitoneal radioactive chromium phosphate and external beam therapy to the abdomen and pelvis. Patients with epithelial carcinoma of the ovary who are selected to receive postoperative irradiation should receive treatment of the entire abdomen plus additional radiation to the pelvis. This broad treatment plan is based on an analysis of postirradiation recurrences of stage I and stage II disease that showed that most of the recurrences were outside the pelvis. There is no lid on the pelvis, and malignant cells are shed from the primary ovarian tumor and circulate throughout the entire abdominal cavity. Lymphatic dissemination is also possible.

Two different radiation treatment techniques have been used for abdominal irradiation. Large portals may be employed, and a dose of 2500 to 3000 cGy can be delivered over 4-5 weeks to the entire abdomen. The kidneys and possibly the right lobe of the liver are shielded with lead to limit the dose to 2000 to 2500 cGy. Nausea and vomiting may be associated with this procedure, and therapy is frequently interrupted. In some centers the abdominal irradiation is delivered by the so-called moving strip tech-

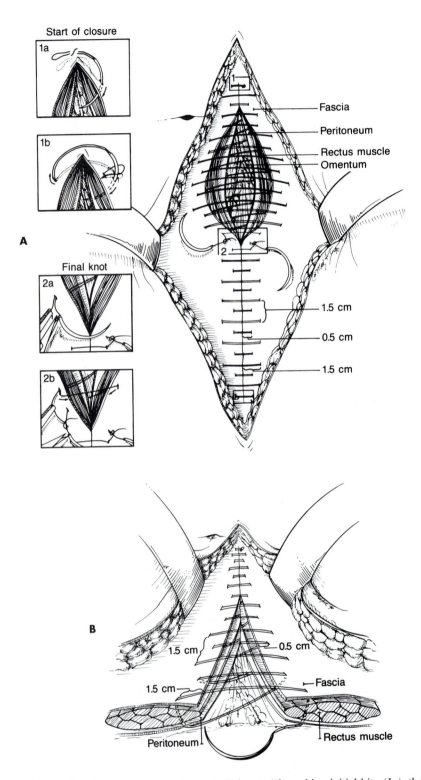

Figure 11-22 A, Running Smead-Jones closure techniques. After taking initial bite *(1a)*, the needle, with double strand suture, is pulled through the open loop end *(1b)*. At completion of the fascial closure, one of the two strands of the looped suture is cut from the needle *(2a)*. A bilateral bite through both anterior fascial layers is taken, and the suture is tied to itself *(2b)*. **B,** A mass closure technique utlizing 0 Maxon loop suture in a running Smead-Jones technique has the value of speed and security in our experience.

nique. The abdomen, or the area to be irradiated, is divided into contiguous segments or strips 2.5 cm wide. Both front and back are treated daily, and the treatment field is increased by one strip every 2 days until four strips (10 cm) have been treated. The 10 cm segment is moved up 2.5 cm every 2 days until the last strip is reached. The field is then reduced progressively one strip at a time, and on the last 2 days of treatment a single 2.5 cm strip is irradiated. Again the kidneys are shielded with lead, as is the upper portion of the liver, in an effort to reduce the dose to these organs. With this technique, each strip of the abdomen is irradiated from front and back for 8 days by the main beam and for 4 days by the penumbra (scatter), for a total of 12 days of irradiation. This treatment is often delivered by a cobalt 60 machine, and a tumor dose of 2600 to 2800 cGy, measured at the midline along a sagittal plane, can be delivered safely. It is calculated that this is biologically equivalent to approximately 4000 cGy given by the whole-abdomen technique. The fact that the dose is administered in a shorter time is the justification for this equivalent, and it is thought that because only a small portion of the abdominal cavity is irradiated at any one time, the treatment may be better tolerated. The occurrence of nausea and vomiting is not infrequent when the upper abdomen is being treated, and diarrhea is common when the beam is low in the abdomen. Both the whole-abdomen and the moving strip techniques usually finish with a pelvic boost of approximately 2000 to 3000 cGy.

As a better understanding of the effects of chemotherapeutic agents in ovarian cancer has been gained, the role of radiation therapy in this disease has diminished in prominence. The spread pattern of ovarian cancer and the normal tissue bed involved in the treatment of this neoplasm make effective radiation therapy difficult. Some special problems are listed in the box below. When the residual disease after laparotomy is bulky, radiation therapy is particularly ineffective. The entire abdomen must be considered at risk, and therefore the volume that must be irradiated is very large, resulting in multiple limitations for the radiotherapist. Dose restrictions are listed in the top box right.

As long as three decades ago, several institutions abandoned the use of irradiation as postoperative therapy in patients with bulky residual epithelial cancers of the

ovary (see box bottom). However, these same institutions continued to test the applicability of irradiation in patients with minimal residual disease after surgery. A study was reported by Smith et al. from the MD Anderson Hospital that gave the results of a randomized prospective study of patients with minimal residual disease (no nodule larger than 2 cm) who were randomized between recipients of single-drug alkylating agent chemotherapy and those who received whole-abdomen irradiation (moving strip technique) with a pelvic boost. This study showed no advantage to the irradiation therapy and showed a significant increase in morbidity. On the basis of this study, the role of radiation therapy in many institutions has become limited for stage III and stage IV disease. The GOG tested the feasibility of using radiation therapy in conjunction with chemotherapy. A prospective randomized study using four arms and assessing radiation therapy alone, radiation therapy before chemotherapy (melphalan), chemotherapy alone, and chemotherapy before radiation therapy was recently completed, with no significant difference found in any of the four arms. It thus becomes difficult to justify the morbidity of extensive radiation therapy for this disease process.

Dembo et al. reported a prospective randomized stratified trial involving 231 patients with stages I and II and asymptomatic stage III ovarian carcinoma who received radiation therapy with or without chlorambucil. Chlorambucil, 6 mg daily, was given for 2 years, and patients receiving abdominal and pelvic irradiation were given 2250 cGy in 10 fractions to the pelvic portal followed immediately by 2250 cGy of cobalt given in 10 fractions to a downward moving abdominal pelvic strip. The upper border of this field was at least 1 cm above the

---

DOSE RESTRICTIONS

Tolerance of small intestine
Limited tolerance of kidneys
Bone marrow depression
Radiation enteritis caused by large volume of intestine
   irradiated
Adhesive peritonitis

SPECIAL PROBLEMS IN OVARIAN CANCER

Limits of tumor spread often unknown
Variability of radiosensitivity
Total tumor burden usually very large
Free mobility of tumor cells within the abdominal cavity
Radiation dosage restricted by neighboring organs
Infrequent detection of early disease

CORRELATION OF TUMOR SIZE WITH TUMORICIDAL DOSE LEVELS IN OVARIAN CARCINOMA

Tumor size (cm)	Tumoricidal dose level (cGy)
>2	5000-6000
0.5-2.0	4500-5000
Microscopic	2500-3000

domes of the diaphragm, and no liver shielding was employed. The lower border extended below the obturator foramina. Posterior renal shields were used throughout the treatment. For patients with stage I or II disease, pelvic irradiation alone at a dose level of 4500 cGy was used. These investigators concluded that for patients who had stage Ib, II, or asymptomatic stage III disease, an incomplete initial pelvic operation correlated with poor survival. For patients in whom the operation was completed, abdominal and pelvic irradiation was superior to pelvic irradiation alone or pelvic irradiation followed by chlorambucil, with respect to long-term survival and control of abdominal disease. The effectiveness of abdominal and pelvic irradiation was independent of stage or histology. The value of abdominal and pelvic irradiation was most strikingly seen in patients with no visible residual tumor. These investigators also concluded that pelvic irradiation alone constituted inadequate and inappropriate postoperative treatment for patients with stage Ib or II disease. Abdominal pelvic irradiation, which encompassed both domes of the diaphragm without liver shielding, significantly reduced tumor failure outside the pelvis and improved survival. However, adjuvant chemotherapy with daily chlorambucil after pelvic irradiation was ineffective in the management of these patients. The authors also concluded that in selecting postoperative therapy, the presence of small amounts of disease in the upper abdomen should not result in the selection of chemotherapy over radiation therapy. They seemed convinced that radiation therapy appears to be effective, even when small amounts of disease exist in the upper abdomen. These studies by Dembo et al. reported good 5-year survival rates such as 58% for stage II and 43% for stage III patients. In addition, Martinez et al. reported a 54% 5-year survival rate in 42 stage II and III patients. Further studies to corroborate these findings are needed before renewed enthusiasm for radiotherapy in stages III and IV epithelial cancers of the ovary is justified.

The role of radiation therapy in localized disease also needs discussion. A prospective randomized study of stage I epithelial cancer of the ovary conducted by the GOG had the following results. Patients were randomized among three arms: (1) no further therapy, (2) melphalan (Alkeran), and (3) pelvic radiation. Hreshchyshyn et al. reported these results, which indicate that patients who received melphalan did the best, with no appreciable benefit being noted from the use of pelvic radiation. On the other hand, the role of pelvic radiation in stage II ovarian cancer has yet to be defined. Indeed, many institutions use pelvic radiation in conjunction with systemic chemotherapy as the customary treatment of stage II disease. Retrospective studies suggest that pelvic radiation improves survival over and above the use of surgery alone (Table 11-20). The efficacy of pelvic radiation, as compared with chemotherapy, in stage II disease has yet to be tested in a prospective randomized

study. The GOG study reported by Young (Table 11-17) compared chemotherapy to intraperitoneal colloidal ^{32}P. It is our opinion that the designation of stage II epithelial ovarian cancer mandates that the entire abdomen be considered at risk. Thus if postoperative radiation therapy is prescribed, it seems appropriate that a technique be used in which the entire abdomen and pelvis are optimally treated. Such an approach has been reported by Menczer and Piver.

There are no phase III data comparing platinum-based chemotherapy with radiation therapy in low and intermediate risk patients with epithelial ovarian cancer. The limitations of comparisons of radiation therapy and chemotherapy results from retrospective studies are many. In many instances, the radiation therapy studies are older and staging procedures were not done with the same accuracy. Several prospective studies have been attempted but failed due to low accrual. The two treatment methods are so different that investigator bias usually prevents reasonable patient accrual. Radiation therapy techniques have advanced, lowering toxicity. This combined with better data for patient selection, makes a strong argument for another attempt at a phase III trial of this modality in ovarian carcinoma.

Radioisotopes

Radioisotopes have been widely used for the treatment of ovarian cancer. Both the pure beta emitter radioactive chromic phosphate (half-life of 14.2 days) and radioactive gold (10% gamma, half-life of 2.7 days) have been used. These isotopes emit radiation with an effective maximal penetration of 4-5 mm and therefore are useful only with minimal disease. Both agents are taken up by the serosal macrophages and transported to the retroperitoneal and mediastinal lymph nodes. The likelihood that the radioactive colloid will eradicate nodal metastases by selective lymphatic uptake is in considerable doubt, since studies suggest that malignant nodes do not take up the isotope, but tumor-free nodes do. It has been estimated that 6000 cGy are delivered to the omentum and peritoneal surfaces and 7000 cGy to some retroperitoneal structures. If a free

Table 11-20 Radiotherapy in FIGO stage II disease

Series	Number of patients		5-year survival rate (%)	
	Surgery alone	Surgery/ irradiation	Surgery alone	Surgery/ irradiation
Van Orden et al.	8	22	25	36.4
Barr, Cawell, and Chatfield	27	91	33	48
Kent and McKay	32	36	28.2	52.8
Munnell	16	61	0	40
Clark et al.	6	51	16.7	31.4

intraperitoneal distribution can be assured, chromic phosphate with a longer half-life and no gamma irradiation is the agent of choice. Decker et al. have demonstrated radioactive colloids (using radiogold) to be advantageous in a selected group of patients with ruptures of ovarian tumors at surgery (80% 5-year survival rate vs 43% 5-year survival rate). Radioactive gold for intraperitoneal use is no longer available in the United States.

Radiotherapy with curative intent was used by Pezner to treat 104 patients with limited epithelial carcinomas of the ovary. All these patients received intraperitoneal radioactive colloid therapy, optimally scheduled 3-6 weeks after laparotomy. The initial four patients received colloidal $_{198}$Au (dose between 140 and 250 mCi). Subsequently, 94 patients received 15 mCi of ^{32}P, and 6 patients received between 11.8 and 16.9 mCi of ^{32}P. Pelvic radiotherapy was given to 56 of 104 patients beginning approximately 6 weeks after intraperitoneal radioactive colloid therapy. The addition of pelvic radiotherapy did not appear to affect survival in limited disease stages and could not be shown to decrease the incidence of local recurrence in the pelvic region. The 5-year actuarial (no evidence of disease) survival rates, according to the FIGO staging classifications, were 95% for stage Ia1, 82% for Ia2, 73% for Ib, 67% for Ic, 67% for IIa, 67% for IIb without gross residual tumor, 25% for IIb with gross residual tumor, and 50% for III with minimal or no residual tumor. In the limited stages, the 5-year recurrence rate was 24% for patients treated with colloid alone and 31% for those treated with colloid plus pelvic radiotherapy. The incidence of small-bowel complication was related to the use of pelvic radiotherapy; these complications occurred in 24% of the patients treated with colloid therapy and pelvic radiotherapy, compared with only 2.2% of the patients treated with colloid therapy alone.

In an Italian study (Bolis et al) of stage I, grade 3 or grades 1 and 2 with ascites, rupture, or capsule penetration, 104 of 124 patients entered were randomized to receive intraperitoneal ^{32}P or six courses of cisplatin. There were no significant differences between the two treatment modalities. The dosimetry and distribution problems inherent in the use of a colloid such as ^{32}P make it difficult to assure consistency in application. Although retrospective reports on cure rates in patients with early stage disease completely resected in combination with ^{32}P appear to be comparable to those treated with whole abdominal irradiation, a direct comparison has never been reported. Two trials by the GOG and the clinical trials group of the National Cancer Institute of Canada have compared the use of ^{32}P with other forms of therapy, including whole abdominal irradiation or single agent Melphalan with very similar results.

Experiments by Rosenshein et al. in the rhesus monkey suggest that adequate distribution of a radioactive colloidal substance instilled into the peritoneal cavity requires a volume of vehicle sufficient to slightly distend the peritoneal cavity. This function appears to be independent of multiple position changes. This may be particularly critical when it is desirable for therapeutic agents to reach the subdiaphragmatic area, where early microscopic metastasis from carcinoma of the ovary may exist. Myers et al. have shown the importance of position change and the value of Trendelenburg position for even distribution. Based on these observations, the following procedure for instillation of radioactive colloidal substances into the peritoneal cavity is suggested.

Technique

Radioactive colloidal chromic phosphate is injected through a multiple-perforated catheter (or catheters) that has been placed in the peritoneal cavity at surgery or inserted through a needle postoperatively. Proper placement of the catheter in the peritoneal cavity is confirmed by the instillation of 500 ml of normal saline solution. If there is free flow of saline, then technetium or Hypaque is instilled. After this, the patient is moved about to maximize distribution. Appropriate radiographs or fluoroscopy is obtained to confirm adequate distribution. Through a closed system similar to that shown in Figure 11-23, 15 mCi of ^{32}P premixed in 500 ml of saline is allowed to run into the abdomen at a rapid rate. The patient is instructed to change her position frequently so that a wide dispersion of the ^{32}P is obtained. The patient should be turned frequently to different positions to facilitate this distribution during the ensuing 90-120 minutes (e.g., Trendelenburg, 10 minutes; right side; left side; feet down).

Chemotherapy
Single-agent chemotherapy

Since relatively high response rates have been traditional with alkylating agent chemotherapy (Table 11-21) there have been few trials with other single agents in patients who have not previously received chemotherapy. Because previous drug therapy lessens the likelihood of response, response rates from nonalkylating agent chemotherapy, as often reported in the literature, may be falsely low (Table 11-22).

Hexamethylmelamine (HMM) has been shown to be a very active alkylating agent in epithelial ovarian cancer. The most extensive experience with HMM alone as primary therapy has been that of the MD Anderson Hospital, reported by Stanhope et al., where a total of 22 previously untreated patients with stages III and IV epithelial cancer of the ovary were treated; 7 complete and 3 partial responses were obtained, for an overall response rate of 45%. A study by the GOG for stages III and IV and recurrent epithelial cancer of the ovary with randomization prospectively between melphalan and (1) cyclophosphamide and doxorubicin and (2) hexamethylmelamine has shown a 32% complete response rate and

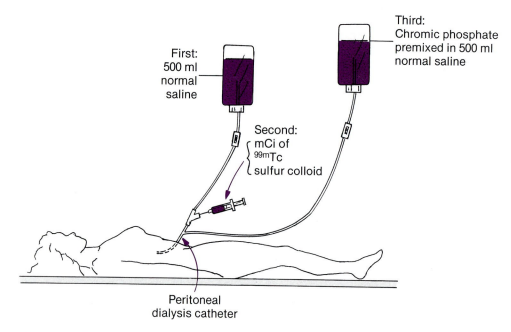

Figure 11-23 Method of administration of radioactive colloidal chromic phosphate into peritoneal cavity.

Table 11-21 Alkylating agent chemotherapy in stage III/IV ovarian cancer

Agent	Number of patients treated	% response
L-PAM	541	47
Cyclophosphamide (conventional dose)	335	43
Cyclophosphamide (intensive dose)	36	61
Chlorambucil	388	51
Triethylenethiophosphoramide (thiotepa)	337	48
Nitrosoureas	26	12

Reprinted by permission of Tobias JS, Griffiths CT: Management of ovarian carcinoma, *N Engl J Med* 294:818, 1976.

Table 11-22 Nonalkylating single-agent chemotherapy in stages III and IV ovarian cancer

Agent	Average % response
Hexamethylmelamine	42
Doxorubicin	36
Methotrexate	30
Cisplatin	35
5-Fluorouracil	20

a 22% partial response rate for patients receiving the latter regimen. HMM is an encouraging agent for further studies of combination chemotherapy in advanced epithelial ovarian cancer in spite of its moderately severe toxicity, consisting primarily of gastrointestinal toxicity, myelosuppression, and/or neurotoxicity with parkinsonian symptoms and abnormalities of gait.

Manetta reported on 52 patients with advanced ovarian carcinoma treated with single-agent HMM. All patients had previously received chemotherapy, and 8 patients (15%) had no evidence of disease at the completion of treatment with HMM. The median survival for the 52 patients was 11 months, 9 months for patients who did not respond and 41 months for patients with no evidence of

disease following therapy. Caution should be used in the administration of this agent to patients who have already had extensive chemotherapy because severe bone marrow suppression may occur.

Doxorubicin also has a broad spectrum of antineoplastic activity, with demonstrated effectiveness in the treatment of epithelial cancer of the ovary. A review by Blum and Carter suggests that this drug had an 18% response rate in a collective group of patients with ovarian cancers, but in all series reviewed the majority of patients had failed with other chemotherapy. Second-line chemotherapy in epithelial cancer of the ovary is notoriously ineffective. De Palo et al. carried out a prospective randomized study done primarily on previously untreated patients with stages III and IV ovarian cancer. Thirty-five patients were treated with doxorubicin (75 mg/m² every 3 weeks) or L-PAM (6 mg/m²/day for 5 days every 4-5 weeks), and treatment was continued until relapse. Tumor regression occurred in 8 of 13 patients treated with doxorubicin and in 4 of 10 patients treated with L-PAM. After treatment failure, crossover was performed, doxorubicin produced regression in 2 of 2 patients, and L-PAM was effective in 1 of 4.

Bolis et al. reported on the use of doxorubicin for the treatment of 38 women with stages III and IV ovarian carcinomas who had previously been treated with surgery and cyclophosphamide. Twelve patients relapsed after response to cyclophosphamide, and 26 patients did not respond initially. Of the 38 patients, 3 responded to doxorubicin therapy—all 3 patients from the group of 12 who had initial responses to cyclophosphamide. None of the 26 patients who failed to respond to cyclophosphamide subsequently responded to doxorubicin. Single-agent doxorubicin is not effective in patients who have progressed on previous chemotherapy containing an alkylating agent.

Of the antimetabolites, 5-fluorouracil has shown low but consistent efficacy in several trials. A review of these trials reveals 18 objective responses in 92 evaluable patients, for a response rate of 29%. In the opinion of most, 5-fluorouracil should not be considered as primary therapy; but because it has some activity, can be administered orally, and has acceptable toxicity, it should be considered as a second-line agent or as a possible member of combination therapy.

Methotrexate, the most widely used of the antifolate drugs, has been used only sporadically as a single agent in ovarian cancer. Sullivan et al. reported four responses in 16 patients, but this response rate has not been confirmed. Interest in methotrexate was stimulated by the observation that high doses of methotrexate followed by citrovorum factor "rescue" may have a higher therapeutic potential for several tumors. A report by Barlow and Piver in a randomized study of 55 patients with advanced-stage epithelial ovarian cancer with progressive disease after prior chemotherapy evaluated the efficacy of high-dose methotrexate with citrovorum factor rescue. All the patients studied had had prior chemotherapy when treated with methotrexate with citrovorum factor rescue plus cyclophosphamide, with or without pretreatment with vincristine. Vincristine did not enhance the efficacy of methotrexate with citrovorum factor rescue plus cyclophosphamide in terms of response rate. Objective responses lasting from 3-12 months were observed in 30% of the evaluable cases. The incidence of serious toxicity was acceptable in this group of patients, who had had extensive prior chemotherapy.

In 1976, the report by Wiltshaw and Kroner on the efficacy of cisplatin in ovarian cancer produced the modern era of combination chemotherapy. A response rate of 26% as a second-line therapy prompted the conclusion that cisplatin appeared to be the most active agent in ovarian cancer. Several cisplatin-containing regimens soon became available, resulting in response rates as high as 90% and complete responses of 40%-50%.

Taxol, a new chemotherapeutic agent that acts by promoting microtubular assembly and stabilizes tubulin polymer formation, has a great deal of activity in ovarian cancer. The initial interest in this agent related to its activity against refractory ovarian cancer, where response of 25%-35% were achieved as a single agent. Although it has primarily been used for salvage therapy, it is currently moving into trials of first-line therapy in combination with other active agents. There is little doubt that it will also be active in fresh postoperative patients.

Navelbine (Vinorelbine Tartrate) is another emerging chemotherapeutic agent that has demonstrated some activity in ovarian cancer in a salvage role. A 30% response rate was obtained in a small group of patients with both platinum resistant and platinum sensitive recurrences of epithelial ovarian cancer. A larger trial is needed before more definitive estimates of the activity of this drug can be made.

Combination chemotherapy

The relatively low rates of response seen with most agents other than alkylating agents have stimulated investigators to search for combination schedules. Smith et al. reported one of the largest initial series, which consisted of 97 patients with stages II through IV epithelial cancers of the ovary, all of whom had residual masses of at least 2 cm and/or ascites after initial laparotomy. Patients were randomized into two groups, those who received L-PAM and those who received a combination of cyclophosphamide, 5-fluorouracil, and dactinomycin (ActFUCy). Fifty patients received single agents, and 47 patients received combinations. A stratification for stage of disease was carefully carried out. Despite a larger number of clinically complete responses in the combination group (30% compared with 20%), the survival times for the two groups were essentially the same (L-PAM, 51.5% at 1 year and 17% at 2 years; ActFUCy 40.6% at 1 year and 17% at 2 years). The toxicity was much greater with the combination therapy. Young et al. reported on 80 patients with advanced (FIGO stages III and IV) untreated epithelial ovarian cancer who were randomized to receive melphalan (PAM) (0.2 mg/kg/day orally for 5 days every 4-6 weeks) or combination chemotherapy (HEXA-CAF: 5-fluorouracil [600 mg/m^2] and methotrexate [40 mg/m^2] intravenously on days 1 and 8 plus cyclophosphamide and hexamethylmelamine [150 mg orally daily for 14 days]). Thirty-seven of 39 patients receiving PAM and 40 of 41 patients receiving HEXA-CAF were receiving therapy longer than 6 months at the time of the report and were evaluable for response. The two groups were similar in stage, age, histologic type, initial surgery, and residual disease. Approximately 80% of each group had residual disease greater than 2 cm after surgery. For patients receiving PAM, the complete response rate was 16%, partial response rate 38%, and no response 46%. For patients receiving HEXA-CAF the complete response rate was 33%, partial response rate 43%, and no response rate 25%. The difference between the 33% complete response rate with HEXA-CAF and the 16% complete response rate with PAM is statistically significant ($p = .02$). The overall response rate was 76% with HEXA-CAF vs 54% with PAM. In summary HEXA-CAF showed a higher percentage of complete responses (33% vs 16%) and longer overall survival (29 months vs 17 months).

Other reports, such as one by De Palo et al., suggest a less optimistic response rate. De Palo studied the effect of combination chemotherapy with HEXA-CAF in 33 patients with advanced epithelial ovarian carcinoma who had not received prior chemotherapy. Of the 33 patients, 31 were evaluable, and a response rate of 42% that included 7 complete responders and 6 partial responders was noted. Seven patients had stable disease, and 11 patients had progressive disease. The authors also reported moderate to severe toxicity with the regimen.

Cisplatin, a heavy metal coordination compound with unique antitumor properties, is the first of its class to undergo extensive clinical testing. As are doxorubicin and hexamethylmelamine, it is a very active agent against epithelial cancer of the ovary. However, the duration of response is often short. In 1976, Vogl et al. introduced the combination of cisplatin and doxorubicin. In their report, 1 of the 5 patients with advanced ovarian carcinoma responded. Briscoe et al. reported 24 women treated with cisplatin, 60 mg/m^2, and doxorubicin, 60 mg/m^2, every 3-4 weeks. There were 10 responses (4 complete responses and 6 partial responses). A 69% response rate was reported by Ehrlich et al. Their combination consisted of doxorubicin, 50 mg/m^2; cisplatin, 50 mg/m^2, or 20 mg/m^2/day for 5 days; and cyclophosphamide, 750 mg/m^2. The combination was repeated every 3-4 weeks. The patients treated were women with previously untreated advanced (stage III or IV) epithelial adenocarcinomas of the ovary. All treatments with cisplatin were given to patients in the hospital with posttreatment intravenous hydration. Cisplatin was discontinued at a cumulative dose of 300 mg/m^2, and doxorubicin was discontinued at a cumulative dose of 450 mg/m^2. Thereafter cyclophosphamide was increased by 20% and given orally every 4 weeks. Of 39 patients entered into this study, 35 were evaluable. The overall response rate was 69%, the complete response rate was 37%, and the partial response rate was 32%. The interval to response was 4-12 weeks. Nausea, vomiting, and alopecia were seen in all patients but no significant neurotoxicity or ototoxicity was observed. No progressive nephrotoxicity was observed after discontinuation of cisplatin, and cardiotoxicity was seen in only 1 patient.

Ehrlich et al. also reported an interesting follow-up of patients treated with cisplatin, doxorubicin, and cyclophosphamide (PAC). In the follow-up report, 58 patients had been entered into the study, but 2 were excluded, leaving 56 who were evaluable. There were 44 of 56 (79%) objective responses, with 23 of 56 (41%) complete

remissions in this group of patients. Of the 56, 29 (52%) patients underwent a second-look laparotomy. Of these, 10 (34%) were negative. Five of the 17 (30%) patients in the good-risk category (residual tumor less than 3 cm), compared with 5 of 39 (12.8%) patients in the poor-risk category, had negative second-look operations. Grade and histology did not appear to strongly influence the induction of complete response documented by laparotomy. These investigators concluded that the combination was very effective against advanced epithelial ovarian carcinoma.

A study by the GOG comparing doxorubicin (Adriamycin) and cyclophosphamide (A-C) with A-C and cisplatin indicated improvement with the three-drug combination. A 26% complete response was obtained with A-C and a 51% complete response was achieved with CAP. Response duration was 9 months vs 15 months, and progression-free interval was 7 months vs 13 months. Median survival was 16 months vs 20 months for CAP.

Four trials were considered in a meta-analysis that specifically addressed the question of the role of doxorubicin in ovarian cancer. Considering only pathologic complete responses, the study shows a constant small benefit for CAP, higher for the GONO and DACOVA studies. By pulling together these data in a meta-analysis, it was possible to detect a statistically significant benefit of 6% in the percentage of pathologic complete responses achieved with CAP. Moreover, this meta-analysis demonstrated a significant survival advantage of 7% at 6 years with CAP. However, because in three trials the dose intensity was greater in CAP than in CT, to what extent the benefit of CAP is from greater dose intensity or from doxorubicin itself remains unsolved (Table 11-23).

A total of 422 patients took part in this latter GOG study. Progression-free interval was significantly longer in patients receiving the cisplatin-based regimen, but survival was not significantly different. Patients with measurable disease who had the three-drug combination

---

Table 11-23 Role of Anthracycline: Pathologic complete responses according to treatment in four different trials

	CP (%)	CAP (%)	Benefit (%)	
GICOG*, 1987	22	26	4	
GOG†, 1989	21	26	5	
DACOVA§, 1987	22	32	10	
GONO‡, 1986	19	28	9	
OVERALL	21	27	6	$P = 0.01$

From Colombo N et al: *Gynecol Oncol* 55:S108-S113, 1994.
*GICOG: Gruppo Interregionale Cooperativo in Oncologia Ginecologica.
†GOG: Gynecologic Oncology Group.
§DACOVA: Danish Ovarian Cancer Group.
‡GONO: Gruppo Oncologico Nord-Ovest.

achieved statistically significant superiority in response rate, progression-free interval, and survival. Thus it would appear from this study that the addition of cisplatin significantly improves the outcome for patients with bulky residual disease. Long-term follow-up is necessary for conclusions regarding "cures." It is important to realize that the number of clinical complete responses in the three-drug arm is virtually double that of the two-drug arm. Other drug combinations in patients who have advanced disease have been studied by other investigators (Table 11-24). Virtually all of the successful combinations are cisplatin based. Whether the three-drug regimen tested

---

Table 11-24   Results of multiagent chemotherapy in advanced ovarian cancer

	Regimen	Patients (number)	Complete response (%)	Total response (%)	Median survival (months)
Young (1978)	Hexacaf vs	41	33	75 } $p < .05$	29 } $p < .02$
	Melphalan	39	6	54	17
Carmo-Pereira (1981)	Hexacaf vs	28	14	36 } $p < .05$	10
	Cytoxan	29	24	62	11
Barker, Wiltshaw (1981)	CbP vs	46	31	56	NG
	CAP	39	34	54	NG
DePalo (1981)	Hexacaf	31	22	42	16
Bell (1982)	Chlorambucil vs	19	NG	23 } $p = .04$	18
	CP	17	NG	69	16
ECOG (1982)	M vs	119	20	43 } $p = .002$	17 } $p = ns$
	CHAD	127	41	64	18
Vogl (1983)	CHAD	26	42	92	NG
Edwards (1983)	MP vs	82	28	38	30 } $p = ns$
	HAC	71	33	31	26
GOG (1983)	M vs	96	20 }	38	12
	MH vs	154	28 } $p = 0.04$	52	14
	AC	119	32 }	49	14
Neijt (1984)	HexaCaf vs	94	19	50 } $p = .0001$	20 } $p < .002$
	Chap-5	92	40	79	31
Williams (1985)	Cb vs	43	15	26 } $p = .0004$	11 } $p = ns$
	PAC	42	26	68	13
Neijt (1985)	CHAP-5 vs	94	34	78	26
	CP	97	37	76	26
Edmonson (1985)	CP vs	89	NG	NG	25
	HCAP	92	NG	NG	25
GOG (1986)	CA vs	215	26 } $p < .001$	48	16 } $p = ns$
	CAP	225	51	76	19
COSA (1986)	CB → P vs	186	18	64 } $p = ns$	13
	CbP	183	17	53	14
GICOG (1987)	P vs	174	22	51	19 }
	CP vs	182	25	62 } $p < .007$	21 } $p = ns$
	CAP	175	30	71	24 }
Alberts/SWOG (1989)	Cis/C vs	110	27		20.0 } $p = ns$
	Carbo/C	115	34		16.8
Hakes (1992)	CAP-5 vs	41	34 } $P = ns$		
	CAP-10	37	35		
McGuire/GOG 111 (1993)	Cis/CTX vs	117	33 } $P = 0.02$	69	13.6
	Cis/Taxol	102	54	74	18.1
Bertelsen/DACOVA (1993)	CAP-6 vs	136	23 } $P = 0.45$	64	23
	CAP-12	66	25	56	27
Alberts/SWOG (1995)	CIS (IV)/CTX vs	279	—	—	41 } $P = 0.02$
	CIS (IP)/CTX	267	—	—	49

Modified from Vogl SE, Kaplan B, Pagano M: *Proc Am Assoc Clinic Onc* 1:119, 1982; Neijt JP, ten Bokkel Huinink WW, van der Berg ME: *Proc Am Soc Clin* 4:114, 442, 1985 (abstract); Carmo-Pereira J, Oliveira Costa F, Henriquez E: *Proc Am Soc Clin Oncl* 1:107, 414, 1982; Edmonson JH et al: *Cancer Treat Rep* 69:1243, 1985; Alberts D et al: *Carboplatin—current perspectives and future directions*, Philadelphia, 1990, Saunders, pp 163-164.
C, Cyclophosphamide; *H,* hexamethylmelamine; *A,* doxorubicin; *D or P,* cisplatin; *F,* 5-fluorouracil; *Cb,* chlorambucil; *NG,* not given; *NS,* not significant.

by the GOG represents the optimal combination of commonly available drugs for patients with bulky advanced disease is unknown, but data supporting the superiority of this combination over non-cisplatin regimens are solid. Patients with minimal residual disease seem to respond best to cisplatin combination chemotherapy.

A SWOG study of stages III (suboptimal) and IV ovarian epithelial carcinoma utilizing cyclophosphamide plus cisplatin vs cyclophosphamide plus carboplatin has been reported by Alberts et al. This study of 342 patients utilized carboplatin at 300 mg/m^2 and cisplatin at 100 mg/m^2 while cyclophosphamide was given at a dose of 600 mg/m^2 every 4 weeks for six courses. The median survival durations were 17.4 and 20.0 months, and estimated 3-year patient survivals were 21% for cisplatin-cyclophosphamide and 20% for carboplatin-cyclophosphamide. Clinical response rates in patients with measurable disease were 31/60 and 39/64 on the cisplatin-cyclophosphamide and carboplatin-cyclophosphamide arms, respectively. The authors claim that the toxicity with the carboplatin arm was much reduced, especially in the areas of nausea, renal toxicity, hearing loss, and neuromuscular toxicities.

Cisplatin analogs such as carboplatin and iproplatin appear to have fewer marked side effects at doses equivalent to 100 mg/m^2 of cisplatin. Silverstone reported on 120 patients with epithelial ovarian cancer who were randomly assigned to receive carboplatin or iproplatin every 4 weeks as initial therapy. The response rates were 63% for carboplatin and 39% for iproplatin. The median survival was 114 weeks for carboplatin patients and 68 weeks for iproplatin patients. Few responses to cyclophosphamide occurred following either drug, implying resistance to the alkylating agent. Gill and others attempted to use carboplatin and cisplatin together, since they do not have overlapping toxicities. Therapeutic doses of each drug were used with no nephrotoxicity and only mild neurotoxicity noted in the phase II study. Additional work with this combination is under way.

A very promising new drug is Taxol, which has proven to be very active when used even as a single agent. Taxol is thought to exert its antineoplastic effect by enhancing polymerization of tubulin monomers into stable microtubules by a direct, high-affinity binding to the polymerized tubulin. The resulting unusual stability prevents dissembling, which is necessary for normal cellular function. A phase II trial at Johns Hopkins noted 16 respondents among 40 patients with measurable disease who had prior chemotherapy. Based on the activity demonstrated for Taxol in advanced and recurrent ovarian cancer, combinations were felt to be a rational next step in developing this drug. Although neurotoxicity was originally thought to be a potentially serious effect of the combinations, mild to modest neurotoxicity occurred. Instead, neutropenia was the principal toxicity. With

Table 11-25 GOG Protocol 111: a comparison of cisplatin plus either cyclophosphamide or Taxol

Clinical response and survival		
Study end point N = 218	Taxol plus cisplatin	Cyclophosphamide plus cisplatin
Overall response	77%*	64%
Pathologic response	26%	19%
Median progression-free interval (mo)	18.0†	12.9
Median survival (mo)	37.5‡	24.4

McGuire WP et al: *Proc Am Soc Clin Oncol* 14:275, Abstract 771, 1995.
McGuire WP et al: *NEJM* 334:1, 1996.
*P = .025
†P = .0002
‡P = .0001

starting doses of Taxol ranging from 170 mg/m^2 to 250 mg/m^2 over 24 hours every three weeks, myelosuppression manifested primarily as neutropenia was the dose limiting toxicity in almost 75% of the patients who experienced neutrophil counts of less than 1000 per deciliter. Significant cardiac problems were rare. The only other major problem was neuropathy seen primarily in patients receiving doses higher than 200 mg/m^2.

The GOG has randomized patients with large volume disease to six cycles of cisplatin 75 mg/m^2 plus cyclophosphamide 750 mg/m^2 every 3 weeks or Taxol 135 mg/m^2 over 24 hours followed by cisplatin 75 mg/m^2 every three weeks. In the Taxol arm, administration of Taxol prior to the cisplatin was important to optimize response and minimize toxicity. A total of 388 patients were entered on to the study. In terms of therapeutic efficacy (Table 11-25), the Taxol arm produced a significantly greater overall response rate (77% vs 64%) and also clinical complete response rate (54% vs 33%) while the frequency of pathological complete response was similar between the two arms (25% in the Taxol arm vs 20%). The % of patients achieving a state of no gross residual disease on the Taxol arm was significantly higher (41%) than seen with the control arm (25%). Progression free survival was significantly greater on the Taxol arm. The risk of progression was 32% lower among those treated with the Taxol regimen as compared to the cyclophosphamide regimen. The risk of death was 39% lower among those treated with the Taxol regimen. How the rate of complete pathological response will affect long term survival is uncertain at this time. However, a combination of Taxol and Cisplatin has emerged as the "gold standard" for combination first-line chemotherapy for the treatment of epithelial ovarian carcinoma. Studies are now evaluating the role of Taxol for large and small volume disease. Patients are also being randomized between a 24-hour vs a 3-hour infusion of the drug.

Toxicity is much reduced with the 3-hour infusion, and the effectiveness of this infusion rate has been proven. Bristol-Myers Squib, New York, reported a study of 300 patients and compared the response rates, time to progression, and toxicity of four different regimens of Taxol for refractory ovarian cancer. The four different regimens of Taxol for refractory ovarian cancer were: 175 mg/m^2 at 24 hours, 175 mg/m^2 at 3 hours, 135 mg/m^2 at 24 hours, and 135 mg/m^2 at 3 hours. There were about 75 patients in each arm of the study, and the 3-hour infusions were given on an outpatient basis. The study results indicated that, when administered with premedication, the 3-hour infusion regimen was safer than the commonly utilized 24-hour infusion in terms of significant hypersensitivity reactions. Three-hour infusions also significantly reduced the incidence of grade IV neutropenia in patients studied. The 175 mg/m^2 dosage had a higher response rate than the 135 mg/m^2 dosage, but the higher dosage resulted in more neutropenia and peripheral neuropathy; these symptoms were reversible when the treatment was discontinued. Patients receiving 175 mg/m^2 over 3 hours showed an improved response rate over the commonly recommended 135 mg/m^2 over 24 hours. There was a highly significant improvement in the time to progression in the patients receiving 175 mg/m^2 compared to those receiving 135 mg/m^2.

In summary, the results of GOG protocol 111, a comparison of cisplatin plus cyclophosphamide or Taxol (Table 11-25) strongly suggest that a combination of Taxol 135 mg/m^2 over 24 hours followed by cisplatin 75 mg/m^2 should be considered the treatment of choice for advanced ovarian carcinoma. The optimal duration of therapy for Taxol administration and the possibility of substituting cisplatin with carboplatin are currently under study. A recently approved new agent, Topotecan, has shown some activity in ovarian cancer. In 1996, Kudelka et al. reported on 28 patients with ovarian cancer. The response rate was 14% in previously treated patients with recurrent or persistent epithelial ovarian cancer. The major toxicity was myelosuppression.

Care must always be taken in interpreting response rates as a definite indicator of trends in survival rates. Too often a chemotherapeutic regimen will produce excellent response rates but not affect the overall survival rate. Therefore, the clinician must await longer studies of cisplatin-based combination chemotherapy to accurately understand its impact on patient survival.

Omura et al. reported a very sobering analysis of two large GOG studies of multi staging chemotherapy in epithelial ovarian cancer. In this analysis of 726 women with stage III or IV disease, excellent follow-up had been obtained. The authors concluded that the impact of chemotherapy to date had been rather modest. Less than 10% of their patients were progression free at 5 years, and late failures continued to occur, even beyond 7 years. Sutton reported a 7% disease-free survival at 10 years.

With respect to specific prognostic factors, Omura et al. found that clear cell and mucinous tumors had significantly worse prognoses than other cell types. They concluded that the reports in the literature of relatively good survival among those with mucinous tumors were the result of reports being limited to women with less advanced disease. If mucinous and clear cell were excluded, cell type and grade were not significant predictors of survival. The analysis also indicated that long-term follow-up resulted in adjustment for several prognostic factors. There appears to be no statistically significant evidence that the effect of cisplatin on survival is different between measurable and nonmeasurable suboptimal disease. Performance status, age, ascites, stage, and residual tumor volume were positive prognostic factors for predicting survival. A negative second-look laparotomy was favorable, but the survival patients eligible for second-look surgery who refused it was similar to that of those who had second-look laparotomies. Omura et al. concluded that further study designs should consider the potential heterogeneity of the study sample with respect to those prognostic factors. Cisplatin treatment is significantly favorable for overall survival.

Marsoni et al. analyzed 852 stage III and IV cases from our consecutive trials, including optimal and suboptimal stage III cases. Residual tumor size, age, stage, and cell type (serous vs other) were independent determinants of survival. In the subset of 721 patients for whom information about performance status was available, tumor size, cell type, and performance were significant but stage and age were no longer significant. Cisplatin-based therapy was favorable for overall survival but not in the subgroup with residual tumors less than 2 cm in diameter.

Swenerton et al. reviewed 556 cases of all stages. Tumor grade, presence of residual disease, and performance status were significant prognostic factors. However, grade was significant only for stage I and II cases; residual disease was the only significant independent prognostic factor in stage III. It showed there is considerable variation from study to study regarding the most significant prognostic factors.

There have been scattered reports of responses to progestin therapy in the treatment of ovarian carcinoma. Unfortunately, studies cited in the literature have been done with small numbers of patients and there has been inadequate evaluation of these patients. There have been many anecdotal reports of benefits from combining alkylating agents with progestin therapy for epithelial carcinoma of the ovary. No prospective randomized trial has been performed to date. However, the use of progestins often creates an anabolic-like effect (e.g., increased appetite) in the patient and undoubtedly contributes to a subjective response. Whether they potentiate or improve the response to chemotherapeutic agents has yet to be proven.

This section on nonalkylating-agent chemotherapy is particularly long and complex. Unfortunately, the superiority of any particular combination of chemotherapeutic agents as reflected by statistically significant improvement in long-term survivors remains unproved. Although cisplatin appears to be the most active agent in epithelial cancer of the ovary, there is still lack of clear evidence that combining it with other agents improves outcome. A study by Mangioni from the Italian Cooperative Group, in which patients who had advanced epithelial cancer of the ovary were randomized among treatments of cisplatin, cisplatin and doxorubicin, and cisplatin, doxorubicin, and cyclophosphamide, showed no superiority of the two- and three-drug regimen over cisplatin alone. The availability of Taxol creates a new set of questions. The current "gold standard" appears to be a combination of Taxol and a platinum analog. Yet, clear evidence that the combination results in more long-term survivors than just platinum alone does not currently exist. Every clinician who uses chemotherapy to treat patients who have epithelial cancers of the ovary must keep informed of the latest literature that could shed additional light on this very complex set of data.

High-dose chemotherapy with autologous bone marrow support

Dose intensity refers to the amount of chemotherapy to which a cancer is exposed per unit of time; this is generally assumed to be reflected by the dose of drug in mg/m^2 body surface area per unit of time. The theory is well grounded in preclinical work that shows that as the concentration of drug in culture medium increases, the fraction of surviving cancer cells decreases logarithmically. To determine if dose intensity is important clinically, randomized trials are needed. The GOG did design such trial in patients with large volume, advanced disease. A total of 458 patients were entered onto the study and were randomized to low dose cisplatin 50 mg/m^2 plus cyclophosphamide 500 mg/m^2 every 3 weeks for 8 cycles or high dose cisplatin 100 mg/m^2 plus cyclophosphamide 1,000 mg/m^2 every 3 weeks for 4 cycles. Each regimen delivered the same total dose of chemotherapy, but the high dose schedule was delivered in half the time. On the low dose arm, the overall response rate of the 130 measurable disease patients was 65% vs 59% for the high dose arm; clinical complete response rates were 26% and 27% respectively. These differences were not significant. There was no difference in progression free survival in the measurable or the nonmeasurable subsets of patients; similarly, no difference in overall survival in either patient subset was noted. The results of this study did not support the concept that increased dose intensity will produce greater therapeutic effect. Colombo reported a randomized trial in patients with advanced disease who were given cisplatin 50 mg/m^2 per week for 9 weeks or cisplatin 75 mg/m^2 every 3 weeks for 6 cycles. The

weekly arm delivered the same total dose of cisplatin in half the time but each arm received the total dose of drug. Within the small volume and large volume disease patient subsets, no significant differences were observed with regard to either response rates or pathologic complete response rates. No overall differences were noted in either of these parameters, nor in regards to progression free or overall survival. While neither of these randomized trials of pure dose intensity showed an advantage for a higher dose intensity across a clinically relevant range of doses, other lines of evidence have been cited to support the use of higher dose schedules. Conducted by the National Cancer Institute (NCI) of the United States, trials of even higher dose intensities of cisplatin in conjunction with hypertonic saline to protect the kidneys have been stated to yield higher response rates than more standard doses. A closer examination of this data reported by Rothenberg shows confusing results. In patients with large volume disease, the NCI results can be compared to GOG results with PAC, as reported by Omura, regimens with a 3.3 fold difference in dose intensity of cisplatin. The pathologic complete response rates for the two regimens were 12% and 11% respectively. In patients with small volume disease, the NCI results can be compared to GOG results with a two-drug combination of cisplatin plus cyclophosphamide, as reported by Omura in 1989. The pathologic complete response rates in this second study for the two regimens are 38% and 30% respectively, not significantly different. There appears to be no evidence from these data to support the importance of dose intensity of cisplatin over a 3.3-fold range of doses.

In the last decade, high dose chemotherapy with autologous bone marrow transplant (ABMT) has been reported for several solid tumors, and there has been a tendency for improved response rates but a relatively short period of disease free survival in most of the reports reviewed. There have been no reports of 5-year survival studies in patients with malignant ovarian tumors treated with high dose chemotherapy followed by ABMT. Murakami reported on 42 patients treated between 1984 and 1989. Twenty eight of the patients were stage III or IV and 14 of the patients were stage I and II. All patients underwent primary cytoreductive surgery but had no prior chemotherapy before entering this study. All 42 patients received two sequential courses of chemotherapy with ABMT after primary surgery. The high dose chemotherapy consisted of cyclophosphamide 1,600-2,400 mg/m^2, doxorubicin 80-100 mg/m^2, and cisplatin 100-150 mg/m^2. All of these drugs were administered intravenously on two consecutive days. Bone marrow was aspirated under general anesthesia from the bilateral posterior iliac crests on the fourth day after the start of the high dose chemotherapy, half of the cryopreserved bone marrow was thawed and immediately infused intravenously into the patients. The overall 5-year survival rates in patients with stage I, II, III, and IV disease were 100%,

66.7%, 53.9%, and 0% respectively. In patients treated in an adjuvant setting after a curative primary operation, the 5-year survival rate was good (78%) compared with patients in the therapeutic setting, i.e., those who had macroscopic residual disease after cytoreductive surgery (26%). These results seem to show that in even advanced cases, the most important factor for long term survival after high dose chemotherapy was the completeness of the primary cytoreductive surgery.

The study by Murakami is unusual in that patients received no prior chemotherapy. Most of the reports in the literature with high dose chemotherapy with ABMT have been phase II trial in patients who have failed first line chemotherapy. Stiff and colleagues provided us with another phase II trial of high dose chemotherapy with ABMT support in patients with recurrent epithelial ovarian carcinoma. Twenty two of the 30 had large volume disease defined as residual >1 cm in diameter upon entry into the study. Response rates were 89% overall with 59% clinical complete responders. The overall median survival of 29 months is very impressive even in a highly selected group of patients, most of whom reportedly had large volume disease. Larger studies are needed before this becomes standard therapy. The toxicity of high dose chemotherapy is a serious concern, as is the additional expense.

Immunochemotherapy

In the last three decades, there has been considerable interest in combining chemotherapy with immunotherapy for better results in patients with epithelial cancer of the ovary.

Creasman et al. reported a series of patients treated with melphalan (Alkeran) plus C-Parvum immuno-therapy. The immunomodulating agent chosen for this study was a gram-positive bacterium, *Corynebacterium parvum*. This agent has been shown to increase nonspecific tumor resistance, to potentiate specific tumor rejections, to effect bone marrow proliferation, and to have additive antitumor effects when combined with alkylating agents. The pilot study done by Creasman et al. on 48 previously untreated stage III epithelial ovarian cancer patients showed a definite suggestion of improved response with the combination of chemotherapy and immunotherapy. The response rate in the group given melphalan alone was 55%, whereas the response rate in the combination group was 65%. Further analysis of the material revealed that 44% of the patients in the melphalan group had minimal residua at the start of therapy, whereas only 23% of the patients in the combination group had this favorable clinical finding. Many concluded that this was a promising combination, and a prospective randomized study comparing similar treatment groups was conducted by the GOG (Table 11-26). All patients had minimal residual advanced disease and participated in a randomized study comparing

Table 11-26 Gynecologic Oncology Group protocol 25

Procedure: Exploratory laparotomy, plus total abdominal hysterectomy and bilateral salpingo-oophorectomy, plus omentectomy with debulking of tumor

Regimen A	**Regimen B**
Melphalan alone, 7 mg/m^2/day PO for 5 days; repeat every 4 weeks	Melphalan alone, 7 mg/m^2/day PO for 5 days; repeat every 4 weeks *plus* C. parvum, 4 mg/m^2/day IV on day 7 following chemotherapy

From Creasman WT et al: *Cancer Treat Rep* 63:319, 1979.

the effectiveness of melphalan, with or without *Corynebacterium parvum*. There were no significant differences between effects of the two regimens. The study did show, however, that the progression-free interval for patients with optimal disease was 16 months, compared with only 7 months in an earlier study of patients with bulky, advanced disease, and that survival was likewise strikingly better in patients with minimal residual disease (31 to 33 months vs 12 months).

Alberts et al. used a combination of doxorubicin and cyclophosphamide, with or without Pasteur Institute BCG, in 121 patients with stage III and IV disease or recurrent ovarian carcinoma who had not previously received chemotherapy. The effects of treatment were evaluable in 121 patients who had received two or more courses. The most striking difference in the two arms of the study was seen in the median duration of survival in patients receiving doxorubicin and cyclophosphamide plus BCG (22.3 months) vs that of those receiving doxorubicin and cyclophosphamide alone (13.7 months) (p <0.03). These investigators concluded that nonspecific immunostimulation therapy combined with chemotherapy could improve the results in advanced epithelial carcinoma of the ovary. The GOG studied doxorubicin, cyclophosphamide, and cisplatin, with or without BCG, to follow up on the study by Alberts et al. There were no significant differences between the two regimens, and the GOG study (Table 11-27) failed to confirm the previous report by Alberts et al.

The potential role of biologic agents in the treatment of ovarian cancer was reviewed by Bast. Ovarian cancer is a suitable model for biologic therapies for other reasons. The peritoneal cavity is capable of mounting an inflammatory response to many stimuli, and this response has been shown to induce an antitumor effect. The identification, cloning, and mass production of the mediators of such responses are in progress. Preliminary data of intraperitoneal administration of Interleukin II have

Table 11-27   Chemoimmunotherapy—epithelial ovarian carcinoma, stages III and IV: response distribution

Response category	CAP(2)		CAP + BCG*		Total
	Number	%	Number	%	
Complete response	37	45.7	40	51.3	77
Partial response	22	27.2	16	20.5	38
Stable disease	17	21.0	19	24.4	36
Increasing disease	5	6.2	3	3.8	8
TOTAL	81	(100.1)	78	(100.0)	159

*CAP, Cyclophosphamide + doxorubicin + cisplatin; BCG, bacillus Calmetta-Guérin.

demonstrated that lymphokines cause the egress into the peritoneal cavity of a large number of lymphocytes, neutrophils, and macrophages, as well as the cytokines those cells produce. The peritoneal cavity is also an attractive site to consider the administration of antibodies as well as adoptive cellular therapies. It has been demonstrated that the intraperitoneal administration of large-molecular-weight molecules may actually lead to a deeper penetration into tumor nodules than can be achieved with small-molecular-weight chemotherapeutic agents such as doxorubicin and cisplatin. The depth of penetration into a tumor mass is a function of the rate of diffusion of the drug through the tissue and its capillary permeability. Although both factors are proportional to molecular weight, the capillary permeability is more vulnerable relative to molecular weight than is tissue diffusion. Consequently, larger-molecular-weight compounds that are allowed to have a long intraperitoneal dwell time may lead to an increased depth of tissue penetration because there may be less clearance through the capillary microcirculation. It is also possible that adoptive cellular therapy may be more effective when administered intraperitoneally to localized tumors because monocytes or lymphocytes when administered in the peritoneal cavity may remain localized for an extended period. These experimental observations indicate that ovarian cancer is a suitable prototype tumor in which to evaluate novel immunotherapeutic and chemo immunotherapeutic approaches.

It has been reported by Berek that recombinant Interferon alfa has clinical activity in patients with small-volume residual disease. This study included only patients who had smaller than 5 mm tumor masses. Four of 11 patients evaluated by restaging laparotomy were found to be disease-free after treatment with Interferon alpha intraperitoneally. However, three of these patients initially had only positive cytologic findings. Nonetheless, the study demonstrates that intraperitoneal administration of a biologic agent has antitumor activity in ovarian cancer. Attempts to use biologic response modifiers (BRM) in phase III trials with chemotherapy have been stalled in recent years until such time as more

effective BRMs are at hand. Numerous phase II trials, utilizing substances such as tumor necrosis factor, IL-2, and the like, are under way, along with other studies using combinations of cytokines. Combining BRMs with standard chemotherapy has proved to be more difficult than initially conceived, because of overlapping toxicities. In view of this, it seems prudent to await proven efficacy before attempting to launch the phase III trials utilizing biologic response modifiers.

Investigators at University of California, Irvine (UCI) have investigated the potential of ovarian cancer vaccines. Genetically engineered autologous cells are rendered capable of secreting large amounts of cytokines, theoretically enhancing the ability of surface antigens to evoke an immune response. Vaccines such as this are a very active area of research into the therapeutic trials of immunochemotherapy. To date, the results of limited clinical trials have been disappointing in humans. However, the need for new modalities must be a stimulus for current and future investigations.

Extraovarian Peritoneal Serous Papillary Carcinoma

Extraovarian peritoneal serous papillary carcinoma is now a recognized clinical-pathological entity in which peritoneal carcinomatosis of ovarian serous type is found in the abdomen and/or pelvis. Similar tumor deposits may be found on the surface of the ovary, but histologic evidence of primary or in-situ ovarian carcinoma is either absent or insignificant. The tumor deposits in all sites are rarely noninvasive (borderline) but are usually frankly invasive. This entity was first reported as "Mesothelioma resembling papillary ovarian adenocarcinoma" by Swerdlow in 1959. Experience with extraovarian serous neoplasia of this type has been too scarce to compare clinical outcome with homologous ovarian tumors of equivalent stage and grade. Some have contested the concept of an extraovarian ideology. The traditional view that these are advanced serous papillary carcinoma from minimally involved ovaries is still maintained by many. The traditional view is supported by the knowledge that some small undifferentiated carcinomas, of both the ovary and many other sites, give rise to bulky metastases. Fromm reported on a series of 74 patients identified as having papillary serous carcinoma of the peritoneum. The average age at diagnosis was 57 years and the majority of the patients were white. Clinical presentation was similar to that of ovarian carcinoma. Clinical response to chemotherapy was seen in 64% of the patients, with 41% having partial responses and 23% having complete responses. Thirty-three patients came to a second assessment surgery, and 27% were negative. Median survival for the total group was 24 months. Dalrymple reported on 31 cases of extraovarian peritoneal serous papillary carcinoma. Their medial survival was 11.3 months for patients with this entity, compared to 13.5 months for patients with the equivalent primary ovarian neoplasms.

Our experience has been that these patients generally respond to therapy in a manner similar to that of patients with serous papillary carcinoma of the ovary. More large series comparing outcome stage for stage are needed to bring out subtle differences. A summary of the key authors suggests that this entity of extraovarian peritoneal serous papillary carcinoma is characterized by (1) an absence of symptoms pointing to ovarian involvement; (2) ovaries normal in size or slightly enlarged; (3) bilateral ovarian involvement; and (4) widespread peritoneal tumor.

Small Cell Carcinoma of the Ovary

Small cell carcinoma of the ovary has been identified as a specific histopathologic entity. This rare and highly aggressive malignancy primarily affects children and young women between the ages of 10 and 40 years. Few, if any, long-term survivors have been reported. The first 11 cases were documented by Dickerson et al. in 1982. Various chemotherapeutic agents have been suggested with minimal success. Senekjian reported on a combination of vinblastine, cisplatin, cyclophosphamide, bleomycin, doxorubicin, and etoposide for this entity. One of their five patients was alive and disease-free at 29 months. Many patients with this lesion, but not all, have an associated hypercalcemia. The authors have had some preliminary success with this same combination. Obviously, further study of this devastating group of lesions is necessary.

FOLLOW-UP TECHNIQUES AND TREATMENT OF RECURRENCES

As stated earlier, ovarian cancer is fast growing and insidious in that it is late to cause symptoms, and thus follow-up examinations are imperative to detect early recurrence. Even then, implants many centimeters in diameter can be hidden in the many crevices of the abdominal cavity and escape physical detection. There is a reasonable limit to the use of such sophisticated techniques as computer tomography in the surveillance of

a patient who has had ovarian cancer. Some have suggested that the proper assessment of the extent of disease is periodic monitoring of serum CA-125 levels and liberal use of surgical procedures (laparoscopy and laparotomy) to assay the contents of the abdominal and pelvic cavities.

In truth, at present the optimal follow-up strategy for the asymptomatic patient who has advanced ovarian cancer after initial treatment remains undecided. Important considerations are divided between a more passive or active approach to follow-up. There is an absence of good data on the benefit of second-line (salvage) therapy and these techniques are expensive, at times morbid, and certainly an inconvenience to the patient. Currently, there is no evidence that intensive investigative monitoring efforts in the symptomatic patient exerts a significant positive impact on the overall survival, symptom free survival, or quality of life. However, each patient should be individualized as to her needs in constructing such a plan of follow-up. Trials of salvage therapy are underway throughout the country, and intuitively, it appears that early recognition of recurrent disease followed by effective salvage therapy will result in improved outcomes. Whether this is real or just intuitive remains to be proven. In an era of cost containment, these considerations are even more relevant. Our practice has been to monitor these patients following negative reassessment laparotomy with physical examination, serum CA-125, and liberal use of imaging on a quarterly basis for 2 years. At the 2-year anniversary, the frequency of follow-up visits is decreased to every six months. For patients who do not undergo reassessment laparotomy, it has been our practice to follow a similar monitoring regime increasing the frequency of visits to every 2 months in the first 2 years. Many patients request even more frequent examinations, in that they are greatly relieved by negative results. These practices are not based on good science and, as stated above, the optimal strategy is unknown.

Use of CA-125 Levels

CA-125 is an antigenic determinant defined by Bast by a murine Igl monoclonal antibody that was raised against an epithelial ovarian carcinoma cell line. Multiple CA-125 determinants are associated with a mucin-like glycoprotein of more than 200,000 daltons. Traces of the antigen are expressed in adult tissues derived from coelomic epithelium, including mesothelial cells lining the pleura, pericardium, and peritoneum, as well as the epithelial component of the fallopian tube, endometrium, and endocervix. CA-125 is not found in fetal or adult ovaries. Determinants are, however, expressed in more than 80% of nonmucinous epithelial ovarian cancers.

The radioimmune assay has been developed by Bast to detect CA-125 in serum and body fluids. The day-to-day coefficient of variability for the assay is approximately 15%. Consequently, a doubling or halving of antigen levels has been considered significant. If a cutoff of 35 units per milliliter is chosen for the upper limit of normal, elevated CA-125 levels should be found in 1% of apparently normal blood bank donors, 6% of patients who have benign disease, 28% of individuals who have nongynecologic malignancies, and 82% of patients who have surgically demonstrable epithelial ovarian cancer. Niloff reported elevated CA-125 detection in sera from patients who have advanced fallopian tube, endometrial, and endocervical adenocarcinomas. In epithelial ovarian carcinoma, rising or falling levels of CA-125 have correlated with disease progression or regression in more than 90% of patients. In a report by Niloff, when CA-125 levels are returned to below 35 units per milliliter, findings of second-look surveillance procedures were in fact negative in 14 of 36 cases but in no instances was a nodule larger than 1 cm found. Persistently elevated CA-125 levels have been associated consistently with persistence of disease. Recurrence of disease has been heralded by elevations of CA-125 in 85% of patients whose tumors shed the antigen. Elevated CA-125 preceded disease recurrence by 1 to 14 months with a mean of 5 months in one study reported by Knapp. Elevation of CA-125 in hepatocellular disease and in chronic peritonitis is important to note but should not compromise the utility of CA-125 as a marker for monitoring ovarian cancer.

Virtually all patients with elevated serum CA-125 levels prior to second-look surgery have residual ovarian cancer at laparotomy or develop disease within the next 4 to 6 months. Normal serum CA-125 levels prior to second-look surgery are of limited value. Over 50% of the patients with such findings (normal CA-125 and negative clinical exam) have persistent disease. Residual disease, less than 2 cm in diameter, rarely elevates serum CA-125 levels. Although elevated serum CA-125 levels before second-look surgery allow the oncologist to counsel the patient with some assurance, the degree of elevation by itself does not precisely predict the amount of residual disease or the outcome. Normal levels may also accompany disease, with tumors of 2 cm or greater, in one third or more of cases. A rapid regression of the serum CA-125 level to normal limits shortly after commencement of chemotherapy is associated with a higher frequency of negative second-assessment surgery. Levin reported that almost all patients who subsequently come to a negative second-look laparotomy have serum CA-125 levels within normal ranges within 3 months of primary cytoreductive surgery. Buller has shown that a favorable outcome is definitely associated with a steep regression curve of serum CA-125 levels following cytoreductive surgery and commencement of chemotherapy. This author has demonstrated that patients in whom the CA-125 level reverts sharply to within the normal range by the third course of chemotherapy following surgery have a survival that is markedly and significantly improved over the

patients who have an elevation of CA-125 levels prior to their fourth course of chemotherapy. Buller described the regression curve of the serum CA-125 level as "s." Indeed, he has suggested that patients with a delayed "s" (regression of the elevated value) possibly should be considered for alternative therapy rather than persisting with the same chemotherapeutic regimens. Hogberg demonstrated that 23 patients, with a serum CA-125 half-life shorter than 16 days during induction chemotherapy, had an estimated survival of 68% at 59 months after second-look operation. This compared with survival of 18% in 49 patients with a serum CA-125 half-life of more than 16 days.

All patients who have successfully completed therapy for ovarian cancer require follow-up examinations at least every 3 months. Serum CA-125 determination should be made at each visit. Patients whose clinical exam and tumor markers remain normal are at a lower risk for recurrence. Those whose serum CA-125 values rise markedly have a 70% or higher chance of developing clinical recurrence. Two questions must be addressed: (1) What constitutes a significant increase in serum CA-125, and (2) Should there be a treatment recommendation based on the new serum CA-125 elevation alone or is histologic proof of recurrent disease required? Serum CA-125 levels should be measured every month—more frequently when there is an elevation—to confirm a newly elevated value and exclude confounding medical conditions, such as renal insufficiency, which may falsely elevate serum CA-125. At present, a 50% rise in the CA-125 level above normal ranges on two separate occasions is considered by the authors as a likely indication of recurrence, especially if the value exceeds 100 units. Histological confirmation is necessary before any salvage chemotherapy is offered. Short of performing a full surgical exploration, one could consider an open diagnostic laparoscopy, although small retroperitoneal disease may be missed with this technique. Many times a paracentesis will yield cytologically positive fluid, confirming the suspected diagnosis of recurrence. Patients whose serum CA-125 levels rise and then plateau and who remain clinically disease-free should be followed (particularly if levels are only minimally elevated, e.g., <100 units) until recurrence is confirmed clinically or a more definitive pattern in serum CA-125 levels is apparent.

Second-look Operation (Reassessment Surgery)

The so-called second-look operation was first defined by Owen Wangensteen in the late 1940s with reference to exploratory laparotomy procedures in colon cancer patients from whom he had previously removed all gross tumor but in whom there was a high risk of recurrence. At varying intervals, usually 6 months initially, he would explore these patients in the hope of detecting early recurrence at a time when secondary resection still offered

Table 11-28   Ovarian cancer: initial stage relative to negative second-look findings

Stage	% with no evidence of disease
I	60-79
II	45-68
III	16-48
IV	33-45

From collected series: Smirz, Cain, Copeland, Gershenson, and Roberts.

STEPS TAKEN IN REASSESSMENT LAPAROTOMY

1. Midline incision
2. Cytologic washings from several areas of the abdomen and pelvis
3. Inspection of the omentum (take biopsies liberally)
4. Visualization of all peritoneal surfaces, including the undersurface of the diaphragm, serosa, and mesentery of the bowel (take biopsies of suspicious areas)
5. Submission of all excised adhesions for histologic review
6. Careful inspection of all pelvic organs and pelvic peritoneum (take biopsies liberally)
7. Retroperitoneal inspection of pelvic and periaortic nodes (take selected biopsies)

---

a chance of cure. Since then, the term *second-look* has been used to describe many procedures. With reference to ovarian cancer, it appears that a second-look (or reassessment) procedure may have three main indications: (1) to restage a patient who probably has localized disease but who has not had an optimal staging procedure as defined previously (see box on p. 300); (2) to evaluate the effect of chemotherapy in patients receiving both standard and investigational regimens; in this regard, some centers have instituted serial laparoscopic examinations to assess the extent of regression or progression of bulk disease several months after beginning chemotherapy, with the option to offer therapy if a poor response is noted (less frequently necessary now when the malignancy expresses CA-125); and (3) to evaluate patients who are clinically free of disease after receiving what is considered a sufficient course of chemotherapy and are then eligible for assessment as to possible "cure" and discontinuation of therapy (Table 11-28). This last indication has been the most widely used and has resulted in small numbers of patients, even with advanced disease, who are free of detectable malignant cells at the second procedure. The most difficult second-look procedure is that in which no evidence of disease apparently exists, because very thorough surgery with multiple biopsies must be performed to establish lack of disease. In essence, an optimal staging procedure must be repeated.

Second-look procedures are often begun with a laparoscopic examination to rule out widespread disease. If this lesser procedure reveals diffuse miliary studding (that was not clinically detectable), a laparotomy is not necessary. It is obvious that these patients need to continue receiving therapy of some sort and are not candidates for a second attempt at surgical resection. On the other hand, at the present state of knowledge, a negative laparoscopic examination is not sufficient evidence for classifying the patient as without evidence of disease and a laparotomy must be performed. At the time of laparotomy, a detailed exploration of the abdominal cavity must be done in a manner similar to the initial staging procedures previously described. Should focal residual disease be encountered, it should be surgically resected and the area marked with metal clips for possible

regional radiation therapy. Careful inspection of the entire abdominal cavity, including the under surface of the diaphragm, the root of the mesentery, and all parietal and visceral peritoneal surfaces, must be tediously carried out with liberal use of biopsy for suspicious areas.

Creasman et al. reported four patients with ovarian cancer who, after chemotherapy or combined immunochemotherapy, were found to have retroperitoneal disease at the time of second-look exploratory laparotomy, even though there was no evidence on intraabdominal residual cancer. Ovarian cancer can metastasize to pelvic and periaortic lymph nodes, and therefore these areas must be evaluated to appropriately assess the true extent of disease in patients with ovarian cancer.

With the conscientious use of a second-look operation (see box above), one can expect a relatively low subsequent recurrence rate if the results are negative. Earlier reports outlining the fate of patients with a negative second-look procedure after surgery and chemotherapy with single-agent alkylating agents suggested that the subsequent recurrence rate was about 10% to 20%. In the last two decades, more and more patients have been treated with platinum-based combination chemotherapy, and the fate of patients with negative second-look procedures has been somewhat altered. Roberts et al. reported on a series of second-look procedures and analyzed the subsequent outcome for the patient with regard to stage. Whereas patients with stages I and II disease continued to have a high correlation between a negative second-look operation and subsequent disease-free survival, as many as 50% of the patients with negative second-look operations after combination chemotherapy have experienced subsequent recurrences of their disease. This 50% figure for patients with stages III and IV epithelial cancers of the ovary has been confirmed by many others in our personal communications. This discouraging statistic suggests that (1) even a very thorough exploration does not reveal microscopic residuals in many patients, and (2) this group of patients should be strongly considered for an adjuvant program using another modality such as radioactive colloids or intraperitoneal immunotherapy. The high subsequent recurrence rate following negative second-look operations after combination chemotherapy, as compared with single-agent therapy, is also difficult to explain. Many have rationalized that since a greater percentage of patients have a negative second-look operation after combination therapy, the apparent difference is not real. Combination therapy appears to increase the number of patients who have regression to the point of having clinically undetectable residual disease. The fact remains: many patients are being treated almost to the point of "cure," and an additional stroke of some sort is needed.

Although second-look laparotomy to ascertain primary therapeutic effect on ovarian cancer has been generally accepted, laparoscopy for this purpose had been controversial. Visually directed biopsy of unresectable residual tumor masses via a laparoscope can spare some patients a laparotomy and provide a safe and easy route for assessment of intra-abdominal disease. One method to ensure a safe entry route for the Verres needle at laparoscopy is achieved with a needle attached to a syringe and careful aspiration of the peritoneal cavity. After injection of 10 cc of air into the peritoneal cavity, free flow of air back into the syringe suggests a safe placement for the Verres needle. The trocar should be inserted lateral to the previous abdominal wall incision. When the introduction site is in doubt, the open technique, in which the laparoscope is inserted under direct vision through a small incision into the peritoneal cavity, ensures accurate placement. Berek et al. reported on a series of 110 laparoscopic examinations of 57 patients with ovarian cancers. Successful procedures were 73%. Fourteen percent of the patients had major complications requiring laparotomy, most of which involved bowel perforation.

Because as many as 40%-50% of patients with a negative second-look will subsequently have recurrence some 1-10 years later, should a second-look procedure be performed on a patient who is not on a clinical trial? This question has been posed by many. The primary contribution of second-assessment surgery appears to be to define prognosis, effect therapeutic selection, and possibly alter survival. It does define a group of patients who have a reasonably high probability of remaining disease free. The authors' experience has been that many patients want this knowledge. In this era of intraperitoneal chemotherapy with both cytotoxic agents and biological response modifiers, second-assessment surgery helps considerably in selecting patients for these trials, and thus it may have some impact on survival when definitive salvage therapies have been identified. Second-look surgery thus provides the managing physician with important information for selecting salvage therapy. Most patients are anxious to proceed with further therapy and insist on knowing their disease status before considering their options. For these reasons, second-assessment surgery continues to be valuable. A positive impact on survival has not yet been proven. On the other hand, the possible benefits of current salvage therapy protocols will not be known for 5-10 years. Should not these patients be offered an opportunity to join such protocols in the hope that such therapies will prove to be effective?

It does not appear that patients with low risk disease (stage I, grades 1 and 2) who are subjected to a full staging operation at their initial surgery will benefit from a reassessment laparotomy. In addition, there is no evidence that patients who progress during primary therapy benefit from the procedure.

Salvage Therapy

Advanced epithelial ovarian cancer is a highly chemosensitive solid tumor with responses in the range of 70%-80% to first-line chemotherapy, including a high proportion of complete responses. The majority of patients, however, eventually relapse and ultimately die of chemo-resistant disease. Even with platinum-based chemotherapy, less than a quarter of the patients with an initial advanced disease diagnosis are alive at 5 years. In all forms of ovarian epithelial cancer, second-line chemotherapy has to date been disappointing. When effective drug combinations are initially used and fail, there is virtually no chance of inducing a significant response with a second drug or combination of drugs. A partial response and control of malignant effusions can be achieved on occasion but these are usually short-lived. However, most gynecologic oncologists attempt to treat these drug-failure patients using a reasonable second-line regimen usually consisting of active chemotherapeutic agents that have not been used in the first treatment plan (Table 11-29). It is hoped that as new agents evolve, a more

Table 11-29 Agents used in epithelial ovarian cancer

Active agents	Inactive agents	Not known
Alkylating agents	BCNU	Procarbazine
Hexamethylmelamine	Vincristine	Mithramycin
Doxorubicin	6-MP	Bleomycin
Cisplatin	Dactinomycin	Dacarbazine (DTIC)
Carboplatin		Mitomycin C
5-Fluorouracil		Hydroxyurea
Methotrexate		
VP-16		
Taxol		
Navelbine		
Gemcitabine		
Topotecan		

effective second echelon of drugs will become available for use. Although second-line surgery is not generally advocated, every experienced gynecologic oncologist has a group of patients who have responded well to a second surgical attack on local or regional recurrent disease that initially had not responded to chemotherapy. This is especially relevant to the patient who, at the time of second-look operation following chemotherapy, has what appears to be localized persistent disease.

Platinum sensitivity, which is defined by a response to first line platinum-based therapy, has been found to predict the response to subsequent retreatment with a platinum containing treatment frequently used for salvage therapy. In general, patients who progress during treatment or have stable disease in response to initial platinum-based therapy or who relapse within 6 months of said therapy are considered to have platinum based refractory disease. Patients who respond and have a progression-free interval of greater than 6 months off treatment are defined as platinum-sensitive. The response rates to salvage therapy are strikingly different in these two groups of patients. Blackledge et al. in an analysis of 92 patients on five different salvage regimens, found that the interval off platinum-based therapy was a strong predictor of response. This observation held for both platinum based and nonplatinum based salvage regimens. A response rate of less than 10% was observed for patients with a treatment-free interval of less than 6 months with the observed response rate rising as the treatment-free interval lengthened, up to 90% for those with an interval greater than 21 months (Table 11-30).

Seltzer et al. reported a 72% response rate, including a 36% complete response rate to salvage cisplatin in 11 patients who had achieved complete response to platinum-based, front line chemotherapy. Markman et al. reported a 77% response rate to cisplatin in patients who had received no treatment for more than 24 months, compared to 27% in women whose treatment-free interval remains from 5-12 months. Similarly, Eisenhauer reported a 43% response rate to carboplatin in patients whose treatment-free interval was more than 2 months compared to 10% in those whose treatment-free interval was 2 months or less. These findings make it mandatory that we define the patient populations in clinical trials of salvage therapy. Phase II trials should include multiple adequately sized cohorts, such as patients with platinum-sensitive disease and those with platinum-refractory disease. In addition, patients probably should be stratified by the length of their treatment-free interval.

Several studies have demonstrated a clinically important dose/response relationship with cisplatin. Bruckner gave 120 mg/m^2 cisplatin to patients who had refractory ovarian cancer and observed responses in 4 of 20 patients who had failed standard cisplatin therapy. Similar results were reported by Barker and Wiltshaw, who treated patients who had refractory ovarian cancer with 100 mg/m^2 cisplatin and observed responses in 21% of patients who had progressed on lower-dose cisplatin regimens. Initially, escalation of cisplatin dose to levels more than 100 to 120 mg/m^2 were not possible because of the dose-limiting nephrotoxicity. The demonstration that cisplatin nephrotoxicity could be greatly reduced by maintenance of a tubular diuresis in experimental animals led to clinical studies of high-dose cisplatin (200 mg/m^2 per cycle) in advanced ovarian cancer. High-dose cisplatin is administered after intensive hydration with 250 ml/hour of normal saline (with each liter containing 20 mEq KC1) started 12 hours before the first cisplatin dose and continuing uninterrupted until 12-24 hours after the last cisplatin dose on day 5. Cisplatin (40 mg/m^2) was dissolved in 250 ml of 3% saline and infused over a 30-minute period on 5 consecutive days. Before each cisplatin dose, 20 mg of furosemide was administered intravenously. Cycles of high-dose cisplatin can be administered every 28 to 35 days as determined by hematologic recovery. Ozols, reporting on this technique, studied 19 previously treated patients and achieved a 32% overall response rate. Unfortunately, the toxicity of high-dose cisplatin in this heavily pretreated group of patients will be substantial. Not only was severe myelosuppression observed but also significant neurotoxicity. Renal toxicity of high-dose cisplatin was well controlled. The major dose-limiting toxicity of high-dose cisplatin appears to be neurotoxicity. Some degree of peripheral neuropathy will develop in all patients who receive more than 2 cycles of high-dose cisplatin, and a third of patients will develop a grade III neuropathy.

High dose chemotherapy regimens with hematological support have achieved substantial response rates. Traditionally, chemotherapy has been associated with short response durations in a salvage setting. The longest response durations have been in patients with platinum sensitive disease with minimal residual disease, where standard doses would likely produce substantial response rates. These findings suggest that trials of high dose chemotherapy with hematologic support would be most appropriate with patients with minimal disease following

Table 11-30   Response rate vs interval from previous treatment with platinum based regimen

Interval (months)	Total no	No responding	% responding
<3	39	4	10
4-6	11	1	9
7-9	11	4	36
10-12	6	1	17
13-15	4	2	50
16-18	4	3	75
19-21	1	1	100
>21	16	15	94

Blackledge G et al: *Br J Cancer* 59:650:1989.

first-line therapy but are unlikely to benefit patients with platinum resistant or bulky disease. A recent survey reported by Stiff of eleven transplant centers in the United States identified 146 patients with ovarian cancer who had undergone high dose chemotherapy with hematologic support. Eighty two patients were evaluable for response. Overall response rates of 73% in patients with platinum-sensitive disease and 34% in patients with platinum-resistant were observed. A median time to progression, however, was only 6 months. Only 14% were free of disease at 1 year.

Carboplatin as second-line therapy in epithelial ovarian cancer has resulted in 14%-38% response rates, with one quarter to one half of the patients having complete response. Response rates increased progressively from between 6% and 13% in CDDP (cisplatin) and alkylator refractory patients to 31% in prior CDDP responders and 45% in previously untreated patients (radiation failures). Patients who progress on CDDP will not respond to carboplatin.

Standard dose Paclitaxel has been shown to produce response rates of 22%-23% in patients with platinum-resistant disease. Kohn et al. evaluated higher doses of Paclitaxel, which required hematologic support, and observed a 48% response rate in platinum-refractory patients. As with other agents, these responses were generally of short duration. Nonetheless, Paclitaxel should figure prominently in the consideration of salvage therapy for patients who have platinum-resistant disease. The importance of dose intensity in this setting is being explored in randomized studies throughout the world. The results will have important implications for Paclitaxel dose in combination regimens, which are being evaluated both as first-line therapy and as second-line therapy (Table 11-31).

The use of Hexamethylmelamine as second-line therapy in ovarian cancer was reported by Manetta in 1990 with encouraging results. In 1992, Vergae reported 61 patients with recurrent or persistent clinical measurable platinum-resistant epithelial ovarian carcinoma who were treated with oral Hexamethylmelamine daily for 14 days repeated at 4-week intervals. Fifty patients were evaluable for response and 57 were evaluable for toxicity. The objective response rate was 14%. The response rate was higher in patients with relapse within 6 months than in patients with progression or stable disease on platinum-based therapy. This observation underscores the importance of defining response and time to progression after first-line platinum-based chemotherapy. The median duration of response was 8 months, and the median survival in responding patients was over 9 months vs 5 months for patients with progression on Hexamethylmelamine. Nausea and vomiting requiring antiemetic treatment occurred in 8 patients (14%) and reversible neuropathy occurred in 3 patients.

Twenty nine patients with recurrent advanced stage ovarian cancer were treated with 5-Fluorouracil (5-FU) and leucovorin by intravenous bolus on 5 consecutive days, repeated every 3 weeks. Twenty one of these patients had experienced disease progression while receiving a cisplatin or carboplatin-based regimen. There were two clinical responders and one partial responder to therapy (10% response rate) and 11 individuals who experienced stable disease for periods ranging 5-27 months. 5-FU and leucovorin appear to have some activity in platinum-refractory ovarian cancer and form a very well tolerated regimen for most patients.

Intraperitoneal therapy (discussed elsewhere in this chapter) has been employed utilizing several antineoplastic agents as salvage therapy in ovarian cancer. Activity is essentially limited to patients with very small volume residual disease (≤0.5 cm in maximum diameter) when the salvage therapy program is initiated. In the absence of a randomized phase III trial, the ultimate impact of these surgically documented responses on survival is difficult to evaluate, although long-term disease free survival (>4 years) has been reported following intraperitoneal therapy in this clinical setting.

There is limited evidence of sustained benefit from salvage therapy in patients with ovarian cancer. Overall only modest response rates with short durations of response have been reported. In addition, there has been a lack of consistency in these studies with regard to key definitions such as platinum sensitivity vs platinum resistance. Future salvage trials should clearly define their patients in these two categories. It may be necessary to also discuss paclitaxel-sensitive vs paclitaxel-resistant lesions in the future. Platinum-sensitive patients are appropriate for pilot studies of platinum combinations incorporating different cytotoxic mechanisms of action and dose schedule investigations. Patients with platinum-resistance are good candidates for novel investigational approaches and studies of drug resistance.

Hoskins, Coltart, and Menczer have all studied whole-abdomen irradiation with a pelvic boost in patients with minimal disease at second-look surgical reassessment for

Table 11-31 Paclitaxel as salvage therapy for patients with ovarian cancer

Author	No of assessable patients	CR + PR	Median duration (months)
Kohn	44 (42R)	6 + 15 (48% R)	6
McGuire	40	1 + 11 (40% S, 30% R)	6
Thigpen	41 (27R)	5 + 10 (36%)	nr
Trimble	652 R	23 + 118 (22% R)	5

Christian MC: *Gynecol Oncol* 55:S143, 1994.

R, platinum resistant; *S*, platinum sensitive; *nr*, not reported.

ovarian carcinoma. They noted that aggressive cytoreductive surgery followed by combination chemotherapy for stage III ovarian carcinoma has resulted in a significant percentage of complete clinical responses. However, 30%-50% of patients with no clinical evidence of disease are found to have residual carcinomas at second-look surgical reassessment. Because recent reports indicate a high degree of effectiveness utilizing abdominal and pelvic irradiation as primary therapy for ovarian carcinomas with small residual disease, these authors treated patients who were found to have residual disease smaller than 1 cm at second-look reassessment with either open-field or split-field abdominal and pelvic irradiation. With rather limited follow-up, as many as 30% of such patients have remained in remission, according to some reports. However, our experience is that with longer follow-up periods more than 90% of patients will have recurrence, even in this optimal group. There appears to be overlap in the resistance of cells to chemotherapy and radiotherapy.

Intraperitoneal Chemotherapy (Figure 11-24)

For a chemotherapeutic agent to kill a malignant cell, it must be delivered to the tumor in the highest concentration possible. As previously mentioned, drugs administered systemically have access to well-vascularized organs such as bone marrow or intestines. Because of longer diffusional distances, however, it is likely that chemotherapeutic agents given intravenously will have much lower penetration into extravascular cavities, such as the pleural space, peritoneal cavity, and central nervous system. From theoretic modeling, a major possible

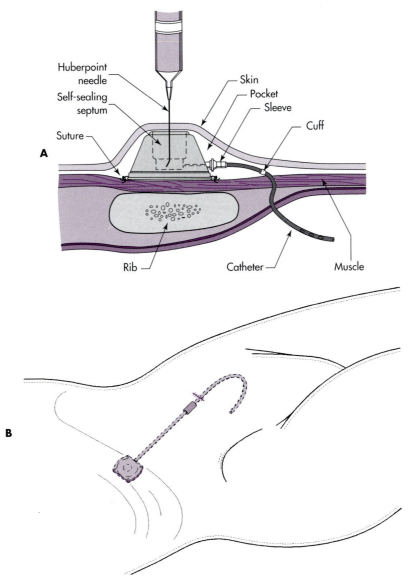

Figure 11-24 A, Implanted peritoneal access catheter with subcutaneous self-sealing port providing a path for intraperitoneal therapy. **B,** Intraperitoneal chemotherapy.

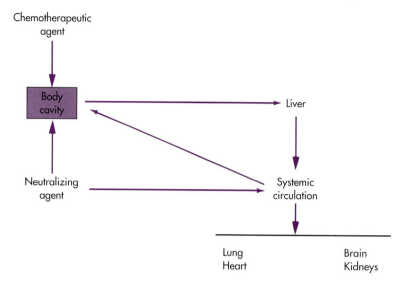

Figure 11-25 Diagrammatic representation of basic principles of intracavitary chemotherapy. Drug administered via intracavitary route will be absorbed into systemic circulation at rate determined by its physical and chemical characteristics. Drug administered intraperitoneally can be metabolized in liver into nontoxic form before entering systemic circulation. Systemically delivered neutralizing aspects of this treatment approach further enhance pharmacokinetic advantages.

pharmacokinetic advantage has been suggested for drugs administered directly into body cavities. Although the details of such mathematical modeling studies are complex, the basic principles they define are important to understand because they form the rationale behind direct intracavity administration of chemotherapeutic agents (Figure 11-25).

When a drug is infused into an extravascular cavity, the steady-state concentration in the cavity and the plasma is a function of the rate of clearance from the cavity and the plasma. For drugs that demonstrate low clearance from the cavity and high systemic clearance, there will be a pharmacokinetic advantage for the cavity into which the drug has been instilled compared with the systemic circulation. Important determinants of clearance include the molecular weight of the drug, its charge, lipid solubility, and the volume of fluid in which the drug is administered. A drug with a low clearance from a body cavity would be one that has a high molecular weight, is ionized and water soluble, and is administered in a large treatment volume.

A second important issue relates to the metabolism of the drug administered. Molecules the size of chemotherapeutic agents are principally taken up in the portal circulation when instilled in the peritoneal cavity. Thus a drug administered intraperitoneally that is hepatically metabolized might show a major pharmacokinetic advantage when administered by this route if it can be converted into a nontoxic metabolite before entering the systemic circulation.

A third principle for successful application of intracavitary chemotherapy is the importance of treatment volume. When drugs are delivered for their sclerosing properties, high concentrations are administered in small volumes. To prevent sclerosis and ensure adequate exposure of all tumor in the cavity to the drug, it is important to deliver the treatment in large volumes. This is a particularly important issue in many patients who have intra-abdominal malignant lesions, because extensive adhesion formation induced by prior surgical procedure or by the tumor itself can possibly prevent access of the drug to the entire abdominal cavity. Markman et al. reported in 1992 a study of 70 patients in which the authors evaluated the influence of the severity of adhesions (observed at the time of laparotomy and found immediately preceding installation of intraperitoneal chemotherapy) on the ability to achieve a surgically defined complete response. Markman retrospectively reviewed the operative reports of these 70 patients with small residual ovarian cancer treated on one of the phase II salvage intraperitoneal trials conducted at their institution. The authors concluded that the presence of extensive adhesions observed within the peritoneal cavity at the time of a laparotomy performed immediately prior to the initiation of intraperitoneal therapy did not have a negative impact on the potential to achieve a surgically defined complete response, assuming it is technically feasible to lyse all significant adhesions prior to the completion of the operative procedure.

An additional question concerning the applicability of intracavitary chemotherapy is that of drug penetration. Little is known about the ability of most chemotherapeutic agents to penetrate solid tumors. Ozols et al. were able to examine the penetrability of doxorubicin into a

Table 11-32 Pharmacologic advantage of intraperitoneal chemotherapy*

Drug	Pharmacologic advantage
Methotrexate	7-36
Fluorouracil	111-898
Adriamycin	474-550
Melphalan	63-93
Cisplatin	21-72
Cytosine arabinoside	300-1000

*Ratio of peak peritoneal level to plasma level.

transplantable murine ovarian teratoma because of its intrinsic fluorescence. Even though doxorubicin was found only in the outermost five to six cell layers of tumor when administered by the intraperitoneal route, this form of treatment was successful in curing 70% of the mice treated. When mice with this tumor were similarly treated with a regimen of intravenously administered doxorubicin, there were no long-term survivors. Theoretically, the intracavitary form of therapy will be most effective against free-floating tumor cells or thin tumor nodules. Free surface diffusion is unlikely to kill a large fraction of tumor in cases of advanced disease where large tumor masses are present. However, if drugs are used at or near their maximum tolerated doses, the combination of drug delivery by capillary flow (from drug absorbed into the systemic circulation) and free surface diffusion may still be more effective than intravenous dosing alone. In addition, the large concentration differences achieved between the body cavity and the plasma (Table 11-32) enables the use of neutralizing agents delivered into the systemic circulation to reduce the toxicity while allowing high levels of drug to be present in the cavity treated. Two examples of this technique that have been clinically useful are the use of systemically delivered folinic acid and sodium thiosulfate administered to neutralize the toxicities of methotrexate and cisplatin, respectively.

Several investigators have utilized intraperitoneal chemotherapy for patients who have minimal residual disease after second-assessment surgery. Single-agent and combination-agent chemotherapy has been used, and results are mixed. An encouraging combination has been reported by Howell utilizing intraperitoneal high-dose cisplatin (200 mg/m^2) together with thiosulfate rescue intravenously and VP-16. Phase II trials utilizing this regimen and other platinum based IP therapy have demonstrated a 25%-35% surgically documented complete response rate. These trials suggest that IP cisplatin-based therapy may be effective in eradicating disease in some patients who responded to systemic platinum and have small residual recurrent disease at the time of IP therapy initiation. In other series, only 2 of 50 patients

(4%) with disease greater than 1 cm at the start of IP therapy experienced a surgically defined complete response. Additionally, patients who fail to respond to systemic platinum therapy have a surgically defined complete response rate of only 7% despite having small disease residual. An intergroup study has been conducted comparing the use of cisplatin (100 mg/m^2) administered intraperitoneally plus cyclophosphamide (600 mg/m^2) administered intravenously with the use of cisplatin (100 mg/m^2) and cyclophosphamide (100 mg/m^2) both administered intravenously as first-line postoperative therapy. Pathologically proven complete response in patients undergoing second look was documented in 31% (52/168) in the intravenous (IV) arm and 40% (62/156) in the intraperitoneal (IP) arm ($p = 0.10$). Adjusting for age, race, tumor type, tumor grade, and stratification factors, patient survival on the IP arm was significantly longer ($p = 0.03$) than the IV arm. Critical hearing loss and neutropenia was significantly more frequent and more severe in the IV treated patients.

Other agents used intraperitoneally in ovarian carcinoma are 5-fluorouracil, carboplatin, mitoxantrone, doxorubicin and Taxol. More study of these agents as compared to or in combination with cisplatin is warranted. Additionally, biological agents are currently undergoing intraperitoneal trials—e.g., gamma interferon, tumor necrosis factor, and interleukin-2.

The field of intracavitary chemotherapy is really in its infancy. Much work remains to define optimum drug combinations and schedules for treatment of various tumors by this route. In addition, improved methods of delivery must be developed to assure adequate drug distribution and reduce the risk of chemical irritation and bacterial infection. Braly reported on the technical aspects of intraperitoneal chemotherapy in abdominal carcinomatosis, outlining difficulties encountered in a series of 41 patients. Clear guidelines are presented for future use. Finally, eventually it will be necessary to show in controlled clinical trials whether the pharmacokinetic advantage of intracavitary drug administration can be translated to improved response rates and survival as both second-line and first-line therapy.

After more than a decade of active clinical research with intraperitoneal therapy in ovarian cancer, it is reasonable to suggest that this form of therapy is an acceptable option in patient management. Patients with persistent minimal residual ovarian cancer (microscopic disease ≤0.5 cm lesions) following initial intravenous platinum-based chemotherapy who have demonstrated a response to the systemically diluted regimen are appropriate candidates for an intraperitoneal platinum-based treatment program. No alternative strategy has yielded superior clinical results, and a subset of patients treated with this approach appears to experience prolonged disease-free survival. For now, the use of intraperitoneal therapy in other clinical settings in ovarian cancer or intraperitoneal therapy with non-platinum-based regimens cannot be recommended as standard practice, simply because the data to support the effect of such an approach are inadequate. Studies under way at this time may alter this statement.

Malignant Effusions

The cause of malignant effusions is not known. The most common explanations are (1) an irritant effect of the tumor on normal serous membranes, (2) lymphatic obstruction, and (3) venous obstruction. Graham et al. studied ascites circulating in patients with peritoneal carcinomatosis. They noted a large increase in the production of fluid by noncancer-bearing peritoneal surfaces that was most marked from the omentum and small-bowel surfaces. They also noted a significant elevation of portal pressure in the presence of ovarian cancer with ascites, as compared with portal pressure in women without disease and in patients with ovarian cancer without ascites. We have observed that clinically troublesome ascites is rare in the absence of diffuse disease on the peritoneal surfaces underlying the right diaphragm, suggesting that large ascitic pools result from severe derangement of this absorptive surface as fluid produced in the peritoneal cavity migrates into lymphatic capillaries in its path to the thoracic duct.

Some concepts regarding the fluid kinetics of the peritoneal cavity have been relatively well substantiated. It is known that lymph vessels can carry molecules away from the tissues. The molecules can be protein, particulates, or cells. Some water also flows through the lymph vessels of tissues: it is a vehicle or solvent for the transported molecules. Removing water in bulk from tissues is a function of the blood capillaries, not of the lymphatics. Filtration and diffusion appear to be the two main processes in the exchange of substances between the blood and tissues. As blood pressure forces fluid from capillaries, the osmotic pressure of the plasma protein sucks the fluid back into the capillaries. The tissue tension tends to inhibit the exodus of fluid and to promote its reentry into capillaries. This small amount of fluid retained in tissues exits via lymphatics.

Although diffusion accounts for the exchange of molecules across a semipermeable membrane, independent of the movement of fluid, the semipermeability restricts the process. Generally, large molecules diffuse more slowly than smaller ones. This process may depend on pores in the capillaries. Large tissue molecules that cannot transgress the capillary pores can still be carried away in lymphatics. When a condition results in accumulation of large particles in the fluid outside capillaries, the osmotic pressure rises to counteract the effect of plasma proteins inside the capillaries, thus increasing filtration and hindering reabsorption. The imbalance reverses only when the tissue tension becomes high enough to counteract the filtering pressure of the capillaries. Oxygen and nutrients are diffused throughout the period of imbalance. When diffusion cannot occur, necrosis begins. In the peritoneal cavity, lymph can accumulate without diffusing and still maintain tissue viability. The constant mixing of ascitic fluid caused by the diaphragmatic contractions and intestinal peristalsis facilitates diffusion. This perhaps accounts for the continued viability of malignant cells in tissue cultures taken from ascitic fluid associated with malignancies. In neoplasia, the absorbing lymphatics may be blocked by cells or by the by-products of cancer cells, such as large molecular mucopolysaccharides. The net effect reduces the absorption of lymph from the peritoneal cavity, resulting in accumulation of lymph fluid (ascites) in the peritoneal cavity. Normal peritoneal lymphatics can also be blocked by fluid that is too tenacious to permit absorption, predisposing mucinous ascites of pseudomyxoma peritonei. Blockage of lymphatics may also contribute to the localization of neoplastic cells in the peritoneal cavity; this generally occurs with pseudomyxoma peritonei.

Malignant effusions are much more effectively managed than they were several decades ago. Chemotherapeutic regimens control 90% of these troublesome situations. The patient who has a distended abdomen, and probable ascites, often presents for diagnosis. There is a tendency to do paracentesis for diagnostic purposes in such situations . We recommend *not* doing paracentesis in patients who are highly suspect of ovarian malignancy for the following reasons:

1. Cytologic examination of fluid may be negative in the presence of malignancy, and laparotomy is still indicated.
2. Even when cytologic examination of the fluid is positive, it seldom provides a definitive clue as to the origin of the primary tumor, and laparotomy is indicated.
3. If the patient has a large fluid-filled cyst (Figure 11-26) rather than ascites, rupture of the cyst and seeding into the peritoneal cavity may occur, often long before laparotomy (Figure 11-27).
4. Paracentesis may be associated with complications other than seeding, such as rupture of an intra-abdominal viscus bleeding infection and severe depletion of electrolytes and proteins. We therefore recommend that these patients be investigated short of paracentesis and that the disease be defined at laparotomy, when the situation can be controlled with more ease.

Our comments are intended to discourage paracentesis as a diagnostic tool but in instances where intra-abdominal pressure causes respiratory embarrassment or severe pain the procedure should be performed as therapy. Often, improved gastrointestinal function and relief of nausea and vomiting, as well as constipation, may be noted following therapeutic paracentesis. Ultrasound may

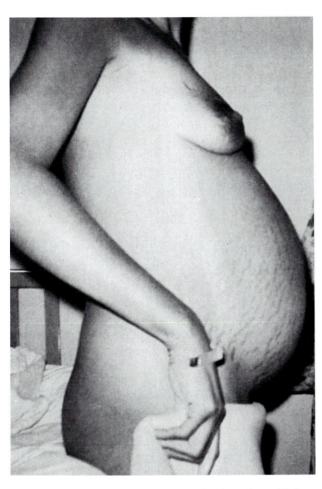

Figure 11-26 Marked abdominal distension in patient with large grade 2 mucinous adenocarcinoma of ovary.

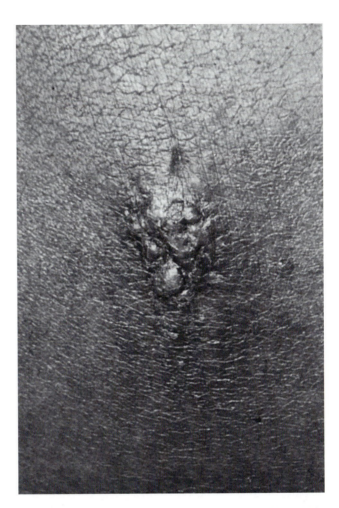

Figure 11-27 Skin implant in patient seen in Figure 11-26. This was found at side of abdominal paracentesis performed 4 weeks earlier and represented the only disease identified outside the large self-contained neoplasm.

be helpful in locating large pockets of fluid and directing the site for needle puncture.

Agents such as bleomycin, tetracycline, quinacrine (Atabrine), *Corynebacterium parvum*, and nitrogen mustards, have an effect on effusions by producing an adhesive serositis that will partially obliterate the peritoneal or pleural cavity, making the accumulation of ascites more difficult. However, these agents also create a situation in which further surgical intervention is almost impossible. When ascites reaccumulates after surgery, it is almost always a problem associated with unresectable carcinoma, and patients usually can be controlled with systemic chemotherapy of one form or the other. If one drug fails, combinations should be tried; they are sometimes successful. Unfortunately, there are some patients whose ascites cannot be completely controlled by systemic chemotherapy, and often they can be kept comfortable by periodic paracentesis. This can be done on an outpatient basis at intervals determined by the patient's symptoms. The site of paracentesis is usually at the lateral border of the rectus muscle and at the level of the umbilicus. The site may be selected by ultrasound scanning to locate the largest pockets of fluid. The midline is avoided because tumor or adhesions are often present and complications can result. It is advisable to infiltrate the abdominal wall with a small amount of local anesthetic and then, using the same syringe and needle, explore for a clear spot in the peritoneal cavity. A larger trocar can then be inserted over the exact area of exploration. In this way, one can avoid the complication of inserting a trocar into an adherent segment of bowel. Measurements of weight and abdominal girth are recorded before and after paracentesis, and the volume of fluid is also noted. Sometimes fluid will continue to leak out of the trocar sites and attaching a urostomy bag to the area will provide some comfort for the patient. Because of this leakage from trocar sites, many physicians prefer to use a 16-gauge needle attached to the type of tubing that is used for blood donors. A needle attached to the other end of the tubing is inserted into a vacuum bottle and the fluid is aspirated under negative pressure, eliminating the need for a large puncture site. Irradiation techniques are usually not recommended in the management of ascites because systemic chemotherapy is so effective. Instillation of ^{32}P is often difficult because of the need to obtain a uniform distribution of the radioactive substance. In addition, large individual tumor masses are usually present and the beta emission of radioactive ^{32}P is effective for only 2-4 mm. There are situations in which a diffuse miliary spread of disease is suspected, and ascites is only partially controlled with chemotherapy. In these instances radioactive chromium phosphate (a beta emitter) may be beneficial and provide minimal chance of severe injury to the bowel.

Pleural effusion is another problem in the management of ovarian cancer. Approximately one third of the patients with ascites will have pleural effusions. They usually respond to systemic chemotherapy, as does ascites. Pleural effusion in the absence of ascites usually indicates involvement of the pleura with disease. The same techniques that have been outlined for the management of ascites can be used. A nitrogen mustard, tetracycline, *Corynebacterium parvum*, or quinacrine (Atabrine) injection into the pleural cavity is associated with a high success rate. Obliteration of the pleural cavity prevents the accumulation of fluid in that space. A dose of 10-15 mg of a nitrogen mustard creates enough pleural reaction to cause obliteration of the space, resulting in relief of this troublesome symptom for patients who are not responding optimally to systemic chemotherapy. Another method employed with some success is the instillation of bleomycin (60-120 mg) into the pleural cavity after thoracentesis. This drug can be used with systemic chemotherapy because of its minimal myelosuppressive effect. Kennedy reported on a technique of pleurodesis using talc slurry with an 81% success rate. The slurry was instilled through a chest tube at the bedside. A febrile episode frequently followed but respiratory difficulties were rare.

Thoracentesis Technique

The site of the thoracentesis is selected by chest x-ray, fluoroscopy, sonography, CT-scan, or physical examination. When there is a large effusion of total hydrothorax, the best site of aspiration is usually the seventh or eighth interspace in the posterior axillary line. The most frequent error performed is to decide on an interspace that is too low. The physician should be aware that with pneumonia or trauma there is an elevation of the diaphragm and a loss of lung volume and appropriately higher interspace levels should be selected. The patient is placed in a comfortable sitting position, leaning slightly forward on a padded stand or supported by an attendant. Premedication with narcotic or Diazepam is often prudent. The skin of the chest wall is prepared with an antiseptic technique and then draped.

The chest wall is anesthetized with 5-10 ml of 1% Xylocaine, using a number 22 gauge needle. Care should be taken to be sure that the skin, rib, rib periosteum, and parietal pleura are thoroughly infiltrated. Thoracentesis is virtually painless if the patient is properly anesthetized with Xylocaine. A short-bevel needle (7-10 cm long, 18-30 gauge) is attached by way of a three way stopcock to a 20-50 ml syringe. Other clinicians prefer to use a needle through which is passed a soft plastic catheter. With firm but steady pressure, the needle is passed into the pleural space. In an effort to avoid injury to the intercostal nerve and vessels, the needle should be passed through the chest wall at the lower margin of the intercostal space (Figure 11-28). A clamp may be placed on the needle to steady it on the chest wall. Care should be taken throughout the procedure to prevent air from entering the chest.

The amount of fluid removed at one setting often approaches 2000-3000 ml. If the aspiration is done slowly, the lung will accommodate to the evacuation. Where the pleural has resulted from malignant implants

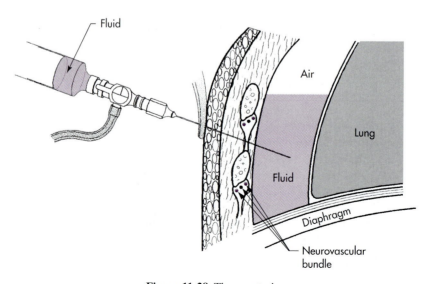

Figure 11-28 Thoracentesis.

on the pleura, the lung tissue becomes much less pliable and a thoracostomy tube may be necessary. A small incision is made in the skin surrounding the needle entry site and a trocar is passed percutaneously into the pleural space. This technique can often be accomplished with a small tube (#12-14). At times the tube must be inserted utilizing a hemostat after an incision of the skin has been made with scalpel at a previously determined site of the thoracentesis. The tube, which has been clamped during insertion, should then be immediately connected to water-sealed drainage after it is secured to the chest wall with suture. These thoracostomy tubes are often left in place several days and removed 24 hours following attempts at pleurodesis. The techniques of pleurodesis are described above.

The surgical approach to recurrent malignant effusions has been somewhat limited. Peritoneovenous shunts for all palliation of malignant ascites refractory to conventional medical management have recently received renewed interest, since the development of the pressure-sensitive peritoneovenous valve first reported by LeVeen et al. Qazi and Savlov reported achieving palliation in 70% (28/40) of their patients.

For pleural effusion, decortication of the lung and pleurectomy have been used with varying results. Instillation of a nitrogen mustard and similar caustic compounds has essentially replaced these procedures. Other agents, including hypertonic glucose and talc, have been used to create pleuritis. Again, they have variable success rates, depending on the investigator. A surgical procedure for uncontrollable ascites called ileoentectropy was promoted by Brunschwig at Memorial Sloan-Kettering Hospital. Effusion was controlled by this method in some of the patients with ascites caused by ovarian cancer, but it has not proved to be a practical approach.

CURRENT AREAS OF RESEARCH

Most of the advances that have been made in the treatment of cancers of the ovary in the last 20 years have resulted from the multimodality approach proven effective in phase III trials. A combination of modalities used in a logical and flexible manner can achieve notable success on an individual basis. It is hoped that this approach, combined with improved chemotherapeutic agents, better understanding of drug resistance, and the possible addition of biologic response modifiers as a new modality, will result in improved outcome for this devastating group of malignancies (see box right).

By far the greatest advance on the horizon is in early detection by immunodiagnostic techniques. Several experimental procedures have strongly suggested the presence of several commonly shared tumor-associated antigens in epithelial cancers of the ovary. One such antigen has resulted in the CA-125 tumor marker assay described earlier. Unfortunately, isolation of these anti-

gens, which has been more difficult than initially conceived, is essential to the creation of a clinically useful immunodiagnostic tool. Given that there are commonly shared tumor-associated antigens in epithelial cancer of the ovary and that a small amount of this antigen or an antibody to it is detectable in the sera of patients with subclinical disease, all the ingredients for a dramatic improvement in the battle against this disease are at hand. Unfortunately, CA-125 serum levels do not appear to be elevated in most patients with subclinical disease. Other antigens are under investigation.

Some phase II studies with leukocyte interferon suggest possible activity for cytokines in carcinoma of the ovary. One study has been reported by Abdulhay of 35 patients who had recurrent epithelial adenocarcinomas of the ovary after failure of cisplatin-based combination chemotherapy. This study showed a 12% response rate and a large number of patients who had unusually long periods of stable disease. A subsequent study was conducted by DiSaia using the same dose of interferon in addition to standard CAP chemotherapy immediately after surgery of patients with stages III and IV disease. The myelosuppressive effect of the interferon and the chemotherapy caused unacceptable toxicity. Further study is needed to explore methods by which interferon-alfa and other cytokines might be utilized in this disease.

Although vigorous saline diuresis eliminates the nephrotoxicity of high-dose cisplatin, it has not eliminated the other toxicities. Peripheral neuropathy has now become the dose-limiting toxicity associated with cisplatin, and it limits the duration of high-dose therapy. In an effort to retain the therapeutic effect of high-dose platin while decreasing the toxicity, a cisplatin analog called carboplatin was developed. Carboplatin used in trials was

---

CLINICAL TRIALS: PHASES AND GOALS

Phase I
- To determine the maximally tolerated dose of drug
- To determine the schedule for administration
- To define toxic effect to normal tissue
- To generate data about the clinical pharmacology of the agent

Phase II
- To identify antitumor activity in a spectrum of common metastatic tumors
- To explore ability to achieve increased rates or response with changes of dose or schedule
- To extend phase I data on toxicity

Phase III
- To compare the investigational therapy against an established form of treatment in previously untreated patients

not associated with any significant neuropathy or nephrotoxicity. A phase III trial of single-agent carboplatin vs cisplatin in previously untreated patients suggests that carboplatin and cisplatin are therapeutically similar. Clinical responses were noted in 53% of patients receiving carboplatin and 64% of those receiving cisplatin. Duration of responses in overall survival was similar, although an analysis of responses of survival is complicated by the crossover design of the trial. Thirty recurrent ovarian cancer patients, all of whom received prior cisplatin therapy, were treated with high-dose carboplatin with cycles administered every 35 days. Objective responses were achieved in 8 of 30 (27%). However, no responses were seen in patients who had progressive disease during previous therapy with high dose cisplatin. The primary toxicity of high-dose carboplatin is myelosuppression. High dose carboplatin did not result in any clinically apparent neurotoxicity. The dose-limiting toxicity of cisplatin is neurotoxicity, whereas the dose-limiting toxicity of carboplatin is myelosuppression. It is anticipated that future manipulations of cisplatin and its analogues will achieve greater effectiveness for this very active family of drugs in epithelial ovarian cancer.

Chemotherapy has proven curative in some types of advanced cancers and useful as an adjunct to surgery and radiotherapy in many others. The fact that 90% of the cures with chemotherapy occur in 10% of the tumors that afflict humans has been a perplexing biological problem that appears to be related to the greater propensity of some tissue to develop specific and permanent resistance to chemotherapy of a broad nature. A discussion of tumor cell resistance is beyond the scope of this section. However, a few general comments can be made. The capacity to develop drug resistance is in fact an inherent and important property of malignant cell populations. It is basically not expressed by normal cell populations. It is an inherent property of malignant cells, similar to the capacity to metastasize and to invade. There appear to be two types of clinical problems. The first occurs when the malignancy is clearly sensitive at the beginning to at least some chemotherapeutic agents. There is a regression of the disease, but then the tumor recurs with treatment that was initially effective. The situation is most easily explained by the selection phenomenon, whereby killing off the population of sensitive cells leaves behind a small core of resistant cells that then proliferate. The second problem is that of so-called intrinsic resistance; namely, tumors that appear to be resistant de novo to the application of therapy, or at least to show a high level of resistance to a broad range of chemotherapeutic agents.

Three commonly accepted mechanisms of drug resistance include (1) diminished drug uptake by the cell, (2) decreased drug activation, and (3) alteration of target proteins. Most investigators feel that many mechanisms of resistance have yet to be identified. Many studies have suggested that p-glycoprotein may mediate clinical multidrug resistance. A consensus is developing that p-glycoprotein functions as an energy-dependent efflux pump. Strong laboratory evidence suggests that the enhanced expression of the p-glycoprotein is a contributing factor to multidrug resistance. The cell literally pumps the drug out. Glutathione, a ubiquitous tripeptide also found in all normal cells, has been of interest in chemotherapy for several years, since increased levels were first shown in some alkylating-resistance tumor cells. The clinical interest in this mechanism of drug resistance increased with the development of potentially clinically feasible ways of lowering glutathione levels with a variety of drugs. Many substances, such as toremifene and cyclosporin-A, are under study as a possible mechanism for such reversal of multidrug resistance.

Pilot studies of dose-intensive chemotherapy with autologous bone marrow transplantation for patients with advanced epithelial ovarian cancer are now under way. Alkylating agents are logical choices for high-dose chemotherapy because they have a steep dose-responsive curve, both in vitro and in vivo, and this response is maintained through multiple logs of tumor cell kill. Of all the solid tumors, epithelial cancer of the ovary should be an excellent model for testing the efficacy of this technology. The toxicity associated with this type of therapy makes a careful analysis of these studies, as well as the life and quality of survival, very important before widespread use can be suggested.

Dose intensity of chemotherapy appears to be a critical factor in many solid tumors, including possibly ovarian cancer. Several retrospective analyses demonstrated that superior results can be achieved in patients treated with higher dose intensities of cisplatin. The same may be true of other drugs, including carboplatin. Ozols et al. demonstrated that carboplatin could safely be administered (at a dose of 800 mg/m^2) to patients with refractory ovarian cancer. This was accomplished by simultaneous administration of GM-CSF. These studies suggested that GM-CSF can only partially decrease the neutropenic complications associated with high-dose carboplatin and that thrombocytopenia remains a problem. However, other cytokines, such as interleukin-3 (IL-3), may have substantial impact on the severe thrombocytopenia associated with chemotherapy and the use of high-dose carboplatin. It remains to be established whether such combinations can markedly increase the dose intensity of platinum compounds. Trials are under way studying dose escalation of platinum with the use of IL-3 and/or GM-CSF to decrease the myelosuppression, particularly thrombocytopenia.

Flow cytometry has been performed on specimens from patients with all stages of disease, although the majority come from patients with advanced (FIGO stages III and IV) ovarian carcinoma. The majority of specimens have elevated S-phase fraction, and aneuploidy is present in one half to three quarters of tumors. In these studies, ploidy and proliferative indices correlate directly with stage and inversely with prognosis in patients with invasive cancer. In contrast, the majority of borderline tumors are diploid. This correlates well with the good prognosis of patients with borderline tumors, as previously discussed. There appears to be clear differences in the flow cytometric features between noninvasive and invasive ovarian cancer. These observations, and the correlation of ploidy with clinical outcome, suggest that flow cytometry provides some insight into ovarian cancer biology and should be investigated further.

The National Institute of Health Consensus statement on ovarian cancer from 1994 listed the following important directions for future research:

- Currently available imaging techniques and tumor markers should be utilized in clinical trials to determine whether ovarian cancer can be identified at an earlier stage, whether this can reduce mortality from ovarian cancer, and whether this can be done without increasing morbidity and mortality for those women who have abnormal screening results but do not have ovarian cancer. Study of this question should include both pre- and postmenopausal women.
- New serum markers (e.g., OVX-1, M-CSF) and imaging techniques should be investigated to see if a more sensitive and specific panel of screening parameters can be identified.
- Researchers should more clearly evaluate and quantitate the benefits of currently used oral contraceptives in reducing the risk of ovarian cancer, evaluate the necessary duration of use and the benefits of prolonged use, and evaluate the other benefits and risks and long-term outcome.
- A national serum and tissue bank should be established.
- Identification of women at increased risk for ovarian cancer should be improved. Studies should focus on genetic research, such as BRCA-1. In addition, environmental and epidemiologic research should be continued.
- The safety and efficacy of laparoscopy for women with ovarian cancer should be studied.
- The combination of platinum compounds and paclitaxel should be further investigated in earlier stage disease. In addition, the ideal dose and schedule of paclitaxel must be evaluated in clinical trials.
- A prospective randomized study is needed to identify optimal treatment of various subsets of stage I ovarian cancer.
- Whole abdominal radiation should be reevaluated and newer radiation techniques evaluated in the treatment of optimally debulked stage II and III disease.

- Innovative approaches to the treatment of advanced primary as well as recurrent ovarian cancer must be identified and studied. Examples include new molecular targets, agents to overcome resistance, and drugs that inhibit signal transduction pathways.
- Clinical trials exploring the role of consolidation therapy in patients with a complete response to primary therapy should be given higher priority.
- Measures of the quality of life in women with ovarian cancer must be identified, evaluated, and then utilized in optimizing the care of patients.

REHABILITATION

The nature of ovarian cancer is such that the major vital organs (lungs, heart, liver, and kidneys) remain unaffected. The disease itself and its therapy appear primarily to attack the gastrointestinal tract. Indeed, the terminal event for most patients who succumb to this disease is electrolyte imbalance caused by prolonged gastrointestinal obstruction, malnutrition, and significant protein and electrolyte loss from repeated paracentesis and thoracentesis. It is necessary to support these patients with various forms of alimentation during therapy to sustain them sufficiently to tolerate the somewhat vigorous therapy often prescribed. The placement of semipermanent Silastic intravenous catheters (e.g., Hickman, Broviac, or Groshong) greatly facilitates the ability to support these patients (Figure 11-29). Some clinicians prefer to gain intravenous access by means of a device (Port-o-Cath) implanted in the subcutaneous tissue. Many centers can arrange intravenous alimentation at home for patients who are unable to take sufficient nourishment by mouth. Home pharmacy services are available in many areas, and intravenous medications, including analgesics, can be administered at home on pump infusion devices via these semipermanent intravenous catheters.

Intermittent episodes of partial small- and large-bowel obstruction are common, and they must be initially treated conservatively and ultimately surgically if the patient is to continue to fight. The issue as to whether a patient with a high-grade small-bowel obstruction from ovarian cancer carcinomatosis should be explored for a possible bypass procedure to reestablish the continuity of the alimentary tract is a subject that has been long debated. Management of these patients is extremely difficult because of the intactness of their vital organs and their alert mental status. Although most patients will not survive 6 months from the time of the bowel obstruction, surgical intervention should be considered because of the difficulty that all people have observing the slow process of death by starvation. Any procedure that can result in the patient's returning to her home and family seems to be worthy of consideration even in these desperate cases. If nothing else, the performance of a gastrostomy to avoid uncomfortable nasogastric intubation or the persistent

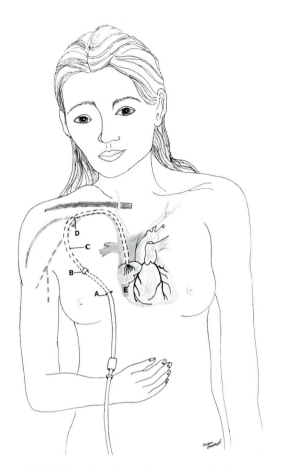

Figure 11-29 Silicone rubber catheter tunneled subcutaneously and positioned in right atrium. *A*, Incision site; *B*, dacron cuff, *C*, subcutaneous tunnel; *D*, insertion into subclavian vein; *E*, right atrium.

agony of constant vomiting is in itself humane and allows more easy return of the patient to a home setting, where the gastrostomy can be used to decompress the gastrointestinal tract as needed.

In general, the most discouraging aspect in the management of ovarian cancer patients is the apathy of many physicians. In truth, these diseases are discouraging, but a determined attitude is medically sound and reassuring to the patient. Significant numbers of patients referred to oncologic centers as "unresectable" have not only been debulked but responded nicely to postoperative therapy. Still other patients have survived complicated combinations of multiple surgical and adjuvant therapies. A positive approach to the disease, which restores hope in the patient with this devastating illness, is justified on that basis alone.

CONCLUSIONS ON MANAGEMENT

Although adenocarcinoma of the ovary remains one of the solid tumors most sensitive to chemotherapeutic regimens, the mortality from this disease remains high. There

appears, however, to be great promise with newer developments in the management of this disease. The following general principles should be kept in mind:

1. An optimal surgical procedure should be carried out whenever possible. This is defined as the removal of all bulk tumor with the intent to leave minimal residua (no individual mass larger than 1-2 cm in diameter). It is not possible to advocate any one operation for all patients, and the clinician must make a judgment at the time of surgery. Unquestionably, patients with small residual tumor volumes have a better prognosis with any postoperative therapy. Even when optimal debulking is not possible, bilateral salpingo-oophorectomy, total abdominal hysterectomy, and omentectomy may afford significant palliation for the patient. Resection of a portion of the bowel should be considered only when such a resection will result in removal of all gross tumor. A careful exploration of the entire abdomen, including the diaphragmatic surfaces and retroperitoneal spaces must be carried out by a methodical surgeon to ensure proper staging of the disease.

2. The conventional view of radiation therapy as the most important postoperative modality for gynecologic cancer must be reexamined with respect to adenocarcinoma of the ovary. In advanced (stages III and IV) disease there is little evidence that radiation therapy has significant value over chemotherapy. A major limiting factor with radiotherapy in advanced disease is the hepatic and renal toxicity that follows adequate doses of whole-abdomen radiation. Shielding these vital organs will lead to undertreatment, especially in commonly involved areas such as the under surface of the diaphragm. The utilization of radiotherapy appears at present to be limited to earlier disease and to patients with minimal residual disease after surgery, although even here there is need of well designed prospective phase III trials. There are too few valid studies comparing radiotherapy with chemotherapy for stages I and II disease.

3. A large number of reports in the literature confirm that chemotherapy with alkylating agents can produce responses in 30%-60% of patients with advanced disease. Experience with other solid tumors suggest strongly that an improved complete response rate with any particular chemotherapeutic regimen correlates well with eventual improved survival rate. Several nonalkylating-agent chemotherapeutic drugs have been identified with considerable activity in ovarian cancer, such as hexamethylmelamine, doxorubicin, and cisplatin, carboplatin, and Taxol. Several reports have confirmed significant improvement in complete response and negative second-look laparotomy rates

when a combination of drugs containing two or more of these active agents was used. It is hoped that, as in other solid tumors, these reports of improved complete response rates will eventuate in later reports of improved overall survival rates.

4. Prognosis depends very much on stage, but other factors are also pertinent. Undifferentiated lesions have a worse prognosis regardless of stage. Patients with bulk residual disease following laparotomy are much less likely to respond to subsequent therapy.

5. Chemotherapy appears to be the most effective method of controlling ascites and pleural effusions. First-line chemotherapy will be effective for varying periods in 90% of patients.

6. The use of intraperitoneal colloidal isotopes such as ^{32}P has great theoretic value for patients with microscopic residual disease after laparotomy. However, maldistribution of the drug within the peritoneal cavity in a patient postoperatively may buffer the theoretical advantages. No positive prospective randomized study comparing intraperitoneal colloidal isotopes with other modalities such as chemotherapy has yet been reported.

7. The efficacy of intraperitoneal chemotherapy for salvage therapy and as first-line postoperative therapy needs further investigation. Randomized trials comparing intraperitoneal with systemic chemotherapy will be necessary to answer the question. Although there appear to be theoretic advantages in achieving high drug concentrations in the peritoneal cavity, only clinical trials can translate this into a clinical advantage.

8. There appears to be a reasonable explanation of the paradox of the invariable inverse relationship between cell number and curability with drugs on one hand, and the difficulty in achieving better results when treating micrometastasis on the other. The explanation resides in the hypothesis put forth by Goldie and Coldman. They propose that, as in bacteria, mutation toward resistance to drugs is an inherent property of the unstable cancer cell, and resistance occurs often by virtue of change in the cell membrane. As proposed, this tendency to mutate occurs at very low cell numbers, well below the level of clinical detectability, and increases dramatically with small increases in tumor mass. Depending on the mutation rate, a tumor can go from sensitive to resistant in 6 doublings or a 2-log increase in cell number. The use of multiple effective drugs covers more cell lines resistant to one drug. This hypothesis is the best explanation for the effectiveness of combination chemotherapy in most human neoplasms. It is hoped this will apply also to epithelial ovarian cancer.

BIBLIOGRAPHY

Incidence, epidemiology, and etiology

Amos CI, Struewing JP: Genetic epidemiology of epithelial ovarian cancer, *Cancer* 71(2):566, 1993.

Amos CI et al: Age at onset for familial epithelial ovarian cancer, *JAMA* 268(14):1896, 1992.

Berchuck A, Kamel A, Whitaker R et al: Overexpression of Her-2/neu is associated with poor survival in advanced epithelial ovarian cancer, *Cancer Res* 50:4087, 1990.

Borrie PM, Thomson JD: Familial ovarian carcinoma, *NZ Med J* 95:147, 1982.

Buller RE et al: Familial ovarian cancer, *Gynecol Oncol* 51:160, 1993.

Casagrande JT et al: "Incessant ovulation" and ovarian cancer, *Lancet* 2:170, 1979.

Chen KTK, Schooley JL, Flam MS: Peritoneal carcinomatosis after prophylactic oophorectomy in familial ovarian cancer syndrome, *Obstet Gynecol* 66:935, 1985.

Cramer DW et al: Ovarian cancer and talc: a case-control study, *Cancer* 50:372, 1982.

Enomoto T, Inoue M, Perantoni AO et al: K-ras activation in neoplasms of the human female reproductive tract, *Cancer Res* 50:6139, 1990.

Finlay C, Hinds P, Levine A: The p53 protooncogene can act as a suppressor of transformation, *Cell* 57:1083, 1989.

Franceschi S, La Vecchia C, Mangioni C: Familial ovarian cancer: eight more families, *Gynecol Oncol* 13:31, 1982.

Genadry R et al: Primary, papillary peritoneal neoplasia, *Obstet Gynecol* 58:730, 1981.

Greene MH, Clark JW, Blayney DW: The epidemiology of ovarian cancer, *Sem Oncol* 11:209, 1984.

Gross TP, Schlesslman JJ: The estimated effect of oral contraceptive use on the cumulative risk of epithelial ovarian cancer, *Obstet Gynecol* 83(3):419, 1994.

Hankinson SE et al: A quantitative assessment of oral contraceptive use and risk of ovarian cancer, *Obstet Gynecol* 80(4):708, 1992.

Harlow BL et al: Perineal exposure to take and ovarian cancer risk: *Obstet Gynecol* 80(1):19, 1992.

Heintz APM, Hacker NF, Lagasse LD: Epidemiology and etiology of ovarian cancer: a review, *Obstet Gynecol* 66:127, 1985.

Henderson BE, Ross RK, Pike MC: Hormonal chemoprevention of cancer in women, *Science* 259:633, 1993.

Jacobs I, Oram D: Prevention of ovarian cancer: a survey of the practice of prophylactic oophorectomy by fellows and members of the Royal College of Obstetricians and Gynaecologists, *Br J Obstet Gynaecol* 96:510, 1989.

Kerlikowske K, Brown JS, Grady DG: Should women with familial ovarian cancer undergo prophylactic oophorectomy? *Obstet Gynecol* 80(4):700, 1992.

Koch M, Gaedke H, Jenkins H: Family history of ovarian cancer patients: a case-control study, *Int J Epidemiol* 18:782, 1989.

Longo DL, Young RC: Cosmetic talc and ovarian cancer, *Lancet* 2:349, 1979.

Lurain JR, Piver MS: Familial ovarian cancer, *Gynecol Oncol* 8:185, 1979.

Lynch HT, Conway T, Lynch J: Hereditary ovarian cancer, *Cancer Genet Cytogenet* 52:161, 1991.

Lynch et al: Hereditary ovarian cancer: heterogeneity in age at onset, *Cancer* 71:S74, 1993.

Lynch HT, Fitzsimmons ML, Conway TA et al: Hereditary carcinoma of the ovary and associated cancers: a study of two families, *Gynecol Oncol* 36:48, 1990.

Lynch HT, Severin MJ, Mooney MJ et al: Insurance adjudication favoring prophylactic surgery in hereditary breast–ovarian cancer syndrome, *Gynecol Oncol* 57:23, 1995.

Lynch HT, Watson P, Bewtra C, et al: Hereditary ovarian cancer, *Cancer* 67(5):1460, 1991.

Matheson JAB, Matheson H, Anderson SA: Familial ovarian cancer: how rare is it? *J Royal Coll Gen Prac* 312:743, 1981.

McGowan L et al: The women at risk for developing ovarian cancer, *Gynecol Oncol 7:325, 1979.*

Menczer J et al: Possible role of mumps virus in the etiology of ovarian cancer, *Cancer* 43:1375, 1979.

Mori M, Harabuchi I, Miyake H et al: Reproductive, genetic, and dietary risk factors for ovarian cancer, *Am J Epidemiol* 128:771, 1988.

O'Brien TJ, Bannon GA, Bard DS et al: Expression of the ras oncogene in gynecologic tumors, *Am J Obstet Gynecol* 160:344, 1989.

Parazzini F, La Vecchia C, Negri E et al: Menstrual factor and the risk of epithelial ovarian cancer, *J Clin Epidemiol* 42(5):443, 1989.

Piver MS et al: Familial ovarian cancer registry, *Obstet Gynecol* 64 (2):195, 1984.

Piver MS et al: *Familial ovarian cancer registry*, Newsletter of the Gilda Radner Ovarian Cancer Registry, April 1989.

Piver MS et al: Familial ovarian cancer, a report of 558 families from the Gilda Radner familial ovarian cancer registry 1981-1991, *Cancer* 71(2):582, 1993.

Riggs JE: Rising ovarian cancer mortality in the elderly: a manifestation of differential survival, *Gynecol Oncol*, 58:64, 1995.

Rosenburg L et al: Epithelial ovarian cancer and combination oral contraceptives, *JAMA* 247:3210, 1982.

Rossing MA et al: Ovarian tumors in a cohort of infertile women, *N Engl J Med* 771:1994.

Schildkraut JM, Thompson WD: Familial ovarian cancer: a population-based case-control study, *Am J Epidemiol* 128:456, 1988.

Stanford JL: Oral contraceptives and neoplasia of the ovary, *Contraception* 43:543, 1991.

Storms R, Bose H: Oncogenes, protooncogenes, and signal transduction: toward a unified theory? *Adv Virus Res* 37:1, 1989.

Tobacman JK et al: Intra-abdominal carcinomatosis after prophylactic oophorectomy in ovarian cancer-prone families, *Lancet* 2(8302):795, 1982.

Venter PF: Ovarian epithelial cancer and chemical carcinogenesis, *Gynecol Oncol* 12:281, 1981.

Whittemore AS: The risk of ovarian cancer after treatment for infertility 331:805, 1994.

Whittemore AS et al: Characteristics relating to ovarian cancer risk: collaborative analysis of 12 US case control studies, *Am J Epidemiol* 136:1184, 1992.

Yancik R, Ries LG, Yates JW: Ovarian cancer in the elderly: an analysis of surveillance, epidemiology, and end-results program data, *Am J Obstet Gynecol* 154:639, 1986.

Signs, symptoms, and attempts at early detection

Alagoz T et al: What is a normal CA 125 level? *Gynecol Oncol* 53:93, 1994.

Aure JC, Hoeg K, Kolstad P: Psammoma bodies in serous carcinoma of the ovary: a prognostic study, *Am J Obstet Gynecol* 109:113, 1971.

Bast RC et al: Coordinate elevation of serum markers in ovarian cancer but not in benign disease, *Cancer* 68:1758, 1991.

Bergman F: Carcinoma of the ovary: a clinicopathological study of 86 autopsied cases with special reference to mode of spread, *Acta Obstet Gynecol Scand* 45:211, 1966.

Bourne TH et al: Ultrasound screening for familial ovarian cancer, *Gynecol Oncol* 43:92, 1991.

Bourne TH et al : Screening early familial ovarian cancer with transvaginal ultrasonography and color flow imaging, *Br Med J* 306:1025, 1993

Bret PM et al: Transvaginal US-guided aspiration of ovarian cysts and solid pelvic masses, *Radiology* 185:377, 1992.

Buchsbaum HJ et al: Surgical staging of carcinoma of the ovaries, *Surg Gynecol Obstet* 169:226, 1989.

Burghardt E et al: Patterns of pelvic and para-aortic lymph node involvement in ovarian cancer, *Gynecol Oncol* 40:103, 1991.

Burghardt E, Girardi F, LaHousen M et al: Patterns of pelvic and paraaortic lymph node involvement in ovarian cancer, *Gynecol Oncol* 40(2):103, 1991.

Campbell S et al: Transabdominal ultrasound screening for early ovarian cancer, *Br Med J* 299 (6712):1363, 1989.

Campbell S et al: Novel screening strategies for early ovarian cancer by transabdominal ultrasonography, *Br J Obstet Gynecol* 97:304, 1990.

Carlson KJ, Skates SJ, Singer DE: Screening for ovarian cancer, *Annal Intern Med* 121:124, 1994.

Chung A, Birnbaum SJ: Ovarian cancer associated with pregnancy, *Obstet Gynecol* 41:211, 1973.

Cohen CJ, Jennings TS: Screening for ovarian cancer: the role of noninvasive imaging techniques, *Am J Obstet Gynecol* 170:1088, 1994.

Crade M: Long Beach Memorial Medical Center Program in early detection of ovarian carcinoma with transvaginal sonography. Potentials and limitations. AC Fleischer and HW Jones, eds, Raven Press, New York, pp 177-182, 1993.

Creasman WT, Abu-Ghazaleh S, Schmidt HJ: Retroperitoneal metastatic spread of ovarian cancer, *Gynecol Oncol* 6:447, 1978.

Creasman WT, DiSaia PJ: Screening in ovarian cancer, *Am J Obstet Gynecol* 165:7, 1991.

DePriest PD et al: Ovarian cancer screening in asymptomatic postmenopausal women, *Gynecol Oncol* 51:205, 1993.

Droegemueller W: Screening for ovarian carcinoma: hopeful and wishful thinking, *Am J Obstet Gynecol* 170:1095, 1994.

Einhorn N: Early diagnosis and screening, *Ovarian Cancer* 6:843, 1992.

Graham JB, Graham RM, Schueller EF: Pre-clinical detection of ovarian cancer, *Cancer* 17:1414, 1964.

Hermann VJ et al: Sonography and ovarian cancer, *Obstet Gynecol* 69:777, 1987.

Higgins RV et al: Transvaginal sonography as a screening method for ovarian cancer, *Gynecol Oncol* 34:402, 1989.

Hirabayashi K, Graham J: Genesis of ascites in ovarian cancer, *Am J Obstet Gynecol* 106:492, 1970.

Jacobs I et al: Multimodal approach to screening for ovarian cancer, *Lancet* 1:268, 1988.

Jacobs I et al: Prevalence screening for ovarian cancer in postmenopausal women by CA-125 measurement and ultrasonography, *Br Med J* 306:1030, 1993.

Johansson H: Clinical aspects of metastatic ovarian cancer of extragenital origin, *Acta Obstet Gynecol Scand* 39:681, 1960.

Karlan BY et al: A multidisciplinary approach to early detection of ovarian cancer: rational, protocol design, and early results, *Am J Obstet Gynecol* 169:494, 1993.

Knapp RC, Friedman EA: Aortic lymph node metastases in early ovarian cancer, *Am J Obstet Gynecol* 119:1013, 1974.

Koch M, Gaedke H, Jenkins H: Family history of ovarian cancer patients: a case-control study. *Int J Epidemiol* 18(4):782, 1989.

Kurjak A et al: Transvaginal ultrasound, color flow, and Doppler wave form of the postmenopausal adnexal mass, *Obste Gynecol* 80:917, 1992.

Layfield LJ, Heaps JM, Berek JS: Fine Needle aspiration cytology accuracy with palpable gynecologic neoplasms, *Gynecol Oncol* 40:70, 1991.

Lifshitz S: Ascites pathophysiology and control measures, *Int J Radiat Oncol Biol Phys* 8:1423, 1982.

McGowan L: Ovarian cancer after hysterectomy, *Obstet Gynecol* 69(3):386, 1987.

Nieminen V, Purola E: Stage and prognosis of ovarian cystadenocarcinomas, *Acta Obstet Gynecol Scand* 49:49, 1970.

Olt GJ, Burchuck A, Bast RC: Gynecologic tumor markers, *Sem Sur Oncol* 6:305, 1990.

Ovarian Cancer: Screening, treatment, and follow-up. NIH Census Statement 12:1, 1994.

Piver MS, Barlow JJ, Lele SB: Incidence of subclinical metastasis in stage I and II ovarian carcinoma, *Obstet Gynecol* 52:100, 1978.

Purola E, Nieminen V: Does rupture of cystic carcinoma during operation influence the prognosis? *Am Clin Gynecol Fenn* 57:615, 1968.

Sampson JA: Endometrial carcinoma of ovary arising in endometrial tissue in that organ, *Arch Surg* 10:1, 1925.

Schwartz PE et al: Early detection of ovarian cancer: background, rationale, and structure of the Yale early detection program, *Yale J Biol Med* 64:557, 1991.

Trimble EL et al: Diagnosing the correct ovarian cancer syndrome, *Obstet Gynecol* 78:1023, 1991.

Trimbos JB, Bolis B, Pecorelli S: The surgical staging of ovarian cancer: current practice in 15 European countries, *Int J Gynecol Cancer* 1:89, 1991.

van Nagell JR et al: Ovarian cancer screening in asymptomatic postmenopausal women by transvaginal sonography, *Cancer* 68:458, 1991.

Young RC et al: Staging laparotomy in early ovarian cancer, *Proc Am Assoc Cancer Res* 20:399, 1979.

Borderline malignant epithelial neoplasms

Bell DA, Scully RE: Serous borderline tumors of the peritoneum, *Am J Sur Pathol* 14:230, 1990.

Bell DA, Weinstock MA, Scully RE: Peritoneal implants of ovarian serous borderline tumors, *Cancer* 62:2212, 1988.

Carter J et al: Pseudomyxoma peritonei: a review, *Int J Gynecol Cancer* 1:243, 1991.

Carter J et al: Borderline and invasive epithelial ovarian tumors in young women, *Obstet Gynecol* 82:752, 1993.

Drescher CW: DNA content of borderline tumors: a new marker, *Contemporary OB/GYN* 63, March 1995.

Fort MG et al: Evidence for the efficacy of adjuvant therapy in epithelial ovarian tumors of low malignant potential, *Gynecol Oncol* 32:69, 1989.

Kærn J, Trope CG, Abeler VM: A retrospective study of 370 borderline tumors of the ovary treated at the Norwegian radium hospital from 1970 to 1982, *Cancer* 71:1810, 1993.

Kurman RJ, Trimble CL: The behavior of serous tumors of low malignant potential: are they ever malignant? *Int J Gynecol Pathol* 12:120, 1993.

Link CJ, Kohn E, Reed E: Review, The relationship between borderline ovarian tumors and epithelial ovarian carcinoma: epidemiologic, pathologic, and molecular aspects, *Gynecol Oncol* 60: 347, 1996.

Manchul LA et al: Borderline epithelial ovarian tumors: a review of 81 cases with an assessment of the impact of treatment, *Int J Rad Oncol Biol Phys* 22:867, 1992.

Menzin AW et al: The accuracy of a frozen section diagnosis of borderline ovarian malignancy, *Gynecol Oncol* 59:183, 1995.

Nikrui N: Survey of clinical behavior of patients with borderline epithelial tumors of the ovary, *Gynecol Oncol* 12:107, 1981.

Shanks HGI: Pseudomyxoma peritonei, *J Obstet Gynaecol Br Commonw* 68:212, 1961.

Sutton GP et al: Stage III ovarian tumors of low malignant potential treated with cisplatin combination therapy (A Gynecologic Oncology Group study), *Gynecol Oncol* 41:230, 1991.

Treatment of malignant epithelial neoplasms

Alberts D et al: Improved efficacy of carboplatin (CarboP) cyclophosphamide (CPA) vs Cisplatin (CisP)/CPA: preliminary report of a phase III randomized trial in stages III-IV suboptimal ovarian cancer (OV CA), *Proc Amer Soc Clin Oncol* 8:151, 1989.

Alberts DS et al: Combination chemotherapy for alkylator-resistant ovarian carcinoma: a preliminary report of a Southwest Oncology Group trial, *Cancer Treat Rep* 63:301, 1979.

Alberts DS et al: Randomized study of chemoimmunotherapy for advanced ovarian carcinoma: a preliminary report of a Southwest Oncology Group study, *Cancer Treat Rep* 63:325, 1979.

Alberts DS et al: Improved efficacy of carboplatin plus cyclophosphamide versus cisplatin plus cyclophosphamide: preliminary report by the Southwest Oncology Group of a phase III randomized trial in stages III and IV suboptimal ovarian cancer. In Bunn PA et al, editors: *Carboplatin (JM-8): current perspectives and future directions*, Philadelphia, 1990, Saunders.

Altaras MM et al: Primary peritoneal papillary serous adenocarcinoma: clinical and management aspects, *Gynecol Oncol* 40:230, 1991.

Aure JC, Hoeg K, Kolstad P: Clinical and histologic studies of ovarian carcinoma: long-term follow-up of 990 cases, *Obstet Gynecol* 37:1, 1971.

Bales G et al: Adriamycin ovarian cancer patients resistant to cyclophosphamide, *Eur J Cancer* 14:1401, 1978.

Behrens BC et al: Characterization of a cisplatin-resistant human ovarian cancer cell line and its use in evaluation of cisplatin analogs, *Cancer Res* 47:414, 1987.

Benedry R et al: Primary, papillary peritoneal neoplasia, *Obstet Gynecol* 58:730, 1981.

Bertelsen K et al: A randomized study of cyclophosphamide and cisplatin with or without doxorubicin in advanced ovarian carcinoma, *Gynecol Oncol* 28:161, 1987.

Blum RH, Carter SK: Adriamycin: a new anticancer drug with significant clinical activity, *Ann Intern Med* 80:249, 1974.

Brady L et al: Radiotherapy, chemotherapy, and combined therapy in stage III epithelial ovarian cancer, *Proc Am Assoc Cancer Res* 20:218, 1979.

Braly P, Doroshaw J, Hoff S: Technical aspects of intraperitoneal chemotherapy in abdominal carcinomatosis, *Gynecol Oncol* 25:319, 1986.

Briggs MH, Caldwell ADS, Pitchford AG: The treatment of cancer by progestogens, *Hosp Med Lond* 2:63, 1967.

Briscoe KE et al: Cis-dichlorodiammineplatinum (II) and Adriamycin treatment of advanced ovarian cancer, *Cancer Treat Rep* 62:2027, 1978.

Bruckner HW et al: Cis-platinum (DDP) for combination chemotherapy of ovarian carcinoma: improved response rate and survival, *Proc Am Assoc Cancer Res* 19:373, 1978.

Bruckner HW et al: Prospective controlled randomized trial comparing combination chemotherapy of advanced ovarian carcinoma with adriamycin and cis-platinum ± cyclophosphamide and hexamethylmelamine, *Proc Am Assoc Cancer Res* 20:414, 1979.

Bruckner HW et al: Improved chemotherapy for ovarian cancer with cis-diamminedichloroplatinum and Adriamycin, *Cancer* 47:2288, 1981.

Bruckner HW et al: Modulation and intensification of a cyclophosphamide, hexamethylmelamine, doxorubicin, and cisplatin ovarian cancer regimen, *Obstet Gynecol* 73 (3):349, 1989.

Canetta R, Bragman K, Smaldone L et al: Carboplatin: current status and future prospects, *Cancer Treat Rev* 15(suppl B):17, 1988.

Conte PF et al: A randomized trial comparing cisplatin plus cyclophosphamide versus cisplatin, doxorubicin and cyclophosphamide in advanced ovarian cancer, *J Clin Oncol* 4:965, 1986.

Creasman WT et al: Chemoimmunotherapy in the management of primary stage III ovarian cancer: a Gynecologic Oncology Group study, *Cancer Treat Rep* 63:319, 1979.

Creasman WT et al: A randomized trial of cyclophosphamide, doxorubicin, and cisplatin with or without bacillus Calmette-Guérin in patients with suboptimal stage III and IV ovarian cancer: a Gynecologic Oncology Group study, *Gynecol Oncol* 39:239, 1990.

Crozier MA et al: Clear cell carcinoma of the ovary: a study of 59 cases, *Gynecol Oncol* 35:199, 1989.

Decker DG et al: Cyclophosphamide plus cis-platinum in combination: treatment program for stage III or IV ovarian carcinoma, *Obstet Gynecol* 60:481, 1982.

Delgato G et al: Single agent vs combination chemotherapy for ovarian cancer, *Am J Clin Oncol* 8:33, 1985.

De Palo G, Demicheli R, Valagussa P: Prospective study with HEXA-CAF combination in ovarian carcinoma, *Cancer Chemother Pharmacol* 5:157, 1981.

De Palo GM, De Lena M, Bonadonna G: Adriamycin versus Adriamycin plus melphalan in advanced ovarian carcinoma, *Cancer Treat Rep* 61:355, 1977.

Dylrymple JC et al: Extraovarian peritoneal serous papillary carcinoma: a clinicopathologic study of 31 cases, *Cancer* 64:110, 1989.

Edelmann DZ et al: Carboplatin and etoposide as first line chemotherapy in advanced epithelial ovarian cancer, *Int J Gynecol Oncol* 5:443, 1995.

Ehrlich CE et al: Chemotherapy for stage III-IV epithelial ovarian cancer with cis-dichlorodiammineplatinum (II), Adriamycin, and cyclophosphamide: a preliminary report, *Cancer Treat Rep* 63:281, 1979.

Ehrlich CE et al: Treatment of advanced epithelial ovarian cancer using cisplatin, Adriamycin, and Cytoxan—the Indiana University experience, *Clin Obstet Gynecol* 10:325, 1983.

Einhorn H, Williams SD: The role of cis-platinum in solid-tumor therapy, *N Engl J Med* 300:289, 1979.

Einhorn H et al: Ondansetron: a new antiemetic for patients receiving cisplatin chemotherapy, *J Clin Oncol* 8(4):731, 1990.

Foyle A, Al-Jaba M, McCaughey WTE: Papillary peritoneal tumors in women, *Am J Surg Pathol* 5:241, 1981.

Frei E et al: New approaches to cancer chemotherapy with methotrexate, *N Engl J Med* 292:846, 1975.

Fromm G, Gershenson DM, Silva EG: Papillary serous carcinoma of the peritoneum, *Obstet Gynecol* 75(1):89, 1990.

Gaver RC et al: The disposition of carboplatin in ovarian cancer patients, *Cancer Chemother Pharmacol* 22:263, 1988.

Geisler HE, Minor JR, Eastlund ME: Treatment of advanced ovarian carcinoma with high dose, intravenous cyclophosphamide, *Gynecol Oncol* 4:43, 1976.

Gershenson DM et al: Combined Cisplatin and carboplatin chemotherapy for treatment of advanced epithelial ovarian cancer, *Gynecol Oncol* 58:349, 1995.

Gill I et al: Carboplatin (CBDCA): clinical tolerance and kinetics of platinum-DNA adduct formation, *Clin Res* 37:143, 1989.

Goff BA et al: Clear cell carcinoma of the ovary: a distinct histologic type with poor prognosis and resistance to platinum-based chemotherapy in stage III disease, *Gynecol Oncol* 60:412, 1996.

Gooneratne S, Sassone M, Blaustein A, et al: Serous surface papillary carcinoma of the ovary: a clinicopathologic study of 16 cases, *Int J Gynecol Pathol* 1:258, 1982.

Gray LA, Barnes ML: Endometrioid carcinoma of the ovary, *Obstet Gynecol* 29:694, 1967.

Greene MH et al: Acute nonlymphatic leukemia after therapy with alkylating agents for ovarian cancer: a study of five randomized clinical trials, *N Engl J Med* 307:1416, 1982.

Gruppe Interregionale Cooperativo Oncologico Ginecologia: Randomized comparison of cisplatin with cyclophosphamide/cisplatin and with cyclophosphamide/doxorubicin/cisplatin in advanced ovarian cancer, *Lancet* 11:353, 1987.

Gruppo Interregionale Cooperativo Oncologia Ginecologica: Long-term results of a randomized trial comparing cisplatin with cisplatin and cyclophosphamide with cisplatin, cyclophosphamide and adriamycin in advanced ovarian cancer, *Gynecol Oncol* 45:115, 1992.

Hainsworth JD et al: Advanced ovarian cancer: long-term results of treatment with intensive cisplatin-based chemotherapy of brief duration, *Ann Intern Med* 108:165, 1988.

Hainsworth JD et al: The role of hexamethylmelamine in the combination chemotherapy of advanced ovarian cancer: a comparison of hexamethylmelamine, cyclophosphamide, doxorubicin, and cisplatin (H-CAP) versus cyclophosphamide, doxorubicin, and cisplatin (CAP), *Am J Clin Oncol* 13(5):410, 1990.

Hansen HH et al: New cystostaxic drugs in ovarian cancer, *Annal Oncol* 4:S63, 1993.

Harris CC: The carcinogenicity of anticancer drugs: a hazard to man, *Cancer* 37:1014, 1976.

Hoskins WJ: The influence of cytoreductive surgery on progression-free interval and survival in epithelial ovarian cancer, *Clin Obstet Gynecol* 3:59, 1989.

Hreshchyshyn MM et al: The role of adjuvant therapy in stage I ovarian cancer, *Am J Obstet Gynecol* 138:139, 1980.

Imachi M et al: Clear cell carcinoma of the ovary: a clinicopathologic analysis of 34 cases, *Int J Gynecol Cancer* 1:113, 1991.

Izquierdo MA et al: Ovarian Carcinoma preceded by cerebral metastasis: review of the literature, *Gynecol Oncol* 45:206, 1992.

James CA et al: Pharmacokinetics of intravenous and oral sodium 2-mercaptoethane sulfonate (mesna) in normal subjects, *Br J Clin Pharm* 23(5):561, 1987.

Jenison EL et al: Clear cell adenocarcinoma of the ovary: a clinical analysis and comparison with serous carcinoma, *Gynecol Oncol* 32:65, 1989.

Johnson BL et al: Hexamethylmelamine in alkylating agent-resistant ovarian carcinoma, *Cancer* 42:2157, 1978.

Johnson CE et al: Advanced ovarian cancer: therapy with radiation and cyclophosphamide in a random series, *AJR* 114:136, 1972.

Kannerstein M, Churg J, McCaughey WTE: Mesothelioma or papillary carcinoma, *Am J Obstet Gynecol* 127:306, 1977.

Kaslow RA, Wisch N, Glass JL: Acute leukemia following cytotoxic chemotherapy, *JAMA* 219:75, 1972.

Katzenstein AL et al: Proliferative serous tumors of the ovary: histologic features and prognosis, *Am J Surg Pathol* 2:339, 1978.

Kurman RJ, Craig JM: Endometrioid and clear cell carcinoma of the ovary, *Cancer* 29:1653, 1972.

Lele SB et al: Peritoneal papillary carcinoma, *Gynecol Oncol* 31:315, 1988.

LeRoux PE et al: Cerebral metastases from ovarian carcinoma, *Cancer* 67:2194, 1991.

Levi MM: Antigenicity of ovarian and cervical malignancies with a view toward possible immunodiagnosis, *Am J Obstet Gynecol* 109:689, 1971.

Levin L, Hryniuk WM: Dose intensity analysis of chemotherapy regimens in ovarian carcinoma, *J Clin Oncol* 4:965, 1986.

Manetta A et al: Hexamethylmelamine as a single second-line agent in ovarian cancer, *Gynecol Oncol* 36:93, 1990.

Mangioni C et al: Chemotherapy with cis-platinum, Adriamycin, cyclophosphamide or hexamethylmelamine, Adriamycin and Cytoxan in ovarian cancer, *Proc Am Assoc Cancer Res* 21:149, 1980.

Mangioni C et al: Randomized trial of cisplatin versus cisplatin plus cyclophosphamide versus platin plus cyclophosphamide plus doxorubicin in advanced epithelial ovarian cancer. Paper presented at Society of Gynecologic Oncologists, Palm Springs, 1986.

Marchetti DL et al: Treatment of advanced ovarian carcinoma in the elderly, *Gynecol Oncol* 49:86, 1993.

Marsoni S et al: Prognostic factors in advanced epithelial ovarian cancer, *Br J Cancer* 62:444, 1990.

McGuire WP et al: Taxol: a unique antineoplastic agent with significant activity in advanced ovarian epithelial neoplasms, *Ann Intern Med* 111(4):273, 1989.

McGuire WP et al: A phase III trial comparing cisplatin/Cytoxan and cisplatin/Taxol in advanced ovarian cancer, *Proc. ASCO* 12:255, 1993.

Mills SE, Andersen WA, Fechner RE, Austin MB: Serous surface papillary carcinoma: a clinicopathologic study of 10 cases and comparison with stage III-IV ovarian serous carcinoma, *Am J Surg Pathol* 12:827, 1988.

Munnell EW: Is conservative therapy ever justified in stage I (Ia) cancer of the ovary? *Am J Obstet Gynecol* 103:641, 1969.

Myers RA et al: Combination chemotherapy of ovarian carcinoma, *Proc Am Assoc Cancer Res* 20:405, 1979.

Neijt JP et al: Hexa-CAF combination chemotherapy and other multiple-drug regimens in advanced ovarian carcinoma: present and future, *Neth J Med* 22:38, 1979.

Norris HJ, Robinowitz M: Ovarian adenocarcinoma of mesonephric type, *Cancer* 28:1074, 1971.

Omura G et al: A randomized trial of cyclophosphamide and doxorubicin with or without cisplatin in advanced ovarian carcinoma, *Cancer* 57:1725, 1986.

Omura GA et al: Randomized trial of melphalan vs. melphalan plus hexamethylmelamine vs. Adriamycin plus cyclophosphamide in advanced ovarian adenocarcinoma, *Proc Am Assoc Cancer Res* 20:358, 1979.

Omura GA et al: A randomized trial of cyclophosphamide plus cisplatin with or without Adriamycin in ovarian carcinoma, *Proc Am Soc Clin Oncol* 6:112, 1987.

Omura GA et al: Randomized trial of cyclophosphamide plus cisplatin with or without doxorubicin in ovarian cancer: a Gynecologic Oncology Group study, *J Clin Oncol* 7:457, 1989.

Omura GA et al: Long-term follow-up and prognostic factor analysis in advanced ovarian carcinoma: the Gynecologic Oncology Group experience, *J Clin Oncol* 7:1138, 1991.

Ovarian cancer meta-analysis project. Cyclophosphamide plus cis-platin versus cyclophosphamide, doxorubicin and cis-platin chemotherapy of ovarian carcinoma: a meta-analysis, *J Clin Oncol* 9:1668, 1991.

Ozols RF: Optimal dosing with carboplatin, *Sem Oncol* 16(Suppl 2):14, 1989.

Ozols RF et al: Phase I and pharmacologic studies of Adriamycin administered intraperitoneally to patients with ovarian cancer, *Cancer Res* 42:4265, 1982.

Parker LM et al: High-dose methotrexate with leucovorin rescue in ovarian cancer: a phase II study, *Cancer Treat Rep* 63:275, 1979.

Parker LM et al: Combination chemotherapy with Adriamycin- cyclophosphamide for advanced ovarian carcinoma, *Cancer* 46:669, 1980.

Piccart MJ et al: Intraperitoneal chemotherapy: technical experience at five institutions, *Sem Oncol* 12:90, 1985.

Ransom DT et al: Papillary serous carcinoma of the peritoneum: a review of 33 cases treated with platin-based chemotherapy, *Cancer* 66:1091, 1990.

Reimer RR et al: Acute leukemia after alkylating agent therapy of ovarian cancer, *N Engl J Med* 297:177, 1977.

Rosen GF, Lurain JR, Newton M: Hexamethylmelamine in ovarian cancer after failure of cisplatin-based multiple-agent chemotherapy, *Gynecol Oncol* 27:173, 1987.

Runowicz CD et al: Catheter complications associated with intraperitoneal chemotherapy, *Gynecol Oncol* 24:41, 1986.

Slayton RE, Pagano M, Creech RH: Progestin therapy for advanced ovarian cancer: a phase II Eastern Cooperative Oncology Group trial, *Cancer Treat Rep* 65:895, 1981.

Smith JP, Day TG: Review of ovarian cancer at the University of Texas Systems Cancer Center, MD Anderson Hospital and Tumor Institute, *Am J Obstet Gynecol* 135:984, 1979.

Sotrel G et al: Acute leukemia in advanced ovarian carcinoma after treatment with alkylating agents, *Obstet Gynecol* 47:67S, 1976.

Sutton GP et al: Ten-year follow-up of patients receiving cisplatin, doxorubicin, and cyclophosphamide chemotherapy for advanced epithelial ovarian carcinoma, *J Clin Oncol* 7:223, 1989.

Tobias JS, Griffiths CT: Management of ovarian carcinoma, *N Engl J Med* 294:818, 1976.

Trask C et al: A randomized trial of carboplatin versus iproplatin in untreated advanced ovarian cancer, *J Clin Oncol* 9(7):1131, 1991.

Trope C et al: High-dose medroxyprogesterone acetate for the treatment of advanced ovarian carcinoma, *Cancer Treat Rep* 66:1441, 1982.

Unzulman RF: Advanced epithelial ovarian carcinoma: long term survival experience at the community hospital, *Am J Obstet Gynecol* 166:1663, 1992.

van Houwelingen JC et al: Predictability of the survival of patients with advanced ovarian cancer, *J Clin Oncol* 7:769, 1989.

Vogl SE, Greenwald E, Kaplan BH: The CHAD regimen (cyclophosphamide, hexamethylmelamine, Adriamycin and diamminedichloroplatinum) in advanced ovarian cancer, *Proc Am Assoc Cancer Res* 20:384, 1979.

Vogl SE et al: The CHAD and HAD regimens in advanced ovarian cancer: combination chemotherapy including cyclophosphamide, hexamethylmelamine, Adriamycin, and cis-dichlorodiammineplatinum (II), *Cancer Treat Rep* 63:311, 1979.

Ward HWC: Progestogen therapy for ovarian carcinoma, *J Obstet Gynaecol Br Commonw* 79:555, 1972.

Weeth JB: Large dose progestin palliation: valuable in solid tumor patients, *Proc Am Soc Clin Oncol* 15:165, 1974.

Wharton JT, Edwards CL, Rutledge FN: Long-term survival after chemotherapy for advanced epithelial ovarian carcinomas, *Am J Obstet Gynecol* 148:997, 1984.

Wharton JT et al: Hexamethylmelamine: an evaluation of its role in the treatment of ovarian cancer, *Am J Obstet Gynecol* 133:833, 1979.

Williams TJ, Symmonds RE, Litwak O: Management of unilateral and encapsulated ovarian cancer in young women, *Gynecol Oncol* 1:143, 1973.

Wiltshaw E, Kroner T: Phase II study of cis-dichorodiammineplatinum (II) (NSC-119875) in advanced adenocarcinoma of the ovary, *Cancer Treat Rep* 60:55, 1976.

Woodruff JD et al: Mucinous cystadenocarcinoma of the ovary, *Obstet Gynecol* 51:483, 1978.

Young RC: Mechanisms to improve chemotherapy effectiveness, *Cancer* 65:815, 1990.

Young RC et al: Adjuvant therapy in stage I and stage II epithelial ovarian cancer: results of two prospective randomized trials, *N Engl J Med* 322:1021, 1990.

Young RE, et al: Advanced ovarian adenocarcinoma: a prospective clinical trial of melphalan (L-PAM) versus combination chemotherapy, *N Engl J Med* 299:1261, 1978.

Maximal surgical effort

Barakat RR, Benjamin I: Surgery for malignant gynecologic disease, *Curr Opin Obstet Gynecol* 5:311, 1993.

Bertelsen K, Hansen MK, Pederson PH: The prognostic and therapeutic value of second-look laparotomy in advanced ovarian cancer, *Br J Obstet Gynaecol* 95:1231, 1988.

Brand E, Pearlman N: Electrosurgical debulking of ovarian cancer: a new technique using the argon beam coagulator, *Gynecol Oncol* 39:115, 1990.

Burghardt E et al: Pelvic lymphadenectomy in operative treatment of ovarian cancer, *Am J Obstet Gynecol* 155:315, 1986.

Carson LF, Rubin SC: Secondary Cytoreduction—Thoughts on the "Pro" side, *Gynecol Oncol* 51:127, 1993. de Gramon A: Survival after second look laparotomy in advanced ovarian endothelial cancer, *Eur J Cancer Clin Oncol* 25:451, 1989.

Delgato G, Aram DH, Petrilli ES: Stage III epithelial ovarian cancer: the role of maximal surgical reduction, *Gynecol Oncol* 18:293, 1984.

Deppe G, Malviya VK, Malone JM: Debulking surgery for ovarian cancer with the Cavitron ultrasonic surgical aspirator (CUSA): a preliminary report, *Gynecol Oncol* 31:223, 1988.

Deppe G et al: Surgical approach to diaphragmatic metastases from ovarian cancer, *Gynecol Oncol* 24:258, 1986.

Edmonson JH et al: Different chemotherapeutic sensitivities and host factors affecting prognosis in advanced ovarian carcinoma versus minimal residual disease, *Cancer Treat Rep* 63:241, 1979.

Golberg GL et al: Lymph node sampling in patients with epithelial ovarian carcinoma, *Gynecol Oncol* 47:143, 1992.

Goodman HM et al: The role of cytoreductive surgery in the management of stage IV epithelial ovarian carcinoma, *Gynecol Oncol* 46:367, 1992.

Griffiths CT, Fuller AF: Intensive surgical and chemotherapeutic management of advanced ovarian cancer, *Surg Clin North Am* 58:1978.

Griffiths CT, Parker LM, Fuller AF: Role of cytoreductive surgical treatment in the management of advanced ovarian cancer, *Cancer Treat Rep* 63:235, 1979.

Guidozzi F, Ball JHS: Extensive primary cytoreductive surgery for advanced epithelial ovarian cancer, *Gynecol Oncol* 53:326, 1994.

Hacker NF et al: Primary cytoreductive surgery for epithelial cancer, *Obstet Gynecol* 61:413, 1983.

Heintz APM: Surgery in advanced ovarian carcinoma: is there proof to show the benefit? *Eur J Surg Oncol* 14:91, 1988.

Heintz APM, Hacker NF, Berek JS: Cytoreductive surgery in ovarian carcinoma: feasibility and morbidity, *Obstet Gynecol* 67:783, 1986.

Hoskins WJ: Influence of secondary cytoreduction at the time of second-look laparotomy on the survival of patients with epithelial ovarian carcinoma, *Gynecol Oncol* 34:365, 1989.

Hoskins WJ: The effect of diameter of largest residual disease on survival after primary cytoreductive surgery in patients with suboptimal residual epithelial ovarian carcinoma, *Am J Obstet Gynecol* 170:974, 1994.

Hoskins W, Rubin S, Dulaney E: The influence of secondary cytoreduction at the time of second-look laparotomy on the survival of patients with epithelial ovarian carcinoma, *Gynecol Oncol* 34:365, 1989.

Hoskins WJ et al: The influence of cytoreductive surgery on recurrence free interval and survival in small volume stage III epithelial ovarian cancer: a Gynecologic Oncology Group study, *Gynecol Oncol* 47:159, 1992.

Hunter RW, Alexander NDE, Soutter WP: Meta-analysis of surgery in advanced ovarian carcinoma: is maximum cytoreductive surgery an independent determinant of prognosis? *Am J Obstet Gynecol* 166, 1992.

Jänicke F et al: Radical surgical procedure improves survival time in patients with recurrent ovarian cancer, *Cancer* 70:2129, 1992.

Markman M, et al: Characteristics of patients with small volume residual ovarian cancer unresponsive to cisplatin based IP chemotherapy: lessons learned from a Gynecologic Oncology Group phase II trial of IP cisplatin and recombinant a-interferon, *Gynecol Oncol* 45:3, 1992.

Montz FJ, Schlaerth JB, Berek JS: Resection of diaphragmatic peritoneum and muscle: role in cytoreductive surgery for advanced ovarian cancer, *Gynecol Oncol* 35:338, 1989.

Morris M, Gershenson DM, Wharton JT: Secondary cytoreductive surgery in epithelial ovarian cancer: non-responders to first-line therapy, *Gynecol Oncol* 33:1, 1989.

Parker LM, et al: Adriamycin/cyclophosphamide and surgical treatment of advanced ovarian cancer, *Proc Am Assoc Cancer Res* 19:399, 1978.

Pecorelli S: Intervention debulking surgery improves survival in advanced epithelial ovarian cancer: EORTC Gynecologic Cancer Cooperative Groups Study, *Eur J Cancer*. Presented at the Society of Gynecologic Oncology 1996.

Potter ME: Secondary cytoreduction in ovarian cancer: Pro or Con? *Gynecol Oncol* 51:131, 1993.

Rubin SC: Surgery for ovarian cancer, *Ovarian Cancer* 6:851, 1992.

Segna RA et al: Secondary cytoreduction for ovarian cancer following cisplatin therapy, *J Clin Oncol* 11:434, 1993.

Stehman FB et al: Long-term follow-up and survival in stage III-IV epithelial ovarian cancer treated with cisplatin, Adriamycin and cyclophosphamide (PAC), *Proc Am Soc Clin Oncol*, C-593, 1983 (abstract).

Vaccarello L et al: Cytoreductive surgery in ovarian carcinoma patients with a documented previously complete surgical response, *Gynecol Oncol* 57:61, 1995.

Van der Burg MEL et al: The effect of debulking surgery after induction chemotherapy on the prognosis in advanced epithelial ovarian cancer, *N Engl J Med* 332:629, 1995.

Vogl SE et al: "Second-Effort" surgical resection for bulky ovarian cancer, *Cancer* 54:2220, 1980.

Williams L: The role of secondary cytoreductive surgery in epithelial ovarian malignancies, *Oncology* 6:25, 1992.

Role of radiation therapy

Carey M et al: Testing the validity of a prognostic classification in patients with surgically optimal ovarian carcinoma: a 15 year review, *Int J Gynecol Cancer* 3:24, 1993.

Clark DGC et al: The role of radiation therapy in the treatment of cancer of the ovary: results of 614 patients, *Prog Clin Cancer* 5:227, 1973.

Decker DG, Webb MJ, Holbrook MA: Radiogold treatment of epithelial cancer of the ovary: late results, *Am J Obstet Gynecol* 115:751, 1973.

Delclos L, Fletcher GH: Postoperative irradiation for ovarian carcinoma with the cobalt-60 moving strip technique, *Clin Obstet Gynecol* 12:993, 1969.

Delgado G et al: Paraaortic lymphadenectomy in gynecologic malignancies confined to the pelvis, *Obstet Gynecol* 50:418, 1977.

Dembo AJ: Abdominopelvic radiography in ovarian cancer: a 10 year experience, *Cancer* 55:2285, 1985.

Dembo AJ: Epithelial ovarian cancer: the role of radiotherapy, *Int J Radiat Oncol Biol Phys* 22:835, 1992.

Dembo AJ et al: The Princess Margaret Hospital study of ovarian cancer: stages I, II and asymptomatic III presentations, *Cancer Treat Rep* 63:249, 1979.

Dembo AJ et al: Prognostic factors in patients with stage I epithelial ovarian cancer, *Obstet Gynecol*, 75:263, 1990.

Hacker NF et al: Whole abdominal radiation as salvage therapy for epithelial ovarian cancer, *Obstet Gynecol* 65:60, 1985.

Hoskins WJ et al: Whole abdominal and pelvic irradiation in patients with minimal disease at second-look surgical reassessment for ovarian carcinoma, *Gynecol Oncol* 20:271, 1985.

Kottmeier HL: Ovarian cancer with special regard to radiotherapy, *AJR* 111:417, 1971.

Martinez A, Schram MS, Howes AE, Bagshaw MA: Postoperative radiation therapy for epithelial ovarian cancer: the curative role based on a 24-year experience, *J Clin Oncol* 3(7):901, 1985.

Menczer J et al: Abdominopelvic irradiation for stage II-IV ovarian carcinoma patients with limited or no residual disease at second-look laparotomy after completion of cis-platinum-based combination chemotherapy, *Gynecol Oncol* 24:149, 1986.

Mychalczak BR, Fuks Z: The current role of radiotherapy in the management of ovarian cancer, *Ovarian Cancer* 6:895, 1992.

Pezner RD: Limited epithelial carcinoma of the ovary treated with curative intent by the intraperitoneal instillation of radioactive colloids, *Cancer* 42:2563, 1978.

Piver MS et al: Intraperitoneal chromic phosphate in peritoneo-scopically confirmed stage I ovarian adenocarcinoma, *Am J Obstet Gynecol* 144:836, 1982.

Piver MS et al: Stage II invasive adenocarcinoma of the ovary: results of treatment by whole abdominal radiation plus pelvic boost versus pelvic radiation plus oral melphalan chemotherapy, *Gynecol Oncol* 23:168, 1986.

Rosenshein N, Leichner P, Vogelsang G: Radiocolloids in the treatment of ovarian cancer, *Obstet Gynecol Surg* 34:708, 1979.

Rosenshein N et al: The effect of volume on the distribution of substances instilled into the peritoneal cavity, *Gynecol Oncol* 6:106, 1978.

Sell A et al: Randomized study of whole-abdomen irradiation versus pelvic irradiation plus cyclophosphamide in treatment of early ovarian cancer, *Gynecol Oncol* 37:367, 1990.

Spanos WJ et al: Complications in the use of intra-abdominal ^{32}P for ovarian carcinoma, *Gynecol Oncol* 45:243, 1992.

Thomas GM: Radiotherapy in early ovarian cancer, *Gynecol Oncol* 55:S73, 1994.

Unzelman RF: Advanced epithelial ovarian carcinoma: long term survival experience at the Community Hospital, *Am J Obstet Gynecol* 166:1663, Abstract, 1992.

Vergae IB et al: Randomized trial comparing cisplatin with radioactive phosphorous or whole abdominal irradiation as adjuvant treatment of ovarian cancer, *Cancer* 69:741, 1992.

Vider M, Deland FH, Maruyama Y: Loculation as a contraindication to intracavitary ^{32}P—chromic phosphate therapy, letter, *J Nucl Med* 17:150, 1976.

Radioisotopes

Bolis G et al: Multicenter controlled trial in patients with epithelial ovarian cancer stage I, *Proc Int Gynecol Cancer Soc* 157, Abstract, 1989.

Chemotherapy

Alberts DS et al: Phase III study of intraperitoneal cisplatin-intravenous cyclophosphamide versus intravenous cisplatin-intravenous cyclophosphamide in patients with optimal disease stage III ovarian cancer: a SWOG-GOG-ECOG Intergroup study, *Int K Gynecol Cancer 6* (supplement) 1:28, 1996.

Alberts D: Cisplatin versus carboplatin in advanced ovarian cancer: an economic analysis, *Pharmacy & Therapeutics*, July 1994.

Alberts DS et al: Phase III study of intraperitoneal cisplatin-intravenous cyclophosphamide versus intravenous cisplatin-intravenous cyclophosphamide in patients with optimal disease stage III ovarian cancer: a SWOG-GOG-ECOG Intergroup study, *Int K Gynecol Cancer 6* (supplement) 1:28, 1996.

Bertelsen K, Bastholt L: High dose platinum chemotherapy in advanced ovarian cancer: a phase II study, *Gynecol Oncol* 44:79, 1992.

Bertelsen K et al: A prospective randomized comparison of 6 and 12 cycles of cyclophosphamide, adriamycin, and cisplatin in advanced epithelial ovarian cancer: a Danish ovarian study group trial (DACOVA), *Gynecol Oncol* 49:30, 1993.

Burger RA et al: Phase II trial of Navelbine in the treatment of women with advanced epithelial ovarian cancer, *Gynecol Oncol* 50:265, 1993.

Canetta R et al: Future directions for paclitaxel (Taxol\R) in gynecologic malignancies, *Int J Gynecol Cancer* 4:23, 1994.

Cavaletti G et al: Cisplatin induced peripheral neurotoxicity is dependent on total dose intensity and single dose intensity, *Cancer* 69:203, 1992.

Colombo N et al: Cisplatin dose intensity in advanced ovarian cancer: a randomized study of conventional dose versus dose intense cisplatin monochemotherapy, *Proc ASCO* 12:255, 1993.

Colombo N et al: Multimodality therapy of early-stage (FIGO I-II) ovarian cancer: review of surgical management and postoperative adjuvant treatment, *Int J Gynecol Cancer 6* (supplement) 1:13, 1996.

Dauplat J: High dose melphalan and autologous bone marrow support for treatment of ovarian carcinoma with positive second look operation, *Gynecol Oncol* 34:294, 1989.

Einzig AI et al: Phase II study and long term follow up of patients treated with Taxol for advanced ovarian adenocarcinoma, *J Clin Oncol* 10:1748, 1992.

Gershenson DM et al: The effect of prolonged cisplatin based chemotherapy on progression free survival in patients with optimal epithelial ovarian cancer; "maintenance" therapy reconsidered, *Gynecol Oncol* 47:7, 1992.

Hakes T et al: Randomized prospective trial of 5 versus 10 cycles of cyclophosphamide, doxorubicin, and cisplatin in advanced ovarian carcinoma, *Gynecol Oncol* 45:284, 1992.

Kotz KW, Schilder RJ: High dose chemotherapy and hematopoietic progenitor cell support for patients with epithelial ovarian cancer, *Semin Oncol* 22:250, 1995.

Kudelka AP et al: Phase II study of intravenous Topotecan as a 5-day infusion for refractory epithelial ovarian carcinoma, *J Clin Oncol* 14 (5):1552, 1996.

Markman M et al: Late effects of cisplatin-based chemotherapy on renal function in patients with ovarian cancer, *Gynecol Oncol* 41:217, 1991.

Markman M et al: Second-line platinum therapy in patients with ovarian cancer previously treated with cisplatin, *J Clin Oncol* 9(3):389, 1991.

Markman M et al: Control of carboplatin-induced emesis with a fixed low dose of granisetron (0.5 mg) plus dexamethasone, *Gynecol Oncol* 60: 435, 1996.

McGuire WP et al: Comparison of combination therapy with paclitaxel Taxol and cisplatin versus cyclophosphamide and cisplatin in patients with suboptimal stage III and stage IV ovarian cancer: a Gynecologic Oncology Group study, *Int J Gynecol Cancer 6* (supplement) 1:2, 1996.

McGuire WP et al: Cyclophosphamide and cisplatin compared with Paclitaxel and Cisplatin in patients with stage III and stage IV ovarian cancer, *NEJM* 334:1, 1996.

McGuire WP et al: A phase III trial of dose intense versus standard dose cisplatin and Cytoxan in advanced ovarian cancer, *Proc ASCO* 11:226, 1992.

Morgan DP Thigpen T: Chemotherapy in gynecologic cancer: celomic epithelial carcinoma of the ovary, *Clin Consult Obstet Gynecol* 4:144, 1992.

Murakami M et al: High dose chemotherapy with autologous bone marrow transplantation for the treatment of malignant ovarian tumors, *Semin Oncol* 21:29, 1994.

Ozols RF: High dose therapy with cisplatin and its analogs in ovarian cancer: current status and future studies, *Educational Booklet of ASCO*:69, 1987.

Ozols RF: Carboplatin and paclitaxel (Taxol\R) for the treatment of advanced ovarian cancer, *Int J Gynecol Cancer* 4:13, 1994.

Ozols RF: Chemotherapeutic dose intensity in ovarian cancer, *Advan Oncol* 11:24, 1995.

Ozols RF: Paclitaxel (Taxol) plus carboplatin as first-line treatment for advanced ovarian cancer, *Int. J Gynecol Cancer 6* (supplement 1) 1996.

Rothenberg M et al: Dose intensive induction therapy with cyclophosphamide, cisplatin, and consolidative abdominal radiation in the advanced stage epithelial ovarian cancer, *J Clin Oncol* 10:727, 1992.

Rowinsky EK, Cazenave LA, Donehower RC: Taxol: a novel investigational antimicrotubule agent, *J Natl Ca Inst* 82:1247, 1990.

Santin AD et al: Development and characterization of a GM-CSF secreting human ovarian tumor vaccine, *Int J Gynecol Cancer* 5:401, 1995.

Santin AD et al: Development and characterization of an IL-4 secreting human ovarian carcinoma cell line, *Gynecol Oncol* 58:230, 1995.

Stiff P et al: A phase II trial of high dose Mitoxantrone, carboplatin, and cyclophosphamide with autologous bone marrow rescue for recurrent epithelial ovarian carcinoma: analysis of risk factors for clinical outcome, *Gynecol Oncol* 57:278, 1995.

Sutton G: Ifosfamide and Mesna in epithelial ovarian carcinoma, *Gynecol Oncol* 51:104, 1993.

Swenerton KD, Peter JL: Carboplatin in the treatment of carcinoma of the ovary: The National Cancer Institute of Canada experience, *Semin Oncol* 19:114, 1992.

Swenerton KD et al: Cisplatin cyclophosphamide versus carboplatin cyclophosphamide in advanced ovarian cancer: a randomized phase III study of the National Cancer Institute of Canada Clinical Trial Group, *J Clin Oncol* 10:718, 1992.

Thigpen, JT: Chemotherapy for ovarian carcinoma, Cancer Update 1994: Ovarian Cancer; Lehigh Valley Hospital Regional Symposium, 1994.

Thigpen T: Editorial: High dose chemotherapy with autologous bone marrow support in ovarian carcinoma: the bottom line, more or less, *Gynecol Oncol* 57:275, 1995.

Trope C et al: A phase II, non randomized study of single agent paclitaxel (Taxol\R) in patients with previously untreated FIGO stage III, suboptimally resected ovarian cancer: a preliminary report, *Int J Gynecol Cancer* 4:7, 1994.

Van der Burg MEL et al: The role of intervention debulking surgery in advanced epithelial ovarian cancer: an EORTC Gynecological Cancer Cooperative Group study, *Int J Gynecol Cancer 6* (supplement) 1:30, 1996.

Vergae IB et al: Randomized trial comparing cisplatin with radioactive phosphorus or whole abdomen irradiation as adjuvant treatment of ovarian cancer, *Cancer* 69:741, 1992.

Warner E: Neurotoxicity of cisplatin and Taxol, *Int J Gynecol Cancer* 5:161, 1995.

Wiernik PH et al: Hexamethylmelamine and low or moderate dose cisplatin with or without pyridoxine for treatment of advanced ovarian carcinoma: a study of the Eastern Cooperative Oncology Group, *Cancer Investig* 10:1, 1992.

Extraovarian peritoneal serous papillary carcinoma

Dalrymple JC et al: Extraovarian peritoneal serous papillary carcinoma, a clinicopathologic study of 31 cases, *Cancer* 64:110, 1989.

Fowler JM et al: Peritoneal adenocarcinoma (serous) of Müllerian type: a subgroup of women presenting with peritoneal carcinomatosis, *Int J Gynecol Cancer* 4:43, 1994.

Killackey MA, Davis AR: Papillary serous carcinoma of the peritoneal surface: matched-case comparison with papillary serous ovarian carcinoma, *Gynecol Oncol* 51:171, 1993.

Weber AM et al: Serous carcinoma of the peritoneum after oophorectomy, *Obstet & Gynecol* 80:558, 1992.

Small cell carcinoma of the ovary

Berek JS, Hack NF, Lichtenstein A et al: Intraperitoneal recombinant a-interferon for "salvage" immunotherapy in stage III epithelial ovarian cancer: a Gynecologic Oncologic Group study, *Cancer Res* 45:4447, 1985.

Dickersin GR, Kline IW, Scully RE: Small cell carcinoma of the ovary with hypercalcemia: a report of 11 cases, *Cancer* 49:188, 1982.

Greene MGH, Boice JD, Greer BE et al: Acute non-lymphocytic leukemia after therapy with alkylating agents for ovarian cancer, *N Engl J Med* 307:1416, 1982.

Hoskins WJ, Rubin SC, Dulaney E et al: Influence of secondary cytoreduction at the time of second-look laparotomy on the survival of patients with epithelial ovarian carcinoma, *Gynecol Oncol* 34:365, 1989.

Howell SB, Kirmani S, Lucas WE et al: A phase II trial of intraperitoneal cisplatin and etoposide for primary treatment of ovarian epithelial cancer, *J Clin Oncol* 8:137, 1990.

Howell SB, Zimm S, Markman M et al: Long-term survival of advanced refractory, ovarian carcinoma patients with small-volume disease, treated with intraperitoneal chemotherapy, *J Clin Oncol* 5:1607, 1987.

Mackintosh J, Buckley CH, Tindall VR et al: The role of postoperative alkylating agent therapy in early-stage epithelial ovarian cancer, *Br J Obstet Gynaecol* 96:353, 1989.

Markman M, Hakes T, Reichman B et al: Intraperitoneal therapy in the management of ovarian carcinoma, *Yale J Biol Med* 62:393, 1989.

Patsner B, Piver MS, Lele SB et al: Small cell carcinoma of the ovary: a rapidly lethal tumor occurring in the young, *Gynecol Oncol* 22:233, 1985.

Piver MS, Malfetano J, Baker TR et al: Adjuvant cisplatin-based chemotherapy for stage I ovarian adenocarcinoma: a preliminary report, *Gynecol Oncol* 35:69, 1989.

Podratz KC, Schray MF, Wieand HS et al: Evaluation of treatment and survival after positive second-look laparotomy, *Gynecol Oncol* 31:9, 1988.

Pruett KM, Gordon AN, Estrada G et al: Small-cell carcinoma of the ovary: an aggressive epithelial cancer occurring in young patients, *Gynecol Oncol* 29:365, 1988.

Reichman B, Markman M et al: Intraperitoneal cisplatin and etoposide in the treatment of refractory/recurrent ovarian carcinoma, *J Clin Oncol* 7:1327, 1989.

Senekjian EK, Weiser PA, Talerman A, Herbst AL: Vinblastine, cisplatin, cyclophosphamide, bleomycin, doxorubicin, and etoposide in the treatment of small cell carcinoma of the ovary, *Cancer* 64(6):1183, 1989.

Taraszewski R et al: Case report: small cell carcinoma of the ovary, *Gynecol Oncol* 41:149, 1991.

Ulbright TM, Roth LM, Stehman FB et al: Poorly differentiated (small cell) carcinoma of the ovary in young women: evidence supporting a germ cell origin, *Hum Pathol* 18:175, 1987.

Young RH, Dickersin GR, Scully RE: Small-cell carcinoma of the ovary: an analysis of 75 cases of a distinct ovarian tumor commonly associated with hypercalcemia, *Lab Invest* 56:89, 1987 (abstract).

Follow-up techniques

Use of CA-125 levels

Alagoz T et al: What is a normal CA 125 level? *Gynecol Oncol* 53:93, 1994.

Alvarez RD et al: CA 125 as a serum marker for poor prognosis in ovarian malignancies, *Gynecol Oncol* 26:284, 1987.

Bast RC, Knapp RC: Immunologic approaches to the management of ovarian carcinoma, *Sem Oncol* 11:264, 1984.

Bast RC, et al: Elevation of serum CA 125 in carcinoma of the fallopian tube, endometrium, and endocervix, *Am J Obstet Gynecol* 148:1057, 1984.

Bast RC et al: Monitoring human ovarian carcinoma with a combination of CA 125, CA 19-9, and carcinoembryonic antigen, *Am J Obstet Gynecol* 149:553, 1984.

Di-Xia C, Schwartz PE, Fan-Qin L: Saliva and serum CA 125 assays for detecting malignant ovarian tumors, *Obstet Gynecol* 75:701, 1990.

Finkler NJ et al: Comparison of serum CA 125, clinical impression, and ultrasound in the preoperative evaluation of ovarian masses, *Obstet Gynecol* 72(4):659, 1988.

Gard GB, Houghton RS: An assessment of the value of serum CA 125 measurements in the management of epithelial ovarian carcinoma, *Gynecol Oncol* 53:283, 1994.

Grover S et al: Screening for ovarian cancer using serum CA 125 and vaginal examination: report on 2550 females, *IGCS* 5:291, 1995.

Herbst A: The epidemiology of ovarian carcinoma and the current status of tumor markers to detect disease, *Am J Obstet Gynecol* 170:1099, 1994.

Hising C, Anjegard IM, Einhorn N: Clinical relevance of the CA 125 assay in monitoring of ovarian cancer patients, *Am J Clin Oncol* 14:111, 1991.

Hogberg T, Kagedal B: Serous half-life of the tumor marker CA 125 during induction chemotherapy as a prognostic indicator for survival in ovarian carcinoma, *Acta Obstet Gynecol Scand* 69:423, 1990.

Loy TS, Quesenberry JT, Sharp SC: Distribution of CA 125 in adenocarcinomas, *ACJP* 98:175, 1992.

Maggino T et al: Prospective multicenter study on CA 125 in postmenopausal pelvic masses, *Gynecol Oncol* 54:117, 1994.

Mogensen O, Mogensen B, Jakobsen A: Predictive value of CA 125 during early chemotherapy of advanced ovarian cancer, *Gynecol Oncol* 37:44, 1990.

Niloff JM et al: Predictive value of CA 125 antigen levels in second-look procedures for ovarian cancer, *Am J Obstet Gynecol* 151:981, 1985.

Olt G, Berchuck A, Bast RC: The role of tumor markers in gynecologic oncology, *Obstet Gynecol Surv* 45(8):570, 1990.

Onsrud M: Tumour markers in gynaecologic oncology, *Scand J Clin Lab Invest* 51:60, 1991.

Podczaski E et al: Use of CA 125 to monitor patients with ovarian epithelial carcinomas, *Gynecol Oncol* 33:193, 1989.

Potter ME et al: Value of serum (125) CA levels: does the result preclude second look? *Gynecol Oncol* 33:201, 1989.

Vasilev SA et al: Serum CA 125 levels in preoperative evaluation of pelvic masses, *Obstet Gynecol* 71(5):751, 1988.

Zurawski VR Jr et al: Elevated serum CA 125 levels prior to diagnosis of ovarian neoplasia: relevance for early detection of ovarian cancer, *Int J Cancer* 42:677, 1988.

Zurawski VR Jr et al: Prospective evaluation of serum CA 125 levels in a normal population, phase I: the specifications of single and serial determinations in testing for ovarian cancer, *Gynecol Oncol* 36:299, 1990.

Second look operation (reassessment surgery)

Berek JS, Griffiths CT, Leventhal JM: Laparoscopy for "second-look" evaluation in ovarian cancer, *Obstet Gynecol* 58:192, 1981.

Chambers SK, Chambers JT, Kohorn EI et al: Evaluation of the role of second-look surgery in ovarian cancer, *Obstet Gynecol* 72:1, 1988.

Childers JM, Brzechffa PR, Surwit EA: Laparoscopy using the left upper quadrant as the primary trocar site, *Gynecol Oncol* 50:221, 1993.

Cohen CJ, Bruckner HW, Goldberg JD et al: Improved therapy with cisplatin regimens for patients with ovarian cancer as measured by surgical end-staging—the Mount Sinai experience, *Clin Obstet Gynecol* 10:307, 1983.

Coin TM et al: A review of second-look laparotomy for ovarian cancer, *Gynecol Oncol* 23:14, 1986.

Copeland LJ: Second-look laparotomy for ovarian carcinoma, *Clin Obstet Gynecol* 28:816, 1985.

Creasman WT, Gall S, Bundy BN et al: Second-look laparotomy in the patient with minimal residual stage III ovarian cancer (a Gynecologic Oncology Group study), *Gynecol Oncol* 35:378, 1989.

Ehrlich CE et al: Response, second-look status and survival in stage III and IV epithelial ovarian cancer treated with cis-platinum, Adriamycin, and cyclophosphamide, *Proc Am Assoc Cancer Res* 21:423, 1980.

Ho AG, Beller U, Speyer JL et al: A reassessment of the role in second-look laparotomy in advanced ovarian cancer, *J Clin Oncol* 5:1316, 1987.

Lippman SC, Alberts DS, Slymen DJ et al: Second-look laparotomy in epithelial ovarian carcinoma, *Cancer* 61:2571, 1988.

Miller DS et al: Critical reassessment of second look exploratory laparotomy for epithelial ovarian carcinoma, *Cancer* 69:502, 1992.

Peters WA et al: Intraperitoneal ^{32}P is not an effective consolidation therapy after a negative second look laparotomy for epithelial carcinoma of the ovary, *Gynecol Oncol* 47:146, 1992.

Podczaski ES, Stevens CW, Manetta A et al: Use of second-look laparotomy in the management of patients with ovarian epithelial malignancies, *Gynecol Oncol* 28:205, 1987.

Podratz KC, Kinney WK: Second look operation in ovarian cancer, *Cancer* 71:1551, 1993.

Roberts W et al: Second-look laparotomy in the management of gynecologic malignancy, *Gynecol Oncol* 133:345, 1982.

Smirz LR et al: Second-look laparotomy after chemotherapy in the management of ovarian malignancy, *Am J Obstet Gynecol* 152:661, 1985.

Soper JT et al: Intraperitoneal chromic phosphate ^{32}P as salvage therapy for persistent carcinoma of the ovary after surgical restaging, *Am J Obstet Gynecol* 156:1153, 1987.

Tarraza HM et al: Consolidation intraperitoneal chemotherapy in epithelial ovarian cancer patients following negative second look laparotomy, *Gynecol Oncol* 50:287, 1993.

Van Lith JMM, Bouma J, Aalders JG et al: Role of an early second-look laparotomy in ovarian cancer, *Gynecol Oncol* 35:255, 1989.

Walton L, Ellenberg SS, Major F Jr et al: Results of second-look laparotomy in patients with early-stage ovarian carcinoma, *Obstet Gynecol* 80:770, 1987.

Salvage Therapy

Abdulhay G et al: Human lymphoblastoid interferon in the treatment of advanced epithelial ovarian malignancies (a GOG study), *Am J Obstet Gynecol* 152:418, 1985.

Adams M: Salvage treatment for ovarian cancer, *Clin Oncol* 2:1, 1990.

Barker GH, Wiltshaw E: Use of high dose cis-dichlorodiammine platinum (II) following failure on previous chemotherapy for advanced carcinoma of the ovary, *Br J Obstet Gynaecol* 88:1192, 1981.

Blackledge G et al: Response of patients in phase II studies of chemotherapy in ovarian cancer: implications for patient treatment and the design of phase II trials, *Br J Cancer* 59:650, 1989.

Brenner DE: Intraperitoneal chemotherapy: a review, *J Clin Oncol* 4:1135, 1986.

Bruckner HW, Wallach R: High-dose cis-platinum for the treatment of refractory ovarian cancer, *Gynecol Oncol* 12:64, 1984.

Covens A et al: Phase II study of Mitomycin C and 5 Fluorouracil in platinum resistant ovarian cancer, *Eur J Gynecol Oncol* 13:1992.

Cruikshank DP, Buchsbaum HJ: Effects of rapid paracentesis: cardiovascular dynamics and body fluid composition, *JAMA* 225:1361, 1973.

Davis T et al: Cis-platinum and hexamethylmelamine in combination for ovarian cancer after failure of alkylating agent therapy—a phase I-II pilot trial, *Proc Am Assoc Cancer Res* 21:428, 1980.

Dougherty J et al: Recurrence pattern of advanced ovarian carcinoma after negative laparotomy, *Proc Am Soc Clin Oncol* 4:122, 1985.

Eisenhauer S et al: Carboplatin therapy for recurrent ovarian cancer: National Cancer Institute experience and review of the literature. In *Carboplatin (JM-8): Current perspectives and future directions* (PA Bunn, R Canetta, RF Ozols, and M Rozencweig, Eds.), Saunders, Philadelphia, 1990.

Fanning J, Hilgers RD, Hutson E: Carboplatin, Etoposide, and Ifosfamide as second line treatment for ovarian cancer, *Am J Clin Oncol* 17:335, 1994.

Fromm GL et al: Sequentially administered ethinyl estradiol and medroxyprogesterone acetate in the treatment of refractory epithelial ovarian carcinoma in patients with positive estrogen receptors, *Cancer* 68:1885, 1991.

Gershenson DM et al: Prognosis of surgically determined complete responders in advanced ovarian cancer, *Cancer* 55:1129, 1985.

Halpin TF, McCann TO: Dynamics of body fluids following the rapid removal of large volumes of ascites, *Am J Obstet Gynecol* 110:103, 1971.

Hoskins PJ, McMurtrie E, Senerton KD: A phase II trial of intravenous etoposide (VP-16-213) in epithelial ovarian cancer resistant to cisplatin or carboplatin: clinical and serological evidence of activity, *Int J Gynecol Cancer* 2:35, 1992.

Howell SB, Kirmani S, McClay EF et al: Intraperitoneal cisplatin-based chemotherapy for ovarian carcinoma, *Sem Oncol* 18(1 suppl 3):5, 1991.

Kavanagh JK, Nicaise C: Carboplatin in refractory epithelial ovarian cancer, *Sem Oncol* 16:45, 1989.

Kirmani S et al: A comparison of intravenous versus intraperitoneal chemotherapy for the initial treatment of ovarian cancer, *Gynecol Oncol* 54:338, 1994.

Kohn EC et al: Dose intense Taxol: high response rate in patients with platinum resistant ovarian cancer, *J Natl Cancer Inst* 86:18, 1994.

Lawton F et al: A randomized trial comparing whole abdominal radiotherapy with chemotherapy following cisplatin cyto-reduction in epithelial ovarian cancer: West Midlands Ovarian Cancer Group trial II, *Clin Oncol* 2:4, 1990.

LeVeen HH, Cristoudias G, Moorn IP: Peritoneovenous shunting for ascites, *Ann Surg* 180:580, 1974.

Long HJ et al: Phase II evaluation of 5-Fluorouracil and low dose leucovorin in cisplatin refractory advanced ovarian carcinoma, *Gynecol Oncol* 54:180, 1994.

Lucas WE, Markman M, Howell SB: Intraperitoneal chemotherapy for advanced ovarian cancer, *Am J Obstet Gynecol* 152:474, 1985.

Manetta A et al: Hexamethylmelamine as a single second line agent in ovarian cancer, *Gynecol Oncol* 36:93, 1990.

Manetta A et al: Analysis of prognostic factors and survival in patients with ovarian cancer treated with second-line hexamethylmelamine (altretamine), *Cancer Treat Rev* 18(suppl A):23, 1991.

Markman M: Intraperitoneal chemotherapy as treatment of ovarian carcinoma: why, how, and when? *Obstet Gynecol Surv* 42:533, 1987.

Markman M: Salvage intraperitoneal therapy of small volume residual ovarian cancer: impact of pretreatment finding of peritoneal carcinomatosis on the surgical complete response rate, *J Cancer Res Clin Oncol* 118:232, 1992.

Markman M: Salvage therapy in ovarian cancer: is there a role for intraperitoneal drug delivery? *Gynecol Oncol* 51:86, 1993.

Markman M: Follow-up of the asymptomatic patient with ovarian cancer, *Gynecol Oncol* 55:S134, 1994.

Markman M, Hoskins W: Responses to salvage chemotherapy in ovarian cancer: a critical need for precise definitions of the treated population, *J Clin Oncol* 10:513, 1992.

Markman M et al: Combination intraperitoneal chemotherapy with cisplatin, cytarabine, and doxorubicin for refractory ovarian carcinoma and other malignancies principally confined to the peritoneal cavity, *J Clin Oncol* 2:1321, 1984.

Markman M et al: Intraperitoneal chemotherapy with high-dose cisplatin and cytosine arabinoside for refractory ovarian carcinoma and other malignancies prinicpally involving the peritoneal cavity, *J Clin Oncol* 3:925, 1985.

Markman M et al: Responses to second line cisplatin based intraperitoneal therapy in ovarian cancer: influence of a prior response to intravenous cisplatin, *J Clin Oncol* 9:1801, 1991.

Markman M et al: Second-line platinum therapy in patients with ovarian cancer previously treated with cisplatin, *J Clin Oncol* 9:389, 1991.

Markman M et al: Association between pretreatment CA-125 levels and surgically documented complete responses in patients with ovarian cancer treated with second-line intraperitoneal therapy, *J Cancer Res Clin Oncol* 118:391, 1992.

Markman M et al: Impact of laparotomy finding of significant intra-abdominal adhesions on the surgically defined complete response rate to subsequent salvage intraperitoneal chemotherapy, *J Cancer Res Clin Oncol* 118:163, 1992.

Markman M et al: Phase I trial of intraperitoneal Taxol: a Gynecologic Oncology Group study, *J Clin Oncol* 10:1485, 1992.

Markman M et al: Evidence supporting the superiority of intraperitoneal Cisplatin compared to intraperitoneal carboplatin for salvage therapy of small volume residual ovarian cancer, *Gynecol Oncol* 50:100, 1993

Markman M, et al: Rationale for the intraperitoneal administration of Paclitaxel (Taxol\R) in the treatment of ovarian cancer, *Int J Gynecol Cancer* 4:19, 1994.

McGuire WP et al: A unique antineoplastic agent with significant activity in advanced ovarian epithelial neoplasms, *Ann Int Med*: 111:273, 1989.

Menczer, J: Use of the Veress Needle for instillation of intraperitoneal chemotherapy, *Gynecol Oncol* 59:249, 1995.

Menczer J et al: Intraperitoneal chemotherapy versus No treatment in patients with ovarian carcinoma who are in complete clinical remission, *Cancer* 70:1956, 1992.

Miller DS, Brady FB, Barrett RJ: A phase II trial of Leuprolide Acetate in patients with advanced epithelial ovarian carcinoma, *Am J Clin Oncol* 15:125, 1992.

Moore DH et al: Hexamethylmelamine chemotherapy for persistent or recurrent epithelial ovarian cancer, *Am J Obstet Gynecol* 165:573, 1991.

Ozols RF et al: High-dose cisplatin in hypertonic saline in refractory ovarian cancer, *J Clin Oncol* 3:1246, 1985.

Ozols RF et al: High-dose carboplatin in refractory ovarian cancer patients, *J Clin Oncol* 5:197, 1987.

Pfeifle CE et al: Totally implantable system for peritoneal access, *J Clin Oncol* 2:1277, 1984.

Piver MS et al: Evaluation of survival after second line intraperitoneal cisplatin bases chemotherapy for advanced ovarian cancer, *Cancer* 73:1693, 1994.

Qazi R, Savlov ED: Peritoneovenous shunt for palliation of malignant ascites, *Cancer* 49:600, 1982.

Reed E et al: 5-Fluorouracil (5-FU) and Leucovorin in platinum refractory advanced stage ovarian carcinoma, *Gynecol Oncol* 46:326, 1992.

Rosen GF, Lurain JR, Newton M: Hexamethylmelamine in ovarian cancer after failure of cisplatin based multiple agent chemotherapy, *Gynecol Oncol* 27, 173, 1987.

Seltzer V, Vogl S, Kaplan B: Recurrent ovarian cancer: retreatment utilizing combination chemotherapy including cis-diamminedichloroplatinum, *Gynecol Oncol* 21:167, 1985.

Sherman AI, Rosenberg R, Fink D: Use of intraperitoneal chemotherapy for treatment of ovarian cancer, *Eur J Gynaec Oncol* 13:295, 1992.

Spencer TR et al: Intraperitoneal P-32 after negative second-look laparotomy in ovarian carcinoma, *Cancer* 63(12):2434, 1989.

Stanhope RC et al: Second trial drugs in ovarian cancer, *Gynecol Oncol* 5:52, 1977.

Stehman FB, Ehrlich CE, Callangan MF: Failure of hexamethylmelamine as salvage therapy in ovarian epithelial adenocarcinoma resistant to combination chemotherapy, *Gynecol Oncol* 17:189, 1984.

Thigpen T et al: Phase II trial of Taxol as second-line therapy for ovarian carcinoma: a Gynecologic Oncology Group study, *Proc Am Soc Clin Oncol* 9:156, 1990 (Abstract)

Trimble EL et al: Paclitaxel for platinum refractory ovarian cancer: results from the first 1,000 patients registered to national Cancer Institute treatment referral center 9103, *J Clin Oncol* 11: 2405, 1993.

Vergae J et al: Hexamethylmelamine as second line therapy in platin resistant ovarian cancer, *Gynecol Oncol* 47:282, 1992.

Zimm S et al: Phase I pharmacokinetic study of intraperitoneal (ip) cisplatin (DDP) and etoposide (VP-16), *Proc Am Soc Clin Oncol* 5:49, 1986.

Malignant effusions

Kennedy L et al: Pleurodesis using Talc slurry, *Chest* 106:342, 1994.

Nagy JA et al: Pathogenesis of ascites tumor growth: fibrinogen influx and fibrin accumulation in tissues lining the peritoneal cavity, *Cancer Research* 55:369, 1995.

Nagy JA et al: Pathogenesis of ascites tumor growth: vascular permeability factor, vascular hypermeability, and ascites fluid accumulation, *Cancer Research* 55:360, 1995.

Nagy, JA et al: Pathogenesis of ascites tumor growth: angiogenesis, vascular remodeling, and stroma formation in the peritoneal lining, *Cancer Research* 55:376, 1995.

Pasquale MD, Campbell JM, Magnant CM: Groshong\R versus Hickman\R catheters, *Surgery Gynecol Obstet* 174:408, 1992.

Ruckdeschel JD et al: Intrapleural therapy for malignant pleural effusions, *Chest* 100:1528, 1991.

Current areas of research

Alberts DS et al: Chemotherapy of ovarian cancer directed by the human tumor stem cell assay, *Cancer Chemother Pharmacol* 2:279, 1981.

Berchuck A et al: Overexpression of Her-2/neu is associated with poor survival in advanced epithelial ovarian cancer, *Cancer Res* 50:4087, 1990.

Berek JS et al: Intraperitoneal immunotherapy of epithelial ovarian carcinoma with *Corynebacterium parvum*, *Am J Obstet Gynecol* 152:1003, 1985.

Bishop J: Trends in oncogenes, *Trends Genet* 1:245, 1985.

Bogden AE et al: Chemotherapy responsiveness of human tumors as first transplant generation xenographs in the normal mouse: six-day subrenal capsule assay, *Cancer* 48:10, 1981.

Bodgen AE et al: Human tumor xenographs implanted under the renal capsule of normal immune competent mice, *Exp Cell Biol* 47:281, 1979.

Bogden AE et al: Chemotherapy responsiveness of human tumors as first transplant generation xenographs in the normal mouse: six-day subrenal capsule assay, *Cancer* 48:10, 1981.

Corbett TH et al: Cyclophosphamide-Adriamycin combination chemotherapy in transplantable murine tumors, *Cancer Res* 35:1568, 1975.

Creasman WT et al: Chemoimmunotherapy in the management of primary stage III ovarian cancer: a Gynecologic Oncology Group study, *Cancer Treat Rep* 63:319, 1979.

DeGregorio MW et al: Toremifene: Pharmacologic and pharmacokinetic basis of reversing multidrug resistance, *Am Soc Clin Oncol* 7(9):1359, 1989.

Einhorn N et al: Human leukocyte interferon therapy for advanced ovarian carcinoma, *Am J Clin Oncol* 5:167, 1982.

Finlay C, Hinds P, Levine A: The p53 protooncogene can act as a suppressor of transformation, *Cell* 57:1083, 1989.

Foxwell BMJ et al: Identification of the multidrug resistance-related p-glycoprotein as a cyclosporine binding protein, *Molecular Pharm* 36:543, 1989.

Friedlander M et al: Prediction of long-term survival by flow-cytometric analysis of cellular DNA content in patients with advanced ovarian cancer, *J Clin Oncol* 6:282, 1988.

Goldie JH, Coldman AJ: A mathematical model for relating the drug sensitivity of tumors to their spontaneous mutation rate, *Cancer Treat Rep* 63:1727, 1979.

Goldie JH, Coldman AJ: The genetic origin of drug resistance in neoplasms: implications for systemic therapy, *Cancer Res* 44:3643, 1984.

Hamburger AW, Salmon SE: Primary bioassay of human tumor stem cells, *Science* 107:461, 1977.

Heintz A, Hacker N, Lagasse L: Epidemiology and etiology of ovarian cancer: a review, *Obstet Gynecol* 66:127, 1985.

Hunter RE et al: Responsiveness of gynecologic tumors and chemotherapeutic agents in the 6-day subrenal capsule assay, *Gynecol Oncol* 14:298, 1982.

Iverson O: Prognostic values of the flow cytometric DNA index in human ovarian carcinoma, *Cancer* 61:971, 1988.

Kern DH, Weisenthal LM: Highly specific prediction of antineoplastic drug resistance with an in vitro assay using suprapharmacologic drug exposures, *J Natl Ca Inst* 82(7):582, 1990.

La Vecchia C et al: Dietary factors and the risk of epithelial ovarian cancer, *J Natl Ca Inst* 79:663, 1987.

National Institute of Health, Office of the Director: NIH consensus statement, ovarian Cancer: screening, treatment, and follow-up 12:20, 1994.

Ozols RF, Young RC: Patterns of failure of chemotherapy in gynecologic malignancy: implications for future clinical trials, *Cancer Treat Symp* 2:233, 1983.

Ozols RF et al: Chemotherapy for murine ovarian cancer: a rationale for ip therapy with Adriamycin, *Cancer Treat Rep* 63:269, 1979.

Ozols RF et al: High-dose carboplatin in refractory ovarian cancer patients, *J Clin Oncol* 5:197, 1987.

Plaxe SC et al: Ovarian intraepithelial neoplasia demonstrated in patients with stage I ovarian carcinoma, *Gynecol Oncol* 38:367, 1990.

Saburi Y et al: Increased expression of glutathione S-transferase gene in cis-diaminodichloroplatinum (II)-resistance variants of a Chinese hamster, *Cancer Treat* 49:7020, 1989.

Slater LM et al: Cyclosporin A corrects daunorubicin resistance in Ehrlich ascites carcinoma, *Br J Cancer* 54:235, 1986.

Slater LM et al: Cyclosporin A reverses vincristine and daunorubicin resistance in acute lymphatic leukemia in vitro, *J Clin Invest* 77:1405, 1986.

Storms R, Bose H: Oncogenes, protooncogenes, and signal transduction: toward a unified theory? *Adv Virus Res* 37:1, 1989.

Stratton JA, Braly PS, DiSaia PJ: A comparison of three assays for prediction of clinical response to chemotherapy, *J Clin Lab Anal* 1:67, 1987.

Trope C, Sigurdsson K: Use of tissue culture in predictive testing of drug sensitivity in human ovarian cancer: correlation between in vitro results and the response in vivo, *Neoplasm* 29:309, 1982.

Widder KJ, Senyei AE, Ranney DF: Magnetically responsive microspheres and other carriers for the biophysical targeting of anti-tumor agents, *Adv Pharmacol Chemother* 16:213, 1979.

Widder KJ et al: Selective targeting of magnetic albumin microspheres containing low-dose doxorubicin: total remission in Yoshida sarcoma-bearing rats, *Eur J Cancer Clin Oncol* 19:135, 1983.

Conclusions on management

Eeles RA, Tan S, Wiltshaw E et al: Hormone replacement therapy and survival after surgery of ovarian cancer, *Br Med J* 302:262, 1991.

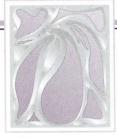

Germ Cell, Stromal, and Other Ovarian Tumors

GERM CELL TUMORS
Classification

This group of ovarian neoplasms is composed of several histologically different tumor types and embraces all the neoplasms considered to be ultimately derived from the primitive germ cells of the embryonic gonad (Figure 12-1). This concept of germ cell tumors as a specific group of gonadal neoplasms has evolved in the last four decades and become generally accepted. This is based primarily on the common histogenesis of these neoplasms, on the relatively common presence of histologically different tumor elements within the same tumor mass, on the presence of histologically similar neoplasms in extragonadal locations along the line of migration of the primitive germ cells from the wall of the yolk sac to the gonadal ridge, and on the remarkable homology between the various tumor types in men and women. In no other group of gonadal neoplasms has this homology been better illustrated. An example of this is the striking similarity between the testicular seminoma and its ovarian counterpart, the dysgerminoma. These were the first neoplasms to become accepted as originating from germ cells. A number of classifications of germ cell neoplasms of the ovary have been proposed over the past few decades. The box on p. 352 shows a modification of a classification originally described by Teilum and is similar to that proposed by the World Health Organization, which divides the germ cell tumors into several groups and also includes neoplasms composed of germ cells and "sex" stroma derivatives.

Clinical Profile

Germ cell tumors represent a relatively small proportion (about 20%) of all ovarian tumors (Table 12-1) but are becoming increasingly important in the clinical practice of obstetrics and gynecology. Most of these neoplasms occur in young women, and extirpation of the disease involves decisions concerning childbearing and probabilities of recurrence. Recent developments in chemotherapy have dramatically changed the prognosis for many patients who develop the more aggressive types of germ cell tumors. Knowing the classification of these lesions and how the pathologist arrives at the diagnosis, as well as the

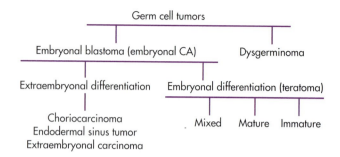

Figure 12-1 Classification schema of germ cell tumors of ovary.

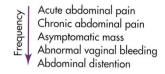

Figure 12-2 Initial symptoms in young patients with malignant germ cell tumors.

CLASSIFICATION OF GERM CELL NEOPLASMS OF THE OVARY

I. Germ cell tumors
  A. Dysgerminoma
  B. Endodermal sinus tumor
  C. Embryonal carcinoma
  D. Polyembryoma
  E. Choriocarcinomas
  F. Teratoma
    1. Immature (solid, cystic, or both)
    2. Mature
      a. Solid
      b. Cystic
        (1) Mature cystic teratoma (dermoid cyst)
        (2) Mature cystic teratoma (dermoid cyst) with malignant transformation
    3. Monodermal or highly specialized
      a. Struma ovarii
      b. Carcinoid
      c. Struma ovarii and carcinoid
      d. Others
  G. Mixed forms (tumors composed of types A through F in any possible combination)

II. Tumors composed of germ cells and sex cord stroma derivative
  A. Gonadoblastoma
  B. Mixed germ cell–sex cord stroma tumor

Table 12-1 Relative frequency of ovarian neoplasms

Type	%
Coelomic epithelium	50-70
Germ cell	15-20
Specialized gonadal stroma	5-10
Nonspecific mesenchyme	5-10
Metastatic tumor	5-10

Dysgerminoma

Dysgerminoma is an uncommon tumor accounting for 1% to 2% of primary ovarian neoplasms and for 3% to 5% of ovarian malignancies. Dysgerminoma may occur at any age, from infancy to old age; reported cases range between the ages of 7 months and 70 years but the majority of cases occur in adolescence and early adulthood (Figure 12-3). Dysgerminoma is composed of germ cells that have not differentiated to form embryonic or extraembryonic structures (Figure 12-4). Its stroma is almost always infiltrated with lymphocytes and often contains granulomas similar to those of sarcoid. Occasionally dysgerminoma contains isolated gonadotropin producing syncytiotrophoblastic giant cells. An elevated serum LDH or hCG level may be present in these patients. Grossly, the tumor may be firm or fleshy and cream colored or pale tan; both its external and its cut surfaces may be lobulated. A small proportion of dysgerminomas arise in sexually abnormal females, particularly those with pure or mixed gonadal dysgenesis or testicular feminization. In such cases the dysgerminoma often develops in a previously existing gonadoblastoma.

The symptoms of dysgerminoma are not distinctive, and they are similar to those observed in patients with other solid ovarian neoplasms. The duration of symptoms is usually short, and despite this the tumor is often large, indicating rapid growth. The most common initial symptoms are abdominal enlargement and the presence of a mass in the lower abdomen. In a number of cases, the tumor has been found incidentally at cesarean section or as a cause of dystocia. Dysgerminoma is one of the two most common ovarian neoplasms observed in pregnancy, the other being serous cystadenoma. The relatively common finding of dysgerminoma in pregnant patients is

---

clinical significance of that diagnosis, has great practical value for the practicing obstetrician/gynecologist. Most of these lesions are found in the second and third decades of life and are frequently diagnosed by finding a palpable abdominal mass, often associated with pain (Figure 12-2). Except for the benign cystic teratoma, ovarian germ cell tumors are usually rapidly enlarging abdominal masses that often cause considerable abdominal pain. At times the pain is exacerbated by rupture or torsion of the neoplasm. One of the classic initial signs of a dysgerminoma is hemoperitoneum from rupture of the capsule of the lesion as it rapidly enlarges.

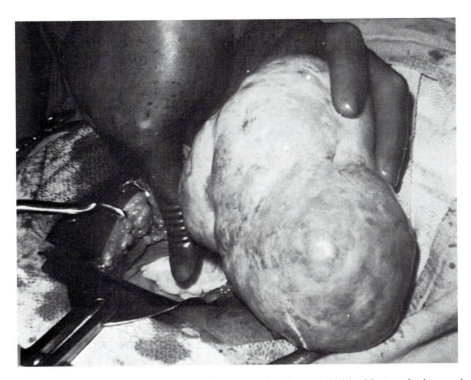

Figure 12-3 Large (25 cm) solid mass of right ovary in 16-year-old girl with stage Ia dysgerminoma.

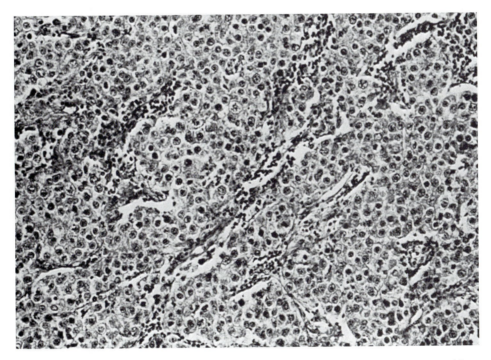

Figure 12-4 Dysgerminoma is characterized histologically by presence of large, round, ovoid, or polygonal cells with stroma infiltrated by lymphocytes.

nonspecific and relates to the age of the patient rather than the pregnant state. Dysgerminoma may also be discovered incidentally in patients investigated for primary amenorrhea, and in these cases it is frequently associated with gonadal dysgenesis and a gonadoblastoma. Occasionally menstrual and endocrine abnormalities may be the initial symptoms, but this tends to be more common in patients with dysgerminoma combined with other neoplastic germ cell elements, especially choriocarcinoma. Dysgerminoma is the only germ cell tumor in which the opposite

Table 12-2   Results of conservative and nonconservative surgery in stage Ia dysgerminoma of the ovary

	10-year survival	
	Conservative surgery	Nonconservative therapy†
Asadourian and Taylor	42/46 (91%)	21/25 (84%)
Gordon et al.	68/72 (94%)	11/14 (79%)
Malkasian and Symmonds	23/27 (85%)	13/14 (93%)
TOTAL	133/145 (92%)*	45/53 (85%)

*Includes those salvaged after recurrence (23/25–92%)
†Surgery plus radiation

ovary may be involved with the tumor process (approximately 10%-15%).

Dysgerminomas are notable by their predilection for lymphatic spread and their acute sensitivity to irradiation. Historically, surgery followed by radiation (in both early- and late-stage disease) has resulted in an excellent cure rate. More recently the use of multiple-agent chemotherapy has been advocated and has produced good results. In the young woman with a unilateral encapsulated dysgerminoma who is desirous of future childbearing, conservative management is indicated. In a review of the recent literature, more than 400 cases of dysgerminoma were reported. Seventy percent of patients were stage I at diagnosis and only 10% involved both ovaries. Because 85% of all patients with dysgerminomas are younger than 30 years, conservative therapy and preservation of fertility are certainly major considerations. Conservative surgery without radiation in stage Ia lesions has resulted in excellent outcomes (Table 12-2). In patients in whom unilateral salpingo-oophorectomy is performed, careful inspection of the other ovary and exploration to rule out disseminated disease are mandatory. Our routine is not to wedge or bivalve the opposite ovary if it is normal size, shape, and consistency. These patients should be followed closely and have periodic examinations because approximately 90% of recurrences will appear in the first 2 years after initial therapy. Fortunately, the majority of recurrences can be successfully eradicated by radiation therapy or chemotherapy. This knowledge permits the conservative management of patients. It should be noted that recurrences can occur in the opposite ovary, although this observation was noted after conservative surgery without careful staging surgery.

Several prognostic factors in dysgerminoma have been suggested as important because they might influence conservative therapy in early-staged disease. Some authors suggest that in patients with large tumors (>10 cm) there is a greater chance of recurrence, and therefore adjuvant therapy should be given. Today, most agree that tumor size is not prognostically important and that these patients do not require additional therapy. The long-term survival is almost 90% in patients who have stage I lesions. Some recent series are reporting 100% survival with conservative surgery in stage Ia patients. These data strongly support initial conservative approach with the preservation of fertility. More extensive surgery and radiation therapy were not beneficial when patients had disease limited to one ovary. Schwartz reported four patients with metastasis to the contralateral ovary and preservation of that ovary with subsequent chemotherapy. All are alive without disease 14-56 months after diagnosis.

De Palo et al. reported on 56 patients who had pure dysgerminomas. In their study 44 patients underwent lymphangiography, and a positive study resulted in the restaging of 32% of patients. Diaphragmatic implants were not found in any patients, and positive cytologic findings were obtained in only 3 patients. The 5-year relapse-free survival rates were 91% in patients with stages Ia, Ib, and Ic; 74% in those with stage III retroperitoneal disease; and 24% in patients who had stage III peritoneal disease. Peritoneal involvement of any kind was associated with a poor prognosis if disease had extended to the abdominal cavity. All patients with stage III disease received postoperative radiation therapy.

Recurrences should be treated aggressively with reexploration and tumor reduction. The removed tissue should be examined carefully for evidence of germ cell elements other than dysgerminoma. Some presumed recurrent dysgerminomas have been found to be mixed germ cell tumors and should be treated accordingly.

Although radiation therapy has been successful in treating dysgerminomas, more recently chemotherapy appears to have become the treatment of choice. Its success rate is as good as that of radiation, and preservation of fertility is possible in many patients, even those with bilateral ovarian disease. Weinblatt and Ortega reported on five children with extensive disease who were treated with chemotherapy as the primary therapeutic modality. Three of the five were alive and free of disease at the time of the report, suggesting a therapeutic approach to extensive childhood dysgerminoma that spares pelvic and reproductive organs.

Chemotherapy is also being used more frequently with significant success in patients who have advanced disease. Bianchi et al. reported 18 patients (6, stage Ib or c, and 12, stage IIb, III, IV, or recurrent) who were treated with doxorubicin and cyclophosphamide or cisplatin, vinblastine, and bleomycin. Doxorubicin and cyclophosphamide were highly effective: 7 of 10 patients were disease-free, 2 of 3 relapsing patients were salvaged with cisplatin, vinblastin, and bleomycin (VBP). Of the 8 patients treated with VBP, one had recurrence in the brain and was salvaged with radiation therapy. Four patients who had no residual disease in the remaining ovary or in the uterus are all free of disease, and one has had a successful pregnancy. The optimal drug combination has not yet been determined. Because bleomycin can cause pulmonary fibrosis with resultant death, it is being used less frequently. Etoposide also appeared to be an effective drug in the treatment of dysgerminomas. More recently, patients with advanced disease have received multiple-agent chemotherapy with results equal to or better than results for those treated with radiation. Complete responses in the 80%-100% range are being reported in patients with stage II to IV disease. This is not surprising—the cure rates for stage III germinomas treated with effective chemotherapy are over 90%. Today, chemotherapy appears to be the treatment of choice after surgery in patients with advanced disease.

The common association of dysgerminoma with gonadoblastoma, a tumor that nearly always occurs in patients with dysgenetic gonads, indicates that there is a relationship between dysgerminoma and genetic and somatosexual abnormalities. The treatment of normal patients with dysgerminoma should be conservative if possible. Historically, the treatment of patients with dysgerminoma associated with gonadoblastoma is radical because of the frequent occurrence of bilateral tumors and the absence of normal gonadal function. Investigation of the genotypes and karyotypes of all patients with this neoplasm is recommended by some, especially if any history of virilization or other developmental abnormalities is elicited. In vivo fertilization (IVF) can occur without gonads. Therefore it does not appear prudent to remove the uterus in these patients only because the ovaries must be removed. In this situation we leave the uterus. This may be particularly important in prepubertal patients, because in these patients other signs of abnormal function, such as primary amenorrhea, virilization, and absence of normal sexual development, are lacking.

Often lesions that consist primarily of dysgerminoma elements will contain small areas of more malignant histology (e.g., embryonal carcinoma or endodermal sinus tumor). When the dysgerminoma is not pure and these more malignant components are present, the prognosis and therapy are determined by the other germ cell elements, and the dysgerminoma component is disregarded.

Endodermal Sinus Tumor

The endodermal sinus tumor is the second most common form of malignant germ cell tumor of the ovary, accounting for 22% of germ cell lesions in one large series. Three fourths of the patients are initially seen with a combination of abdominal pain and abdominal or pelvic mass; the median age of the patients is 19 years. Alpha-fetoprotein (AFP) levels are often elevated in this group of tumors. The endodermal sinus tumor is characterized by extremely rapid growth and extensive intraabdominal spread; nearly half the patients seen by a physician initially for symptoms of 1 week's duration or less.

Schiller called these neoplasms *mesonephroma*, but most pathologists now consider them to be various germ cell tumors unrelated to the mesonephros. They were thought to originate from germ cells that differentiate into the extraembryonal yolk sac, since the tumor structure is similar to that in the endodermal sinuses of the rat yolk sac. The tumors consist of scattered tubules or spaces lined by single layers of flattened cuboidal cells, loose reticular stroma, numerous scattered paraaminosalicylic-positive globules, and, within some spaces or clefts, a characteristic invaginated papillary structure with a central blood vessel (Schiller-Duval body) (Figure 12-5).

Historically, the prognosis for patients with endodermal sinus tumor of the ovary has been unfavorable: most patients have died of the disease within 12-18 months of diagnosis. Until multiple-agent chemotherapy was developed, there were only a few known 5-year survivors. The majority of these patients had tumors confined to the ovary; and in several cases, the tumor was composed of endodermal sinus tumors admixed with other neoplastic germ cell elements, frequently dysgerminoma. The clinical course in most patients with tumors composed of endodermal sinus tumor associated with dysgerminoma or other neoplastic germ cell elements does not differ greatly from that in patients with pure endodermal sinus tumors. Frequently, intracellular and extracellular hyaline droplets that represent deposits of alpha-fetoprotein can be identified throughout the tumor. Mixed germ cell lesions often contain endodermal sinus tumors as one of the types present.

In the past, the treatment of patients with endodermal sinus tumor of the ovary has been frustrating. Kurman and Norris reported no long-term survivals in 17 stage I patients receiving adjunctive radiation and/or single alkylating agent, dactinomycin, or methotrexate. Gallion reviewed the literature in 1979 and found only 27% of 96 patients with stage I endodermal sinus tumors alive at 2 years. The tumor is not sensitive to radiation therapy, although there may be an initial response. Optimal surgical extirpation of the disease has been advocated but this alone is unsuccessful in producing a significant number of cures. In recent years, there have been optimistic reports of sustained remissions in some patients treated by surgery and chemotherapy using a combination of dactinomycin, 5-fluorouracil, and cyclophosphamide (ActFUCy) or VAC. Forney et al. and Smith et al. reported long-term survival in patients with advanced disease treated with these vigorous chemotherapeutic regimens. Creasman et al. have had comparable results using a combination of methotrexate, dactinomycin, and chlorambucil (MAC). In addition, they suggest that the VAC or MAC regimen is effective when administered for a period no longer than 6 months.

The GOG used VAC chemotherapy to treat 24 patients who had pure endodermal sinus tumors (EST) that were completely resected and 7 whose diseases were partially

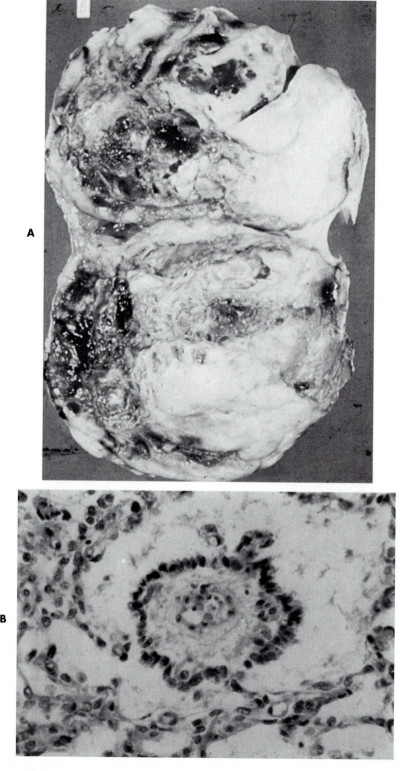

Figure 12-5 Endodermal sinus tumor. **A,** Gross appearance with areas of hemorrhage and gelatinous necrosis. **B,** Microscopic appearance with isolated papillary projections containing single blood vessels and having peripheral lining of neoplastic cells (Schiller-Duval body).

Table 12-3   VAC, VBP, and BEP regimens

Regimen	Dosage schedule
VAC	
Vincristine, 1.5 mg/m² (maximum dose 2.5 mg)	Weekly IV administration for 12 weeks
Dactinomycin, 0.5 mg	5-day IV course every 4 weeks
Cyclophosphamide, 5-7 mg/kg	
VBP	
Vinblastine, 12 mg/m²	IV every 3 weeks for 4 courses
Bleomycin, 20 U/m² (maximum dose 30 U/m²)	IV weekly for 7 courses; eighth course given in week 10
Cisplatin, 20 mg/m²	Daily × 5 every 3 weeks for 3-4 courses
BEP	
Bleomycin, 20 U/m² (maximum dose 30 U)	IV weekly × 9
Etoposide, 100 mgm/m²	IV days 1-5 q 3 weeks × 3
Cisplatin, 20 mgm/m²	IV days 1-5 q 3 weeks × 3

resected. Of 31 patients, 15 (48%) failed, including 11 of 24 (46%) who had complete resection. Of 15 patients with mixed germ cell tumors containing EST elements treated with VAC, 8 (53%) failed. Subsequently, GOG treated 48 patients with stage I to III completely resected endodermal sinus tumors with VAC for 6 to 9 courses. The disease-free patients were 35 (73%) with a median of 4-year follow-up. More recently, 21 similar patients were treated with BEP (bleomycin, etoposide, and cisplatin), the first 9 being without evidence of disease. BEP was given for 3 courses over 9 weeks. Gershenson et al. reported that 18 of 26 (69%) patients who had pure EST were free of tumor after VAC therapy. Gallion et al. reported 17 of 25 (68%) patients with stage I disease alive and well 2 or more years after treatment with VAC. Sessa et al. treated 13 patients who had pure EST of the ovary, 12 of whom had initial unilateral oophorectomy. All received VBP and are alive at 20 months to 6 years (Table 12-3). Three patients relapsed but were salvaged. This experience is important because 9 of these patients had stage IIb or more advanced disease.

Schwartz et al. has used VAC for stage I disease but prefers VBP for stage II-IV patients. Of 15 patients, 12 are alive without evidence of disease. Their routine is to treat at least one course beyond a normal alpha-fetoprotein titre (this has become routine in many centers). One recurrence was treated successfully with BEP. Two early VAC failures were not salvaged with VBP. The GOG evaluated VBP in stage III and IV and in recurrent malignant germ cell tumors, many with measureable disease after surgery. Sixteen of 29 (55%) ESTs were long-term disease-free survivors. VBP induced a substantial number of durable complete responses, even in patients with prior chemotherapy. Toxicity was significant. Although a second-look laparotomy was part of this protocol, not all patients underwent (for various reasons) second-look surgery. The role of second-look surgery in germ cell tumors certainly has not been established. Some investigators, including the authors, feel the role of second-look laparotomy in germ cell tumors is very limited if indicated at all. The GOG is currently evaluating BEP in advanced germ cell tumors. Smith et al., at Duke, reported 3 patients whose diseases were resistant to MAC and VBP who were put into complete remission with regimens that contained VP-16-213 and cisplatin. All patients have remained free of tumor for 4 years or longer. Williams noted that in disseminated germ cell tumors (primarily of the testes) BEP was more effective and had less neuromuscular toxicity than VBP.

Fujita from Japan reported 41 patients with endodermal sinus tumors, either pure or mixed. Although this covered a long time interval (1965-1992), 21 of their patients were treated surgically with unilateral oophorectomy. More aggressive surgery did not increase survival. Survival was similar whether VAC or PBV were used. None of the stage I patients died if postoperative VAC or PBV was given.

From a practical point of view, serum AFP determination is considered to be a useful diagnostic tool in patients who have endodermal sinus tumors and in fact should be considered an ideal tumor marker. It can be of value in monitoring the results of therapy and in detecting metastasis and recurrences after therapy. As previously noted, many investigators use AFP as a guide to the number of courses needed for an individual patient. In many instances, only 3 or 4 courses have placed patients into remission with long-term survival. Conservative surgery plus chemotherapy have resulted in an appreciable number of successful pregnancies after treatment. Curtin has nevertheless reported two patients with normal AFPs but positive second-look laparotomies, although this finding currently must be considered the exception. Recent reports suggest that there may be recurrences in the retroperitoneal nodes in the absence of recognizable intraperitoneal disease.

Levels of human chorionic gonadotropin (hCG) and its beta subunit (β-hCG) have been found to be normal in patients with endodermal sinus tumor.

Embryonal Carcinoma

Embryonal carcinoma is one of the most malignant cancers arising in the ovary (Figure 12-6). The neoplasm, only recently described, closely resembles the embryonal carcinoma of the adult testes, where it is relatively

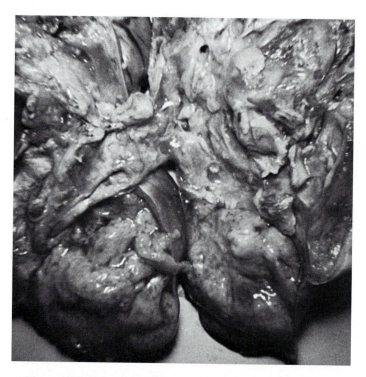

Figure 12-6 Gross photograph of embryonal carcinoma of ovary.

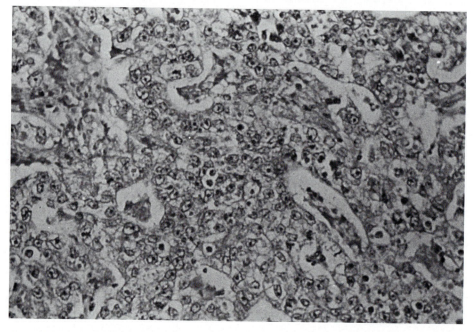

Figure 12-7 Microscopic appearance of large primitive cells with occasional papillary or gland-like formations characteristic of embryonal carcinoma.

common. However, it represents only 4% of the malignant ovarian germ cell tumors. in the ovary and its confusion with choriocarcinoma and endodermal tumors in the past account for its late identification as a distinct entity. It usually manifests as an abdominal mass or pelvic mass occurring at a mean age of 15 years. More than half the patients have hormonal abnormalities, including precocious puberty, irregular uterine bleeding, amenorrhea, or hirsutism. The tumors consist of large primitive cells with occasional papillary or glandlike formations (Figure 12-7). The cells have eosinophilic cytoplasm with distinct borders and round nuclei with prominent nucleoli.

Table 12-4   Comparison of embryonal carcinoma with endodermal sinus tumor

	Endodermal sinus tumor (71 cases)	Embryonal carcinoma (15 cases)
Median age	19 years	15 years
Prepubertal status	23%	47%
Precocious puberty	0	43%
Positive pregnancy test	None (0/15)	All (9/9)
Vaginal bleeding	1%	33%
Amenorrhea	0	7%
Hirsutism	0	7%
Survival, stage I patients	16%	50%
Human chorionic gonadotrophin	Negative (0/15)	Positive (10/10)
Alpha-fetoprotein	Positive (15/15)	Positive (7/10)

From Kurman RJ, Norris HJ: *Cancer* 38:2404, 1976.

Numerous mitotic figures, many atypical, are seen; and scattered throughout the tumor are multinucleated giant cells that resemble syncytial cells.

These tumors contain hCG, syncytiotrophoblast-like cells, and AFP in the large primitive cells. This tumor probably arises from primordial germ cells, but it develops before there is much further differentiation toward either embryonic or extraembryonic tissue. In a review of 15 patients Kurman and Norris reported an actuarial survival rate of 30% for the entire group; for those with stage I tumors, it was 50% (Table 12-4). This is significantly better than survival with the endodermal sinus tumor for the same period of time and before the advent of vigorous multiple-agent adjuvant chemotherapy. With modern therapy, survivals should be much improved. Optimal therapy, although not yet established, is probably similar to that for endodermal sinus tumor.

The VAC regimen is definitely active in this disease but does not appear to be as reliable for advanced cases as the VBP regimen. It is suggested that patients receiving VAC be watched closely for progression, and the more toxic VBP regimen can be used at that point in the hope of salvage. The total number of courses of VAC therapy needed to achieve optimal numbers of disease-free patients is really not known.

The GOG has evaluated the effectiveness of the VBP regimen in stages III and IV recurrent malignant germ cell tumors of the ovary, including embryonal carcinoma. Ninety-four patients have been treated, and this therapy has produced a substantial number of durable complete responses in patients who previously received chemotherapy. The overall progression-free interval at 24 months is approximately 55%. The GOG is currently evaluating bleomycin, etoposide, and cisplatin (BEP) in

this group of patients. Progress can be monitored by measuring hCG and AFP levels.

Polyembryoma

Polyembryoma is a rare ovarian germ cell neoplasm composed of numerous embryoid bodies resembling morphologically normal embryos. Similar homologous neoplasms occur more frequently in the human testes. To date, only a handful of ovarian polyembryomas have been reported. In most instances the polyembryoma has been associated with other neoplastic germ cell elements, mainly immature teratoma.

Polyembryoma is a highly malignant germ cell neoplasm, and in the majority of cases it has been associated with invasion of adjacent structures and organs and extensive metastases that are mainly confined to the abdominal cavity. The tumor is not sensitive to radiotherapy and its response to chemotherapy is unknown.

Choriocarcinoma

Choriocarcinoma, a rare, highly malignant tumor that may be associated with sexual precocity, can arise in one of three ways: (1) as a primary gestational choriocarcinoma associated with ovarian pregnancy; (2) as a metastatic choriocarcinoma from a primary gestational choriocarcinoma arising in other parts of the genital tract, mainly the uterus; and (3) as a germ cell tumor differentiating in the direction of trophoblastic structures and arising admixed with other neoplastic germ cell elements. Choriocarcinomas of the ovary may also be divided into two broad groups: gestational choriocarcinoma, encompassing the first two groups mentioned above, and nongestational choriocarcinoma, a germ cell tumor differentiating toward trophoblastic structures. Only nongestational choriocarcinoma of the ovary are discussed here. In the majority of cases the tumor is admixed with other neoplastic germ cell elements, and their presence is diagnostic of nongestational choriocarcinoma, except for the remote possibility of the tumor being a gestational choriocarcinoma metastatic to an ovarian germ cell tumor. The tumor, in common with other malignant germ cell neoplasms, occurs in children and young adults. Its occurrence in children has been emphasized; in some series, 50% of cases occurred in prepubescent children. This high incidence in children may result from the previous reluctance of investigators to make the diagnosis in adults.

These neoplasms secrete hCG. This is particularly noticeable in prepubescent children, who show evidence of isosexual precocious puberty with mammary development, growth of pubic and axillary hair, and uterine bleeding. Adult patients may have signs of ectopic pregnancies, because the nongestational choriocarcinoma, like its gestational counterpart, is associated with an increased production of hCG. Estimation of urinary or plasma hCG levels is a useful diagnostic test in these cases. Historically, the prognosis of patients with choriocarcinoma of the ovary was unfavorable, but modern chemotherapy regimens appear to be effective. Prolonged remissions have been achieved by Creasman et al. in four cases using the MAC combination chemotherapy. Some responses have been seen with combination chemotherapy using methotrexate as one of the drugs in the regimen. In most instances the other drugs used in the combinations have been dactinomycin and an alkylating agent.

Mixed Germ Cell Tumors

Mixed germ cell tumors contain at least two malignant germ cell elements. Dysgerminoma is the most common component (80% in Kurman and Norris's report and 69% in material from MD Anderson Hospital). Immature teratoma and EST are also frequently identified; embryonal carcinoma and choriocarcinoma are seen only occasionally. It is not unusual to see three or four different germ cell components. In 42 patients treated at MD Anderson Hospital, 9 were treated with surgery alone, and another 6 received radiation therapy—all developed recurrences. Of 17 patients who received VAC, 9 were placed into remission. Five received primary treatment of VBP after surgery, and 4 are alive and well. Twenty patients (48%) are alive and well. Eleven underwent second-look laparotomies after various chemotherapeutic courses, and all were negative. Of 14 patients who had stage I disease and were treated with combination chemotherapy after surgery, 11 (79%) survived. Creasman et al. treated five stage I lesions with MAC chemotherapy for three courses or fewer. Three patients also received pelvic radiation, and all 5 are alive at 12 to 14 months. The GOG treated 10 completely resected mixed germ cell tumors with VAC, and 7 are long-term survivors. Four of five patients who had incompletely resected disease and who were treated with VAC developed recurrences. Schwartz treated 8 patients with mixed tumors with VAC and 7 are long-term survivors. Only 1 patient did not respond to PVB therapy. Because the most significant component of mixed tumors usually predicts results, it should determine therapy and follow-up.

Teratoma

Mature cystic teratoma

Accounting for more than 95% of all ovarian teratomas, the dermoid cyst, or mature cystic teratoma, is one of the most common ovarian neoplasms. Teratomas account for approximately 15% of all ovarian tumors. They are the most common ovarian tumors in women in the second and third decades of life. Fortunately, the overwhelming majority of benign cystic lesions contain mature tissue of ectodermal, mesodermal, and/or endodermal origin. The most common elements are ectodermal derivatives such as skin, hair follicles, and sebaceous or sweat glands, accounting for the characteristic histologic and gross appearance of teratomas (Figure 12-8). These tumors are usually multicystic and contain hair intermixed with foul-smelling, sticky, keratinaceous and sebaceous debris. Occasionally, well-formed teeth are seen along with cartilage or bone. If the tumor is composed of only ectodermal derivatives of skin and skin appendages, it is a true dermoid cyst. A mix of other, usually mature tissues (gastrointestinal, respiratory) may be present.

The clinical manifestation of this slow-growing lesion is usually related to its size, compression, or torsion, or to a chemical peritonitis secondary to intra-abdominal spill of the cholesterol-laden debris. The latter event tends to occur more commonly when the tumor is large. Torsion is the most frequent complication, observed in as many as 16% of the cases in one large series, and it tends to be more common during pregnancy and the puerperium. Mature cystic teratomas are said to comprise 22%-40% of ovarian tumors in pregnancy, and 0.8%-12.8% of reported cases of mature cystic teratomas have occurred in pregnancy. In general, torsion is more common in children and younger patients. Severe acute abdominal pain is usually the initial symptom, and the condition is considered an acute abdominal emergency. Rupture of a mature cystic teratoma is an uncommon complication, occurring in approximately 1% of cases, but it is much more common during pregnancy and may manifest during labor. The immediate result of rupture may be shock or hemorrhage, especially during pregnancy or labor, but the prognosis even in these cases is favorable. Rupture of the tumor into the peritoneal cavity may be followed by a chemical peritonitis caused by the spill of the contents of the tumor. This may result in a marked granulomatous reaction and lead to the formation of dense adhesions throughout the peritoneal cavity. Infection is an uncommon complication of mature cystic teratoma and occurs in approximately 1% of cases. The infecting organism is usually a coliform, but *Salmonella* species infection causing typhoid fever has also been reported. Removal of the neoplasm by ovarian cystectomy or, rarely, oophorectomy appears to be adequate therapy.

Mature solid teratoma

Mature solid teratoma is a very rare ovarian neoplasm and a very uncommon type of ovarian teratoma. The histologic components in it are similar to those found in immature solid teratoma, which occurs mainly in children and young adults. The presence of immature elements immediately excludes the tumor from this group, and by definition only tumors composed entirely of mature tissues may be included. The tumor is usually unilateral and therefore adequately treated by unilateral oophorectomy. Although this neoplasm is considered benign, occasionally mature solid teratomas may be associated with peritoneal implants composed entirely of mature glial tissue, and in spite of the extensive involvement that may be present, the prognosis is excellent.

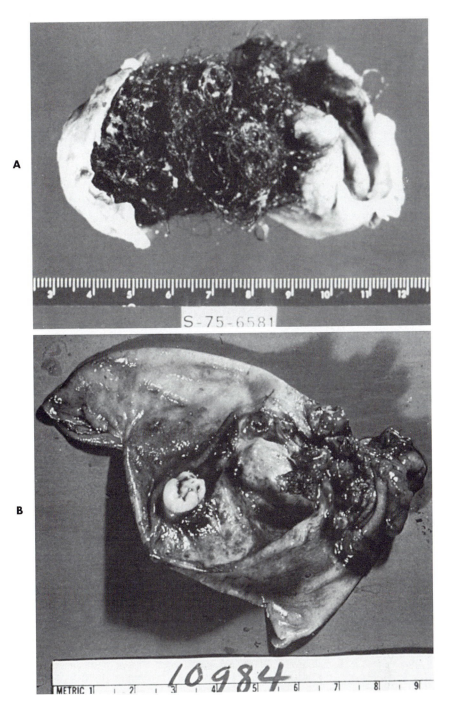

Figure 12-8 Benign cystic teratoma. **A** and **B,** Gross appearance.   *Continued.*

Immature teratoma

Immature teratomas are composed of tissue derived from the three germ layers—ectoderm, mesoderm, and endoderm—and, in contrast to the much more common mature teratoma, they contain immature or embryonal structures. These tumors have had a variety of names: solid teratoma, malignant teratoma, teratoblastoma, teratocarcinoma, and embryonal teratoma. These names have arisen because immature teratomas have been incorrectly considered mixed germ cell tumors or secondary malignant tumors originating in mature benign teratomas. Mature tissues are frequently present and sometimes may predominate. Immature teratoma of the ovary is an uncommon tumor, comprising less than 1% of ovarian teratomas. In contrast to the mature cystic teratoma, which is encountered most frequently during the reproductive years but occurs at all ages, the immature teratoma has a specific age incidence, occurring most commonly in the first two decades of life and almost unknown after menopause. By definition, an

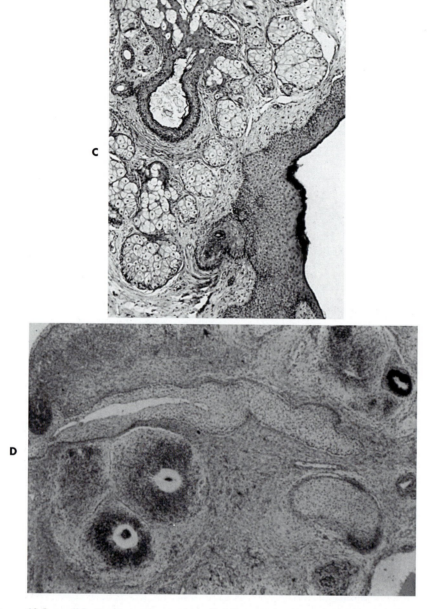

Figure 12-8, cont'd. Benign cystic teratoma. **C,** Microscopic view of ectodermal elements (skin and skin appendages). **D,** Immature neural elements evident with squamous epithelium and cartilage.

immature teratoma contains immature neural elements. According to Norris et al. the quantity of immature neural tissue alone determines the grade.

Neuroblastomatous elements, glial tissue, and immature cerebellar and cortical tissue may also be seen. These tumors are graded histologically on the basis of the amount and degree of cellular immaturity. The range is from grade 1 (mature teratoma containing only rare immature foci) through grade 3 (large portions of the tumor consist of embryonal tissue with atypicality and mitotic activity). Generally, older patients tend to have lower grade primary tumors than younger patients. When

the neoplasm is solid and all elements are well differentiated histologically (solid mature teratoma), a grade 0 designation is given (Table 12-5).

Immature teratomas are virtually never bilateral, although occasionally a benign teratoma is found in the opposite ovary. These tumors may have multiple peritoneal implants at the time of initial surgery, and the prognosis is closely correlated with the histologic grade of the primary tumor and the implants. Norris et al. studied 58 patients with immature teratomas and reported an 82% survival rate for patients who had grade 1 primary lesions, 63% for grade 2, and 30% for grade 3 (Table

Table 12-5   Immature teratoma—grading system

Grade	Thurlbeck and Scully	Norris et al.
0	All cells well differentiated	All tissue mature; rare mitotic activity
1	Cells well differentiated; rare small foci of embryonal tissue	Some immaturity and neuroepithelium limited to low magnification field in any slide (× 40)
2	Moderate quantities of embryonal tissue; atypia and mitosis present	Immaturity and neuroepithelium does not exceed 3 low power microscopic fields in any one slide
3	Large quantities of embryonal tissue; atypia and mitosis present	Immaturity and neuroepithelium occupying 4 or more low magnification fields on a single slide

Table 12-6   Immature (malignant) teratomas

Grade	n	Tumor deaths	%
1	22	4	(18)
2	24	9	(37)
3	10	7	(70)

From Norris HJ, Zirkin HJ, Benson WL: *Cancer* 37:2356, 1976.

12-6). Multiple sections of the primary lesion and wide sampling of the peritoneal implants are necessary to properly grade the tumor. In the majority of cases the implants are better differentiated than the primary tumors. Both the primary lesion and the implants should be graded according to the most immature tissue present.

Because the lesion is rarely bilateral in its ovarian involvement, the present method of therapy consists of unilateral salpingo-oophorectomy with wide sampling of peritoneal implants. Total abdominal hysterectomy with bilateral salpingo-oophorectomy does not seem to be indicated, since it does not influence the outcome for the patient. Radiotherapy has also been shown to be of little value. If the primary tumor is grade 1 and all peritoneal implants (if they exist) are grade 0, no further therapy is recommended. However, if the primary tumor is grade 2 or 3 or if implants or recurrences are grade 1, 2, or 3, triple-agent chemotherapy has recently been shown to be helpful. The VAC regimen has proved to be highly effective. DiSaia et al. have reported on several patients with disseminated disease treated with this chemotherapeutic regimen. At second-look laparotomy these patients were free of immature elements but retained peritoneal

implants containing exclusively mature elements. This was labeled chemotherapeutic retroconversion of immature teratoma of the ovary. All these patients have had uneventful follow-ups with the mature implants apparently remaining in static states. Apparently this is a common occurrence.

Experience with the treatment of 25 patients (mean age at diagnosis 19 years) with immature teratomas of the ovary was reported by Curry et al. In their study, 4 patients received postoperative external radiation therapy to the pelvis and/or abdomen, either alone or with a single chemotherapeutic agent, 2 were treated with postoperative single-agent chemotherapy, and 2 had no treatment other than surgical removal of the tumors. All 8 patients died of their disease; the longest survival time was 40 months, and 6 of the 8 patients survived less than 12 months after the initial treatment. Five patients received postoperative combination chemotherapy, with MAC or ActFUCy. Two were surviving at 73 and 50 months after the initiation of chemotherapy. The combination of vincristine (1.5 mg/m^2), dactinomycin (0.5 mg), and cyclophosphamide (500 mg) was administered to 12 patients. The drugs were administered intravenously every week for 12 consecutive weeks, and then a 5-day intravenous course was given every 4 weeks for 2 years. At the time of their report, all of the 10 patients who initially responded were surviving 16 to 28 months after the initiation of chemotherapy. Of the 12 patients, 1 died at 3 months and 1 died at 26 months.

The GOG treated 20 completely resected immature teratomas with VAC. Only one patient failed, and she was treated primarily at the time of recurrence. Of 8 advanced or recurrent lesions that were incompletely resected, only 4 responded to VAC. The group at MD Anderson Hospital reported that 15 of 18 patients (83%) with immature teratomas had sustained remission with primary VAC chemotherapy. VBP has been used by the GOG in patients with advanced or recurrent immature teratomas. They treated 26 patients, of whom 14 (54%) were disease-free survivors. Creasman treated 6 patients who had immature teratomas with MAC, and all are long-term survivors. Schwartz usually treats stage I patients with 6 cycles of VAC. Those with more advanced disease are given 12 cycles and a second-look operation. Of 29 patients, 24 were successfully treated. Four of the five patients with persistent lesions were successfully salvaged. Today, most investigators treat stage Ia grade 1 immature teratomas with unilateral oophorectomy alone. Patients with stage Ia grade 2 or 3, as well as more advanced lesions, are treated postsurgically with VAC. Three courses appear to be as effective as longer chemotherapy regimens, particularly in patients with completed resected disease.

Bonazzi and colleagues from Italy reported their experience with 32 patients with pure immature teratomas. This represents 28% of all germ cell tumors seen by these investigators. Twenty-nine patients were stage I or II and 24 had grade 1 or 2 tumors. Twenty-two patients were treated with conservative surgery only (unilateral oophorectomy or cystectomy). Thirty of 32 patients had fertility-sparing surgery performed. Five of 6 patients wishing subsequent pregnancies had 7 pregnancies with delivery of 7 normal infants. Chemotherapy was given after surgery only in stage I and II grade 3 tumors or in stage III. Ten patients received a cisplatin-based regimen. All 32 patients are alive and disease free at a median of 47 months (11-138 months).

It should be noted that conservative therapy for germ cell tumors is now the norm. Even with advanced disease, unilateral oophorectomy and complete surgical staging with preservation of the uterus and other ovary may be considered. Fortunately, most germ cell tumors are early staged and with the exception of dysgerminomas are almost always limited to one ovary. Length of chemotherapy is also being given with fewer courses and excellent results. This is important because menstrual irregularity (even amenorrhea) during chemotherapy may be related to length of chemotherapy. Subsequent fertility may be affected. Fortunately many patients with germ cell tumors have had many successful subsequent pregnancies after therapy. Although this appears to be age related in that the earlier the age at treatment the less vulnerable to menstrual irregularities and infertility, most germ cell patients are young and have apparent minimal infertility. This is in contrast to older patients (e.g., breasts cancer) who are premenopausal. Most become amenorrheic during chemotherapy, and very few will have resumption of their menstrual periods and therefore have premature ovarian failure.

Monodermal or highly specialized teratomas

Struma ovarii. Another tumor thought to represent the unilateral development of benign teratoma is struma ovarii, which is composed totally or predominantly of thyroid parenchyma. This is an uncommon lesion and should not be confused with benign teratomas that contain small foci of thyroid tissue. Between 25%-35% of patients with strumal tumors will have clinical hyperthyroidism. The gross and microscopic appearance of these lesions is similar to that of typical thyroid tissue, although the histologic pattern may resemble that in adenomatous thyroid. These ovarian tumors may undergo malignant transformation but they are usually benign and easily treated by simple surgical resection.

Carcinoid tumors. Primary ovarian carcinoid tumors usually arise in association with gastrointestinal or respiratory epithelium present in mature cystic teratoma. They may also be observed within a solid teratoma or a mucinous tumor, or they may occur in an apparently pure form. Primary ovarian carcinoid tumors are uncommon. Approximately 50 cases have been reported. The age distribution of patients with ovarian carcinoid tumors is similar to that of patients with mature cystic teratoma, although the average age may be somewhat higher in ovarian carcinoid tumors. Many patients are postmenopausal.

One third of the reported cases have been associated with the typical carcinoid syndrome, in spite of the absence of metastasis. This is in contrast to intestinal carcinoid tumors, which are associated with the syndrome only when there is metastatic spread to the liver. Excision of the tumor has been associated with the rapid remission of symptoms in all of the described cases and the disappearance of 5-hydroxyindoleacetic acid from the urine. The primary ovarian carcinoids are only occasionally associated with metastasis; metastasis was observed in only 3 of 47 reported cases in one review. The prognosis after excision of the primary tumor is favorable and in the majority of cases a cure results.

Strumal carcinoid is an even rarer entity. It represents a close admixture of the previously discussed struma ovarii and carcinoid tumors and may actually represent medullary carcinoma resulting in thyroid tissue. Most cases follow a benign course.

Gonadoblastoma

Gonadoblastoma is a rare ovarian lesion composed of germ cells resembling those of dysgerminoma and gonadal stroma cells resembling those of a granulosa or Sertoli tumor. Sex chromatin studies usually show a negative nuclear pattern (45, X) or a sex chromosome mosaicism (45, X/46, XY). Patients who have a gonadoblastoma usually have primary amenorrhea, virilization, or developmental abnormalities of the genitalia. The discovery of gonadoblastoma is made in the course of investigation of these conditions. Another not infrequent initial symptom is the presence of a pelvic tumor. The majority of patients with gonadoblastoma (80%) are phenotypic women, and the remainder are phenotypic men with cryptorchidism, hypospadias, and internal female secondary sex organs. Among the phenotypic women, 60% are virilized, and the remainder are normal in appearance.

The prognosis of patients with gonadoblastoma is excellent if the tumor and the contralateral gonad, which may be harboring a macroscopically undetectable gonadoblastoma, are excised. When gonadoblastoma is associated with or overgrown by dysgerminoma, the prognosis is still excellent. Metastases tend to occur later and more infrequently than in dysgerminoma arising de novo. Complete agreement has not been reached on whether the uterus should be excised with the gonads. In the opinion of many the uterus should be retained for psychologic reasons and exogenous estrogen therapy given for periodic bleeding. It is our practice to leave the uterus even after removing both gonads. Cyclic hormone therapy is indicated in these young women. Ovum transfer has been successful in patients with both ovaries removed.

Second Look Laparotomy and Recurrences in Germ-Cell Tumors

The role of the second look laparotomy (SLL) in carcinoma of the ovary is currently being debated. Experience in germ-cell tumors of the ovary is even less well defined. Williams reporting the experience of the GOG noted that in patients with complete tumor resection followed by chemotherapy, 43 of 45 patient had no evidence of tumor or mature teratoma at the time of the SLL. Two patients had immature teratomas. There were 72 patients with advanced incompletely resected tumors who received chemotherapy followed by SLL. Of 48 patients who did not have teratomatous lesions in their primary surgery, 45 had no tumor. The 3 with persistence died from their disease despite aggressive therapy. There were 24 patients with teratomatous elements in their primary tumor and 16 immature elements at SLL. These authors feel that the role of SLL is rarely, if ever, beneficial if the tumor is primarily resected followed by adequate chemotherapy. Other authors in small series have suggested that there is a role for SLL, particularly in patients initially seen with advanced unresected disease.

Recurrences in many instances can be successfully treated. The group at MD Anderson noted 42 primary therapy failures in 160 germ-cell patients. Using different chemotherapeutic regimens, 12 of 42 (29%) are currently disease free. Surgical debulking may have a role in the management of recurrences. Twenty-four patients had surgery and 12 are alive, all with less than 2 cm residual disease. None of the 7 patients with disease greater than 2 cm residual survived.

TUMORS DERIVED FROM SPECIAL GONADAL STROMA

Classification

This category of ovarian tumors includes all those that contain granulosa cells, theca cells and luteinized derivatives, Sertoli cells, Leydig cells, and fibroblasts of gonadal stromal origin. Sex cord-stromal tumors as a group account for approximately 5% of all ovarian tumors, but functioning neoplastic groups of this variety comprise only 2%. Five percent to 10% of ovarian cancers belong in the sex cord-stromal group; most of these are granulosa cell tumors, which are low-grade malignancies.

Granulosa-Stromal Cell Tumors

Granulosa and theca cell tumors occur about as frequently in women in the reproductive age group as they do in women who are postmenopausal. Only about 5% of granulosa cell tumors occur before puberty (Table 12-7). Most granulosa and theca cells produce estrogen, but a few are androgenic. The exact proportion of these neoplasms that have function is really not known because the endometrium is often not examined microscopically and appropriate preoperative laboratory tests are not done.

Table 12-7   Granulosa cell tumor—age distribution of 118 cases

Age	Number
Child	3
12-40	27
41-50	28
51-60	32
60-79	28
TOTAL	118

Based on data from Evans AJ III et al: *Obstet Gynecol* 55:213, 1980.

Table 12-8   Granulosa cell tumor (76 patients)

Endometrial histology	Number	%
Proliferative endometrium	19	25
Atrophic endometrium	5	7
Hyperplastic endometrium	42	55
Adenocarcinoma	10	13

Based on data from Evans AJ III et al: *Obstet Gynecol* 55:213, 1980.

About 80%-85% of granulosa cell and theca cell neoplasms are palpable on abdominal or pelvic examination, but occasionally an unsuspected tumor is found when a hysterectomy is done on a patient who has abnormal bleeding as a result of endometrial hyperplasia or endometrial carcinoma. A study by Evans et al. from the Mayo Clinic of 76 patients who had granulosa cell tumors and in whom endometrial tissue was available shows a high incidence of endometrial stimulation (Table 12-8). In another study, one third of patients had atypia of endometrial cells noted.

Granulosa cell tumors vary greatly in gross appearance (Figure 12-9). Sometimes they are solid tumors that are soft or firm, depending on the relative amounts of neoplastic cells and fibrothecomatous stroma they contain, and are yellow or gray, depending on the amount of intracellular lipid in the lesion. More commonly, the granulosa cell tumor is predominantly cystic and, on external examination, may resemble mucinous cystadenoma or cystadenocarcinoma. However, when sectioned, this cyst is generally found to be filled with serous fluid or clotted blood. About 15% of patients with cystic granulosa cell tumors are first examined for acute abdomens associated with hemoperitoneum.

Granulosa cell tumors occur in two subtypes: adult and juvenile. Adult granulosa cell tumors account for approximately 95% of all granulosa cell tumors. They occur more commonly in the postmenopausal patient and are the most common tumor that produces estrogen. Abnormal en-

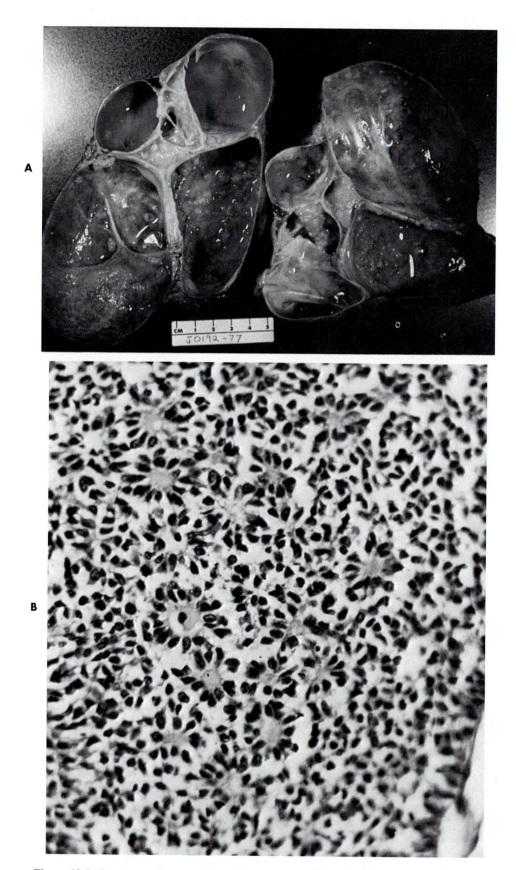

Figure 12-9 Granulosa cell tumor of ovary. **A,** Gross appearance. **B,** Microscopic appearance with Call-Exner bodies.

dometria in these patients are not uncommon such as hyperplasia or even carcinoma of the endometrium. The latter, which is usually well differentiated has been reported as high as 25% of cases in some reports, although they probably occur in 5% or less of cases. Other estrogenic effects may also be noted such as tenderness or swelling of the breast, and vaginal cytology may show an increase in maturation of the squamous cells. Rarely, androgenic effects may be present in which hirsute changes may be present. Histologically, fibrothecomatous components are common and the cytoplasm is usually scant. The typical coffee-bean grooved cells are present. Mature follicles and Call Exner bodies are common.

In juvenile granulosa cell tumors, the great majority are in young adults with the most occurring in the first three decades of life. Most of the juvenile granulosa cell tumors that occur in children result in sexual precocity with the development of breasts and pubic and axillary hair. Irregular uterine bleeding may also be present. Thyroidmegaly may also occur. The vast majority of these tumors are limited to one ovary. Histologically, thecomatous components are common; cytoplasm is abundant. Mitosis may be numerous, and the nuclei are dark and usually do not have the grooved coffee bean appearance. Pleomorphism may also be present. Even though these tumors appear to be less well differentiated than the adult type, nevertheless, the cure rate is quite high.

On the basis of their differentiation, granulosa cell tumors should be divided into two general categories: well differentiated and moderately differentiated. The former pattern may have various presentations, including microfollicular, macrofollicular, trabecular, solid-tubular, and watered-silk. Tumors in the moderately differentiated category have a diffuse pattern that has also been designated "sarcomatoid." Although attempts have been made by many authors, no distinct correlation between histologic structure and prognosis has yet been substantiated. It is important that undifferentiated carcinomas, adenocarcinomas, and carcinoids not be misdiagnosed as granulosa cell tumors, which they may superficially resemble. Each of these tumors has a strikingly different prognosis. One characteristic feature is the appearance of the nuclei. Oval or angular, grooved nuclei are typical of granulosa cell tumors ("coffee bean appearance"). Call-Exner bodies are also of diagnostic importance but unfortunately are not often sharply defined.

True granulosa tumors are low-grade malignancies, the majority of which are confined to one ovary at the time of diagnosis. Only 5%-10% of the stage I cases will subsequently recur, and they often appear more than 5 years after initial therapy. The prognosis for these patients is excellent: long-term survival rates from 75%-90% have been reported for all stages. These lesions are adequately managed during the reproductive years by removing the involved ovary and ipsilateral tube. The uterus and uninvolved adnexa should be removed in the perimeno-

pausal and postmenopausal age groups, which is the treatment for other benign or low malignant potential tumors. In a series from the Mayo Clinic 92% of the patients had survived 5-10 years (76 patients, 82% of whom had stage I lesions). The recurrence pattern in this same series (18.6% overall recurrence rate) revealed that 23% of the recurrences were more than 13 years after initial therapy. Most of the recurrences occurred in preserved genital tract structures. These kinds of data have prompted our recommendation that the preserved internal genitalia be removed in the perimenopausal patient in whom preservation may have been appropriate during the childbearing period.

Several studies address prognostic factors in granulosa cell tumor of the ovary. Other than stage, mitotic activity, DNA ploidy and S-phase fractions have been evaluated. In a study of 54 patients from Sweden, patients with mitotic rates of ≤4/10 HPF had no deaths while all patients with ≥10/10 HPF died, with the longest survival being 4 years. Patients with mitotic rate of 4-10/10 HPF had a median survival of 9 years. Fortunately, most patients had mitotic counts of ≤4/10 HPF. In a small study, about two thirds of the patients studied were found to have euploid tumors and only 1 patient died of disease while 4 of 5 patients with aneuploidy tumors died of disease. S-phase fraction was not correlated with any clinical or histologic parameters.

Inhibin is a glycoprotein secreted by granulosa cells of the ovary. It secretes throughout the menstrual cycle and during pregnancy but not in the postmenopausal woman. As a result, inhibin has been suggested as a tumor marker for granulosa cell tumors. In collective series, albeit in small numbers, the relationship of tumor to the level of inhibin appears to be very good.

Often, recurrent tumors have been effectively treated by means of reoperation, radiation therapy, chemotherapy, or a combination thereof. Although radiation therapy has been advocated for these tumors by many authors, careful search of the literature shows a paucity of evidence relating enhanced curability to the use of radiation therapy. There has never been a prospective study comparing one form of therapy with another for patients who have advanced or recurrent disease. The question of adjuvant radiotherapy in the postmenopausal woman found to have granulosa cell tumor is often an issue.

Our practice has been to recommend no further therapy in patients who have stage I lesions. Stage II or III or recurrent granulosa cell tumors are probably best treated with systemic chemotherapy. Although the optimal chemotherapeutic regimen has not yet been determined, the following drugs have been used singly or in combination and appear to be effective: Adriamycin, bleomycin, cisplatin, and vinblastine. Colombo and associates reported 11 previously untreated women with recurrent and/or metastatic granulosa cell tumor of the ovary who were treated with VBP. Nine patients responded; 6 with complete pathological response. Patients received between 2 and 6 courses of chemotherapy. The GOG is currently evaluating BEP in a nonrandomized study of advanced or recurrent granulosa cell tumors of the ovary.

Thecomas are not quite as frequent as granulosa cell tumors but have similar appearances. They are solid fibromatous lesions that show varying degrees of yellow or orange coloration. Whereas granulosa cell tumors are found to be bilateral in 2%-5% of patients, thecomas are almost always confined to one ovary. On microscopic examination most tumors in the granulosa-theca cell category are found to contain both cell types. If more than a very small component of granulosa cells is present, the term *granulosa cell tumor*, rather than *granulosa-theca cell tumor*, is generally applied. The designation theca cell tumor or thecoma should be reserved for neoplasms consisting entirely of benign theca cells.

Thecomas consist of neoplastic cells of ovarian stromal origin that have accumulated moderate to large amounts of lipid. Sometimes such tumors contain clusters of lutein cells, in which case the term *luteinized thecoma* is often used. Occasionally, tumors fall into a gray zone between thecomas and fibromas. Although the latter also arise from ovarian stromal cells, they differentiate predominantly in the direction of collagen-producing fibroblasts. Tumors in the gray zone may be designated thecoma-fibroma. They are almost always unilateral and virtually never malignant. Several tumors have been reported in the literature as malignant thecomas but at least some of these are better interpreted as fibrosarcomas or diffuse forms of granulosa cell tumors. In cases in which preservation of fertility is important, a thecoma may be treated adequately by unilateral oophorectomy. However, total hysterectomy with bilateral salpingo-oophorectomy is recommended in most postmenopausal and perimenopausal women.

Sertoli-Leydig Cell Tumors

Sertoli-Leydig cell tumors contain Sertoli cells and/or Leydig cells in varying proportions and varying degrees of differentiation. These tumors are thought to originate from the specialized gonadal stroma. The cells were able to differentiate into any of the structures derived from the embryonic gonadal mesenchyme. Because less well-differentiated neoplasms within this category may recapitulate the development of the testes, the terms *andro-blastoma* and *arrhenoblastoma* have been used as synonyms for Sertoli-Leydig cell tumors. However, their connotation of associated masculinization is misleading, since some of these tumors have no endocrine manifestation and others may even be accompanied by an estrogenic syndrome. Nevertheless, the World Health Organization has selected *androblastoma* as an alternate term for Sertoli-Leydig cell tumor. These neoplasms account for less than 0.5% of all ovarian tumors but are

among the most fascinating from pathologic and clinical viewpoints. They occur in all age groups but are most often encountered in young women, who usually become virilized (Figure 12-10). In immunocytochemical studies testosterone appears to be localized predominantly within the Leydig cells. Estrogen and androstenedione appear in many of the same cells. Thus one can see the multifaceted clinical presentation of this fascinating neoplasm. Classically there is progressive masculinization that is heralded by hirsutism, temporal balding, deepening of the voice, and enlargement of the clitoris.

Sertoli-Leydig cell tumors with heterologous elements may contain a variety of unusual cell types but the degree of differentiation of the tumors is probably of greater importance in determining its prognosis than is its content of unexpected tissue. In the report by Young and Scully, only 29 of 220 tumors of this type have been clinically malignant. None of the 27 well-differentiated tumors and only 4 of 100 tumors of intermediate differentiation were known to be clinically malignant. Zaloudek and Norris reported on 64 intermediately and poorly differentiated neoplasms. Only 3 of 50 patients with stage I disease developed recurrence. The 5-year survival in all of their patients was 92%.

The overall 5-year survival rate of patients with Sertoli-Leydig cell tumors has been reported to be slightly over 70% to slightly over 90%. Because these tumors occur predominantly in young women and are bilateral in fewer than 5% of cases, conservative removal of the tumor and adjacent fallopian tube is justifiable, if

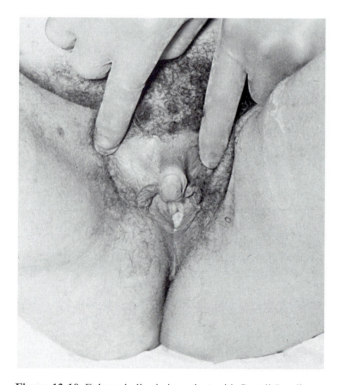

Figure 12-10 Enlarged clitoris in patient with Sertoli-Leydig cell tumor (arrhenoblastoma).

preservation of fertility is an important consideration and if there is no evidence of extension beyond the involved ovary. Like granulosa cell tumors, they are considered to have low malignant potential. Once again the VAC regimen of chemotherapy is often recommended for patients who have advanced or recurrent lesions. In the unusual patient who has advanced or recurrent Sertoli-Leydig cell tumor, it seems that chemotherapy appears to be effective, although the experience is very limited. The combination of cisplatin and vinblastine and bleomycin appears to be active in this disease. There is at least one case report that has noted an elevated serum alpha-fetoprotein as an early indication of recurrence.

Gynandroblastoma

Rarely, a gonadostromal tumor contains unequivocal granulosa cell elements combined with tubules and Leydig cells characteristic of arrhenoblastomas. Designated as gynandroblastomas, these mixed tumors may be associated with either androgen or estrogen production, and they can be expected to behave as low-grade malignancies similar to the individual components.

Lipid Cell Neoplasms

Lipid cell neoplasms are a heterologous group of tumors that have in common a parenchyma composed of polygonal cells containing lipid. They include neoplasms that have been designated as hilus cell tumors, Leydig tumors, adrenal rest tumors, stroma luteomas, or masculinovoblastomas. Leydig cell tumors are unilateral and are commonly found in the medulla or hilus regions of the ovaries. Tumors that have spread to contiguous organs or have a microscopic cellular pleomorphism with high mitotic activity should be considered malignant. Reinke crystals, normally occurring in mature Leydig cells of the testes, are often found in these neoplasms, and their presence may be interpreted as signifying a benign lesion. Regardless of the presence or absence of Reinke crystals, neoplasms smaller than 8 cm in diameter can be expected to act benignly.

TUMORS DERIVED FROM NONSPECIFIC MESENCHYME

Benign and malignant tumors, including fibromas, hemangiomas, leiomyomas, soft-tissue sarcomas, lymphomas, and rare neoplasms, may arise in the ovaries from nonspecific supporting tissues that are common to most organs. The most common and most important tumors in this category are the fibroma and the lymphoma.

The mixed mesodermal sarcoma of the ovary (analogous to its uterine counterpart) has been more widely recognized in the last decade. It is an extremely rare neoplasm and one that is invariably fatal. A recent review by Hernandez et al. suggested that 50% of the patients have stage III tumors when first seen, and the patients are

most commonly diagnosed in the sixth decade of life. Various forms of combination chemotherapy, including a vigorous regimen with VAC, have been advocated with varied results.

METASTATIC TUMORS TO THE OVARY

Roughly 6% of ovarian cancers encountered by surgeons exploring pelvic or abdominal masses are metastases, most often either metastatic breast tumors or metastatic adenocarcinomas of large intestine origin. Metastases from carcinomas of the breast are among the more common surgical specimens of the ovary, especially if one includes those found incidentally. They are almost always incidental findings in therapeutic oophorectomy and rarely form symptomatic masses that require surgical removal. The term *Krukenberg tumor* should be reserved for metastases that contain significant numbers of signet ring cells in a cellular stroma derived from the ovarian stroma. This restriction is important because tumors with these microscopic characteristics also have distinctive gross pathologic and clinical features. Almost all metastasize from the stomach but some arise in the breast, intestine, or other mucous gland-containing organs. Krukenberg tumors form a solid, often uniform mass, the sectioned surface of which typically exhibits gelatinous necrosis and hemorrhage.

Metastatic adenocarcinomas of large intestinal origin have become more common than Krukenberg tumors in the past two decades with the gradual decline in the incidence of carcinoma of the stomach. These lesions are characterized microscopically by the presence of large acini similar to those of primary intestinal carcinomas. Grossly, they may form solid metastases but more often appear as large, partly cystic tumors with areas of hemorrhage and necrosis (Figure 12-11). In such instances they are easily confused with cystic forms of primary ovarian cancers.

The ovary is frequently the site of metastasis from certain primary carcinomas. Approximately 10% of ovarian tumors are not primary in origin. The most common metastasis is in the form of a carcinoma arising in the endometrium. There is no doubt that cancer of the endometrium metastasizes to the ovaries but it may be difficult to distinguish metastasis of an endometrial cancer from a separate ovarian tumor. This is particularly true in the case of ovarian endometrioid carcinoma, which according to Scully is associated with a similar tumor in the endometrium in one third of cases.

There are four possible pathways of spread to tumors to the ovary: (1) direct continuity, (2) surface papillation, (3) lymphatic metastasis, and (4) hematogenous spread. Lymphatic metastasis is undoubtedly the most common pathway for spread to the ovary. The rich network of lymph nodes and lymphatic channels in the pelvis readily explains the metastatic pathway of tumors in the uterus

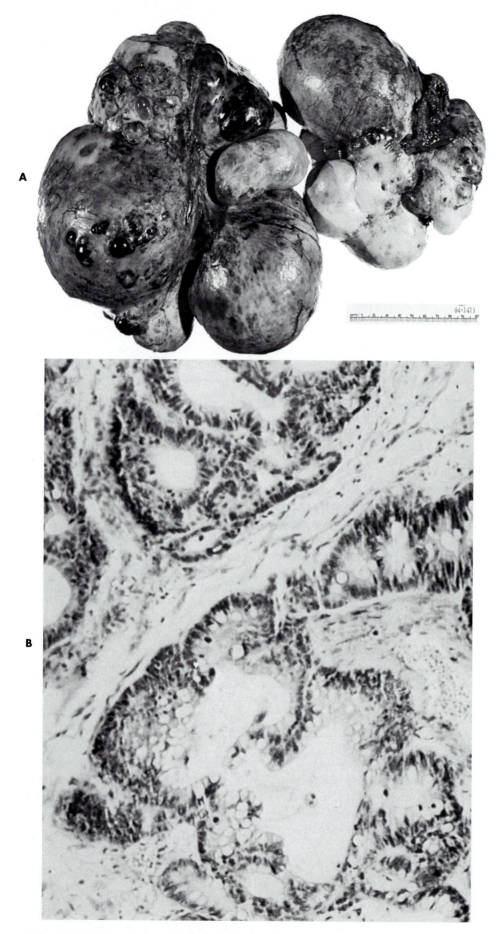

Figure 12-11 Metastatic tumor to ovary from adenocarcinoma of colon. **A,** Gross appearance. **B,** Histologic appearance. Note large acini similar to those of intestinal carcinoma.

and contralateral ovary. The rare finding of clusters of tumor cells limited to lymphatics in the medulla of the ovary in cases of breast carcinoma confirms that this is the pathway of spread to the ovary. As yet, no one has convincingly described the pathway of metastasis to the ovaries from cancer of the stomach. It is known that the lymphatic channels that drain the upper gastrointestinal tract ultimately link up with the lumbar chain of lymph nodes. Ovarian lymphatics drain into the lumbar nodes. This could well be the route of spread to the ovaries in these cases.

There have been cases of metastatic ovarian carcinoma in which there was a clinical presentation consistent with hormonal activity. Both androgen and estrogen excretion have been described. Endometrial hyperplasia has been described in postmenopausal patients with metastatic ovarian carcinomas, presumably indicating estrogen activity within the metastatic lesion or its normal tissue capsule.

MALIGNANT OVARIAN TUMORS IN CHILDREN

Ovarian tumors, cysts, and torsion are more frequent indications for surgical intervention in infancy and childhood than is commonly realized. They may produce symptoms similar to appendicitis and it is not always appreciated how often they mimic this condition. Pain is the most frequently reported symptom. The proportion of all tumors of the abdomen in this age group that are ovarian in origin has not been reported. A palpable abdominal mass is found in half of the patients with neoplasms. Roughly 10% of the patients have isosexual precocity, which includes patients who demonstrate precocious puberty and those with an early onset of sexual development. The initial signs are areolar pigmentation and breast development. Some patients have vaginal discharge or bleeding, and others have pubic hair. These changes usually completely regress after surgical extirpation of the responsible endocrine-secreting tumor. Granulosa-theca cell tumors are by far the most common ovarian neoplasms found in these patients with isosexual precocity and adnexal enlargement.

Most ovarian cancers in children are of germ cell origin. Cangir et al. reported on 21 girls younger than 16 years, with a median age of 13.5. Of the 21 patients, 8 had malignant teratomas, 6 had mixed germinal tumors, 6 had endodermal sinus tumors, and 1 had a stromal cell tumor (Sertoli-Leydig type). There were 8 stage I, 1 stage II, 7 stage III, and 5 stage IV patients. Ablin reported on a study of 17 children with ovarian germ cell tumors treated with multiple-agent chemotherapy. Of the 17 patients, 13 showed complete responses to therapy, suggesting that survival rates in this group of patients have improved significantly with modern chemotherapy. Lack et al. reported that granulosa-theca cell tumors in the premenarche patient accounted for 4% of childhood ovarian tumors at their institution from 1928 to 1979. The average age of diagnosis of their 10 patients was 5 years, and precocious "pseudopuberty" was the most common presentation. These 10 lesions were solitary; 5 were on the right side and 5 were on the left side, with an average diameter of 12 cm. All 10 patients survived at least 10 years, and salpingo-oophorectomy was curative despite tumor spill in 2.

Fortunately the most common germ cell neoplasm is the benign teratoma. A significant number of other patients have benign functional cysts of the ovary. All patients are treated in a manner similar to that of the adolescent, or the older patient in the early reproductive age period.

BIBLIOGRAPHY

Germ cell tumors

Abell MR, Johnson VJ, Holtz F: Ovarian neoplasms in childhood and adolescence. I. Tumors of germ cell origin, *Am J Obstet Gynecol* 92:1059, 1965. Albites V: Solid teratoma of the ovary with malignant gliomatosis peritonei, *Int J Gynaecol Obstet* 12:59, 1974.

Arias-Bernal L, Jones HW: Chromosomes of a malignant ovarian teratoma, *Am J Obstet Gynecol* 100:785, 1968.

Asadourian LA, Taylor HB: Dysgerminoma: an analysis of 105 cases, *Obstet Gynecol* 33:370, 1969.

Ashley DJB: Origin of teratomas, *Cancer* 32:390, 1983.

Bianchi UA, Sartori E, Favallin G: New trends in treatment of ovarian dysgerminoma, *Gynecol Oncol* 23:246, 1986.

Boczkowski K, Teter J, Sternadel Z: Sibship occurrence of XY gonadal dysgenesis with dysgerminoma, *Am J Obstet Gynecol* 113:952, 1972.

Bonazzi C, Peccatori F, Colombo N et al: Pure ovarian immature teratome, a unique and curable disease: 10 year's experience of 32 prospectively treated patients, *Obstet Gynecol* 84:598-604, 1994.

Bradof JE et al: Germ cell malignancies of the ovary, treatment with vinblastine, actinomycin D, bleomycin, and cis-platin containing chemotherapy combinations, *Cancer* 50:1070, 1982.

Breen JL, Neubecker RD: Malignant teratoma of the ovary: an analysis of 17 cases, *Obstet Gynecol* 21:669, 1963.

Creasman WT, Soper JT: Assessment of contemporary management of germ cell malignancies of the ovary, *Am J Obstet Gynecol* 153:828, 1985.

Creasman WT et al: Germ cell malignancies of the ovary, *Obstet Gynecol* 53:226, 1979.

Curry SL, Smith JP, Gallagher HS: Malignant teratoma of the ovary: prognostic factors and treatment, *Am J Obstet Gynecol* 131:845, 1978.

Curtin JP, Morrow CP, Ablaing GD, Schlaerth JB: Malignant germ cell tumors of the ovary: 20- year report of LAC-USC Women's Hospital, *Int J Gynecol Cancer* 4:29-35, 1994.

Curtin JP, Rubin SL, Hoskins WJ et al: Second look laparotomy in endodermal sinus tumor: a report of two patients with normal levels of alphafetoprotein and residual tumor at re-exploration, *Obstet Gynecol* 73:93, 1989.

De Palo G et al: Natural history of dysgerminoma, *Am J Obstet Gynecol* 143:799, 1982.

DiSaia PJ et al: Chemotherapeutic retroconversion of immature teratome of the ovary, *Obstet Gynecol* 49:346, 1977.

Emig OR, Hertig AT, Rowe FJ: Gynandroblastoma of the ovary: review and report of a case, *Obstet Gynecol* 13:135, 1959.

Favara BE, Franciosi RA: Ovarian teratoma and neuroglial implants on the peritoneum, *Cancer* 31:678, 1973.

Felmus LB, Pedowitz P: Clinical malignancy of endocrine tumors of the ovary and dysgerminoma, *Obstet Gynecol* 29:344, 1967.

Forney JP, DiSaia PJ, Morrow CP: Endodermal sinus tumor: a report of two sustained remissions treated postoperatively with a combination of actinomycin D, 5-fluorouracil and cyclophosphamide, *Obstet Gynecol* 45:186, 1975.

Freel JH et al: Dysgerminoma of the ovary, *Cancer* 43:798, 1979.

Fujita M, Inque M, Tanizawa et al: Retrospective review of 41 patients with endodermal sinus tumor of the ovary, *Int J Gynecol Cancer* 3:329-335, 1993.

Gallion HH, Van Nagell JR, Donaldson ES et al: Ovarian dysgerminoma: report of seven cases and review of the literature, *Am J Obstet Gynecol* 158:591, 1988.

Gallion H, Van Nagell JR, Pall BF: Therapy of endodermal sinus tumors of the ovary, *Am J Obstet Gynecol* 135:447, 1979.

Gerbie MV, Brewer JI, Taminni H: Primary choriocarcinoma of the ovary, *Obstet Gynecol* 46:720, 1975.

Gershenson DM: Menstrual and reproductive function after treatment with combined chemotherapy for malignant ovarian germ cell tumors, *J Clin Oncol* 6:270, 1988.

Gershenson DM, Del Junco G, Copeland LJ: Mixed germ cell tumors of the ovary, *Obstet Gynecol* 64:200, 1985.

Gershenson DM et al: Endodermal sinus tumor of the ovary, *Obstet Gynecol* 61:194, 1983.

Goldstein DP, Piro JA: Combination chemotherapy in the treatment of germ cell tumors containing choriocarcinoma, *Surg Gynecol Obstet* 134:61, 1972.

Gordon A, Lipton D, Woodruff JD: Dysgerminoma: a review of 158 cases from the Emil Novak Ovarian Tumor Registry, *Obstet Gynecol* 58:497, 1981.

Hart WR, Burkons DM: Germ cell neoplasms arising in gonadoblastomas, *Cancer* 43:669, 1979.

Hay DM, Stewart DB: Primary ovarian choriocarcinoma, *J Obstet Gynaecol Br Commonw* 76:941, 1969.

Jacobs A et al: Treatment of recurrent and persistent germ cell tumors with cis-platin, vinblastine and bleomycin, *Obstet Gynecol* 59:129, 1982.

Jimerson GK, Woodruff JD: Ovarian extra-embryonal teratoma. I. Endodermal sinus tumor, *Am J Obstet Gynecol* 127:73, 1977.

Koller O, Gjonnaess H: Dysgerminoma of the ovary: a clinical report of 20 cases, *Acta Obstet Gynecol Scand* 43:268, 1964.

Kosloske AM et al: Management of immature teratoma of the ovary in children by conservative resection and chemotherapy, *J Pediatr Surg* 11:839, 1976.

Krepart G et al: The treatment of dysgerminoma of the ovary, *Cancer* 41:986, 1978.

Kurman RJ, Norris HJ: Embryonal carcinoma of the ovary—a clinico-pathologic entity distinct from endodermal sinus tumor resembling embryonal carcinoma of the adult testis, *Cancer* 38:2420, 1976.

Kurman RJ, Norris HJ: Endodermal sinus tumor of the ovary: a clinical and pathological analysis of 71 cases, *Cancer* 38:2404, 1976.

Kurman RJ, Norris HJ: Malignant germ cell tumors of the ovary, *Hum Pathol* 8:551, 1977.

Kurman RJ, Norris HJ: Malignant mixed germ cell tumors of the ovary: a clinical and pathological analysis of 30 cases, *Obstet Gynecol* 48:579, 1976.

La Polla JP, Bende J, Vigliotti AP et al: Dysgerminoma of the ovary, *Obstet Gynecol* 69:859, 1987.

Lucraft HH: A review of 33 cases of ovarian dysgerminoma emphasizing the role of radiotherapy, *Clin Radiol* 30:585, 1979.

Messing MJ, Gershenson DM, Morris M et al: Primary treatment failure in patients with malignant ovarian germ cell neoplasms, *Int J Gynecol Cancer* 2:295-300, 1992.

Morris HHB, La Vecchia C, Draper GJ: Endodermal sinus tumor and embryonal carcinoma of the ovary in children, *Gynecol Oncol* 21:7, 1985.

Neubecker RD, Breen JL: Gynandroblastoma: a report of five cases, with a discussion of the histogenesis and classification of ovarian tumors, *Am J Clin Pathol* 38:60, 1982.

Newlands ES et al: Potential for cure in metastatic ovarian teratomas and dysgerminomas, *Br J Obstet Gynaecol* 89:555, 1982.

Nogales FF Jr et al: Immature teratoma of the ovary with a neural component ("solid" teratoma): a clinicopathologic study of 20 cases, *Hum Pathol* 7:625, 1976.

Nogales-Fernandez F et al: Yolk sac carcinoma (endodermal sinus tumor): ultrastructure and histogenesis of gonadal and extragonadal tumors in comparison with normal human yolk sac, *Cancer* 39:1462, 1977.

Norris HJ, Zirkin HJ, Benson WL: Immature (malignant) teratoma of the ovary: a clinical and pathologic study of 58 cases, *Cancer* 37:2359, 1976.

Parvez D et al: Long-term disease-free survival in immature teratoma of the ovary, *Cancer* 50:159, 1982.

Robboy SJ, Scully RE: Ovarian teratoma with glial implants on the peritoneum: an analysis of 12 cases, *Hum Pathol* 1:643, 1970.

Rosenshein NB et al: Pregnancy following chemotherapy for an ovarian immature embryonal teratoma, *Gynecol Oncol* 8:234, 1979.

Roth LM, Panganiban WG: Gonadal and extragonadal yolk sac carcinomas: a clinicopathologic study of 14 cases, *Cancer* 37:812, 1976.

Russell P, Pointer DM: The pathologic assessment of ovarian neoplasms. V. The germ cell tumors, *Pathology* 14:47, 1982.

Santesson L, Marrubini G: Clinical and pathological survey of ovarian embryonal carcinomas, including so-called "mesonephromas" (Schiller) or "mesoblastomas" (Teilum), treated at the Radiumhemmet, *Acta Obstet Gynecol Scand* 36:399, 1957.

Schellhas HF et al: Germ cell tumors associated with XY gonadal dysgenesis, *Am J Obstet Gynecol* 109:1197, 1971.

Schwartz PE, Chambers SK, Chambers JT et al: Ovarian germ cell malignancies: the Yale University experience, *Gynecol Oncol* 45:26, 1992.

Scully RE: Gonadoblastoma: a review of 74 cases, *Cancer* 25:1340, 1970.

Scully RE: Ovarian tumors: a review, *Am J Pathol* 87:686, 1977.

Scully RE: Special ovarian tumors and their management, *Int J Radiat Oncol Biol Phys* 8:1419, 1982.

Sessa C et al: Cisplatin, vinblastine, and bleomycin combination chemotherapy in endodermal sinus tumors of the ovary, *Obstet Gynecol* 70:220, 1987.

Slate RE et al: Vincristine, dactinomycin and cyclophosphamide in treatment of germ cell tumors of the ovary, *Cancer* 56:243, 1985.

Slayton RE et al: Treatment of malignant ovarian germ cell tumors; response to vincristine, dactinomycin, and cyclophosphamide (preliminary report), *Cancer* 42:390, 1978.

Slayton RE, Park RC, Schenberg SG et al: Vincristine, dactinomycin and cyclophosphamide in the treatment of malignant germ cell tumors of the ovary, *Cancer* 56:243, 1985.

Smith EB, Clarke-Pearson DL, Creasman WT: A VP16-213- and cisplatin-containing regimen for treatment of refractory ovarian germ cell malignancies, *Am J Obstet Gynecol* 150:927, 1984.

Takeda A et al: Polyembryoma of ovary producing alpha-fetoprotein and HCG: immunoperoxidase and electron microscopic study, *Cancer* 49:1878, 1982.

Talerman A, Haije WG, Baggerman L: Serum alpha fetoprotein (AFP) in the diagnosis and management of endodermal sinus (yolk sac) tumor and mixed germ cell tumor of the ovary, *Cancer* 41:272, 1978.

Teilum G: Endodermal sinus tumors of the ovary and testes: comparative morphogenesis of the so-called mesonephroma ovarii (Schiller) and extraembryonic (yolk sac allantoic) structure of the rat placenta, *Cancer* 12:1029, 1959.

Teilum G: Classification of endodermal sinus tumor (mesoblastoma vitellinum) and so-called "embryonal carcinoma" of the ovary, *Acta Pathol Microbiol Scand* 64:407, 1965.

Tewfik HH, Tewfik FA, Latourette HB: A clinical review of seventeen patients with ovarian dysgerminoma, *Int J Radiat Oncol Biol Phys* 8:1705, 1982.

Thomas EM, Dembo AJ, Hacker NF et al: Current therapy for dysgerminoma of the ovary, *Obstet Gynecol* 70:268, 1987.

Thomas GM et al: Current therapy for dysgerminoma of the ovary, *Obstet Gynecol* 70:268, 1987.

Thurlback WM, Scully RE: Solid teratoma of the ovary: a clinicopathic analysis of 9 cases, *Cancer* 13:804, 1960.

Ungerleider RS et al: Endodermal sinus tumor: the Stanford experience and the first reported case arising in the vulva, *Cancer* 41:1627, 1978.

Williams SD: Current management of ovarian germ cell tumors, *Oncol* 8:53-67, 1994.

Williams SD, Birch R, Einhorn LH et al: Treatment of disseminated germ-cell tumors with cisplatin, bleomycin and either vinblastine or etoposide, *N Engl J Med* 316:1435, 1987.

Williams SD, Blessing JA, DiSaia PJ et al: Second look laparotomy in ovarian germ cell tumors: The Gynecologic Oncology Group Experience, *Gynecol Oncol* 52:287-291, 1994.

Williams SD, Blessing JA, Moore DM et al: Cisplatin, vinblastine and bleomycin in advanced and recurrent ovarian germ cell tumors, *Ann Int Med* 111:22, 1989.

Wiltshaw E et al: Chemotherapy of endodermal sinus tumour (yolk sac tumor) of the ovary: preliminary communication, *J R Soc Med* 75:888, 1982.

Stromal tumors

Anderson WR, Levine AJ, MacMillan D: Granulosa-theca cell tumors: clinical and pathologic study, *Am J Obstet Gynecol* 110:32, 1971.

Burger HG: Clinical utility of inhibin measurements, *J Clin Endocrin Metab* 76:1391-1395, 1993.

Camlibel FT, Caputo TA: Chemotherapy of granulosa cell tumors, *Am J Obstet Gynecol* 145:763, 1983.

Chalvardjian A, Scully RE: Sclerosing stromal tumors of the ovary, *Cancer* 31:664, 1973.

Colombo N, Essa C, Landonin F et al: Cisplatin, vinblastine and bleomycin combination chemotherapy in metastatic granulosa cell tumor of the ovary, *Obstet Gynecol* 67:265, 1986.

Dinnerstein AJ, O'Leary JA: Granulosa-theca cell tumors: a clinical review of 102 patients, *Obstet Gynecol* 31:654, 1968.

DiSaia PJ et al: A temporary response of recurrent granulosa cell tumor to Adriamycin, *Obstet Gynecol* 52:355, 1978.

Evans AJ III et al: Clinicopathologic review of 118 granulosa and 82 theca cell tumors, *Obstet Gynecol* 55:213, 1980.

Finan MA, Roberts WS, Kavanagh JJ: Ovarian Sertoli-Leydig cell tumor: success with salvage therapy, *Int J Gynecol Cancer* 3:189-91, 1993.

Gillibrand PN: Granulosa-theca cell tumors of the ovary associated with pregnancy: case report and review of the literature, *Am J Obstet Gynecol* 94:1108, 1966.

Goldstein DP, Lamb EJ: Arrhenoblastoma in first cousins: report of 2 cases, *Obstet Gynecol* 35:444, 1970.

Gusberg SB, Kardon P: Proliferative endometrial response to theca-granulosa cell tumors, *Am J Obstet Gynecol* 111:633, 1971.

Healy DL, Burger HG, Mamers P et al: Elevated serum inhibin concentrations in postmenopausal women with ovarian tumors, *New Engl J Med* 329: 1539-42, 1993.

Jacobs AJ, Deppe G, Cohen CJ: Combination chemotherapy of ovarian granulosa cell tumor with cisplatinum and doxorubicin, *Gynecol Oncol* 14:294, 1982.

Lack EE et al: Granuloa-theca cell tumors in premenarchal girls: a clinical and pathologic study of ten cases, *Cancer* 48:1846, 1981.

Malstrom H, Hogberg T, Risberg B, Simonsen E: Granulosa cell tumors of the ovary: prognostic factors and outcome, *Gynecol Oncol* 52:50-55, 1994.

Norris HJ, Taylor HB: Prognosis of granulosa-theca tumors of the ovary, *Cancer* 21:255, 1968.

Norris HJ, Taylor HB: Virilization associated with cystic granulosa tumors, *Obstet Gynecol* 34:629, 1969.

Novak ER, Long JH: Arrhenoblastoma of the ovary: a review of the Ovarian Tumor Registry, *Am J Obstet Gynecol* 92:1082, 1965.

Novak ER, Mattingly RF: Hilus cell tumor of the ovary, *Obstet Gynecol* 15:425, 1960.

Novak ER et al: Feminizing gonadal stromal tumors: analysis of granulosa-theca cell tumors of the Ovarian Tumor Registry, *Obstet Gynecol* 38:701, 1971.

Pedowitz P, O'Brien FB: Arrhenoblastoma of the ovary: review of the literature and report of 2 cases, *Obstet Gynecol* 16:62, 1960.

Roush GR, El-Nagger AK, Abdul-Karim FW: Granulosa cell tumor of the ovary: a clinicopathologic and flow cytometric DNA analysis, *Gynecol Oncol* 56:430-434, 1995.

Sjostedt S, Wahlen T: Prognosis of granulosa cell tumors, *Acta Obstet Gynecol Scand* 49(suppl 6):1, 1961.

Stenwig JT, Hazekamp J, Beecham J: Granulosa cell tumors of the ovary: a clinicopathological study of 118 cases with long term follow-up, *Gynecol Oncol* 7:136, 1979.

Teilum G: Classification of testicular and ovarian androblastoma and Sertoli cell tumors, *Cancer* 11:769, 1958.

Young RH, Scully RE: Ovarian Sertoli-Leydig cell tumors with a retiform pattern: a problem in histopathologic diagnosis: a report of 25 cases, *Am J Surg Pathol* 7:755, 1983.

Zaloudek C, Norris HJ: Granulosa tumors of the ovary in children: a clinical and pathological study of 32 cases, *Am J Surg Pathol* 6:503, 1982.

Zaloudek C, Norris HJ: Sertoli-Leydig tumors of the ovary: a clinicopathologic study of 64 intermediate and poorly differentiated neoplasms, *Am J Surg Pathol* 8:405, 1984.

Children and/or pregnancy

Abell MR, Holtz F: Ovarian neoplasms in childhood and adolescence. II. Tumors of non-germ cell origin, *Am J Obstet Gynecol* 93:850, 1965.

Ablin AR: Malignant germ cell tumors in children, *Front Radiat Ther Oncol* 16:141, 1982.

Acosta A, Kaplan AL, Kaufman RH: Gynecologic cancer in children, *Am J Obstet Gynecol* 112:944, 1972.

Barber HRK: Ovarian cancers in childhood, *Int J Radiat Oncol Biol Phys* 8:1427, 1982.

Barber HRK, Graber EA: Gynecological tumors in childhood and adolescence, *Obstet Gynecol Surv* 28:357, 1973.

Breen JL, Bonamo JF, Maxson WS: Genital tract tumors in children, *Pediatr Clin North Am* 28:355, 1981.

Breen JL, Neubecker RD: Ovarian malignancy in children with special reference to the germ cell tumors, *Ann NY Acad Sci* 142:208, 1962.

Cangir A, Smith J, van Eys J: Improved prognosis in children with ovarian cancers following modified VAC (vincristine, sulfate, dactinomycin, and cyclophosphamide) chemotherapy, *Cancer* 42:1234, 1978.

Carlson DH, Griscom NT: Ovarian cysts in the newborn, *AJR* 116:664, 1972.

Creasman WT, Rutledge FN, Smith JP: Carcinoma of the ovary associated with pregnancy, *Obstet Gynecol* 38:111, 1971.

Groeber WR: Ovarian tumors during infancy and childhood, *Am J Obstet Gynecol* 86:1027, 1963.

Hernandez W et al: Mixed mesodermal sarcoma of the ovary, *Obstet Gynecol* 49:59, 1977.

Holtz F, Hart WR: Krukenberg tumors of the ovary: a clinicopathologic analysis of 27 cases, *Cancer* 50:2438, 1982.

Kase N, Conrad S: Steroid synthesis in abnormal ovaries. I. Arrhenoblastoma, *Am J Obstet Gynecol* 90:1251, 1964.

Kempers RD et al: Struma ovarii-ascitic, hyperthyroid and asymptomatic syndromes, *Ann Intern Med* 72:883, 1970.

Marshall JR: Ovarian enlargement in the first year of life: review of 45 cases, *Ann Surg* 161:372, 1965.

Moore JC, Schifrin BS, Erez S: Ovarian tumors in infancy, childhood and adolescence, *Am J Obstet Gynecol* 99:913, 1967.

Norris HJ, Jensen RD: Relative frequency of ovarian neoplasms in children and adolescents, *Cancer* 39:713, 1972.

Smith JP, Rutledge F, Sutow WW: Malignant gynecologic tumors in children: current approaches to treatment, *Am J Obstet Gynecol* 116:261, 1973.

Weinblatt ME, Ortega JA: Treatment of children with dysgerminoma of the ovary, *Cancer* 49:2608, 1982.

Other ovarian tumors

Azoury RS, Woodruff JD: Primary ovarian sarcomas: report of 43 cases from the Emil Novak Ovarian Tumor Registry, *Obstet Gynecol* 37:920, 1971.

Blackwell WJ et al: Dermoid cysts of the ovary, their clinical and pathologic significance, *Am J Obstet Gynecol* 51:151, 1946.

Dehner LP, Norris HJ, Taylor HB: Carcinosarcomas and mixed mesodermal tumors of the ovary, *Cancer* 27:207, 1971.

Einhorn LH, Donohue J: Cis-diamminedichloro-platinum, vinblastine, and bleomycin combination chemotherapy in disseminated testicular cancer, *Ann Intern Med* 87:293, 1977.

Ferenczy A, Okagaki T, Richart RM: Para-endocrine hypercalcemia in ovarian neoplasms: report of mesonephroma with hypercalcemia and review of literature, *Cancer* 27:427, 1971.

Fox LP, Stamm WJ: Krukenberg tumor complicating pregnancy: report of a case with androgenic activity, *Am J Obstet Gynecol* 92:702, 1965.

Genadry R, Parmley T, Woodruff JD: Case report—secondary malignancies in benign cystic teratomas, *Gynecol Oncol* 8:246, 1979.

Hale RW: Krukenberg tumor of the ovaries: a review of 81 records, *Obstet Gynecol* 22:221, 1968.

Joshi VV: Primary Krukenberg tumor of ovary: a review of literature and case report, *Cancer* 22:1199, 1968.

Judd HL et al: Maternal virilization developing during a twin pregnancy: demonstration of excess ovarian androgen production associated with theca-lutein cysts, *N Engl J Med* 288:118, 1973.

Krumerman MS, Chung A: Squamous carcinoma arising in benign cystic teratoma of the ovary, *Cancer* 29:1237, 1977.

Peterson WF et al: Benign cystic teratomas of the ovary: a clinico-statistical study of 1007 cases with a review of the literature, *Am J Obstet Gynecol* 70:568, 1955.

Qizilbach AH et al: Functioning primary carcinoid tumor of the ovary, *Am J Clin Pathol* 62:629, 1974.

Robboy SJ, Scully RE, Norris HJ: Carcinoid metastatic to the ovary; a clinicopathologic analysis of 35 cases, *Cancer* 33:798, 1974.

Robboy SJ, Scully RE, Norris HJ: Primary trabecular carcinoid of the ovary, *Obstet Gynecol* 49:202, 1977.

Spadoni LR et al: Virilization coexisting with Krukenberg tumor during pregnancy, *Am J Obstet Gynecol* 92:981, 1965.

Woodruff D, Noli Castillo RD, Novak ER: Lymphoma of the ovary: a study of 35 cases from the Ovarian Tumor Registry of the American Gynecological Society, *Am J Obstet Gynecol* 85:912, 1963.

Woodruff JD, Novak ER: The Krukenberg tumor: a study of 48 cases from the Ovarian Tumor Registry, *Obstet Gynecol* 15:351, 1960.

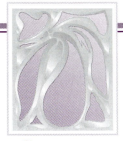

Carcinoma of the Fallopian Tube

SIGNS AND SYMPTOMS
DIAGNOSIS
THERAPY
PROGNOSIS
SARCOMAS

Adenocarcinoma of the fallopian tube is one of the rarest malignancies of the female genital tract. Its frequency in relationship to all gynecologic cancers is usually considered to be 1% or less. In review of nine population-based cancer registries in the United States between 1973 and 1984, the average annual incidence of fallopian tube neoplasms was 3.6/1,000,000 women. More recent data confirms this rare occurrence. Therefore, the experience of any one physician (even at a large cancer referral institution) is limited. As a result, it is not at all surprising that the diagnosis is infrequently made preoperatively. In many instances, this lesion is initially seen as an unexpected operative finding, and cases have been reported in patients who were undergoing tubal sterilization. At one time, chronic tubal inflammation was said to be associated with fallopian tube carcinoma. The initial connection was with tuberculosis; however, more recent reports fail to note this association. Although histologic features of old pelvic inflammatory disease are frequently noted on gross or histologic examination of the tube, it is impossible to determine whether such changes preceded the development of the carcinoma. Chronic inflammation is no longer considered a predisposing factor. Primary infertility in more than 70% of patients has been reported in some series. Bilateral occurrence of tubal cancer is seen much more frequently in infertile patients. Mei-Lin noted a fivefold greater bilateral incidence. As a result, almost one half of patients reported in some series are nullipa-

rous. Several studies noted a higher frequency rate of other gynecologic malignancies, as well as breast cancer, in patients with tubal cancer. Age incidence resembles the pattern seen among women who develop ovarian or endometrial malignancies, with the average age at the time of diagnosis in the 50s. It should be noted that a patient in her teens has been reported with this malignancy.

SIGNS AND SYMPTOMS

Most patients who have these malignancies will have symptoms such as vaginal bleeding or discharge, lower abdominal pain, abdominal distention, and pressure. In many instances these symptoms are vague and nonspecific. Vaginal bleeding is the most common symptom of tubal carcinoma and is present in more than 50% of the patients. Because this lesion occurs most frequently in the postmenopausal patient, postmenopausal bleeding is common, and as a result, carcinoma of the endometrium is the first consideration in the differential diagnosis. One must seriously consider the diagnosis of fallopian tube carcinoma when the D&C is negative and symptoms persist. Vaginal bleeding is caused by blood that accumulates from the lesion in the fallopian tube, which subsequently passes into the uterine cavity, and finally exits into the vagina. Pain is frequently a symptom in tubal carcinoma, is usually colicky, and often accompanies the vaginal bleeding. The pain is caused by distention of the tubal wall and stimulation of peristaltic activity. This pain, in many instances, is relieved with the passage of blood or watery discharge. Vaginal discharge, which is usually clear, is a common finding in tubal carcinoma.

Pain combined with a profuse, watery vaginal discharge is referred to as hydrops tubae profluens. Although the triad of pain, menorrhagia, and leukorrhea is considered pathognomonic for tubal carcinoma, it occurs infrequently. Pain with bloody vaginal discharge is a more common finding. If a patient is examined during the time that hydrops tubae profluens is present, a palpable pelvic mass is frequently found. The mass can actually decrease during the examination while the watery discharge continues. With the cessation of watery discharge and decrease in pelvic mass, the pain also decreases. Hydrops tubae profluens is caused by the effusion produced by the tumor that accumulates within the tube and causes the distention, which in turn produces the colicky pain. The same symptoms are present when bleeding occurs into the tubal lumen. Ascites as well as positive peritoneal cytologic findings are being reported at an increasing frequency. The mass is usually adnexal in location, and in most instances it is interpreted as a pedunculated fibroid or ovarian neoplasm (Figure 13-1).

Delay of symptoms appears to be commonplace. In a study by Eddy et al. symptoms have been present for as long as 48 months. One half the patients had symptoms 2 months or longer. Only 6% of patients were asymptomatic. Semrad et al. noted a delay from onset of symptoms to diagnosis of an average of 4 months in about one half of their patients.

Malignant cells in cervical cytologic preparations have been said to be present in as many as 60% of patients with tubal carcinomas, although that is probably a very optimistic statistic. In a study of 115 patients, Peters found that 23% had positive cervical cytology. The identification of psammoma bodies in cervical cytology should increase the suspicion of tubal or ovarian cancer being present. Certainly, in patients with hydrops tubae proflu-

ens the chances of obtaining malignant cells should be relatively high.

DIAGNOSIS

As previously noted, the diagnosis of this malignancy preoperatively is unusual, if not rare. In 1943 McGoldrick et al. reviewed 376 cases and found only 1 diagnosed correctly preoperatively. In a review of the recent literature, this has not improved substantially. In 71 patients reported by Eddy et al., only two were correctly diagnosed preoperatively. Three of 47 patients reported by Podratz were diagnosed correctly before surgery; however, 2 had prior diagnostic procedures that identified the process. A lack of high index of suspicion probably accounts for not considering this diagnosis preoperatively.

More than 80% of patients have either a pelvic or an abdominal mass noted before surgery. Between 10% and 25% will have abnormal cervical cytology suggestive of adenocarcinoma. Since uterine and ovarian pathology are much more common than tubal disease, it is not surprising that patients with pelvic masses are thought to have abnormalities other than tubal. Patients with abnormal cytology are likewise believed to have cervical or uterine malignancy instead of primary tubal.

Ultrasound, both abdominal and vaginal, is reported to be very accurate in noting changes in adnexal size and and its morphology. Reports have appeared in the literature using this technique as a preoperative diagnosis of tubal cancer. In the large cancer screening project of the Royal

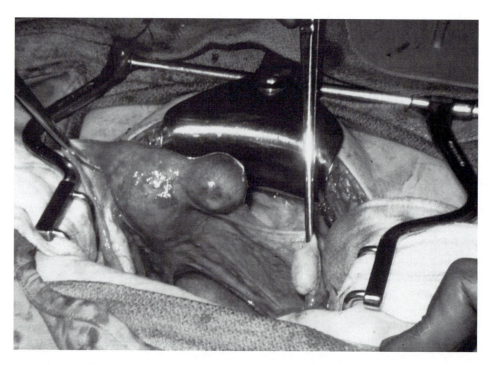

Figure 13-1 Primary tubal carcinoma. The right ovary is normal.

London Hospital 22,000 have been screened with CA125, and if elevated, ultrasound. Of 15 patients with pelvic malignancies identified through the elevated CA125 screening, 3 (20%) were primary fallopian tube cancers. The ratio of epithelial ovarian cancer to fallopian tube cancers was 6:1, a 25-fold greater than expected ratio. Two of the patients had stage I disease and one patient had stage II. Whether this is a true incidence or a selection bias in regard to the woman being screened is unknown. The authors suggest that possibly patients diagnosed with late stage ovarian cancer, in fact, may have had a fallopian tube primary that could not be distinguished from late stage ovarian disease.

Roberts and Lifshitz reported 102 evaluable cases (28 of their own and 74 from the recent literature). Although tubal carcinoma appeared similar to ovarian carcinoma, these authors believed that tubal carcinomas were seen often in early, more curable stages. Recent manuscripts show that more than 50% of patients have stage I or II disease. Certainly this is a more favorable situation than that of ovarian cancer in which two thirds of the patients have stage III or IV disease when the diagnosis is established.

Histologic diagnosis may be difficult. The carcinoma should arise in the mucosa of the endosalpinx and have a papillary pattern with histologic characteristics of the endosalpinx. A transition between the benign and malignant tubal epithelium should be demonstrated. When the ovaries are involved, differentiation between a primary tubal or primary ovarian malignancy should be attempted. When ovarian cancer extends to the tube, serosal involvement is usually quite evident, and the mucosa of the endosalpinx may not be involved. In such situations, the correct diagnosis is apparent. Interestingly, in tubal carcinoma there is usually intraperitoneal involvement before the ovaries are affected. Because of the possibility of early intraperitoneal cytologic spread even with only mucosal involvement, the role of peritoneal cytology is extremely important in this disease entity. In patients with disease limited to the tube, the exact extent should be ascertained. If only the mucosa is involved, an in situ lesion is present, and the prognosis is quite good. When the muscularis is invaded, the prognosis worsens, even with disease limited to the tube.

Hu has suggested diagnostic criteria for the histologic diagnosis of tubal cancer: 1) the main tumor grossly should be in the tube, 2) histologically, the tubal mucosa should be involved with a papillary pattern, and 3) if the tubal wall is involved to a large extent, transition from benign to malignant tubal epithelium should be identified. As previously noted, this distinction in early staged disease should be easily accomplished but may be very difficult in advanced disease.

Late stage disease mimics late staged ovarian cancer with intraperitoneal spread. It appears that fallopian tube cancer, like ovarian cancer, also has a propensity for lymph node metastasis. Klein and associates from Austria noted no nodal metastasis if disease was limited to the tube. Three of 7 patients with clinical stage II disease had lymph node metastasis. Rate of lymph node metastatis increased with intra-abdominal disease. Six of 8 stage III patients had lymph node metastasis. Only 2 patients had only pelvic node metastasis; all others had both pelvic and para-aortic involvement. None of the well-differentiated tumors had nodal metastasis. Patients with nodal metastasis had a worse prognosis than patients without metastasis.

Metastasis to retroperitoneal lymph nodes has been noted in as many as one third of patients.

Nearly all carcinomas of the tube are adenocarcinomas. Endometrioid, clear cell carcinomas, as well as adenocarcinomas and adenosquamous carcinomas, have been reported. Sarcomas have been removed and several case reports have been recently published (see p. 380).

Both tubes are equally effected. Bilaterality has been noted in 10%-25% of patients. Tumors are usually large and noted on pelvic exam; however, the smallest reported adenocarcinoma measured 2.3 mm. Meticulous histologic evaluation of the fallopian tube in apparent benign cases is obligatory.

THERAPY

Because the diagnosis is rarely established preoperatively, one must be prepared to proceed with definitive therapy at the time of exploratory laparotomy for any adnexal mass or when this lesion is found coincidently with other disease. In 1991, FIGO established a staging classification for tubal carcinoma for the first time. It follows the general outline of ovarian carcinoma (Table 13-1).

Therapy guidelines should be essentially the same as those for ovarian carcinoma, and a total abdominal hysterectomy with bilateral salpingo-oophorectomy is minimal therapy. The safety of unilateral salpingo-oophorectomy in young patients desiring fertility whose disease apparently is confined to one tube has not been established. In patients with stage 0, which may be identified at the time of tubal ligation, definitive therapy may be a salpingectomy. Data in this regard is limited. Since fertility is no longer a consideration, bilateral salpingectomy and hysterectomy appears to be a reasonable therapy.

Even with apparent early disease, this malignancy can be bilateral. Peritoneal cytologic specimens should be obtained on opening the peritoneal cavity, not only from the pelvis but also from the lateral paracolonic gutters and supradiaphragmatic areas. Prognostic correlation with peritoneal cytologic findings has been noted in a report from the Mayo Clinic. Patients with negative cytologic findings had a 5-year survival of 67% vs 20% in patients with positive cytologic findings. A partial omentectomy should be performed as well. Any disease outside the

Table 13-1   FIGO fallopian tube staging

Stage 0	Carcinoma in situ (limited to tubal mucosa)
Stage I	Growth limited to the fallopian tubes
Stage Ia	Growth is limited to one tube, with extension into the submucosa and/or muscularis but not penetrating the serosal surface; no ascites
Stage Ib	Growth is limited to both tubes with extension into the submucosa and/or muscularis but not penetrating the serosal surface; no ascites
Stage Ic	Tumor stage Ia or Ib but with tumor extension through or onto the tubal serosa; or with ascites present containing malignant cells, or with positive peritoneal washings
Stage II	Growth involving one or both fallopian tubes with pelvic extension
Stage IIa	Extension and/or metastasis to the uterus and/or ovaries
Stage IIb	Extension to other pelvic tissues
Stage IIc	Tumor stage IIa or IIb, with ascites present containing malignant cells or with positive peritoneal washings
Stage III	Tumor involves one or both fallopian tubes, with peritoneal implants outside the pelvis and/or positive retroperitoneal or inguinal nodes. Superficial liver metastasis equals stage III. Tumor appears limited to the true pelvis but with histologically proven malignant extension to the small bowel or omentum
Stage IIIa	Tumor is grossly limited to the true pelvis, with negative nodes but with histologically confirmed microscopic seeding of abdominal peritoneal surfaces
Stage IIIb	Tumor involving one or both tubes, with histologically confirmed implants of abdominal peritoneal surfaces, none exceeding 2 cm in diameter. Lymph nodes are negative
Stage IIIc	Abdominal implants greater than 2 cm in diameter and/or positive retroperitoneal or inguinal nodes
Stage IV	Growth involving one or both fallopian tubes with distant metastases. If pleural effusion is present, there must be positive cytology to be stage IV. Parenchymal liver metastases equals stage IV

NOTE: Staging for fallopian tube is by the surgical pathological system. Operative findings designating stage are determined prior to tumor debulking.

areas already extirpated should be removed if technically feasible. Debulking as described in ovarian carcinoma would also be applicable to this malignancy: carcinomatous reduction to 1 cm or smaller was feasible in two thirds of patients reported by Podratz. Optimal debulking appears to enhance survival as in ovarian cancer. Obviously, patients with an earlier stage and complete surgical removal have a better survival than patients with advanced disease and suboptimal removal. Barakat et al. noted in their patients undergoing second-look laparotomy that the absence of gross residual disease following primary surgery was the best predictor of disease free status at second-look laparotomy. These patients also had a significantly better 5-years survival (83%) than those with gross residual disease (28%). Yoonessi, in reporting 47 patients, noted that 12 had autopsy data. Nine of these 12 patients had positive retroperitoneal nodes. Six patients had positive pelvic and periaortic nodes, and 2 of these had metastases in the supraclavicular lymph nodes. Three patients had positive periaortic nodes but negative pelvic nodes. In addition, 2 patients developed recurrences in the groin and supraclavicular nodes, 3 patients were reported as having positive periaortic nodes, and 1 had positive pelvic nodes at the time of surgery. It has been established that lymphatic metastasis can also occur at the pelvic lymph nodes in both early ovarian and uterine cancer, and therefore these areas should also be carefully evaluated. Postoperative therapy is needed, as in ovarian carcinoma. There may be a group of patients with

early tubal cancer in whom no further therapy is needed. Five-year survival of 90% has been reported in patients with stage I ovarian cancer. Adjunctive therapy in stage I tubal cancer has not been determined. Alkylating-agent chemotherapy and/or pelvic radiation has not improved survival in this group of patients. In instances of tubal carcinoma where disease is limited to the tube and ovary or uterus but no gross residua is left behind, radioactive chromic phosphate has been used and appears to be efficacious (Figure 13-2). Radiation therapy after surgery has probably been used in more patients than any other subsequent therapy. In a study by Roberts and Lifshitz, data on survival for stage I and II (approximately 60% over 5 years) suggested that further therapy other than surgery is needed; however, the use of pelvic irradiation did not improve survival. Yoonessi found that only about one third of stages I and II patients survived, and the use of pelvic radiotherapy did not improve survival. Some data, however, suggest an improvement in survival of women with limited disease if whole abdominal radiation is used. Peters, in his evaluation of stage I fallopian tube cancers, noted a long-term survival difference of 30%-75% with different adjuvant therapies. Because of the small numbers, however, no statistical difference was present.

In four studies, the role of adjunctant therapy in early-stage disease (I and II) has not shown a benefit in survival. The fact that stages I and II have similar survival (and only in the 50%-60% range) indicates that there was

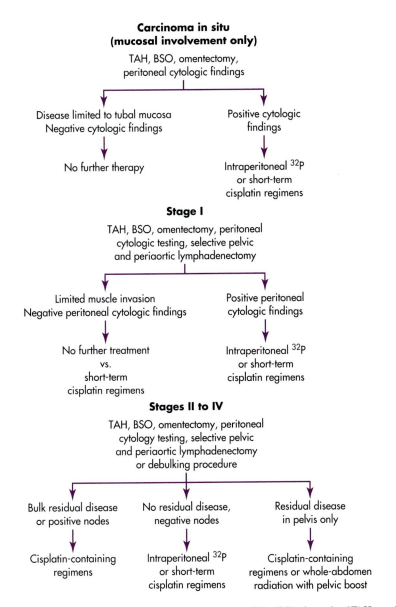

Figure 13-2 Suggested management for adenocarcinoma of the fallopian tube (*TAH*, total abdominal hysterectomy; *BSO*, bilateral salpingo-oophorectomy).

probably undetected disease outside the pelvis. Early experience with stage I carcinoma of the ovary showed that survival was approximately 60%. With more intense surgical staging, survival has increased to 85%-90% in many series. Adjuvant therapy may have played a role in this improved survival in ovarian cancer, but in some instances surgery only accounted for survival equal to that of those who received adjunctant therapy. Obviously adjunctant therapy can be more optimally and judiciously utilized if exact extent of the disease is identified surgically.

The role of chemotherapy, particularly cisplatin based regimens, appears to have an increasing importance in this disease. On an empiric basis, alkylating agents have been used, because they have been the primary treatment for ovarian carcinoma. Studies utilizing alkylating agents report an objective response rate of 17% and a complete response rate of 11%. Most of the complete responders have had subsequent recurrences. Progestin has been added in many circumstances because the endosalpinx is anatomically, embryologically, and histologically similar to the uterine endometrium. Deppe et al. reported two patients with advanced fallopian tube adenocarcinoma who were treated with cisplatin, doxorubicin (Adriamycin), and progestins, with one patient also receiving cyclophosphamide (Cytoxan). Both patients had negative second-look operations and remained tumor free.

Cisplatin-containing regimens are reportedly producing complete responses and long-term survivals. In a recent series of 12 evaluable patients with measurable tubal cancers treated with cisplatin and Cytoxan, with or without Adriamycin, 9 experienced a complete response. Peters reported 11 stage III patients treated with multiple-agent chemotherapy and noted a significantly improved survival compared to that of 14 stage III patients receiving other forms of adjuvant therapy. All patients surviving more than 2 years had received cisplatin. The group at MD Anderson Hospital treated 18 patients with CAP (cisplatin, Adriamycin, and Cytoxan). There were 16 grade II lesions and 2 grade III. At the completion of surgery, 9 had no gross disease, 2 had <1 cm, and 7 had more than 2 cm residual. Of the latter 7 patients, 2 had complete responses to chemotherapy. Of the 15 patients with stages II to IV disease, 8 underwent second-look and 4 had negative findings. Excluding the 3 stage I patients, the mean survival was 44 months. No patient responded to second-line therapy. In a recent report by Barakat, 38 patients were treated with cisplatin-based combination chemotherapy. The overall survival was 51% at 5 years. Patients with stages II to IV who had completed resected tumors had a 5-year survival of 83% compared with 28% if gross disease remained after surgery. It appears that cisplatin-based chemotherapy does improve long-term survival in patients with advanced disease. The role in early staged disease (I and II) is undetermined at the present time. The place of second-look laparotomy certainly has not been defined in tubal carcinoma. Eddy et al. noted their experience with 8 patients. Their results mimic those of ovarian cancer. The procedure may be prognostic although 2 of 5 patients with negative second-look had recurrence. One patient who had microscopic disease only is alive and without disease, but the 2 patients who had macroscopic disease are dead from disease despite additional chemotherapy. The group at Memorial Sloan-Kettering evaluated 35 patients with 2LL following cytoreductive surgery and platinum-based chemotherapy. Twenty-one patients were tumor free at the time of 2LL. None of 5 patients with stage I and/or grade 1 tumors had disease at 2LL. The absence of gross disease at the completion of primary surgery was the best predictor of disease free status at 2LL. Of the patients who were negative at 2LL, only 4 (19%) had a recurrence of their tumor (mean follow up of 50 months). Combined series in the literature also note this low recurrence rate. This, of course, is much better than in ovarian cancer. About 30% of those found to have persistent disease at 2LL were alive at 5 years. Whether or not a 2LL has any appreciable effect on long-term survival is unknown.

PROGNOSIS

Because this disease is rare and the treatment varies, prognosis may be prejudiced. Sedlis noted that the 5-year survival rate for all cases of tubal carcinoma was 38% regardless of stage. Other authors noted 5-year survival rates as high as 88% in stage I fallopian tube carcinoma,

with diminishing survival rates as the stage increases. In fact, prognosis mimics ovarian carcinoma when stage is used as a discriminating factor. Hellström, in a review of 128 patients at the Radiumhemmet, noted in a multivariate analysis that stage followed by tumor grade were important prognostic factors. Although grade did not achieve statistical significance in Rosen's retrospective review of 66 patients, patients with grade I tumor had a survival of 45 months compared to 29 months if G2 or G3 was present (p = 0.25). They also noted a significant improvement in survival by stage of disease. Inflammatory reaction also correlated survival (p = 0.004). In the Hellström study, patients receiving cisplatin chemotherapy had a superior survival rate (p = 0.006) compared with those not receiving chemotherapy. Tumor volume, as noted by stage, and amount of residual tumor are important prognostic factors. Peters, in his review of 115 patients, evaluated potentially significant prognostic factors using multivariant analysis. He found that the only statistically significant variables were stage II compared with stage I and the amount of residual disease. When patients with disease limited to fallopian tube were analyzed separately, the only statistically significant variable was depth of invasion within the tubal wall. In patients with invasion of more than 50% of the tubal muscularis, there was a statistically significant increase in the risk of death from tumor. In these patients, the long-term survival was only 20%, compared with 80% survival among patients who had no muscle involvement and 60% among patients who had less than 50% muscle invasion. Peritoneal cytologic studies appear to be prognostically important, and if malignant cells are present based on uterine and ovarian studies, ^{32}P appear to be a worthwhile adjunctant. Recurrences appear to a lesser degree than ovarian cancer, particularly if platinum therapy is given. Recurrences can be intra- as well as extraperitoneally.

SARCOMAS

Sarcomas are extremely rare. Although mixed mesodermal tumor of the fallopian tube represents the largest number of sarcomas, fewer than 30 have been reported. Only one patient is surviving longer than 5 years. She had a stage Ia cancer treated with surgery and multiple-agent chemotherapy. Sarcomas have been reported in adolescents as well as in the elderly. Most patients present with symptoms similar to those of adenocarcinoma. Most patients are in the sixth decade of life and have low parity. Prognosis is guarded. Treatment should be surgery initially, as in adenocarcinoma of the fallopian tube. Adjunctive chemotherapy with doxorubicin would appear to be treatment of choice after surgery. Prognosis in MMT is certainly guarded. Weber, in a review of the literature, noted a survival of 63% at 1 year and only 47% at 2 years. Imachi noted a mean survival of all patients of only 16 months. Carlson reported 5 patients with MMT of the tube. Only 1 died of cancer at 51 months with the other 4 alive NED at 58 to 205 months. All patients had earlier stage disease with no residual gross disease and were treated with radiation alone, chemotherapy alone, or a combination thereof. Interestingly, only 1 patient was treated with cisplatin and she died of disease. Leiomyosarcoma of the tube has been reported but is more rare than MMT. Optimal surgery plus adjuvant therapy seems appropriate. Adjuvant therapy has yet to be defined.

BIBLIOGRAPHY

Backelandt M, Kocky M, Wesling F et al: Primary adenocarcinoma of the fallopian tube. In *J Gynecol Cancer* 3:65, 1993.

Barakat RR, Rubin SC, Saigo PE et al: Cisplatin-based combination chemotherapy in carcinoma of the fallopian tube, *Gynecol Oncol* 42:156, 1991.

Barakat RR, Rubin SC, Saigo PE et al: Second look laparotomy in carcinoma of the fallopian tube, *Obstet Gynecol* 82:748, 1993.

Benedet JL et al: Adenocarcinoma of the fallopian tube, *Obstet Gynecol* 50:654, 1977.

Boronow RC: Chemotherapy for disseminated tubal cancer, *Obstet Gynecol* 42:62, 1973.

Boutselis J, Thompson J: Clinical aspects of primary carcinoma of the fallopian tube, *Am J Obstet Gynecol* 111:98, 1971.

Carlson JA, Ackerman BL, Wheeler JE: Malignant mixed müllerian tumor of the fallopian tube, *Cancer* 71:187, 1993.

Deppe G, Bruckner HW, Cohen CJ: Combination chemotherapy for advanced carcinoma of the fallopian tube, *Obstet Gynecol* 56:530, 1980.

Dodson MG, Ford JH, Averette HE: Clinical aspects of fallopian tube carcinoma, *Obstet Gynecol* 36:935, 1970.

Eddy GL, Copeland LG, Gershenson DN: Second-look laparotomy in fallopian tube carcinoma, *Gynecol Oncol* 19:182, 1984.

Eddy GL et al: Fallopian tube carcinoma, *Obstet Gynecol* 64:546, 1984.

Erey S, Kaplan AL, Wall TA: Clinical staging of carcinoma of the uterine tube, *Obstet Gynecol* 30:547, 1967.

Harrison CR, Averette HE, Gerald MA et al: Carcinoma of the fallopian tube: clinical management, *Gynecol Oncol* 32:357, 1989.

Hellström AC, Silfversward C, Nilsson B et al: Carcinoma of the fallopian tube: a clinical histopathologic review, *Int J Cancer* 4:395, 1994.

Henderson SR et al: Primary carcinoma of the fallopian tube: difficulties of diagnosis and treatment, *Gynecol Oncol* 5:168, 1977.

Hu CY, Taylor ML, Hertig AJ: Primary carcinoma of the fallopian tube, *Am J Obstet Gynecol* 59:58, 1950.

Imachi M, Tsukamoto N, Shigematsu T et al: Malignant mixed müllerian tumor of the fallopian tube, *Gynecol Oncol* 47:114, 1992.

Jacoby AF, Fuller AF, Thor AD et al: Primary leiomyosarcoma of the fallopian tube, *Gynecol Oncol* 51:404, 1993.

Jones OV: Primary carcinoma of the uterine tube, *Obstet Gynecol* 26:122, 1965.

Kawase N et al: Primary carcinoma of the fallopian tube, *Acta Obstet Gynaecol Jap* 22:20, 1975.

Kinoshita M, Asano S, Yamashita M et al: Mesodermal mixed tumor primary in fallopian tube, *Gynecol Oncol* 32:331, 1989.

Kinzel GE: Primary carcinoma of the fallopian tube, *Am J Obstet Gynecol* 125:816, 1976.

Klein M, Rosen A, Labousen M et al: Lymphogenous metastasis in the primary carcinoma of the fallopian tube, *Gynecol Oncol* 55:336, 1994.

Maxson WZ, Stehman FB, Ulbright TM et al: Primary carcinoma of the fallopian tube: evidence for activity of cisplatin combination therapy, *Gynecol Oncol* 26:305, 1987.

McGoldrick JL, Strauss H, Rao J: Primary carcinoma of the fallopian tube, *Am J Surg* 59:559, 1943.

McMurray EH et al: Carcinoma of the fallopian tube, *Cancer* 58:2070, 1986.

Mei-Liu M, Gan-Gao, Schong-Sun et al: Diagnosis of primary adenocarcinomas of the fallopian tube, *N Cancer Res Clin Oncol* 110:136-40, 1985.

Momtazee S, Kempson RL: Primary adenocarcinoma of the fallopian tube, *Obstet Gynecol* 32:649, 1968.

Moore DH, Woosley JT, Reddick RL et al: Adenosquamous carcinoma of the fallopian tube, *Am J Obstet Gynecol* 157:903, 1987.

Morris M, Gershenson DM, Burke TW et al: Treatment of fallopian tube carcinoma with cisplatin, doxorubicin and cyclophosphamide, *Obstet Gynecol* 76:1020, 1990.

Muntz HG, Tarraza HM, Goff BA et al: Combination chemotherapy in advanced adenocarcinoma of the fallopian tube, *Gynecol Oncol* 40:268, 1989.

Peters WA, Anderson WA, Hopkins MD et al: Prognostic factors of carcinoma of the fallopian tube, *Obstet Gynecol* 71:757, 1988.

Peters WA et al: Results of chemotherapy in advanced carcinoma of the fallopian tube, *Cancer* 63:836, 1989.

Phelps HM, Chapman KE: Role of radiation therapy in treatment of primary carcinoma of the uterine tube, *Obstet Gynecol* 43:669, 1974.

Podratz KC et al: Primary carcinoma of the fallopian tube, *Am J Obstet Gynecol* 154:1319, 1986.

Roberts JA, Lifshitz S: Primary adenocarcinoma of the fallopian tube, *Gynecol Oncol* 13:301, 1982.

Rosen AC, Reiner A, Klein M et al: Prognostic factors in primary fallopian tube carcinoma, *Gynecol Oncol* 53:307, 1994.

Rosenblatt KA, Weiss NS, Schwartz SM: Incidence of malignant fallopian tube tumors, *Gynecol Oncol* 35:326, 1989.

Schiller HM, Silverberg SG: Staging and prognosis in primary carcinoma of the fallopian tube, *Cancer* 28:389, 1971.

Sedlis A: Carcinoma of the fallopian tube, *Surg Clin North Am* 58:121, 1978.

Semrad N et al: Fallopian tube adenocarcinoma: common extraperitoneal recurrence, *Gynecol Oncol* 24:230, 1986.

Seraz IM, King A, Close D: Malignant mixed müllerian tumor of the fallopian tube, *Gynecol Oncol* 37:296, 1990.

Weber AM, Hewett WF, Gajewski et al: Malignant mixed müllerian tumor of the fallopian tube, *Gynecol Oncol* 50:239, 1993.

Woolas R, Jacob I, Davis AP et al: What is the true incidence of primary fallopian tube carcinoma? *Int J Gynecol Cancer* 4:384, 1994.

Yoonessi N: Carcinoma of the fallopian tube, *Obstet Gynecol Surv* 34:257, 1979.

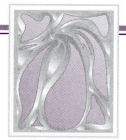

Breast Diseases

Despite some arguments to the contrary, the obstetrician/gynecologist functions as the primary care physician for women, especially during the reproductive and perimenopausal years. Therefore, the diagnosis of breast cancer in its most curable forms lies within this specialty for large numbers of women. Breast cancer is the most common neoplasm in women. One of every 9 women, or about 11%, will develop breast cancer. In 1995, there were nearly 182,000 new cases in the United States alone. Breast cancer incidence rates increased by about 3% every year from 84.8 per 100,000 in 1980 to 111.9 in 1987 and then recently leveled off at a rate of 110 per 100,000 per year. It is possible that some, but not all, of the earlier increase was due to screening programs detecting subclinical disease. Breast cancer is also the leading cause of cancer death in women, as well as the leading cause of death from all causes in women 40 to 44 years old. Deaths caused by breast cancer occur at the rate of one every 15 minutes. Nearly 46,000 deaths in the United States during 1995 were attributed to breast cancer. These startling statistics clearly call for an immediate attack against this dread disease. Obviously, the most direct approach would be to find its cause and eradicate its inception. Unfortunately, the cause of breast cancer seems to be multifactorial, a constellation of risk factors rather than a single factor. Among many suggested causes of breast cancer are genetic predisposition, loss of the host's immunologic defense mechanism, and viruses, as well as other carcinogens. Hormones, especially estrogens, were once considered to be primary carcinogenic agents, but they are now believed to be possible promoters in carcinogenesis. Therefore, despite all the research aimed at finding the cause of breast cancer, this avenue does not seem to hold promise for the near future.

Other than finding the cause of breast cancer, the most important aspect in combating the disease is diagnosis at an early stage when the prognosis for cure with appropriate therapy is excellent. By instructing the patient in the art of monthly breast examination, by performing careful periodic breast examinations in the office, and by judiciously using diagnostic aids, especially in patients with increased risk for the disease, the physician has a golden opportunity to detect breast cancer at an early and highly curable stage. The 5-year survival rate for localized breast cancer (which includes all women living at 5 years after diagnosis, whether the patient is in remission, disease-free or under treatment) has risen to 94%.

ANATOMY OF THE ADULT BREAST

The adult breast lies between the second and the sixth ribs in the vertical axis and between the sternal edge and the midaxillary line in the horizontal axis. The average breast is 10-12 cm in diameter and its average thickness is 5-7 cm. Breast tissue also projects into the axilla as the axillary tail of Spence. The contour of the breast varies but is usually dome-like with a conical configuration in the nulliparous woman and a pendulous configuration in the parous woman. The breast is composed of three major structures: skin, subcutaneous tissue, and breast tissue; the breast tissue contains both parenchyma and stroma. The parenchyma is divided into 15 to 20 segments that converge at the nipple in a radial arrangement. The collecting ducts draining each segment are 2 mm in diameter with subareolar lactiferous sinuses 5-8 mm in diameter. Five to ten major collecting milk ducts open at the nipple and another 5 to 10 ducts at the nipple are, in reality, blind pits. Each duct drains a lobe made up of 20 to 40 lobules. Each lobule consists of 10 to 100 alveoli or tubulosaccular secretory units. The stroma and subcutaneous tissues of the breast contain fat, connective tissue, blood vessels, nerves, and lymphatics (Figure 14-1).

The skin of the breast is thin and contains hair follicles, sebaceous glands, and eccrine glands. The nipple, which is located over the fourth intercostal space in the nonpendulous breast, contains abundant sensory nerve endings, as well as sebaceous and apocrine sweat glands, but no hair follicles. The areola is circular and pigmented, and 15-60 mm in diameter. Morgagni's tubercles, located near the periphery of the areola, are elevations formed by the openings of the ducts of Montgomery's glands. Montgomery's glands are large sebaceous glands capable

of secreting milk; they represent an intermediate stage between the sweat and the mammary glands. Fascial tissues envelope the breast; the superficial pectoral fascia envelopes the breast and is continuous with the superficial abdominal fascia of Camper. The under surface of the breast lies on the deep pectoral fascia, covering the pectoralis major and the anterior serratus muscles. Connecting these two fascial layers are fibrous bands (Cooper's suspensory ligaments) that are the natural means of support of the breast.

The principal blood supply to the breast is from the internal mammary and the lateral thoracic arteries. Approximately 60% of the breast, mainly the medial and central parts, is supplied by the anterior perforating branches of the internal mammary artery. About 30% of the breast, mainly the upper outer quadrant, is supplied by the lateral thoracic artery. There are subepithelial or a papillary plexus of lymphatics of the breast that are confluent with the subepithelial lymphatics over the surface of the body. These valveless lymphatic vessels communicate with subdermal lymphatic vessels and merge with Sappey's subareolar plexus. The subareolar plexus receives lymphatic vessels from the nipple and the areola and communicates by way of the vertical lymphatic vessels that are equivalent to those connecting the subepithelial and subdermal plexus elsewhere in the body. Lymph flows unidirectionally from the superficial to the deep plexus and from the subareolar plexus via the lymphatic vessels of the lactiferous duct to the perilobular

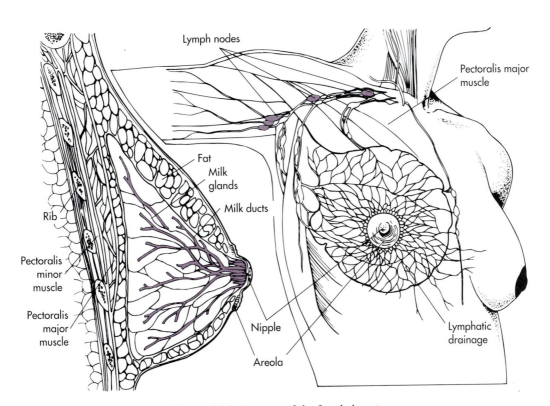

Figure 14-1 Anatomy of the female breast.

and deep subcutaneous plexus. Lymph flow from the deep subcutaneous and intramammary lymphatic vessels moves centrifugally toward the axillary and internal mammary lymph nodes. It is estimated that about 3% of the lymph from the breast flows to the internal mammary chain, whereas 97% flows to the axillary nodes. Drainage of the lymph to the internal mammary chain may be observed after injection of any quadrant of the breast.

The anatomic arrangement of the axillary lymph nodes has been subject to many classifications. Axillary lymph nodes may be divided into (1) the apical or subclavicular nodes, which lie medial to the pectoralis minor muscle; (2) the axillary vein lymph nodes, which are along the axillary vein from the pectoralis minor muscle to the lateral limit of the axilla; (3) the interpectoral nodes, which lie between the pectoralis major and minor muscles along the lateral pectoral nerve; (4) the scapula group, which lie along the subscapular vessels; and (5) the central nodes, which are beneath the lateral border of the pectoralis major muscle and below the pectoralis minor muscle.

An alternative method of delineating metastatic spread, for the purposes of determining pathologic anatomy and metastatic progression, is to divide the axillary lymph nodes into arbitrary levels. Level I lymph nodes lie lateral to the lateral border of the pectoralis minor muscle, level II lymph nodes lie behind the pectoralis minor muscle, and level III lymph nodes are medial to the medial border of the pectoralis minor muscle. These levels can be determined accurately only by marking them with tags at the time of surgery.

BENIGN CONDITIONS OF THE BREAST
Epidemiology

It is impossible to estimate the incidence of benign breast disorders. The subjectivity in any woman's evaluation of her own breasts, as well as a variation in the physician's designation of breast disease, invalidates any clinical estimates. To gain some degree of reproducibility, most studies rely on data from women who have had biopsies for benign conditions. This approach, too, is subject to bias, because not every woman with lumpy breasts will have a biopsy, and because the decision to do a biopsy is influenced by the presence of other risk factors for malignant disease.

Clinically defined, benign breast symptoms are common and have been estimated to occur in 50% of women. In a case-controlled study by Cole in Boston from 1968 to 1969, the age-standardized incidence rates for histologically diagnosed fibrocystic disease and fibroadenoma were 89.4% and 32.8% per 100,000 women years, respectively. Cole found that the incidence increased in women 45 years of age or younger and then declined sharply. The results of this study are influenced by the bias inherent in using biopsies, however, and possibly under-

estimates the incidence in younger women. Hislop and Elwood conducted a 30-year cohort study of nurses in British Columbia and found that by the age of 50, the subjects' cumulative risk for benign breast disorders was 17% for those undergoing biopsy and 31% for those who had symptomatic disease. In autopsy studies, the incidence of histologic fibrocystic disease may be determined with only slightly greater accuracy. Davis summarized eight autopsy studies conducted before 1964 and found evidence of cystic disease in 58.5% of a total of 725 breasts in women who had had no symptoms of breast disease. Cystic disease was bilateral in 43% of these women. The average incidence of gross cysts was 21%, whereas the average incidence of coexisting gross and microscopic cysts and of cystic disease with epithelial hyperplasia was 58.3% and 30.6% respectively. Kramer and Rush studied the breasts of women older than 30 years and found histologic evidence of fibrocystic disease in 67%. Thus, although the incidence of clinical features may decrease in the postmenopausal period, histologic features persist.

Physiologic Changes

Most women discover their own breast tumors by chance or by periodic self-examination. Two thirds of the tumors found by all methods during a woman's reproductive years are benign and represent cystic changes, dysplasia, fibroadenomas, and papillomas. However, 50% of the palpable masses in perimenopausal women and the majority of lesions in postmenopausal patients are malignant.

Cystic breast changes and mammary dysplasia are common, often symptomatic, and require considerable judgment on the part of the physician in choosing the appropriate therapy. The incidence of these benign changes peaks in women 30-50 years of age and may be the result of estrogen stimulation in the absence of cyclic corpus luteum formation and the cyclic production of progesterone. Continued estrogen stimulation may be a factor in the development of the so-called macrocyst. The fact that breast tenderness often occurs premenstrually suggests that progesterone may also play a role in the development and symptoms of cystic alterations in breast tissue. However, the proportional effect of each of these hormones on the cause of benign breast conditions is unclear and needs further clarification.

A more thorough understanding of the embryologic and prepubertal development of the breast will aid in the study of benign breast lesions. The mammary glands are highly specialized skin derivatives of ectodermal origin. The epithelial ridge that will develop into breast tissue undergoes a series of proliferations to form the lactiferous ducts. Primitive breast tissue is under the gonadal control of fetal androgen production, which causes a suppression of breast growth during the period of gestation, when the tissue is under the simultaneous influence of increasing levels of growth-promoting estrogen and progesterone. Following birth, breast tissue remains dormant until adolescence, when estrogen produces a proliferation of ductal epithelium and progesterone produces rapid growth of the acini. However, breast growth and development are not totally dependent on estrogen and progesterone levels. Insulin, cortisol, thyroxine, growth hormone, and prolactin are also required for complete functional development. Minor deficiencies in any one of these hormones can be compensated for by an excess of prolactin, the interesting hormone found in mammals that suckle their young.

During pregnancy, increasing amounts of estrogen, progesterone, and human placental lactogen produce active growth of functional breast tissue. Serum prolactin rises from nonpregnant levels of 10 ng/ml to term levels of 200 ng/ml. Amniotic fluid prolactin levels are more than 100 times greater than the levels seen in maternal or fetal blood early in pregnancy. It is not known whether the fetal pituitary gland or the trophoblast secretes the hormone into the amniotic fluid, but one hypothesis suggests that prolactin may help the embryo survive its aquatic environment such as it helps the teleost fish in its journey from salt to fresh water to spawn. Elevated levels of estradiol parallel those of prolactin and indicate that estriol may be responsible for increases in prolactin. Although estrogen may initiate prolactin secretion, high levels block its physiologic effects. Prolactin secretion is also controlled by the prolactin-inhibiting factor. A decrease of estrogen level following delivery and suppression of the prolactin-inhibiting factor by suckling increases prolactin levels. If breast-feeding does not occur, serum prolactin levels decrease to nonpregnant levels in about 1 week. The final episode in nature's plan to provide the newborn with milk from its mother's breast is the contraction of the duct system by the release of oxytocin from the posterior pituitary and the delivery of milk to the nipples. After 3-4 months of breast-feeding, suckling appears to be the only stimulus required for lactation.

Physical Examination

Although the techniques and importance of breast examination are taught in nearly every medical school, the current trends of clinical specialization and subspecialization may cause clinicians to lose expertise in or, even worse, to forget to include adequate breast examination as part of the assessment of their patients. To omit breast evaluation from routine examinations or to neglect to advise appropriate patients to undergo mammography may result in missed opportunities for early detections. This is tantamount to performing a gynecologic examination without a Papanicolaou smear, or to neglecting to perform an examination for occult blood in a stool specimen. In diseases in which early detection is so clearly related to improved survival, the

value of these relatively simple techniques cannot be overemphasized.

Examination of the patient in the sitting position

Physical examination of the breasts should always begin with the patient in the sitting position. In this position, obvious asymmetry, bulging of the skin, skin or nipple retraction, or nipple ulceration should be most apparent (Figure 14-2, *A*). When the patient's arms are raised (Figure 14-2, *B*), skin changes in the lower half of the breast, or in the inframammary fold, will become accentuated. Contraction of the pectoralis major muscle, effected by the patient pushing her hands against her hips (Figure 14-2, *C*), may demonstrate an otherwise undetected skin retraction. Next, palpation of the breast with the patient still upright may allow detection of subtle lesions that would be more difficult to palpate if she were supine (Figure 14-2, *D*). This is particularly true for masses high in the breast or in the axillary tail region, which are more apparent when the surrounding breast tissue is displaced inferiorly while the patient is in the sitting position. The use of talc on the fingers of the examiner's hand reduces friction between the skin of the hand and the skin of the breast, facilitating palpation. For this same reason patients should be advised to begin self-examination in the shower, using soap on their fingers. Examination of the supraclavicular areas and both sides of the neck for purposes of detecting suspicious lymphadenopathy also is best done when the patient is in the upright position. The axilla is examined with the patient's right arm fixed at the elbow and held there by the physician's right hand, a position that allows relaxation of the chest wall musculature (Figure 14-2, *E*). Palpation with the left hand permits assessment of the lower axilla, and with extension higher toward the clavicle, the middle and upper portions of the axilla can be assessed. The left axilla is examined with the right hand, after relaxation of the patient's left arm in the physician's left hand. If lymph nodes are palpable, the clinician must assess their level and size, as well as whether they are single or multiple and/or mobile or fixed to underlying structures. Nodes are considered suspicious for metastases that are larger than 1 cm in diameter, firm, irregular, and multiple or matted together. Many women, especially those subject to low-grade inflammatory processes of the hands or arms (from paper cuts, hang nails, minor abrasions, or burns) will have small, soft, mobile, and palpable axillary lymph nodes caused by lymphadenitis. These nodes are generally smaller than 1 cm in diameter and are recorded as being palpable but clinically uninvolved.

Close inspection of the skin and nipple of the breast may reveal abnormalities suggesting an underlying malignant process (Figure 14-3, *A* and *B*). Edema of the skin of the breast (peau d'orange) is occasionally subtle but is more often extensive. This condition is frequently more

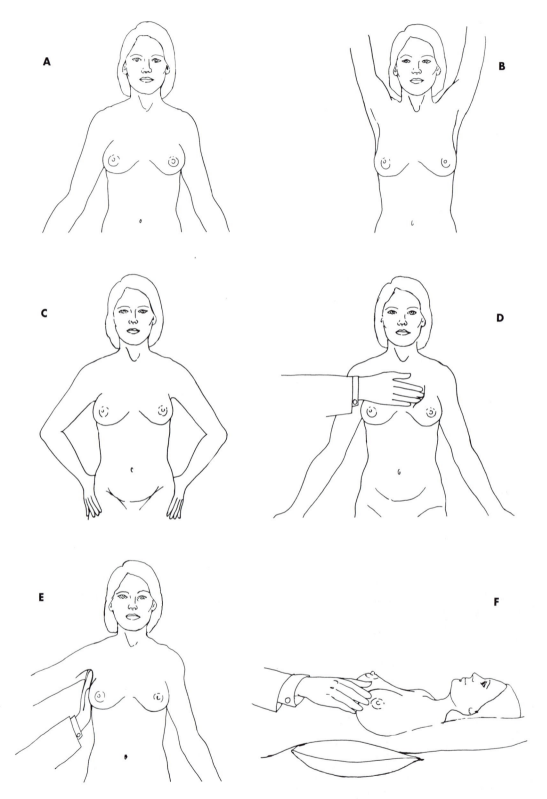

Figure 14-2 Physical examination of the breast. **A,** Upright position. **B,** Arms raised. **C,** Pushing hands against hips. **D,** Palpation in upright position. **E,** Palpation of the axilla. **F,** Palpation in supine position.

Skin dimpling

Dimpling of skin over a carcinoma is caused by involvement and retraction of Cooper's ligaments. Pectoralis contraction may enhance dimpling if fascia is involved.

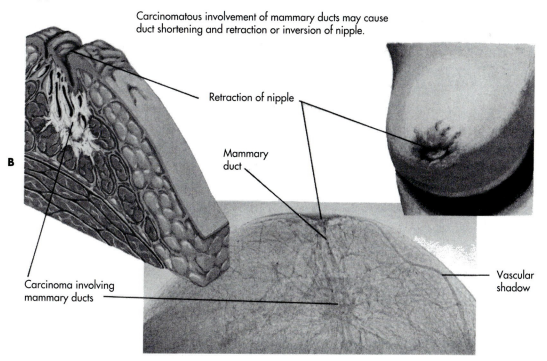

Skin dimple over carcinoma

Carcinoma

Edema of skin

Connective tissue shadows

Cooper's ligament

Cooper's ligament

Pectoralis fascia

JOHN A. CRAIG—AD
© CIBA

A

Nipple retraction

Carcinomatous involvement of mammary ducts may cause duct shortening and retraction or inversion of nipple.

Retraction of nipple

Mammary duct

Carcinoma involving mammary ducts

Vascular shadow

B

Figure 14-3 Clinical signs of cancer. **A,** Retraction of skin. **B,** Retraction of nipple. (Reprinted from *Clinical Symposia CIBA,* vol. 32, no. 2, 1980. Townsend CM Jr: Breast lumps. Art by John A Craig.)

prominent in the lower half of the breast than in any other region, and it is most noticeable when the patient's arms are raised. Although this edema is often attributable to lymphatic obstruction from a deep-seeded carcinoma in the breast, it may also be caused by extensive axillary lymph node involvement with metastatic disease. Retraction of the skin and nipple may be accentuated by contraction of the pectoralis major muscle. Erythema of the skin of the breast is an ominous sign. Although the cause may be inflammation such as periductal mastitis or even abscess formation, inflammatory carcinoma should be considered a possibility. Inspection of the nipple for either retraction or ulceration is important. The latter, which may begin as a minimal process involving a portion of the nipple, raises the suspicion of Paget's disease. This early form of breast carcinoma, which originates in and extends along the major ducts and which expresses itself as nipple abnormality, can involve the entire nipple.

Examination of the patient lying supine

The patient is subsequently asked to assume a supine position. The breast is best examined when it is positioned on top of and splayed out over the chest wall. This position is accomplished with a small pillow placed beneath the ipsilateral shoulder to elevate the breast and with the ipsilateral arm raised above the patient's head (Figure 14-2, *F*). Breast examination is most accurate when the least possible amount of breast tissue is present between the skin and the chest wall; it is least accurate when the converse is true. The examiner must assess the entire breast, with the examination extending from the sternum to the midaxillary line and superiorly from the clavicle to the lower rib cage. Usually the examiner uses the flat of the hand or running fingers technique, remembering that the changes being sought are very subtle. All quadrants are examined. Because of the proclivity for malignant lesions to occur in the upper outer quadrant of the breast (Figure 14-4), we make it a practice to begin in that quadrant, palpating clockwise and returning to examine the upper outer quadrant a second time. Carcinomas smaller than 1 cm in diameter are palpated in some women; in others, very large lesions may be hidden. The examiner must assess the background consistency of the breast; in premenopausal patients who are examined premenstrually, clumps of engorged glandular tissue may seem impossible to assess. A repeat examination 1-2 weeks after a menstrual period may reveal a marked improvement, with decreased glandular elements. Postmenopausal patients have a higher ratio of fat to glandular elements, making palpation and mammographic examination more accurate. No cyclic changes occur in these patients, so indiscreet thickening may be more significant in them than it is in premenopausal patients.

The examiner searches for three-dimensional masses or significant thickenings. On palpation, firm masses or

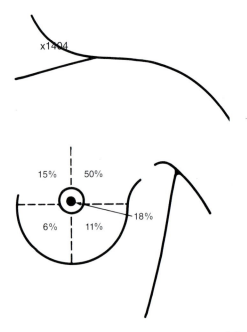

Figure 14-4 Relative location of malignant lesions of the breast.

areas that are three-dimensional, irregular, and fixed to the skin or underlying fascia are characteristic of carcinomas. Benign lesions tend to be softer and smoother, to have more regular borders, and to be freely movable. Fibroadenoma, the most common benign disease of the breast occurring in younger women, is the easiest condition to appreciate. These lesions are clearly demarcated and feel like marbles despite the dense, glandular, parenchymal tissue present in these young women. Gross cysts are soft and circumscribed, and the fluid may be ballottable occasionally. Sclerosing adenitis tends to produce firm, small (less than 1 cm in diameter), peripherally located nodules that frequently appear close to the skin.

After the physical examination, the physician should explain to the patient the importance and technique of self-breast examination (SBE). The physician should advise a monthly SBE at a time in her menstrual cycle when the breasts are neither engorged nor tender. A postmenopausal woman may be instructed to select her birth date each month as the time for her examination. Many physicians instruct their patients to examine themselves while bathing, because a mass is more easily felt when the hand and breasts are wet. Next, the physician should have the patient sit before a mirror and inspect her breasts when her arms are at her sides and then when her arms are raised. She should be told to look for changes in contour, dimpling, or nipple abnormality. Next, the patient should lie in the supine position with a small pillow under her shoulder on the side to be examined; she should then palpate the entire right breast with the flat of the fingers of the left hand and vice versa. A mass should be reported to the physician; often the patient's concerns are ill-founded, and only reassurance is

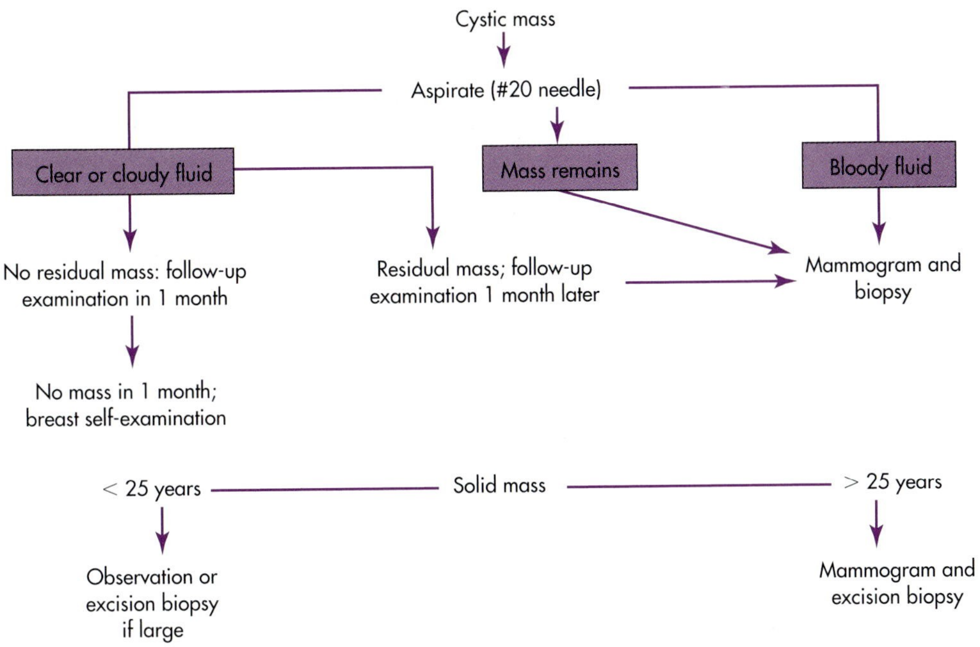

Figure 14-5 Management of probable benign breast masses. (Modified from Marchant DJ: *Female patient*, 4(3), 1979, PW Communications, Inc.)

required. For this reason, it is our practice to advise morning SBE so that a patient need not spend a sleepless night with undue concern if she palpates a "lump."

Diagnosis and Management (Figure 14-5)

Fibrocystic changes (fibrocystic disease) (Figure 14-6)

A variety of histologic conditions have been included under the heading of "fibrocystic disease" of the breast. From a pathologic point of view there is no such entity. Histologically, the term encompasses a spectrum of change, some normal variance, and some abnormal conditions. The breast is an inhomogeneous organ, and the nonlactating normal breast is composed primarily of adipose and fibrous tissue that is often unevenly distributed. This lack of even distribution leads to physiologic inhomogeneity, irregularity, and/or lumpiness. Biopsy of a lumpy area may show primarily fibrous tissue and mammary epithelium. Although normal, this finding would, in most institutions, be reported as fibrocystic disease, fibrocystic change, mammary dysplasia, chronic cystic mastitis, or any of a number of other entities.

The lesions are commonly bilateral and multiple. They are characterized by dull, heavy pain, a sense of fullness, and tenderness. These symptoms increase premenstrually, as does lump size. In the case of a cyst the patient will often report that there was a sudden appearance of a tender lump and that she or her doctor recently examined her breast and did not notice a lump. The lumps are cystic to palpation, tender, well delineated, slightly mobile, and clear on transillumination. Aspiration reveals a typical turbid, nonhemorrhagic fluid that has a yellow, green, or brown tint (Figure 14-7). Deeply embedded cysts, a cluster of cysts, or dominant areas caused by sclerosing adenosis or dense fibrous dysplasia can produce a mass that clinically mimics cancer.

There are three basic reasons for considering treatment of fibrocystic changes:

1. To control troublesome clinical symptoms
2. To normalize dense and nodular breasts before a woman reaches the age when breast cancer is most prevalent in an effort to facilitate periodic breast examination and avoid unnecessary repeated biopsies
3. To reduce the risk of cancer in patients who have benign lesions that may have premalignant potential

A number of methods that have emerged for the treatment of fibrocystic disease can be broadly characterized into two groups: (1) diet and vitamin therapy and (2) hormone manipulation.

Perhaps the simplest methods are advocated by those who maintain that dimethylxanthines (caffeine, theophylline) and nicotine stimulate the formation of fibrocystic changes in the breasts. Advocates of this philosophy suggest that patients stop consuming coffee, tea, cola, and chocolate; stop using certain respiratory drugs containing dimethylxanthines; and quit smoking.

Others have suggested that vitamin E is helpful in relieving symptoms and causing regression of fibrocystic changes of the breast. Its mechanism of action is unknown, although an alteration in serum gonadotropins and adrenal tropines has been shown to occur in patients

Fibrocystic disease

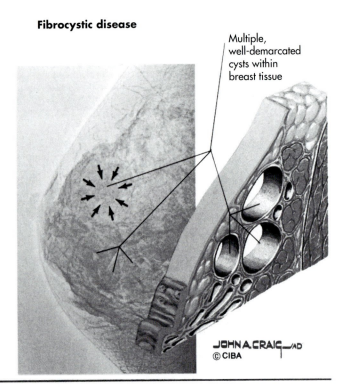

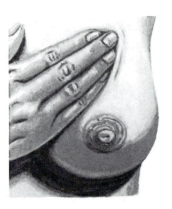

Often detected on self-examination as a mass that may fluctuate in size in different phases of the menstrual cycle.

Multiple, well-demarcated cysts within breast tissue

JOHN A. CRAIG AD
© CIBA

Figure 14-6 Fibrocystic disease. (Reprinted from *Clinical Symposia CIBA*, vol. 32, no. 2, 1980. Townsend CM Jr: Breast lumps. Art by John A Craig.)

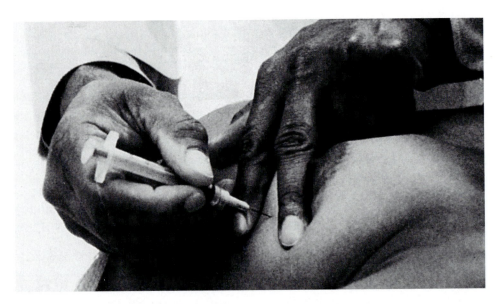

Figure 14-7 Fine-needle aspiration of a breast mass.

taking high doses of vitamin E. As reported by Gonzales, a double-blind study consisted of the treatment of 20 patients and 8 control subjects receiving placebos for 4 weeks, followed by 600 IU of vitamin E per day for 8 weeks. Vitamin E induced a 40% complete response rate and a 46% partial response rate for a total response rate of 86%. There was no response seen in the placebo group.

Ariel has used norethynodrel (Enovid), and Jern has had success with norethindrone acetate (Norlutate), a progestin. It is likely that the resolution of fibrocystic disease induced by these agents is mediated via the direct effect of the progestin on cystic breasts, although the exact method remains unknown.

Recently danazol, an "impeded androgen" derived from 17-ethinyl testosterone, has received a great deal of attention in the treatment of endometriosis and of fibrocystic disease of the breast. As with other progestogens, the mechanism of its effect on fibrocystic disease is unclear. It has been shown to alter several parameters of endocrine function that could have bearing on the breast:

1. Antigonadotropin prevents the midcycle luteinizing hormone surge
2. Antireceptor finds and translocates androgen receptors but not estrogen or progesterone receptors
3. Antiestrogen inhibits several enzymes involved in ovarian steroidogenesis

Bookshaw reported 514 patients who had benign breast disease treated with varying doses of danazol for as long as 6 months. For the best results, treatment was necessary for 4-6 months at a dose of 200-400 mg/day, with a complete response rate of 68%.

The effectiveness of tamoxifen has been studied by Ricciardi and Ianniruberto using 10 mg/day from day 5 to day 25 of the menstrual cycle for 4 months. The response rate was 72%.

A recent medical treatment advocates the use of bromocriptine. Blichert-Toft et al., in Copenhagen, performed a double-blind crossover study in 10 women with diffuse fibrocystic disease. During treatment with 2.5 mg/day during the first week of each menstrual cycle and 5 mg/day during the next 3 weeks or identical placebos for 2 months, 8 of the 10 women had complete relief of mastalgia and 2 had definite improvements, but only 1 had relief with the placebo.

There is considerable controversy as to whether the patient with benign cystic changes in the breast is a greater risk for the development of cancer. Some authorities believe that the risk of cancer is 2 to 4 times greater in the patient who has cystic changes. Other authorities disagree. The simplest and most common studies evaluate the coexistence of benign pathology in mastectomy specimens removed because of malignant conditions. These studies show that there is no greater incidence of microscopic "fibrocystic disease" in cancerous breasts than in noncancerous breasts studied at autopsy. "Fibrocystic disease" was found in 58% of autopsied noncancerous breasts, but was found in only 26% of cancerous breasts. In addition, epithelial hyperplasia, often thought to be a precursor of malignant disease, was at least as common in the noncancerous breast as in the cancerous breast (32% and 23%, respectively). Davis et al. concluded that the mere finding of coexistent cystic disease was not adequate evidence that cystic change had predisposed to breast carcinoma.

Two other types of epidemiologic studies have been used to assess the relationship of "fibrocystic disease" to

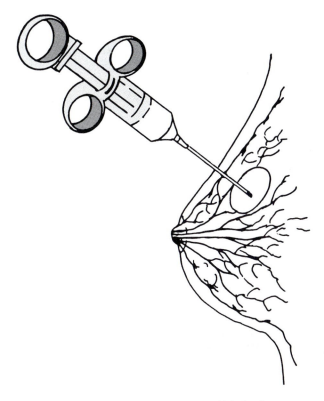

Figure 14-8 Aspiration of a gross cyst. Hold lesion between fingers; pass needle through lesion four or five times; push air through needle onto slide; fix slide after smearing.

cancer: a retrospective analysis of the number and histology of previous biopsy specimens in patients who subsequently had breast cancer (retrospective case-controlled study), and a retrospective cohort study of patients in whom biopsy specimens showed benign disease (Figure 14-8) and who developed cancer later.

In the retrospective, case-controlled study, the percentage of previous biopsies in patients who had cancer was quite low (about 8%) compared with the percentage of previous biopsies done in patients who had benign disease (about 14%). DeVitt and Chetty showed that when a woman has a biopsy for benign disease, she is more likely to have a second biopsy, perhaps because of the increased surveillance or even anatomic distortion caused by the previous surgery.

Evaluation of retrospective cohort studies, in which women who had benign biopsy specimens were followed to determine the subsequent incidence of cancer, poses even greater problems. There are statistical difficulties, including unspecified age distributions and periods of follow-up. In addition, only some of the investigators revealed the original histology to substantiate the diagnosis; others relied on the pathology reports as adequate evidence of fibrocystic disease. Finally, each study used a different control to establish the expected risk of cancer.

Although the epidemiologic risk of developing cancer after biopsy has been somewhat discounted, the pathologic precursors have been clarified. Several studies have demonstrated that the most important pathologic risk factors for the subsequent development of carcinoma are the degree and nature (typical or atypical) of epithelial proliferation. The relative risks vary from study to study and depend to a great extent on the classification used on various benign lesions. When biopsy results are categorized as showing nonproliferative lesions, proliferative lesions without atypia, or atypical proliferative lesions, populations with low risk of developing breast cancer may be isolated (Table 14-1). When additional factors such as family history and age are considered, subgroups that are at significantly greater risk of developing breast cancer may be identified.

In 1985 the Cancer Committee of the College of American Pathologists published a consensus statement and discouraged the use of the term *fibrocystic disease.* Their preference was use of the terms *fibrocystic changes* or *fibrocystic condition.* Epithelial hyperplasias were assigned to risk categories (see box). Mild hyperplasia was defined as the epithelium being more than two but not more than four cells deep. Moderate and florid hyperplasia referred to more extensive degrees of epithelial proliferation. In the absence of atypical hyperplasia, mild hyperplasia was not associated with an increased risk for invasive carcinoma. Moderate or florid hyperplasia without atypical hyperplasia was associated with slightly increased risk (1½ to 2 times) for invasive carcinoma. Atypical hyperplasia referred to lesions that have some of the features of carcinomas in situ but not enough to make unequivocal diagnoses of carcinomas in situ. Although there is a moderately increased risk for invasive cancer in women who have atypical hyperplasia, the relative risk of lesser degrees of atypia (mild and moderate) has not yet been established. Carcinoma in situ was considered the end point for atypical hyperplasia. Women who have carcinomas in situ established by breast biopsies who have no further treatment are at high risk for developing invasive carcinomas (8 to 10 times) relative to comparable women who do not have breast biopsies. Thus it seems that the utilization of a classification consisting of nonproliferative lesions, proliferative lesions with atypia, or atypical proliferative lesions, has relevance to the malignant potential of these lesions. The following benign conditions (Table 14-2) are commonly found.

Fibroadenoma (Figure 14-9)

Another common benign lesion is the fibroadenoma, which appears predominantly in young women and occasionally in adolescents. It is initially seen as a firm, painless, mobile mass and may be very large, particularly in adolescents. Fibroadenomas are multiple and bilateral in about 14%-25% of patients. They are the most common benign tumors of the breast. Fine-needle aspiration

---

BREAST DIAGNOSIS GROUPED BY CANCER RISK

No increased risk
Adenosis, sclerosing or florid
Apocrine metaplasia
Cysts, macro and/or micro
Duct ectasia
Fibroadenoma
Fibrosis
Hyperplasia (mild)
Mastitis
Periductal mastitis
Squamous metaplasia

Slightly increased risk
Hyperplasia
    Moderate or florid
    Solid or papillary
Papilloma
    with fibrovascular core

Moderately increased risk
Atypical Hyperplasia
    Ductal
    Lobular

Table 14-1 Proliferative breast disease and breast cancer risk

Characteristic	Risk
Proliferative disease—no atypia	1.9
Atypical hyperplasia (AH)	4.5
AH + positive family history (FH)	11.0
Cysts alone	1.5
Cysts + FH	3.0
70% of women—no increased risk	

From Dupont WD: *N Engl J Med* 312:146, 1985.

Table 14-2 Benign breast lesions (70% of all lesions removed)

	Age (median)	%
Fibrocystic disease	29-49 (30)	34
Carcinoma	40-71 (54)	27
Fibroadenoma	20-49 (30)	19
Intraductal papilloma	35-55 (40)	6
Ductal ectasia	35-55 (40)	4
Other		10

cytologic testing is accurate and dependable for diagnosing fibroadenomas. Cytologic criteria for distinguishing fibroadenomas from cancers and phylloides tumors have been well established.

Management of fibroadenomas, especially in young women, has been controversial. The choice of treatment should be a shared decision between the patient and her physician. Fear of cancer and death is a paramount anxiety in women with breast tumors, but benign lesions can be monitored with regular clinical breast examinations and mammography. As with all dominant breast masses, a definitive diagnosis must be established by fine-needle aspiration cytology testing or by histologic features on open surgical biopsy. Hindle reviewed 498 cases of biopsy-proven fibroadenomas and found no cases of co-incident carcinoma within the fibroadenomas. He concluded that monitoring definitely has a role in the management of some of these lesions.

Histologically, fibroadenomas have both an epithelial and a stromal component. The histologic classification depends on which of these components predominates. In general, the epithelial component consists of well-defined, gland-like, and duct-like spaces lined by cuboidal or columnar cells. Varying degrees of epithelial hyperplasia have been noted. The stromal component consists of connective tissue that has a variable content of collagen. Infrequently carcinoma may occur in association with fibroadenoma. The prognosis of carcinoma limited to fibroadenoma is excellent. Treatment should follow the same principle used in the management of in situ or infiltrating carcinomas that occur in breast tissue in the absence of fibroadenomas. The most common carcinoma involving fibroadenomas is lobular carcinoma in situ, but intraductal, infiltrating ductal, and infiltrating lobular carcinoma have also been observed.

Phylloides tumor

Phylloides tumor is an uncommon, generally slow-growing lesion representing both epithelial and stromal proliferation. Although it can occur in women of any age, it is most common in premenopausal patients. Like a fibroadenoma, it is a fibroepithelial tumor but generally it is larger and contains a different type of connective tissue. In general, this connective tissue is hypercellular and has increased pleomorphism and mitotic activity. The cellularity of the connective tissue is the distinguishing characteristic of this tumor.

The clinical course of a phylloides tumor is variable and often unpredictable. Attempts to determine the degree of potential malignancy by evaluating cellularity and pleomorphism have not met with uniform success. Approximately 10% of all phylloides tumors contain some characteristics suggestive of a frankly malignant process. Most demonstrate equivocal histopathologic characteristics or appear benign. Phylloides tumors should be treated by a total excision with a wide margin

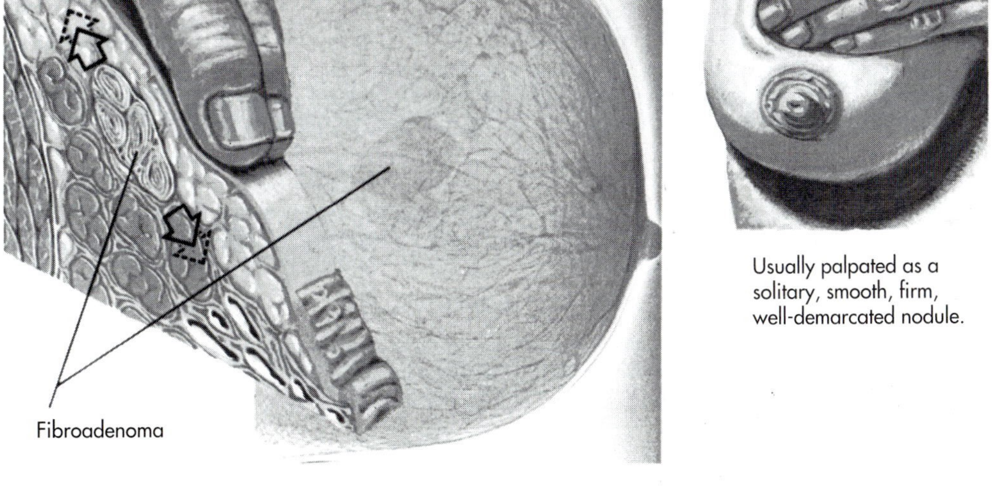

Fibroadenoma

Vascular shadow

Connective tissue shadows

Fibroadenoma

Usually palpated as a solitary, smooth, firm, well-demarcated nodule.

Figure 14-9 Fibroadenoma. (Reprinted from *Clinical Symposia CIBA*, vol. 32, no. 2, 1980. Townsend CM Jr: Breast lumps. Art by John A Craig.)

of healthy tissue. Radical mastectomy or modified radical procedures are not indicated.

Intraductal papilloma (Figure 14-10)

Intraductal papilloma manifests as a serous, serosanguineous, or watery type of nipple discharge. In the absence of a mass, the most common cause of bloody nipple discharge is an intraductal papilloma. The discharge is usually spontaneous and from a single duct and is commonly unilateral. Pressure on one area of the areola will result in the discharge, and that area usually contains the lesion. Intraductal papillomas are generally smaller than 1 cm in diameter, usually 3-4 mm. Occasionally these lesions may be as large as 4-5 cm. On gross examination, papillomas are tan or pink viable tumors within dilated ducts or cysts. A frankly papillary configuration may or may not be apparent. The tumor is usually attached to the wall of the involved duct by a delicate stalk, but it may be sessile. To identify the papilloma, the physician should use a pair of fine scissors and carefully open the involved duct until the tumor is exposed. Microscopically, these tumors are composed of multiple branching and anastomosing papillae, each with a central fibrovascular core and a covering layer of cuboidal to columnar epithelial cells. There has been considerable debate in the literature regarding the malignant potential of solitary intraductal papillomas. Available evidence suggests that these lesions rarely undergo malignant transformation. Therefore the risk of breast carcinoma in a woman who has had an intraductal papilloma appears to be no greater than that in the general population.

Most nipple discharges are a result of benign conditions and do not require surgical intervention. The color and consistency of the discharge is important, however, and cytologic examination of the nipple discharge and, occasionally, mammography are important diagnostic aids. Even bloody nipple discharge is associated with the finding of a malignancy only 20%-30% of the time. Tranquilizers, particularly the phenothiazines, may cause bilateral nipple discharge, principally because they decrease prolactin-inhibiting factor and thus elevate prolactin levels.

Ductal ectasia (Figure 14-11)

Ductal ectasia is also commonly manifested by nipple discharge. However, this discharge is usually multicolored and sticky, bilateral, and from multiple ducts. Frequently a patient experiences a burning, itching, or dull drawing type of pain around the nipple and areola, and there are palpable tortuous tubular swellings under

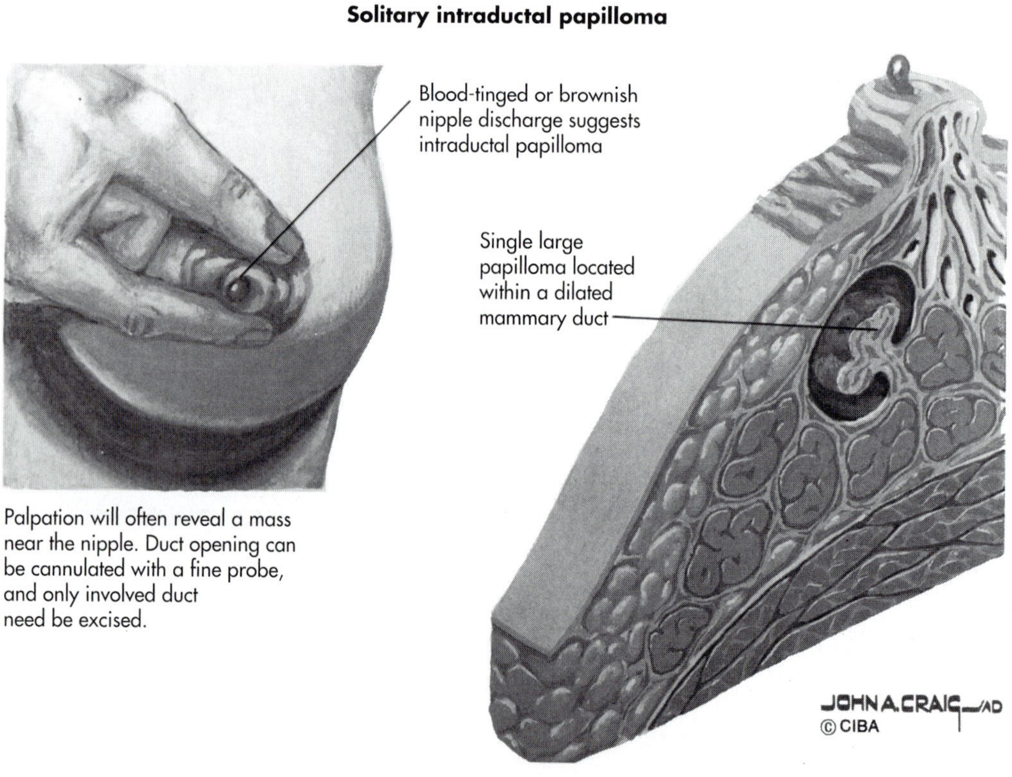

Solitary intraductal papilloma

Blood-tinged or brownish nipple discharge suggests intraductal papilloma

Single large papilloma located within a dilated mammary duct

Palpation will often reveal a mass near the nipple. Duct opening can be cannulated with a fine probe, and only involved duct need be excised.

JOHN A. CRAIG—AD
© CIBA

Figure 14-10 Solitary intraductal papilloma. (Reprinted from *Clinical Symposia CIBA*, vol 32, no. 2, 1980. Townsend CM Jr: Breast lumps. Art by John A Craig.)

the areola. When the condition is more advanced, a mass can develop that may resemble a locally advanced clinical stage III breast carcinoma.

The pathogenesis of this condition has not been fully established. Available evidence suggests, however, that the primary event is periductal inflammation and that duct ectasia is the ultimate outcome of this disorder. The postulated sequence of events in the evolution of this disease is that periductal inflammation leads to periductal fibrosis that subsequently results in ductal dilation. It should be noted, however, that the etiology of the initial inflammatory response remains obscure. Treatment consists of local excision of the inflamed area of the breast tissue. On microscopic examination, many cases show prominence of a lipid-rich material within ducts, accompanied by periductal inflammation. Rupture or leakage of these ducts may result in release of this material into the adjacent stroma, with subsequent inflammation and fat necrosis.

Adenoma

Adenoma of the breast is a well-circumscribed tumor composed of benign epithelial elements with sparse, inconspicuous stroma. This last feature differentiates this lesion from fibroadenoma, in which the stroma is an integral part of the tumor. For practical purposes, adenomas may be divided into two major groups: tubular adenomas and lactating adenomas. Tubular adenomas in young women are well-defined, freely movable nodules that clinically resemble fibroadenomas. Lactating adenomas manifest as one or more freely movable masses during pregnancy or the postpartum period. They are grossly well circumscribed and lobulated, and on cut section appear tan and softer than tubular adenomas. On microscopic examination, these lesions have lobulated borders and are composed of glands lined by cuboidal cells with secretory activity, identical to the lactational changes normally observed in the breast tissue during pregnancy and the puerperium.

Sclerosing lesions

Sclerosing lesions have been described by a variety of names, including sclerosing, papillary proliferation, non-encapsulated sclerosing lesion, indurative mastopathy, and radial scar. Their importance lies in that they may on mammographic, gross, and microscopic examinations simulate carcinoma. These lesions are typically smaller than 1 cm in diameter and on gross examination are irregular, gray or white, and indurated with central retraction, and have an appearance identical to that of scirrhus carcinoma. Microscopically, the lesion has a stellate configuration and consists of a central, fibrotic core containing entrapped glandular elements. The surrounding breast tissue typically shows varying degrees of

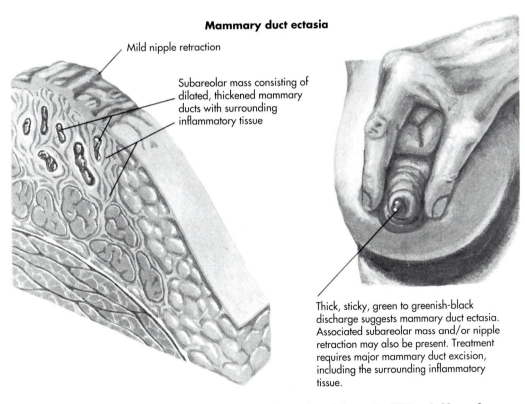

Figure 14-11 Mammary duct ectasia. (Reprinted from *Clinical Symposia CIBA*, vol. 32, no. 2, 1980. Townsend CM Jr: Breast lumps. Art by John A Craig.)

intraductal hyperplasia and adenosis. The significance of this lesion relative to subsequent development of carcinoma is controversial. Available evidence suggests that these lesions are part of the fibrocystic complex. It is likely that their premalignant potential is the same as that of the constituent parts. Local excision of these lesions is the treatment of choice.

Nipple discharge

Nipple discharge is usually noted to be bloody, milky, serous, or purulent. The great majority of cases of spontaneous nipple discharge are due to benign conditions. Galactorrhea presents as bilateral milky nipple discharge consisting of lipid droplets; the condition is usually idiopathic but can be found following discontinuation of oral contraceptive or a persistent discharge after pregnancy. Plasma prolactin levels should be obtained because of the possibility of a prolactin-producing pituitary adenoma. Bloody discharge is usually produced by a solid papilloma; green sticky discharge is characteristic of duct ectasia (Table 14-3).

Breast mass during pregnancy/lactation

Benign lesions during pregnancy include the following:
  Fibroadenomas
  Lipomas
  Papillomas
  Fibrocystic changes
  Galactoceles
  Inflammatory lesions

Byrd in a series of 105 benign biopsies found that 71% of patients had conditions found in non-pregnant women, and 29% had changes particular to gestation (e.g., lobular hyperplasia, galactocele, lactational mastitis). As pregnancy progresses, the breasts become firmer, more nodular, and hypertrophic. This is of course also true of the post partum lactation period. A subtle palpable mass may disappear as pregnancy progresses and the breast becomes more engorged. Whereas a breast mass in a menstruating woman can be re-examined just after the next menstrual period, the hormonal milieu will continue to intensify in the pregnant woman, making subsequent examinations more difficult. Fine-needle aspiration of a mass that yields fluid and causes the mass to disappear readily differentiates the fluid-filled cyst or galactocele from a solid tumor. However, cytology from fine-needle aspiration is not as accurate in the pregnant as in the nonpregnant woman. The hyperproliferative cellular state of the pregnant breast increases the possibility of a false positive diagnosis. Excisional biopsy under local anesthesia may be difficult during pregnancy because of the hypervascularity and edema but it remains the best diagnostic tool. Many clinicians attribute the advanced state and poor prognosis of breast cancer in pregnancy to delayed diagnosis. More recent theories of cancer in pregnancy have shown improved survivals undoubtedly

Table 14-3 Characteristics of nipple discharge

Color	Likely cause	% caused by cancer
Milky (galactorrhea)	Pituitary adenoma Pregnancy Oral contraceptives	Rare
Green, yellow, sticky	Ductal ectasia	Rare
Clear, watery	Ductal carcinoma	30-50
Bloody, sanguineous	Fibrocystic disease Ductal papillomas	25
Pink, serosanguineous	Fibrocystic disease Ductal papillomas	10
Yellow, serous	Fibrocystic disease Ductal papillomas	5
Purulent	Bacterial infection	Rare

as a result of less reluctance to biopsy the breasts of pregnant women.

Breast biopsy in a pregnant or a lactating woman calls for meticulous hemostatis because of the increased vascularity and risk of a postoperative hematoma. The lactating breast is predisposed to postoperative infection, since milk is a good culture medium. Anesthesia by local injection may be difficult in the enlarged breast but is the method of choice. Incisional biopsy under local anesthesia is an option when excisional biopsy is problematic. Because of the significant risk of infection and milk fistula, the patient who is lactating should cease lactating before biopsy is performed.

Guidelines for management

The American Cancer Society, the National Cancer Institute, and the American College of Obstetricians and Gynecologists have agreed on guidelines for early detection of breast cancer. These guidelines state as follows:

"Physicians should encourage their female patients in doing monthly breast self-examinations. Physicians should be encouraged to do clinical breast examinations on all female patients in whom they are doing a periodic examination. A baseline mammogram should be obtained between the ages of 35 and 40. Thereafter, a mammography is suggested every one to two years for women age 40-50 years and annually for women over 50 years of age."

Most patients discover their own breast masses and then consult their physicians. It is essential that an active diagnosis be made and proper treatment be initiated with minimal delay. Definitive treatment of cystic alterations and mammary dysplasia depends on the age of the patient and the size and characteristics of the lesion (Figure 14-12). An obvious fibroadenoma may be safely observed in patients younger than the age of 25, but large dominant masses should be removed, even if the mammogram is

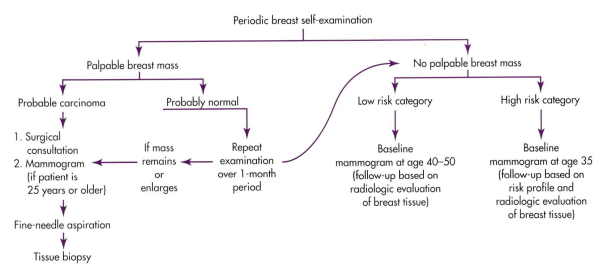

Figure 14-12 Flow diagram of breast surveillance. (Modified from Logan WW: *J Contin Ed Ob/Gyn*, July 1979.)

negative, because continued growth may cause local destruction of functioning breast tissue. Solid masses should be excised by means of a circumareolar circumalveolar incision. Obvious cystic masses can be aspirated and the fluid sent for cytologic analysis. Some authorities feel that cytologic examination of clear breast fluid is unnecessary, but it would seem that pathologic analysis of the fluid is prudent in all other circumstances. The presence of serosanguineous or bloody fluid demands further tissue biopsy. Women older than the age of 25 who have dominant masses should have a baseline mammogram with any biopsy or aspiration. Since breast cancer is exceedingly rare in patients younger than 25 years, a mammogram need not be done in this age group.

ESTROGEN THERAPY AND BREAST CANCER INCIDENCE

It is well known that estrogens influence the growth of normal breast tissue. It is also true that estrogens, extracts of estrogen-producing endocrine glands, and antihormones have been used to impede the growth of and to control established human and animal breast cancers. The estrogen-endometrial cancer link that began in the mid-1970s has led to considerable interest in the relationship of estrogen replacement therapy in breast cancer. A few epidemiologic studies implied a slight increase in the incidence of breast cancer among patients receiving estrogens. The many benefits of estrogen therapy during and after the menopause make it imperative that clinicians understand all the risks involved in exogenous estrogen therapy. Does giving a patient estrogen increase the risk of breast cancer? What is the prognosis for patients who develop breast cancer while taking exogenous estrogens?

Gambrell reported on studies from the Wilford Hall United States Air Force Medical Center. These were prospective studies done from 1975 to 1979, and they showed no evidence that estrogen replacement therapy for menopausal women increased the risk of breast cancer. As a matter of fact, their data indicated that estrogen therapy may even provide some protection, particularly when it is combined with a progestogen. Gambrell followed 5563 postmenopausal women for a total of 24,599 patient-years of observation. During the 5 years of the study he found 43 patients with breast cancer, for an overall incidence of 174.8/100,000 women per year. This incidence is similar to the incidence of 188.3/100,000 for women ages 55 to 59 reported in the Third National Cancer Survey. The mean age of his postmenopausal breast cancer patients was 57.5 years. During 7322 patient-years of observation he found 7 breast cancers in the women treated with estrogen and progestogens, for an annual incidence of 95.6/100,000. During 3799 patient-years of observation 19 women in the untreated group had breast cancer—an incidence of 500/100,000. The differences appear to be statistically significant. A similar study done by Nachtigall et al. was statistically significant, with a p value less than 0.05. These findings correlate well with Korenman's "estrogen window" hypothesis, which proposes that the risk of breast cancer is related to the duration of unopposed estrogen exposure during the reproductive years of a woman's life. This suggests that progestogen-treated postmenopausal women are at lower risk for breast cancer, just as progestogen-treated women seem to be protected from endometrial cancer. However, more clinical experience with progestogen therapy after menopause is needed before firm recommendations can be made for hysterectomized women.

Korenman's "estrogen window" hypothesis implies that unopposed endogenous estrogens, caused by progesterone deficiency or luteal dysfunction, may provide a state favorable to the induction of breast cancer by carcinogens in a susceptible mammary gland. Although this hypothesis may indeed be correct, no abnormalities in progesterone production have been reported in breast cancer patients; thus confirmation is lacking. Some support for this hypothesis comes from the report of Nachtigall et al., which suggests that progestins may provide protection from the incidence of breast cancer. In addition, epidemiological data suggest that groups of patients likely to have undergone long periods of unopposed estrogen (e.g., nulligravida, infertile patients, polycystic ovarian disease) are at higher risk to develop the disease. Others attempt to link prolactin to breast cancer. Most of this has come from the indirect improvement noted in some patients with metastatic breast disease treated by prolactin-suppressing drugs such as l-dopa or bromocriptine. Higher levels of prolactin and estriol have been found in daughters of women with breast cancer, although no differences in estrogen or prolactin production have ever been found in patients with breast cancer. An association between thyroid hormone and breast cancer has been suggested, especially since increased levels of thyrotropin-releasing hormone can increase prolactin levels. Breast cancer is more common in patients who are hypothyroid and uncommon among those who are hyperthyroid.

Many scientists have done extensive studies to clarify the role of endogenous estrogen in breast cancer but as yet no clear pattern has emerged. Indeed, the issue is full of paradoxes such that some patients with metastatic breast disease respond to endocrine ablation while others go into remission when estrogen therapy is given. Indeed, many years of extensive investigation of endocrine factors have thus far failed to link endogenous hormones, including androgen, estrogen, progesterone, prolactin, and thyroid, with breast cancer in a cause-and-effect relationship.

In 1990, Colditz et al. published material from the Nurses Health Study in which they examined the use of estrogen replacement therapy in relation to breast cancer incidence in a cohort of women 30 to 55 years of age beginning in 1976. During the 376,000 person-years of follow-up among postmenopausal women, 722 incident cases of breast cancer were documented. Overall, past users of estrogen replacement therapy were not at increased risk. Relative risk (0.98), included even those with more than 10 years of use. Colditz et al. also found that the risk of breast cancer was significantly elevated among current users, who had a relative risk of 1.36 (Table 14-4). Among current users, a stronger relationship was observed with increasing age, but not with increasing duration of use. They felt that their data suggest that long-term past use of estrogen replacement therapy was not related to increased risk of breast cancer but that current use may modestly increase risk.

A meta-analysis reported by Steinberg suggests that breast cancer risk increased to an estimated 1.3 after 15 years of estrogen use. Risk did not appear to increase at

Table 14-4 Nurses' Health Study 1976 to 1992

Hormone use	Cases of breast cancer	Person-years of F/U	Adjusted relative risk (95% CI)
None	972	374,197	1.0
Current			
1-23 months	82	31,966	1.14 (0.91-1.45)
24-59 months	140	49,672	1.20 (0.99-1.44)
60-119 months	150	44,112	1.46 (1.22-1.74)
≥120 months	141	37,454	1.46 (1.20-1.76)
Past			
1-23 months	193	81,047	0.90 (0.77-1.05)
24-59 months	120	54,046	0.86 (0.71-1.05)
60-119 months	89	34,952	1.00 (0.80-1.26)
≥120 months	48	18,104	1.03 (0.76-1.41)

From Colditz GA et al: Use of estrogens and progestins and risk of breast cancer in postmenopausal women, *N Engl J Med* 332:1589, 1995.
F/U, Follow-up; CI, confidence interval.

all until after at least 5 years of use. The authors admit that this discrepancy could result from publication bias in that authors are more likely to report analyses of stratified data if the analyses show differences between cases and control.

Another meta-analysis, by Dupont and Page concerning breast cancer and estrogen replacement therapy reported an overall risk of breast cancer associated with this therapy at 1.07. Women who took 0.625 mg or less of conjugated estrogens had a risk of breast cancer 1.08 times the risk of women who did not receive this therapy. Women who took 1.25 mg or more per day of conjugated estrogens had a breast cancer relative risk 2.0 or less in all studies. The relative risk of breast cancer associated with estrogen replacement therapy among women with histories of benign breast disease was 1.16. Dupont and Page concluded that the combined results from multiple studies provided strong evidence that menopausal therapy consisting of 0.625 mg per day or less of conjugated estrogens did not increase breast cancer risk (Table 14-5).

A much-publicized article by Bergkvist, published in the *New England Journal of Medicine* in 1989, examined the risk of breast cancer after noncontraceptive treatment with estrogen. A relative increase in risk was noted for some subsets using synthetic estrogen but no increase was found with the use of conjugated estrogens.

The results of the 3-year prospective postmenopausal estrogen/progestin intervention (PEPI) trial, published in the *Journal of the American Medical Association* in January of 1995, indicated no increased risk of breast cancer in study participants. A total of 875 healthy postmenopausal women aged 45-64 years who had no contraindication to hormone therapy were given placebo, unopposed estrogen, or one of three estrogen/progestin

Table 14-5 Meta-analyses of breast cancer incidence among HRT users vs nonusers

Reference	Effects of ever-use RR (95% CI)	Use more than 15 yr RR (95% CI)	Special risk group? RR (95% CI)
Armstrong	0.96 (0.98-1.05)	1.04 (0.88-1.24)	Nil identified
Dupont and Page	1.08 (0.96-1.2)	No conclusion	Nil identified
Steinberg et al.	1.0	1.3 (1.2-1.6)	Family history 3.4
Grady and Ernster	No increase	1.25	Nil identified

HRT, Hormone replacement therapy; RR, risk ratio, CI, confidence interval.

regimens in a 3-year, multicenter, randomized, double blind, placebo-controlled trial. Although the goals of the study were directed toward the analysis of effects on heart disease, all patient subsets were closely monitored for any disease process, including breast cancer. The results are reassuring regarding the risks of breast cancer in users of HRT.

What about the woman who develops the disease while receiving estrogen? Is her prognosis altered? Gambrell's study suggested that hormone users have a better prognosis than non-hormone users. At the time of his report 57 of the total group of 199 postmenopausal women with breast cancer had died. Among the women using hormones when breast cancer was diagnosed, 14 of 63 died, for a mortality rate of 22%. In women who had breast cancers who had never taken hormones 75 of 165 had died, for a mortality rate of 46% (Table 14-6). This difference was statistically significant, with a p value less than 0.01. Gambrell concluded that the better prognosis was a result of earlier diagnosis of the estrogen-treated women. This was suggested in the statistic that 51% of the estrogen users with breast cancer had negative nodes, whereas only 45% of the nonusers were found to have negative nodes. Even more suggestive was the fact that 35% of nonusers had four or more positive axillary nodes as compared with only 22% of the hormone users. Bergkvist (1989) studied the prognosis after the diagnosis of breast cancer in women exposed to estrogen and estrogen-progestin replacement therapy. The article looked directly at the outcome for patients who developed breast cancer while receiving HRT. The relative survival rate at 8 years was significantly higher by approximately 10% in patients who had received estrogen treatment (Figure 14-13), corresponding to an approximately 40% reduction in mortality. This more favorable outcome was observed in patients aged 50 years or older at diagnosis and was most pronounced in recent users, i.e., in women whose treatment was ongoing or had been discontinued within 1 year before diagnosis of breast cancer was made. There are at least three additional reports (see Table 14-6) that come to the same conclusions regarding improved

Table 14-6 Breast cancer survival in current users of ERT

Report	Results
Bergkvist (*Am J Epidemiol* 130(2):221, 1989)	10% improvement
Gambrell (*AJOG* 150:119, 1984)	Mortality rates 22% users 46% non-users
Hunt (*Br J OG* 94:620, 1987)	Mortality rate—RR 0.55 study of 4544 ERT users
Henderson (*Ar Int Med* 151:75, 1991)	19% reduction in mortality 4988 users—3865 non-users

From Cobleigh MA et al: Estrogen replacement therapy in breast cancer survivors, *JAMA* 272(7):540, 1994.

survival outcome in HRT users who develop breast cancer.

Ovarian Stimulation and Breast Cancer

Over the past decade, many women have undergone follicular stimulation, especially during assisted reproductive technology procedures. Brezezinski reported 16 women who were treated by induction ovulation and subsequently were diagnosed with breast cancer. These women were drawn out of 950 cases of infertile women who had undergone induction of ovulation at their fertility clinic. The author presents a possible association between ovarian stimulation and promotion of breast cancer and recommends that a controlled study be performed.

Progestin Use

If a decision is made to give estrogen-replacement therapy (ERT) to a patient at risk of breast cancer a common query is whether the patient also should receive progestin with the estrogen even in the hysterectomized patient. There is little definitive clinical data on this issue. However, one large study suggested that the addition of progestin conferred significant protection against the development

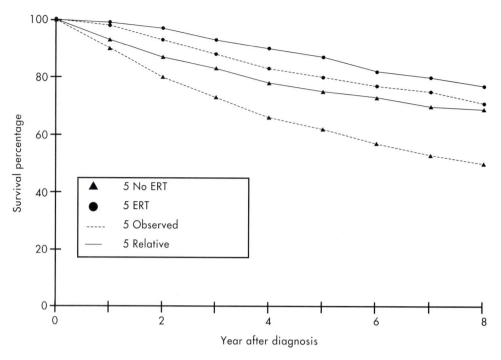

Figure 14-13 Observed (*dashed line*) and relative survival (*solid line*) in 261 patients with breast cancer with previous estrogen therapy (*circles*) and 6617 such patients without previous estrogen therapy (*triangles*). (Uppsala Health Care Region, Sweden, 1977-1986. Modified from Bergkvist L, Adami HO, Persson I, Bergstrom R, Krusemo UB: Prognosis after breast cancer diagnosis in women exposed to estrogen and estrogen-progestogen replacement therapy, *Am J Epidemiol* 130:221, 1989.)

of breast cancer compared with the control population in patients receiving estrogens alone. These data have been reanalyzed; it was found that a significant portion of the control group consisted of patients with benign breast disease who may or may not have been at higher risk for the development of breast cancer. A more important question is whether the progestin confers an additional therapeutic effect if there are occult foci of malignant breast tissue in the patient. In an elegant study using human breast cells obtained at the time of reduction mammoplasty and grown in long-term culture, estrogen-stimulated growth could be turned off or abrogated by the addition of progestin to the culture medium. Pharmacologic doses of megestrol acetate and progesterone had a direct effect on these human breast cells, including a decrease in the cell number. These agents were able to modify and abrogate the stimulation of estrogen on the breast cell lines studied. Others report similar findings. Normal human breast epithelial cells were cultured from tissue taken at the time of reduction mammoplasty and used to study the actions of estrogen, progesterone, and estrogen-progesterone combinations. When estrogen stimulation of cell growth was detected, a progestin inhibited cell manipulation, favored differentiation, and abrogated the stimulation of the estrogen on the cells in culture.

Nachtigall reported on a 22-year prospective study of the incidence of breast cancer in 84 continuously matched pairs of institutionalized women receiving HRT or placebo. During the first 10 years, 4 placebo users developed breast cancer compared with none of the HRT users. During the entire 22-year period, there were 6 cases of breast cancer in 52 never-users, whereas none of the 116 women who used HRT at any time developed breast cancer ($p = .01$). The author advocates HRT using conjugated estrogens, 0.625 mg/d, with medroxyprogesterone acetate, 2.5 mg/d, in a continuous regimen with patients who have a history of breast cancer.

Progestins are a group of compounds once considered ineffective for the treatment of breast cancer, but more recent studies have shown that both medroxyprogesterone acetate and megestrol acetate are as active as any other endocrine therapy commonly used. Although there are no direct comparisons of these two forms of progestin therapy, they appear to be equally effective. Medroxyprogesterone acetate is used more frequently in Europe; megestrol acetate is used more frequently in the United States. Each has been compared in randomized trials with tamoxifen, and there was no difference in the response rates. Preliminary data suggest that receptor status is unimportant in the selection of patients for the use of progestins. More studies are needed to test this point. Thus this author does not believe that one should hesitate to administer progestins to patients with breast cancer because of any concern of an adverse effect on an occult metastatic focus.

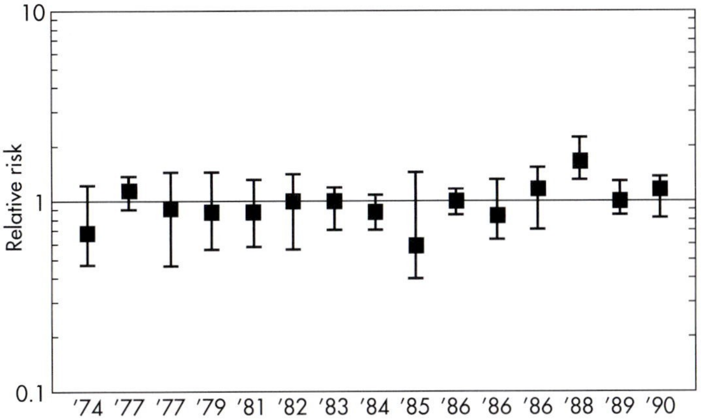

Figure 14-14 Relative risks of breast cancer in women in developed countries who have ever used OCs. Case-control studies of women of all ages at risk of exposure. (From Thomas DB: *Oral contraceptives and breast cancer*, Washington, DC, 1991, National Academy Press.)

The long-acting injectable progestational contraceptive Depot-medroxyprogesterone acetate (DMPA) is used around the world. This drug has been recently approved by the FDA as a contraceptive in the United States. Research in beagles linked mammary tumors to the drug, accounting for several years of delay prior to approval. Eleven million women in more than 80 countries who have used DMPA for many years were shown not to have an increased risk of breast cancer.

In summary, the in vitro data (and at least two clinical studies) suggest that the administration of progestin with estrogen may be prudent for any patient and especially for the patient with a history of breast cancer who has decided to receive HRT. This author has made it a practice to use conjugated estrogens 0.625 mg with medroxyprogesterone acetate 2.5 mg daily in a continuous regimen for patients with a history of breast cancer.

Menopause

Another fascinating hypothesis is found in the influence of iatrogenic menopause on the incidence of breast cancer. As in early natural menopause, an early surgically induced menopause was found to have a protective effect. The protection afforded by iatrogenic menopause is greater the earlier the surgery is done. According to Hirayama and Wynder, this protection applies only if oophorectomy is done before the patient is 44 years of age. Protection appears to be more pronounced in the case of surgically induced menopause than in the natural menopause. This is understandable, in that 90% of women have natural menopause between the ages of 45 and 55 years, whereas a comparatively far larger portion of the oophorectomized women experience induced menopause before 40 years of age. A very extensive study of the influence of artificial menopause on the prognosis of breast cancer was done by MacKay and Sellers, who observed a 5-year survival of 61% in a population of 237 women with iatrogenic menopause compared with 49% for patients with natural menopause. They suggest that

this difference is a result of the tendency of natural menopause to suppress ovarian activity later than iatrogenic menopause.

Breast Cancer and Oral Contraceptives

The use of oral contraceptives (OC) for long periods or the use of them in the presence of other risk factors has been hypothesized to increase the risk of breast cancer. Oral contraceptives, which are potent combinations of estrogen and progestin, have been used by more than 25 million women in the United States and 150 million women worldwide. The net hormonal effect of oral contraceptives could plausibly either increase or decrease the risk of breast cancer.

Of interest is a study by Matthews et al. of breast cancer developing in women who have used oral contraceptives, including those who have taken them but not currently, and the finding of a significantly improved survival rate. The authors concluded that not only was earlier diagnosis and improved prognosis a result of pill usage but also that the contraceptive steroids may have some beneficial biologic effect on the host.

In a 1991 review of the literature, Thomas summarized the data from 15 case-control studies of breast cancer and oral contraceptive use in women of all ages in developed countries (Figure 14-14). Relative risk estimates are shown by year of study in Figure 14-14. A summary relative risk of 1.0 in women who ever used oral contraceptives was estimated from the published results of these studies. Only one study found a significant trend of increasing risk with duration of exposure. Thomas also estimated the relative risk for the published results of five cohort studies. A summary relative risk of 1.06 in women who ever used OCs was found. The conclusion derived from his overview of case-control and cohort studies was that there appeared to be no overall association between the use of oral contraceptives and breast cancer.

Schlesselman concluded that the risk of breast cancer through 59 years of age was not affected appreciably by the use of oral contraceptives. He recognized that concern continues to be expressed about the effects of early age at first use, long-term duration of use, formulation, and various other factors thought to influence breast cancer risk in the presence of oral contraception. He recognized that a number of recent studies restricted to young women suggested that long-term use may increase the risk of disease occurring very early, but the present lack of consistent findings in well-conducted epidemiological studies prevents any certain conclusion with regard to cause and effect. Increased risks were indeed present. The most plausible interpretation is that long-term oral contraception promotes earlier clinical manifestation of breast cancer in some women but has no net impact on their lifetime risk of the disease.

Given the long natural history of this neoplasm, it is inevitable that a large number of patients subsequently diagnosed with breast cancer would have been exposed to oral contraceptive use during the initiation and progression of their neoplasms. Unfortunately, most data in the literature are relevant to the incidence of breast cancer and oral contraceptive use, and there is a paucity of information about the outcome of patients who may have been exposed to OCs while harboring a malignant breast neoplasm. We suggest an assumption that if OCs do not increase the risk for breast cancer development it is unlikely they would adversely affect the outcome in patients harboring breast cancer. Also, with the realization that breast cancer may originate and remain occult for years before its presentation as a mass, large numbers of women with primary breast cancer may have been exposed inadvertently to OCs during the inception and evolution of their tumors. When these women were studied by Rosner and compared with other patients with breast cancer of similar age who have never used OCs, a trend toward an earlier stage of presentation in users of OCs was observed. The authors attributed this trend to surveillance bias; women receiving regular medical care were scrutinized more carefully than those not using OCs.

Women who used OCs in the past were intermediate for the stage at presentation compared with current users and women who never used OCs. Generally, the trend toward an earlier stage at detection did not translate into better survival for recent users of OCs and no adverse effect on the survival rates for users was noted.

A larger study that showed no increase in breast cancer incidence in young women associated with OC use was the Cancer and Steroid Hormone Study, which was conducted simultaneously in eight areas of the United States. For women younger than age 45 years, no increased risk was found for any duration of OC use or for use before the first full-term pregnancy. An excess risk associated with OC use was reported among the small subgroup of nulliparous women younger than age 45 years who underwent menarche before the age of 13 years.

Yet, other studies by Pike suggest that the starting age of OC use is associated significantly with breast cancer. The exposure-response relationship between the duration of OC use and the risk of breast cancer depended on the age when the first doses of these drugs were administered. Given a fixed duration of use, the risk increased with the younger starting age of OC use. Currently, however, no one has translated this into a poor outcome for patients who, unfortunately, have clinical disease.

At the same time, one must consider that the health benefits of OCs include not only protection from endometrial and ovarian cancers but also reduction in the incidence of dysmenorrhea, iron-deficiency anemia, pelvic inflammatory disease, functional ovarian cysts, benign breast disease, and ectopic pregnancy. A study from the Allen-Guttmacher Institute reports that the risk of developing cancer (breast, endometrial, ovarian, or liver) for OC users actually would be less than if OCs were never used (Figure 14-15). The greatest protection is conferred after age 40. The data indicated that the overall risk of developing breast cancer is no greater for OC users up to age 55 than the risk for those who never used OCs.

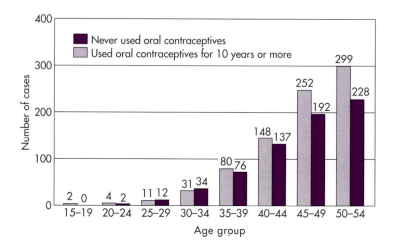

Figure 14-15 Estimated annual number of newly diagnosed cases of ovarian, endometrial, breast, and liver cancer per 100,000 women. (Modified from Thomas DB: *Oral contraceptives and breast cancer*, Washington DC, 1991, National Academy Press.)

In addition, it does not appear that OCs increase the risk for women with other risk factors for breast cancer, such as family history of breast cancer or nulliparity. There remain some unanswered questions regarding early long-term OC use and the risk of breast cancer, but on balance, the evidence available at this time does not warrant any change in prescribing patterns for OCs. Furthermore, the potential risk must always be weighed against the known health benefits of OCs and the prevention of unwanted pregnancy.

BREAST CANCERS
Epidemiology

Considering the epidemiology of breast cancer, it must be kept in mind that while populations at high risk can be identified, the majority of breast cancers occur in women whose only defined risk factors are sex and increased age. The risk that a 30-year-old woman will have breast cancer is 7% that of a 60-year-old woman. There is no combination of risk factors that will match this 14-fold increase produced by advancing age. Eighty five percent of all breast cancer occurs in women without a meaningful family history of breast cancer. Breast cancer appears to have a complex etiology, with many of its causes and preventative factors operating over a long period of time. Some individual risk factors are relatively weak (see box below), a major increase in risk over most of the population occurs only when there are two or more factors. In a woman's lifetime, she has a 1 in 9 chance of developing breast cancer. Breast cancer now accounts for 28% of all newly diagnosed cancers in women and 18%

of female cancer deaths. The age-adjusted mortality rate for breast cancer has changed very little in the last two decades.

A hereditary predisposition to breast cancer plays an important role in perhaps 5% of all breast cancers in the United States. The relative risk in individuals with a first-degree relative with breast cancer is given in Table 14-7. This risk is increased if more than one relative has breast cancer. The relative risk of second-degree relatives approximates 1.5. These familial factors that increase risk may be joined by other factors, such as the presence or absence of proliferative disease within the breast tissue (see Table 14-1).

Several protective factors have been suggested in the literature. They are as follows:
1. Early pregnancy (If the first birth is before age 18 years, the risk is only one third the risk of a first pregnancy after 35 years)
2. Prolonged lactation (Controversial effect on cancer incidence)
3. Castration (Significant decrease in risk in women having oophorectomy before age 35)
4. Exercise (Physically active women have fewer ovulatory menstrual cycles and have a lower incidence)
5. Abstinence from alcohol
6. Low-fat diet (Controversial)
7. Chemopreventives such as retinoids or antiestrogens (Experimental)

Some data suggest that dietary factors may have a major influence on breast cancer incidence. This has often been suggested as an explanation for wide differences in breast cancer incidence among various countries of the world (Table 14-8). There is strong epidemiological evidence associating dietary fat and, perhaps, low dietary fiber with increased risk of breast cancer. The National Cancer Institute and the American Cancer Society recommend a low-fat, high-fiber diet for the prevention of breast cancer. However, there are no prospective studies to demonstrate that modification of diet decreases risk. Kritchevsky reported that case-control studies carried out

---

BREAST CANCER—NONFAMILIAL RISK FACTORS

1. Sex (99% in women)
2. Age (85% over age 40)
3. Proliferative fibrocystic changes with and without atypia (2–5/1)
4. Previous cancer of one breast (5/1)
5. Nulliparous vs parous (3/1)
6. First birth after age 34 (4/1)
7. Menarche before age 12 (1.3/1)
8. Menopause after age 50 (1.5/1)
9. Affluent vs poor (2/1)
10. Jewish vs non-Jewish (2/1)
11. Western Hemisphere vs Eastern Hemisphere (1.5/1)
12. Cold climate vs warm climate (1.5/1)
13. Chronic psychologic stress (2/1)
14. Obesity (2/1)
15. Triad of obesity, hypertension, and diabetes (3/1)
16. High dietary fat intake (3/1)
17. White vs Asian (5/1)

Table 14-7   First-degree relative with breast cancer—relative risk for patient

Index case	Relative risk
Premenopausal	
Unilateral	1.8
Bilateral	8.8
Postmenopausal	
Unilateral	1.2
Bilateral	4.0

Table 14-8 Age standardized mortality rates from breast cancer

Country	Rate per 100,000 females
England and Wales, 1982	28.4
Scotland, 1981	27.7
Nothern Ireland, 1980	27.7
Netherlands, 1982	26.4
USA, 1982	22.1
Iceland, 1983	19.9
France, 1981	19.2
Sweden, 1984	18.6
Finland, 1983	16.8
Yugoslavia, 1982	13.0
Venezuela, 1982	9.2
Mauritius, 1982	6.9
Japan, 1982	5.8

Source: *World Health Statistics Annual* 1985.

in several countries show no real association between fat intake and breast cancer. There is some evidence that vitamin A or beta-carotene may exert a protective effect. Alcohol intake, on the other hand, seems to be positively associated with breast cancer risk. Elevated body fat, body mass, stature, and frame size have also been found to be associated as risk factors for breast cancer in women. Animal studies found that caloric restriction inhibits growth of spontaneous induced mammary tumors, an observation that remained valid even when the calorie-restricted animals ingested more fat than the liberally fed controls. College women who exercise have a lower incidence of breast cancer than their more sedentary classmates. Exercise is another means of reducing caloric availability.

Several publications address breast cancer incidence in pregnant women who ingested DES. Two of these studies were randomized clinical trials reporting the long-term follow-up results of the use of DES during pregnancy. In one (Beral), 80 diabetic women received hormonal treatment and 76 women received placebos. After 29 years of follow-up, 4 cases of breast cancer had occurred among the exposed women and none among the unexposed group. In another study (Vessey), 10 cases of breast cancer were found among 319 DES-exposed women and 9 cases were found among 331 unexposed women, suggesting there was no excess risk. Still, other studies quoted an overall relative risk of breast cancer among the exposed women between 1.2 and 1.5. The 1985 DES Task Force, sponsored by the US Department of Health, Education, and Welfare, concluded that women who used DES during their pregnancies may subsequently experience an increased risk of breast cancer. However, a causal relationship is still unproved and the observed level of

excess risk is similar to that for a number of other breast cancer risk factors.

Although breast cancer is primarily a postmenopausal condition, it also affects a small proportion of women in their 20s and 30s. This patient population may be small but their prospects for long-term survival are significantly worse than their older counterparts (age |Lf40). In a SEER program of 77,368 subjects, 26% of white women diagnosed with breast cancer in their 20s will die from the disease in the first 5 years after diagnosis, compared to 20% diagnosed in their 30s and 15% diagnosed in their 40s. Doubling time studies also demonstrate shorter intervals in younger women, implying more aggressive lesions.

The enormous popularity of silicone mammoplasty and its rapidly increasing use has placed silicone again under scrutiny for its potential long-term adverse effects. At this time, with patients now exposed to breast implants for more than 20 years and a large number of patients now reaching the age of high breast cancer incidence, carefully planned review studies may be necessary. Further epidemiological research, including scientific clinical and animal studies, may be required to determine the short- and long-term safety of breast implants. In 1991, the FDA ordered the makers of all breast implants to demonstrate the safety of their products or remove them from the market. The FDA also recommended that any new implantation procedure involving these products be delayed until risk assessment analysis is completed. The ultimate fate of the polyurethane in implant capsule walls has not been clinically determined. It is suggested by some that the hazards associated with these implants outweigh their advantages and, therefore, that their use may not be justifiable. More data are necessary.

Early Detection and Diagnosis

The gynecologist should recognize that there are special groups of women at added risk for development of breast cancer (see box below).

HIGH-RISK FACTORS IN BREAST CANCER

1. Older than 40 years of age
2. Family history: first-degree relatives
3. Obstetric history: late parity (older than age 35)
4. Previous cancer in one breast
5. Other organ cancer, such as endometrium and ovary
6. Fibrocystic changes—proliferative type
7. Obesity
8. Lower immunologic competence
9. Excess exposure of the breast to radiation
10. High dietary fat intake

Breast cancer doubling times

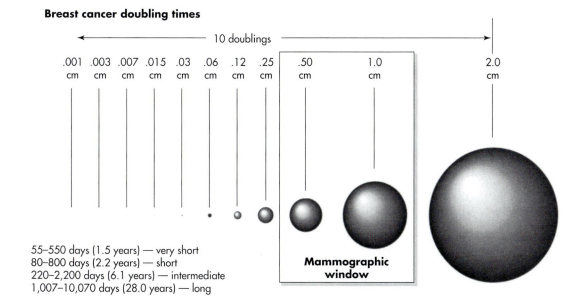

Figure 14-16 Breast cancer doubling time.

First, occurrence of development of breast cancer is twice as frequent among those who have family histories of breast cancer (grandmother, mother, aunt, or sister) as in the control group. Second, patients who have had cancer in one breast are five times more likely to develop cancer in the remaining breast as are those in the control group. Third, there is a group of patients who have severe cystic disease (proliferative type) in whom subsequent breast cancer (apparently unrelated to the cysts themselves) is reported to occur two to four times more frequently than in the control group. Women in each of these groups should have breast examinations every 4-6 months for the duration of their lives. Women between the ages of 40 and 44 and those older than 60 have a higher risk, especially if they have not been pregnant or have not borne their first child before the age of 34. Whites are at higher risk than blacks and Asians. In addition, patients who experience early menarche and late menopause are apparently at higher risk. Most malignant breast lesions are in the breast several years prior to clinical detection (Figure 14-16), allowing ample opportunity for early diagnosis.

Outpatient biopsy has become increasingly popular and inconveniences the patient minimally. A biopsy is not an office procedure and is best performed in an operating room with a team of assistants. Local anesthesia can be used, and in most instances a circumareolar incision is made. Meticulous hemostasis must be achieved during these biopsies to minimize postoperative complications. Limited biopsy and definitive diagnosis are becoming more popular, even for lesions that appear to be malignant. Available data suggest that a 12-week delay in treatment does not adversely influence survival in breast cancer, so diagnostic and therapeutic procedures need not be combined in the same surgical procedure.

More than 50% of all breast cancers are accidentally detected by the patient. Masses found by patients in this manner are likely to be sizable, and methods are needed for detection of earlier disease. The signs and symptoms of breast cancer, such as localized skin edema, nipple retraction, localized erythema, swelling, skin retraction, changes in contour, ulceration, and enlargement of the axillary nodes, represent manifestations of locally advanced disease. Minimal breast cancer is occasionally found accidentally when an abnormality actually caused by benign breast disease leads to the performance of a biopsy and minimal carcinoma is found in adjacent tissue by histologic examination. Such fortuitous events are obviously unusual and not the main method of diagnosis. To detect breast cancer before the development of signs of advanced disease, mass population screening is necessary. The modalities commonly available for screening are physical examination, mammography, and ultrasonography.

Physical examination of the breast in a screening center consists of rigidly systematic palpation and inspection, usually carried out by physicians or trained paramedical specialists. In one or two earlier attempts at breast cancer screening, physical examination alone was used and was found to be effective in increasing the frequency of node-negative breast cancer cases. More productive, however, is a combination of mammography and physical examination. The examination period also provides an opportunity for instruction of the patient in SBE. The patient is shown how to perform the examination and introduced to the variations that may be present

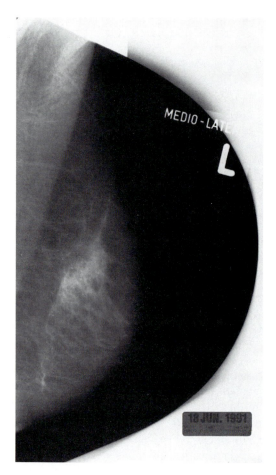

Figure 14-17 Mammogram showing an irregular configuration characteristic of malignancy.

in her own breast. A good instructor in SBE attempts to instill strong motivation in the woman to do a monthly assessment of her own breasts. Although some reports suggest that carefully performed SBE avoids only the development of advanced-stage breast cancers, its continued use should be encouraged.

Mammographic examination usually consists of two views of each breast. In most of the breast cancer detection centers a screen-film apparatus is used. Images are obtained by trained radiographic technicians and interpreted by radiologists who have special training and experience in this radiographic discipline (Figure 14-17).

Cyrlak noted that increasing numbers of postmenopausal women were undergoing hormone replacement therapy, and this was having an effect on mammographic findings. She found that the changes included symmetric and asymmetric increases in breast density, increases in the size of fibroadenomas, and the development or increase in the size of cysts. Her article demonstrates examples of all of these findings. She and her colleagues also noted that the addition of progesterone to the regimen resulted in diffuse increase in density but fewer breast cysts. This author stresses the need for documentation of

the commencement of hormone replacement therapy when ordering a mammographic study.

Thermography as a means of breast cancer detection is unproved. Early studies gave hope that it might be useful in prescreening to identify a group of women most at risk. Experience in most centers, however, has been disappointing. The number of false negative and false positive results obtained by thermography has been unacceptably high, and the examination has been dropped from the screening routine in all but a few centers, where it is retained as a research tool.

Recently technical improvements in ultrasonic imaging techniques have led to the suggestion that this modality might also be used in breast cancer detection. The proposal is attractive because ultrasonography exposes the breast to only trivial levels of energy, on the order of a few milliwatt-seconds. Although much preliminary work has been done that indicates there are differences in the absorption of ultrasound by normal and neoplastic tissue, neither the practical aspects of application nor the specific diagnostic parameters for its use as a screening tool have, as yet, been accurately defined. Its clinical use at present has been limited to distinguishing the nature of a detected mass (solid vs cystic) as it bears on the malignant potential of a given lesion.

The HIP Trial is the oldest significant study of breast screening by mammography. Previous analyses of this trial, after follow-up periods of 5 to 16 years, have shown significantly decreased mortality from breast cancer in screened women aged 50-64 years but not for screened women aged 40-49 years. Chu et al. evaluated breast cancer mortality after at least 18 years of follow-up in the HIP Trial using a statistical method different from those previously chosen for analyzing by age-at-entry cohort. They found that significant mortality benefited for both age cohorts (Figure 14-18). The author's analysis of these cohorts demonstrated a significant decrease in mortality for all stages combined at the end of the follow-up. This effect was observed 4 years after entry into the 50-64 year cohort and 9 years after entry into the 40-49 year cohort. In the Breast Cancer Detection Demonstration Project (BCDDP) study, the average sensitivity of the combination of clinical examination and mammography in the 5 years of close follow-up was 71%. Other studies have shown this to range from 70%-80%, with increased sensitivity reported among older patients. The specificity of mammography overall is 94%-99%.

The experience gained through the BCDDP (Table 14-9) has been helpful in drawing some conclusions. Analysis of their data suggests that screening for breast cancer leads to earlier detection. Although the high yield encountered in that project may in part be a result of self-detection of the patient population, a significant number of the cancers detected were small. The women involved in the screening project were volunteers, and it had been hoped that they would be primarily asymptom-

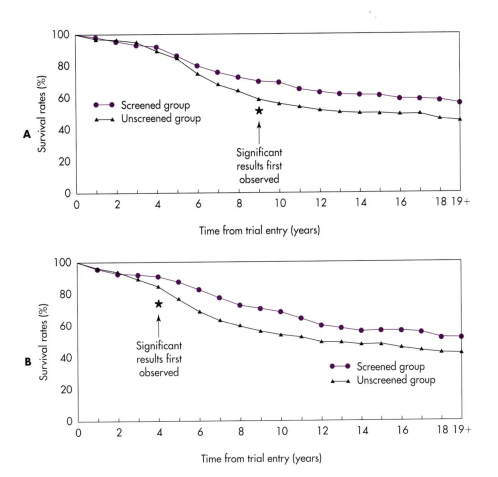

Figure 14-18 A, Survival rates for women in HIP study aged 40-49 years at entry (all stages). **B,** Survival rates for women in HIP study aged 50-64 years at entry (all stages). (Modified from Chu KC, Smart CR, Tarone RE: *J Natl Ca Inst* 80:1125, 1988.)

Table 14-9   Breast cancers detected by modality of detection (BCDDP), 1981

Modality	Ages 40-49 at surgery		Ages 50-59 at surgery	
Mammography only	270	(35%)	540	(42%)
Mammography and physical examination	381	(50%)	638	(50%)
Physical examination only	100	(13%)	86	(7%)
Unknown	11	(2%)	19	(1%)
TOTAL	762	(100%)	1283	(100%)

From American Cancer Society: Breast Cancer Demonstration Project, September 1981, *Cancer Journal for Clinicians* 32:216, 1982.

atic; however, it appeared that there was a significant factor of self-detection because of individual concerns about breast disease. Until 1981, approximately 4443 carcinomas had been discovered by biopsy on the basis of initial recommendations through the screening programs.

Many of these tumors were very small, and it can be concluded that at least part of the increase in survival was a result of early recognition of tumors that under ordinary circumstances would have been undetectable until later. Mammography proved to be highly successful in early breast detection in this program. Physical examination is less likely to be effective in influencing end results but plays an important role in detection of cancers missed by radiographic examination. Until mammography can achieve total accuracy of diagnosis, physical examinations must remain an integral part of the screening examination.

Since the BCDDP data are weakened by the absence of a control group, a high detection rate of early cancer in women younger than 50 years merits further evaluation. However, some risks are associated with repeated mammography in patients in this age group. The report of Upton and his National Cancer Institute group, issued in February 1977, on the risks associated with mammography in mass screening for the detection of breast cancer noted that epidemiologic studies reveal an excess of breast cancers in three groups: American women treated with x-irradiation of the breast for postpartum mastitis, American and Canadian women subjected to multiple fluoroscopic examinations of the chest during artificial pneumothorax treatment of pulmonary tuberculosis, and Japanese women surviving atomic bomb irradiation who were more than 10 years old at the time of the exposure. From these observations, it was possible for Upton and his group to estimate the carcinogenic risk to the breast associated with the far lower doses of mammography—if the dose-response relationship was assumed to remain linear, irrespective of dose, dose rate, and age at irradiation. On the basis of this assumption, along with the adjustment for the effects of age difference and susceptibility, the risk was assumed to be approximately 3.5 to 7.5 cases of breast cancer per million women of ages 35 or older at risk per year per cGy to both breasts, from the tenth year after irradiation throughout the remainder of life (Figure 14-19). According to this model, a single mammographic examination performed with a technique that involves an average dose to the breast of less than 1 cGy should be expected to increase a woman's subsequent risk of developing breast cancer by much less than 1% of the natural risk of 7% at the age of 35 and by a progressively smaller percentage with increasing age at examinations thereafter, that is, from a risk of 7% (because 1 of 13 American women developed breast cancer at the time of Upton's report) to a risk of 7.07%.

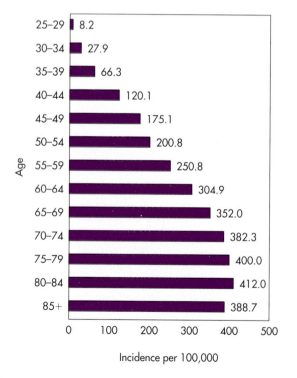

Figure 14-19 Breast cancer frequency by age. (Based on data from *Cancer statistics review 1973-1986*, Washington DC, 1989, National Cancer Institute.)

Projecting from that estimate, a 50-year-old woman getting a mammogram with a midline exposure of 1 cGy every year for 20 years would theoretically increase her risk from 7% to 8.4%, disregarding all beneficial factors. Whether the risk is greater in women affected by other high-risk factors (see box on p. 404) remains to be determined. With newer technology and less exposure to the breast from high-quality mammograms we can expect that these estimates would be greatly reduced. Among recent developments in mammographic technique is a large reduction of radiation doses because of improved image receptors. Any of the several techniques now widely used produce a technically satisfactory image with mean average tissue doses between 0.06 and 0.45 cGy per exposure. There is a corresponding decline in risk. Obviously, the risk-benefit factor for an individual is altered by the clinical or familial indications that increase the patient's risk for breast cancer. The risk-benefit factor also was affected by the recent demonstrations of the effectiveness of mammography in finding early cancers in the absence of palpable masses or other overt physical symptoms.

A 1993 report from the Canadian National Breast Screening Study (CNBSS) addresses the effectiveness of screening for women ages 40-49 and the benefit of adding mammography to a standard clinical examination in women aged 50-59. The CNBSS results did not show reductions in breast cancer mortality after 7 years of follow-up in either age group. The CNBSS is a major study from which all data must be taken seriously. On the other hand, there are methodological questions about this study that have arisen. Concerns focus on the unexplained presence of more women with poor prognosis breast cancers in the screened group, the combined effects of technical deficiencies (mammographic equipment), and incomplete patient compliance.

Based on this type of reasoning, the following recommendations are made for the use of mammography:

1. Mammography should be performed at any age when clinical findings indicate a significant suspicion of cancer.
2. Mammography should not be performed in women younger than the age of 35 except when there is a specific strong clinical indication. The incidence of carcinoma in this age group is very low. In addition, breast tissue in a woman younger than the age of 35 is generally too dense and radiopaque to reveal pathologic abnormalities by mammography.
3. A baseline mammogram should be considered in women ages 35-40 because a baseline study provides the groundwork for assessing subtle changes in subsequent mammograms that may indicate mammary cancer. Many authorities argue with this indication for mammography, preferring to await clinical indications.

4. Periodic mammography with low-level radiation may be performed in women between the ages of 35-49 only after the risk factors have been thoroughly evaluated. Patients who are at high risk or who are clinically suspect would of course be included in this category. Frequency of screening mammography may be variable and often relates to the characteristics of the breast parenchyma.

5. For women 50 years of age or older, annual or other periodic mammography is statistically justified to screen asymptomatic women for breast cancer.

There is no single 100% effective method of diagnosing all breast carcinomas. The major value of mammography lies in the detection of nonpalpable, hitherto totally unsuspected, lesions (for example, on a baseline mammogram in a woman who is at high risk or in the left breast of a woman who has had palpable mass or cyst in the right breast) (Table 14-10). Another valuable role lies in prompting the surgeon to operate earlier, instead of observing a breast mass of borderline significance over a period of time, when the radiologic diagnosis is that of a definite malignancy. The undesirable situation in which a surgeon delays biopsy or the gynecologist delays referral of the patient to a surgeon based on a report of a "normal" mammogram should not occur if the decision to obtain a biopsy or to refer the patient is carried out despite the mammogram report. The gynecologist must remember that mammography is not the first step one takes in evaluating a breast mass: it is an additional step. Table 14-9 underlines the improved accuracy of combining mammography with a physical examination of the breasts. When a heightened suspicion exists, the patient should be further evaluated regardless of the mammogram report.

Mammography is the most accurate technique for the detection of early-stage breast cancers. However, a false negative rate of 5%-15% has been reported for clinically palpable masses. Indications for needle aspiration of palpable masses vary, depending on the clinician and the institution. The authors encourage liberal use of this procedure, described earlier in this chapter. Fine-needle

aspiration is ideal for evaluating multiple and/or recurrent breast lesions—it avoids disfigurement with numerous open biopsy scars. The equipment required is available in most physician offices. When the diagnostic triad of physical examination, fine-needle aspiration, and mammography is employed for multiple or recurrent breast masses, open biopsy is rarely needed. In any case, *a fine-needle aspiration or open biopsy should be performed on a clinically suspicious mass whether the mammogram is suspicious or not.* Some cancers, particularly the medullary type, appear well circumscribed on the mammogram and mimic cysts or fibroadenomas. It is much more common, however, for a palpable carcinoma to possess the classic characteristics of irregular or spiculated borders, with or without microcalcifications (see Figure 14-17).

The American College of Radiology (ACR) Breast Imaging Reporting and Data System (BI-RADS) is the product of a collaborative effort between the ACR, the National Cancer Institute, the Centers for Disease Control and Prevention, the Food and Drug Administration, the American Medical Association, the American College of Surgeons, and the College of American Pathologists. The system is a quality assurance tool designed to standardize mammographic reporting, reduce confusion in breast imaging interpretations and facilitate outcome monitoring. There is no test or groups of tests that can ever ensure that a woman does not have breast cancer, but mammography has become a very useful tool for diagnosis. The boxed excerpt from the BI-RADS guidelines lists the recommendations for a reporting system (pp. 410-411). This system is clear and concise and should be adopted by physicians treating breast disease in the interest of uniformity.

When an open biopsy is to be performed, basic plastic surgery techniques and principles can provide a minimum of disfigurement and a nearly undetectable scar, at the same time meeting all the requirements necessary. Breast mobility allows the nipple to be rotated to any point of the breast. A peri-areolar incision circumscribing one half the circumference of the areola will allow for a linear wound 3.14 times the diameter of the areola (Figure 14-20).

Breast cancer accounts for 28% of all nondermatologic cancers and 18% of all cancer deaths in women. The incidence of breast cancer has increased steadily since 1930, but the mortality has remained between 35% and 50%, although the death rate does increase with age (Figure 14-21; Table 14-11). After an improvement in the 5-year survival rate from 53% for patients diagnosed between 1940 and 1949 to 60% during the next decade, further gains were modest. The 5-year survival rate for localized breast cancer has risen from 78% in the 1940s to 91% today. If the cancer has spread regionally, however, the survival rate is 69%; with distant metastases, it is 18%. In children younger than 15 years, breast cancer

Table 14-10   Mammography and reduced mortality from breast cancer

Study	Schedule	Results
HIP	Every year for 4 years	Mortality ↓ 30%
Verbec	Every 2 years for 4 years	Mortality ↓ 33%
Colette	At 1, 12, 18 and 24 months	Mortality ↓ 50%
Tabar	Every 2 years (age 40-49) Every 33 months (>50 years)	Mortality ↓ 31%

REPORT ORGANIZATION

The reporting system should be concise and organized using the following structure. A statement indicating that the present examination has been compared to previous mammograms should be included. If this is not included, it should be assumed that no comparison has been made.

1. A succinct description of the overall breast composition.

   This is an overall assessment of the attenuating tissues in the breast to help indicate the relative possibility that a lesion could be hidden by the normal tissues. Generally, this includes fatty, mixed or dense.

   Since mammography cannot detect all breast cancers, physical examination is always a key element of screening. It is important to alert the clinician that in the radiographically dense breast the ability of mammography to detect small cancers is reduced. Although mammography is still useful in these women, the physical examination (which is always important) is increased in importance. The available data do not support the use of mammographic patterns for determining screening frequency (i.e., risk for breast cancer).

   For consistency, this should be included for all patients using the following patterns:

   1. The breast is almost entirely fat.
   2. There are scattered fibroglandular densities that could obscure a lesion on mammography.
   3. The breast tissue is heterogeneously dense. This may lower the sensitivity of mammography.
   4. The breast tissue is extremely dense, which lowers the sensitivity of mammography.

   If an implant is present, it should be stated in the report and an implant description code added as appropriate.

2. A clear description of any significant finding. (It is assumed that most significant findings are new.)

   a. Mass:

   Size
   Lesion type and modifiers

   Associated calcifications
   Associated findings
   Location
   How changed, if previously present

   b. Calcifications:

   Morphology—type or shape and modifiers
   DistributionAssociated findings
   Location
   How changed, if previously present

   The Clinical location of the abnormality as extrapolated from the mammographic location (based on the face of a clock).

3. An overall (summary) impression:

   All final impressions should be complete with eachlesion fully categorized and qualified. An indeterminate reading should be given only in the screening setting where additional imaging evaluation is recommended before a final opinion can be rendered.

   In the screening situation a suggestion for the next course of action should be given if the study is not conclusive (magnification, ultrasound, etc.).

   Interpretation is facilitated by recognizing that most mammograms can be categorized under a few headings. These are listed below and suggested codes are included for computer use.

   If a suspicious abnormality is detected, the report should indicate that biopsy should be considered. This is an assessment where the radiologist has sufficient concern that biopsy is warranted unless there are other reasons why the patient and her physician might wish to defer the biopsy.

REPORT ORGANIZATION—cont'd

a. Assessment is Incomplete

Category 0   Need Additional Imaging Evaluation:

Finding for which additional imaging evaluation is needed. This is almost always used in a screening situation and should be used rarely after a full imaging workup. A recommendation for additional imaging evaluation includes the use of spot compression, magnification, special mammographic views, ultrasound, etc. Whenever possible, the present mammogram should be compared to previous studies. The radiologist should use judgment in how vigorously to pursue previous studies.

b. Assessment is Complete—**Final** Categories

Category 1   Negative:

There is nothing on which to comment. The breasts are symmetrical and no masses, architectural disturbances, or suspicious calcifications are present.

Category 2   Benign Finding:

This is also a negative mammogram, but the interpreter may wish to describe a finding. Involuting, calcified fibroadenomas; multiple secretory calcifications; fat-containing lesions such as oil cysts, lipomas, galactoceles, and mixed density hamartomas all have characteristic appearances and may be labeled with confidence. The interpreter might wish to describe intramammary lymph nodes, implants, etc. but still conclude that there is no mammographic evidence of malignancy.

Category 3   Probably Benign Finding—Short Interval Follow-up Suggested:

A finding placed in this category has a very high probability of being benign. It is not expected to change over the follow-up interval, but the radiologist would prefer to establish its stability. Data are becoming available that show importance on the efficacy of short interval follow-up. At the present time, most approaches are intuitive. These will likely undergo future modification as more data accrue as to the validity of an approach, the interval required, and the type of findings that should be followed.

Category 4   Suspicious Abnormality—Biopsy Should Be Considered:

These are lesions that do not have the characteristic morphologies of breast cancer but have a definite probability of being malignant. The radiologist has sufficient concern to urge a biopsy. If possible, the relevant probabilities should be cited so that the patient and her physician can make the decision on the ultimate course of action.

Category 5   Highly Suggestive of Malignancy—Appropriate Action Should Be Taken:

These lesions have a high probability of being cancer.

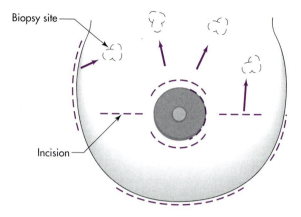

Figure 14-20 Location of incisions for breast biopsy with good cosmetic result. (From Keen G et al: *Operative surgery and management,* 1987, Macmillan.

Table 14-11	Breast cancer frequency by age		
Age	Incidence per 100,000	Age	Incidence per 100,000
25-29	8.2	55-59	250.8
30-34	27.9	60-64	304.9
35-39	66.3	65-69	352.0
40-44	120.1	70-74	382.3
45-49	175.1	75-79	400.0
50-54	200.8	80-84	412.0
		85+	388.7

Based on data from *Cancer statistics review,* 1973-1986, Washington, DC, 1989, National Cancer Institute.

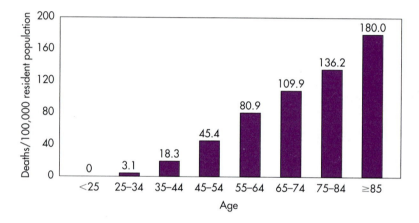

Figure 14-21 Breast cancer death rates by age in the United States, 1986. (Source: US Department of Health and Human Services.)

is relatively rare and appears to follow a favorable course. Between 1% and 3% of all female mammary cancers occur in women younger than 30 years, 5% occur in women younger than 35 years, and 10%-15% occur in women younger than 41 years. At age 45 the incidence curve approaches its first peak. More than 70% of breast cancers are self-detected and are merely confirmed by physicians. Early diagnosis, which greatly improves the results of breast cancer treatment, would be possible if all women were taught to examine their breasts; at present, regular self-examination is practiced by fewer than 20% of American women. Physical findings characteristic of malignant disease often occur relatively late. Moreover, in young women palpable masses are notoriously difficult to evaluate clinically and radiographically.

Clinical staging of patients with suspected operable mammary cancer begins with measurement of the primary tumor in two or three diameters and with a description of its location and attachments (Table 14-12). Palpation of regional lymph node areas should be thorough. Although about one fourth of the patients with enlarged axillary nodes (clinical stage II) are without nodal metastasis, about 40% of those without palpable nodes (stage I) have nodal metastasis. The clinical staging, nevertheless, correlates well with the 5- to 10-year survival rate and is the basis for selection of therapy in many cases. Biopsy should be done on enlarged supraclavicular nodes before mastectomy, and other signs of local spread of tumor outside the breasts (stage III) should be sought (see box, Chapter 16, p. 470 for staging).

The number of positive axillary nodes definitely affects survival, with the 10-year disease-free survival rate being 38% for one to three positive nodes and 13% for four or more positive nodes. Size and histopathologic character of the neoplasms are correlated with curability. All patients with suspected progression of disease beyond clinical stage I, on the basis of the history and physical examination, require careful radiologic search for distant metastasis as well. The most useful tests are bone scans and x-ray films of bones with abnormal uptake on the scan, as well as films of the chest and contralateral breast.

Differences in the extent of the disease in the presence of asymptomatic but possibly detectable metastasis at the time of initial diagnosis may explain much of the variability in the results of therapy. Large clinical series indicate a frequency of clinical stage IV disease of between 2% and 13% at the time of presentation. Without including the number of patients who did not have scans or x-ray examinations, Roberts et al. reported that 18% of new breast cancer patients with normal bone radiographs had scans with evidence of bone metastasis. Such a frequency of bone involvement in patients with clinically localized and operable breast cancer appears extensive in view of the 17% total recurrence rate at all sites observed by others in the first 18 months after surgery in patients

Table 14-12   Staging for breast cancer (American Joint Commission on Cancer, American Cancer Society, American College of Surgeons Committee on Cancer)

Stage	Characteristics
Definition of TNM	
TX	Primary tumor cannot be assessed
T0	No evidence of primary tumor
Tis	Carcinoma in situ: intraductal carcinoma, lobular carcinoma in situ, or Paget's disease of the nipple with no tumor
T1	Tumor 2 cm or less in greatest dimension
T1a	Tumor 0.5 cm or less in greatest dimension
T1b	Tumor more than 0.5 cm but not more than 1 cm in greatest dimension
T1c	Tumor more than 1 cm but not more than 2 cm in greatest dimension
T2	Tumor more than 2 cm but not more than 5 cm in greatest dimension
T3	Tumor more than 5 cm in greatest dimension
T4	Tumor of any size with direct extension to the chest wall or skin
T4a	Extension to the chest wall
T4b	Edema (including peau d'orange) or ulceration of the skin of the breast or satellite skin nodules confined to the same breast
T4c	Both T4a and T4b
Regional lymph nodes	
NX	Regional lymph nodes cannot be assessed (e.g., previously removed)
N0	No regional lymph node metastasis
N1	Metastasis to movable ipsilateral axillary lymph node(s)
N2	Metastasis to ipsilateral axillary lymph node(s), fixed to one another or to other structures
N3	Metastasis to ipsilateral internal mammary lymph node(s)
MX	Presence of distant metastasis cannot be assessed
M0	No evidence of distant metastasis
M1	Distant metastasis, including metastasis to ipsilateral supraclavicular lymph node(s)

Stage groupings			
Stage	Tumor size	Lymph node metastases	Distant metastases
0	Tis	N0	M0
I	T1	N0	M0
IIa	T0	N1	M0
	T1	N1	M0
	T2	N0	M0
IIb	T2	N1	M0
	T3	N0	M0
IIIa	T0	N2	M0
	T1	N2	M0
	T2	N2	M0
	T3	N1, N2	M0
IIIb	T4	Any N	M0
	Any T	N3	M0
IV	Any T	Any N	M1

From the American Joint Committee on Cancer: *Manual for staging of cancer,* ed 3, Philadelphia, 1988, JB Lippincott, pp 146-147.

with operable breast cancer. With a trend toward less radical surgery and more systemic adjuvant therapy, the importance of proper staging becomes crucial. One objective of adjuvant chemotherapy is eradication of minimal "microscopic" disease. If patients with detectable primary metastatic disease contaminate the true adjuvant population, results of such therapy may be obscured. Moreover, patients with primary metastatic disease should be considered for alternative therapeutic options, such as endocrine therapy before or in combination with chemotherapy.

Chemo Prevention

An increasing body of data suggest that tamoxifen can suppress the development of preclinical breast cancer. Intervention clinical trials are underway to address whether tamoxifen can prevent breast cancer development. Consideration of tamoxifen as a potentially human breast cancer prevention receives substantial impetus from controlled clinical trials of adjuvant tamoxifen used in patients with early stage resected breast cancer. A review of the clinical trials involving nearly 10,000 patients with resected breast cancer showed a 40% reduction in contralateral breast cancer development in the tamoxifen treated group. The lower frequency of contralateral breast cancer was seen in seven of the eight clinical trials making up these 10,000 patients. This consistent pattern and substantial magnitude of contralateral breast cancer inhibition provided the major support for a clinical trial of tamoxifen in breast cancer prevention (Table 14-13). Clinical trials addressing these hypotheses have begun in the United States and Great Britain and Italy.

Treatment

Carcinoma in Situ

Ductal Carcinoma In Situ (DCIS) is also known as intraductal carcinoma and is a proliferation of malignant epithelial cells within the mammary ductal system. There is a similar distribution of lesions with respect to location in the breast as is seen with invasive lesions. On light microscopy, there is no evidence of invasion into the surrounding tissue. The increased use of screening mammography over the past two decades has led to a marked increase in the number of patients diagnosed with DCIS (Figure 14-22), and today in many centers one DCIS is diagnosed for every two or three mammographically detected invasive breast cancers. Age specific time trends illustrate that the greatest rise has been in women over 40 who are more likely to have mammography (Figure 14-23). As a matter of fact, autopsy series suggest that latent DCIS is relatively common, ranging from 6%-18% of women who died of causes other than breast cancer.

Traditionally, DCIS was treated with mastectomy. However, this treatment approach has recently come

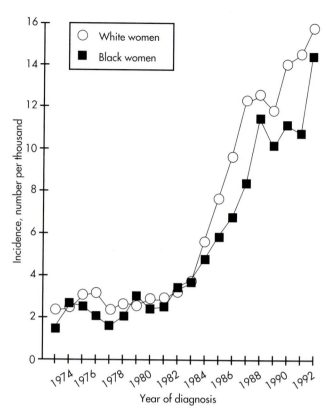

Figure 14-22 Age-adjusted incidence rates for ductal carcinoma in situ of the breast from 1973 to 1992 for white and black women in the United States. (Adapted from National Cancer Institute SEER tapes.)

Table 14-13 Cumulative frequency of occurrence of contralateral breast cancer in eight clinical trials of adjuvant tamoxifen therapy compared with no therapy

Adjuvant therapy group	No. of patients	Contralateral cancers
Tamoxifen	4975	79 (1.6%)
Control	4971	121 (2.4%)

From Nayfield SG et al: Potential role of tamoxifen in prevention of breast cancer, *J Natl Cancer Inst* 83:1450, 1991.

under scrutiny. First, many patients with invasive breast cancer are currently treated with breast conserving therapy, making it difficult to justify the generalized use of mastectomy for patients with DCIS. In addition, the natural history of DCIS is only partially understood, particularly for small mammographically detected lesions. The microcalcifications in DCIS are most often secondary to calcification of necrotic cellular debris within the involved ducts, and their extent and characteristics are better defined with magnification views of the microcalcification. Suspicious mammographic microcal-

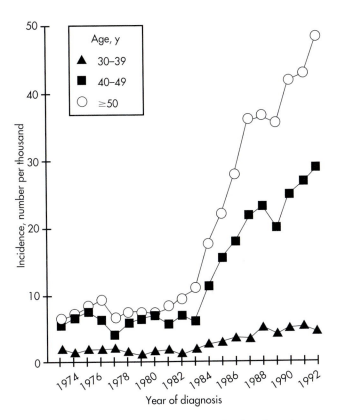

Figure 14-23 Age-specific incidence rates for ductal carcinoma in situ of the breast from 1973 to 1992 for US women, all races combined. (Adapted from National Cancer Institute SEER tapes.)

cification are generally differentiated from benign calcium deposits by their number, distribution, and appearance. Coarse granular or linear calcifications are larger clusters of varying shapes and are regarded as the most suspicious.

The potential of DCIS to progress to invasive breast cancer is an unresolved issue. Because DCIS has historically been treated with mastectomy, little information on the risk of progression to invasive disease is available. Page's retrospective study of benign breast biopsies revealed 25 patients who were subsequently identified with DCIS; 7 (28%) had progressed to invasive disease during the period of observation.

Most patients with DCIS have nonpalpable, mammographically detected lesions, and careful mammographic and pathological evaluation is necessary to formulate treatment recommendations. Patients who are found to have suspicious calcifications should have magnification views performed to clearly define the full extent of the calcifications. Needle localization should be used to guide biopsy of the area. Pathological evaluation of the specimen should be carefully oriented and inked, with particular attention being paid to the nuclear grade, architectural subtype, the extent of disease, and the distance between DCIS and the resection margins. Breast

conserving treatment should require removal of all microcalcification and negative microscopic margins of resection; a wide excision may be necessary to achieve this. Not every patient with DCIS who desires breast conserving treatment will be an appropriate candidate. In general, simple mastectomy is recommended for women in whom the DCIS is too extensive to be adequately removed. Axillary resection is not routinely performed; however, a limited dissection is commonly performed in patients with extensive lesions particularly if these are high grade. A prospective randomized study of DCIS was conducted by the NSABP (Protocol B-17) in which patients were randomized to lumpectomy alone or lumpectomy followed by breast irradiation. Histologically negative surgical margins were a study requirement. With a median follow-up of 43 months, event-free survival was found to be higher in women treated with breast irradiation (84% vs 74%), and this was primarily due to fewer ipsilateral breast recurrences developing in the irradiated group.

Lobular Carcinoma in Situ

There are important differences (Table 14-14) between intraductal carcinoma and lobular carcinoma in situ. Intraductal carcinoma has rates of local recurrences that are similar to invasive carcinoma with breast preserving surgery. These recurrences appear in the vicinity of the original surgery and probably represent malignant foci that persisted after the initial treatment, rather than a second primary. Approximately 50% of the recurrences will be frankly invasive ductal carcinoma; the other half will again be intraductal.

Lobular carcinoma in situ (LCIS) does not uniformly recur at the original excision site, and the recurrences are as likely to appear in the opposite breast as in the ipsilateral breast. The rate of recurrence of LCIS following excision alone is approximately equal to that of atypical ductal hyperplasia with a positive family history of breast cancer. Cancers that develop following excision of LCIS may be intraductal carcinoma, invasive ductal carcinoma, or lobular carcinoma. Indeed, some authorities consider LCIS as only a risk factor for subsequent development of a true malignancy and not a true cancer.

Invasive disease

In recent years a change in attitude has created controversies concerning the extent of surgery for primary operable tumors, and at present there is no one best operation for breast cancer. Radical mastectomy had been the standard procedure since Halsted published his first series in 1894. There was universal acceptance of his concept of wide en bloc resection of the primary tumor together with the lymphatic pathway of spread to the axillary lymph nodes. This mode of treatment was dominant for about 50 years in spite of undesirable cure rates. Thereafter, dissatisfaction with the standard radical

Table 14-14   Comparison of ductal carcinoma in situ (DCIS) and lobular carcinoma in situ (LCIS)

Characteristic	DCIS	LCIS
Age	Pre and post menopausal	Predominantly premenopausal
Mammographic appearance	Microcalcification	Usually invisible
Diagnosis	Needle-localization biopsy or excision of palpable lesion	Incidental finding on biopsy of benign disease
Multicentric	Infrequent	Common
Bilateral	Rare	Common
Site of recurrence	Near original site	Anywhere in either breast
Histology of recurrence	50% invasive 50% DCIS	Usually invasive ductal carcinoma
Rate of recurrence	5% per year	1% per year

mastectomy began to gain momentum, and the trend toward less radical procedures has been widespread in the past two decades. The surgical world is now in a dilemma, and the enlightened public is well aware of the controversies over the extent of surgery for the cure of primary operable breast cancer. There are proponents for essentially three types of treatment: standard radical mastectomy, modified radical mastectomy, and local excision plus radiation. Statistical data gathered on a worldwide basis from each of these groups indicate that all arrive at essentially similar survival figures.

There are several reasons for the gradual decline of use of the radical mastectomy. The cosmetic defect produced by loss of the pectoral muscles was unacceptable to many women, and the morbidity included a 30% incidence of chronic arm edema. It also became apparent that increasing the extent of the surgery to include the internal mammary chain of nodes did not improve the salvage rates. For primary operable lesions, the 10-year survival rate stayed at about 50%. Early critics indicated that the radical operation was not necessary if a small lesion was localized and furthermore it was uselessly destructive if there were metastases that ruled out cure. They also questioned the simplistic explanation of tumor spread from tumor site to regional nodes and then to distant sites. The concept of breast cancer as a systemic disease developed and led to the reevaluation of the role of axillary node dissection. Is it therapeutic or simply a diagnostic maneuver? Those who limit the extent of surgery to primary excision rely on radiation therapy to sterilize not only regional node areas but also multicentric foci that might remain in the involved breast. Increasing knowledge of chemotherapy and the kinetics of cancer kill and growth is having a major impact on ideas concerning the total management of primary operable breast cancer. There is good evidence that micrometastases can be handled by immune mechanisms and/or multiple-agent chemotherapy.

The trend toward less radical surgery really began when the concept of removing the breast and axillary

contents and leaving the chest wall muscles intact was first introduced. It was demonstrated that simple mastectomy followed by radiation resulted in salvage rates equal to those of radical mastectomy. The trend was completed with recent reports advocating local excision and radiation. The present dilemma stems from the fact that absolute data on survival in randomized control series are almost impossible to obtain. There are many operative control studies now in progress but increasing restrictions of an ethical and legal nature are making it difficult to gather significant data. In most studies, survival figures are compared with those of studies based on the Halsted radical mastectomy. It is significant that all lesser procedures reveal similar end results but none surpass those obtained with radical surgery. Accordingly, many proponents of Halsted's radical mastectomy will continue to use that operation until offered an alternative that will yield better 10-year salvage rates.

Several trials demonstrated favorable results with conservative treatment of breast cancer, but not all patients are candidates for this technique of minimal surgery and postoperative radiation therapy. Hellman reported on 255 patients with stages I and II disease who were treated in this way. The tumor was controlled locally for 97% of stage I women and 87% of stage II women. The survival rate was 93% for stage I and 84% for stage II. Patients were treated with excisional biopsy to remove the tumors, followed by 4500-5000 cGy in 23 treatments for 5 weeks to the entire breast and a booster dose of an additional 2000-2200 cGy to the primary tumor area using interstitial $_{192}$Ir. Lumpectomy (tylectomy) should be reserved for tumors less than 2 cm, and postoperative irradiation can be expected to achieve an 80%-85% local control rate with comparable survivals.

Montague reported on 1073 patients with clinically favorable breast cancer who were treated at the University of Texas MD Anderson Hospital between 1955 and 1980. Of this group, 355 were treated with conservative surgery and radiation, and 728 were treated with radical or modified radical mastectomy alone. The local regional recurrence in patients treated with conservative surgery was 4.9%; local regional recurrence in patients who had radical or modified radical mastectomy was 5.6%. In essence there was no significant difference in the 10-year disease-free survival rates between the two groups. Although this was a nonrandomized study, there is remarkable agreement with results found in other studies.

Lichter reported a randomized trial in 1992 from the National Cancer Institute where mastectomy was compared to breast-conserving therapy in the treatment of stages I and II carcinomas of the breast. Two hundred and thirty seven women were randomized between mastectomy and excisional biopsy plus radiation. All women in both groups underwent full axillary lymph node dissection; node positive patients in both groups received adjuvant chemotherapy with cyclophosphamide and doxorubicin every 28 days for 1 year and tamoxifen 40 mg/day for 5 years. Overall survival and disease-free survival were not significantly different in the two treatment arms. They also summarized six solid prospective randomized trials with more than 3800 patients comparing mastectomy and lumpectomy plus radiation in the treatment of stages I and II breast cancer. All these studies have come to the same conclusion. It would appear that the clinician can now be confident recommending lumpectomy plus radiation to patients, since it appears to be equivalent to mastectomy in terms of survival and optimal local-regional control.

Probably no area of medical therapy queries the appropriateness of the en bloc dissection for cancer more than that of surgery for breast cancer. Since the introduction of the en bloc concept by Halsted in 1894 that advocated routine removal of the pectoralis major muscle to ensure a more adequate excision of the large tumors he treated, there have been a series of modifications. The modified radical mastectomy has been very popular: the entire breast, but not the pectoralis major muscle, is removed, thus avoiding the concave configuration of the anterior chest wall. Even the axillary dissection varies from complete (levels I, II, and III with the pectoralis minor muscle), to partial (levels I and II with sparing of the pectoralis minor muscle). Retrospective studies found that survivals were similar regardless of the extent of the operative procedure when comparing the Halsted radical mastectomy with any of the modified approaches; thus a modified approach was accepted in 1979 by the National Cancer Institute Consensus Conference.

Prophylactic removal of regional axillary lymph nodes was next questioned. With the observation that clinical examination alone was not sufficiently accurate to detect small metastases, axillary node dissection quickly became routine, not only to rid the patient of clinically occult nodal metastasis, but, by removal of nodes, to eliminate a secondary source of further metastases. Handley was among the first to observe that recurrence in axillary nodes after simple mastectomy was less frequent than one would expect in light of the frequency of occult metastases at this site and suggested that some metastases were destroyed in the nodes by host defenses. In 1971, the National Surgical Adjuvant Breast Project (NSABP) began a trial designed to answer the question of the value of prophylactic regional node dissection. Patients with clinically uninvolved axillary nodes (clinical stage I) were randomized for treatment among radical mastectomy, total mastectomy plus irradiation of the chest wall and regional lymphatics, and total mastectomy alone. Women who had clinically involved axillary nodes (clinical stage II) were randomized to treatment with either radical mastectomy or total mastectomy and irradiation to the chest wall and all lymph node drainage areas for the breast. If ignoring occult axillary metastases permitted continuing dissemination, the patients treated with total mastectomy alone should fare poorly; if having still-functioning nodes improves host defenses, the patients treated with total mastectomy alone should fare better than the others. A total of 1665 patients were entered and followed for 72 months with no difference observed among the three treatment arms in stage I. Overall, stage II patients survived less well, but again there was no difference between the two treatment alternatives. Only 60 (16%) of the 365 patients who did not undergo prophylactic axillary dissection developed progression in the axilla as a first sign of failure and underwent axillary dissections, predominantly in the first 30 months of follow-up but also as long as 112 months after surgery. In the group in which prophylactic axillary dissection was done, the incidence of positive nodes was 39%. More than half of the patients who should have had positive axillary nodes did not develop clinical evidence of such. In 1985, Fisher reported on this same group of 1665 women followed for a mean of 126 months. There were no significant differences among the three groups of patients who had clinically positive nodes treated by radical mastectomy or by total mastectomy without axillary dissection but with regional irradiation. Survival at 10 years was about 38% in both groups.

After the report by Moore in 1967 relating the frequency of local recurrence after partial mastectomy, removal of the entire breast became routine surgical practice. The problem of incomplete excision is compounded by the multifocal origin of breast: almost 50% of breast cancers have origin in more than one quadrant of the breast, and that frequency does not appear to be diminished by early detection. More recent studies of less than total mastectomy have sought to determine whether irradiation of the breast can control these residua if just the primary lesion is removed. Obviously, this approach would not improve survival nor preserve the function of the breast, but it may improve the cosmetic result and the patient's body image. A trial of breast preservation was conducted by the Cancer Institute of Milan in which women with tumors smaller than 2 cm in diameter and without palpable axillary nodes were randomized between radical mastectomy and a wide "quadrantectomy" of the breast with a complete axillary dissection followed by 5000 cGy of irradiation to the breast alone (an additional 1000 cGy to the tumor site). After 7 years, 701 patients could be analyzed, and there were no significant differences in local control, survival, or interval to recurrence. This study demonstrated that high-dose irradiation makes breast preservation possible for patients with small clinically localized breast cancers. Cosmetic results were said to be satisfactory to more than 70% of the patients. Some radiation fibrosis and arm edema was reported, and the long-term carcinogenic effects on the breast from the radiation are yet to be determined.

Another study by Fisher and the NSABP reports the results of a randomized trial comparing total mastectomy and segmental mastectomy with or without radiation in the treatment of breast cancer (stages I and II breast tumors no larger than 4 cm). In segmental resection the surgeon removed tissue sufficient only to ensure that margins of the resected specimens were free of tumor. Women were randomly assigned to total mastectomy, segmental mastectomy alone, or segmental mastectomy followed by breast irradiation. All patients had axillary dissections, and patients with positive nodes received chemotherapy. Life table estimates based on data from 1843 women indicated that treatment by segmental mastectomy, with or without breast irradiation, resulted in disease-free, distant disease-free, and overall survival at 5 years that was no worse than that after total breast removal. In fact, disease-free survival after segmental mastectomy plus irradiation was better than disease-free survival after total mastectomy and overall survival after total mastectomy. However, a total of 92% of women treated with radiation remained free of breast tumor at 5 years, compared with 72% of those receiving no irradiation, indicating the value of breast irradiation for reducing the incidence of tumor in the ipsilateral breast after segmental mastectomy.

The Halstedian concept of tumor spread is that breast cancer starts as a local disease and spreads in an orderly, chronologic fashion from the original site to the regional lymph nodes, which serve as temporary barriers to spread, and then to distant sites such as the lung, liver, and bones. The cancer was believed to be always surgically curable if the breast, pectoral muscles, and axillary lymph nodes could be removed before the tumor had metastasized beyond that region. The findings of the NSABP and others suggest that the spread of cancer is not nearly as orderly as Halsted proposed. Cancer may metastasize to a distant site before, during, or after it spreads to the lymph nodes. The rationale for Halsted's radical surgical procedure becomes untenable if the cancer cannot be stopped at some distinct point on a supposedly orderly pathway. Breast cancer is often a systemic disease, even in its early stages.

Trials of management of primary breast cancer are long-term studies that may need at least 10 years before definitive analysis can be made. Although an early relapse rate may be helpful in an analysis, only data on long-term survival will give the final answer. Analysis of these trials must also include consideration of the heterogeneity of primary breast cancer. Subset analysis requires adequate numbers, with the various categories occurring as a result of important prognostic variables, such as size of the primary tumor, clinical and pathologic status of the axillary lymph nodes, menopausal status, and estrogen receptor content. A detailed discussion of the advantages and disadvantages of the alternatives for primary therapy in patients with potentially curable breast cancer is beyond the scope of this text. The reader is referred to the bibliography at the end of the chapter for more detailed information concerning this interesting current controversy.

In June 1990, the National Institutes of Health Consensus Development Conference was held on early-stage breast cancer, and the following conclusions were reached:

1. Breast conservation treatment is an appropriate method of primary therapy for the majority of women with stages I and II breast cancer. It is preferable because it provides survival equivalent to that provided by total mastectomy and axillary dissection while preserving the breast. In general, primary therapy for stages I and II cancer consists of either breast conservation treatment or total mastectomy. The breast conservation treatment is defined as excision of the primary tumor and adjacent breast tissue (this procedure is also referred to as lumpectomy, segmental mastectomy, or partial mastectomy) followed by radiation therapy.

2. Total mastectomy is an appropriate primary therapy when breast conservation treatment is not indicated or selected. Both surgical therapies are accompanied by axillary dissection, which provides important prognostic information. Prospective randomized trials comparing breast conservation treatment to total mastectomy, with maximum follow-up of 17 years, have demonstrated equivalent results as measured by overall patient survival.

3. In the selection of women for breast conservation treatment or mastectomy, certain women are not candidates for breast conservation treatment. They are women with multicentric breast malignancies, including those with gross multifocal disease or diffuse microcalcification detected by mammography. Others are patients for whom breast conservation treatment would produce an unacceptable cosmetic result. Examples include women whose tumors are large relative to breast size and those with certain collagen vascular diseases.

4. Local control is the major goal of breast conservation treatment.

5. Another goal of primary breast cancer treatment is to produce the best cosmetic result consistent with achievement of local-regional control.

6. Women should be educated about treatment choices and clinical trial options in order to make informed decisions in consultation with their physicians. The diagnosis should be established by fine-needle aspiration cytology, limited incisional biopsy, or definitive wide local excision.

7. The type and place of incisions can greatly influence the quality of cosmesis. It is appropriate to excise the primary lesion with a normal tissue margin of approximately 1 cm. Because nodal status is the most important available prognostic factor, a level I-II axillary node dissection should be routine, both for staging and for prevention of axillary recurrence. Separate incisions should usually be employed to permit the primary tumor excision and the axillary dissection to enhance functional and cosmetic results.

8. Megavoltage radiation therapy to the whole breast to a dose of 4500-5000 cGy (180-200 cGy/fraction) should routinely be used. If a level I-II axillary dissection has been performed, axillary node irradiation is not routinely indicated. No data indicate any increase of secondary malignancies or contralateral breast cancers resulting from breast irradiation. Although local control can be obtained in some patients through local excision alone, no subgroups have been identified in which radiation therapy can be avoided.

9. In patients receiving adjuvant chemotherapy, no precise recommendations regarding the sequence and timing of radiation therapy and chemotherapy can be made.

10. A small percentage of patients will develop a local recurrence following breast conservation therapy. Total mastectomy is effective salvage therapy for a substantial percentage of these patients.

The treatment of locally advanced breast cancer (stages III and IV) is often palliative. Many of these patients have detectable distant metastases by the time they seek medical treatment, and their prognoses are poor (10-year survival rate of 14%). For palliation, systemic endocrine therapy or chemotherapy is necessary. In addition, several groups reported good results with aggressive preoperative radiotherapy, reducing the frequency of local recurrences after mastectomy. Removal of tumor bulk by mastectomy is usually recommended but the value of postoperative radiotherapy is equivocal. Preoperative or postoperative radiotherapy does not appear to improve the 5- or 10-year survival rates, and radiation to regional lymph nodes may have detrimental immunosuppressive effects. Any local control achieved is usually not appreciated, since there is subsequent appearance of distant metastasis.

The treatment of metastatic breast cancer includes a cooperative effort on the part of surgeons, radiotherapists, endocrinologists, and medical oncologists to produce a systemic therapy supplemented by local palliative measures to lesions in immediate need of palliation.

Estrogen receptors are proteins found in hormonally dependent tissue, both malignant and nonmalignant. The amount of receptor present in the breast cancer specimen is predictive of the success or failure of endocrine therapy. The identification of the estrogen receptor protein in certain human mammary cancers and the subsequent explanation of the role of estrogen in tumor growth clarified a clinical relationship that had been observed for a century. In 1896, Beatson produced regression of mammary cancer by oophorectomy. Huggins and Bergenstal demonstrated in 1952 that some mammary and prostatic cancers were not autonomous but were under the partial control of the endocrine system. Regressions of mammary cancers were continually obtained by removing the source of endogenous circulating hormones via oophorectomy, adrenalectomy, and hypophysectomy. Alternatively, breast cancer regressions were also achieved by administering large doses of estrogen, androgen, progesterone, and glucocorticoids. The choice of a particular endocrine therapy has been in large part empirical, guided by certain clinical features such as menopausal status, disease-free interval, site of dominant lesion, and response to previous therapy. Regardless of the method of endocrine therapy employed, objective regressions were obtained in no more than one third of breast cancer patients. As a result of basic investigations by Jensen, Smith, and DeSombre of steroid hormone metabolism, there have developed a series of assays that can identify with considerable accuracy breast cancers that are not autonomous and will respond to endocrine manipulation. Such a method of predicting a priori those cancers that will be responsive to changes in endocrine milieu greatly enhances the usefulness of hormonal therapy and allows recommendation of such treatments on a plausible biochemical basis.

Knowledge of the estrogen receptor content of either the primary or the recurrent mammary cancer must be viewed within the proper clinical perspective. This one determination is but a single piece in the mosaic of the subcellular biochemistry of breast cancer. To deprecate the clinical importance of this determination because some patients with significant estrogen receptor content will not respond to hormonal treatment (because of eventual escape from hormonal regulation or because of lack of understanding of the role of other steroid or protein hormone receptors) begs the question. Knowledge of the estrogen receptor content of either a primary or a metastatic tumor does not allow the physician to predict the hormonal dependency of a tumor with enough accuracy to be rationally employed in the selection of appropriate palliative treatment. It does, however, allow for a good assessment of the likelihood that the breast cancer patient would benefit from endocrine therapy.

On behalf of the NSABP, Ravdin et al. reported the results of a multicenter study of prophylactic oophorectomy in premenopausal women with operable carcinomas of the breast. The results of this study showed no benefit from prophylactic oophorectomy in terms of survival or recurrence at 3, 4, or 5 years. Ten-year follow-up of these patient groups continued to show no benefit in the surgery group. In addition, no evidence was found to indicate that prophylactic oophorectomy lengthened the time from operation to recurrence, nor did it delay death. This study concluded that there was no justification for the use of prophylactic oophorectomy in the treatment of operable breast cancer. In 1981, Bryant and Weir reported a prospective randomized study done in Canada in which 240 patients had been followed for 10 years. The overall results of the oophorectomy group were superior to those of the control group not undergoing oophorectomy. Bryant and Weir contended that patients had not been followed long enough in the Ravdin et al. report. Bryant and Weir also reported that patients who had cancer confined to the breast showed no significant benefit from oophorectomy. When one to three axillary nodes were involved, women younger than 50 years were found to benefit significantly from prophylactic oophorectomy in relapse-free status at 5 years and in survival and relapse-free status at 10 years. Patients 50 years of age and older showed no advantage from oophorectomy. This suggests that there may be a place for prophylactic oophorectomy in patients younger than 50 years with operable carcinoma of the breast and with positive axillary nodes; however, the NSABP results were derived from a much larger series and cannot be disregarded. The final word on this issue, like many others on breast cancer management, is not available. In fact, this issue will be very difficult to study given the frequent use of adjuvant chemotherapy in premenopausal breast cancer patients and the chemical menopause that results from the use of these drugs.

Bilateral oophorectomy at the time of documented metastatic locally recurrent disease appears to be the most useful treatment for a premenopausal patient with an estrogen receptor-containing tumor. Castration is also indicated when the receptor status cannot be assessed, whereas patients with negative analyses should benefit more from chemotherapy. Responses are less frequent in patients younger than the age of 35 and are rare if the disease-free interval is shorter than 24 months. Soft-tissue and bone lesions respond more frequently than visceral and metastatic lesions and inoperable primary disease.

Chemotherapy

For decades the primary therapy for women with breast cancer has been surgery or radiation or a combination of both. At present many women are being treated with steroid hormones and cytotoxic agents for advanced or metastatic breast cancer. However, these two classifications of drugs have different modes of action and toxic effects. Both are most effective when these differences are taken into account and chemotherapy is employed selectively. The choice depends essentially on whether breast cancer in a given patient is a hormone-dependent neoplasm. It has been established that about half of all breast cancers are somewhat hormone dependent, and it is also evident that hormone dependence is associated with specific estrogen receptors, or cytoplasmic estrogen-binding proteins, in neoplastic cells. Equating hormone dependence with the presence of estrogen receptors in neoplastic cells is fraught with uncertainty. The presence of an estrogen-receptor protein is just one determination in a constellation of subcellular biochemistry that determines the overall effectiveness of manipulating the endocrine system. It should be reemphasized that some patients with significant estrogen-receptor content will not respond to hormone treatment. On the other hand, the likelihood that hormonal therapy will be effective is significantly increased if the patient has a neoplasm with estrogen-receptor sites demonstrated. On this basis one can first determine the presence or absence of estrogen receptors and proceed accordingly. Hormonal therapy is the treatment of choice in hormone-related breast cancer. Judicious use of cytotoxic agents is indicated if an assay proves receptor negative or if initial hormone treatment is unsuccessful.

Several cytotoxic agents have commonly been used, either singly or in combination, for the treatment of advanced breast cancer. Agents that have been found to be active are the antimetabolites 5-fluorouracil and methotrexate, alkylating agents such as cyclophosphamide and melphalan, vincristine, and cytotoxic antibiotics such as doxorubicin and mitomycin C (Table 14-15).

Table 14-15 Useful single agents in the treatment of breast cancer

Drug	Dosage	Response rate (%)
Doxorubicin	60-75 mg/m^2 IV every 3 weeks	37
Cyclophosphamide	100 mg/m^2/day PO 500 mg/m^2/week IV	34
L-phenylalanine mustard	6 mg/m^2/day PO for 5 days every 4-6 weeks	23
5-Fluorouracil	600 mg/m^2/week IV	26
Methotrexate	20 mg/m^2 IV or IM 2 times a week	34
Vincristine	1 mg/m^2/week IV	21
Dibromodulcitol	180 mg/m^2/day PO for 10 days every 4 weeks	27
Mitomycin C	20 mg/m^2 IV every 4-6 weeks	38

The use of multiple-drug combinations in cancer chemotherapy was introduced more than three decades ago. Although superior clinical results with combination therapy have been reported, acceptance of the use of multiple-drug therapy has been slow, mainly because of the fear of increased toxicity. Most combination programs were designed empirically, and it appears well proved that combination chemotherapy yields clinical results superior to those achieved with single-agent therapy. The various combinations that are commonly used in the treatment of breast cancer are cyclophosphamide and 5-fluorouracil; cyclophosphamide, prednisone, and 5-fluorouracil; cyclophosphamide, methotrexate, and 5-fluorouracil; doxorubicin (Adriamycin) and cyclophosphamide; and cyclophosphamide, methotrexate, 5-fluorouracil, vincristine, and prednisone (Table 14-16).

Adjuvant chemotherapy

The rationale for adjuvant chemotherapy is based on the premise that minimal residual disease after primary resection of a carcinoma (which may account for subsequent development of metastasis) may be eliminated by early systemic therapy with cytotoxic chemotherapeutic drugs. The goal is to improve cure rate. An early study using thiotepa as adjuvant therapy after mastectomy has suggested a delay in recurrence in patients receiving this drug. This finding, however, was observed only in premenopausal patients. A more recent study using melphalan (L-PAM) as adjuvant therapy for an extended period (more than 1 year after mastectomy) again demonstrated a beneficial effect (delay of recur-

rence) in premenopausal women with high-risk cancer. Interestingly, the postmenopausal patients receiving postoperative melphalan treatment showed no significant increase in the recurrence-free period as compared with the control group, in which patients were not given adjuvant chemotherapy. A trial with drug combinations such as cyclophosphamide, methotrexate, and 5-fluorouracil as adjuvant therapy after mastectomy in women with high-risk breast cancer has yielded results similar to those seen in the study using melphalan. Again, an increase in the recurrence-free period was observed in the premenopausal but not the postmenopausal women. Clinical and laboratory studies have shown that cytotoxic alkylating agents and antimetabolites induce marked suppression of ovarian function and cessation of menstruation. It is conceivable that the beneficial effect of adjuvant chemotherapy in premenopausal patients is partially the result of a suppression of ovarian activity by these drugs, although studies of surgical castration of premenopausal patients suggest that this is not a mechanism. Some authors used cytotoxic chemotherapeutic agents as adjuvant therapy only in high-risk breast cancer patients whose tumors were found to be negative for estrogen receptors (Table 14-17). These same investigators recommend endocrine ablation as adjuvant therapy in high-risk patients whose tumors contain estrogen receptors.

One of the most impressive adjuvant studies in breast cancer is that reported by Bonadonna from the Milan Cancer Institute. The Bonadonna study of 12 cycles of cyclophosphamide, methotrexate, and 5-fluorouracil

---

Table 14-16   Useful drug combinations in the treatment of breast cancer

	Regimen	Dosage	Response rate (%)
CMFVP	Cyclophosphamide	80 mg/m²/day PO	62
	Methotrexate	20 mg/m²/week IV	
	5-Fluorouracil	500 mg/m²/week IV	
	Vincristine	1 mg/m²/week IV	
	Prednisone	30 mg/m²/day PO for 15 days, *then taper*	
CMF	Cyclophosphamide	100 mg/m² PO days 1 through 4	53
	Methotrexate	60 mg/m² IV days 1 and 8	
	5-Fluorouracil	600 mg/m² IV days 1 and 8 *Repeat cycles every 4 weeks*	
CMF (P)	Cyclophosphamide	100 mg/m² PO days 1 through 14	63
	Methotrexate	60 mg/m² IV days 1 and 8	
	5-Fluorouracil	600 mg/m² IV days 1 and 8	
	Prednisone	40 mg/m² PO days 1 through 14 *Repeat cycles every 4 weeks*	
CA	Cyclophosphamide	200 mg/m² PO days 3 through 6	74
	Doxorubicin	40 mg/m² IV day 1 *Repeat cycles every 3-4 weeks*	
CAF	Cyclophosphamide	100 mg/m² PO days 1 through 14	82
	Doxorubicin	30 mg/m² IV days 1 and 8	
	5-Fluorouracil	500 mg/m² IV days 1 and 8 *Repeat cycles every 4 weeks*	
DAV	Dibromodulcitol	150 mg/m² PO days 1 through 10	71
	Doxorubicin	45 mg/m² IV day 1	
	Vincristine	1.2 mg/m² IV day 1 *Repeat cycles every 4 weeks*	

Table 14-17   Summary of benefit from adjuvant treatment reported in prospectively randomized clinical trials of patients with axillary node metastasis

	Evidence of benefit	
Clinical situation	Disease-free interval	Survival
Premenopausal		
1-3 nodes		
ER* positive	Yes	Yes
ER negative	Yes	?Yes
4 or more nodes		
ER positive	Yes	Yes
ER negative	Yes	?Yes
Postmenopausal		
1-3 nodes		
ER positive	Yes	No
ER negative	?Yes	No
4 or more nodes		
ER positive	Yes	?Yes
ER negative	?Yes	No

*ER, Estrogen receptor.

Table 14-18   British Columbia Cancer Agency adjuvant systemic therapy guidelines for patients with operable breast cancer

Eligible women have any one of the following:

- Primary tumor 32 cm diameter
- Lymphatic or vascular invasion
- Axillary lymph node metastases

Age	Estrogen receptors	Treatment recommendation
<50	Positive or unknown	AC or CMF chemotherapy (tamoxifen investigational)
	Negative	AC or CMF chemotherapy
	Positive or unknown	Tamoxifen for 5 years (chemotherapy may be of small additional benefit)
50-65		
>65	Positive or negative	Tamoxifen for 5 years

Neville AM et al: *J Clin Oncol* 10:696, 1992.
AC, IV adriamycin, 60 mg/m², and cyclophosphamide, 600 mg/m², every 3 weeks for 4 doses.
CMF, Oral or IV cyclophosphamide, methotrexate, and fluorouracil for 6 months.

(CMF) showed an overall relapse-free survival at 5 years of 63.5% for the treated patients vs 48% for the controls. This difference was accounted for largely by the effect in premenopausal patients (69.4% vs 44.3%), relapse-free survival being virtually identical in the postmenopausal group. Bonadonna suggested that the apparent lack of effect of CMF on postmenopausal patients may have been a result of the lower doses that many of the more elderly patients received. Although this observation should be interpreted cautiously, it suggests that aggressive full-dose therapy may be necessary for maximal therapeutic effect. Tancini et al. reported that six cycles of CMF give equivalent results.

The addition of hormones to cytotoxic therapy as an adjuvant is somewhat controversial. Studies are currently being performed in which chemotherapy is preceded by either surgical or radiation-induced oophorectomy in premenopausal women. The initial trial of Hubay et al. studied the addition of the antiestrogen tamoxifen to low-dose CMF alone in patients who had tumors positive for estrogen receptor (ER). Similar results from adding tamoxifen to the combination of L-PAM plus 5-fluorouracil have been reported by Fisher et al. from the NSABP.

The possible advantage of adjuvant chemotherapy in patients who have negative nodes is open to question, especially if the lesion is smaller than 3 cm and ER positive. These patients have a good prognosis; therefore,

the long-term physical and emotional effects of the chemotherapy must be considered.

The 1990 Consensus Development Conference on Early-Stage Breast Cancer also addressed the role of adjuvant therapy for patients with node-negative breast cancer. Their conclusions were as follows: The many unanswered questions in adjuvant systemic treatment of node-negative breast cancer make it imperative that all patients who are candidates for clinical trials be offered the opportunity to participate. All node-negative patients should be aware of the benefits and the risks of adjuvant systemic therapy. The decision to use adjuvant treatment should follow a thorough discussion with the patient regarding the likely risk of recurrence without adjuvant therapy, the expected reduction in risk with adjuvant therapy, the toxicities of therapy, and its impact on the quality of life. Some degrees of improvement may be so small that they are outweighed by the disadvantages of therapy. Adjuvant therapy should consist of combination chemotherapy or tamoxifen (20 mg/day for at least 2 years) (Table 14-18). The Early Breast Cancer Trials Collaborative Group (EBCTCG) meta-analysis suggested that the addition of tamoxifen to standard adjuvant chemotherapy provided an increased benefit, in terms of both relapse-free and overall survival for patients aged 50 years and older. Similar comparisons in women younger than 50 years failed to demonstrate an improvement in relapse-free survival or a significant overall survival

FACTORS INFLUENCING RISK OF RECURRENCE AND SURVIVAL IN PATIENTS WITH APPARENTLY LOCALIZED BREAST CANCER*

1. Axillary lymph node metastasis
2. Hormone receptor content of tumor
3. Tumor size and extent
4. Tumor grade or vascular invasion
5. Anatomic site of tumor

*Listed in approximate decreasing order of significance.

benefit. Tamoxifen has less acute toxicity than chemotherapy but no statement is possible regarding chronic toxicity or comparative efficacy. The results of current and future trials concerning the safety of tamoxifen in premenopausal patients must be followed more carefully. Prognostic factors should be used to provide an estimate of risk or recurrence in women with early-stage breast cancer (see box above). Although no individual patient can be assured that she has no risk of recurrence, the majority of women will be cured with local/regional therapy. There is a strong correlation between tumor size and risk of recurrence. Tumors of 1 cm or less have a particularly good prognosis. Patients with receptor-positive tumors have a better prognosis than those with the receptor-negative tumors. Nuclear grade is a well-documented factor in discriminating between favorable and unfavorable prognostic groups. Measurements of cellular proliferation in breast cancer specimens using a variety of techniques have shown a strong correlation with outcome. Several well-characterized histologic subtypes are part of a favorable prognosis, although they are a distinct minority of all breast cancer cases. The subtypes include tubular, colloid (mucinous), and papillary types.

Suggested treatment recommendations on Adjuvant Chemotherapy and Endocrine Therapy for Breast Cancer are as follows:

1. For premenopausal women with positive nodes, regardless of hormone-receptor status, treatment with established combination chemotherapy has become standard care.
2. For premenopausal patients with negative nodes, adjuvant therapy is not always recommended. For certain "high-risk" patients (see box above) in this group, adjuvant chemotherapy should be considered. Trials are underway to better define this "high risk" patient group.
3. For postmenopausal women with positive nodes and positive hormone-receptor levels, tamoxifen is the treatment of choice. Chemotherapy may be added for "high risk" patients.
4. For postmenopausal women with positive nodes and negative hormone-receptor levels, chemotherapy is usually recommended.
5. Between the ages of 50-69, direct comparisons show that poly-chemotherapy plus tamoxifen is better than chemotherapy alone for both recurrence and for mortality and better than tamoxifen alone for recurrence. The 30%-40% proportional risk reductions that can be produced by combined chemo-endocrine therapy in middle age is similar for node positive and for node negative patients, but the absolute improvement in 10-year survival is about twice as great for the former than for the latter.

Trials of 2 years of tamoxifen vs 5 years or more of the drug are currently in progress. The most widely tested regimen is 20 mg/day for 2 years.

Conclusions. It has been demonstrated that adjuvant chemotherapy and adjuvant endocrine therapy will prolong the survival at 10 years of patients who have early breast cancers.

The standard adjuvant therapy for premenopausal women with histologically proven positive lymph nodes is 6 months of CMF. Longer durations of therapy have not been shown to be advantageous and may be detrimental. It is plausible that some combinations, especially those that include doxorubicin, may eventually prove superior to CMF, but it has not yet been demonstrated that any regimen will reproducibly improve the long-term survival of premenopausal women beyond that achieved with CMF.

At least 2 years of adjuvant tamoxifen may be considered the standard treatment for estrogen receptor positive postmenopausal patients. Adjuvant chemotherapy is also effective in this group, but the side effects of chemotherapy need to be weighed against the risk of relapse.

Adjuvant therapy may prolong the survival of patients who do not have histologic lymph node involvement. The 10-year data (EBCTCG) suggest that the smaller the risk of relapse for the individual patient, the smaller will be the absolute benefit of adjuvant therapy, and so the greater will be the relative importance of any toxic side-effects of that therapy.

About four in every five new patients with breast cancer are aged 50 or more, and among such women, tamoxifen has little toxicity and definite benefits. The choice of which of these women to treat is made easier by the fact that the effects of tamoxifen on survival are to be seen in women of different ages and different stages of disease (I or II). These effects are seen regardless of whether these patients are receiving concurrent chemotherapy or not, whether premenopausal or postmenopausal, and whether their tumors are estrogen receptor positive or estrogen receptor negative. Among younger women the effects of tamoxifen are less definite, but both

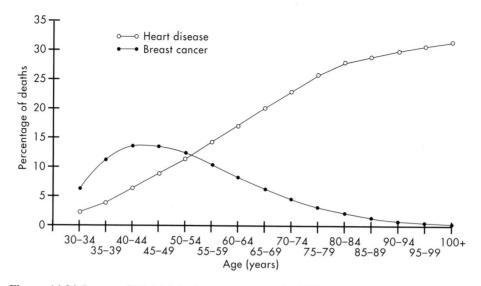

Figure 14-24 Percent of US total deaths among women in 1988 due to breast cancer or heart disease by age. (From Public Health Service Publication # 90-1102, Washington DC, US Government Printing Office, 1990.)

ovarian ablation and cytotoxic chemotherapy improve survival, and these benefits are likewise discernible in several subgroups.

The EBCTCG study also revealed that postmenopausal women who are estrogen receptor negative also derive benefit from tamoxifen therapy, and this benefit appears to be equivalent to chemotherapy. Furthermore, in premenopausal women the studies of tamoxifen in the absence of chemotherapy show distinct risk reduction, even though tamoxifen induces very high levels of unopposed estradiols.

Since the publication of the first randomized trials of adjuvant chemotherapy in early breast cancer, cytotoxic drugs have become the standard treatment for node positive premenopausal women. Reports on adjuvant ovarian ablation in the same group of women were sporadic and apparently contradictory, some indicating no significant delay even in recurrence, some indicating a significant delay of recurrence but not death, and some indicating a significant delay of death but only in certain subgroups. The real effect of ovarian ablation seems to have been obscured by the small sample size of the many studies and by the increasing popularity of chemotherapy for breast cancer as medical oncology became a major subspecialty. Few groups have made a direct comparison of adjuvant ovarian ablation or other hormonal approaches with adjuvant chemotherapy. There have been no comparisons of ovarian ablation alone vs ovarian ablation plus chemotherapy. The EBCTCG also suggests that adjuvant chemotherapy has a greater effect in premenopausal than in postmenopausal women (25% compared to a 12% reduction in annual odds of death). At least some of the benefits gained from adjuvant chemotherapy in the premenopausal women is likely to be

obtained through an endocrine effect. Many women receiving this therapy become amenorrheic and prematurely menopausal. It is not likely, however, that all of the benefits of adjuvant chemotherapy in premenopausal women is obtained through a hormonal mechanism.

Hormonal Replacement Therapy

Previously treated breast cancer patients are denied the benefit of menopausal hormone replacement therapy (HRT) on the basis of traditional, untested beliefs that breast cancer will be exacerbated by renewed hormonal exposure. Breast cancer becomes less important as a cause of death as a woman ages, and heart disease rises dramatically as the number one cause of death (Figure 14-24). New information regarding the prevention of osteoporosis and cardiovascular disease by HRT, as well as issues concerning improved quality of life, require re-examination of this matter. Wile and DiSaia reviewed the recent literature referable to patients, with or without breast cancer, who are exposed to high levels of estrogen. These included women with breast cancer who were pregnant, patients with breast cancer who were current and/or previous users of oral contraceptives, and postmenopausal women on HRT who had breast cancer. After reviewing the studies, the authors concluded that there was no hard evidence that estrogen had an adverse effect on outcome for patients with established breast cancer. DiSaia et al. published their experience with 77 patients who received hormone replacement therapy following therapy for breast cancer. With a median follow-up of 5 years, the authors reported seven recurrences in their series of 77 unselected patients who presented with the request for replacement therapy. Forty one of these patients were from a region that employed a population based tumor registry. When the 41 were matched with 82 controls from that same population base, no difference in outcome of the HRT treated patients vs the controls could be demonstrated. Although this indirect evidence is reassuring, the fact remains that there is no large series of patients who have received HRT following treatment of breast cancer. Obviously, undertaking such a prospective and randomized study would be very difficult, and the accumulation of adequate prospective evidence to document safety would take a very long time (Table 14-19).

A somewhat related issue deals with endometrial carcinoma associated with tamoxifen in postmenopausal breast cancer patients. The occurrence of endometrial cancer in patients with breast cancer has been reported in many studies. In 1987, Adami reported on 60,000 women with breast cancer in a case-controlled study in Sweden: 151 cases of endometrial carcinoma were expected and 260 were observed for a calculated risk ratio of 1.7. A number of reports in the more recent literature suggest that the addition of tamoxifen entails a still higher risk of endometrial carcinoma. A large prospective study will be necessary to determine whether women on tamoxifen therapy have an increased risk of endometrial hyperplasia and endometrial cancer and to estimate the magnitude of such a risk. In the meantime, several questions come to mind. Should this group of patients be treated in a manner similar to that used with patients on estrogen replacement therapy? Should regular endometrial sampling be done, cyclic progesterone given, or low-dose progesterone given in a continuous fashion? There are controversies regarding the use of progesterones in patients with breast carcinoma, even though some progesterones have been used to treat such patients. It is to be hoped that future studies will answer these questions. In the mean time, the authors recommend that patients on tamoxifen be monitored closely and endometrial sampling be reserved for patients on tamoxifen who demonstrate uterine bleeding. Routine use of endometrial sampling appears to be an inappropriate recommendation at this time. In the authors'

Table 14-19   Regimens for hormone replacement therapy

	Dosage	Dosage
Conjugated estrogen 0.625-1.250 g + MPA 2.5-5.0 mg		Daily
or		
Estradiol 1-2 mg		
or		
Conjugated estrogen 0.625-1.250 mg		Day 1-25 each
or		
Estradiol 1-2 mg + MPA 5 or 10 mg-		Day 16-25 each

MPA, Medroxyprogesterone acetate.

experiences, the type of endometrial carcinoma that patients on tamoxifen develop is similar to the general population, and the incidence appears to be quite low. Routine use of progestins in combination with tamoxifen for patients who are not on simultaneous estrogen replacement therapy appears excessive given our current knowledge. The clinician may wish to see patients on tamoxifen at 6-month intervals instead of annually to have an opportunity to elicit a history of uterine bleeding. Some authorities suggest that patients on tamoxifen be monitored with periodic transvaginal ultrasound with particular attention being paid to the thickness of the endometrial stripe. Transvaginal ultrasound is certainly less invasive than periodic endometrial biopsies. It has been well established that endometrial stripe less than 5 mm in thickness is rarely associated with neoplasia, whereas the risk of neoplasia increases dramatically as the thickness of the endometrial stripe exceeds 8 mm in postmenopausal women. The cost of periodic transvaginal ultrasonography is high and there has been no studies to date demonstrating a distinct advantage in terms of lowered mortality from endometrial neoplasia in this group of patients.

BIBLIOGRAPHY

Benign conditions of the breast

ACOG Technical Bulletin: Nonmalignant conditions of the breast, 156:1, 1991.

American College of Obstetricians and Gynecologists: Report of task force on routine cancer screening, ACOG Committee Opinion Number 68. Washington, DC: ACOG 1989.

American College of Radiology: Breast Imaging Reporting and Data System, ed. 2, 1995.

Ariel IM: Enovid therapy for fibrocystic disease, *Am J Obstet Gynecol* 117:453, 1973.

Baker HW, Snedecor PA: Clinical trial of danazol for benign breast disease, *Am J Surg* 45:727, 1979.

Blichert-Toft M et al: Treatment of mastalgia with bromocriptine: a double-blind crossover study, *Br Med J* 1:237, 1979.

Byrd BF et al: Treatment of breast tumors associated with pregnancy and lactation, *Ann Sur* 155:940, 1962.

Chetty U et al: Benign breast disease in cancer, *Br J Surg* 67:789, 1979.

Cole P, Elwood JM, Kaplan SD: Incidence rates and risk factors of benign breast neoplasms, *Am J Epidemiol* 108:112, 1978.

Davis HH, Simmonds M, Davis JB: Cystic disease of the breast: relationship to cancer, *Cancer* 17:957, 1964.

DeVitt JE: Fibrocystic disease of the breast is not premalignant, *Surg Gynecol Obstet* 134:803, 1972.

Donegan WL: Pregnancy and breast cancer, *Obstet Gynecol* 50:244, 1977.

Gonzales ER: Vitamin E relieves most cystic breast disease; may alter lipids, hormones (news), *JAMA* 244:1077, 1980.

Hindle WH, Alonzo LJ: Conservative management of breast fibroadenomas, *Am J Obstet Gynecol* 164:1647, 1991.

Hislop TJ, Elwood JM: Risk factors for benign breast disease: a 30 year cohort study, *Can Med Assoc J* 124:283, 1981.

Kramer WM, Rush BF: Mammary duct proliferation in the elderly, *Cancer* 31:130, 1973.

Leis HP Jr: *Diagnosis and treatment of breast lesions*, New York, 1970, Medical Examination Publishing.

Nezhat C et al: Danazol for benign breast disease, *Am J Obstet Gynecol* 137:604, 1980.

Petrek JA: Surveillance and diagnosis of breast masses in pregnancy and lactation, *The Female Patient* 18:16, 1993.

Petrek JA, Dukoff R, Rogatko A: Pregnancy-associated breast cancer, *CA* 67:869, 1991.

Ricciardi I, Ianniruberto A: Tamoxifen-induced regression of benign breast lesions, *Obstet Gynecol* 54:80, 1979.

Sitruk-Ware R, Thalabard JC, Benotmane A et al: Risk factors for breast fibroadenoma in young women, *Contraception* 40(3):251, 1989.

Wilkinson S, Anderson TJ, Rifkind E et al: Fibroadenoma of the breast: a follow-up of conservative management, *Br J Surg* 76:390, 1989.

Estrogen therapy and breast cancer incidence

Allegra JC, Kiefer SM. Mechanisms of action of progestational agents. *Semin Oncol* 2:3-5, 1985.

Armstrong BK; Oestrogen therapy in menopause—boon or bane? *Med J Aust* 148:213, 1988.

Barrett A et al: A breast carcinoma dependent on human placental lactogen, letter, *Lancet* 1:1347, 1975.

Beral V, Colwell L: Randomized trial of high doses of stilbestrol and ethisterone in pregnancy; long-term follow-up of mothers, *Br Med J* 281:1098, 1980.

Bergkvist L, Adami HO, Persson I et al: The risk of breast cancer after estrogen and estrogen-progesterone replacement, *N Engl J Med* 5:293, 1989.

Brezezinski A et al: Ovarian stimulation and breast cancer: is there a link? *Gynecol Oncol* 52:292, 1994.

Brookshaw JD: Danazol treatment of benign breast disease: a survey of USA Multicenter Studies, *Postgrad Med J Suppl* 5:58, 1979.

Bryant AJS, Weir JA: Prophylactic oophorectomy in operable instances of carcinoma of the breast, *Surg Gynecol Obstet* 153:660, 1981.

The Centers for Disease Control Cancer and Steroid Hormone Study. Long-term oral contraceptive use and the risk of breast cancer, *JAMA* 249:1591, 1983.

Chan L, O'Malley BW: Mechanism of action of the sex steroid hormones, *N Engl J Med* 294:1322, 1372, 1430, 1976.

Colditz GA, Stampfer MJ, Willett WC et al: Prospective study of estrogen replacement therapy and risk of breast cancer in postmenopausal women, *JAMA* 264(20):2648, 1990.

DiSaia PJ: Estrogen replacement therapy for patients with a history of breast or endometrial cancer, *Clin Consult Obstet Gynecol* 3(2):112, 1991.

Dupont WD, Page DL: Menopausal estrogen replacement therapy and breast cancer, *Arch Intern Med* 151:67, 1991.

Grady D, Ernster V: Does postmenopausal hormone therapy cause breast cancer? *Am J Epidemiol* 134:1396, 1991.

Gambrell RD Jr: Breast disease in the postmenopausal years, *Sem Reprod Endocrinol* 1:1, 1983.

Gambrell RD Jr: Proposal to decrease the risk and improve the prognosis of breast cancer, *AJOG* 150:119, 1984.

Gambrell RD Jr, Maier RC, Sanders BI: Decreased incidence of breast cancer in postmenopausal estrogen-progestogen users, *Obstet Gynecol* 62:435, 1983.

Gambrell RD Jr., Vasquez JM. Estrogen therapy and breast cancer: is the verdict in? *Contemp Obstet Gynecol* 19:38-45, 1982.

Gambrell RD Jr et al: Estrogen therapy and breast cancer in postmenopausal women, *J Am Geriatr Soc* 28:251, 1980.

Gompel A, Malet C, Spritzer P et al: Progestin effect on cell proliferation and 17 β-hydroxysteroid dehydrogenase activity in normal human breast cells in culture, *J Clin Endocrin Metab* 63:1174-80, 1986.

Harlap S et al: Estimated annual number of newly diagnosed cases of ovarian, endometrial, breast and liver cancer per 100,000 women, The Alan Guttmacher Institute, *The Contraception Report* 2(3):8, 1991.

Henderson IC: Endocrine therapy of metastatic breast cancer. In Harris JR, Hellman S, Henderson IC, Kinne DW, editors, *Breast diseases*, Philadelphia: JB Lippincott, 398-428, 1987.

Hirayama T, Wynder EL: Protective effect of surgical menopause on the incidence of breast cancer, *Cancer* 15:28, 1962.

Horwitz KB et al: Predicting response to endocrine therapy in human breast cancer: a hypothesis, *Science* 189:726, 1975.

Jensen EV, Smith S, DeSombre E: Hormone dependency in breast cancer, *J Steroid Biochem* 7:911, 1976.

Jick H et al: Replacement estrogens in breast cancer, *Am J Epidemiol* 112:586, 1980.

Jern HZ: *Hormone therapy of the menopause and aging*, Springfield, Illinois, 1973, Charles C. Thomas.

Kiang D, Kennedy B: Estrogen receptor assay in the differential diagnosis of adenocarcinoma, *JAMA* 238:32, 1977.

Korenman SG: The endocrinology of breast cancer, *Cancer* 46:874, 1980.

Lipsett MB: Hormones, nutrition, and cancer, *Cancer Res* 35:3359, 1975.

MacKay EN, Sellers AH: Artificial menopause and prognosis in breast cancer, *Can Med Assoc J* 92:647, 1965.

Matthews PN, Mills RR, Haywood JL: Breast cancer in women who have taken oral contraceptive steroids, *Br Med J* 282:774, 1971.

McGuire WL et al: Current status of estrogen and progesterone receptors in breast cancer, *Cancer* 39:2934, 1977.

Nachtigall LE et al: Estrogen replacement to a prospective study in the relationship to carcinoma and cardiovascular and metabolic problems, *Obstet Gynecol* 54:74, 1979.

Nachtigall MJ, Smilen SW, Nachtigall RAD et al: Incidence of breast cancer in a 22-year study of women receiving estrogen progestin replacement therapy, *Obstet Gynecol* 80:827-830, 1992.

Olsson H, Moller TR, Ranstma J: Early oral contraceptive use and breast cancer among premenopausal women: final report from a study in southern Sweden, *J Natl Ca Inst* 82:1000, 1989.

The PEPI Trial Group: Effects of estrogen or estrogen/progestin regimens on heart disease risk factors in postmenopausal women, *JAMA* 273:199-208, 1995.

Pike MC et al: Breast cancer in young women and use of oral contraceptives: possible modifying effect of formulation and age at use, *Lancet* 2:926, 1983.

Ravdin RG et al: Results of a clinical trial concerning the worth of prophylactic oophorectomy for breast carcinoma, *Surg Gynecol Obstet* 131:1005, 1970.

Rosner D, Lane W: Oral contraceptive use has no adverse effect on the prognosis of breast cancer, *Cancer* 57:591, 1986.

Ross K et al: A case-control study of menopausal estrogen therapy in breast cancer, *JAMA* 243:1635, 1980.

Schlesselman JJ: Cancer of the breast and reproductive tract in relation to use of oral contraceptives, *Contraception* 40:1, 1989.

Schlesselman JJ: Oral contraceptives and breast cancer, *Am J Obstet Gynecol* 163(4):1379, 1990.

Sherman B, Wallace R, Bean J: Estrogen use and breast cancer, *Cancer* 51:1527, 1983.

Spicer D, Pike MC, Henderson BE: The question of estrogen replacement therapy in patients with a prior diagnosis of breast cancer, *Oncology* 12:49, 1990.

Steinberg KK, Thacker SB, Smith SJ et al: A meta-analysis of the effect of estrogen replacement therapy on the risk of breast cancer, *JAMA* 265(15):1985, 1991.

Tagman H: Antiestrogen in treatment of breast cancer, *Cancer* 39:2959, 1977.

Thomas DB: Update on breast cancer and oral contraceptives, *The Contraception Report* 2:3, 1991.

US Department of Health and Human Services: Long-term oral contraceptive use and the risk of breast cancer, *JAMA* 249:1591, 1983.

Vessey M, Baron J, Doll R et al: Oral contraceptives and breast cancer: final report of an epidemiological study, *Br J Cancer* 47:455, 1983.

Vessey MP, Fairweather DVI, Norman-Smith B, Buckley J: A randomized double-blind controlled trial of the value of stilbestrol therapy in pregnancy: long-term follow-up of mothers and their offspring, *Br J Obstet Gynaecol* 90:1007, 1983.

WHO Collaborative study of neoplasia and steroid contraceptives: breast cancer and depot-medroxyprogesterone acetate: a multinational study, *Lancet* 338:833, 1991.

Wile AG, DiSaia PJ: Hormones and breast cancer, *Am J Surg* 157:438, 1989.

Epidemiology

ACOG Technical Bulletin: Carcinoma of the breast, 158:1, 1991.

American Joint Committee on Cancer: *Manual for staging of cancer*, ed 3, Philadelphia, 1988, JB Lippincott.

American Joint Committee on Cancer, American Cancer Society, American College of Surgeons Commission on Cancer. Am Cancer Society, Inc. 1989;89-12M-No. 3485.01.

Glass AG, Hoover RN: Rising incidence of breast cancer: relationship to stage and receptor status, *J Natl Ca Inst* 82:693, 1990.

Howe GR, Hirohata T, Hislop TG et al: Dietary factors and risk of breast cancer: combined analysis of 12 case-control studies, *J Natl Ca Inst* 82:561, 1990.

Kritchevsky D: Diet, nutrition, and cancer, *Cancer* 58(8):1830, 1986.

Kritchevsky D: Nutrition and breast cancer, *Cancer* 66(6):1321, 1990.

Mettlin C: Diet and the epidemiology of human breast cancer, *Cancer* 53:605, 1984.

Early detection and diagnosis

Anderson DE, Badzioch MD: Risk of familial breast cancer, *Cancer* 56:383, 1985.

Boyd NF et al: Mammographic patterns and breast cancer risk: methodologic standards and contradictory results, *J Natl Ca Inst* 72:1253, 1984.

Byrne R: Utilization of thermography as a risk indicator in the detection of breast cancer, *Bull NY Acad Med* 52:741, 1976.

Chu KC, Smart CR, Tarone RE: Analysis of breast cancer mortality and stage distribution by age for the health insurance plan clinical trial, *J Natl Ca Inst* 80:1125, 1988.

Cook DC, Dent O, Hewitt D: Breast cancer following multiple chest fluoroscopy: the Ontario experience, *Can Med Assoc J* 111:406, 1974.

Council on Scientific Affairs: Mammographic screening in asymptomatic women ages 40 years and older, *JAMA* 261:2535, 1989.

Cutler SJ: Classification of extent of disease in breast cancer, *Sem Oncol* 1:91, 1974.

Cyrlak D, Wong CH: Mammographic changes in postmenopausal women undergoing hormonal replacement therapy, *AJR* 161:1177, 1993.

Dent DM, Kirkpatrick AE, McGoogan E et al: Stereotaxic localization and aspiration cytology of impalpable breast lesions, *Clin Radiol* 40:380, 1989.

Dodd GD: Mammography, *Breast Cancer* 25, 1989.

Ersek RA, Denton DR: Breast biopsy technique: a plea for cosmesis, *South Med J* 79:167, 1986.

Fisher B et al: Cancer of the breast: size of neoplasm and prognosis, *Cancer* 24:1071, 1969.

Gogas J, Skalkeas G: Prognosis of mammary carcinoma in young women, *Surgery* 78:339, 1975.

Hindle WH: Changing concepts in the evaluation of dominant breast masses, *Female Patient* 15:43, 1990.

Holleb AI: The technique of breast examination. In Holleb AI, editor: *Breast cancer: early and late*, Chicago, 1970, Year Book Medical.

Holleb AI: Restoring confidence in mammography, *CA* 26:376, 1976.

Leis HP Jr: Breast lesions with malignant transformation potential. Proceedings of the nineteenth European Federation Congress of the International College of Surgeons, Amsterdam, 1976, American College of Surgeons.

Lester RG: Risk versus benefit in mammography, *Radiology* 124:1, 1977.

Locker AP, Stickland V, Manhire AR et al: Mammography in symptomatic breast disease, *Lancet* 1:887, 1989.

Lyon JL et al: Cancer incidence in Mormons and non-Mormons: Utah 1966-1970, *N Engl J Med* 294:129, 1976.

Martin JW: Xeromammography—an improved diagnostic method: review of 250 biopsied cases, *AJR* 117:90, 1973.

Mettlin C: Diet and the epidemiology of human breast cancer, *Cancer* 53:605, 1984.

Mitchell GW Jr, Homer MJ: Outpatient breast biopsies on a gynecologic service, *Am J Obstet Gynecol* 144:127, 1982.

Nayfield SG et al: Potential role of tamoxifen in prevention of breast cancer, *J Natl Cancer Inst* 83:1450, 1991.

Newcomb PA, Weiss NS, Storer BE et al: Breast self-examination in relation to the occurrence of advanced breast cancer, *J Natl Ca Inst* 83:260, 1991.

Nyirjesy I, Billingsely FS: Detection of breast carcinoma in gynecologic practice, *Obstet Gynecol* 64:747, 1984.

Ostrum BJ, Becker W, Isard HJ: Low dose mammography, *Radiology* 109:323, 1973.

Pike MC et al: Breast cancer in young women and the use of oral contraceptives: possible modifying effect of formulation in agent use, *Lancet* 2:926, 1983.

Strax P: Results of mass screening for breast cancer in 50,000 examinations, *Cancer* 37:30, 1976.

Tabor L et al: Reduction of mortality from breast cancer after mass screening with mammography, *Lancet* 1:829, 1985.

Vacheir H: Breast aspiration biopsy, *Am J Obstet Gynecol* 148:127, 1984.

Verbeek ALM et al: Reduction of breast cancer mortality through mass screening with modern mammography: first results of Nijmegen project, 1975-1981, *Lancet* 1:1222, 1984.

Vogel VG, Graves DS, Vernon SW et al: Mammographic screening of women with increased risk of breast cancer, *Cancer* 66:1613, 1990.

Winchester DP: Evaluation and management of breast abnormalities, *Cancer* 66(6):1345, 1990.

Wolfe JN: Developments in mammography, *Am J Obstet Gynecol* 124:312, 1976.

Treatment

Adami HO, Krusemo UB, Bergkvist L et al: On the age-dependent associations between cancer of the breast and of the endometrium: a nationwide cohort study, *Br J Cancer* 47:77, 1987.

Barth A et al: Current management of ductal carcinoma in situ, *West J Med* 163:360, 1995.

Berg JW, Hutter RVP: Breast cancer, *Cancer* 75:257, 1995.

Blichert-Toft M, Andersen J, Dyreborg U: In situ carcinomas of the female breast, *Acta Chir Scand* 156:113, 1990.

Bonadonna G, Valagussa P: Dose response: effect of adjuvant chemotherapy in breast cancer, *N Engl J Med* 304:10, 1981.

Bonadonna G et al: 10-year experience with CMF-based adjuvant chemotherapy in resectable breast cancer, *Breast Cancer Res Treat* 5:95, 1985.

Canellos GP et al: Combination chemotherapy for advanced breast cancer: response and effect on survival, *Ann Intern Med* 84:389, 1976.

Dorr FA, Friedman MA: The role of chemotherapy in the management of primary breast cancer, *CA* 41(4):231, 1991.

Ernster VL et al: Incidence of and treatment for ductal carcinoma in situ of the breast, *JAMA* 275 (12):913, 1996.

Fisher B, Fisher ER, Redmond C: 10-year results from the NSABP clinical trial evaluating the use of l-phenylalanine mustard (L-PAM) in the management of primary breast cancer, *J Clin Oncol* 4:929, 1986.

Fisher B, Wolmack N: Current status of systemic adjuvant therapy in the management of primary breast cancer, *Surg Clin North Am* 61:1347, 1981.

Fisher B et al: l-Phenylalanine mustard (L-PAM) in the management of primary breast cancer: a report of early findings, *N Engl J Med* 292:117, 1975.

Fisher B et al: Treatment of primary breast cancer with chemotherapy and tamoxifen, *N Engl J Med* 305:1, 1981.

Fisher B et al: Five-year results of a randomized clinical trial comparing total mastectomy and segmental mastectomy with or without radiation in the treatment of breast cancer, *N Engl J Med* 312:665, 1985.

Fisher B et al: Ten-year results of a randomized clinical trial comparing radical mastectomy and total mastectomy with or without radiation, *N Engl J Med* 312:674, 1985.

Fisher B, Constantino J, Redmond C et al: Lumpectomy compared with lumpectomy and radiation therapy for the treatment of intraductal breast cancer, *N Engl J Med* 328:1581, 1993

Gelber RD, Goldhirsch A: The concept of an overview of cancer clinical trials with special emphasis on early breast cancer, *J Clin Oncol* 4:1696, 1986.

Gelber RD, Goldhirsch A: A new end-point for the assessment of adjuvant therapy in postmenopausal women with operable breast cancer, *J Clin Oncol* 4:1772, 1986.

Gusberg SB: Tamoxifen for breast cancer: associated endometrial cancer, *Cancer*, 65:1463, 1990.

Haagensen CD: The choice of treatment for operable carcinoma of the breast, *Surgery* 76:685, 1974.

Halsted WS: The results of radical operations for the cure of carcinoma of the breast, *Ann Surg* 46:1, 1907.

Handley WS: *Cancer of the breast and its treatment*, ed 2, London, 1922, John Murray.

Harris JR, Recht A, Connolly J et al: Conservative surgery and radiotherapy for early breast cancer, *Cancer* 66(6):1427, 1990.

Hayes DF, Henderson IC: Adjuvant therapy for node-negative breast cancer patients, *Adv Oncol* 6(4):8, 1991.

Hellman S: Controversies in breast cancer, Conference sponsored by the MD Anderson Hospital and Tumor Institute, Chicago, 1983, Year Book Medical.

Hubay CA et al: Antiestrogen, cytotoxic chemotherapy and BCG vaccination in Stage II breast cancer, *Surgery* 87:494, 1980.

International Breast Cancer Study Group: Late effects of adjuvant oophorectomy and chemotherapy upon premenopausal breast cancer patients, *Ann Oncol* 1:30, 1990.

Jones SE, Durie BGM, Salmon SE: Combination chemotherapy with Adriamycin and cyclophosphamide for advanced breast cancer, *Cancer* 36:90, 1975.

Kerlikowski K et al: Efficacy of screening mammography: a meta analysis, *JAMA* 273:149, 1995.

Killacey MA, Hakes TB, Pierce UK: Endometrial adenocarcinoma in breast cancer patients receiving antiestrogens, *Cancer Treat Rep* 69:237, 1985.

Lichter AS et al: mastectomy versus breast-conserving therapy in the treatment of stage I and II carcinoma of the breast: a randomized trial at the national Cancer Institute, *J Clin Oncol* 10:976, 1992.

Lippman ME: The NIH consensus development conference on adjuvant chemotherapy for breast cancer: a commentary, *Breast Cancer Res Treat* 6:195, 1985.

Malfetano JH: Tamoxifen-associated endometrial carcinoma in postmenopausal breast cancer patients, *Gynecol Oncol* 39:82, 1990.

Mathew A, Chabon AB, Kabakow B et al: Endometrial carcinoma in five patients with breast cancer on tamoxifen therapy, *NY State J Med* 90:207, 1990.

Montague ED: Conservative surgery and radiation therapy in the treatment of operable breast cancer, *Cancer* 53:700, 1984.

Moore CM: On the influence of inadequate operations on the theory of cancer: Royal Medical and Chirurgical Society, London, *Med Chir Trans* 32:245, 1967.

Neville AM et al: Factors predicting treatment responsiveness and prognosis in node-negative breast cancer, *J Clin Oncol* 10:696, 1992.

Nielsen M et al: Breast cancer and atypia among young and middle-aged women: a study of 110 medicolegal autopsies, *Br J Cancer*, 56:814, 1987.

Page DL et al: Continued local recurrence of carcinoma 15-25 years after a diagnosis of low grade ductal carcinoma in situ of the breast treated only with biopsy, *Cancer* 76:1187, 1995.

Pritchard KI: Systemic adjuvant therapy for node-negative breast cancer: proven or premature? *Ann Intern Med* 111:1, 1989.

Roberts JG et al: Evaluation of radiography and isotopic scintigraphy for detecting skeletal metastases in breast cancer, *Lancet* 1:237, 1976.

Schwartz FG et al: Multicentricity of nonpalpable breast cancer, *Cancer* 45:2913, 1980.

Shingleton WW, McCarty KS: Breast carcinoma: an overview, *Gynecol Oncol* 26:271, 1987.

Silverstein MJ et al: Prognostic classification of breast ductal carcinoma-in-situ, *Lancet* 345:1154, 1995.

Surveillance, epidemiology, and end results (SEER program public use CD-ROM (1973-1992). Bethesda, Md: National Cancer Institute, DCPC, Surveillance program, Cancer Statistics Branch, July 1995.

Tancini G et al: Adjuvant CMF in breast cancer: comparative 5 year results of 12 vs. 6 cycles *Proc Am Soc Clin Oncol* 1:86, 1982 (abstract).

Taylor HC Jr: The coincidence of primary breast and uterine cancer, *Am J Cancer* 15:277, 1931.

Tormey DC, Gray R, Gilchrist K et al: Adjuvant chemohormonal therapy with cyclophosphamide, methotrexate, 5-fluorouracil, and prednisone (CMFP) or CMFP plus tamoxifen compared with CMF for premenopausal breast cancer patients, *Cancer* 65:200, 1990.

Torres JE, Mickal A: Carcinoma of the breast in pregnancy, *Clin Obstet Gynecol* 18:219, 1975.

Veronesi U et al: Comparing radical mastectomy with quadrantectomy, axillary dissection, and radiotherapy in patients with small cancers of the breast, *N Engl J Med* 305(1):6, 1981.

Westberg SV: Prognosis of breast cancer for pregnant and nursing women: a clinical statistical study, *Acta Obstet Gynecol Scand* 25:1, 1946.

Hormonal replacement therapy in breast cancer patients

Beatson GT: On the treatment of inoperable cases of carcinoma of the mammary glands: suggestions for a new method of treatment with illustrative cases, *Lancet* 11:104, 1896.

Bergkvist L, Adami HO, Persson I et al: Prognosis after breast cancer diagnosis in women exposed to estrogen and estrogen-progestogen replacement therapy, *Am J Epidemiol* 130:221, 1989.

Brinton LA, Hoover R, Fraumeni JF Jr: Menopausal oestrogens and breast cancer risk: an expanded case-control study, *Br J Cancer* 54:825, 1986.

Buchanan RB, Blamey RW, Durrant KR et al: A randomized comparison of tamoxifen with surgical oophorectomy in premenopausal patients with advanced breast cancer, *J Clin Oncol* 4 (9):1326, 1986.

DiSaia PJ et al: Replacement therapy for breast cancer survivors, a pilot study, *Cancer* 476(10), 1995.

Dupont WD, Page DL: Risk factors for breast cancers in women with proliferative breast disease, *N Engl J Med* 312:146, 1985.

Dupont WD, Page DL: Menopausal estrogen replacement therapy and breast cancer, *Arch Intern Med* 151:67, 1991.

Dupont WD, Page DL, Rogers LW et al: Influence of exogenous estrogens, proliferative breast disease and other variables on breast cancer risk, *Cancer* 63:948, 1989.

Fornander T, Rutqvist LE, Cedermark B et al: Adjuvant tamoxifen in early breast cancer: occurrence of new primary cancers, *Lancet* 1:117, 1989.

Hardell L: Tamoxifen as risk factor for carcinoma of corpus uteri, *Lancet* 2:563, 1988.

Hulka BS: Hormone replacement therapy and the risk of breast cancer, *Cancer* 40:289, 1990.

Ingle JN, Ahmann DL, Green SJ et al: Randomized clinical trial of diethylstilbestrol versus tamoxifen in postmenopausal women with advanced breast cancer, *N Engl J Med* 304:16, 1981.

Love RR, Newcomb PA, Wiebe DA: Effects of tamoxifen therapy on lipid and lipoprotein levels in postmenopausal patients with node-negative breast cancer, *Articles* 82:1327, 1990.

Parente JT, Amsel M, Lerner R et al: Breast cancer associated with pregnancy, *Obstet Gynecol* 71(6):861, 1988.

Patterson JS: Clinical aspects and development of antiestrogen therapy: a review of endocrine effects of tamoxifen in animals and man, *J Endocrinol* 89:67, 1981.

Sullivan JM, VanderZwagg R, Hughes JP et al: Estrogen replacement and coronary artery disease, *Arch Intern Med* 150:2557, 1990.

Villarino CB & Fenster PE: Coronary heart disease, *Prim Care Update Ob/Gyn* 1:150, 1994.

Wile AG, DiSaia PJ: Hormones and breast cancer, *Am J Surg* 157:438, 1989.

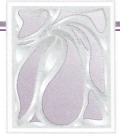

Colorectal and Bladder Cancer

COLORECTAL CANCER
Epidemiology
Screening
Polyps
Staging
Chemoprevention
Surgical Therapy
Adjuvant Therapy
Recurrence Patterns
Therapy of Recurrence
BLADDER CANCER
Pathology
Diagnosis and Staging
Treatment and Results

Table 15-1   Patients at high risk for colorectal neoplasms

Personal history of	Family history of
Breast cancer	Colorectal polyp
Endometrial cancer	Colorectal cancer
Crohn's disease	
Visceral irradiation	
Uterosigmoidostomy	
Colorectal polyp	
Colorectal cancer	

From Gryska PV, Cohen AM: *Dis Colon Rectum* 30:18, 1987.
Ulcerative colitis predisposes to malignancy but is not usually considered asymptomatic; screening is not useful in patients with familial polyposis or Gardner's syndrome.

COLORECTAL CANCER

Epidemiology

Although the epidemiology of rectal cancer differs in some respects from that of colon cancer, the two share so many features that most investigators regard all large bowel cancers as a single entity. Colorectal cancer is the Western World's most common internal malignancy and one of its leading causes of cancer deaths. During 1995 about 68,000 new cases of colorectal cancer were diagnosed in women in the United States alone, and 28,000 women died of this disease. In the United States, slightly over 50% of colon cancers and slightly under 45% of rectal cancers occur in women (Table 15-1). The US overall incidence has remained fairly constant during the past five decades but for unknown reasons the proportion of cases involving the rectum and the colon has changed. About 70% of the incidence and 80% of deaths now involve the colon. More lesions involve the right colon (Figure 15-1).

Colorectal cancer is the second leading cause of death from cancer in the United States. Fortunately, mortality from colorectal cancer has fallen 29% for women and 7% for men over the last 30 years. There is a trend toward earlier stage disease, even though the majority of patients are still diagnosed with regional or distant disease. The majority of colorectal cancers are diagnosed in patients over 50 years of age (Figure 15-2). A patient younger than 50 years of age is likely to belong to a high-risk group. Adenomatous polyps are the most common precursor lesion; they are estimated to occur in 93% of cases. Adenomatous polyps occur in 30% of older individuals, however, and less than 10% progress to malignancy.

Because of the numbers of patients and the long periods of observation required, it has been extraordinarily difficult to mount large-scale prospective studies of dietary intervention in colorectal cancer. However, observations of the epidemiologic patterns of this cancer suggest potential changes in dietary habits that may lead

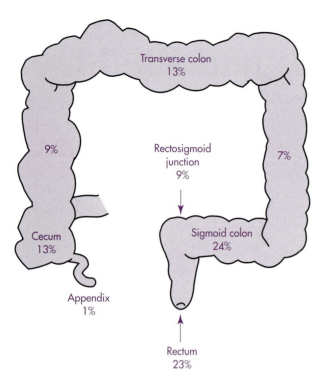

Figure 15-1 Distribution of colorectal cancer.

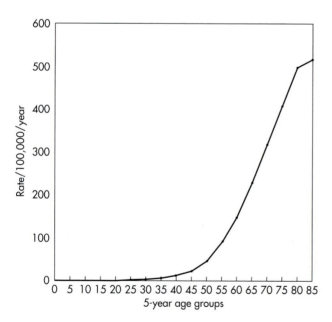

Figure 15-2 Colorectal cancer; age-specific incidence.

to a reduction in risk for populations with high incidence of disease. The observations of Burkitt and others in African populations have led many investigators to conclude that the low risk in these populations was largely attributable to high-fiber diets, which resulted in high-bulk stools in rapid transit time. Theoretically, slow stool transit and low-bulk stools may be prone to higher

concentrations of carcinogens adjacent to the bowel wall. Not all fiber may be beneficial, however, and there are no prospective intervention studies that prove the ability of fiber alone to decrease the risk of colorectal cancer.

Other epidemiologic studies of the low risk of colon cancer in the Far East (compared with Western societies) suggest that diets that are low in unsaturated fats may be associated with a reduction in the incidence of colorectal cancer. Changes in the diet of the traditionally low-risk cultures, such as Japan, toward a diet that has a higher fat content typical of that of Western countries have been associated with a rising incidence of colorectal cancer. Although the exact mechanism by which fats (and fiber) affect colon carcinogenesis is not clearly understood, these epidemiologic studies leave little doubt that there are environmental risk factors in the development of this common tumor. This conclusion is supported by the alterations of risk patterns for colorectal cancer in migrating cultures who experience changing environments. For example, the migration of Japanese persons to the United States is associated with an increasing incidence of colorectal cancer in successive generations, until their risk is equivalent to that of the native-born population.

Certain micronutrients found in cruciferous vegetables (cabbage, broccoli, cauliflower, and Brussels sprouts) may reduce the risk of colon cancer. Figure 15-3 demonstrates some theories about how these agents act to interfere with initiation of malignant changes. Some of these micronutrients may directly inhibit carcinogen formation or function by binding carcinogens within the intestine; others may exert a more general systemic effect. Table 15-2 is a list of some of the foods and chemicals in foods that inhibit cancer in laboratory animals. Calcium and wheat bran have been used in various preventative trials. It has been reported that 1.5-2.0 g/day of calcium significantly decreases DNA synthesizing cells of high risk patients. Chronic wheat bran supplementation appears to decrease both rectal mucosal DNA synthesis and polyp recurrence.

The action of bile acids appears to be related to the development of colon cancer. Patients who have undergone cholecystectomy have a higher incidence of right-sided colon cancer. Cholecystectomy results in an increased concentration of secondary bile acids, particularly in the right colon. This effect of bile acids may also explain the action of dietary fiber, since the breakdown of carbohydrates (dietary fiber) by anaerobic bacteria results in the lowering of fecal pH, which inhibits conversion of the bile acids to deoxycholic acid, a potential carcinogen.

In addition to the average-risk patients, that is, men and women age 40 and older, there are subgroups in the population at increased risk for colorectal cancer. These include:

1. Patients who have been cured of colorectal cancer
2. Patients who have previously had adenomas

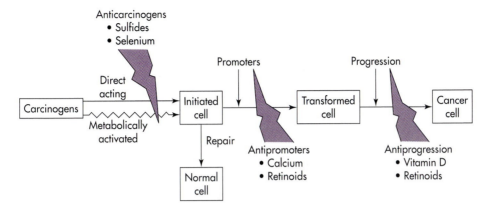

Figure 15-3 Mechanism of action of select dietary anticarcinogens and antipromoters. (From Wargovich MJ: New dietary anticarcinogens and prevention of gastrointestinal cancer, *Dis Colon Rectum* 31:72, 1988.)

Table 15-2   Food and food chemicals that inhibit gastrointestinal cancer in laboratory animals

Food source	Chemical
Grapes, strawberries, apples	Plant phenols
Cabbage, broccoli, Brussels sprouts, cauliflower	Dithiothiones, flavones
Garlic, onions, leeks	Thioethers
Citrus fruits	Terpenes
Carrots, yams, watermelon	Carotenoids

3. Patients who have had universal ulcerative colitis for longer than 7 years
4. Women who have had genital cancer
5. Individuals who have a family history of one of the polyposis syndromes
6. Individuals who have inherited colon cancer syndromes

Although much work needs to be done to clarify further these high-risk subgroups, especially those with familial factors, a much clearer picture exists today of those who are at increased risk for colorectal cancer compared with the average-risk population. Technologic advances have also occurred recently: new methods for fecal occult blood testing, flexible sigmoidoscopy, colonoscopy, and refinement of the double-contrast barium enema.

A desirable goal based on these improvements is early diagnosis for improved survival. This concept is in keeping with the current emphasis on preventive measures for cancer in general and for colorectal cancer specifically. Prevention of colorectal cancer can be defined as primary or secondary. Primary prevention is the identification of factors, either genetic or environmental, responsible for colorectal cancers and their eradication. Secondary prevention may be defined as early detection of colorectal cancer before its more advanced, devastating, and fatal consequences, as well as detection and eradication of premalignant disease before its transformation into cancer.

The terms *hereditary*, *sporadic*, and *familial colorectal cancer* (CRC) have been used by many authors. These terms are defined operationally on the basis of a family history of cancer and possibly other phenotypic information. The sporadic type occurs in the absence of a family history of CRC in a first-degree relative. The familial type occurs when at least one first-degree relative has CRC. In the case of hereditary CRC, there is a family history of CRC occurring in a pattern that indicates autosomal-dominant inheritance. Although this classification does not produce etiologically homogenous groups, it has utility in planning surveillance and management strategies. The long-term objective of study on the genetic epidemiology of CRC is primary and secondary prevention through specific management and surveillance recommendations.

In 1995, Calle and colleagues confirmed earlier studies reporting that ERT decreases risk of developing colon cancer. Every use of ERT was associated with significantly decreased risk of fatal colon cancer (RR=0.71). The reduction in risk was strongest among current users (RR=0.55) and there was a significant trend of decreasing risk with increasing years of use among all users. These associations were not altered in multi-variate analysis controlling for other risk factors.

Screening

The rationale for screening is based on the widely held view that most colorectal cancers are the product of a slow and orderly progression from normal colonic mucosa to adenomatous polyp, early and surgically curable cancer, and, finally, advanced and incurable cancer. Screening is intended to detect and remove cancer in its earliest stages, as well as polyps thought to be precancerous. (e.g., adenomatous polyps measuring more than 1 cm in diameter). However, recommendations for screening vary considerably because of the uncertainty about whether any type of screening is efficacious in reducing the morbidity or mortality of colorectal cancer.

The common clinical manifestations of colorectal cancer are bleeding and anemia, pain, and obstructive symptoms. These manifestations are most common with the advanced lesions. Effective screening implies the examination of asymptomatic persons at high risk to detect early, highly curable lesions. Unlike the detection of many other cancers, detection of colorectal cancer at an early stage is possible with already existing resources. This includes digital examination of the rectum, examination for occult blood in the stool, and radiographic and endoscopic procedures. A large number of rectal cancers occur in the most distal 10 cm of this organ and can be easily palpated by a digital rectal examination. There are few studies that have prospectively or retrospectively evaluated the usefulness of this examination in affecting morbidity or mortality of rectal cancer. However, because of the low cost and ease with which it may be performed, this procedure is to be routinely recommended in all patients. No gynecologist should do a pelvic examination without including an examination of the rectum. Rectovaginal examination affords an excellent opportunity to accomplish an examination of the rectum and a thorough pelvic examination with more adequate evaluation of the cul-de-sac and its contents, as well as other obvious advantages.

The testing of stool for the presence of occult blood as an indicator of gastrointestinal cancer is an old concept. Seventy percent of all colorectal cancer can be detected using fecal occult blood screening; however, 30% of patients do not bleed and are not detected in this manner. In the past, patients were given no dietary restrictions and asked to bring stool samples to be tested with guaiac and hydrogen peroxide solutions. There was no quality control of the stability of the reagents used. Because of the high percentage of false positives and false negatives, this approach fell into disfavor. Benzidine was used in a similar matter but it too was discarded because of an extremely high sensitivity that resulted in a high percentage of false positives and subsequently unnecessary diagnostic workups. Greegor reintroduced the guaiac test for occult blood in the stool: patients, while on high-fiber meat-free diets, were asked to smear onto paper slides impregnated with guaiac two samples of stool per day for 3 days (a total of six smears). The slides were then tested with a reagent of hydrogen peroxide in denatured alcohol. Colorectal cancers were detected in several patients at an early pathologic stage. Following Greegor's reintroduction of the occult blood test in the form of an impregnated guaiac test, several studies and programs were initiated

around the world using this technique in the screening of colorectal cancer. Initial observations were confirmed in other studies in the United States and in Germany. Two control trials were initiated, and these studies demonstrated the feasibility of screening patients with fecal occult blood testing. The rate of positive slides reported by Winawer has been low (2%-5%); the false positivity, low (1%-2%); the predictive value for neoplasia, high (30%-50%); and the Dukes' staging, favorable for cancers detected by screening. The false negative rate and the long-term impact of screening on mortality have not yet been established. Patient compliance and cost effectiveness are major unresolved issues. Currently the American Cancer Society recommends that a fecal occult blood test be done annually after the age of 50. Although hemorrhoids are common in women who have borne children, blood in the stool should never be assumed to be hemorrhoidal unless the source is visualized.

The American Cancer Society, the American College of Obstetricians and Gynecologists, and the National Cancer Institute have similar guidelines for the screening of colorectal cancer. These guidelines are as follows.

Colorectal examination should be included as part of the periodic health examination. At age 50, fecal occult blood testing should be done annually, and a sigmoidoscopy should be performed every 3-5 years. The physician should identify for special surveillance high-risk patients, including those with a strong family history of colon cancer or with personal history of polyps, colon cancer, or inflammatory bowel disease.

Carcinoembryonic antigen (CEA) is not considered to be a screening or diagnostic test for colon cancer, and is used only to monitor disease activity. For monitoring, most investigation using serial values report that this predictor can anticipate recurrence in about one third of patients by approximately 3-6 months. Serial values measured at 2-month intervals the first 2 years after definitive surgery in patients with B2, C1, and C2 lesions and continuing quarterly for an additional 2 years appear useful. Endoscopic procedures have aided significantly in both colon cancer screening and therapy. In addition to assisting in the diagnosis of polyps and early cancers, the removal of polyps may be effected by the endoscopist. This may lead to a total reduction of cancer incidence. Proctosigmoidoscopy, which examines the terminal 25 cm of large bowel, has been technically the easiest for physicians to master, and it has been associated with a finding of unsuspected cancer in 1 of every 435 persons. However, it has been observed that fewer than 20% of physicians routinely use this procedure in their practices. Recently, flexible sigmoidoscopes, which examine up to 60 cm of bowel, have been introduced that may improve routine endoscopic screening procedures.

Objections to the flexible 60 cm colonoscope for screening include cost and an examination time often exceeding 30 minutes. Moreover, advanced training is required to use it effectively. Subsequently, a flexible 35 cm instrument has been developed to overcome these objections: the 35 cm flexible fiber-optic proctosigmoidoscope appears ideally suited for office use. Its cost is relatively low, and the training required is minimal. Although examination of the entire sigmoid colon is feasible, examination to a depth of 30 cm should reveal nearly 65% of bowel cancers and polyps, and pathology yield should be at least twice as great as with the rigid scope. In one investigation involving 26 women, average examination time using a 35 cm two-way tip deflection instrument was 4.3 minutes and a mean insertion depth was 29 cm. The instrument's small cross-sectional diameter and ability to conform to normal bowel curvature minimized patient discomfort. The following guidelines should be observed when screening for colorectal cancer using the fiber-optic sigmoidoscope:

1. Perform fiber-optic sigmoidoscopy examination every 3-5 years on women 50 years or older who have had two initial negative examinations 1 year apart.
2. Identify high-risk patients (those with familial polyposis, ulcerative colitis, polyps, history of carcinoma of the colon, or family history of colon cancer [Table 15-3]) and begin sigmoidoscopy examinations on these patients when they are younger and examine them more frequently.
3. Instruct the patient to prepare herself shortly before the examination with a Phospho-soda enema.
4. After the rectovaginal examination, the patient should be assisted to the dorsal lithotomy position for the sigmoidoscopy examination.
5. Promptly refer any abnormalities that are revealed by screening to a gastroenterologist for diagnosis.

Polyps

The risk of carcinogenesis for an individual who has polyps has been debated for decades. Whether cancer arises in an observable premalignant lesion or whether it arises spontaneously in normal colonic mucosa has great implications for the prevention of colon cancer. Dukes'

Table 15-3   Cancer risk factors

Patient history	Family history	Associated disease
Breast cancer	Colorectal cancer	Granulomatous
Colorectal adenoma	Colorectal polyp	colitis
		Ulcerative colitis
Colorectal cancer	Familial polyposis	
	Gardner's syndrome	
	Juvenile polyposis	

original analysis of 1000 cases of rectal cancer supported the concept of malignant degeneration of polyps but the details of this event have never been fully described. Circumstantial evidence supports the concept that colorectal cancer can arise in a benign polyp: benign adenomatous tissue is frequently observed to be contiguous to frank cancer; cancer risk increases with increasing numbers and sizes of polyps; and animal-human models (familial polyposis) demonstrate that transition does occur. Significantly, intervention studies have demonstrated that removal of benign polyps decreases the incidence of malignancies in large populations. Gilbertsen and his coworkers demonstrated that, in 21,150 persons undergoing proctosigmoidoscopy with polyps removal, the subsequent development of colorectal cancer was 15% of the risk predicted for the general population.

The classifications of adenomatous polyps include tubular adenomas, villotubular or mixed adenomas, and villous adenomas. These polyps occur in all sizes and shapes, and during endoscopy they can be identified as pedunculated, sessile, or semisessile. Regardless of their gross appearance, these polyps all have cytologic characteristics of neoplasia and illustrate a serious disturbance in cell renewal where there is a loss of growth-control mechanism. Mitosis is unrestricted and is observed at all levels of the adenomatous crypt. Cellular differentiation is abnormal, and differentiation into mature goblet cells is incomplete or absent. Therefore, the crypts are lined with tall cells with prominent, elongated, hyperchromatic nuclei arranged in characteristic pseudostratification or picket-fence pattern. The increased cellular mass produces the characteristic villous, tubular, or mixed villotubular growth pattern. One of the most important distinctions to be made by the pathologist and the surgeon in examining adenomatous polyps is whether carcinomatous foci are confined to the area above the muscularis mucosae (in situ) or whether the lesion has traversed this boundary and invaded the submucosa, and as such would be classified as invasive. Intramucosal carcinomas, that is, carcinomas that do not extend beyond the muscularis mucosae, do not metastasize (lymphatics are located in the submucosal layer). However, if left untreated these lesions will progress to invasive carcinoma. Approximately, two thirds of adenomas are tubular; tubular adenomas have less premalignant potential than adenomas with villous features (Figure 15-4). Villous features are more common with increasing size (Figure 15-5). Roughly 5% of patients with adenomas have high-grade dysplasia, and 2%-3% have invasive cancer at time of presentation. Patients presenting with an adenoma have a 40%-50% likelihood of developing another adenoma in the future.

It is agreed that complete polypectomy is a definitive procedure for an in situ carcinoma in an adenomatous

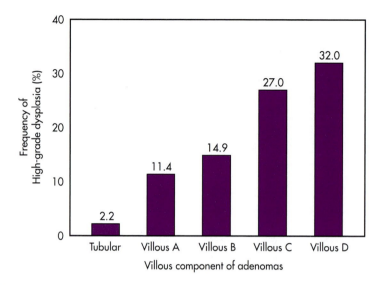

Figure 15-4 The frequency of high-grade dysplasia in adenomas according to histologic classification was determined by the National Polyp Study. (From O'Brien MJ, Winawer SJ, Zauber AG, et al: *Gastroenterology* 98(2):371, 1990.)

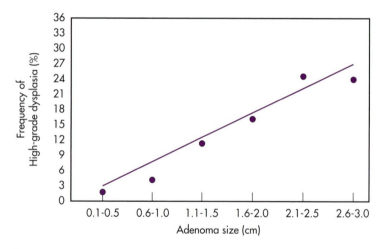

Figure 15-5 The frequency of high-grade dysplasia (severe dysplasia or carcinoma in situ) in adenomas according to size was determined from National Polyp Study data (•, observed; ——, expected regression line). (From O'Brien MJ, Winawer SJ, Zauber AG, et al: *Gastroenterology* 98(2):371, 1990.)

polyp (Figure 15-6). However, there is controversy about treatment of an adenomatous polyp that is found to have an invasive carcinoma (penetration into the submucosa). Several investigators advocate treatment by radical surgical resection when the diagnosis of invasive malignancy has been made, whereas others advocate a more conservative approach. Other factors that should be taken into account are the type of adenomatous polyp and its size. For example, a villous adenoma is the least common of neoplastic polyps. However, it has the highest tendency toward malignant degeneration. In a collected series of cases reviewed by Coutsoftides et al., the overall incidence of invasive malignancy was 30%. In the same

reports, the incidence of positive lymph nodes ranged from 16%-39%. In view of this, most surgeons advise radical surgical treatment of villous adenomas, once invasive malignancy has been confirmed. Another consideration regarding the type of surgery (polypectomy vs radical surgical resection) is the degree of differentiation of the tumor in the presence of lymphatic invasion and/or angioinvasion. For the majority of patients, management of colorectal polyps should be individualized. The therapeutic decision concerning the treatment of invasive carcinomas arising in adenomatous polyps should be based on the polyp's malignant potential and its ability to metastasize. The burden of the surgeon is to confirm the

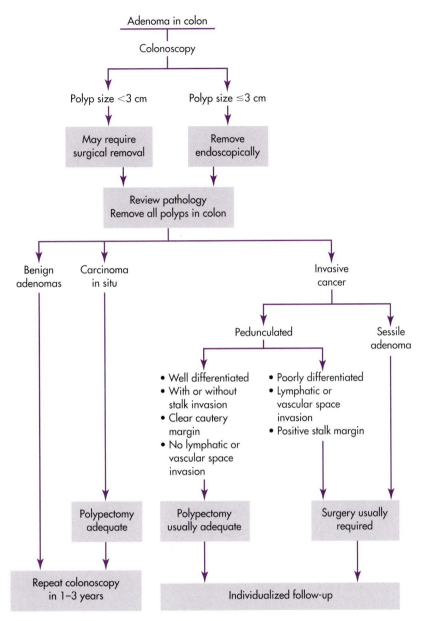

Figure 15-6 Management of adenomas. (Modified from Hornsby-Lewis L et al: *Oncology* 4:142, 1990.)

presence of invasive malignancy by an excisional biopsy examination and to weigh the risks of the presence of involved lymph nodes against the risks of radical surgery.

Staging

Considerable thought should be given to staging. Final staging should depend on histology, the depth of penetration, the involvement of the nodes, differentiation, mucinous content, signet-ring appearance, pushing vs infiltrating margins, venous or perineural invasion, and lymphoplasmacytosis. Ideally, to assure reasonably accurate staging, at least a dozen lymph nodes should be found in the specimen. Various staging classifications have been proposed (see box on p. 436).

Among the most commonly used staging classifications is that of Dukes and its modifications. These modifications are based on the ability of two pathologic features of rectal cancer to predict prognosis: lymph node involvement and depth of tumor penetration. The Astler-Coller modification of this system stresses the depth of penetration as an independent variable in prognosis (Table 15-4).

In addition to surgical staging, there are other variables that have adverse effects on the prognosis of patients who have primary colorectal cancers: ulceration of the primary tumor, fixation to adjacent organs, rectal origin, colonic perforation or obstruction, younger age, and elevated preoperative carcinoembryonic antigen (CEA). Most

---

STAGING FOR COLORECTAL CANCER OF THE AMERICAN JOINT COMMITTEE ON CANCER, AMERICAN CANCER SOCIETY, AND AMERICAN COLLEGE OF SURGEONS COMMISSION ON CANCER

Primary tumor (T)

TX	Primary tumor cannot be assessed
T0	No evidence of primary tumor
Tis	Carcinoma in situ
T1	Tumor invades submucosa
T2	Tumor invades muscularis propria
T3	Tumor invades through the muscularis propria into the subserosa, or into non-peritonealized pericolic or perirectal tissues
T4	Tumor perforates the visceral peritoneum or directly invades other organs or structures.*

Regional lymph nodes (N)

NX	Regional lymph nodes cannot be assessed
N0	No regional lymph node metastasis
N1	Metastasis in 1-3 pericolic or perirectal lymph nodes
N2	Metastasis in 4 or more pericolic or perirectal lymph nodes
N3	Metastasis in any lymph node along the course of a named vascular trunk

Distant metastasis (M)

Mx	Presence of distant metastasis cannot be assessed
M0	No distant metastasis
M1	Distant metastasis

Stage grouping

				Dukes†
Stage 0	Tis	N0	M0	
Stage 1	T1	N0	M0	A
	T2	N0	M0	
Stage II	T3	N0	M0	B
	T4	N0	M0	
Stage III	Any T	N1	M0	C
	Any T	N2, N3	M0	
Stage IV	Any T	Any N	MI	

T, Primary tumor; N, regional lymph nodes; M, distant metastasis
*Direct invasion of other organs or structures includes invasion of other segments of colorectum by way of serosa (e.g., invasion of the sigmoid colon by a carcinoma of the cecum).
†Dukes' B is a composite of better (T3, N0, M0) and worse (T4, N0, M0) prognostic groups, as is Dukes' C (any T, N1, M0 and any T, N2, N3, M0).

Table 15-4   Dukes' classification: Astler-Coller modification

Stage	Extension	5-year survival (%)
A	Mucosa only	95
B	Bowel wall involvement	
B₁	Within wall	85-90
B₂ (m)	Microscopically through wall	60-70
B₂ (g)	Grossly through wall	50
B₃	Adjacent structures involved	30
C	Lymph nodes positive for tumor	
C₁	Within wall	40-50
C₂ (m)	Microscopically through wall	40-50
C₂ (g)	Grossly through wall	15-25
C₃	Adjacent structures involved	10-20
D	Distant metastatic disease	<5

clinical studies indicate that the Dukes staging system, or its variations, is the single most important prognostic variable.

Chemoprevention

Several research disciplines working together in the area of chemoprevention research are contributing to the identification of effective cancer inhibitors, both synthetic and naturally occurring chemical compounds. The chemoprevention program of the National Cancer Institute is studying these basically nontoxic chemical agents that may inhibit the development of cancer in asymptomatic, mostly high risk subjects. This program is systematically pursuing the development of effective agents through:

1. Information management of research leads from laboratory and epidemiology studies
2. Biochemical and in vitro screening of new chemo preventive agents

3. In vivo animal model screening
4. Chemopreventative agent procurement
5. Toxicology testing
6. Clinical chemoprevention trials

The National Cancer Institute is supporting several phase III colon cancer prevention trials that are designed to evaluate the effects of vitamin C and E, beta carotene, and calcium in subjects with adenomatous polyps. In addition, smaller phase I and II trials are being conducted in high risk subjects at various institutes to study the effectiveness of calcium citrate, calcium carbonate, wheat bran, Beta carotene, piroxicam (a prostaglandin synthesis inhibitor), difluoromethylornithine, and Ibuprofen.

Surgical Therapy

The only curative therapy for colorectal cancer is surgical resection of the primary tumor and regional mesentery lymph nodes. The extent of colorectal surgery is determined by anatomic landmarks. These include lymphatic drainage of the colon and rectum, location of the superior mesenteric artery, the middle and left colic arteries, the marginal artery, the inferior mesenteric artery, and the superior hemorrhoidal vessels. As stated by Stearns, the essential elements of resection are (1) wide removal of the cancer-bearing colon or rectal segments, (2) wide excision of the lymphatics draining the cancer-bearing segment of the bowel, and (3) accomplishing (1) and (2) with a minimum of cancer-cell contamination and embolization. The extent of surgery is well standardized for lesions draining into the superior mesenteric artery: a right colectomy is a well-established practice. However, as one approaches the rectosigmoid and rectum, there is controversy about treatment, and alternative procedures arise. The basic trend has been for more conservative surgery and the use of sphincter-saving approaches for lesions of the proximal two thirds of the rectum. Another consideration for treatment of these tumors is the extension of the lymph node dissection to the retroperitoneal or pelvic nodes. Most studies of these approaches show no gain in survival but show increased morbidity and mortality. On the other hand, considerable evidence suggests that when a tumor extends to adjacent structures, particularly in rectosigmoid and rectal cancer, en bloc resection is preferable to other approaches and results in a higher level of salvage. The reason is that a significant percentage of tumors, although involving adjacent structures, do not show lymph node or distant metastases. The bladder, ureter, vagina, small bowel, abdominal wall, uterus, and ovary may all be involved contiguously with tumor and may require resection. The margin in the bowel wall itself is classically 5 cm from the gross tumor edge. This is of particular importance in rectal surgery. However, there is evidence that a 2-3 cm margin may be adequate in some patients. In general, the stage of colorectal cancer relates closely to prognosis (Figure 15-7).

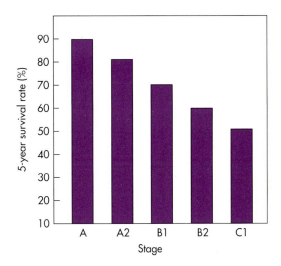

Figure 15-7 The stage of colorectal cancer relates closely to prognosis.

Adjuvant Therapy

Although colorectal cancers are among the most highly curable neoplasms, almost half of the patients will relapse. The potential benefits of adjuvant therapy for colorectal cancer must therefore be seriously considered. The goals of such therapy are to prevent or delay the recurrence of the disease and to increase the percent of patients who survive. For lesions at high risk for local recurrence, adjuvant radiation therapy has been studied. Both preoperative and postoperative radiation has been used. The goal of preoperative radiation therapy is to decrease the dissemination of cancer at surgery and to downstage the primary tumor. Postoperative radiation is used for patients at high risk for local recurrence, for example, those with transmural invasion, known metastasis, and direct invasion of adjacent organs. Nonrandomized studies of postoperative therapy have suggested that such treatment has potential for decreasingly local recurrences.

Adjuvant chemotherapy programs have generally utilized 5-FU or 5-FU plus methyl-CCNU. Cooperative group studies have demonstrated a 5%-10% benefit in 5-year survival for patients receiving adjuvant 5-FU. For Dukes C colon cancer, a significant disease-free survival benefit was noted: 40% of adjuvantly treated patients had recurrence at 5 years vs 52% of controls. Several studies of large numbers of patients with Dukes stages B and C tumors suggest that adjuvant chemotherapy may delay recurrence without necessarily prolonging survival in all treated patients. In other studies, certain subgroups of patients appear to benefit more than others but consistent overall benefits have not been demonstrated. However, investigators have attempted to improve the therapeutic index of 5-FU by incorporating biochemical modulators or synergistically acting agents to their drug regimens. Agents such as levamisole and streptozotocin have been used in combination with 5-FU. Doses were administered to optimize objective response rates. None of the regimens demonstrated a significant statistical difference over that achieved by 5-FU alone.

The immunomodulatory agent levamisole plus 5-FU has demonstrated improved disease-free survival when compared to survival of a similar group of patients receiving no adjuvant therapy for Dukes C lesions. Three randomized clinical trials involving more than 400 patients have evaluated the addition of levamisole to 5-FU chemotherapy for patients with metastatic disease with no positive results in favor of the levamisole containing treatment arms. Based on this trial and the earlier positive results with levamisole, two adjuvant chemotherapy trials were reported in 1989. The North Central Cancer Treatment Group at the Mayo clinic reported the results of a randomized study containing levamisole alone to a combination of levamisole plus 5-FU to no further therapy after surgery. A total of 101 eligible patients were randomized: 21 patients had primary rectal cancer and the remaining patients had colon cancer; 40% had tumors invading through the bowel wall that spread to regional lymph nodes. With a median follow-up in excess of 7 years, the levamisole plus 5-FU combination demonstrated a significant improvement in disease free survival compared to no further therapy (P=0.02). Overall, however, there was no improvement in survival. Subset analysis by stage demonstrated a significant decreased disease-free survival advantage for 5-FU and levamisole only in stage C patients. Subsequent studies were conducted by other cooperative groups, and in 1990 the National Cancer Institute Consensus Development Conference recommended that stage II patients unable to participate in clinical trials be offered adjuvant 5-FU and levamisole.

Several non-randomized trails of adjuvant preoperative radiation suggested a possible survival benefit with a dose of 5000 rads. Memorial Hospital/Sloan-Kettering Cancer Center performed the first randomized prospective study and refuted their own retrospective results in that no survival advantage was seen in any subgroup. Although the rate of local recurrence was decreased by therapy, the incidence of blood borne metastasis increased. A large scale cooperative trial of the VA Surgical Adjuvant Group found otherwise. Utilizing 2000-3000 rads in 2 weeks, there was a significant improvement in 5-year survival among patients undergoing abdominal peritoneal resections. From 28.4% for controls to 40.8% in treated patients. Similar studies are underway with conflicting preliminary results.

Combined modality for colorectal cancer has frequently been used in adjuvant settings. The relapse rate for combined-modality therapy appears to be significantly lower than that of surgery alone. Several randomized and non-randomized studies have been done to evaluate the impact of adjuvant therapy on both the local recurrence rate and the overall rates in patients with rectal cancer. These studies included radiotherapy administered preop-

eratively, postoperatively, both pre- and postoperatively, and, more recently, with concomitant chemotherapy in single and multi drug regimens. In general, these studies indicated the incidence of local recurrence can be reduced by approximately 50% with the use of moderate dose radiation. However, there is no demonstrable survival benefit for this adjuvant treatment approach.

Certainly, the selection of patients likely to benefit from adjuvant therapy of colorectal cancer is based primarily on accurate surgical staging. The application of new techniques to assess the biologic aggressiveness of a tumor may allow identification of patients with particularly poor prognosis. Continued progress in understanding the molecular genetics of initiation and progression of colorectal cancer may ultimately enable the use of molecular staging to further refine our clinical prognostic ability.

Recurrence Patterns

Recurrence patterns for colorectal cancer are the result of local extension or implantation, as well as lymphatic or hematogenous dissemination. Distant failures to the lung or liver are the most dramatic but local and regional failures also occur frequently. As an initial pattern of failure from colorectal cancer, distant metastases alone are distinctly uncommon. Autopsy studies confirm that abdominal failure is common and almost 75% of patients will die from intra-abdominal causes. Although lung and liver metastases are also common, they account for fewer than 25% of all deaths. Patients who have isolated liver metastases form a small but highly interesting and extensively studied group of patients. Early detection of such patients by CT scan has led to a new appreciation of the long median survivals that may be achieved in patients who have disease limited to a single or a few unilobular metastases—18-24 months in many series. Small numbers of patients treated by direct infusion of 5-FU into the portal system have had impressive remissions, although follow-up is still brief. This type of approach seems beneficial for this subgroup of patients. The use of CEA as a tumor marker has helped in monitoring patients for recurrent cancer. Often an elevated CEA level is the earlier sign of recurrence. Minton has reported on the use of CEA values to direct second-look surgery. The goal of such surgery was to determine whether early detection, thus early intervention, would lead to improved survival in patients who had recurrent disease. Although 5-year survivals of approximately 30% have been reported in such patients when they are resected with curative intent, control studies of CEA-directed second-look surgery are lacking, and further studies are indicated.

Approximately 35% of colon cancer patients who have surgery will have disease spread to regional lymph nodes, and about 25%-35% of these patients will survive 5 years. After surgical resection for colorectal carcinoma, about 60% of tumor recurrences are within the first 2 years, and 90% occur within 5 years of the surgical resection.

Despite these recurrence rates, a potential for cure remains in a select population of patients who develop recurrent colorectal carcinomas after definitive resection. For example, the recurrence of adenocarcinoma of the colon or rectum at a site of previous anastomosis is a failure of the primary surgical treatment, which in some patients can be managed successfully by additional operative procedures. In this particular group of patients, when complete resection of the recurrent tumor can be performed, the survival rates are surprisingly high.

Close follow-up and evaluation of patients who have colorectal carcinoma must be priorities. Some guidelines for clinical application may be drawn from knowledge of the patterns of tumor spread of colorectal carcinoma. High-risk areas for recurrence can be identified, and clinical attention must be focused on these sites for early detection of recurrence and subsequent palliative or curative resection. Obviously, a complete history and a complete physical examination are important elements of such evaluation. The value of rectal examinations and subsequent stool guaiac testing cannot be overemphasized. One must be aware of the conditions that can produce false readings on stool guaiac testing. The physician must make sure that the patient has not been on a diet containing rare meat, turnips, or horseradish for 48 hours. No aspirin or vitamin supplements containing vitamin C in excess of 250 mg per day should be taken. A history of bleeding from the rectum or a positive stool guaiac test should be followed by rigid proctosigmoidoscopy or flexible sigmoidoscopy examination. If the endoscopy is negative, the patient should undergo a double-contrast barium enema or colonoscopy. Colonoscopy also plays an important role in the patients being followed for tumor detection. Many physicians recommend colonoscopy every 6 months for the first year or two and then yearly thereafter (Table 15-5).

Therapy of Recurrence

For purposes of therapy, patients who have recurrent colorectal carcinomas may be divided into three groups:

1. Those who have local or regional recurrences
2. Those who have hepatic metastasis
3. Those who have widely disseminated disease

Surgery for local or regional recurrences may result in secondary cure in selected groups of patients, although control trials are lacking. External beam irradiation for recurrent colorectal cancer has been associated with palliation of symptoms in a reasonably large proportion of patients, but low survival rates can be expected. Detection of recurrence at the anastomotic site by barium enema remains the most favorable pattern of recurrence in terms of secondary cure.

Patients with apparently localized hepatic metastasis may survive for 2 years, even without therapy. Uncontrolled studies of surgical resection of hepatic metastases have demonstrated 5-year survivals of approximately 25% in selected patients. In some series, 25% of patients

Table 15-5   Postoperative follow-up in colorectal carcinoma

First year after resection of primary tumor

Physical examination (including stool guaiac testing)	Every 3 months
Liver function tests	Every 3 months (CT scan if abnormal)
Carcinoembryonic antigen	Every 3 months (begin 6 weeks after surgery)
Colonoscopy	Every 6 months
Chest roentgenogram	Every 6 months

Second year after resection of primary tumor

Physical examination (including stool guaiac testing)	Every 6 months
Liver function tests	Every 6 months
Carcinoembryonic antigen	Every 3 months
Colonoscopy	Every 6 months
Chest roentgenogram	Every 6 months

Third year and yearly thereafter

Physical examination and stool guaiac testing
Liver-function tests
Carcinoembryonic antigen
Colonoscopy
Intravenous pyelogram (rectal carcinoma)
Chest roentgenogram

who have liver metastases have resectable disease, and 25% of that group will benefit from resection. This means that 7% of patients who have hepatic metastases will benefit from surgical resection. This is a small number, and its merits have to be closely evaluated with future studies. For patients who have unresectable hepatic metastases, infusional chemotherapy has been advocated. Hepatic-directed infusional therapy via the hepatic artery circulation results in drug concentrations to the liver that are significantly higher than those achieved by systemic infusion of the same drug. Nonrandomized studies suggest that the response rates are indeed higher than those seen with systemic chemotherapy. This approach has received renewed interest because of totally implantable infusion pumps. Phase II studies with such devices indicate response rates of more than 80% with median survivals as long as 26 months. One drug favored for such infusion therapy is floxuridine (FUDR). The drug 5-fluorouracil (5-FU) has been the most widely tested for systemic therapy with a 20% partial objective response rate in most studies. The optimum dose and schedule has not been determined, although numerous studies of standard bolus therapy indicate that some moderate degree of systemic toxicity is necessary to achieve objective response. Clinical trials are under way to evaluate response rates and survival with continuous infusion 5-FU therapy compared with standard bolus therapy. In addition to 5-FU, only mitomycin-C and the nitrosoureas (CCNU, BCNU, methyl-CCNU) are generally considered to have any degree of activity. The most extensively evaluated combination of 5-FU and methyl-CCNU was initially reported to have a response rate of greater than 40%, but later trials failed to confirm this superiority to 5-FU alone.

In general, benefits from systemic chemotherapy are limited by low partial-response rate with generally low durations of response. Although some patients may achieve palliation of symptoms, prolongation of survival has to date been an illusive goal. Further investigations of new agents and promising combinations are needed.

BLADDER CANCER

More than 90% of the bladder tumors accruing in the Northern Hemisphere are transitional cell lesions, with adenocarcinoma, squamous carcinoma, and sarcomas making up the remainder. Tumors originating from the urothelial lining of the bladder in women have an occurrence of 13,200 cases in the United States in 1995. Thirty-seven thousand occurred in men. Bladder cancer is the ninth most common form of cancer in women and the fourteenth leading cause of cancer deaths in women. Hematuria, usually associated with increased frequency of urination are the usual warning signals promoted by the American Cancer Society and others. Smoking is the greatest risk factor for bladder cancer, with smokers experiencing twice the risk of non-smokers. Smoking is estimated to be responsible for approximately 37% of the bladder cancer deaths among women. Overall, the incidence of bladder cancer is four times greater among men than among women and it is higher in whites than in blacks. People living in urban areas and workers exposed to dye, rubber, or leather also are at higher risk. Surgery alone or in combination with other treatments is used in over 90% of cases.

Pathology

Over 90% of urothelial tumors are transitional (epidermoid) cell carcinoma; the remainder are squamous cell (6%-8%) carcinoma, adenocarcinoma, or urachal carcinoma. The majority of epidermoid tumors originate in the lateral and posterior bladder wall, whereas adenocarcinoma is found in the dome of the bladder and the trigone. Lesions can occur within bladder diverticula. Urachal cancer originates from the urachus, an embryonic remnant of the gut, and is similar to colonic adenocarcinoma, producing carcinoembryonic antigen (CEA).

The urinary bladder is lined with five to seven avascular layers of transitional cells attached to a lamina propria that separates mucosa from muscle. Adipose tissue surrounds the bladder, and the parietal peritoneum covers the cephalad portion of the bladder. Nerves, blood vessels, and lymphatics invade muscle and lamina propria, explaining lymphatic and hematogenous patterns of dissemination with high-grade lesions. Metastases can involve the hypogastric lymph node chain, as well as the obturator nodes at the junction of the internal and external iliac vessels. Nodal metastases may drain from this point to the aortic bifurcation and further up the aortic chain. Common sites for metastases include, in addition to regional lymph nodes, lung, liver and bone.

Diagnosis and Staging

Cystoscopy under anesthesia with bimanual palpation and appropriate biopsies is mandatory for diagnosis. Urinary cytology is extremely useful and more often is positive

Table 15-6 Bladder cancer staging systems

AJC*	Bladder cancer	JSM†
Primary tumor		
TX	Cannot be assessed	—
T0	No tumor clinically	—
Tis	Carcinoma in situ (flat)	0
Ta	Papillary non invasive tumor	0
T1	No microscopic invasion beyond lamina propria; induration on bimanual examination; freely mobile mass that disappears after resection	A
T2	Microscopic invasion of superficial bladder muscle; mobile induration of bladder on bimanual examination that disappears after resection	B1
T3	Tumor invades into muscle or perivesical fat; induration or nodular mobile mass that persists after transurethral resection	
	• T3a Deep muscle invasion	B2
	• T3b Perivesical fat invasion	C
T4	Tumor fixed or invades neighboring structures	
	• T4a Prostate, uterus, vagina invasion	D1
	• T4b Tumor fixed to pelvic walls or invades abdominal wall	D1
N	**Regional lymph nodes**	
NX	Cannot be assessed	—
N0	No tumor	—
N1	Single homolateral regional lymph node	D1
N2	Contralateral, bilateral, multiple regional nodes	D1
N3	Fixed mass on pelvic wall with space between mass and tumor	D1
N4	Tumor involves just regional lymph nodes	D2
M	**Distant metastasis**	
MX	Cannot be assessed	
M0	No known distant metastasis	
M1	Distant metastases	D2

*AJC, American Joint Commission.
†JSM, Jewett-Strong-Marshall.

after cystoscopy. Flow cytometry is being used increasingly for diagnosis and to better define the extent of tumor aneuploidy as a possible prognostic sign. Additional tests include an intravenous urogram to evaluate the upper tracts, as well as the urinary bladder, and a pelvic and abdominal CT scan. The role of transvaginal and abdominal ultrasonography is still uncertain. While the Jewett-Strong-Marshall staging system has been used in the United States, the American Joint Commission system outlined in Table 15-6 is more precise. Stage 0 indicates superficial mucosal tumors, both SIS (TIS) and exophytic papillary (TA) lesions. Invasion into the lamina propria is stage A (T1); stage B-1 (T2) denotes tumor confined to less than half of the bladder muscle; B-2 (T3a) denotes tumor involving more than half of the bladder muscle. Anaplastic tumors are deeply infiltrating in the muscle, whereas Grade 1 well-differentiated lesions tend to be B-1. Stage C (T3b) tumors involve perivesical fat. Stage D-1 involves adjacent local extension to prostate (T4a) or lymph nodes below the sacral promontory (N1-3), and D-2 (N4) denotes nodal involvement above the sacrum. Superficial tumors (Ta, TIS, T1), represent about 70% of newly diagnosed cases. Muscle infiltrating tumors (T2, T3, T4), represent about 25% and metastatic tumors (N$^+$ or M$^+$) represent about 5% of cases.

Treatment and Results

Therapy for superficial lesions (Stages 0, A, and sometimes B-1) is in most cases endoscopic resection and fulguration with cystoscopy repeated every 3 months. When lesions recur frequently or are diffuse, another therapy utilized is thiotepa 60 mg/60 ml normal saline instilled intravesically for 2 hours and then weekly for 6 consecutive weeks. Approximately 30%-40% of patients will respond, particularly those with low-grade papillary lesions. Since this drug is absorbed following intravesical administration, severe myelosuppression can occur. BCG 120 mg/50 ml normal saline has been found to be extremely efficacious when given weekly for 6 weeks, resulting in 60% of cases achieving complete remission following intravesical administration. Although three randomized studies find similar response rates with BCG and a marked delay in time to cystectomy when compared with a control arm, this agent is still not licensed in the United States for this indication. Other agents utilized include mitomycin-C, 20-60 mg/20-40 ml, and doxoru-

bicin 20-60 mg; both of these agents can cause serious bladder irritation after intravesical administration. Radical cystectomy is utilized for diffuse or recurrent superficial lesions, a procedure resulting in a 5-year survival rate of 70%-90%. Clinicians vary in their judgment of precisely what existing circumstances constitute indications for radical therapy. Standard therapy for stages B-C disease is radical cystectomy with resection of local pelvic nodes. If local organ invasion has occurred, the prostate, seminal vesicle, urethra, and part of the ureters may have to be removed. Recent modifications of urinary diversion have resulted in the contingent pouch as an option for these patients. Segmental or partial cystectomy should only be used in selected patients presenting with a single lesion outside the trigone, and without areas of TIS. Most data for preoperative and postoperative radiation therapy suggest little benefit in preventing tumor dissemination. Overall 5-year survival rates for stages B-C range from 30%-50%; in patients presenting with papillary low-grade lesions, survival is 60%-75%. When surgery is medically contraindicated, supervoltage irradiation, 6000 cGy to 7000 cGy in 6-8 weeks, can produce 5-year survival rates for approximately 20%-30% or higher for B1-1 and C disease. A major difficulty in evaluating the efficacy of irradiation is the high clinical staging error with large bladder tumors.

For chemotherapy, the most active single agents are cisplatin and methotrexate, and to a lesser extent, doxorubicin, vinblastine, and mitomycin-C. Single agents induce response in 15%-30% of cases; few responses are complete. Most combinations employ cisplatin and doxorubicin, frequently with cyclophosphamide. Lymph node involvement (stage D2, N1-4) is an extremely poor prognostic sign, with 50% of the patients undergoing radical cystectomy and lymph node dissection dying in less than 1 year; 87% die in less than 2 years. The 5-year survival rate is 0%-7% with most patients dying from disseminated disease.

Follow-up of patients after therapy consists of a chest film at 2-3 month intervals, urine cytology, and an intravenous urogram at 6-12 month intervals. Abdominal and pelvic CT scans need to be performed within the first 2 months following radical cystectomy to serve as a baseline for future examination at 5-6 month intervals during the first 1-2 years.

BIBLIOGRAPHY

Achkar E, Carey W: Small polyps found during fiberoptic sigmoidoscopy in asymptomatic patients, *Ann Intern Med* 109:880, 1988.

ACOG Committee Opinion: Routine cancer screening, 128: Oct 1993.

American College of Obstetricians and Gynecologists: Report of task force on routine cancer screening, ACOG Committee Opinion Number 68, Washington, DC: ACOG 1989.

American Joint Committee on Cancer: *Manual for staging of cancer*, ed 3, Philadelphia, 1988, JB Lippincott.

Astler VB, Coller FA: The prognostic significance of direct extension of cancer of the colon and rectum, *Ann Surg* 139:846, 1954.

Balslev JB et al: Postoperative radiotherapy in Dukes' B and C carcinoma of the rectum and rectosigmoid. A randomized multicenter study, *Cancer* 58:22, 1986.

Beart RW Jr: Colon, rectum, and anus, *Cancer* 33:684, 1990.

Bohlman TW, Katon BM, Lipshutz GR: Fiberoptic pansigmoidoscopy: an evaluation and comparison with rigid sigmoidoscopy, *Gastroenterology* 72:644, 1977.

Bostick RM et al: Sugar, meat, and fat intake, and non-dietary risk factors for colon cancer incidence in Iowa women, *Cancer Causes Control* 5:38, 1994.

Burkitt DP: Some neglected leads to cancer causation, *J Natl Ca Inst* 47:913, 1971.

Buroker TR et al: A controlled evaluation of recent approaches to biochemical modulation of enhancement of 5-fluorouracil therapy in colorectal carcinoma, *J Clin Oncol* 3:1624, 1985.

Calle EE, Miracle-McMahill HL, Thun MJ, Health CW: Estrogen replacement therapy and risk of fatal colon cancer in a prospective cohort of postmenopausal women, *J Natl Cancer Inst* 87(7):51, 1995.

Coutsoftides T et al: Malignant polyps of the colon and rectum: a clinicopathologic study, *Dis Colon Rectum* 22:82, 1979.

Davis HL: Chemotherapy of large bowel cancer, *Cancer* 50(11):2638, 1982.

Decosse JJ, Tsioulias GJ, Jacobson JS: Colorectal cancer: detection, treatment, and rehabilitation, *Ca J Clin* 44:27, 1994.

Decosse JJ, Tsioulias GJ, Jacobson JS: Colorectal cancer: detection, treatment, and rehabilitation, *Ca J Clin* 44:27, 1994.

DeVita VT, Hellman S, Rosenberg SA, editors: *Cancer: principles and practice of oncology*, ed 2, Philadelphia, 1985, JB Lippincott.

Division of Cancer Prevention and Control National Cancer Institute: Working Guidelines for early cancer detection: rationale and supporting evidence to decrease mortality, Bethesda, MD: The Institute: 1, 1987.

Dukes CE, Bussey HJR: The spread of rectal cancer and its effect on prognosis, *Br J Cancer* 12:309, 1958.

Dwyer J: Dietary fiber and colorectal cancer risk, *Nutr Rev* 51:147, 1993.

Ehya H, O'Hara BJ: Brush cytology in the diagnosis of colonic neoplasms, *Cancer* 66(7):1563, 1990.

Enblad P, Adami HO, Glimelius B et al: The risk of subsequent primary malignant diseases after cancers of the colon and rectum, *Cancer* 65 (9):2091, 1990.

Fath RB, Winawer SJ: Early diagnosis of colorectal cancer, *Ann Rev Med* 34:501, 1984.

Ferguson LR, Lynch JF: Towards reducing the incidence of colorectal cancer: the role of inheritance and diet, *Mutagenesis* 8:377, 1993.

Fisher HAG: Diagnosis and management of early-stage bladder cancer, *Curr Concepts Oncol* 4:1986.

Gastrointestinal Tumor Study Group: Adjuvant therapy of colon cancer: results of a prospectively randomized trial, *N Engl J Med* 310:737, 1984.

Gerard A et al: Preoperative radiotherapy as adjuvant treatment in rectal cancer, *Ann Surg* 208:606, 1988.

Gilbertsen VA: Proctosigmoidoscopy and polypectomy in reducing the incidence of rectal cancer, *Cancer* 34:936, 1974.

Gilbertsen VA, Nelms JN: The prevention of invasive cancer of the rectum, *Cancer* 41:1137, 1978.

Gilbertsen VA et al: The earlier detection of colorectal cancers: a preliminary report of the results of the occult blood study, *Cancer* 45:2899, 1980.

Grabe JL, Kozarek RA, and Sanowski RA: Flexible versus rigid sigmoidoscopy: a comparison using inexpensive 35 cm flexible proctosigmoidoscopy, *Am J Gastroenterol* 78:569, 1983.

Grage TB, Moss SE: Adjuvant chemotherapy in cancer of the colon and rectum: controlled randomized trial, *Surg Clin North Am* 61:1321, 1981.

Greegor DH: Diagnosis of large bowel cancer in the asymptomatic patient, *JAMA* 201:943, 1967.

Greenwald P: Colon cancer overview *Cancer Supplement* 70(5):1206, 1992.

Grem JL, Allegra CJ: Toxicity of levamisole and 5-fluorouracil in human colon carcinoma cells, *J Natl Cancer Inst* 81:1413, 1989.

Gryska PV, Cohen AM: Screening asymptomatic patients at high risk for colon cancer with full colonoscopy, *Dis Colon Rectum* 30(1):18, 1987.

Gunderson LL, Sosin H: Areas of failure found at reoperation (second or symptomatic look) following "curative surgery" for adenocarcinoma of the rectum, *Cancer* 34:1278, 1974.

Health and Public Policy Committee, American College of Physicians: Clinical competence in colonoscopy, *Ann Intern Med* 107:772, 1987.

Herr HW: Conservative management of muscle-invading bladder cancer: prospective experience, *J Urol* 138:1162, 1987.

Herr HW, Laudone VP, Whitmore WF Jr: Review article: an overview of intravesical therapy for superficial bladder tumors, *J Urol* 138:363, 1987.

Herr HW et al: BCG therapy alters the progression of superficial bladder cancer, *J Clin Oncol* 6:1450, 1988.

Higgins GA et al: The case for adjuvant 5-fluorouracil in colorectal cancer, *Cancer Clin Trials* 1:35, 1978.

Higgins GA et al: Preoperative radiation and surgery for cancer of the rectum, Veterans administration Surgical Oncology Group Trial II, *Cancer* 58:352, 1986.

Hornsby-Lewis L, Winawer SJ: Natural history and current management of colorectal polyps, *Oncology* 4:139, 1990.

Jacobs EJ, White E, Weiss NS: Exogenous hormones, reproductive history, and colon cancer, *Cancer Causes Control* 3:359, 1994.

Kritchevsky D: Diet, nutrition, and cancer: the role of fiber, *Cancer* 58(8):1830, 1986.

Kuo DY, Smith HO, Runwicz CD, Goldberg GL: Cecal cancer in teenager presenting with a pelvic mass: a case report and review of the literature, *Gynecol Oncol* 55(1):149, 1994.

Laurie JA et al: Surgical adjuvant therapy of large-bowel carcinoma: an evaluation of levamisole and the combination of levamisole and 5-fluorouracil, *J Clin Oncol* 7:1447, 1989.

Letsou G, Ballantyne GH, Zdon MJ et al: Screening for colorectal neoplasms: a comparison of the fecal occult blood test and endoscopic examination, *Dis Colon Rectum* 30(11):839, 1987.

Levin B: Colorectal cancer: approach to long-term management, *Adv Oncol* 2(2):16, 1986.

Lipkin M, Newmark H: Effect of added dietary calcium on colonic epithelial cell proliferation in subjects at high risk for familial colonic cancer, *N Engl J Med* 313:1381, 1985.

Lush DT: Screening for colorectal cancer: use of a new protocol may reduce death rates, *Postgrad Med* 96:99, 1994.

Lynch HT et al: Colon cancer genetics, *Cancer Supplement* 70(5):1300, 1992.

Mansour EG et al: Combined modality therapy following resection of colorectal carcinoma in patients with non-measurable intra-abdominal metastases, an ECOG study 3282, *Proc Am Soc Clin Oncol* 9:107, 1990.

Marshall VF, McCarron JP Jr: The curability of vesical cancer: greater now or then? *Cancer Res* 37:2753, 1977.

Metlin C, Cummings KM: The current status of early detection and screening of colorectal cancer, *Sem Surg Oncol* 2(4):215, 1988.

Metlin C et al: Management and survival of adenocarcinoma of the rectum in the United States: results of a national survey by the American College of Surgery, *Oncology* 39:265, 1978.

Minton JP: Colon cancer: special surgical considerations, *Cancer* 50:2624, 1982.

Moertel CG: Chemotherapy for colorectal cancer, *N Engl J Med* 330:1136, 1994.

Mommsen S, Aagaard J: Tobacco as a risk factor in bladder cancer, *Carcinogenesis* 4:335, 1983.

Murphy WM et al: Urinary cytology and bladder cancer: the cellular features of transitional cell neoplasms, *Cancer* 53:1555, 1984.

Nava H, Pagana T: Postoperative surveillance of colorectal carcinoma, *Cancer* 49:1043, 1982.

Neugut AI, Pita S: Role of sigmoidoscopy in screening for colorectal cancer: a critical view, *Gastroenterology* 95:492, 1988.

Niederhuber JE: Colon and rectum cancer, *Cancer* 71(12):4187, 1993.

O'Brien MJ, Winawer SJ, Zauber AG et al: The national polyp study: patients and polyp characteristics associated with high grade dysplasia in colorectal adenomas, *Gastroenterology* 98:371, 1990.

Prout GR Jr, Griffin PP, Shipley WU: Bladder carcinoma as a systemic disease, *Cancer* 43:2532, 1979.

Prout GR Jr et al: Combined therapies in the treatment with muscle-invasive bladder carcinoma: a preliminary report of a bladder-sparing effort (Abstr), *J Urol* 139:268, 1988.

Ransohoff DF, Lang CA: Screening for colorectal cancer, *N Engl J Med* 325:37, 1991.

Reddy BS, Burill C, Rigotty J: Effects of diets in omega-3 and omega-6 fatty acids on initiation and post initiation stages of colon carcinogenesis, *Cancer Res* 51:487, 1991.

Reddy BS et al: Chemoprevention of colon carcinogenesis by concurrent administration of piroxicam, a nonsteroidal antiinflammatory drug with D, l-a-difluoromethylornithine, an ornithine decarboxylase inhibitor in diet, *Cancer Res* 50:2562, 1990.

Rosato FE, Marks SG: Changing site distribution patterns of colorectal cancer at Thomas Jefferson University Hospital, *Dis Colon Rectum* 24:93, 1981.

Shipley WU, Prout GR Jr, Kaufman DS: Bladder cancer: advances in laboratory innovations and clinical management, with emphasis on innovations allowing bladder-sparing approaches for patients with invasive tumors, *Cancer* 65(3):675, 1990.

Shipley WU et al: Full-dose irradiation for patients with invasive bladder carcinoma: clinical and histological factors prognostic of improved survival, *J Urol* 134:679, 1985.

Silverberg E, Lubera JA: Cancer statistics, *Cancer* 38:5, 1988.

Silverberg E, Lubera JA: Cancer statistics, *Cancer* 39(1):3, 1989.

Soloway MS: Surgery and intravesical chemotherapy in the management of superficial bladder cancer, *Semin Urol* 1:23, 1983.

Stearns M: Benign and malignant neoplasms of the colon and rectum: diagnosis and management, *Surg Clin North Am* 58:695, 1978.

Stockholm Rectal Cancer Study Group: Preoperative short-term radiation therapy in operable rectal carcinoma, *Cancer* 66:49, 1990.

Thompson IM: The evaluation of microscopic hematuria: a population-based study, *J Urol* 138:1189, 1987.

Thompson WM, Trenkner SW: Staging colorectal carcinoma, *Radiol Clin North Am* 32:25, 1994.

Vargus PA, Alberts DS: Primary prevention of colorectal cancer through dietary modification, *Cancer Supplement* 70(5):1229, 1992.

Verhoegen H, DeCree J, DeCock W et al: Levamisole therapy in patients with colorectal cancer. In Terry WD, Rosenberg SA, editors: *Immunotherapy of human cancer*, 1982, NY Excerpta Medica.

Wargovich MJ: New dietary anticarcinogens and prevention of gastrointestinal cancer, *Dis Colon Rectum* 31(1):72, 1988.

Waye JD: Techniques of polypectomy: hot biopsy forceps and snare polypectomy, *Am J Gastroenterol* 82:615, 1987.

Whitmore WF Jr: Bladder Cancer: an overview, *CA-A Cancer J Clinicans* 38(4):213, 1988.

Willett W: The search for the causes of breast and colon cancer, *Nature* 338:389, 1989.

Williams JT, Slack WW: A prospective study of sexual function after major colorectal surgery, *Br J Surg* 67:772, 1980.

Winawer SJ et al: Current status of fecal occult blood testing in screening for colorectal cancer, *CA* 32:100, 1982.

Wynder EL, Bandaru SR, Weisburger JH: Environmental dietary factors in colorectal cancer, some unresolved issues, *Cancer Supplement*, 70(5):1222, 1992.

Yagoda A: Chemotherapy for advanced bladder cancer. In Yagoda A, ed., *Bladder Cancer: Future Directions for Treatment*, New York: ParkRow, 87-106, 1986.

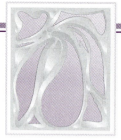

Cancer in Pregnancy

PELVIC MALIGNANCIES
Malignancies of the Vulva
Vaginal Tumors
Cervical Cancer
Uterine Cancer
Fallopian Tube Cancer
Ovarian Cancer
Other Pelvic Malignancies
CHEMOTHERAPY
RADIATION THERAPY
EXTRAPELVIC MALIGNANCIES
Hodgkin's Disease
Non-Hodgkin's Lymphoma
Leukemia
Melanoma
Breast Cancer
Bone Tumors
Thyroid Cancer
FETAL AND PLACENTAL METASTASES

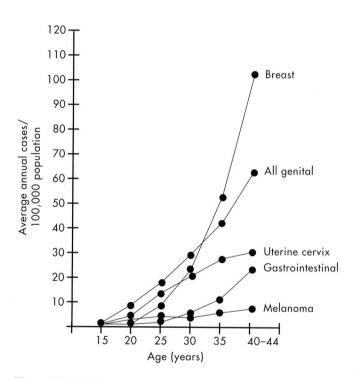

Figure 16-1 Incidence by age of more common malignancies seen in pregnancy. (Data from 1995 American Cancer Society [ACS] facts and figures.)

Cancer in pregnancy appears to challenge the clinician more commonly of late. This is undoubtedly the result of the recent trend to defer childbearing into the fourth decade of life where the incidence of some of the more common malignancies begins to rise (Figure 16-1). The tragedy of the presence of a malignancy discovered during pregnancy raises many issues. Is termination of the pregnancy necessary or advantageous? Will the malignancy or the therapy for the malignancy affect the fetus? Should therapy be deferred and initiated at the termination of the pregnant state? Should patients be advised against future pregnancies? Finding answers to these questions is difficult. Fortunately, the peak incidence years for most malignant diseases do not overlap the peak reproductive

years (Table 16-1). Thus as in any unusual situation that physicians rarely encounter, clear therapeutic decisions are not readily at hand. On the other hand, a significant number of well-studied reviews have been published and can provide some guidance in this dilemma. The largest series ever reported was that of Barber and Brunschwig in 1968, which consisted of 700 cases of cancer in pregnancy. The most common malignancies in that series were breast tumors, leukemia, and lymphomas as a category, melanomas, gynecologic cancer, and bone

Table 16-1   Cancer and young women

Site	Occurrence in women aged 15-44 (%)
Cervix	35
Ovary	15
All genital	18
Lymphomas	23
Thyroid	50
Bones and joints	27
Melanoma	27
Breast	15
Leukemia	10
Soft tissues	20

Table 16-2   Incidence of cancer in pregnancy

Site/type	Estimated incidence per 1000 pregnancies
Cervix uteri	
Noninvasive	1.3
Invasive	1.0
Breast	0.33
Melanoma	0.14
Ovary	0.10
Thyroid	unknown
Leukemia	0.01
Lymphoma	0.01
Colorectal	0.02

From Allen HH, Nisker JA, editors: *Cancer in pregnancy: therapeutic guidelines,* Mt Kisco, New York, 1986, Futura.

tumors, in that order. Other authors suggest that gynecologic malignancies are second only to breast carcinoma and remind us that cancer of the colon and thyroid are also seen in pregnancy (Table 16-2).

The enormous physiologic changes of pregnancy suggest many possible influences on the malignant state. First, it has been assumed by many that malignancies arising in tissues and organs influenced by the endocrine system are possibly subject to exacerbation with pregnancy, and this has often been erroneously extrapolated to a recommendation for "therapeutic" abortion. Second, the anatomic and physiologic changes of pregnancy may obscure the subtle changes of an early neoplasm. Third, the increased vascularity and lymphatic drainage may contribute to early dissemination of the malignant process. Although all of these hypotheses are interesting, the validity of each is variable, even within the same organ. In fact, there is currently no significant clinical data substantiating an adverse effect of pregnancy on any malignancy.

PELVIC MALIGNANCIES
Malignancies of the Vulva

Fewer than 50 cases of invasive cancer of the vulva associated with pregnancy have been reported in the literature. Lutz estimated an incidence of 1 case/8000 deliveries at his institution; our experience has been less frequent at about 1 per 20,000 deliveries. The most common of these are invasive epidermoid carcinomas, followed by melanomas, sarcomas, and adenoid cystic adenocarcinomas. The majority of patients have been between 25 and 35 years of age; the youngest patient diagnosed was 17. With the increasing frequency of the diagnosis of carcinoma in situ of the vulva, the occurrence of pervasive disease with pregnancy is common today. As is the practice with cervical intraepithelial neoplasia, therapy for the vulvar counterpart is delayed until the postpartum period. Adequate biopsies of the most suspicious areas are essential to rule out invasive disease. The presence of intraepithelial neoplasia should not prohibit vaginal delivery.

Invasive vulvar malignancy diagnosed during the first and second trimesters is usually treated by radical vulvectomy with bilateral groin dissection some time after the eighteenth week of pregnancy. When the diagnosis is made in the third trimester, many recommend a wide local excision, with definitive surgery postponed until the postpartum period. This avoids the greatly enhanced vascularity seen in vulvar tissues during the later months of gestation and into the immediate postpartum period. Because this disease occurs more frequently in lower socioeconomic groups, who often do not seek prenatal care, many of these cases are diagnosed at the time of delivery or later. In this group of patients, definitive therapy should be started within 1 week after delivery during the same hospitalization. The pregnant state does not appear to significantly alter the course of the malignant process; survival of these patients stage for stage is similar to that of nonpregnant patients.

There have been several reports of patients treated for carcinoma of the vulva with radical vulvectomy and bilateral inguinal lymphadenectomy who subsequently became pregnant and had normal deliveries. The decision on whether the patient should deliver vaginally or by cesarean section rests with the obstetrician but is heavily influenced by the state of the postsurgical vulva. In most instances the vulva is soft and would not impede a vaginal delivery. In other instances there may be a high degree of vaginal stenosis or other fibrosis, which would make cesarean section the more appropriate means of delivery.

Barclay, in a review of the literature, found 31 women with vulvar cancers associated with pregnancy. Of these women, only 12 were actually diagnosed and treated during pregnancy; another 2 were treated after termination of pregnancy. Lutz reported five vulvar cancers associated with pregnancy, of which three were diagnosed and treated during pregnancy and two within 6 months postpartum.

Vaginal Tumors

Cancer of the vagina has been found mainly in women older than 50 years. The diagnosis of vaginal cancer during pregnancy is exceptionally uncommon, even with the recent rash of clear cell adenocarcinoma of the vagina alleged to be associated with the diethylstilbestrol (DES)-exposed offspring. Although all of these clear cell adenocarcinomas have occurred in women younger than 34 years, the incidence in association with pregnancy fortunately has been rare. Senekjian reported 24 women who were pregnant when they were diagnosed to have clear cell adenocarcinoma of the vagina or cervix: 14 were in the first trimester, 6 in the second, and 4 in the third. Among the stage I and stage II tumors, 16 (73%) were vaginal and 6 (27%) were cervical. Thirteen long-term survivors were reported among the 16 early vaginal lesions. The overall 5- and 10-year actuarial survival rates (age adjusted) for the group pregnant at diagnosis did not differ significantly from the never-pregnant group analyzed concomitantly. Pregnancy did not seem to adversely affect the outcome of clear cell adenocarcinoma of the vagina and cervix. Primary squamous cell carcinoma of the vagina discovered during pregnancy is exceptionally uncommon. Collins and Barclay reported 10 women who had vaginal squamous carcinomas associated with pregnancy collected from the literature, and in those with follow-up the prognosis was poor. Baruah and Lutz reported two additional cases for a total of 12 as of 1986. A few scattered reports of sarcoma botryoides of the cervix and vagina in pregnancy are recorded. When these sarcomatous lesions occur in the upper half of the vagina with or without cervical involvement, the most appropriate therapy has been a radical hysterectomy, upper vaginectomy, and bilateral pelvic lymphadenectomy followed by postoperative adjuvant chemotherapy. Treatment of clear cell adenocarcinoma of the cervix and upper vagina is surgically similar. In both instances the pregnancy is disregarded if the patient is in the first or early second trimester. Should the pregnancy be further along, the decision for appropriate time of intervention depends on the preferences of the patient and the physician. In instances where there is extensive involvement of the vagina by any lesion, including squamous cell carcinoma, one should seriously consider evacuation of the uterus via a hysterotomy or cesarean section and beginning appropriate radiation therapy. Radical surgery appears to be appropriate only for the early lesions involving the upper vagina and/or cervix. The prognosis appears to be unaffected by the pregnancy.

Cervical Cancer

A diversity of opinion abounds in the literature about the cause and effect of carcinoma of the cervix in the pregnant patient. It is said by some that carcinoma of the cervix prevents pregnancy, whereas others claim that pregnancy prevents carcinoma of the cervix. Some reports emphasize the fact that pregnancy accelerates carcinoma of the cervix; other authors believe that pregnancy actually slows the growth of carcinoma of the cervix. Young age at discovery of the carcinoma is thought to be a good prognostic indicator in some people's opinion; others believe that youth is a detriment. High estrogen levels during pregnancy have been considered to predispose to cancer of the cervix by some; others believe that the high estrogen content actually controls carcinoma of the cervix. Numerous articles in the literature state that radiotherapy is the treatment of choice for this lesion, but others feel that primary radical surgical therapy is the best treatment. These controversies have been well outlined by Waldrop and Palmer from the Roswell Park Memorial Institute and by Bosch and Marcial from the I. Gonzales Martinez Oncology Hospital in Puerto Rico. Unfortunately, these controversies have been perpetuated over the years. One reason for the different opinions may be that this lesion is somewhat uncommon; it is unusual for a report in the literature to contain more than 30 or 40 cases.

Since the peak age incidence for carcinoma of the cervix is in the mid-40s, one would not expect many cervical cancer patients to be concomitantly pregnant. Reports in the literature show an overall incidence ranging from 1-13 cases in 10,000 pregnancies. Reports from large maternity hospitals give average incidences of 1 cervical cancer per 1000-2500 pregnancies. Reports from large cancer centers reveal that about 1% of the women who have carcinomas of the cervix are pregnant at the time of diagnosis. In the younger patients (younger than 50 years) who had carcinomas of the cervix, however, Creasman et al. found that 9% were pregnant or had been pregnant within 6 months when a diagnosis of carcinoma of the cervix was established. This figure may be distorted by the referral nature of the institution from which they were reporting.

Carcinoma of the cervix is curable, particularly if it is diagnosed and treated in the early stages. The efficacy of the Pap smear in detecting early cervical disease is well documented and is an acceptable part of routine examination of the female patient. Since most women, and particularly young women, do not have an annual pelvic examination and Pap smear, pregnancy offers an added opportunity for cancer surveillance.

Vaginal bleeding is the most common symptom seen in carcinoma of the cervix whether or not the patient is pregnant. Unfortunately, many times this symptom appears only with far advanced disease. Thirty percent of the patients of Creasman et al. had no symptoms when the diagnosis of cervical cancer was established. When bleeding occurs during pregnancy, this symptom must be investigated and not automatically attributed to the pregnancy. Examination during the first trimester will not lead to abortion. Third-trimester bleeding can be adequately assessed in the operating room as a double setup procedure.

The methods for diagnosis and treatment of this lesion in the pregnant or postpartum woman are the same as in the nonpregnant patient. Many times visual inspection is all that is needed for diagnosis of this malignancy.

The Pap smear is reportedly accurate in detecting cervical lesions, particularly in the early occult stages. In more than half of the asymptomatic patients in the study by Creasman et al., the only abnormality noted was that of abnormal Pap smears. Colposcopically directed cervical biopsy is extremely accurate in diagnosing invasive squamous cell carcinoma of the cervix. The cone biopsy is needed only when a microinvasive lesion is found on colposcopically directed biopsy and a frankly invasive lesion must be ruled out.

The age of patients ranged from 19-46 years, with a mean of 33 years, in the series of Creasman et al. In this group of patients, the age when the diagnosis of carcinoma of the cervix was made had no influence on the prognosis of the lesion within a given stage. This is compatible with other reported series previously mentioned.

For many years parity has been considered an important factor in the cause of carcinoma of the cervix. Although early coital activity appears to be the important possible etiologic factor, certainly early pregnancy and multiparity usually go hand in hand. The average parity in the Creasman et al. study group was 5.4. In 1307 patients in the same age group who had carcinomas of the cervix and were not pregnant, the average parity was 3.5. It did not appear that a more advanced lesion was found with increasing parity, and prognosis was not related to parity as long as the patients were compared within a given stage.

Therapy for these lesions is discussed in Chapter 3 and illustrated in Figure 16-5. Choices for therapy depend on the stage of the pregnancy and the desires of the patient and the physician. In multiple reports there has been little difference in maternal survival rate if the pregnancy was terminated by cesarean section or vaginal delivery. This was borne out in the case experience from MD Anderson Hospital. The same appears to be true of fetal survival. This is not to be considered an endorsement of vaginal delivery as the delivery of choice in carcinoma of the cervix, because considerable difficulties can be encountered with this mode of delivery, particularly if there are large lesions. In most of the patients who deliver vaginally, unfortunately, diagnosis of carcinoma is made several weeks postpartum. The major indications for cesarean section in patients with large cervical lesions are bleeding and infection that can result from a vaginal delivery when the cervix is extensively involved with a malignant process.

The general philosophy for diagnosis and treatment of intraepithelial neoplasia of the cervix detected during pregnancy is one of expectant therapy after careful diagnosis. Pregnant patients with abnormal Pap smears should undergo colposcopically directed biopsies of suspicious areas to rule out invasive disease. Depending on the experience of the colposcopist, areas of abnormality that clearly are not invasive, such as those with minimal white epithelium without underlying vascular changes, may be observed without biopsy until the postpartum period (Figure 16-2). It is with great hesitancy that any oncologist suggests deferring a biopsy, and it is important to stress again that this determination be made by an experienced colposcopist who is confident after review of the Pap smear and the colposcopic findings that there is little likelihood of an invasive lesion on the cervix. Nonetheless, the patient should undergo a repeat Pap smear and colposcopy 1 or 2 additional times during the pregnancy. Where suspicion of invasion exists, a carefully directed incisional biopsy of sufficient depth to permit an accurate diagnosis should be done. A diagnosis of microinvasion made by colposcopically directed biopsy must be followed as soon as possible by a cone biopsy to rule out frankly invasive disease. This is the only absolute indication for conization during pregnancy. Conization will distinguish patients who have "early stromal invasion" and who can proceed to term without appreciable risk to their survival from those with frank invasion in whom consideration must be given to early interruption of the pregnancy. Patients with intraepithelial neoplasia of the cervix may deliver vaginally with subsequent reassessment in the postpartum state. Interestingly, many of these patients will not demonstrate persistent intraepithelial neoplasia when reevaluated 6 weeks postpartum. Explanation for this change is obscure but probably results from spontaneous regression or traumatic loss of the epithelium during the birth process.

The performance of a cone biopsy in pregnant patients who are diagnosed as having "microinvasive cancer" by colposcopically directed biopsy is a formidable undertaking with an increased risk of hemorrhage and spontaneous abortion. We recommend using six hemostatic sutures (Figure 16-3) evenly distributed around the

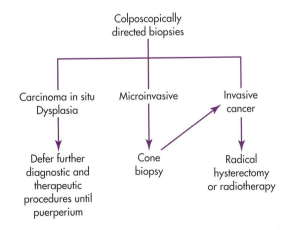

Figure 16-2 Abnormal cytologic findings in pregnancy.

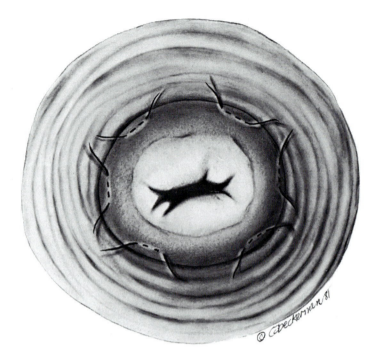

Figure 16-3 Figure shows location of six hemostatic sutures. (From Creasy RK, Resnick R: *Maternal-fetal medicine: principles and practices*, Philadelphia, 1987, WB Saunders.)

Figure 16-4 Demonstration of shallow "coin biopsy" appropriate in pregnancy. (From Creasy RK, Resnick R: *Maternal-fetal medicine: principles and practices*, Philadelphia, 1987, WB Saunders.)

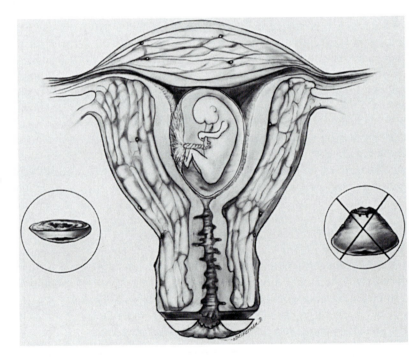

portion of the cervix close to the vaginal reflection. These sutures will reduce blood flow to the cone bed, evert the squamocolumnar junction, and facilitate performing a shallow cone biopsy with little invasion of the endocervical canal. Fortunately, pregnancy itself causes the squamocolumnar junction to be everted, thereby limiting the need for sampling tissue high in the endocervix. The surgical procedure described for pregnancy might be envisioned as excising a "coin" of tissue rather than a cone of tissue (Figure 16-4). Avoiding trauma to the

endocervical canal will minimize the risk of excessive bleeding and disruption of the pregnancy.

Microinvasion or early stromal invasion of the cervix is defined in our opinion as an invasive cancer that does not penetrate the stroma more than 3 mm below the basement membrane of the surface epithelium, does not manifest vascular or lymphatic invasion, is free of confluent tongues of tumor, and does not extend to the margins of the surgical specimen. When these histologic criteria have been met, we advise the patient that

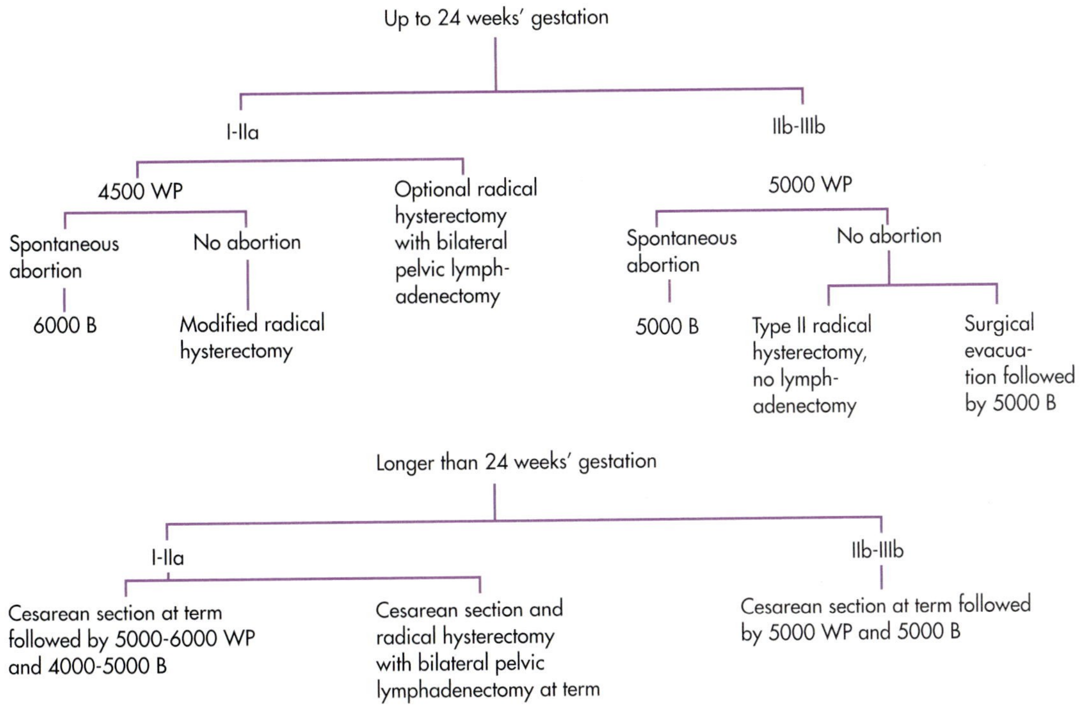

Figure 16-5 Suggested therapy for cervical cancer in pregnancy. *WP*, Whole-pelvis irradiation (cGy); *B*, brachytherapy (mg-hr) vaginal radium in two applications.

pregnancy may continue safely to term. Cesarean section is not thought to be necessary for this group of patients, and the route of delivery should be determined by obstetric indications. Indeed, 14 such patients treated by conization alone at our institution have been followed for intervals of 2-16 years, and none have developed recurrent invasive disease. Two of these patients subsequently developed preinvasive disease and elected to have hysterectomies; no invasion was found in these two specimens. We now believe that a recommendation for postpartum hysterectomy is not essential in patients who have early stromal invasions who desire further childbearing.

In deciding on therapy for invasive cervical cancer in pregnancy, the physician must consider both the stage of disease and the duration of pregnancy. The decision often can be influenced by the religious convictions of the patient and family and the desire of the mother for the child. Because pregnancy has not been shown convincingly to have an adverse effect on cancer of the cervix, short delays of several weeks in definitive therapy, until the fetus has reached viability, are appropriate. The former belief that pregnancy might accelerate tumor growth or that parturition might squeeze viable cells into the vascular system and increase the incidence of metastatic spread has not been substantiated by recent studies. Indeed, stage for stage (the undifferentiated lesion should be considered separately), the outcome for the pregnant patient who has cervical cancer is approxi-

mately that of the young nonpregnant patient. An outline of recommended treatment for cervical cancer in pregnancy is shown in Figure 16-5. For stage I and IIa lesions, radical hysterectomy with bilateral lymphadenectomy is acceptable during any trimester (Figure 16-6). The complication of radical surgery for cervical carcinoma in pregnant patients does not exceed that for nonpregnant patients when normal surgical principles are scrupulously followed. Normal tissue planes are very distinct, facilitating easier dissection. Generally, patients in the first and second trimester are advised to undergo definitive therapy immediately, and thus interruption of the pregnancy usually is advised. Exceptions to this philosophy in patients with early stromal invasion have been discussed earlier.

Radiation therapy is equally efficacious in treating patients with early stage cervical cancer in pregnancy and the treatment of choice in more advanced stages. In the first and second trimesters when the pregnancy is to be disregarded, treatment should begin with whole-pelvis irradiation. Spontaneous abortion usually will occur during therapy, and the treatment then is completed with intracavitary radium or cesium applications. Spontaneous abortion usually occurs at about 35 days in the first trimester and at 45 days in the second trimester following onset of radiotherapy. Some second-trimester patients will go 60-70 days before abortion occurs. If spontaneous abortion does not occur by completion of the external beam therapy, as occurs commonly after the sixteenth

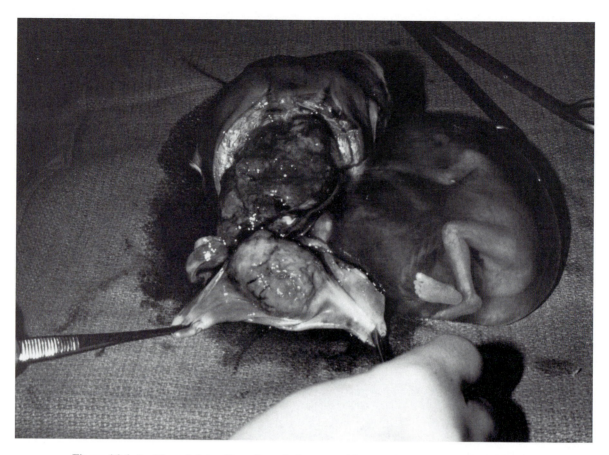

Figure 16-6 An 18-week fetus. Stage 1 cervical cancer with vaginal cuff and extruding placenta are seen in radical hysterectomy specimen from 32-year-old patient treated with radical cesarean hysterectomy. (From Creasy RK, Resnick R: *Maternal-fetal medicine: principles and practices*, Philadelphia, 1987, WB Saunders.)

week of gestation, a modified radical hysterectomy without pelvic lymphadenectomy should be done to excise the remaining central neoplasm. This strategy delivers potentially curative doses of radiation to pelvic lymph nodes with microscopic foci of metastatic tumor followed by surgical resection of the remaining central tumor, since the gravid uterus is not suitable for intracavitary radium or cesium. Although some clinics prefer an extended extrafascial hysterectomy following 5000 cGy of whole-pelvis radiation in patients who have early lesions, we prefer the more extensive modified radical hysterectomy. This approach accomplishes adequate excision of the cervix and accompanying medial parametria and upper vagina, which includes all of the tissues that would have been effectively irradiated by the pear-shaped isodose distribution of a tandem and ovoid application of radium or cesium. Those who advocate an extrafascial hysterectomy centrally often advise further vaginal vault irradiation after the surgical procedure to treat the upper vagina and medial parametria more completely. An alternate approach in the patient who has not aborted is to evacuate the uterus by means of a hysterotomy followed by conventional intracavitary irradiation delivered within 1-2 weeks.

Patients who are at least 24 weeks pregnant may have therapy delayed until fetal viability is reached. Cesarean section is performed when tests of fetal lung maturity indicate viability. If a radical hysterectomy with pelvic lymphadenectomy is not performed at the time of cesarean section, whole-pelvis irradiation is begun immediately after the abdominal incision is healed. Intracavitary radiation can follow completion of treatment to the whole pelvis. The basic treatment plan employed for cancer of the cervix in the nonpregnant patient generally can be used for patients in whom only cesarean section has been performed. Wertheim-type radical hysterectomy at the time of cesarean section can be performed safely and allows the patient to return home with her infant without needing further therapy. Greer reported impressive fetal benefit where definitive radical surgery was deferred 6-17 weeks in a small group of patients with stage Ib cervical carcinoma in pregnancy. This approach also permits preservation of ovarian function, a noteworthy consideration in this group of young patients.

Stages Ib and IIa can be treated with surgery or radiation. The question of which is preferable remains the subject of debate. Although Creasman et al. demonstrated the effectiveness of radiation therapy used exclusively or as an important part of the therapy in 108 pregnant patients with cervical cancer, there is a lack of conclusive evidence that either approach offers increased survival over the other. The choice of therapy often appears to be determined by either the institutional preference or the expertise of the gynecologic or radiation therapy service. We prefer to do a radical hysterectomy with bilateral pelvic lymphadenectomy because of the overall result, which included ovarian preservation, improved sexual function, and elimination of unnecessary delays for the patient.

Cliby reported 4 patients with episiotomy site recurrence of squamous cell carcinoma of the cervix at the Mayo Clinic. The cervical cancers were originally diagnosed at delivery or in the immediate postpartum period and had been treated by radical hysterectomy. Episiotomy site recurrences were detected less than 12 weeks after surgery in 3 patients and at 2 years in 1 patient. Three patients died of recurrent cancer. One patient was disease free at 1 year at the time of the report. The authors concluded that vaginal delivery can be associated with this rare but serious complication, and patients who are delivered vaginally should be monitored closely for this recurrence. The review included 9 patients with stage Ib disease where recurrence occurred in the episiotomy site; six of these recurrences were noted within 12 weeks of primary therapy. Careful monitoring of the perineum in the immediate postoperative period appears to be warranted.

Hacker et al. reported a comprehensive review of carcinoma of the cervix associated with pregnancy. Their conclusions regarding prognosis are as follows. Although limited data are available concerning carcinoma in situ, it is clear that this lesion behaves as in nonpregnant women relative to potential for persistence, progression to invasive cancer, and recurrence. The overall 5-year survival rate for those with invasive carcinoma was 49.2% (Table 16-3), which compares favorably with the 51% rate quoted for nonpregnant patients. The overall prognosis for all stages of cervical cancer in pregnancy, as well as for stage I disease, is similar to that in nonpregnant women. Clinical stage is the most important determinant of prognosis. Although patients with disease diagnosed in the third trimester and postpartum (Table 16-4) do significantly worse than those with disease diagnosed early in pregnancy, this is a result of more advanced disease. Hacker et al. believed that because of the retrospective nature of the material reviewed and the absence of information on lesion size within any given stage of disease, no definite conclusions could be reached regarding the influence of mode of therapy or mode of delivery on prognosis. The perceived favorable survival rate after vaginal delivery may be related to this mode of delivery being used in patients with smaller lesions.

In a report by Allen and Nisker of 96 cases of cervical cancer occurring in pregnancy of which 87 patients were

Table 16-3   Five-year survival by clinical stage

Stage	Treated	Survival	%	Annual report 1987-1989 (%)*
Ib	474	348	73.5	84
II	449	214	47.8	65
III/IV	326	53	16.2	36
TOTAL	1249	615	49.2	62

From Hacker NF et al. Reprinted with permission from The American College of Obstetricians and Gynecologists. (*Obstetrics and Gynecology,* vol 59, 1981, p 735.)
*Survival for all cases of cervical cancer.

Table 16-4   Five-year survival by stage of gestation

Trimester	Treated	Survived	%
First	137	94	68.6
Second	51	32	62.7
Third	87	45	51.7
Postpartum	621	289	46.3
TOTAL	896	460	51.3

From Hacker NF et al. Reprinted with permission from The American College of Obstetricians and Gynecologists. (*Obstetrics and Gynecology,* vol 59, 1981, p 735.)

available for disease-free survival-rate analysis, the following was noted. The disease-free survival rate was 92.3% for stage Ia1, 68.2% for stage Ib, 54.5% for stage II, and 37.5% for stage III. The overall survival rate was 65.5%, which is slightly better than that reported by Hacker. They also observed an association of advanced clinical staging with diagnosis in the third trimester and postpartum. Of 49 cases of stage Ib cervical carcinoma, 64.5% were diagnosed in the third trimester and postpartum. Of 22 cases of stage II cervical carcinoma, 77.3% were diagnosed in the third trimester in postpartum, and all 9 cases of stage III cervical carcinoma were diagnosed in the third trimester and postpartum. Ten of the 32 patients who underwent pelvic lymphadenectomy were noted to have positive nodes. This increase in frequency has not been our experience.

Sivanesaratnam reported in 1993 under surgical management of early invasive cancer of the cervix in a series of 18 patients who underwent radical hysterectomy and pelvic lymphadenectomy with a 5-year survival of 77.7%. A comparable group of nonpregnant patients who also underwent radical surgery had a survival of 92.3%. Nisker also reports that there was a slightly better survival in the nonpregnant group as compared to the pregnant group. These reports contrast to the previous reports by Creasman, Sablinska, and Lee who found no appreciative

Table 16-5 Five-year survival rates of treated cervical cancer in pregnant and nonpregnant patients

Author	Pregnant Survival (%)	Nonpregnant Survival (%)
Creasman (1970)		
Stage I	85	80
Stage II	60	70
Sablinska (1977)		
Stage I	72	76
Stage II	54	56
Lee (1981)		
Stage Ib–surgery	93	91
Stage Ib–radiation	80	88
Nisken and Shubert (1983)		
Stage Ib	70	87
Sivanesaratnam–surgery	78	92

difference in the 5-year survival rates in the pregnant vs nonpregnant patients with cervical cancer (Table 16-5).

Uterine Cancer

Endometrial carcinoma in conjunction with pregnancy is extremely rare. In 1972 Karlen et al. reviewed the literature since 1900, summarized five acceptable cases, and added a sixth. Another case was added by Sandstrom et al. in 1979. This was noted as an incidental finding at therapeutic abortion. The total had reached 10 at the time of the report by Mitchell in 1989. When endometrial carcinoma does occur with pregnancy, it is usually focal, well differentiated, and minimally invasive or not invasive. In the report by Karlen et al. 4 of the 6 women were older than age 35.

Many authorities have argued that adenocarcinoma in pregnancy does not occur and that the reported cases were misdiagnosed Arias-Stella phenomenon. Most of the described cases were diagnosed at examination of uterine content obtained by curettage for elective pregnancy termination or spontaneous abortion. In addition, most of the cases were grade I lesions with minimal or no myometrium invasion. In 1984 Suzuki et al. reported a well-documented case of grade 2 adenocarcinoma of the endometrium with deep myometrial invasion occurring in pregnancy. The recommended therapy is total hysterectomy with bilateral salpingo-oophorectomy and adjuvant radiotherapy where indicated; eight of nine so treated are long term survivors.

Leiomyosarcoma and carcinosarcoma have also been reported during pregnancy. They are usually incidental findings noted in surgical specimens.

Fallopian Tube Cancer

The mean age of women who have cancer of the fallopian tube is between 50 and 55 years. Thus, the possibility of its presence in pregnancy is extremely remote. There have been reported cases associated with pregnancy, and in those instances the neoplasm is usually unilateral and most often adenocarcinoma. The clinical presentation of carcinoma of the tube is quite variable and nonspecific even without an associated pregnancy. The usual watery, blood-tinged vaginal discharge would be obviated in pregnancy because at 12 weeks' gestation the communication between the uterine cavity and the fallopian tube is blocked. In most instances the diagnosis is established at laparotomy, and the treatment is total abdominal hysterectomy with bilateral salpingo-oophorectomy and postoperative radiation therapy or chemotherapy, depending on the operative findings and the residual disease after surgery. Several instances are reported in the literature of incidental findings of carcinoma in situ of the tube noted in specimens submitted following postpartum tubal ligation. In these instances a total abdominal hysterectomy with bilateral salpingo-oophorectomy has been recommended; however, simple removal of the fallopian tubes may be a reasonable alternative.

Ovarian Cancer

Ovarian tumors are relatively uncommon complications of pregnancy, although when they do occur, they present challenging problems in diagnosis and management. The management of ovarian tumors in pregnancy is crucial because of the various complications that may develop, such as pelvic impaction, obstructed labor, torsion of the ovarian pedicle, hemorrhage into the tumor, rupture of the cyst, infection, and malignancy. Malignancy, although relatively uncommon and least acute of the complications in the pregnant patient, should always be foremost in the clinician's mind. Ovarian cancer is reported to occur in from 1:10,000 to 1:25,000 pregnancies. Pregnancy does not alter the prognosis of most ovarian malignancies but complications such as torsion and rupture may increase the incidence of spontaneous abortion or preterm delivery. Eastman and Hellman quoted an incidence of ovarian cysts in pregnancy of 1 in 81, and Grimes et al. stated that in 1 of 328 pregnancies a cyst large enough to be hazardous is present.

Most cysts in pregnant patients are follicular or corpus luteum cysts and are usually no more than 3-5 cm in diameter. Functional cysts as large as 11 cm in diameter have been reported but are rare. More than 90% of these functional cysts will disappear as pregnancy progresses and are undetectable by the fourteenth week of gestation. Our experience has been that patients operated on about the eighteenth week of gestation have negligible fetal wastage associated with the exploration. Therefore 18 weeks' gestation appears to be a judicious period for laparotomy both in terms of its safety for the fetus and for the elimination of functional ovarian cysts. If the cyst is complex and suspicious for malignancy and increases in size, the patient should be explored earlier than 18 weeks (Figure 16-7). Whenever exploration is conducted, our

Management of ovarian mass in pregnancy

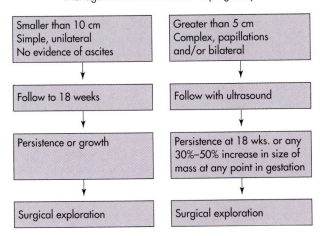

Figure 16-7 Management of ovarian mass in pregnancy.

Table 16-6   Histologic classification of ovarian lesions in pregnancy

Histologic classification	Number	%
Serous cystadenoma	17	25
Mucinous cystadenoma	8	12
Dermoid cyst	25	36
Endometriotic cyst	1	1½
Parovarian cyst	9	13
Corpus luteum cyst	4	5½
Follicular cyst	1	1½
Malignant tumor	3	4
Various	1	1½

From Struyk APHB, Treffers PE: Ovarian tumors in pregnancy, *Acta Obstet Gynecol Scand* 63:421, 1984.

Table 16-7   Histology of adnexal masses removed during pregnancy

Histologic type	No. (%)
Cystadenoma	450 (37.3)
Dermoid	259 (21.5)
Parovarian/paratubal	192 (15.9) (134/228 in one series)
Functional	149 (12.4)
Endometrioma	35 (2.9)
Benign stromal	17 (1.0)
Leiomyoma	12 (1.0)
Luteoma	7 (.6)
Miscellaneous	49 (4.1)
Malignant	36 (3.0)
TOTAL	1206

Hoffman MS: Primary ovarian carcinoma during pregnancy, case report, Clinical consultations in *Obstetric and Gynecology* 7(4):237, 1995.

recommendation is that the uterus not be manipulated during surgery ("hands off the uterus") in an effort to minimize its irritability. Carcinoma of the ovary in pregnancy is relatively rare (the incidence is 2%-5% of all ovarian neoplasms found in pregnancy). Chung and Birnbaum found that fewer than 40 cases of ovarian cancer in pregnancy had been reported between 1963 and 1972. In their report there were an additional 10 cases during pregnancy and 4 cases after pregnancy. Beischer reported 164 ovarian lesions diagnosed during pregnancy at the Royal Women's Hospital in Melbourne from 1947 to 1969. More than 50% were either adult cystic teratomas or mucinous cystadenomas, and only 4 (2.4%) were malignant. They concluded that the size of the neoplasm was not a reliable criterion of malignancy. Novak reported 100 cases of ovarian neoplasms in pregnancy, with an absolute 5-year survival rate of 76%, reflecting the favorable cell types usually found at these times. In comparable-aged nonpregnant patients, about 20% of ovarian tumors are malignant, but during pregnancy this percentage drops to 5%.

Struyk reported on 90 pregnancies complicated by ovarian tumors. The histologic classification of 69 tumors that came to surgery is given in Table 16-6. No functional cysts were noted in patients operated on after the eighteenth week. In 8 patients, ovarian tumor enlargement was noted during a period of observation; 2 were malignant, 1 serous cystadenoma occurred, and 5 were teratomas. Fifty-four percent of the tumors were diagnosed in the first trimester. Severe pain occurred in 26%, torsion in 12%, obstruction of labor in 17%, and rupture in 9%. Only 37% of the patients had no complications. Fetal wastage was high—death in utero in 3 cases and neonatal death in 7 cases.

Thornton reviewed 131 ovarian enlargements in pregnancy, 81 (including one carcinoma and six borderline lesions) were removed. Thirty-nine were larger than 5 cm in diameter and had simple internal echo patterns and

smooth walls; three of these were borderline malignancies. Hoffman reviewed 13 reports of ovarian neoplasms removed in pregnancy and found benign cystadenomas or cystic teratomas most frequently diagnosed (Table 16-7). The Hoffman review also included a summary of 127 malignant ovarian lesions found during pregnancy (Table 16-8). Borderline and frankly malignant epithelial lesions were the most commonly encountered during pregnancy.

The most pressing problems associated with ovarian tumors in pregnancy are the initial diagnosis and the differential diagnosis. When the tumor is palpable within the pelvis, it must be differentiated from a retroverted pregnant uterus, a pedunculated uterine fibroid, carcinoma of the rectosigmoid, pelvic kidney, or a congenital uterine abnormality (e.g., rudimentary uterine horn). In the latter half of pregnancy, ovarian tumors are particularly difficult to diagnose (Figure 16-8). As the tumor ascends into the abdominal cavity and beyond the reach

Table 16-8 History of malignant adnexal masses removed during pregnancy

Histologic type	No. (%)
Epithelial	35 (27.6)
Borderline epithelial	26 (20.5)
Germ cell	7 (5.5)
Dysgerminoma	
Other	
Stromal	20 (15.7) (13/64 from Novak)
Undifferentiated	4 (3.1)
Sarcoma	2 (1.6)
Metastatic	3 (2.4)
TOTAL	127

Hoffman MS: Primary ovarian carcinoma during pregnancy, case report, Clinical consultations in *Obstetric and Gynecology* 7(4):237, 1995.

of vaginal examination, abdominal palpation becomes the chief method of clinical diagnosis. Ultrasonography is particularly helpful in this situation.

Torsion is common in pregnancy, with a reported incidence of between 10%-15% of ovarian tumors in pregnancy undergoing this complication. Most torsions occur when the uterus is rising at rapid rate (8-16 weeks) or when the uterus is involuting (in the puerperium). About 60% of the cases occur at the beginning of the pregnancy and the remaining 40% occur in the puerperium. The usual sequence of events is sudden lower abdominal pain, nausea, vomiting, and in some cases, shock-like symptoms. The abdomen is tense and tender, and there is rebound tenderness with guarding.

In many instances the presence of an ovarian tumor may not be suspected until delivery. The large uterus obscures the growth of the ovarian neoplasm. The tumor may be growing in the abdomen behind the large uterus

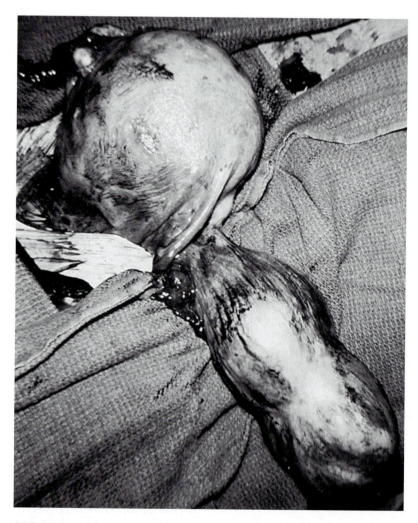

Figure 16-8 Benign cystic teratoma; gross appearance at cesarean section (undiagnosed preoperative).

and may not fall back into the cul-de-sac until it is very large. If there is a mechanical obstruction of the birth canal, exploratory laparotomy is indicated for both delivery of the baby and management of the ovarian neoplasm. Allowing labor to proceed when an ovarian neoplasm is causing obstruction of the birth canal may result in rupture of the ovarian cyst. Even if the cyst is not ruptured, the trauma of labor may cause hemorrhage into the tumor followed by necrosis and suppuration.

Ovarian cancer in pregnancy fortunately is rare, because the disease is most common in the age group older than 50. The incidence for all pregnancies is from 1 in 8000 to 1 in 20,000 deliveries. The diagnosis is usually fortuitous; the patient undergoes laparotomy for an adnexal mass that is subsequently found to be malignant. In many instances the close observation of the pregnant patient has led to the discovery of a lesion in the earlier stages. If an ovarian malignancy is found at the time of abdominal exploration, the surgeon's first obligation is to properly stage the patient as outlined in Chapter 11. In the young pregnant patient one would expect to find germ cell tumors such as dysgerminoma, embryonal carcinoma, immature teratoma, and endodermal sinus tumor. Epithelial cancers such as papillary serous cystadenocarcinoma and papillary mucinous cystadenocarcinoma are more common as the patient approaches 40 years and should be treated appropriately for the stage of the disease regardless of the pregnancy. The majority of these epithelial lesions are of low malignant potential or are stage I, as commonly found in nonpregnant patients in the reproductive age group. Stage I lesions may be treated conservatively as outlined in Chapter 10. Patients with more advanced lesions should not be encouraged to follow a conservative treatment plan. Pregnancy does not appear to adversely affect the prognosis for the patient who has an ovarian malignancy.

Fortunately, ovarian germ cell neoplasms in pregnancy are usually benign. Dermoid cysts are by far the most common neoplastic cysts found in pregnancy. Attempts should be made to remove them in the early part of the second trimester when they are recognized early in pregnancy. Other ovarian germ cell neoplasms that are commonly found are malignant teratoma, endodermal sinus tumor, and embryonal carcinoma. Functioning ovarian tumors such as granulosa-stromal cell tumors and Sertoli-Leydig cell tumors are also found rarely. It is recommended that management be similar to that in the nonpregnant patient.

Malignant germ cell neoplasms (Figure 16-9) usually can be managed with a unilateral salpingo-oophorectomy because they are usually stage Ia and the prognosis for this stage is not improved with more extensive surgery. Adjuvant chemotherapy in this group of highly malignant tumors plays an important role in treating all except the dysgerminoma. Combined chemotherapy has improved survival markedly and can permit preservation of childbearing capacity, as well as maintenance of the existing pregnancy if the disease is stage I. If the diagnosis is made during the first or second trimester, the patient must

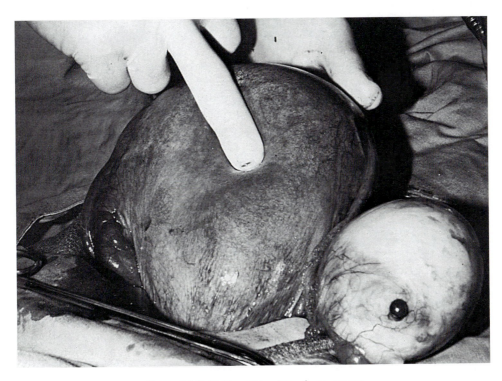

Figure 16-9 Malignant teratoma in pregnancy.

decide whether to permit the pregnancy to continue to viability before instituting adjuvant chemotherapy. Because these tumors characteristically grow rapidly and often recur within months when therapy is withheld, such delays can be harmful. Indeed, the high success rate obtained with adjuvant chemotherapy has been recorded using this modality in the immediate postoperative period. The effect of a treatment-free interval of several months before the commencement of adjuvant chemotherapy has not been tested adequately. Thus the patient with a stage Ia embryonal carcinoma, endodermal sinus tumor, or immature teratoma discovered early in pregnancy is faced with a dilemma for which no data are available. Malone reported a patient with stage Ic endodermal sinus tumor diagnosed in the twenty-fifth week of gestation who received two cycles of combination chemotherapy consisting of vinblastine, bleomycin, and cisplatin, and delivered a healthy boy by cesarean section at 32 weeks' gestation. She subsequently completed three more cycles of chemotherapy and remained well at the time of Malone's report 18 months after initial diagnosis. To our knowledge, this was the first report of a case of a patient who had endodermal sinus tumor treated with combination chemotherapy during pregnancy that apparently had a successful outcome for both mother and infant.

Therapeutic decisions for patients who have more advanced stages of these tumors also are difficult and controversial. Many such patients can be cured with early adjuvant chemotherapy after surgery. As in earlier stages, the uterus and opposite ovary can be preserved if metastatic tumor is not found in these locations. Some clinics preserve the uterus and opposite ovary under all conditions in the hope that postoperative chemotherapy will sterilize those organs as well. No long-term follow-up of this approach is available. Delays in withholding chemotherapy are not warranted, and uterine evacuation is often requested because of fear of potential teratogenic effects.

Initiation of adjuvant chemotherapy during pregnancy is a controversial subject for which little firm data exist. This subject is discussed under the subheading of chemotherapy in pregnancy, but we emphasize that all chemotherapeutic agents are theoretically teratogenic. Although retrospective studies have not shown frequent congenital abnormalities in patients treated in the second and third trimesters, many newer agents have not been used frequently in pregnancy.

Ovarian dysgerminomas are unique among the malignant germ cell tumors because of their overall good prognosis in stage I treated by surgery alone and their exquisite sensitivity to chemotherapy and radiation therapy. Dysgerminoma is particularly common and accounts for 30% of ovarian malignancies in pregnancy. We believe that these tumors can be managed with a unilateral adnexectomy and continuation of the pregnancy without additional therapy in stage Ia. Optimal staging should include a pelvic and periaortic lymphadenectomy on the side of the tumor mass, because dysgerminomas metastasize primarily via the lymphatic system to the ipsilateral pelvic and periaortic lymph nodes. Because lymphangiography and computed tomography (CT) are contraindicated when the pregnancy is to be continued, patients who are not explored adequately at initial surgery should be considered for re-exploration before recommending no further therapy and continuation of the pregnancy. Appropriate diagnostic studies, including lymphangiography and CT scan of the abdomen and pelvis, should be done in the postpartum period. A mass on scan or suspicious lymph node on lymphangiography should be evaluated at re-exploration.

Emergency surgical intervention and obstetric complications are common in patients with dysgerminomas. Karlen et al. reviewed 27 cases of dysgerminoma associated with pregnancy. Torsion and incarceration were found commonly in this group of patients, who had rapidly enlarging neoplasms, averaging 25 cm in diameter. Obstetric complications occurred in nearly half the patients and fetal demise occurred in one quarter of the reviewed cases. There were recurrences in 30% of 23 stage Ia tumors treated by unilateral oophorectomy, questioning the philosophy of treating these patients conservatively. The extent to which the patients were explored was not known in most cases, however, and therefore accuracy of staging cannot be assessed. This information is essential to interpret findings appropriately.

In our experience lesions that are confined to one ovary have a 10% recurrence rate. Although most of these lesions recur in the first 2 years after surgery, we believe that this group of patients can continue their pregnancy safely with completion of their proper evaluation in the puerperium. Because radiation therapy and chemotherapy are successful in curing more than 75% of patients, even those with metastatic and/or recurrent dysgerminoma, and because there is a low incidence of recurrence in patients with stage Ia disease, we maintain a philosophy of conservatism for the treatment of these tumors.

Ovarian tumors of stromal cell origin, such as granulosa-theca cell tumors and Sertoli-Leydig cell tumors, are found rarely in pregnancy. It is recommended that these be managed conservatively as in the young nonpregnant patient because they are neoplasms of low malignant potential. Young reported a series of 17 granulosa cell, 13 Sertoli-Leydig cell, and 6 unclassified sex cord-stromal tumors diagnosed during pregnancy or the puerperium. Eleven patients had abdominal pain or swelling when first seen by a physician, 5 were in shock, 2 had virilization, and 1 had vaginal bleeding. Three asymptomatic patients were explored because of palpable masses and one was explored because of an adnexal mass found on ultrasound examination. In 13 patients the tumors were discovered during cesarean sections; 5

patients had dystocia, and in 8 patients the tumors were incidental findings. All the tumors were stage I, but 13 of the tumors had ruptured. All but one were unilateral. Hemoperitoneum was present in seven cases. On microscopic examination, many of the tumors differed from similar tumors in nonpregnant women by having disorderly arrangements of cells, by lacking recognizable differentiation in many areas, by showing prominent edema, and by containing unusually large numbers of lutein or Leydig cells. The last two features are the most obvious in tumors removed at term. With one exception, the patients were initially treated by conservative surgical procedures. Two of them received chemotherapy and 2 received radiation therapy postoperatively. Hysterectomies and salpingo-oophorectomies were done in second operations in eight cases; no residual tumor was found in any of these specimens. Only 1 patient had a recurrence, which was treated surgically. Follow-up for the average of 4.7 years was available for 30 of the 36 patients; all of them were free of disease at their last examination.

In summary the problem of ovarian tumor in pregnancy is quite simple. One must have a high index of suspicion, make the diagnosis early, and treat promptly. The difficulty arises when both patient and physician resist abdominal exploration during pregnancy because of fear of precipitating fetal wastage. However, the potential danger to the mother far exceeds the imagined danger to the child. Most of the difficulties seen with ovarian tumors are those of omission rather than commission. The probability of ovarian cancer must be kept foremost in the minds of physicians caring for these patients. At laparotomy malignant ovarian tumors confined apparently to one ovary require complete surgical staging; this is recommended for LMP tumors as well. A technique of "hands off the uterus" whenever possible appears to reduce postoperative uterine contractions.

Other Pelvic Malignancies

Cancer of the bladder has been reported in pregnancy. About 95% of the cases are epithelial and start in the region of the trigone and spread by direct extension by the lymphatics, and, less commonly, by the hematogenous route. Metastasis to the bone is common, mostly to the lumbar spine and pelvis. The prognosis depends on the extent of the disease. Superficial and well-differentiated tumors can be managed by local fulguration, whereas others require partial or total cystectomy for cure. Radiation therapy has also been used for lesions occurring in this area. It is obvious that the fetus technically complicates the picture as far as radiation is concerned. In all cases, the mode of delivery must be individualized depending on the length of gestation as well as patient and physician preference.

Colorectal cancer is a rare complication of pregnancy. The incidence is believed to range from 1 in 50,000 to 1 in 100,000 pregnancies. As more women are delaying pregnancy into their late thirties and early forties, the incidence of this disease concomitant with pregnancy may well be increasing. Seventy percent of all colorectal cancer is found in the distal colon and rectum. The distribution of colorectal cancer in the general population is approximately 23% rectal, 9% rectosigmoid, 24% sigmoid colon, and 44% other segments of the colon. The distribution appears to be similar when colorectal cancer is associated with pregnancy. Eight percent of colorectal carcinomas occur in women younger than 40 years. Delay in diagnosis is frequently seen when this disease occurs in pregnancy. Rectal bleeding is often attributed to an increase in hemorrhoidal symptoms and the constipation often associated with pregnancy. Management of these tumors in pregnancy is the same as in the nonpregnant state. The gravid uterus will cause variations only in the mechanics of handling the bowel, not in the principle. Colorectal cancer found in the first trimester generally should be treated as if no pregnancy were present. Radical surgery at this stage is frequently followed by abortion. The tubes, ovaries, and uterus may be resected as dictated by the patient and the findings at the time of laparotomy. If the patient is at 12-20 weeks' gestation, Barber and Brunschwig advocate routine hysterectomy to provide better exposure for an adequate margin of resection around the rectosigmoid tumors.

Modern anesthesia, careful surgery, and good postoperative care afford a good chance of continuing the pregnancy to viability. Multiple successful pregnancies have been reported by O'Leary after definitive surgery for early colorectal carcinoma. Delivery should be carried out according to obstetric indications. Oophorectomy is recommended for all low-lying colonic tumors because of the high incidence of metastasis to the ovaries. According to Graffner, 3%-8% of women operated for colorectal carcinoma have macroscopic evidence of metastasis in their ovaries. Autopsy studies using microscopic review of the ovarian tissue reveal an incidence of about 14%. Tsukamoto reported a case of adenocarcinoma of the descending colon during pregnancy in which the patient had bilateral large ovarian tumors. The treatment of early colorectal cancer during the third trimester is controversial. Some surgeons believe that with adequate exposure the neoplasm can be removed without disturbing the uterus and its content. Others believe that the resection should be done 2 weeks after cesarean section when the patient has regained strength and when the uterus and the vasculature of the pelvis are less troublesome to the surgeon.

Unfortunately, many patients have large lesions, and metastasis is either present or highly suspected. Prognosis for this group of patients is guarded, as it is for most young patients afflicted with colorectal cancer. The fetus becomes of prime importance at this stage of disease. The pregnancy may be allowed to continue to viability but the patient must be a significant participant in this decision.

Delivery should be by cesarean section because of the risk of dystocia caused by the tumor extending into the pelvic basin. A bowel resection should be planned at the time of cesarean section if feasible. If the lesion is above the pelvic brim, obstruction of labor is not probable, and vaginal delivery can occur. Definitive surgery could then be done a few days postpartum because the vaginal vault is not likely to be opened by the removal of this lesion, and the increased morbidity from changes in vaginal flora will not be a factor. The malignant process (both bladder and bowel cancer) does not appear to be significantly influenced by pregnancy itself. The prognosis for the pregnant patient stage for stage is equivalent to that of her nonpregnant control. Colorectal cancer has no known effect on the fetus.

Retroperitoneal sarcomas occur coincident with pregnancy and present technical difficulties for removal. Most of these lesions are neurofibrosarcomas or similar lesions and their courses greatly depend on the grade of the neoplasm. Therapy for low-grade sarcomas can be deferred to the postpartum period, when resection should be technically much easier. High-grade lesions have very poor prognoses, and therapy must be individualized depending on the length of gestation and patient preference.

CHEMOTHERAPY

Many cytotoxic agents useful in chemotherapy for malignant neoplasms are teratogenic in animals and humans receiving these drugs early in pregnancy. The use of these drugs often evokes moral and philosophic, as well as medical and emotional, decisions. Both mother and fetus are at risk. All antineoplastic drugs are theoretically teratogenic and mutagenic; their use can result in abortion, fetal death, malformations, and growth retardation. The long-term effect on the fetus is unknown. The problem of long-term observation has been dramatically emphasized by the occurrence of adenosis of the vagina in young women exposed to DES in utero during the first trimester of pregnancy. A similar long-term effect is possible when chemotherapeutic agents are used in pregnancy. These theoretic dangers to the fetus must be weighed against the possible detrimental effect to the mother of withholding these agents.

Teratology is defined as the study of the causes, mechanisms, and manifestations of abnormal fetal development. Environmental factors, such as infectious diseases, drugs, chemicals, and radiation, have been shown to cause abnormal development by inducing chromosomal abnormalities, specific gene changes, vascular changes, or mechanical disruption. In many instances, the exact cause for a fetal abnormality is unknown. Although different classes of teratogens have been established, there are certain general principles that apply to all. There are three stages of embryonic development. In the first 2 weeks of life, the blastocyst is resistant to teratogens. It is during this period that a large insult is necessary to kill the blastocyst. A surviving blastocyst will not manifest any organ's specific abnormalities as a result of that teratogen. Early embryonic cells have not differentiated sufficiently, so if one cell dies, another can take over. The second stage is organogenesis, or the process of organ differentiation. The most critical period extends from the third to eighth week of development (fifth through tenth week of gestational age) when susceptibility to teratogenic agents is maximum. In the human fetus, the period of organogenesis usually ends by the thirteenth week of gestation. The third and final period of growth is called organ development and is characterized by increase in fetal and organ size. However, brain and gonadal tissue are exceptions because they continue to differentiate beyond the second period. Exposure to the teratogenic agent beyond the third period can affect general fetal growth but will not produce organ-specific morphologic malformations. Drug responses vary among individuals because of differences in absorption, protein binding, and excretion rate, as well as differences in placental transfer and fetal metabolism of the teratogen. Both polygenic and Mendelian factors can be responsible for different responses to identical doses of a teratogen in two fetuses of the same species. Small intermittent doses of teratogen administered over a period of time may enable a system to safely metabolize the teratogen and prevent malformation. The effect would be different if the total dose were administered at one time. On the other hand, small constant doses of a teratogen may interfere with cellular metabolism and cause more serious malformations than might be expected.

Most of the available data suggesting the teratogenicity and mutagenicity of chemotherapeutic agents have been derived from experiments in laboratory animals. These experiments indicate potential danger to the human fetus only. All chemotherapeutic agents profoundly affect rapidly growing tissues, and a high rate of cell division is characteristic of the fetus. Following this reasoning, one would expect a much greater effect than is actually observed. Unquestionably, the first trimester of pregnancy is when the fetus is most vulnerable to cancer chemotherapeutic agents. There are two aspects to the problem of fetal damage: (1) death of the fetus and (2) induction of fetal abnormalities inadequate to cause fetal death. Sokal and Lessman collected 50 reports of pregnant women who received anticancer chemotherapy. In their series there were 8 instances of fetal abnormalities, 16 spontaneous abortions, and 7 therapeutic abortions. They noted that no obvious fetal malformations were observed among these women who received chemotherapy in the second and third trimesters of pregnancy only. Although serious congenital anomalies and spontaneous abortions did occur in patients receiving chemotherapy in the first trimester of pregnancy, such complications were not inevitable. The lack of adequate observation of the long-term status of the fetus or infant prevents any definite conclusions as to the relative safety or danger of anticancer chemotherapy during pregnancy, even in the second and third trimesters. It is surprising how often the detailed status of the fetus is not mentioned in available reports. Often the infant is described as "normal" with few, if any, details on the physical or laboratory profile of the baby. Long-term observation is necessary to establish normalcy, because many of the defects may not be obvious on inspection and may emerge as derangements of growth, development, function, reproduction, and heredity.

Nicholson collected 185 cases of human pregnancies during anticancer chemotherapy. Of 110 women who received such treatment during the first trimester, the status of the fetus or infant was recorded in only 68 patients. Of these there were 15 instances of fetal abnormalities. Ten of these women received folic acid antagonists, 2 had taken busulfan, and 1 each had received 6-mercaptopurine, chlorambucil, and cyclophosphamide. No malformations were reported in the fetuses of 75 women who received chemotherapy during the second and third trimesters of pregnancy, although the status of the fetus or the infant is recorded in only 73 instances. Sweet and Kinzie reported an update of the original article by Nicholson. They gathered the remaining published data on chemotherapy during pregnancy and reviewed 39 pregnancies in which an alkylating agent was used in the first trimester. Malformations were seen in 6 of the 39 pregnancies, but the majority of these patients had also received radiation during pregnancy or just before conception. During the second or third trimester, 27 patients received an alkylating agent, and no congenital anomalies were noted. They concluded that the risk of alkylating agents given during pregnancy appears to be small, with no increased risk if given after the first trimester. Vinca alkaloids were given to 15 patients in the first trimester with only one congenital malformation noted, and no abnormalities were noted in 11 pregnancies so treated after the first trimester. Similar results have been compiled in a review article by Doll (Table 16-9).

There is no doubt that the antifolics aminopterin and methotrexate when given in the first trimester of pregnancy almost invariably result in spontaneous abortion or an abnormal fetus. These drugs should not be given to the pregnant woman in the first trimester unless there is life-threatening disease that can be counteracted by the drug. If an antifolic is used and the mother does not have a spontaneous abortion, therapeutic abortion should be seriously considered. A small amount of data seems to indicate that aminopterin and methotrexate do not cause harm when given after the first trimester of pregnancy.

In 1992, Zemlickis reported his experience with 21 pregnancies after in utero exposure to chemotherapy. Of the 13 women exposed during the first trimester, 2 of 5

Table 16-9   Chemotherapy during first trimester of pregnancy

Class	Number of exposed patients/ number of fetal malformations
Alkylating agents	
Busulfan	22/2
Chlorambucil	5/1
Cyclophosphamide	7/3
TOTAL (%)	34/6 (18)
Antimetabolites	
Aminopterin	52/10
Methotrexate	3/3
Mercaptopurine	20/0
Cytarabine	1/1
Fluorouracil	1/1
TOTAL (%)	77/15 (19)
Plant alkaloids	
Vinblastine sulfate	14/1
Antibiotics	
Daunorubicin hydrochloride	1/1
Miscellaneous	
Procarbazine hydrochloride	1/1
Amsacrine	1/1
Cisplatin	1/0
TOTAL (%)	18/3 (17)
Total	127/24 (19)
Combinations (5)	30/7 (23)

Modified from Doll DC et al: *Arch Intern Med* 148:205, 1988.

whose pregnancies continued to term had major malformations in their infants, 4 had spontaneous abortions, and 4 had therapeutic abortions. Of 4 women with second-trimester exposure to chemotherapy, 2 had normal live births; 1 had a still birth, and 1 had a therapeutic abortion. All four pregnancies exposed to chemotherapy during the third trimester resulted in healthy live births. However, infants exposed to chemotherapy had statistically significantly lower birth weights than match controls, due to significantly lower gestational age and substantial intrauterine growth retardation. The rate of still birth was 1/11; this was too small a series for comparison with matched controls. On the other hand, the authors analyzed 223 births in their community occurring to women who had any form of cancer in the same 30-year time period and found 10 still births among the 223 deliveries, significantly more than in the general population ($p < .0005$). This latter still birth rate was calculated at an R.R. 4.23 (95% confidence interval, 2.0-7.8).

Although most of the other cancer chemotherapeutic agents, including 6-mercaptopurine, azathioprine, 5-fluorouracil, alkylating agents, vinca alkaloids, and procarbazine, are known to be teratogenic in animal experiments, surprisingly there have been very few case reports of human fetal abnormalities resulting from the use of these agents in the first trimester of pregnancy other than the previously mentioned effects of antifolics. On the other hand, there have been isolated reports of fetal abnormalities with every drug. Thus all cancer chemotherapeutic agents should be considered teratogenic and should be avoided in the first trimester of pregnancy if at all possible.

Although the alkylating agents are well-known teratogens in animal experiments, the dose regimen for treating humans is apparently such that the incidence of fetal abnormalities is low. However, because fetal abnormalities have occurred and are an ever present danger, alkylating agents should not be used in the first trimester of pregnancy unless the patient's life is threatened.

Analogous comments can be made about agents such as doxorubicin and cisplatin. Both of these newer agents have been used infrequently during pregnancy, especially during the first trimester. However, no abnormalities have been reported with use of these agents in the second and third trimesters. Roboz reported the use of doxorubicin at 20 weeks' gestation and an attempt to measure amniotic fluid drug levels. He found no measurable quantity of doxorubicin in the two samples taken 4 and 16 hours after treatment. Egan reported a case in which milk and plasma concentrations of doxorubicin (Adriamycin) and cisplatin were measured after IV administration of these agents to a lactating patient who had ovarian cancer. Cisplatin was undetectable in human milk. Although at times the milk concentrations of doxorubicin often exceeded those detected in concomitant plasma samples, the total amount of drug delivered in the milk was negligible. However, the authors concluded that it was prudent to advise lactating women who are receiving these antineoplastic drugs to refrain from breast feeding.

Most reports of combination chemotherapy given during pregnancy have been in patients who had leukemias and Hodgkin's disease. Pizzuto reported 9 cases of acute leukemia treated during pregnancy with multiple chemotherapeutic agents in combination, including prednisone, cytosine arabinoside, 6-mercaptopurine, methotrexate, vincristine, and doxorubicin. Of the 9 fetuses, 8 were born alive and 1 was stillborn. No congenital anomalies were noted, although 1 infant had pancytopenia. Pancytopenia was confirmed in another infant whose mother was treated with combination chemotherapy for acute leukemia. Many other reports about the use of combination chemotherapy for acute leukemia during pregnancy are available. No fetal congenital anomalies have been noted, and live births have resulted.

In 1985, Selevan reported a statistically significant association between fetal loss among nurses and occupational exposure to antineoplastic drugs during the first trimester of pregnancy, the odds ratio equaling 2:30. Most nurses studied in this report handled many drugs, so specific associations were difficult to establish, but caution was advised for all drugs.

In summary, the administration of chemotherapy during the first trimester can be associated with morphologic abnormalities and fetal loss. Chemotherapy administered in the second and third trimester appears not associated with a significant risk of structured anomalies but some reports suggest an association with preterm delivery, fetal death in utero, and intrauterine growth retardation. In these latter reports it is often difficult to separate the effects of the drug from that of what is often an advanced malignancy. The effect of most exogenous cytokines and new drugs such as paclitaxel administered during pregnancy is unknown. The general pharmacokinetics of chemotherapeutic drugs in pregnant women is largely unknown. The data available on in utero exposure is not adequate to analyze the lifetime risk for the offspring in terms of subsequent malignancies, gonadal function, or neurologic dysfunction. When cytotoxic drugs are used in late pregnancy, the nadir should be timed to avoid the interval when delivery is expected. Neonates exposed to chemotherapy 3 weeks before delivery should be assessed for transient bone marrow suppression, and long-term neurologic and developmental follow-up is recommended.

Effects on fertility

Of equal importance are the possible long-term gonadal effects of cytostatic agents, on men and women both. Patients undergoing chemotherapy for choriocarcinoma, testicular tumors, Hodgkin's disease, acute lymphoblastic leukemia, and other tumors are now expected to survive for prolonged periods, and the majority are cured. Most of these patients are in the reproductive age and some are in the prepubertal period. It is not surprising that chemotherapeutic agents could potentially damage gonadal function. Because ovarian and testicular functions are characterized by rapid turnover of cells, these cells are similar to tumor cells in that both are prime targets for anticancer agents. Some of the best evidence on the possible gonadal effects of these drugs can be found in the studies of reproduction after renal transplantation. These patients are maintained on immunosuppressive therapy with azathioprine (Imuran) and prednisone. The literature concerning the effects of this therapy on reproductive capacity and fetal outcome is mixed, with optimistic and pessimistic reports both. Mothers who become pregnant while receiving immunosuppressive therapy appear to deliver healthy babies barring prematurity and other obstetric problems. In addition, Penn et al. reported on 19 men receiving immunosuppressive therapies who fathered 23 children. Three infants were not delivered at the time of the report, 1 spontaneous abortion occurred, and there were 19 live births; only 1 infant had an anomaly (meningomyelocele).

Van Theil et al. reported on 88 pregnancies in 50 women who had previously been treated with chemotherapeutic agents for gestational trophoblastic disease. No increase in fetal wastage, congenital anomalies, or complicated pregnancies was noted, suggesting that these drugs do not damage human oocytes in the doses and time period used. The possibility that recessive mutations were induced but were undetected could not be evaluated definitively and was recognized by the authors.

Several authors have noted that women undergoing chemotherapy often subsequently experience amenorrhea and the menopausal syndrome, especially when drugs such as cyclophosphamide are used. The effects of chemotherapy on female fertility are not only age dependent but dose dependent also, with preovulatory follicles most sensitive to chemotherapy. Because damage to many follicles occurs during prolonged chemotherapy, resultant fertility may depend on the number of oocytes available for maturation at the onset of chemotherapy.

Alkylating agents appear to be a primary cause of a decrease in fertility. These cell cycle nonspecific chemotherapeutic agents include cyclophosphamide, chlorambucil, melphalan, busulfan, and nitrogen mustard. Reports indicate the high incidence of amenorrhea and oligomenorrhea in previously menstruating females. The drugs caused amenorrhea through direct ovarian depression as determined by higher follicle-stimulating hormone (FSH) and luteinizing hormone (LH) levels, with suppressed serum estrogen levels. Ovarian pathologic findings seem to be fairly uniform. There is a depression in follicular maturation without primordial follicle development. Ovarian fibrosis may result with a total lack of follicles on histologic examination. The severity of the follicular depletion seems to be a function of the number and the activity of follicles present at the initiation of chemotherapy. Prepubertal females show almost uniformly normal development of menses after alkylating-agent chemotherapy, but postpubertal females show variable responses. Schilsky reported a recent study of breast carcinoma patients receiving adjuvant chemotherapy with melphalan, or melphalan and 5-fluorouracil. Amenorrhea occurred in 22% of the patients younger than 39 years and in 73% of patients 40 years or older. In summary, quiescent prepubertal ovaries not yet under cyclic hormonal control seem protected against destruction from chemotherapy. Gershenson reported on 40 patients treated with multi-agent chemotherapy for malignant germ cell tumors of the ovary. Median age at onset of therapy was 15 years. Twenty-eight patients who received VAC chemotherapy have resumed regular menses; only 3 of the remaining patients have serious menstrual irregularities. Of the 16 patients attempting pregnancy, 11 delivered 22 healthy infants. The final outcome of reproductive potential appears to be related to age: the younger the patient, the larger the reserve of oocytes that can be recruited after chemotherapy to reestablish the normal ovulatory state. Return of menses and ovulation is therefore the function of age.

The effect of chemotherapy on testicular function is more easily studied than its effect on ovarian function. A thorough review of this is presented by Shalet. Alkylating agents again seem to be the most implicated drugs in testicular failure, especially procarbazine. The loss of testicular function is related to total drug dose and the length of time of administration. The pathologic changes in the testes have been confirmed by biopsy. The testicular germinal epithelium undergoes aplasia with the resultant depletion of the epithelium in the seminiferous tubules. Leydig cell function and appearance remain visibly unchanged. Testicular atrophy, oligospermia, or azoospermia results. Few clinical changes take place because Leydig cell function remains constant, and serum testosterone levels do not significantly decline. The recovery of the germinal epithelium of the testes varies and is a function of dose. Recovery is often delayed for as long as 4 years after chemotherapy. Even then, recovery is not necessarily complete: fewer than 50% of men show normal spermatogenesis. From current information available, the progeny of patients treated with chemotherapy (single agents and multiple agents both) appear to have intact genetic apparatus without recessive congenital anomalies or hidden chromosomal damage.

Sperm cryopreservation before chemotherapy has been advocated in view of the prolonged suppression in sperm production caused by chemotherapy. It is interesting that spermatogenesis may be abnormal before chemotherapy, and the usefulness of sperm preservation has therefore been questioned. In a study by Sanger et al. only 5 of 22 patients who had lymphoma and testicular cancer had semen qualities before initiation of their therapy that met the criteria of fertility. The exact cause of depressed serum count in males with malignancy is unknown but it appears that the chance of future fertility using semen cryopreservation is not as simple as it first appeared.

RADIATION THERAPY

The primary concern of both surgeon and obstetrician regarding radiation therapy during pregnancy is its possible effect on the baby. Will irradiation of the fetal and maternal gonads contribute to reproductive difficulties in the future? The embryo undoubtedly represents the most radiosensitive stage of human life. This radiosensitivity is a combination of factors:

1. Many of the cells in the embryo are differentiating, and differentiating cells are relatively more sensitive
2. There is a high rate of mitotic activity in the cells of the embryo, and the mitotic phase of the cell is the most radiosensitive period in the life cycle of the cell

3. If the embryonic cell is genetically altered or killed during its development, the adult form will be deformed or will not survive

There are varying sensitivities within the tissues in the human embryo. Various abnormalities have been attributed to irradiation of the embryo: microcephaly and associated conditions are most common. Other abnormalities of the central nervous system, the eye, and the skeleton have also been ascribed to irradiation. However, an accurate prediction of incidence with regard to dose has not been possible. It is widely accepted that irradiation of human beings, especially of their gonads, has certain undesirable effects. Any irradiation of gonadal tissue involves possible genetic damage because the photons can cause gene mutation or chromosome breakage with subsequent translocation, loss, deletion, and abnormal fusion of chromosomal material. Basically the effect is additive and cumulative; generally the changes are in direct proportion to the total dose. Unfortunately, there is no threshold for genetic damage, and even relatively small doses of irradiation can cause gene mutations, most of which can be harmful. It is estimated that 1 cGy of radiation produces 5 mutations in every 1 million genes exposed. Fortunately, most mutants are recessive. Mutant effects are not seen in the first generation and may not be expressed for many generations until two people with the same mutation mate. Most estimates of genetic damage are empiric, but it is estimated that to double the rate of gene mutation, 25 to 150 cGy must be given from birth to the end of reproductive age. Constant changes are being made in what is considered the permissible body dose of radiation. Some authorities cite 14 cGy in the first 30 years of life; others cite 10 cGy or less as the maximum. This includes medical and background sources. Radiation doses in excess of 200 cGy during the first 20 weeks of gestation will result in congenital malformations in the majority of fetuses exposed (frequently microcephaly and mental retardation). With doses above 300 cGy there is increasing risk of abortion.

If therapeutic irradiation is necessary for a pregnant patient and therapeutic abortion is refused, delay in the initiation of treatment until at least the mid second trimester is recommended. Irradiation of even supradiaphragmatic structures during pregnancy will deliver fetal doses ranging from 1.2%-7.1% of the total treatment dose. This dose to the fetus is related to interval scatter of radiation after it enters the supradiaphragmatic tissues. Some scatter may also come from the treatment head of the machine and the colli motor. Zucali used a tissue equivalent phantom to measure scatter dose to the uterus. In this study, doses of 1.5% of the total dose were measured at the estimated top of the uterus with less than 1% being measurable in the true pelvis. This occurs even with abdominal shielding.

For the fetus, the most sensitive period is day 18 through day 38. After day 40 primary organ systems have developed, and much larger doses of x-rays or gamma rays are necessary to produce serious abnormalities. Three periods of fetal development are highly significant from a radiologic point of view:

1. Preimplantation. In this phase, radiation produces an all-or-none effect in that it either destroys the fertilized egg or does not affect it significantly.
2. Organ system formation. This is the period from day 18 through day 38, when doses of 10-40 cGy may cause visceral organ or somatic damage. Microcephaly, anencephaly, eye damage, growth retardation, spina bifida, and foot damage are reported with doses of 4 cGy or less. Cause and effect have not been proved with these lower doses.
3. Period of fetal development after day 40, when larger doses are prone to produce external malformations but organ systems, especially the nervous system, may still be undamaged. Doses more than 50 cGy may produce significant mental retardation and microcephaly, even in the second trimester (Figure 16-10). An analysis of children in utero to the atomic bomb in Hiroshima and Nagasaki shows a 30 in 1600 incidence of severe mental retardation. Most of the mentally retarded children were exposed at 8-15 weeks of life with no cases reported before the 8th week of gestation. A rough linear relationship is suggested with a probability of mental retardation occurring at 0.4% per cGy (rad). Although individual doses are highest in association with radiation therapy, the greatest risk to both the general population and the cancer patient comes from diagnostic procedures.

Most radiologic diagnostic procedures should be avoided during the first and second trimesters of pregnancy. The exposure to the fetus and gonads will vary with the procedure performed and the precautions taken. A chest x-ray film will result in an exposure of 300 mcGy per plate, whereas a barium enema will result in a total dose to the gonads and pelvis of 6 cGy. In a pregnant patient the barium enema is obviously a greater threat because of the greater dose and the area irradiated. Any radiation therapy to the abdomen should be postponed until after delivery if at all possible. The exposure dose that is associated with developmental abnormalities remains controversial. Hammer-Jacobsen suggests that 10 cGy received in the first 6 weeks of gestation should be considered a threshold for therapeutic abortion. Others disagree and suggest that the minimum level increases as the pregnancy progresses. Low dose exposure (less than 100 cGy) seems acceptable only in the third trimester. Evidence suggests that even an exposure of 3-5 cGy can result in an increase in benign or malignant tumors in the child after birth. In addition, the possibility that human exposure to ionizing radiation might have detrimental genetic consequence remains a matter of concern and uncertainty. There is concern because recessive mutations

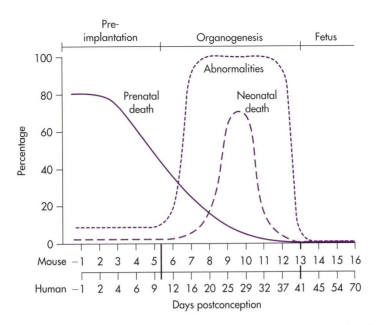

Figure 16-10 Incidence of abnormalities and of prenatal and neonatal death in mice given a dose of 200 cGy at various times postfertilization. The lower scale consists of Rugh's estimates of the equivalent stages for the human embryo. (From Hall EJ: *Radiobiology for the radiologist*, New York, 1973, Harper & Row; adapted from Russell LB et al: *J Cell Comp Physiol* 43:103 [suppl 1], 1954; and Rugh R: *AJR* 87:559, 1962.)

may not become apparent for several generations, and there is uncertainty because, although there are no human data available, experimental animal studies have demonstrated significant radiation-induced genetic effects. There appears to be no apparent threshold dose for genetic damage but the effect of any particular radiation dose is considerably reduced if that dose is administered over a prolonged period. Of importance also for patients planning childbearing after significant exposure of gonadal tissue to irradiation is that the genetic effect of radiation on the gonad may be minimized by delaying conception after exposure. In humans, pregnancy should be delayed 12-14 months after significant exposure.

Multidisciplinary consultation with the pregnant cancer patient who needs radiation therapy is necessary. When the patient wishes to continue her pregnancy, delay of initiation of therapeutic radiation as long as possible without compromising cure is recommended. Most of the data to date on the effects of irradiation on the fetus are from single dose exposure with little data available concerning the effects of fractionated irradiation. Reported cases of fractionated irradiation during pregnancy show a very low incidence of fetal anomalies.

EXTRAPELVIC MALIGNANCIES
Hodgkin's disease

Hodgkin's disease commonly affects young people (peak incidence, ages 18-30). It is now being cured and controlled for long periods with irradiation and chemotherapy. Hodgkin's disease in pregnancy occurs in

approximately 1 in 6000 deliveries. Young women diagnosed with Hodgkin's disease are usually asymptomatic. The nodular sclerosis subtype of Hodgkin's disease is the most common subtype encountered in pregnancy and carries a favorable prognosis. Barry et al. reported on 347 patients with Hodgkin's disease who had a total of 112 pregnancies. Many of the women in the study who had active disease during pregnancy had disease activity above the diaphragm, and this was treated with external radiation while shielding the abdomen. Standard doses were given without apparent adverse effects to the fetus. Most reports suggest that the onset of Hodgkin's disease during pregnancy does not adversely affect survival. Chemotherapy and radiation therapy to the abdomen can usually be postponed until the pregnancy is terminated. The drugs commonly used for Hodgkin's disease are contraindicated in the first trimester of pregnancy and are preferably withheld until the postpartum period. The amazing successes recently achieved with early stages of this disease allow much more flexibility and improved regard for the fetus. Pregnancy itself does not appear to adversely affect the course of the disease, and interruption of pregnancy during the course of the disease is not definitely indicated.

The importance of staging in Hodgkin's disease was recognized by Peters as early as 1950, when she devised the first clinical staging classification. Then lymphangiography made possible the earlier detection of retroperitoneal lymph node involvement, and it became important to distinguish two subgroups: those with widespread disease confined to lymphatic organs and those with spread of disease beyond the lymph nodes, thymus, spleen, and Waldeyer ring to one or more extralymphatic organs or tissues. The latter group is now recognized as stage IV disease (see upper box below). Thorough staging of the pregnant patient is significantly compromised without termination of the pregnancy by one means or another (see lower box below). The major difference in the workup of the pregnant patient lies with the last three diagnostic procedures given in the lower box below.

**CLINICAL STAGING OF HODGKIN'S DISEASE
(ANN ARBOR CLASSIFICATION)**

Stage I Disease localized to a single lymph node, or a single lymph node–bearing area, either above or below the diaphragm

IE Disease confined to a single focus in an extralymphatic organ other than liver or bone marrow

Stage II Disease confined to two or more lymph node–bearing areas on the same side of diaphragm

IIE Involvement of one or more lymph node regions on either side of the diaphragm, plus a localized solitary area of contiguous spread to an extralymphatic organ other than liver or bone marrow

Stage III Disease confined to lymph nodes but involving both sides of the diaphragm

IIIS Stage III involvement of the spleen

IIIE Stage III with solitary area of contiguous spread to an extralymphatic organ other than liver or bone marrow

IIISE Stage IIIS plus IIIE

Stage IV Disease with disseminated extranodal involvement (e.g., to liver, lung, bone marrow, skin)

STAGING WORKUP

1. Careful clinical history
2. Thorough physical examination with careful description of all superficial lymph node areas
3. Roentgenographic examination of chest, including tomograms or CT scan if necessary
4. Liver function tests, particularly alkaline phosphatase
5. Biopsy of bone marrow, needle or open
6. Complete blood counts and urinalysis
7. Serum electrophoresis
8. Lower extremity lymphangiograms
9. Abdominal CT scan with intravenous contrast
10. Bone and liver scans in symptomatic patients

Surgical staging has gained popularity in Hodgkin's disease. Surgical staging of the pregnant patient after the eighteenth week of pregnancy is feasible and often avoids the necessity of many of the diagnostic techniques that might be harmful to the fetus, such as lower extremity lymphangiography, intravenous pyelography, and bone and liver scans. Splenectomy is often performed at these staging procedures, and no contraindication in pregnancy is known. The purpose of staging with this disease is to achieve the best differentiation between those curable with local therapy (radiation) and those who require systemic therapy (chemotherapy and/or radiation) for cure. Once a criterion for systemic therapy has been uncovered, no additional diagnostic procedures are required.

The feature of the disease most helpful in selecting therapy and estimating the prognosis at the time of onset is its clinical extent. In general the more widespread the disease, the poorer the prognosis, even if all apparent disease is confined to the lymphoid regions. The poorer prognosis of patients who have involvement of sites beyond the usual lymphoid tissues is well known. Five-year survival rates of 50% are often reported for patients who have widespread lymph node disease, and rates of 8% are reported for those who have involvement of extranodal sites such as the lung, liver, bone, or bone marrow. It has been shown that the prognosis of patients with limited disease, even if it is extranodal, is more favorable because radiotherapists have been able to adequately treat the limited extranodal disease. Today at least 90% of patients who have disease other than stage IIIE or IV will obtain complete remissions, and approximately 85% will maintain a complete response. Of the 85% or more patients with stage IIIE or IV disease who obtain a complete response from treatment, 55%-65% will remain disease free. This extranodal disease must be limited to extranodal involvement adjacent to or contiguous with nodal disease. It has been well documented that women have a better prognosis than men. This is in part related to the greater frequency of a more favorable nodular sclerosis variety in women. Patients older than the age of 40 have a poorer prognosis than younger patients, which tends to make the prognosis for patients with disease concomitant with pregnancy appear slightly more favorable than one would expect. In the past, pregnancy was thought to have an unfavorable effect on the course of Hodgkin's disease; this cannot be substantiated except inasmuch as diagnostic studies and therapy must be modified during pregnancy.

The treatment of Hodgkin's disease has undergone radical changes in the last 40 years (Table 16-10). Present recommendations are based on the assumptions that radiotherapy is the mainstay of treatment for early stage disease, combination chemotherapy is the primary treatment for advanced stage disease with parenchymal organ involvement, and a combination of the two is required for patients with bulky disease (large mediastinal mass) and/or generalized abdominal nodal involvement. Aggressive therapy has resulted in considerable improvement in overall survival rates for patients with Hodgkin's disease. The most successful and widely tested combination of drugs has been developed at the National Cancer Institute (DeVita et al.) and consists of six 2-week cycles of therapy with nitrogen mustard, vincristine, procarbazine, and prednisone—the so-called MOPP program. The major technical factors that determine the efficacy of radiation therapy in Hodgkin's disease are the total radiation dose per field; the size, shape, and number of treatment fields; and the beam energy. Permanent eradication of any given site of involvement can be achieved consistently with doses of 3500-4500 cGy delivered at a rate of 1000 cGy/week. The desirability of irradiating apparently uninvolved lymph node regions has long been advocated by experienced radiotherapists. This approach is based on the knowledge of the clinical behavior of Hodgkin's disease, the inadequacies of our diagnostic techniques to discover minute or microscopic foci of the disease, the advantage and efficacy of avoiding patchwork and overlapping fields, and the possible reseeding of previously irradiated regions from unrecognized and untreated sites. Extended field irradiation, so-called total lymphoid or total radial therapy, is technically demanding and potentially hazardous (Figure 16-11).

Proper aggressive radiotherapy and chemotherapy for Hodgkin's disease require termination of pregnancy. One must individualize the application of aggressive diagnostic and therapeutic procedures in pregnant patients with Hodgkin's disease. If a patient and her family absolutely refuse any intervention or treatment until the natural termination of the pregnancy, one has no choice but to wait. On the other hand, when one recognizes the potential curability of this disease, and not the concept of

Table 16-10   Recommended treatment for Hodgkin's disease

Treatment group	Patients included	Procedure
1	Ia, IIa, III$_1$a (spleen and/or upper abdominal nodes are the only intra-abdominal involvement); patients must have no mediastinal mass or one that is less than one third of chest diameter; no E stage of lung (may be E stage elsewhere, such as thyroid or bone)	Extended field radiotherapy alone; pelvic nodes need not be treated
2	Any I, II, or IIIa patient with E stage of lung or a mediastinal mass greater than one third of chest diameter; all Ib and IIb patients; all III$_2$a patients (lower abdominal nodal involvement)	Extended field radiotherapy followed by six courses of MOPP with a month between modalities; pelvic nodes irradiated only for stage III$_2$a
3	IIIb, IVa, IVb	MOPP alone

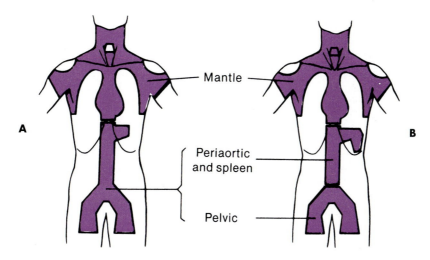

Figure 16-11 Schematic representation of "mantle" and "inverted Y" fields for total lymphoid irradiation. A, Two-field technique, with small extension to include splenic pedicle, used in splenectomized patients. B, Three-field technique usually used when spleen is still present. (From Rosenberg SA, Kaplan HS: *Calif Med* 113:23, Oct 1970.)

palliation prevalent two to three decades ago, one is less inclined to individualize or defer unless the pregnancy takes precedence. In patients with stage I or II disease, with or without symptoms and irrespective of the length of gestation, vigorous therapy is strongly indicated. Delay should be minimal, and termination of pregnancy appears prudent unless the patient is well into her third trimester. Some authors suggest that when the diagnosis of Hodgkin's disease is made before 20 weeks gestation, therapeutic abortion should definitely be considered as an option in the following situations:

1. Presence of intradiaphragmatic disease
2. Histology associated with poor prognosis
3. Visceral involvement
4. Rapid progression during pregnancy
5. Bulky disease in the mediastinum, or patient who refuses therapy while pregnant

Patients in the third trimester can begin the upper portion of the "mantle" technique of radiotherapy with proper shielding of the uterus (see Figure 16-11). Combination chemotherapy, including the MOPP program, is definitely contraindicated in the first trimester and relatively contraindicated in the second and third trimesters. Once again it should be emphasized that termination of the pregnancy before radiotherapy and combination chemotherapy is desirable.

Jacobs reported the results of 15 pregnant women with Hodgkin's disease. Nine were diagnosed during pregnancy. Therapeutic abortions were done on 3 patients who underwent radiotherapy and achieved long term complete remission. Supradiaphragmatic radiotherapy was used in 4 women during pregnancy followed by additional radiotherapy after delivery. These women had prolonged disease free survival. Therapy was delayed in 2 patients. One achieved complete remission with radiotherapy; 1 died postpartum without receiving any therapy. Five pregnancies were diagnosed while the patients were taking chemotherapy. Therapeutic abortions were performed in 3 patients followed by two complete remissions. Spontaneous abortion occurred in 1 patient. One patient treated with chlorambucil had a normal child.

Thomas reported 19 pregnancies in 15 women with Hodgkin's disease. Seven women, (eight pregnancies) were treated with supradiaphragmatic radiation. Complete remission were achieved in six women. Two patients required salvage chemotherapy, and two had therapeutic abortions. The remaining patients delivered normal infants. Therapy was deferred in 7 patients until after delivery, with 5 of these patients subsequently going into complete remission. One infant was born prematurely and died of respiratory distress syndrome.

A report by Holmes and Holmes addresses the reproductive prospects for patients with Hodgkin's disease after therapy. Their study compared the outcome of 93 pregnancies in 48 patients with 228 pregnancies in 69 sibling controls. No statistically significant differences for spontaneous abortions or abnormal offspring were noted when all patients were compared with all controls or when 35 irradiated patients were compared with all controls. The pregnancy outcome of 13 patients who received both radiation and chemotherapy before pregnancy appeared to be compromised when compared with controls. Wives of male patients in this category were more likely to have spontaneous abortions than wives of male controls; female patients in this category were significantly more likely to produce abnormal offspring than were female controls. Thus in this series of patients, therapeutic irradiation alone did not appear to jeopardize posttreatment reproduction in fertile Hodgkin's disease patients. However, in the smaller group of patients who received both irradiation and chemotherapy the reproduction picture was statistically not as good. Horning reported on the probability of maintaining ovarian function after successful therapy for Hodgkin's disease (Figure 16-12), illustrating the importance of age at treatment.

Trueblood et al. emphasized surgical oophoropexy when dealing with young women in whom preservation of ovarian function is desired and pelvic radiation is planned. This procedure is done at the time of staging laparotomy. Le Floch et al. reported a 10-year experience at Stanford University Medical Center where attempts were made to protect ovarian function in young female patients irradiated for Hodgkin's disease by performing oophoropexy at the time of surgical staging as described by Trueblood et al. A lead block 10 cm thick was used to shield the ovaries in the midline. Two thirds of the women retained ovarian function, and many had become pregnant at the time of the report. The minimal radiation dose to the ovaries by this technique was 300-400 cGy in 39-46 days. At the time of the report, no abnormalities were observed in the children born to these women.

Hodgkin's disease does not appear to affect the outcome of pregnancy, and pregnancy does not affect the cause of Hodgkin's disease. The management of the pregnant patient with Hodgkin's disease should be individual-

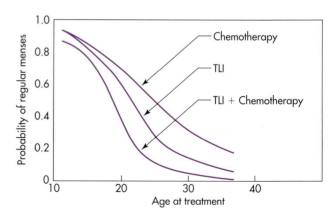

Figure 16-12 Reproductive potential after Hodgkin's disease. *TLI*, Total lymphoid irradiation. (Modified from Horning SJ et al: *N Engl J Med* 304:1377, 1981.)

ized and involve a multidisciplinary team of physicians and other professionals. Three of four patients diagnosed with Hodgkin's disease will be cured.

Non-Hodgkin's Lymphoma

Non-Hodgkin's lymphoma occurs at a mean age of 42 and is less common than Hodgkin's disease in pregnancy. Non-Hodgkin's lymphoma adversely affects the pregnancy because patients usually have an aggressive histology and an advanced stage disease on presentation. As an example, Burkitt's lymphoma is usually rapidly progressive and may involve the breast and ovary. Lymphoma of the breast has a particularly poor prognosis. Ward reviewed 42 patients with non-Hodgkin's lymphoma during pregnancy. Twenty four of the cases were reported from 1976-1985. Three first trimester cases resulted in two surviving infants. Twenty one second and third trimester cases resulted in 15 surviving infants. Infants who were born to mothers who were untreated or treated with surgery had a 38% prenatal mortality rate, while 87.5% of infants of mothers treated with chemotherapy survived. Eight of the 21 second and third trimester patients received single agent or combination chemotherapy. Four of these patients survived. Spitzer reported radiotherapy treatments, given to six women in the second or third trimester of pregnancy resulted in no harm to the fetus; yet four of the mothers died of their disease. Of the four cases with a successful delivery and maternal survival, two were treated with combination chemotherapy, one with chemotherapy and radiotherapy, and one with radiotherapy alone.

High-grade lymphomas have a particularly poor outcome. In the review by Ward, none of the patients diagnosed with Burkitt's lymphoma during pregnancy (n=18) survived; however, only five of the patients were treated with chemotherapy. Only five cases ended with fetal survival. The most important factor influencing the well-being of the fetus is the health of the mother. If the hematologic malignancy is early stage and/or low grade, treatment can be deferred or non-toxic therapy can be employed. However, many non-Hodgkin's lymphomas present with disseminated disease or aggressive histology where the most effective therapy is chemotherapy. The mother deserves the most effective chemotherapeutic regimen despite its teratogenic potential.

Leukemia

The average age of the patient with acute leukemia in pregnancy is 28 years. Premature labor is common in these women, and the average period of gestation is approximately 8 months. Postpartum hemorrhage occurs in 10%-15% of cases. The fibrinogen level in patients with acute leukemia in pregnancy may be reduced from the level anticipated at that stage of gestation. Frenkel and Meyers stated that pregnancy exerts no specific effect on the course of acute leukemia, except that early gestation poses an obstacle to vigorous treatment of leukemia.

Other authors have observed that infants born of leukemic mothers are as well as normal controls. The following factors determine the delivery of a normal baby: (1) antimetabolite drugs are not administered, (2) radiotherapy to the uterus is not given during the first trimester of pregnancy, and (3) the fetus reaches the age of viability. Lilleyman et al. and Bitran and Roth have written comprehensive reports on this subject.

There are many reports of successful chemotherapy treatment of patients who have acute leukemia in pregnancy, and there has been little if any significant increase in fetal wastage or congenital anomalies. In 1984, Catanzarite published a review of management and outcome of acute leukemia in pregnancy for the years 1972-1982. During these years, effective combination chemotherapy was in widespread use. Previous reviews covered cases reported before the introduction of effective combination chemotherapy. There were fewer than 300 reported pregnancies, with a 36%-69% perinatal mortality and a median maternal survival from diagnosis of shorter than 6 months. Advances in the fields of hematology and oncology, maternal and fetal medicine, and neonatology have resulted in marked improvements in both perinatal survival statistics and median maternal survival. Catanzarite collected 14 pregnancies reported in patients cured of acute lymphocytic leukemia, of which there was 1 early spontaneous abortion and 13 term infants. All mothers survived. He also collected 47 reports of pregnancy in association with acute leukemia. In 40 pregnancies in which acute leukemia was treated, there were 5 abortions, 3 perinatal demises, 1 infant "live-born in grave condition," and 31 surviving infants. Median maternal survival was at least 6 and possibly longer than 12 months from delivery. In the remaining 7 cases the leukemia was untreated. In spite of this, there were 2 perinatal deaths, 1 abortion, and 4 living infants. Current chemotherapy results in a 70% remission rate for adult acute leukemia. However, the majority of adult patients who achieve remission subsequently recur, and only 10%-20% survive 5 years. The long-term survival rate seen in children is not obtained in adults.

Chronic myelocytic leukemia comprises approximately 90% of all chronic leukemias in pregnancy. An additional 5% of the chronic leukemias in pregnancy are chronic lymphocytic leukemias. Several reports show that pregnant patients with chronic granulocytic leukemia treated during the first trimester with chemotherapy and radiation therapy to the spleen will usually deliver apparently healthy, viable babies if the uterus is protected with lead shields. Lee et al. reported 12 cases of leukemia associated with pregnancy. Six of seven women with chronic leukemia were treated with radiation therapy and chemotherapy and delivered apparently healthy infants. These authors stressed, however, that chemotherapy should be used with extreme caution, especially in the first trimester of pregnancy. Another study that showed similar results was reported by Levin and Collea. The prognosis for these patients is poor, with a median survival of 45 months.

The decision whether a pregnancy should be interrupted in patients discovered to have leukemia is primarily based on the desires of the patient. Prompt therapy is always advisable for the possibility of obtaining remission. However, the physician's advice to the patient should be influenced by the aggressiveness of the disease process. For instance, patients with chronic myelocytic leukemia are less likely to be harmed by deferring termination of pregnancy than are patients with acute myelocytic leukemia demonstrating symptoms and having a somewhat fulminating course.

Melanoma

It is rare that pregnancy adversely affects a malignant process but malignant melanoma may be in this category. The average age of melanoma is 45 years, and 35% of women will be diagnosed during childbearing years. This is suggested by many case reports in which pregnancy has been incriminated in the induction or exacerbation of a melanoma. Partial or complete regressions of melanoma after delivery have been reported. In contrast, Stewart describes a case in which a tumor recurred three times: each recurrence was a few weeks after the patient delivered a child. Many observations give support to the assumption concerning the adverse effect of pregnancy on malignant melanoma. Melanocyte-stimulating hormone (MSH) of the pituitary has been measured and noted to increase after the second month of pregnancy. Pregnancy is also associated with increased ACTH production, which results in heightened intrinsic MSH activity. Increased pigmentation is characteristic of pregnancy as evidenced in the nipple, vulva, and linea nigra and on occasion by changes in pre-existent nevi. Estrogen itself (which is produced in enormous amounts during pregnancy) has been shown to control melanocyte activity in the guinea pig model. All melanomas masquerade as nevi before diagnosis. The average individual has 15-20 nevi, and removal of all these lesions prophylactically is hardly practical. Potentially dangerous nevi should be removed during childhood; these are the lesions on the feet, palms, genitals, and areas of persistent irritation from clothing.

In 1960, George et al. gave a comprehensive report of 115 cases of melanoma in pregnancy as compared with 330 controls from the same institution. In this report they disagreed with an earlier report from the same institution in that they found that spread to regional nodes appeared to be more rapid in the pregnant patient but that stage for stage there was no significant difference in the outcome for the patient. This was directly contradictory to an earlier philosophy popularized by Pack and Scharnagel that melanoma was indeed aggravated by the pregnant state.

The criteria for staging melanoma have been adopted by the American Joint Committee on Cancer (Table 16-11). Both depth of penetration of the lesion and the extent to which the lesion has involved local and regional

Table 16-11   New staging system for melanoma adopted by the American Joint Committee on Cancer

Stage	Criteria
Ia	Localized melanoma ≤0.75 mm or level II* (T1N0M0)
Ib	Localized melanoma 0.76 mm to 1.5 mm or level III* (T2N0M0)
IIa	Localized melanoma 1.5 mm to 4 mm or level IV* (T3N0M0)
IIb	Localized melanoma >4 mm or level V* (T4N0M0)
III	Limited nodal metastases involving only one regional lymph node basin, or less than 5 in-transit metastases, but without nodal metastases (any T, N1M0)
IV	Advanced regional metastases (any T, N2M0) or any patient with distant metastases (any T, any N, M1 or M2)

From Ketcham AS, Balch CM: *Classification and staging systems.* In Balch CM, Milton GW, editors: *Cutaneous melanoma: clinical management and treatment results worldwide,* Philadelphia, 1985, JB Lippincott.
*When the thickness and level of invasion criteria do not coincide within a T classification, thickness should take precedence.

CLARK'S FIVE LEVELS OF CUTANEOUS INVASION

Level I	Melanoma located above the basement membrane (basal lamina) of the epidermis. These lesions are essentially in situ, are extremely rare, and present no danger.
Level II	Melanoma invades through the basement membrane down to the papillary dermis.
Level III	Melanoma at this level is characterized by filling and widening by melanoma cells of the papillary dermis at its interface with the reticular dermis. Characteristically, there is no invasion of the underlying reticular layer.
Level IV	These lesions show melanoma penetration into reticular dermis.
Level V	Melanoma at this level is evident by its presence in the subcutaneous tissue.

Modified from Goldsmith HS: Melanoma: an overview, *CA—A Cancer Journal for Clinicians,* vol 29, no. 4, July/Aug 1979, American Cancer Society.

tissues are brought into the staging system. It is a blend of the old staging system with the Clark and Breslow micro staging classification discussed in the next two paragraphs.

The Clark micro staging classification (see box above), which has also become widely adopted, provides a histologic staging scheme for classifying melanomas based on the level of penetration of the melanoma under the epidermis and dermis. Prognosis for the patient relates well to this micro staging system. Data indicate that a Clark level I melanoma should be viewed as an in situ lesion requiring no lymph node dissection. Involvement of Clark level II indicates superficial dermal penetration with lymph node metastases seen in 1%-5% of patients not justifying an elective lymph node dissection. At the other end of this pathologic spectrum are melanomas of Clark levels IV and V, which metastasize to regional lymph nodes in approximately 40% and 70% of patients, respectively, necessitating lymphadenectomy as part of initial therapy.

An alternate classification suggested by Breslow (see Figure 8-27) has been used by some clinicians and is a simple micrometer measurement of lesion thickness. Lesions greater than 4 mm have a high incidence of distant metastasis. Lesions from 1.5-4 mm have a 57% incidence of regional node involvement and 15% incidence of distant metastasis. Lesions between 0.76 and 1.5 mm have a 25% incidence of regional node involvement and an 8% incidence of distant metastasis. Lesions less than 0.76 mm are usually not associated with any spread.

Female patients have improved survival compared to age and tumor thickness matched male controls. This suggests that some hormonally based mechanisms are operational in the biologic behavior of melanoma. Contemporary studies fail to substantiate any effect previously attributed to pregnancy.

In 1961, White et al. reported a study of 71 young women (ages 15-39), 30 of whom had melanoma during pregnancy. The 5-year survival rate in this group of 30 pregnant patients was 73%. The 41 patients not pregnant had a survival rate of 54%. They concluded that based on the 5-year survival rates in pregnant and nonpregnant women with age and stage of disease taken into account, survival was equal in the two groups. No deleterious effect of pregnancy on survival of women with melanoma was demonstrated in this series.

Reintgen reported on 58 women who were pregnant when the disease was diagnosed and another 43 patients who became pregnant within 5 years of diagnosis. Control groups were extracted from a total of 1424 women who were registered at the Duke University Melanoma Clinic. The mean age of patients in the series was 28. Both actuarial disease-free intervals and survivals were calculated for the study populations and their respective control. There was no statistical difference in survival between patients who had mole changes and melanomas diagnosed during pregnancy and the control population. The results of the study also indicated no difference in survival for women who became pregnant within 5 years of diagnosis. Despite this, many authorities continue to recommend that patients who have histories of malignant melanomas are best advised to avoid pregnancy for approximately 3 years after complete surgical excision,

because this is the period of highest risk of relapse. Obviously, each case must be individualized, and the recommendation should be heavily influenced by the size, depth of invasion, and any detected dissemination. The role of previous pregnancy as a protective factor in melanomas has been suggested by some but also remains controversial. Patients surviving disease free for 5 years have a 95% chance of long-term cure.

The reported low incidence of metastasis of malignancies to products of conception is probably caused by several factors. One factor is the unexplained resistance of the placenta to invasion by maternal cancer as demonstrated in many animal studies. Metastasis of maternal cancer to products of conception is rare despite the sizable number of pregnancies at risk. However, although melanoma accounts for only a small number of all cancers associated with pregnancy, almost half of all tumors metastasizing to the placenta and nearly 90% metastasizing to the fetus are melanomas. A few cases of transplacental transmission of malignant melanomas with subsequent death of the fetus or newborn child from disseminated melanoma have been described, but this situation is extremely rare and occurs only when the mother has widespread blood borne metastatic disease during pregnancy. Schneiderman reported a case of a primary fetal malignant melanoma fatal to a newborn. Microscopic metastases were present in the lungs and liver, and the placenta showed widespread metastases to the chorionic villi but no evidence of invasion of the intervillous spaces. The mother was NED one year after delivery. To date, there have been no reported instances of fetal to mother metastases documented. On the other hand, maternal to fetal metastases do take place. Moller reported a case of maternal melanoma with metastasis to the placental intervilli sinuses. Tumor cells were also present in the fetal cord blood. The mother died post partum, and the infant survived. Mothers with advanced or recurrent disease should undergo ultrasound examination during pregnancy to assess for any obvious fetal tumor masses. Attention should be directed to placental thickness as well as to fetal liver and spleen size. Cord blood should be examined for malignant cells and placental tissue should be carefully inspected.

If a biopsy is done during pregnancy and a malignant melanoma is found, further therapy is appropriate according to the depth of invasion. Lesions less than 1 mm in depth require a wide local excision with a 1 cm margin. For lesions greater than 1.0 mm in thickness, a 2.0 cm margin is probably as good as the former recommendation of a 4.0 cm margin. The value of a regional lymph node dissection is controversial and probably does not improve survival but most authors recommend it be done with larger lesions.

Reproductive age women who have been diagnosed with melanoma are often encouraged to refrain from a pregnancy for 2-3 years from the date of diagnosis. During this period (depending on tumor thickness), most of the relapses will occur. Patients with melanoma in pregnancy appear to have a shorter disease-free survival, reflecting a higher rate of nodal metastases. However, ultimate survival is the same as compared with populations of women who are not pregnant. After a woman has been diagnosed as having a melanoma (cutaneous). a subsequent pregnancy has no effect on recurrence rates or survival.

Breast cancer

Cancer of the breast in pregnancy is a disaster for all involved. Both patient and physician find it difficult to accept this dread disease in a healthy young pregnant woman. Because breast cancer is rare in women younger than the age of 35, this problem, fortunately, is a rare complication of pregnancy, the incidence being approximately 1 in every 3000 deliveries.

Epidemiologically, it is known that there is an increased incidence of breast cancers in certain families, the risk increasing 5-10 times if a patient's mother and/or sister has had the disease. Although the overall survival rate for breast cancer is over 60%, in pregnancy the overall rate is reported by some to have dropped to 15% or 20%. Pregnant patients tend to have a higher incidence of positive nodes, and with positive nodes the prognosis is poor and in all likelihood the neoplasm has metastasized at the time of the initiation of therapy. The advanced stage of the presentation of disease in the pregnant patient has been attributed to multiple factors. First the engorged breast can successfully obscure a region for a much longer period. Survivals are lower for cases diagnosed late in pregnancy than for those recognized in the first trimester. Others emphasize the 30-50 multiples of increase in serum levels of estrogens and progesterone. In addition, there may be increased vascularity and lymphatic drainage from the pregnant breast, assisting the metastatic process to regional lymph nodes. If a lesion is detected early (present less than 3 months, smaller than 2 cm, histologically non-neoplastic, and no positive nodes), the chance of survival for the pregnant or nonpregnant patient is the same, about 70%-80%. If, on the other hand, there is involvement of the subareolar region, diffuse inflammatory carcinoma, edema or ulceration of the skin, fixation of the tumor to the breast wall, or involvement of the high axillary, supraclavicular, or internal mammary nodes, the prognosis is poor for the pregnant and the nonpregnant patient both. It is often stated that inflammatory carcinoma of the breast is more common in pregnancy. This is false; the incidence of this lesion is equal both before and after menopause and in the pregnant and nonpregnant states.

Early diagnosis has been associated with improved survivals. Patients with negative nodes in pregnancy do as well as nonpregnant patients. Early diagnosis relies on the liberal use of the core and fine-needle biopsy techniques for this group of patients. When necessary, an open biopsy under local anesthesia is also appropriate.

HAAGENSEN CLINICAL STAGING FOR BREAST CANCER

Stage A — No skin edema, ulceration, or solid fixation to chest wall; axillary nodes clinically negative

Stage B — As in stage A, clinically involved nodes not more than 2.5 cm in transverse diameter and not fixed to skin or deeper structures; palpable

Stage C — Any one of five grave signs present:
1. Edema of skin of limited extent (involves less than one third of breast surface)
2. Skin ulceration
3. Solid fixation to chest wall
4. Massive axillary nodes (more than 2.5 cm transverse diameter)
5. Fixation of axillary nodes to skin or deep structures

Stage D — All more advanced carcinomas, including:
1. Any combination of two or more grave signs
2. Extensive edema (more than one third breast surface)
3. Satellite skin nodules
4. Inflammatory carcinoma
5. Clinically involved supraclavicular nodes
6. Parasternal tumor of internal mammary nodes
7. Edema of the arm
8. Distant metastases

From Haagensen CD: *Diseases of the breast*, Philadelphia, 1971, WB Saunders.

Staging of breast cancer currently employs a complicated system jointly recommended by the International Union Against Cancer and the American Joint Committee (see Table 14-10). The Haagensen clinical staging for breast cancer (see box) is more useful in pointing out the unfavorable prognostic indicators in this disease process.

Of all patients with breast cancer, 1%-2% are pregnant at the time of diagnosis (Table 16-12). The best evidence indicates that pregnancy does not augment the rate of growth or distant spread of breast cancer and that abortion for women with breast cancer does not improve the prognosis. Radical mastectomy is well tolerated during pregnancy, and the results of treatment during pregnancy are much the same, stage for stage, as they are in the nonpregnant woman. The treatment of the patient who has cancer of the breast during pregnancy is confusing. Most reports involve small numbers of patients and varying treatment plans. Most authorities recommend a radical mastectomy for patients with Haagensen stage A or stage B disease. The extent of surgery in the treatment of cancer of the breast is being debated throughout the world, and

Table 16-12   Incidence of breast cancer during pregnancy and lactation (selected series)

Author	Years accrued	No. of patients	Average age (yr) (range)	Total breast cancers (%)
Harrington (1936)	1910-1933	92	37	2.0
White (1956)*	1850-1953	1,413†	38	2.8
Treves and Holleb (1958)	1937-1949	108	≤35	
Applewhite (1973)*	1948-1967	2,689 (655 <45 yr)	34	2.0
Riberio and Palmer (1977)	1941-1969	88	(21-47)	0.3
King et al. (1985)	1950-1980	60	35 (22-44)	

Modified from Holmes FA: Breast cancer during pregnancy, *The Cancer Bulletin* 46(5):100, 1994.
*Pregnant and lactating patients were included.
†Age known in 55% of series of 1375 patients.

Table 16-13   Axillary node involvement in pregnancy-associated breast cancer

Investigator	No.	Positive nodes no.	%
Holleb and Farrow, 1962	117	86	74
Rosemond, 1963	37	23	62
Haagensen, 1971	48	33	69
Ribeiro and Palmer, 1977	88	78	89
Clark and Reid, 1978	121	100	83
Donegan, 1979	24	17	71
Petrek and associates, 1991	56	34	61
Ishida and colleagues, 1992	192	110	58
TOTAL	683	482	71

Gilstrap LC et al: *Williams Obstetrics Supplement* 17:1, 1996.

that issue cannot be adequately addressed here. Lumpectomy or partial mastectomy are more commonly utilized especially when the lesion is not large, and total mastectomy with axillary dissection is not always the recommendation. If patients choose a tissue sparing procedure, local irradiation should be deferred until after delivery of the fetus. The doses of internal scatter of irradiation have been calculated: at 12 weeks gestation the fetus would receive 10-15 cGy. In the third trimester, this dose can be as high as 200 cGy. Since the "safe dose" to the fetus is unknown, it is best to avoid irradiation until the postpartum period. Locally advanced disease is difficult to manage with the pregnancy in place. Chemotherapy or local radiotherapy, followed in 6 weeks by mastectomy, is the usual treatment plan for these lesions.

The timing of surgery for cancer diagnosed late in pregnancy is another source of debate. Some reports suggest that patients treated postpartum survive longer than those treated in the second and third trimesters. This suggests that postponement of therapy for patients near term may be of benefit. These reports fail to consider the possibility that patients selected for postponed treatment might have been those with small, more favorable cancers discovered late in pregnancy whereas larger, aggressive, anaplastic cancers with rapid progression received immediate treatment. If such treatment bias exists, prompt treatment would not be expected to correlate with good results, and treatment after delivery would appear favorable because of a preponderance of favorable patients in that group.

The reported overall survival rate for breast cancer in pregnancy is poor, reflecting the more advanced stage of disease at diagnosis (Table 16-13). Holleb and Farrow (Table 16-14) reported a series of 283 patients with carcinomas of the breast in pregnancy, including 73 who were inoperable and 210 who underwent surgery with or without postoperative radiation. Ninety-three percent of inoperable patients died within 2 years of the diagnosis, including all 7 of those who had interruption of pregnancy. The majority of the remaining 210 patients underwent radical mastectomy and were given postoperative radiation therapy. Of 28 patients diagnosed in the first trimester, 7 survived for 5 years. One half of these patients were allowed to deliver normally; the other half underwent termination of pregnancy. The interruption of pregnancy did not seem to affect the survival rate, which was 33% in the group of patients who carried to term and 17% in those who were aborted. Peters reported 70 patients with breast cancer in pregnancy, all of whom were treated with preoperative, postoperative, or palliative radiotherapy in conjunction with radical mastectomy. The overall survival rate in this series was 32.9% at 5 years and 19.5% at 10 years. Three of 12 patients treated during the first and second trimester survived 5 years. Only 1 of the 9 patients treated during the third trimester survived 5 years, and she had active disease at the time of the report. The remaining 49 patients who were treated postpartum had a 39% 5-year survival rate, prompting the author to suggest that a delay in the treatment of breast carcinoma until after delivery should be considered.

Both Rissanen and Ribeiro demonstrated that when pregnant patients with breast cancer are compared with breast cancer patients of similar age and stage of disease, the additional fact of pregnancy did not confer a worse prognosis (Table 16-15). It is now recognized that the independent variable of youth results in an unfavorable

Table 16-14   Effect of interruption of pregnancy on survival from breast cancer

Author (yr)	Years accrued	Normal delivery survival (%)			Therapeutic abortion survival (%)		
		No. pts.	5 yr	10 yr	No. pts.	5 yr	10 yr
Adair (1953)		59	44	—	23	70	—
Holleb and Farrow (1962)	1962	24	33	—	12	17	—
Rissanen (1968)	1940-1961	31	50	—	7	43	—
Clark and Reid (1978)	1931-1975	121	29	23	13	15	8
King (1985)	1950-1980	63	67	—	18	53	—

Table 16-15   Five- and ten-year survival (%) by TNM stage for breast cancer in pregnancy

Author (yr)	No. patients	Survival (yr)	Stage I (%)	Stage II (%)	Stage III (%)	Stage IV (%)	Overall (%)
Rissanen (1968)	33	5 yr	80	80	15	0	38
		10 yr	80	78	22	0	24
Riberio (1977)	88	5 yr	90	37	15	0	50
		10 yr	90	21	10	0	—

prognosis in breast cancer patients, presumably because of the likelihood of more aggressive tumors in these young women. Previously, only young breast cancer patients had an opportunity of having breast cancer coincident with pregnancy, but as women postpone childbearing, pregnancy coincident with breast cancer will become more common. Physicians must treat breast cancer patients in pregnancy aggressively and with curative intent.

Some suggest that the massive endogenous hormonal production in pregnancy might influence the course of breast cancer adversely. The striking rise in estrogen production during pregnancy has been of sufficient concern that pregnancy termination is considered by many to be an important therapeutic objective and future pregnancy avoidance a principle of continuing care. Urinary excretion of all three major fractions—estrone, estradiol, and estriol—rises progressively after the eighth week of gestation, although there is a disproportionate rise in estriol production by the placenta. Serum concentrations of total estrogens rise from 4 μg/dl early in pregnancy to mean values of 8-22 mg/dl at term, at least a 2000-fold increase. The ability of estrogens to promote growth of breast cancer in animals and humans has been amply illustrated. Whether the stimulatory effect of increased estrogen production has an adverse effect on prognosis or whether the disproportionate rise of estriol, a relatively weak estrogen and a possible antagonist of estrone and estradiol, confers some measure of protection is unknown.

Additional hormonal substances secreted in increased quantities in pregnancy that might influence neoplastic growths in the breast include the glucocorticoids and prolactin. Elevated corticosteroid levels are a regular accompaniment of pregnancy and might influence the outcome of breast cancer. Mean production of 17-hydroxycorticosteroids increases from 12 mg/24 hours to approximately 18 mg/24 hours in late pregnancy. Because glucocorticoids can reduce cellular immunity and perhaps promote the implantation and growth of malignant neoplasms, this increased production has grave clinical implications. Similarly, elevated levels of prolactin produced by the hypophysis and human placental lactogen by the placenta late in pregnancy and during milk production might affect breast cancer adversely. Prolactin promotes the growth of dimethyleneanthracene-induced mammary tumors in mice. Its role is not established in humans but it is a subject of current investigation. The levels of prolactin in breast cancer patients are not appreciably different from those of controls, and prolactin suppression with ergot compounds or with l-dopa, has not been proved to be of therapeutic value. However, the observation that women with bone pain from metastatic breast cancer sometimes obtain relief from prolactin suppression implicates prolactin as a possible promotor of breast cancer in humans. Although many clinicians feel that localized breast cancer in the first trimester of pregnancy is a valid reason to recommend termination, therapeutic abortion has not been found to increase survival, and the presence of a fetus does not compromise proper therapy in early stages. Similarly, therapy of localized disease in later pregnancy can be carried out when the diagnosis is made without pregnancy termination. Therapeutic abortion is not currently believed to be an essential component of effective treatment of early disease despite the theoretic advantage of removing the source of massive estrogen production. Reports by Peters and Rosemond illustrate that termination of pregnancy has no effect on patient survival. In addition, there have been no reports of metastasis to the fetus, as in patients with melanomas, lymphosarcomas, and leukemias. Historically, pregnancy was of concern to surgeons primarily because the risk of excess hemorrhage and shock with mastectomy was increased greatly in the gravid state. Billroth advocated premature induction of labor for this reason but did not find that abortion contributed to cure.

In advanced breast cancer, therapeutic abortion is usually a necessity to achieve effective palliation. Surgical castration is generally acknowledged as the appropriate first step in managing premenopausal women with disseminated mammary cancer, and castration would be useless unless accompanied by therapeutic abortion to remove the placental source of hormones. In the first trimester of pregnancy, the termination can be accomplished by suction curettage of the uterus; later in pregnancy, termination is accomplished by Prostin suppositories, Pitocin administration, hysterotomy, or hysterectomy. Chemotherapy will cause a cessation of ovarian hormone production in most patients and castration may not be necessary. When pregnancy enters the third trimester, the decision for preterm delivery depends heavily on the patient's wishes and the urgency for palliation. A short wait until a viable fetus can be obtained might not be accompanied by significant progress of the neoplasm. Continued gestation represents no threat to the fetus, and the risk of cancer passing the placenta and metastasizing to the fetus is negligible.

In many instances hormonal dependence of these tumors does not exist, as determined by estrogen-binding measurements. In this situation the pregnant patient with advanced disease might elect to undergo primary cytotoxic chemotherapy without hormonal ablation by abortion plus castration. When this occurs after the first trimester of pregnancy, the apparent risks of chemotherapy to the fetus are small, and pregnancy can be allowed to proceed. However, when estrogen or progesterone dependency in a premenopausal patient with metastatic carcinoma of the breast is present, termination of pregnancy should be performed.

The value of hormonal ablation in advanced disease has been studied extensively. If distant metastases occur after pregnancy, oophorectomy will produce a remission in 50% of patients. Almost all of these patients will have estrogen receptors as determined by estrogen-binding measurements on the primary tumor. Interestingly, if a patient does not respond to oophorectomy, she will not respond to other hormonal manipulations, including androgen or estrogen administration. On the other hand, if there is a response to ovarian ablation and later relapse, androgen or estrogen administration will result in remission in about 25% of patients. A response to oophorectomy will also determine whether the patient will have a favorable result to a second or third procedure involving adrenal or hypophyseal ablation.

Prophylactic surgical castration in early stage breast cancer has been advocated to prevent further pregnancy, which might cause recrudescence of the disease through hormonal stimulation, and to eliminate the ovarian source of estrogen production, ideally preventing or delaying subsequent recurrence. Neither argument is substantiated by data to support a role for "prophylactic castration." Indeed, pregnancy after mastectomy has no influence on the disease, and a few reports even suggest that future pregnancies might be protective. The rationale for eliminating the ovarian source of estrogens in the primary treatment of early disease is based on the observation that castration in the presence of observable recurrent disease results in partial or complete temporary tumor regression in approximately one third of cases. This argument is refuted by two large clinical trials conducted in the United States that failed to demonstrate a significant benefit from castration and adjuvant therapy. For example, the National Surgical Adjuvant Breast Project conducted a randomized trial of prophylactic castration in premenopausal women involving 129 castrates and 70 controls. After observation for as long as 10 years, there was no evidence that those who were castrated derived any benefit from the procedure.

The incidence of pregnancy after mastectomy for breast cancer is influenced by prior treatment, fecundity, the nature of the recommendation for or against childbearing, the duration of survival, and other factors. As many as 7% of fertile women have one or more pregnancies after mastectomy for breast cancer, 70% of which can be expected within the first 5 years. What should the physician advise the patient who had a mastectomy for breast cancer about future pregnancies? Should pregnancy be avoided; should it be terminated if it occurs? The recommendations should be influenced by two major considerations: whether pregnancy promotes recurrence of cancer and the probability of having been cured. It is generally observed that women who become pregnant after mastectomy survive surprisingly well, far better than those whose pregnancy coexisted with the primary tumor, and often better than mastectomy patients overall. This phenomenon might be a function of selection, since most women will wait at least 1 to 2 years, during which time many patients destined to recur will do so. In addition, only women with good prognoses are likely to achieve counsel recommending subsequent pregnancies. Although on the basis of retrospective studies it may be presumptuous to conclude that pregnancy protects against recurrence after mastectomy, it is reasonably safe to conclude that it does not promote it. Peters found that in 96 patients matched for tumor stage and age, survival was increased by a subsequent pregnancy, including pregnancies during the first 2 years after development of the neoplasm. Similar results were reported by Cooper. Consequently, if a pregnancy occurs, there appears to be no justification for recommending its termination in patients without evidence of recurrence. The converse that pregnancy with recurrence should be terminated in most instances and that an uneventful pregnancy in no way guarantees against a subsequent recurrence also is true. Indeed, there are cases on record in which multiple pregnancies eventually have been followed by recurrence. Our usual recommendations are that women with favorable tumors without regional or distant spread wait at least 3 years (to avoid a recurrence at the time of a subsequent pregnancy) before pregnancy is attempted. All such patients should undergo extensive evaluation before pregnancy, including bone and liver scans, chest x-ray examinations, and mammography of the opposite breast, and all must be followed closely during pregnancy. The study by Holleb and Farrow grouped patients as follows:

Simultaneous pregnancy
Postpartum pregnancy
Subsequent pregnancy

The overall 5-year survival rates for these major groups were 33%, 29%, and 52%, respectively. When there were positive nodes, the rates were 21%, 15%, and 30%, respectively. Their overall incidence of positive nodes was 70%.

Although there is no clear evidence that pregnancy adversely affects the course of this disease, the suspicion persists. It has been established that once the diagnosis is made, stage for stage, the pregnant patient does as well as the nonpregnant patient. However, the low incidence of stage I lesions in pregnancy strongly suggests an acceleration of the disease process in the preclinical period. As stated previously (Chapter 14), many cell kinetic studies of breast cancer suggest that lesions are harbored within the breast for 5-8 years before becoming clinical entities. Since the period of gestation is no longer than 9 months, it is difficult to believe that the sole explanation for the high incidence of advanced disease in pregnancy is related to late diagnosis caused by the engorged breast.

The question of breast-feeding in this group of patients is another difficult issue. Many have postulated that breast cancer is at least in part of viral origin, and the possibility exists that the contralateral breast will be contaminated with the etiologic agent, which will be passed on to the fetus. This theory has never been borne out in fact but most surgeons recommend artificial feeding of the infant, ostensibly to avoid vascular enrichment in the opposite breast, which may also contain a neoplasm.

Reports by Higgins and Tralins suggest that successful lactation in the breast treated by lumpectomy and irradiation is possible. Apparently, location of the breast incision is important. Not surprisingly, circumareolar incisions were associated with diminished ability to lactate, since such incisions interrupt a great number of major milk ducts. Radial incisions in the breast interrupt fewer ducts but may be, on the other hand, cosmetically inferior. In addition, the size, shape, and orientation of the nipple are important to allow its normal mechanical function. Patients whose nipples did not extend sufficiently or were not oriented properly or were not supple found that the infant would not nurse from the treated breast. Finally, concerns have been expressed by some clinicians that attempts to breast-feed following conservative surgery may lead to a greater incidence of mastitis secondary to the disruptions of the ductal system.

For very advanced disease, chemotherapy has been used after the first trimester. Chemotherapy should be administered when the patient is reluctant to have the pregnancy terminated and the disease appears to be progressing at an alarming rate. The issue of whether chemotherapy should be administered to patients with node-positive breast cancer in pregnancy is complicated by recent reports suggesting that both single-agent and combination chemotherapy may significantly improve survival in premenopausal patients when used in an adjuvant setting. Ten-and 15-year follow-ups are always necessary in breast cancer, but it would appear that the premenopausal patient is the best candidate for aggressive adjuvant chemotherapy and a resulting improved survival rate. This is especially pertinent to patients in whom positive nodes are discovered at the time of the initial procedure.

A multidisciplinary approach should be used in planning the treatment of patients who have carcinomas of the breast during pregnancy or lactation. At all stages there should be close liaisons among the patient, her husband, and the therapist, and all options of treatment should be explained in detail. Special attention must be given to the desire of the patient to have a child and to her religious beliefs, especially when discussing termination of pregnancy.

Bone tumors

Benign tumors of the bone rarely are a problem in pregnancy; however, two types of benign tumors can affect pregnancy and delivery: endochondroma and benign exostosis, which can develop at the pelvic brim. These may interfere with the progression of labor and the engagement of the head of the fetus by blocking the pelvic inlet and requiring cesarean section.

The most frequent primary tumors seen in the age group who may become pregnant are Ewing sarcoma, osteogenic sarcoma, and osteocystoma. The usual areas attached are the clavicle, sternum, spine, humerus, and femur. These tumors are associated with local pain, mass, and disability. Signs and symptoms of myelitis can be produced by primary sarcoma of the spine, which is very painful when it involves the nerve roots. Fortunately, metastatic lesions to bone tend to occur in the lower thoracic and lumbar regions, with a lesser incidence of involvement of the sacrum and pelvis. The malignancies that cause most of the metastatic disease in these areas are breast, uterine, thyroid, and adrenal cancers.

Primary bone cancer is treated by surgical excision, usually without regard for pregnancy. X-ray examination and chemotherapy are often delayed until delivery if the neoplasm occurs in a pregnant patient. MRI may be a useful option during pregnancy. Pregnancy does not affect the growth of bone malignancy, nor does the tumor affect the pregnancy, so strong indications for termination of pregnancy are not present. Most recurrences from bone malignancy occur within the first 3 years after initial diagnosis, so the recommendation is often made that future pregnancies be deferred until that interval has passed.

A report by Simon in 1984 confirmed these impressions. Simon reported a retrospective study of 33 patients in an effort to assess the effect of pregnancy on the behavior of primary bone malignancies. He concluded that pregnancy has no effect on the clinical behavior of bone sarcomas, and pregnancy termination was not indicated in the cases of simultaneous occurrence. However, optimum therapy had to be approached with caution because it could cause irreparable harm to the fetus. Simon's recommendation was that a woman who has a high-grade sarcoma during the first trimester of pregnancy should strongly consider abortion if optimum therapy is chemotherapy in addition to surgery. If a high-grade sarcoma was diagnosed in the third trimester, early induced delivery appeared judicious. If a low-grade tumor occurred in the third trimester, spontaneous or early induced delivery was indicated. If radiation therapy to the femur, pelvis, or thoracolumbar spine was indicated, elective abortion or early induced delivery was indicated. Minimum radioisotope imaging should be performed, and special shielding must be used for radiographic imaging.

Thyroid Cancer

Cancer of the thyroid gland is much more common in women than in men, in the same proportion as benign disease of the thyroid. The incidence in women is 5.5 per 100,000 population as compared with 2.4 per 100,000 population in men. The peak in age distribution of the common papillary adenocarcinomas in women occurs in the ages 30 through 34 year group. Although cancer of the thyroid occurs infrequently, there is a preponderance of cases developing in the reproductive age period, and thus it does occur as a complication of pregnancy. The actual incidence of thyroid cancer in pregnancy has not been established.

Clinical enlargement of the thyroid gland is a normal finding in pregnancy; the gland may be enlarged up to 2 times normal size. Histologically, this enlargement is caused by an apparent hyperplasia of the follicular cells

and abundant colloid formation. Although a nontoxic goiter is more typical, even a nodular goiter may occur in pregnancy. Except in the latter situation, these physiologic changes usually do not obscure a thyroid malignancy, which typically causes a single nodule. Serum thyroxin and total triiodothyronine are elevated in normal pregnancy, while TSH levels remain normal. The T_3 uptake test is also usually decreased in pregnancy. These changes in normal values of thyroid function must be kept in mind when interpreting available tests before direct assessment of a solitary thyroid nodule, even though these tests are not directly useful in determining the presence of malignancy in a thyroid nodule.

Papillary, follicular, and anaplastic carcinomas are the most common primary thyroid malignancies. Medullary carcinoma accounts for only 5% of thyroid cancers. Carcinoma of the thyroid gland usually manifests as a relatively asymptomatic nodular mass in the thyroid gland. Because papillary carcinomas are the most common lesions to occur in the reproductive age group, a solitary nodule in an otherwise normal gland would be the most common presentation of thyroid carcinoma in pregnancy. The lesion is multifocal, as seen on careful sectioning in approximately 30%-40% of patients, but in only 5% do these become clinically evident if thyroid tissue remains after surgery. Although studies show that these tumors involve regional lymphatics microscopically in 50%-70% of patients, this subclinical involvement does not affect the prognosis. The growth of papillary carcinoma may depend on TSH, and therefore thyroid hormone administration to suppress TSH is used routinely as an adjuvant in all patients. The prognosis for patients who have this cancer is favorable, especially in the younger age group. Specifically, in women younger than 49 years, a 90%-95% survival at 15 years is consistently reported. A history of radiation therapy to the head, neck, or chest during childhood or a recent onset of hoarseness are high risk factors. Clinical evidence of recent enlargement of an anterior neck nodule, cervical lymphadenopathy, and fixation to local tissues are features suggestive of malignancy. Laboratory indices of thyroid function are contributory only if they indicate a hyperthyroid state, thus supporting the diagnosis of a toxic adenoma. The physiologic changes in serum values that are normal in pregnancy must be incorporated into this interpretation. Radioisotope scanning using any radionuclide is contraindicated. Even though trace doses are used in these uptake studies, there is still a theoretic risk of a destructive effect on the fetal thyroid and a concern for teratogenesis within the fetus. The best diagnostic test of a solitary nodule is cytologic study obtained by fine-needle aspirate. The test is 90% reliable and can be done in pregnancy using standard techniques. If the results of cytologic examination are benign, a course of thyroid suppression using 0.2 mg of l-thyroxine daily is indicated for the duration of the pregnancy. Repeat cytologic evaluation may be necessary if the nodule does not diminish on suppression or if it enlarges during pregnancy because 6% of needle aspirations give a false negative result. The theoretic risk of two false negative diagnoses is about 0.05%, thus providing excellent confirmation of a conservative approach if the aspirate is repeatedly negative. Because this is a relatively new modality, the pathologist must be skilled in cytologic interpretation. This technique rivals that of Pap smear in its ease and usefulness.

Most solitary nodules diagnosed during pregnancy will be handled nonsurgically. If clinical examination, laboratory tests, and needle cytology indicate a benign process, thyroid suppression is indicated (Figure 16-13). If, on the other hand, examination reveals clinical signs of a nodule with fixation, a nonfunctioning vocal cord, the association of obvious lymphadenopathy, or positive cytologic findings, the patient's desires, and the biology of the tumor must be carefully discussed to arrive at an optimal plan. If these latter conditions exist, the options for therapy are best considered in three categories: well-differentiated (papillary and follicular carcinoma), poorly differentiated (anaplastic tumor), and medullary carcinoma, which is relatively rare.

Fortunately, the majority of thyroid cancers in the pregnant patient are well-differentiated tumors. The effect of pregnancy on the growth and spread of these lesions is negligible. Hill et al. reported on 70 women who conceived after the diagnosis of thyroid cancer and compared them with 109 women who remained childless. There was no difference in the overall recurrence rate. The authors concluded that subsequent pregnancy did not alter the course of the disease. Rosvoll reviewed 60 women treated for thyroid carcinoma who subsequently became pregnant and concluded that a history of thyroid cancer is not an indication for avoidance of pregnancy or for therapeutic abortion. Friedman suggested that pregnancy was not contraindicated if the disease-free interval was at least 3-5 years. However, even in patients who had residual or recurrent disease, the prognosis did not appear to be altered by the pregnancy. Because of a 95% survival rate in patients with or without subclinical nodal me-

tastases, aggressive surgery or any surgery in the patient with an inconclusive cytologic examination of a thyroid nodule is not warranted until it is safe to do so, both for the mother and for the baby. In most patients, this will mean that thyroid suppression will be continued until after delivery regardless of the trimester in which the tumor is diagnosed. However, if the tumor is fixed to surrounding tissues, if it rapidly enlarges, or if the lymph nodes develop despite suppressive therapy, surgical management is indicated without delay. A combination of radical surgery and I-131 therapy is most judiciously administered in the postpartum period.

After delivery, the management of the thyroid tumor that does not demonstrate aggressive features involves a hemithyroidectomy for the solitary nodule. Well-differentiated lesions usually manifest as solitary nodules, and local fixation or enlarged lymph nodes usually are associated with poorly differentiated or anaplastic lesions. When a medullary carcinoma is suspected either by history, needle cytology, or elevated thyrocalcitonin levels, one must be more aggressive than when the patient has a well-differentiated lesion. Surgery is the only known effective therapy and results in a 50% survival at 5 years. A prophylactic lymph node dissection on the site of the lesion is indicated. Extensive surgery including neck dissection is associated with a high incidence of fetal wastage. Because of this, one might consider some delay to allow the fetus to mature a few weeks in the third trimester. Induction of labor or cesarean section should be done as soon as fetal viability is ascertained.

The majority of patients who develop undifferentiated lesions face poor prognoses: 90%-95% of patients are dead within 1 year of diagnosis. The standard treatment in these patients would be radical thyroidectomy followed by radiation therapy. This obviously presents a difficult situation for the patient in the first or second trimester, and one must carefully discuss the situation with the patient and the family. Management of pregnant patients who have progressive, local, unresectable, or metastatic thyroid carcinoma has to be individualized and tailored to the wishes of the patient. Surgical removal of these poorly

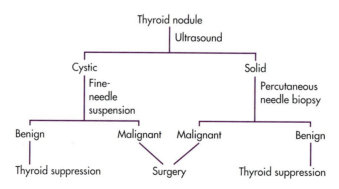

Figure 16-13 Evaluation of thyroid nodule in pregnancy. (From Hod M et al: *Obstet Gynecol Surv* 44:774, 1989.)

differentiated lesions will achieve the best local control. The role of irradiation therapy and chemotherapy remains investigational.

In summary, thyroid cancer associated with pregnancy is rare. The most common lesion is the papillary adenocarcinoma, which fortunately behaves in the least aggressive manner. The diagnostic procedures for women with solitary nodules are essentially the same as for nonpregnant patients, with the exception of the avoidance of radioisotope scanning. Fine-needle biopsy with cytologic evaluation of the specimen is currently the key diagnostic tool. There is no evidence to support a significant detrimental effect of pregnancy on the well-differentiated carcinoma of the thyroid. Thyroid suppression or replacement therapy should be instituted when the diagnosis of any solitary thyroid nodule is made. If the lesion is medullary carcinoma of the thyroid, aggressive surgical treatment is indicated. However, if gestation is in the third trimester, surgery should be delayed a few weeks to ensure the viability of the fetus, since pregnancy loss is common following such surgery. As soon as viability has been reached, labor should be induced or a cesarean section done. In the uncommon situation of poorly differentiated carcinoma of the thyroid, the main concern will be to keep the mother alive until the pregnancy has come to term because these tumors are almost uniformly lethal lesions. In all patients, the biology of a particular tumor determined both clinically and pathologically by cytologic examination must be taken into account to determine the best course for the patient and her fetus.

FETAL AND PLACENTAL METASTASES

Metastatic lesions to the fetus and/or placenta remain a poorly understood subject. Commonly the patient afflicted with cancer in pregnancy asks whether the disease can spread to her child. Fortunately, this complication is extremely rare, and fewer than 50 cases have been reported, of which the most common primary lesions were melanoma, breast cancer, and leukemia-lymphoma types. Rothman reports 35 cases of disseminated maternal malignant disease with either placental or fetal involvement. In only two instances was tumor demonstrated on both the maternal and fetal sides of the placenta and in the fetus. It is rare for the fetus to be involved if there is invasion only of the maternal side of the placenta. Of six cases in the literature when the villus itself was invaded, there was only one case of demonstrable fetal disease. Why have the products of conception been privileged in this way? Several theories have been advanced: (1) the placenta has microscopic disease that goes undetected by the usual gross and histologic examination, (2) the trophoblast acts as a barrier to these allogenic cells, (3) the fetal environment itself will not accept these foreign cells that cross the placental barrier, and (4) multiple unknown factors are involved in the determination of which tumors will metastasize to the fetus and placenta. Holland reported a case in which maternal, placental, and fetal disease were all documented.

There are reports of acute leukemia developing postnatally in the child of a mother with acute leukemia. In one report by Cramblett, the child developed acute leukemia 9 months after delivery, and in another report by Bernard, disease manifestation occurred 5 months after delivery. Hypotheses relating to familial, hereditary, environmental, and viral factors can be advanced in these circumstances but the weight of evidence suggests that acquisition of maternal malignant disease by the fetus is extremely unlikely. In another report by Potter and Schoeneman, 24 cases of maternal cancer metastasizing to the fetus or placenta were reviewed. Malignant melanoma, by far the most common tumor to spread to the fetus or placenta, was found in 11 cases. Breast cancer was found in 4 cases. Eight infants were found to have cancer at birth, and 6 of these subsequently died from their malignancies. Two infants with metastatic melanoma were noted to have complete tumor regression and ultimately survived. Seven of 8 occurrences of metastasis to the fetus were found in cases of maternal malignant melanoma, and there was 1 case of lymphosarcoma.

BIBLIOGRAPHY

Pelvic malignancies

Allen HH, Nisker JA, editors: *Cancer in pregnancy: therapeutic guidelines,* Mt Kisco, New York, 1986, Futura.

Ashkenazy M et al: Ovarian tumors in pregnancy, *Int J Gynecol Obstet* 27:765, 1988.

Baltzer J et al: Carcinoma of the cervix and pregnancy, *Int J Gynecol Obstet* 31:317, 1990.

Barber HRK, Brunschwig A: Gynecologic cancer complicating pregnancy, *Am J Obstet Gynecol* 85:156, 1963.

Barclay DL: Surgery of the vulva, perineum, and vagina in pregnancy. In Barber HRK, Graber EA, editors: *Surgical disease in pregnancy,* Philadelphia, 1974, WB Saunders.

Beischer HA: Growth and malignancy of ovarian tumors in pregnancy, *Aust NZ J Obstet Gynecol* 11:208, 1971.

Benedet JL, Anderson GH, Boyes DA: Colposcopic accuracy in the diagnosis of microinvasive and occult invasive carcinoma of the cervix, *Obstet Gynecol* 65:557, 1985.

Bosch A, Marcial VA: Carcinoma of the uterine cervix associated with pregnancy, *AJR* 96:92, 1966.

Buckley SL et al: Case report: Advanced ovarian carcinoma diagnosed during pregnancy in a patient with human immunodeficiency virus infection, *Gynecol Oncol* 50:352, 1993.

Burke TW et al: Radical wide excision and selective inguinal node dissection for squamous cell carcinoma of the vulva, *Gynecol Oncol* 38:328, 1990.

Chung A, Birnbaum SJ: Ovarian cancer associated with pregnancy, *Obstet Gynecol* 41:211, 1972.

Cliby WA, Dodson MK, Podratz KC: Cervical cancer complicated by pregnancy: episiotomy site recurrences following vaginal delivery, *Obstet Gynecol* 84(No 2), 1994.

Collins CG, Barclay DL: Cancer of the vulva and cancer of the vagina in pregnancy, *Clin Obstet Gynecol* 6:927, 1972.

Creasman WT, Rutledge F, Fletcher G: Carcinoma of the cervix associated with pregnancy, *Obstet Gynecol* 36:495, 1970.

Cruikshank SH, McNellis TM: Carcinoma of the bladder in pregnancy, *Am J Obstet Gynecol* 145:768, 1983.

Eastman NJ, Hellman LM: Ovarian tumors in pregnancy. In Eastman NJ, Hellman KM, editors: *William's Obstetrics*, ed. 13, New York, Appleton-Century Crofts, 1966.

El-Yahia AR et al: Ovarian tumours in pregnancy, *Aust NZ Obstet Gynaecol* 31:327, 1991.

Farahmand SM et al: Ovarian endodermal sinus tumor associated with pregnancy: review of the literature, *Gynecol Oncol* 41:156, 1991.

Gershenson DM et al: Treatment of malignant germ cell tumors of the ovary with bleomycin, etoposide, and cisplatin (BEP), *J Clin Oncol* 8:715, 1990.

Gordon AN, Jensen R, Jones HW III: Squamous carcinoma of the cervix complicating pregnancy: recurrence in episiotomy after vaginal delivery, *Obstet Gynecol* 73:850, 1989.

Greer BE et al: Fetal and maternal considerations in the management of stage I-B cervical cancer during pregnancy, *Gynecol Oncol* 34:61, 1989.

Hacker WF et al: Carcinoma of the cervix associated with pregnancy, *Obstet Gynecol* 59:735, 1982.

Hannigan EV et al: Cone biopsy during pregnancy, *Obstet Gynecol* 60:450, 1982.

Henderson CE et al: Case report: platinum chemotherapy during pregnancy for serous cystadenocarcinoma of the ovary, *Gynecol Oncol* 49:92,1993.

Hoffman MS: Primary ovarian carcinoma during pregnancy, case report, Clinical consultations in *Obstetrica and Gynecology* 7(4):237, 1995.

Hoffman MS et al: Adenocarcinoma of the endometrium and endometrioid carcinoma of the ovary associated with pregnancy, *Gynecol Oncol* 32:82, 1989.

Hoffman MS et al: Recent modifications in the treatment of invasive squamous cell carcinoma of the vulva, *Obstet Gynecol Surv* 44:227, 1989.

Jubb ED: Primary ovarian carcinoma in pregnancy, *Am J Obstet Gynecol*, 83:345, 1963.

Karlen JR, Sternberg LB, Abbott JN: Carcinoma of the endometrium coexisting with pregnancy, *Obstet Gynecol* 40:334, 1972.

Karlen JR et al: Dysgerminoma associated with pregnancy, *Obstet Gynecol* 53:330, 1979.

Kempson RL, Pokorny GE: Adenocarcinoma of the endometrium in women aged forty and younger, *Cancer* 21:650, 1968.

Kim DS, Park MI: Maternal and fetal survival following surgery and chemotherapy for endometrial sinus tumor of the ovary during pregnancy: a case report, *Obstet Gynecol* 73:503, 1989.

King LA et al: Treatment of advanced epithelial ovarian carcinoma in pregnancy with cisplatin-based chemotherapy, *Gynecol Oncol* 41:78, 1991.

Lee RB, Neglia W, Park RC: Cervical carcinoma in pregnancy, *Obstet Gynecol* 58:584, 1981.

Lutz MH et al: Genital malignancy in pregnancy, *Am J Obstet Gynecol*, 129:536, 1977.

Malone JM et al: Endodermal sinus tumor of the ovary associated with pregnancy, *Obstet Gynecol* 68(suppl):865, 1986.

McDonnell JM et al: Colposcopy in pregnancy: a twelve year review, *Br J Obstet Gynaecol* 88:414, 1981.

Melfetona JH, Goldkrand JW: Cisplatinum combination chemotherapy during pregnancy for advanced epithelial ovarian cancer, *Obstet Gynecol* 75:545, 1990.

Monaghan JM, Lindeque G: Commentary: vulvar carcinoma in pregnancy, *Br J Obstet Gynaecol* 93:785, 1986.

Moore DH, Fowler WC Jr, Currie JL: Case report: squamous cell carcinoma of the vulva in pregnancy, *Gynecol Oncol* 41:74, 1991.

Munnell EW: Primary ovarian cancer associated with pregnancy, *Clin Obstet Gynecol* 4:983, 1963.

Nevin J et al: Advanced cervical carcinoma associated with pregnancy, *Int J Gynecol Cancer* 3:57, 1993.

Nevin J et al: Cervical carcinoma associated with pregnancy, *Obstet Gynecol Surv* 50:228, 1995.

Nisker JA, Shubat M: Stage Ib cervical carcinoma and pregnancy report of 49 cases, *Am J Obstet Gynecol* 145:230, 1983.

Novak ER: Ovarian tumors in pregnancy: an Ovarian Tumor Registry overview, *Obstet Gynecol* 46:401, 1975.

O'Leary JA, Pratt JH, Symmonds RE: Rectal carcinoma in pregnancy, *Obstet Gynecol* 30:862, 1967.

Perkins RL, Hernandez E, Miyazawa K: Ovarian endodermal sinus tumor during pregnancy, *Am J Gynecol Health*, 111(3):21, 1989.

Roman LD et al: Unsuspected invasive squamous carcinoma of the vulva in young women, *Gynecol Oncol* 41:182, 1991.

Sablinska RE, Tarlowska L, Stelmachow J: Invasive carcinoma of the cervix associated with pregnancy: correlation between patient age, advancement of cancer and gestation, and result of treatment, *Gynecol Oncol* 5:363, 1977.

Sandstrom RE, Welch WR, Green TH: Adenocarcinoma of the endometrium in pregnancy, *Obstet Gynecol* 53(suppl):73, 1979.

Schumann EA: Observations upon the coexistence of carcinoma fundus uteri and pregnancy, *Trans Am Gynecol Soc* 52:245, 1927.

Schwartz PE, Vidone RA: Pregnancy following combination chemotherapy for a mixed germ cell tumor of the ovary, *Gynecol Oncol* 12:373, 1981.

Schwartz RP et al: Endodermal sinus tumor in pregnancy: report of case and review of literature, *Gynecol Oncol* 15:434, 1983.

Senekjian EK et al: Clear cell adenocarcinoma (CA) of the vagina and cervix in association with pregnancy, *Gynecol Oncol* 24:207, 1986.

Sivanesaratnam V, Jayalakshmi P, Loo C: Surgical management of early invasive cancer of the cervix associated with pregnancy, *Gynecol Oncol* 48:68, 1993.

Sorosky JI et al: Stage I squamous cell cervical carcinoma in pregnancy: planned delay in therapy awaiting fetal maturity, *Gynecol Oncol* 59:207, 1995.

Struyk APHB, Treffers PE: Ovarian tumors in pregnancy, *Acta Obstet Gynecol Scand* 63:421, 1984.

Summer GM et al: A case of endometrial carcinoma of the ovary associated with pregnancy, *Gynecol Oncol* 21:364, 1985.

Suzuki A et al: A case of grade II adenocarcinoma of the endometrium in pregnancy, *Gynecol Oncol* 18:261, 1984.

Thornton JG, Wells M: Ovarian cysts in pregnancy: does ultrasound make traditional management inappropriate? *Obstet Gynecol* 69:717, 1987.

Van Der See AGJ et al: Endodermal sinus tumor of the ovary during pregnancy: a case report, *Am J Obstet Gynecol* 164(2):504, 1991.

Van Voorhis B, Cruikshank DP: Colon carcinoma complicating pregnancy, *J Reprod Med* 34:923, 1989.

Waldrop GM, Palmer JP: Carcinoma of the cervix associated with pregnancy, *Am J Obstet Gynecol* 86:202, 1963.

Wallingford AJ: Cancer of the body of the uterus complicating pregnancy, *Am J Obstet Gynecol* 27:224, 1934.

Waxman J: Cancer, chemotherapy, and fertility, *Br Med J* 290:1096, 1985.

Yazigi R, Cunningham G: Cancer and pregnancy. In *Williams Obstetrics*, Cunningham, Macdonald, Gant 4, 1990.

Young RH, Dudley AG, Scully RE: Granulosa cell, Sertoli-Leydig cell, and unclassified sex-cord stromal tumors associated with pregnancy: a clinical-pathological analysis of 36 cases, *Gynecol Oncol* 18:181, 1984.

Zemlickis D et al: Maternal and fetal outcome after invasive cervical cancer in pregnancy, *J Clin Oncol* 9:1956, 1991.

Chemotherapy

Aviles A et al: Growth and development of children of mothers treated with chemotherapy during pregnancy: current status of 43 children, *Am J Hematol* 36:243, 1991.

Baer MR, Ozer H, Foon KA: Interferon-alpha therapy during pregnancy in chronic myelogenous leukemia and hairy cell leukemia, *Br J Hematol* 81:167, 1992.

Barnicle MM: Chemotherapy and pregnancy, *Semin Oncol Nurs*, 8:124, 1992.

Blatt J et al: Pregnancy outcome following cancer chemotherapy, *Am J Med* 69:828, 1980.

Boros SJ, Reynolds JW: Intrauterine growth retardation following third-trimester exposure to busulfan, *Am J Obstet Gynecol* 129:111, 1977.

Briggs GG, Freeman RK, Yafee SJ: Instructions for use of the reference guide. In Briggs GG, Freeman RK, Yafee SJ, eds: *A reference guide to fetal and neonatal risk: drugs in pregnancy and lactation*. ed 3, Baltimore, Md: Williams & Wilkins, 1990.

Byrne J et al: Effects of treatment on fertility in long-term survivors of childhood or adolescent cancer, *N Engl. J Med* 37:1315, 1987.

Chapman RM, Sutcliffe SB, Malpas JS: Cytotoxic-induced ovarian failure in women with Hodgkin's disease. I. Hormone function, *JAMA* 242:1877, 1979.

Coates A: Cyclophosphamide in pregnancy, *Aust NZ J Obstet Gynecol* 10:33, 1970.

Crump M et al: Successful pregnancy and delivery during interferon therapy for chronic myeloid leukemia, *Am J Hematol* 40:238, 1992. Letter.

Daly H et al: Successful pregnancy during combination chemotherapy for Hodgkin's disease, *Acta Haematol* 64:154, 1980.

Dara PM, Slater LM, Armentrout SA: Successful pregnancy during chemotherapy for acute leukemia, *Cancer* 47:845, 1981.

Daw EG: Procarbazine in pregnancy, letter, *Lancet* 2:984, 1970.

Doll DC et al: Management of cancer during pregnancy, *Arch Intern Med* 148:2058, 1988.

Farney JP: Pregnancy following removal and chemotherapy of ovarian endodermal sinus tumor, *Obstet Gynecol* 52:360, 1978.

Garber JE: Long-term follow-up of children exposed in utero to antineoplastic agents, *Semin Oncol* 16:437, 1989.

Gershenson DM: Menstrual and reproductive function after treatment with combination chemotherapy for malignant ovarian germ cell tumors, *J Clin Oncol* 6:270, 1988.

Gilland J, Weinstein L: The effects of cancer chemotherapeutic agents on the developing fetus, *Obstet Gynecol Surv* 38:6, 1983.

Horning SJ et al: Female reproductive potential after treatment for Hodgkin's disease, *N Engl J Med* 304:1377, 1981.

Kolowski RD et al: Outcome of first-trimester exposure to low-dose methotrexate in eight patients with rheumatic disease, *Am J Med* 88:589, 1990.

Lurain JR et al: Pregnancy outcome subsequent to consecutive hydatidiform moles, *Am J Obstet Gynecol* 142(No 8), 1982.

Meistrich ML et al: Recovery of sperm production after chemotherapy for osteosarcoma, *Cancer* 63:2115, 1989.

Morishata S et al: Acute myelogenous leukemia in pregnancy: fetal blood sampling and early effects of chemotherapy, *Int J Gynaecol Obstet* 44:273, 1994.

Mulvihill JJ et al: Pregnancy outcome in cancer patients, *Cancer* 60:1143, 1987.

Nicholson HO: Cytotoxic drugs in pregnancy, *J Obstet Gynaecol Br Common* 75:307, 1968.

Powis G: Anticancer drug pharmacodynamics, *Cancer Chemother Pharmacol* 14:177, 1985.

Randall T: National registry seeks scarce data on pregnancy outcomes during chemotherapy, *JAMA*, 269:323, 1993.

Roboz J et al: Does doxorubicin cross the placenta? *Lancet* 2:1382, 1972.

Schilsky RL et al: Gonadal dysfunction in patients receiving chemotherapy for cancer, *Ann Intern Med* 93:109, 1980.

Selevan SG et al: A study of occupational exposure to antineoplastic drugs and fetal loss in nurses, *N Engl J Med* 313:1173, 1985.

Shalet SM: Effects of cancer chemotherapy on gonadal function of patients, *Cancer Treat Rev* 7:141, 1980.

Sokal JE, Lessman EM: The effects of cancer chemotherapeutic agents on the human fetus, *JAMA* 172:1765, 1960.

Stillman RJ, Schuff I, Schienfeld J: Reproductive and gonadal functions in the female after therapy for childhood malignancy, *Obstet Gynecol Surv* 37:385, 1982.

Van Thiel DH, Ross GT, Lipsett MB: Pregnancies after chemotherapy of trophoblastic neoplasms, *Science* 169:1326, 1970.

Waxman J et al: Gonadal function in Hodgkin's disease: long-term follow-up of chemotherapy, *Br Med J Clin Res* 285:1612, 1982.

Zemlickis D et al: Fetal outcome after in utero exposure to cancer chemotherapy, *Arch Intern Med* 152:573, 1992.

Zuazu X, Julia A, Sierra J: Pregnancy outcome in hematologic malignancies, *Cancer* 67:703, 1991.

Radiation therapy

Dekaban AS: Abnormalities in children exposed to x-irradiation during various stages of gestation: tentative timetable of radiation injury to the human fetus, *J Nucl Med* 9:471, 1968.

Doll R: Radiation hazards: 25 years of collaborative research, *Br J Radiol* 54:179, 1981.

Grosovsky AJ, Little JB: Evidence for linear response for the induction of mutations in human cells by x-ray exposures below 10 rads, *Proc Natl Acad Sci USA* 82:2092, 1985.

Hahn EW et al: Recovery from aspermia endured by low-dose radiation in seminoma patients, *Cancer* 50:337, 1982.

Hawkins MM, Smith RA: Pregnancy outcomes in childhood cancer survivors: probable effects of abdominal irradiation, *Int J Cancer* 43:399, 1989.

Jacobsen E: Therapeutic abortion on account of x-ray examination during pregnancy, *Dan Med Bull* 6:113, 1959.

Kalter H, Warkany J: Medical progress of congenital malformations: etiologic factors and their role in prevention, *N Engl J Med* 8:424, 1983.

Little JB: Cellular, molecular and carcinogenic effects of radiation, *Hematol/Oncol Clin North Am* 7:337, 1993.

Shimizu Y, Kato H, Schull WJ: Studies of the mortality of A-bomb survivors, 9. Mortality 1950-1985; Part 2, Cancer mortality based on the recently revised doses, *Radiat Res* 121:1990.

Smith PG, Doll R: Mortality from cancer and all causes among British radiologists, *Br J Radiol* 54:187, 1981.

Sneed PK et al: Fetal dose estimates for radiotherapy of brain tumors during pregnancy, *Int J Radiat Biol Oncol Phys* 32:823, 1995.

Stovall M et al: Fetal dose from radiotherapy with photon beams: report AAPM Radiation Therapy Committee Task Group No. 36, *Med Phys* 22:63, 1995.

Sweet DL, Kinzie J: Consequence of radiotherapy and antineoplastic therapy for the fetus, *J Reprod Med* 17:241, 1976.

Taylor G, Blom J: Acute leukemia during pregnancy, *South Med J* 73:1314, 1980.

Wall BF et al: A reappraisal of the genetic consequences of diagnostic radiology in Great Britain, *Br J Radiol* 54:719, 1981.

Woo SY et al: Radiotherapy during pregnancy for clinical stages IA-IIA Hodgkin's disease, *Int J Radiat Oncol Biol Phys* 23:407, 1992.

Nongynecologic malignancies

Anderson JM: Mammary cancers and pregnancy, *Br Med J* 1:1124, 1979.

Aviles A, Diaz-Maqueo JC, Torras V: Non-Hodgkin's lymphomas and pregnancy: presentation of 16 cases, *Gynecol Oncol* 37:335, 1990.

Barber HRK, Brunschwig A: Carcinoma of the bowel: radiation and surgical management and pregnancy, *Am J Obstet Gynecol* 100:926, 1968.

Barni S et al: Weekly doxorubicin chemotherapy for breast cancer in pregnancy: a case report, *Tumori* 78:349, 1992.

Barry RM et al: Influence of pregnancy on the course of Hodgkin's disease, *Am J Obstet Gynecol* 84:445, 1962.

Bitran JD, Roth DG: Acute leukemia during reproductive life: its course, complications and sequelae for fertility, *J Reprod Med* 17:225, 1976.

Boronow R: Extrapelvic malignancy and pregnancy, *Obstet Gynecol Surv* 19:1, 1964.

Bryant AJS, Weir JA: Prophylactic oophorectomy in operable instances of carcinoma of the breast, *Surg Gynecol Obstet* 153:660, 1981.

Bunker ML, Peters MV: Breast cancer associated with pregnancy or lactation, *Am J Obstet Gynecol* 85:312, 1963.

Burrow GW: The thyroid in pregnancy, *Med Clin Wash* 59:1089, 1973.

Byers T, Graham S, Swanson M: Parity and colorectal cancer risk in women, *J Natl Ca Inst* 69:1059, 1979.

Byrd BF Jr, McGanity WJ: The effect of pregnancy on the clinical course of sarcoma of the soft somatic tissues, *Surg Obstet Gynecol* 125:28, 1967.

Catanzarite VA, Ferguson JE: Acute leukemia in pregnancy: a review of the management and outcome, 1972-1982, *Obstet Gynecol Surv* 39:663, 1984.

Cheek JH: Cancer of the breast in pregnancy and lactation, *Am J Surg* 126:729, 1973.

Cohen PJ, Jaffe ES: Current methods used in the diagnosis and classification of malignant lymphomas, Updates 1(8), 1987. In *Cancer, Principles & Practice of Oncology*, DeVita VT, ed. 2.

Cunningham MP, Slaughter DP: Surgical treatment of disease of the thyroid gland in pregnancy, *Surg Gynecol Obstet* 131:486, 1970.

Dein RA et al: The reproductive potential of young men and women with Hodgkin's disease, *Obstet Gynecol Surv* 39(8):474, 1982.

Dein RA et al: The reproductive potential of young men and women with Hodgkin's disease, *Obstet Gynecol Surv* 39:474, 1984.

DeVita VH, Serpick AA, Carbone PP: Combination chemotherapy in the treatment of advanced Hodgkin's disease, *Ann Intern Med* 73:881, 1970.

DiSaia PJ, Creasman WT: *Clinical gynecologic oncology*, ed 3, St. Louis, 1993, Times Mirror/Mosby College Publishing.

Donegan WL: Mammary carcinoma and pregnancy, *Major Prob Clin Surg* 5:448, 1979.

Donegan WL: Cancer and pregnancy, *CA* 33:194, 1983.

Durkin JW: Carcinoid tumor and pregnancy, *Am J Obstet Gynecol* 145:757, 1983.

Egan PC et al: Doxorubicin and cisplatin excretion into human milk, *Cancer Treat Rep* 69:1387, 1985.

Falksen HC, Simson IW, Falksen G: Non-Hodgkin's lymphoma in pregnancy, *Cancer* 45:1679, 1980.

Frenkel EP, Meyers MC: Acute leukemia and pregnancy, *Ann Intern Med* 53:656, 1960.

Friedman EW: Carcinoma of the thyroid. In Rovensky JJ, Gullmacher AF, editors: *Medical, surgical, and gynecologic complications of pregnancy*, Baltimore, Williams and Wilkins, 1965.

Gaetini A et al: Lateral high abdominal ovariopexy: an original surgical technique for protection of the ovaries during curative radiotherapy for Hodgkin's disease, *J Surg Oncol* 39:22, 1988.

Gambardella FR: Pancreatic cancer in pregnancy: a case report, *Am J Obstet Gynecol* 149:15, 1984.

Girard M, Lamarche J, Baillot R: Cancer of the colon associated with pregnancy, *Am Soc Colon-Rectal Surg* 24:473, 1980.

Graffner HOL, Alm POA, Oscarson JEA: Prophylactic oophorectomy in colorectal cancer, *Am J Surg* 146:233, 1983.

Green DM, Hall B, Zevon MA: Pregnancy outcome after treatment for acute lymphoblastic leukemia during childhood or adolescence, *Cancer* 64:2335, 1989.

Green LK et al: Cancer of the colon during pregnancy, *Obstet Gynecol* 46(4):480, 1974.

Haagensen CD: Cancer of the breast in pregnancy and during lactation, *Am J Obstet Gynecol* 98:141, 1967.

Haagensen CD: *Diseases of the breast*, ed 2, Philadelphia, Pa: WB Saunders, 1971.

Hammer-Jacobsen E: Therapeutic abortion on account of x-ray examination during pregnancy, *Dan Med Bull* 6:113, 1959.

Harkin KP et al: Metastatic malignant melanoma during pregnancy, *Ir med J* 83:116, 1990.

Hill CS, Clark RL, Wolf M: The effect of subsequent pregnancy in patients with thyroid carcinoma, *Surg Gynecol Obstet* 122:1219, 1966.

Hill JA et al: Colonic cancer in pregnancy, *South Med J* 77(3):375, 1984.

Hod M et al: Pregnancy and thyroid carcinoma: a review of incidence, course and prognosis, *Obstet Gynecol Surv* 44:774, 1989.

Holleb AI, Farrow JH: The relation of carcinoma of the breast and pregnancy in 283 patients, *Surg Gynecol Obstet* 115:65, 1962.

Holmes GE, Holmes FF: Pregnancy outcome of patients treated for Hodgkin's disease: a controlled study, *Cancer* 41:1317, 1978.

Hoppe RT, Castellino RA: The staging of Hodgkin's disease, PPO updates 4 (7), 1990.

Horning SJ, Hoppe RT, Kaplan HS: Female reproduction after treatment for Hodgkin's disease, *N Engl J Med* 304(23):1377, 1977.

Hunter MCH, Glees JP, Gazet JC: Oophorectomy and ovarian functions in the treatment of Hodgkin's disease, *Clin Radiol* 31:21, 1980.

Jacobs C, Donaldson SS, Rosenberg SA: Management of the pregnant patient with Hodgkin's disease, *Ann Inter Med* 95:669, 1981.

Jafari K, Lash AF, Webster A: Pregnancy and sarcoma, *Acta Obstet Gynecol Scand* 57:265, 1978.

Juarez S et al: Association of leukemia and pregnancy: clinical and obstetric aspects, *Am J Clin Oncol* 11:159, 1988.

Kasdon SC: Pregnancy and Hodgkin's disease with a report of three cases, *Am J Obstet Gynecol* 57:282, 1949.

Klein VR et al: Renal cell carcinoma in pregnancy, *Obstet Gynecol* 69(3), 1987.

Le Floch O, Donaldson SS, Kaplan HS: Pregnancy following oophoropexy and total nodal irradiation in women with Hodgkin's disease, *Cancer* 38:2263, 1976.

Levin B: Aspects of gastrointestinal tumors during the reproductive years, *J Reprod Med* 17(4):223, 1976.

Levine AM, Collea JV: When pregnancy complicates chronic granulocytic leukemia, *Contemp Ob/Gyn* 13:47, 1979.

Lilleyman JS, Hill AS, Anderton KJ: Consequences of acute myelogenous leukemia in early pregnancy, *Obstet Gynecol Surv* 33:393, 1978.

Lishner M et al: Maternal and foetal outcome following Hodgkin's disease in pregnancy, *Br J Cancer* 65:114, 1992.

McKeen EA, Rosner F, Zarrobi MH: Pregnancy outcome in Hodgkin's disease, *Lancet* 2:590, 1979.

Merkatz IR et al: Resumption of female reproductive function following renal transplantation, *JAMA* 216:1749, 1971.

Mestman JH: Management of thyroid diseases in pregnancy, *Clin Perinatol* 7:371, 1980.

Nantel S, Parboosingh J, Poon MC: Treatment of an aggressive non-Hodgkin's lymphoma during pregnancy with MACOP-B chemotherapy, *Med Pediatr Oncol* 18:143, 1990.

Nesbitt JC, Moise KJ, Sawyers JL: Colorectal carcinoma in pregnancy, *Arch Surg* 120:636, 1985.

Nisce LZ et al: Management of coexisting Hodgkin's disease and pregnancy, *Am J Clin Oncol* 9:146, 1986.

O'Dell RF: Leukemia and lymphoma complications of pregnancy, *Clin Obstet Gynecol* 22:859, 1979.

O'Leary JA, Pratt JH, Symonds RE: Rectal carcinoma in pregnancy: a review of 17 cases, *Obstet Gynecol* 30:862, 1967.

Patel M, Dukes IAF, Hill JC: Use of hydroxyurea in chronic myeloid leukemia during pregnancy: a case report, *Am J Obstet Gynecol* 165:565, 1991.

Peters MV, Meakin JW: The influence of pregnancy in carcinoma of the breast, *Prog Clin Cancer* 1:471, 1965.

Petrek JV: Breast cancer in pregnancy, *Cancer* 74:518, 1994 (suppl).

Pizzuto J et al: Treatment of acute leukemia in pregnancy: presentation of nine cases, *Cancer Treat Rep* 64:679, 1980.

Raich PC, Curet LB: Treatment of acute leukemia during pregnancy, *Cancer* 36:861, 1975.

Raydin RG et al: Results of a clinical trial concerning the worth of prophylactic oophorectomy for breast carcinoma, *Surg Gynecol Obstet* 131:1055, 1970.

Ribeiro GG, Palmer MK: Breast carcinoma associated with pregnancy: a clinician's dilemma, *Br Med J* 2:1524, 1977.

Rosemond GP: Carcinoma of the breast during pregnancy, *Clin Obstet Gynecol* 6:994, 1963.

Rosenberg SA: A critique of the value of laparotomy and splenectomy in the evaluation of patients with Hodgkin's disease, *Cancer Res* 31:1737, 1971.

Rosvoll RV, Winship T: Thyroid carcinoma and pregnancy, *Surg Gynecol Obstet* 121:1039, 1965.

Sanger WG, Armitage JO, Schmidt MA: Feasibility of semen cryopreservation in patients with malignant disease, *JAMA* 244:789, 1980.

Simon R: Statistical methods for evaluating pregnancy outcomes in patients with Hodgkin's disease, *Cancer* 45:2890, 1980.

Spitzer M et al: Non-Hodgkin's lymphoma during pregnancy, *Gynecol Oncol* 43:309, 1991.

Sweet DL Jr: Malignant lymphoma: implications during the reproductive years and pregnancy, *J Reprod Med* 17(4):198, 1976.

Taylor S: Endocrine ablation in disseminated mammary carcinoma, *Surg Gynecol Obstet* 115:443, 1962.

Thomas PRM, Peckham MJ: The investigation and management of Hodgkin's disease in the pregnant patient, *Cancer* 38:1443, 1994.

Trueblood WH, Enright LP, Nelsen TS: Preservation of ovarian function with radiotherapy for malignant lymphoma, *Arch Surg* 100:236, 1970.

Tsukamoto N et al: Cancer of the colon presenting as bilateral ovarian tumors during pregnancy, *Gynecol Oncol* 24:386, 1986.

Van Voorhis B, Cruiskshank DP: Colon carcinoma complicating pregnancy, *J Reprod Med* 34:923, 1989.

Vitums VC, Sites JG: Leukemia in pregnancy, *Med Ann DC* 37:588, 1968.

Ward FT, Weiss RB: Lymphoma and pregnancy, *Semin Oncol* 16:397, 1989.

White LP et al: Studies on melanoma: the effect of pregnancy on survival in human melanoma, *JAMA* 117:235, 1961.

Williams SF, Bitran JD: Cancer and pregnancy, *Clin Perinatol* 12(3):609, 1985.

Woo SY et al: Radiotherapy during pregnancy for clinical stages IA-IIA Hodgkin's disease, *Int J Radiat Oncol Biol Phys* 23:407, 1992.

Yazigi R, Driscoll SG: Sarcoma complicating pregnancy, *Gynecol Oncol* 25:125, 1986.

Zuazu J, Julia A, Sierra J et al: Pregnancy outcome in hematologic malignancies, *Cancer* 67:703, 1991.

Melanoma

Breslow A: Tumor thickness, level of invasion, and node dissection in stage I cutaneous melanoma, *Ann Surg* 182:572, 1975.

Campbell WA, et al: Fetal malignant melanoma: ultrasound presentation and review of the literature, *Obstet Gynecol* 70:434, 1987.

Clark WH et al: The histogenesis and biologic behavior of primary malignant melanomas of the skin, *Cancer Res* 29:705, 1969.

Colbourn DS, Nathanson L, Belilos E: Pregnancy and malignant melanoma, *Semin Oncol* 16:377, 1989.

Elwood JM, Coldman AJ: Previous pregnancy and melanoma prognosis, *Lancet* 2(8097):1000, 1978.

George PA, Fortner JG, Pack GT: Melanoma with pregnancy: report of 115 cases, *Cancer* 13:854, 1960.

Hersey P et al: Previous pregnancy as a protective factor against death from melanoma, *Lancet* 1:451, 1977.

Houghton A et al: Malignant melanoma of the skin occurring during pregnancy, *Cancer* 48:407, 1981.

Kjems E, Kraq C: Melanoma and pregnancy: a review, *Acta Oncol* 32:371, 1993.

Lerner AB, Nordlernd JJ, Kirkwood JM: Effects of oral contraceptives and pregnancy on melanoma, *N Engl J Med* 31:47, 1979.

Mackie RM et al: Lack of effect of pregnancy on outcome of melanoma, *Lancet* 337:653, 1991.

McManamny DS et al: Melanoma and pregnancy: a long-term follow-up, *Br J Obstet Gynecol* 96:1419, 1989.

Moller D, Ipsen L, Asschenfeldt P: Fatal course of malignant melanoma during pregnancy with dissemination to the products of conception, *Acata Obstet Gynecol Scand* 65:501, 1986.

Pack GT, Scharnagel LM: The prognosis for malignant melanoma in the pregnant woman, *Cancer* 4:324, 1951.

Reintgen DS et al: Malignant melanoma and pregnancy, *Cancer* 55:1340, 1985.

Reintgen DS et al: The orderly progression of melanoma nodal metastases, *Ann Surg* 220:759, 1994.

Reintgen DS et al: Pregnancy in association with malignant melanoma, *Clinical Consult Obstet Gynecol* 7(4):257, 1995.

Schneiderman H et al: Congenital melanoma with multiple prenatal metastasis, *Cancer* 60:1371, 1987.

Shaw HM et al: Malignant melanoma: influence of site of lesion and age of patient in the female superiority in survival, *Cancer* 46:2731, 1980.

Shiu MH et al: Adverse effect of pregnancy on melanoma, *Cancer* 37:181, 1976.

Shocket EC, Fortner JG: Melanoma and pregnancy: an experimental evaluation of a clinical impression, *Surg Forum* 9:671, 1958.

Simon MA, Phillips WA, Bonfiglio M: Pregnancy and aggressive or malignant primary bone tumors, *Cancer* 53:2564, 1984.

Slingluff CL et al: Malignant melanoma arising during pregnancy: a study of 100 patients, *Ann Surg* 211:552, 1990.

Slingluff CL et al: Malignant melanoma in pregnancy, *Ann Plast Surg* 28:95, 1992.

Sutherland CM et al: Effect of pregnancy upon malignant melanoma, *Surg Gynecol Obstet* 157:443, 1983.

Travers R et al: Increased thickness of pregnancy associated melanoma: a study of the MGH pigmented lesion clinic, *Melanoma Res.* 3(suppl):44, 1993.

Wong JH et al: Prognostic significance of pregnancy in stage I melanoma, *Arch Surg* 124:1227, 1989.

Breast cancer and pregnancy

Adair EA: Cancer of the breast, *Surg Clin North Am* 33:313, 1953.

Applewhite RR, Smith LR, DiVincenti F: Carcinoma of the breast associated with pregnancy and lactation, *Ann Surg* 39:101, 1973.

Aviles A, Diaz Maqueo JC, Talavera A: Growth and development of children of mothers treated with chemotherapy during pregnancy: current status of 43 children, *Am J Hematol* 36:243, 1991.

Barnavon Y, Wallack MK: Management of the pregnant patient with carcinoma of the breast, *Surg Gynecol Obstet* 171:279, 1990.

Barni S et al: Weekly doxorubicin chemotherapy for breast cancer in pregnancy: a case report, *Tumori* 78:349, 1992.

Beatson GT: On the treatment of inoperable cases of carcinoma of the mamma: suggestions for new methods of treatment with illustrative cases, *Lancet* 2:104, 1896.

Bryant AJS, Weir JA: Prophylactic oophorectomy in operable instances of carcinoma of the breast, *Surg Gynecol Obstet* 153:660, 1981.

Bunker ML, Peters MV: Breast cancer associated with pregnancy or lactation, *Am J Obstet Gynecol* 85:312, 1963.

Cheek JH: Cancer of the breast in pregnancy and lactation, *Am J Surg* 126:729, 1973.

Clark RM, Reid J: Carcinoma of the breast in pregnancy and lactation, *Int J Radiat Oncol Biol Phys* 4:693, 1978.

Cooper DR, Butterfield J: Pregnancy subsequent to mastectomy for cancer of the breast, *Ann Surg* 171:429, 1970.

Dildy G et al: Maternal malignancy metastatic to the products of conception: a review, *Obstet Gynecol Surv* 44:535, 1989.

Donegan WL: Cancer and pregnancy, *CA* 33:194, 1983.

Early TK, Gallagher JQ, Chapman KE: Carcinoma of the breast in women under thirty years of age, *Am J Surg* 118:832, 1969.

Egan PC et al: Doxorubicin and cisplatin excretion into human milk, *Cancer Treat Rep* 69:1387, 1985.

Elledge RM et al: Estrogen receptor, progesterone receptor, and HER-2/neu protein in breast cancers from pregnant patients, *Cancer* 71:2499, 1993.

Haagensen CD: Cancer of the breast in pregnancy and during lactation, *Am J Obstet Gynecol* 98:141, 1967.

Harrington SW: Carcinoma of the breast: results of treatment when the carcinoma occurred in the course of pregnancy or lactation and when pregnancy occurred subsequent to operation (1910-1933), *Ann Surg* 106:690, 1937.

Harvey JC et al: The effect of pregnancy on the prognosis of carcinoma of the breast following radical mastectomy, *Surg Gynecol Obstet* 153:723, 1981.

Hassey KM: Pregnancy and parenthood after treatment for breast cancer, *ONF* 15(4), 1988.

Higgins S, Haffty B: Pregnancy and lactation after breast-conserving therapy for early stage breast cancer, *Cancer* 73:2175, 1994.

Holleb AI, Farrow JH: The relation of carcinoma of the breast and pregnancy in 283 patients, *Surg Gynecol Obstet* 115:65, 1962.

Hornstein E, Skornick Y, Rozin R: The management of breast carcinoma in pregnancy and lactation, *J Surg Oncol* 21:179, 1982.

Horsley JS III, Alrich EM, Wright CB: Carcinoma of the breast in women 35 years of age or younger, *Ann Surg* 196:839, 1969.

Hubay CA, Barry FM, Moss CC: Pregnancy and breast cancer, *Surg Clin North Am* 58:819, 1978.

Hulka BS: Replacement estrogens and risk of gynecologic cancers and breast cancer, *Cancer* 60:1960, 1987.

Ishida T, Yoko T, Kasumi F: Clinical pathological characteristics and progress of breast cancer patients associated with pregnancy and lactation: analysis of case-control study in Japan, *Jpn J Cancer Res* 83:1143, 1992.

Kim Y, Pomper J, Goldberg ME: Anesthetic management of the pregnant patient with carcinoma of the breast, *J Clin Anesth* 5:76, 1993.

King RM et al: Carcinoma of the breast associated with pregnancy, *Surg Gynecol Obstet* 160:228, 1985.

Nugent P, O'Connell TX: Breast cancer and pregnancy, *Arch Surg* 120:1221, 1985.

Petrek JA: Breast cancer during pregnancy, *Cancer* 74(1):518, 1994.

Petrek JA, Dukoff R, Rogatko A: Prognosis of pregnancy-associated breast cancer, *Cancer* 67:869, 1991.

Rabdall T: National registry seeks scarce data on pregnancy outcomes during chemotherapy, *JAMA* 269:323, 1993.

Raydin RG et al: Results of a clinical trial concerning the worth of prophylactic oophorectomy for breast carcinoma, *Surg Gynecol Obstet* 131:1055, 1970.

Ribeiro GG, Palmer MK: Breast carcinoma associated with pregnancy: a clinician's dilemma, *Br Med J* 2:1524, 1977.

Rissanen PN: Carcinoma of the breast during pregnancy and lactation, *Br J Cancer* 22:663, 1968.

Robinson DW: Breast carcinoma associated with pregnancy, *Am J Obstet Gynecol* 92:658, 1965.

Saunders CM, Baum M: Breast cancer and pregnancy: a review, *J R Soc Med* 86:162, 1993.

Sutton R, Buzdar AU, Hortobagyi GN: Pregnancy and offspring after adjuvant chemotherapy in breast cancer patients, *Cancer* 65:847, 1990.

Taylor S: Endocrine ablation in disseminated mammary carcinoma, *Surg Gynecol Obstet* 115:443, 1962.

Theriault RL, Stallings CB, Buzdar AU: Pregnancy and breast cancer: clinical and legal issues: clinical case reports from MD Anderson Cancer Center, *Am J Clin Oncol* 15:535, 1992.

Tobon H, Horowitz LF: Breast cancer during pregnancy, *Breast Dis* 6:127, 1993.

Tralins A: Is lactation possible after breast irradiation? *Proc Am Soc Clin Oncol*, Abstract 12:77, 1993.

Treves N, Holleb AI: A report of 549 cases of breast cancer in women 35 years of age or younger, *Surg Gynecol Oncol* 100:661, 1955.

Van der Vange N, Van Donegan JA: Breast cancer and pregnancy, *Eur J Surg Oncol* 17:1, 1991.

Wagner LK, Lester RG, Saldana LR: The amount of radiation absorbed by the conceptus. In *Exposure of the Pregnant Patient to Diagnostic Radiation. A guide to Medical Management.* Philadelphia, PA: LB Lippincott, 52, 1985.

White TT: Cancer of the breast in the pregnant or nursing patient, *Am J Obstet Gynecol* 69:1277, 1955.

White TT: Prognosis of breast cancer for pregnant women: analysis of 1413 cases, *Surg Gynecol Obstet* 100:661, 1955.

White TT, White WC: Breast cancer and pregnancy, *Ann Surg* 144:385, 1956.

Wile AG, DiSaia PJ: Hormones and breast cancer, *Am J Surg* 157:438, 1989.

Willemse PHB, van der Sijde R, Sleijfer DT: Combination chemotherapy and radiation for stage IV breast cancer during pregnancy, *Gynecol Oncol* 36:281, 1990.

Zemlikis D et al: Maternal and fetal outcome after breast cancer in pregnancy, *Am J Obstet Gynecol* 166:781, 1992.

Fetal and placental metastases

Bernard J et al: Leucimi aigue d'une eufqnt de 5 wois nce' de' une me're atteinte de leucemie argu' au moment de l'accouchement, *Nouv Rev Franc Haenatal* 4:140, 1964.

Brodsky I et al: Metastatic malignant melanoma from mother to fetus, *Cancer* 181:48, 1965.

Cavell B: Transplacental metastasis of malignant melanoma, *Acta Pathol* 146(suppl):37, 1963.

Cramblett HG, Friedman JL, Najjao S: Leukemia in an infant born of a mother with leukemia, *N Engl J Med* 259:727, 1958.

Dargeon HW et al: Malignant melanoma in an infant, *Cancer* 3:299, 1950.

Diamondopoulos GT, Hertig AT: Transmission of leukemia and allied diseases from mother to fetus, *Obstet Gynecol* 21:150, 1963.

Holland E: A case of transplacental metastasis of malignant melanoma from mother to fetus, *J Obstet Gynaecol Br Emp* 56:529, 1949.

Potter JF, Schoeneman M: Metastasis of maternal causes to the placenta and fetus, *Cancer* 25:380, 1970.

Rothman LA, Cohen CJ, Asterloa J: Placental and fetal involvement by maternal malignancy: a report of rectal carcinoma and review of the literature, *Am J Obstet Gynecol* 116:1023, 1973.

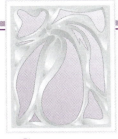

Complications of Disease and Therapy

The physician of a patient who has a gynecologic cancer must realize that complications of the disease and treatment may be the rule rather than the exception. Many of these conditions must be anticipated and recognized early for proper management. Often the complication is what initially prompts the patient to seek medical advice. Even in the 1990s, urinary leakage from bladder fistulae, uremia from bilateral ureteral obstruction caused by cervical cancer, or small bowel obstruction from ovarian cancer can be the initial symptoms. Although some complications have been discussed, it seems appropriate to devote a chapter exclusively to complications of disease and therapy. All possible complications are not catalogued, because that is beyond the scope of this presentation and books have been devoted to these subjects. However, the most common and the occasional unusual complication are discussed with some suggestions for management.

DISEASE-ORIENTED COMPLICATIONS

Common symptoms of a disease are not usually considered complications in the true sense of the word. Hemor-

rhage, for instance, can be a useful symptom because it will bring the patient to the physician for medical attention; however, bleeding can be severe enough to indeed be a true complication.

Hemorrhage

A patient with a lesion on the vulva, vagina, or cervix may initially be seen with massive hemorrhage resulting in hypovolemia and even hypotension requiring immediate intravascular replacement. The patient will usually give a history of increased hemorrhage requiring several pads per day. Some will even relate the use of towels or sheets to manage the flow, and often no good explanation is given for the delay in seeking medical advice. The hemorrhage is usually coming from a large exophytic lesion, and many times an arterial "pumper" can be identified in the tumor mass. On occasion these hemorrhage points can be coagulated with sclerosing agents such as ferric subsulfate (Monsel Solution). Other methods such as cryosurgery have been reported to be successful, but most of the time packing with a large gauze roll will control the hemorrhage. We have frequently soaked the end of the roll in acetone before packing and have found this technique more beneficial than using the pack by itself. Agents such as ferric subsulfate should not be used on the pack because this will result in general sloughing of the normal epithelium of the lower genital tract. When a large pack is used (small packing such as iodoform gauze is usually unsuccessful because a large volume of gauze is necessary), an indwelling catheter should be placed in the bladder. The pack is left in place for 24-48 hours, and if the hemorrhage has not soaked through the pack during this interval, it is unlikely to do so when removed. Suturing bleeders in the tumor mass is usually not successful and not recommended.

For the few patients with hemorrhage in whom conservative methods are unsuccessful, more aggressive management of arterial hemorrhage is required. These situations are more common in patients who have previously had surgery and/or radiation and less common in patients seen for the first time with disease. In the past these patients have been treated with bilateral hypogastric artery ligation with reasonable success when the patient was a good surgical candidate. Today hypogastric ligation is usually limited to the control of intraoperative hemorrhage. In most instances, judicious packing and identification of the specific hemorrhage sites allow control of hemorrhage without difficulty. Blind clamping and suture ligation are usually unsuccessful and have a high complication rate in regard to surrounding structures. Significant arterial hemorrhage can usually be identified and electively ligated; or if a major vessel is involved, the opening can be sutured closed. If hypogastric ligation is required to control hemorrhage, the hemorrhage is usually low in the pelvis where it may be difficult to identify. Unless hemorrhage is predominantly on one side, bilateral ligation should be seriously considered. The lateral pelvic wall vessels can be identified easily by direct visualization or palpation. The ureter crosses at the bifurcation and must be retracted medially. The hypogastric artery divides into anterior and posterior branches 2-3 cm below its origin, and the anterior branch is isolated for ligation with permanent ligature. The right angle clamp should be advanced lateral to medial to decrease the possibility of injuring the internal iliac vein. In most instances the anterior branch ligation is all that is necessary (Figure 17-1). In the previously irradiated patient, fibrosis of the pelvis may make the retroperitoneal dissection difficult,

thereby increasing the surgical risk in an already seriously compromised patient.

Recent advances in selective arteriography have added immensely to our ability to control pelvic and gastrointestinal (GI) arterial hemorrhage and to avoid surgery. Arteriographic techniques are well developed, and specific arterial bleeders can in many instances be identified (Figure 17-2). For hypogastric embolization, access is usually gained through the femoral artery on the opposite side from the hemorrhage if known. The catheter is advanced toward the aortic bifurcation, and an arteriogram usually shows the hemorrhage site. The catheter is advanced to the hemorrhage location, and embolization is performed. Postembolization films confirm success. It is important to remember that there may be hemorrhage from more than one artery at the same time; therefore a search for multiple hemorrhage sites must be made. If the hemorrhage site(s) can be identified, several techniques can be used in an attempt to control hemorrhage:

1. Vasopressin infusion has been successful particularly for GI tract hemorrhage such as in an anastomosis site or from an ulcer. This infusion may take several hours to be successful. Complications of the technique can be associated with fluid and electrolyte imbalance, and these parameters must be monitored closely.

2. Transcatheter embolization techniques using clotted autologous blood and tissue and synthetic material (Gelfoam or Oxycel) have been used. It should be remembered that blood of a patient who has had a major hemorrhage may require thrombin or platelets to maintain an adequate clot. An adequate clot will usually lyse within 12-36 hours after embolization. A gelatin sponge "clot," on the other hand, will last for 20-50 days before recanalization occurs.

3. The balloon catheter technique is indicated for major vessel hemorrhage. The results are usually dramatic and it should be left inflated for 12-24 hours.

4. The Gianturco spring embolus has been used with relative success. It is a stainless steel coil 5 cm long holding multiple strands of Dacron evenly distributed along 4 cm of its length. These coils are available in three widths and are designed for use with the standard angiography catheter and guidewire.

Migration of the embolus and peripheral embolization can be minimized by slowly and carefully positioning the embolus deep into the arterial inlet. High flow rates in the bleeding vessels promote distal spread of the embolus and reflux is prevented. Possible allergic reactions to the dye can usually be kept to a minimum with small injection doses and with the patient well hydrated. This technique has been successful even after failed bilateral hypogastric ligation.

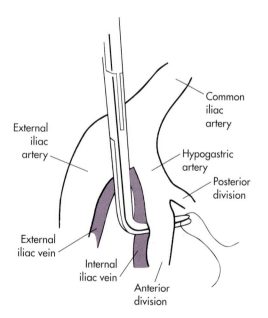

External iliac artery

Common iliac artery

Hypogastric artery

Posterior division

External iliac vein

Internal iliac vein

Anterior division

Figure 17-1 Technique for intraoperative ligation of hypogastric artery. The ligature is placed 2-3 cm below the bifurcation so the posterior branch will not be ligated. The clamp is passed lateral to medial to prevent trauma to internal iliac vein.

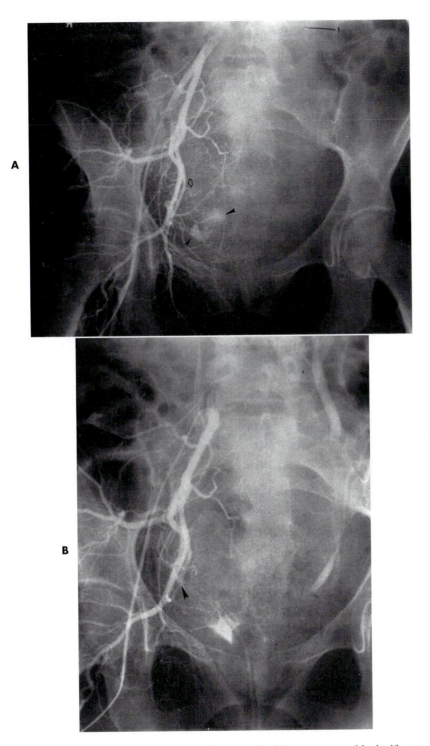

Figure 17-2 A patient who is postoperative from a vaginal hysterectomy with significant vaginal bleeding requiring multiple blood transfusions. Of interest is that she also has von Willebrand's disease. **A,** Note hemorrhage from the internal pudendal artery on the right. **B,** After embolization, no hemorrhage from the internal pudendal artery is seen. Dye in the pelvis is localized to the bladder, and the left ureter can be visualized. (Courtesy Dr. Ivan Vujic and Dr. Keeling Warburton, Medical University of South Carolina.)

Ureteral Obstruction

Ureteral obstruction from a malignant neoplasm may be identified during the course of the patient's initial evaluation. An elevated creatinine or blood urea nitrogen (BUN) level along with the obstruction noted on the intravenous pyelogram (IVP) or computed tomography (CT scan) is not unusual. Unless renal function is markedly compromised or there is significant bilateral involvement, no specific treatment is indicated because the obstruction will often be improved when the primary disease is adequately treated. Carcinoma of the cervix with its lateral parametrial extension is the most common neoplastic cause of ureteral obstruction in the female pelvis. Occasionally, large uteri seen with endometrial carcinomas or sarcomas can cause ureteral obstruction just from the expanding pelvic mass (as can be occasionally seen with fibroids). It is unusual to see ureteral obstruction caused by ovarian cancer even with large masses or ascites, primarily because the masses are not "held" in the pelvis but can find other areas for expansion. Some clinicians have observed that in postirradiated patients large benign ovarian masses can cause ureteral obstruction; possibly radiation fibrosis prevented an upward migration of the mass, which in turn led to the obstruction.

A few patients are seen with anuria and uremia as initial symptoms of cervical cancer. Formerly, operative intervention was the only means for urinary diversion in these patients, and several days were usually required to dialyze the individual so that she was able to tolerate the surgical procedure. With the use of ultrasonically guided percutaneous nephrostomies, this condition can be alleviated rapidly without extensive surgery. Patients will undergo a postobstructive diuresis usually over several days with a rapid fall in BUN and creatinine levels. Adequate intake and electrolyte balance must be obtained during this period. When edema has subsided, catheters can be passed down the ureters into the bladder, and double J stents or other internal devices can replace the nephrostomy catheter (Figure 17-3).

Dudley has reported the experience with percutaneous nephrostomy catheter in 30 patients with 41 nephrostomy catheters at the MD Anderson Hospital. This was for both recurrent and primary gynecologic cancers. Twenty-one of the 30 patients (70%) had at least one urinary tract infection. Hemorrhage was seen in 28% of the patients and blockage of catheter in 65%. Renal function was recovered in 14 of 20 patients (70%) who had elevated creatinine values. Twenty-six of the 28 patients with malignant obstruction were able to receive further therapy. Twenty of 28 patients with malignant obstruction have died, and the only long-term survivors had primary advanced cervical cancer. Three of these patients are alive at 12 to 81 months. The median survival time for patients with recurrent cervical cancer was 4½ months. Similar results have been noted by other investigators.

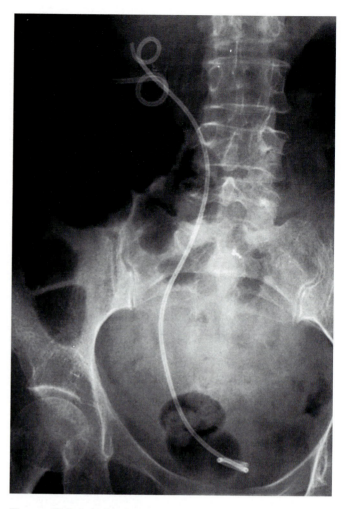

Figure 17-3 A double J stent has been inserted into right kidney, ureter, and bladder through percutaneous nephrostomy.

The role of percutaneous nephrostomy in patients with recurrent disease and ureteral obstruction must be individualized. Unless adequate therapy for recurrence is of benefit, the advisability of diversion must be questioned. On the other hand, the use of percutaneous nephrostomy in the management of benign conditions such as lymphocysts or fistulae has been a major advance and should be considered as first-line management of such conditions. In most instances, complications, including hemorrhage, infection, and catheter obstruction or displacement, are usually minor and can be handled easily.

Genitourinary Fistulae

Although vesicovaginal and/or ureterovaginal fistulae can occur in untreated patients with pelvic malignancies, it is unusual. On initial evaluation for cervical cancer, tumor may be found growing into the bladder with a resultant fistula, but in the majority of instances tumor will be identified in the bladder without a fistula. When a fistula is found concomitant with a primary tumor, therapy aimed at correcting the fistula locally cannot be initiated until therapy for the neoplasm has been completed. Even then repair should be attempted only if tumor is not present in the fistula margin as confirmed by liberal biopsies. Urinary leakage is obviously troublesome and compromises personal hygiene. An indwelling catheter with a leg bag should be used to keep the patient dry. The use of a modified menstrual cup or external appliances has sometimes been helpful in this situation. In the patient with fistula noted primary in advanced cervical cancer, initial surgical staging with urinary diversion may be a reasonable first step in the management.

Occasionally multiple and complex fistulae are encountered. More often these are noted after irradiation therapy but occasionally they can be seen with primary tumor. The fistulae can and usually involve the genitourinary (GU) and GI tracts along with one or more openings into the vagina or anterior abdominal wall. Definitive diagnostic procedures must be initiated to accurately identify these complex fistulae, because surgical correction depends on knowledge of the exact abnormalities. In most instances patients with fistulae caused by neoplasm or therapy should be considered for diversion procedures such as ileal conduit and colostomy.

Gastrointestinal Obstruction

Obstruction caused by a malignant pelvic neoplasm is most commonly seen with ovarian cancer, and the patient usually has classic obstructive signs and symptoms. Conservative management in the form of nothing by mouth, intravenous hydration, and nasogastric suction is initially prudent. The patient will often respond rapidly when these methods are successful; however, surgical management is usually necessary. Bypass surgery is usually the quickest and easiest method of alleviating the obstruction and has proved to be more prudent than attempts at lysis of adhesions or bowel resection. The use of staple instruments has facilitated these bypass procedures considerably, shortening the operative time in these very ill patients. The survival of many of these patients is brief (50% are dead within 3 months) and this should be considered in the decision for surgery. Philosophically, aggressive management has been advocated because GI obstruction is a horrible way to die.

The Duke group reported their experience with the surgical management of intestinal obstruction in 49 known ovarian cancer patients. All had received adjunctive chemotherapy and/or radiation therapy before the bowel obstruction. Thirty patients had small bowel involvement; 16, colonic; and 3, both large and small bowel involvement. Progressive ovarian cancer was ultimately found to be the cause of obstruction in 86% of patients. Major postoperative complications occurred in 49% of the patients and were significantly more common in patients with small bowel obstruction. These complications included wound infection, enterocutaneous fistula, and other sequelae. Median survival rate was 149 days. Patients with colonic obstruction had a median

postoperative survival of 263 days compared to 88 days in the small intestinal obstruction group. Only 14.3% of patients were alive at 12 months. Thirteen patients subsequently developed another intestinal obstruction that was managed medically in 8 preterminal patients and surgically in 5 patients. Complications were similar for handsewn and stapled anastomoses.

Extensive bowel resection with debulking at the time of primary ovarian cancer surgery has been adovcated by some investigators in the past. This recommendation has been challenged because it is unusual for bowel resection during the debulking procedure to leave the patient grossly free of cancer. Patients with measurable disease after extensive debulking and bowel resection have poor prognoses, even with aggressive chemotherapy. Complications from the bowel surgery are appreciable, including postoperative deaths.

In recent years more conservative management in the preterminal patient has been advocated by many to avoid a long postoperative recovery period when the patient's life expectancy is short. This management technique takes the form of 12-hour intravenous alimentation, usually through a Hickman catheter and nasogastric suction as needed, all of which can be arranged on an outpatient basis. The use of a gastrostomy or cecostomy may also be appropriate in some patients.

Percutaneous endoscopic gastrostomy has been successfully performed in patients with upper tract obstruction from malignancy. Adelson reported on 14 tube placements in 12 patients. All catheters decompressed the GI obstruction with good drainage. Complications were low and this technique was effective in eliminating nausea and vomiting and improving quality of life as a palliative procedure.

In the inoperable or terminally ill patient, Octreotide (0.1-0.2 mg tid) has decreased the nausea and vomiting to a considerable degree, thereby allowing removal of the NG tube and allowing the patient to go home.

Gastrointestinal Fistulae

Rectovaginal fistulae secondary to cancer may be seen with cervical, vaginal, or vulvar neoplasias. Involuntary loss of fecal material, gas, and intermittent mucous discharge are the most common symptoms. Because cervical and vaginal cancers with related fistulae will usually be treated with radiation therapy, a primary colostomy for fecal diversion should be suggested to the patient, because radiation-induced diarrhea will compound the symptom of uncontrolled stools through the fistula. To promote good hygiene and reduce local inflammation, a colostomy is recommended if a fistula is present with vulvar cancer, despite the fact that these lesions are customarily treated with primary surgery and a second operative procedure is usually anticipated to initiate the therapeutic plan. Primary diversion will reduce the morbidity of the subsequent procedure. It should be remembered that the anal sphincter can be removed and the patient can remain reasonably fecal continent if the levators remain intact. It is our preference in this latter group of patients to avoid primary colostomy and defer the decision until after definitive therapy when patients who have continued incontinence are clearly defined. Many patients are able to control their stools and prefer not to have a colostomy.

Thromboembolic Disease

Thromboembolic (TE) complications are a major concern for the physician managing gynecologic malignancies. It is one of the leading causes of significant morbidity and mortality after any operation for pelvic malignancy. Many of the conditions commonly associated with TE phenomena are often simultaneously present in the patient with a malignancy: advanced age, obesity, multiple medical problems, previous vascular problems, and certain medications. In addition to the malignant state and the above conditions is the pelvic surgery, which may include extensive retroperitoneal dissection, vessel wall injury, venous stasis, a hypercoagulable state, blood loss, transfusion, and a decreased blood flow in leg veins during and after surgery. It is generally accepted that TE and pelvic surgery are one process, although many times the two are separated clinically into distinct entities. Several studies have found that in patients with DVT who are pulmonary asymptomatic, 40% will have diagnostic evidence of a PE. Conversely, patients with PE will have an 80% documented evidence of DVT. In gynecology, it is thought that a considerable number of postsurgical patients will have DVT in pelvic veins without evidence of leg disease. The relationship of TE in cancer and postsurgical patients is well documented. It should be remembered that chemotherapy, particularly in combination with tamoxifen and progestins, seems to increase the incidence of PE. Patients on tamoxifen have a 1%-3% incidence of thrombosis; 4% of patients on progestins will experience TE. In one study, the incidence of thrombosis was 10.4% when tamoxifen was combined with chemotherapy compared to 2.7% when chemotherapy alone was used and 0% in the control group.

In a thorough review of these patients at Duke University Medical Center, TE conditions were the primary cause of death in patients undergoing treatment for gynecologic cancer. Although this complication is more common after surgery, unsuspected TE disease has been diagnosed at the time of primary evaluation, and unfortunately, patients have developed fatal pulmonary emboli while in the hospital awaiting definitive treatment for malignancy. In a retrospective review at Duke University Medical Center, in 281 patients who had surgery for gynecologic malignancy, 7.8% of patients encountered significant TE complications after surgery, accounting for the only 4 postoperative deaths on this service (Table 17-1). Of interest is that 45% of patients who developed TE disease did so after discharge from the hospital. The preoperative risk factors found to be associated with TE disease in order of significance were weight in excess of 190 pounds, advanced clinical stage of malignancy, and radiation therapy within 6 weeks of the operative procedure. Low-dose heparin therapy and the use of antiembolism stockings as preventive measures did not appear to reduce the incidence of TE complications. In fact, in the obese patient (greater than 190 pounds) who wore antiembolism stockings the risk of TE disease was increased to 23.5% vs 6.8% if her weight was less than 190 pounds and she did not wear stockings.

A prospective controlled trial of low-dose heparin by the Duke group was performed in 185 patients undergoing surgery for gynecologic malignancy. Twelve percent of the patients in the control group and 15% of patients in the low-dose heparin group developed a TE complication (Table 17-2). There was no difference in the incidence of proximal deep vein thrombosis, calf vein thrombosis, or pulmonary emboli between the control and the low-dose heparin groups. Calf vein thrombosis only was present in almost three fourths of these patients, and none of these calf vein thrombi propagated proximally to the popliteal

Table 17-1 Thromboembolic complications after gynecologic oncology surgery

	Surgery patients*
Deep venous thrombosis	11/281
Pulmonary embolus	6/281
Deep venous thrombosis and pulmonary embolus	5/281
TOTAL	22/281

From Clarke-Pearson DL, Jelovsek FR, Creasman WT: Reprinted with permission from the American College of Obstetricians and Gynecologists. (*Obstetrics and Gynecology*, vol 61, 1983, p 87.)
*Radical hysterectomy, pelvic lymphadenectomy (n = 103), abdominal hysterectomy, bilateral salpingo-oophorectomy, and selective pelvic and para-aortic lymphadenectomy (n = 178).

Table 17-2 Prospective study of low-dose heparin in prevention of thromboembolism

	Control (n = 97)	Heparin (n = 88)
Calf vein only	10 (10%)	6 (7%)
Deep venous thrombosis	1 (1%)	3 (3%)
Pulmonary embolus	1 (1%)	4 (4%)
TOTAL	12 (12%)	13 (14%)

Based on data from Clarke-Pearson DL et al: *Am J Obstet Gynecol* 145:606, 1983.

or femoral venous segment. Almost one half of these calf vein thrombi lysed spontaneously while under observation and ^{125}I fibrinogen scanning. Three of the five pulmonary emboli apparently originated in the pelvic veins. Of interest in the control group is that the mean time of occurrence was the third postoperative day compared with the sixth postoperative day in the low-dose heparin group. Of 13 TE complications in the heparin group, 5 occurred after the heparin was discontinued and, in some instances, after the patient had been discharged. Complications of low-dose heparin therapy included increased bleeding during surgery, wound hematomas, thrombocytopenia, and sloughing of tissue at injection sites requiring plastic surgery. According to this study, the use of low-dose heparin prophylaxis does not appear to be of benefit in preventing TE complications in the gynecologic oncology patient. Other studies confirm these observations.

A prospective controlled trial of external pneumatic calf compression (EPC) compared with a control group was done by the Duke group. In 107 patients undergoing surgery for gynecologic cancer those who were in the EPC group had a 13% incidence of TE complication compared with 35% in the control group (Table 17-3). When independently associated risk factors (age older than 60, advanced clinical stage, and varicose veins) were corrected in the two groups, patients in the control group had a significantly higher TE rate than those using EPC ($p < 0.005$).

A high index of suspicion and constant monitoring with impedence plethysmography or ^{125}I fibrinogen scanning appear to be the best means of early diagnosis and treatment. An asymptomatic pelvic vein thrombosis and a pulmonary embolus were recently detected using the ^{111}In-labeled platelet imaging technique.

In a prospective study of 411 gynecologic patients from Duke, all known variables associated with deep venous thrombosis (DVT) were recorded. Deep venous thrombosis was diagnosed by an ^{125}I fibrinogen scan

performed daily. Patients who had increased counting had venography to document the extent of the DVT. The following variables on univariant analysis were significantly related to postoperative DVTs:

> History of DVT
> Leg edema or venous stasis changes
> Venous varicosities
> Degree of preoperative ambulation
> Type of surgery
> Nonwhite race
> Recurrent malignancy
> Prior pelvic radiation therapy
> Age beyond 45 years
> Obesity
> Intraoperative blood loss
> Duration of anesthesia

A stepwise logistic regression analysis of these variables was done. The following preoperative prognostic factors remain significant:

> Type of surgery
> Age
> Leg edema
> Nonwhite patients
> Severity of venous varicosities
> Prior radiation therapy
> History of deep venous thrombosis

Duration of anesthesia was also important when intraoperative factors were considered in analysis. With these factors, a prognostic model was created that allows one to evaluate the risk of postoperative deep venous thrombosis for an individual patient. The Duke group has completed a prospective randomized study that attempted to evaluate the effectiveness of two low-dose heparin regimens as a means for preventing postoperative venous thrombosis in the gynecologic oncology patient. This was a three-arm protocol in which patients received low-dose calcium heparin 5000 units subcutaneously 2 hours preoperatively and every 8 hours for 7 days postoperatively vs those with a heparin "load" who received calcium heparin 5000 units subcutaneously every 8 hours for at least 1 day before surgery and every 8 hours for 7 days postoperatively vs a control no-treatment group. In the control group, 17 of 103 (16%) developed scan-detected calf thromboses vs 8 of 104 (8%) in the low-dose heparin group compared with 2 of 98 (2%) in the "load" heparin group. However, there were no proximal DVTs or pulmonary emboli in the control group. This compared with one pulmonary embolus in the low-dose heparin group and one proximal DVT and one pulmonary embolus in the heparin "load" group. When one evaluates only the cancer patients in this group (not all patients after surgery were found to have cancer) there was a statistically significant difference in the scan-detected thrombi when one compares the control groups with the "load" group; no other significance was present among any of the other groups. Although the scan-detected thrombi are

Table 17-3   Prospective study of external pneumatic calf compression in prevention of thromboembolism

	Control (n = 52)	EPC (n = 55)
Calf vein only	13 (25%)	4 (7%)
Deep venous thrombosis	4 (8%)	1 (2%)
Pulmonary embolism	1 (2%)	2 (4%)
TOTAL	18 (35%)	7 (13%)

From Clarke-Pearson DL et al: Reprinted with permission from the American College of Obstetricians and Gynecologists. (*Obstetrics and Gynecology,* vol 63, 1984, p 92.)

increased in the control group, there was no difference among any of the three groups when one evaluated proximal DVTs or pulmonary emboli.

Dihydroergotamine-heparin has been suggested as a possible prophylaxis for deep venous thrombus. Dihydroergotamine exerts a selective constrictive effect on veins and venula with only minimal effect on arteries and arterioles, thereby counteracting venous stasis and accelerating venous return from the lower extremities. A multicentric trial was carried out in 880 patients undergoing elective abdominal, pelvic, and thoracic surgery and randomized into five treatment groups:

1. Dihydroergotamine-mesylate (DHE) plus 5000 units of sodium heparin
2. DHE plus 2500 units of sodium heparin
3. Sodium heparin 5000 units alone
4. DHE alone
5. Placebo

Treatment was initiated preoperatively and continued twice daily for 5-7 days. Patients were followed with radiofibrinogen uptake tests. With this diagnostic technique, the DVT rates were:

First group	9.4%
Second group	16.8%
Third group	16.8%
Fourth group	19.4%
Fifth group	24.4%

None of the DVTs were confirmed with venography. Two patients developed pulmonary emboli during the study and another two developed pulmonary emboli and apparently died from the emboli during the postsurgical interval but after they had been taken off the study. The combination of DHE and 5000 units of sodium heparin appeared to have protection against radiofibrinogen uptake scan-detected thrombi. There was no significance in prevention of pulmonary emboli. No data were given about DVTs of the upper legs. Only 64 of the patients had gynecologic procedures. One of the major concerns about DHE is that it may produce peripheral arterial vasoconstriction in the presence of severe sepsis or shock and lead to an adverse effect, which appears to be a higher risk in older patients.

If deep venous thrombosis or pulmonary embolism is diagnosed, anticoagulation should be started immediately. Suggested treatment is noted in the box above.

There is an increased interest in the use of low-molecular-weight heparin (LMWH) for the treatment of DVT. Prospective randomized studies with standard unfractionated heparin have been performed with no difference in efficacy and long term effects. Advantages of LMWH include longer half life in plasma, less variability in anticoagulant response to fixed doses, and the ability to treat on an outpatient basis using subcutaneous injections without laboratory monitoring.

SUGGESTED THERAPY FOR DEEP VENOUS THROMBOSIS AND/OR PULMONARY EMBOLUS

1. Aqueous heparin, 5000 U as an IV bolus
2. Aqueous heparin, 1000 U/hr as an IV infusion
3. Heparin may be adjusted to give a partial prothrombin time of 1.5-2.0 times control
4. Continue heparin 7-10 days
5. Begin warfarin (Coumadin) on day 5 or earlier at 10 or 20 mg first day, 10 mg second day, then 5-10 mg every day thereafter until prothrombin time is approximately 1.2-1.5 times normal
6. Discontinue heparin only when anticoagulation is adequate with warfarin
7. Continue warfarin a minimum of 3 months

Superior Vena Cava Syndrome

Superior vena cava syndrome usually occurs with far advanced disease and has been described as one of the true radiation therapy emergencies, although this concept seems to be changing. In most instances superior vena caval obstruction occurs secondary to malignant tumors arising in or invading the mediastinum and impairing venous drainage of the head, neck, and upper thoracic regions. Primary tumors are most commonly the cause of this syndrome, although metastasis to this area from gynecologic malignancies can also present in this manner. Benign tumors can also be the etiology. Thrombosis of the superior vena cava associated with central invasive monitoring, hyperalimentation, and chemotherapy is probably the most common cause of non-malignant syndrome (Figure 17-4). Tumor masses cause embarrassment of the superior vena cava, resulting in edema and plethora of the head, neck, upper extremities, and trunk. The vena cava has a low intravascular pressure and is easily compressed by adjacent masses, and the elevated venous pressures lead to the facial and upper extremity edema. Pleural and pericardial effusions can occur with a decreased venous return to the heart and an associated fall in cardiac output. Diagnosis of the etiologic cause is necessary to adequately treat this syndrome. Chemotherapy may be appropriate particularly for primary tumor management. Expandable wire stents across the constricted portion of the vena cava have been used successfully. For metastatic gynecologic cancers, radiation remains the treatment of choice the majority of times. The use of radiation therapy to the mediastinum in doses of 400 cGy for 3 days, and then 150-180 cGy per day for a total dose of 3000-5000 cGy, has been successful in relieving the vascular compromise with its resultant physical characteristics. Most patients will appreciate a prompt response usually within 3-4 days

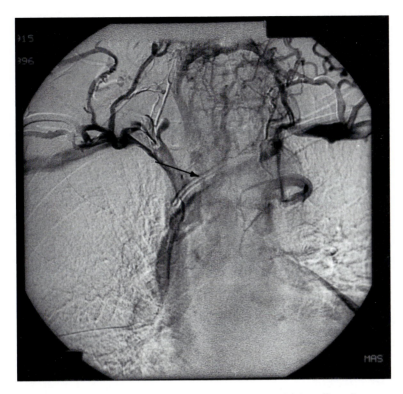

Figure 17-4 Extensive thrombosis of large vessels in thorax. Multiple collaterals are present. Subclavian catheter is evident (*arrow*).

Jaundice

Jaundice may be caused by direct involvement of the liver parenchyma with tumor; however, retroperitoneal lymph node metastasis may also cause obstructive jaundice secondary to compression of the biliary tree. Surgical correction is often impossible because of the far advanced disease. Obstruction of the common bile duct by tumor in either intra- or retroperitoneal compartment can be corrected with resultant disappearance of jaundice by stenting the duct endoscopically. Accompanying the jaundice one may often find a high GI obstruction caused by compression of the duodenum by enlarged lymph nodes. A gastrojejunostomy will correct the immediate problem, although survival is limited.

TREATMENT-RELATED COMPLICATIONS
Surgery

Surgery carries inherent risks that are usually minimal in comparison to the benefits obtained. Because of the extensive surgery required in the treatment of pelvic malignancies and the proximity of the GI and GU systems, complications are naturally increased with regard to these organs. These complications and others that are more specific to pelvic surgery for gynecologic malignancies are addressed. Areas such as anesthesia risk and similar problems are considered.

Vascular complications

Because of the extensive retroperitoneal dissection and radicality of the pelvic surgery, serious damage to adjacent vascular structures can occur. Lacerations of veins or arteries and evulsion of a minor or major vessel can occur. Bleeding from lateral pelvic sidewall veins is always a potential and serious problem. Ligation of compromised vessels is the most time-honored method of controlling hemorrhage. If a laceration is small, many times pressure with a finger or instrument (sponge stick) will control the bleeding. Large vessel injuries will usually need to be closed by arterial suture (5-0 or 6-0 Tevdek or similar suture). The surgeon's finger or an instrument can be used to control the bleeding point while the suture is placed on both sides of the injury. If necessary, occluding vascular clamps may be used on both sides of the injury so that suturing can take place in a blood-free environment. A continuous running suture can be used if necessary, but it is absolutely essential when repairing vessels that the vessel be cleaned of surrounding tissue. It is an unusual situation when a graft or prosthesis is required to correct a surgical injury.

Vessel injury caused by perforation during a laparoscopic examination is fortunately rare but requires speed and experience to control the bleeding. If retroperitoneal vessels are involved, a hematoma in this area occurs rapidly and can interfere with the identification of the bleeding site. The operator's finger can usually control the bleeding, allowing time to evacuate the hematoma and then proceed with proper repair. If a major artery is involved, adequate peripheral perfusion must be proven before terminating the operative procedure.

Venous oozing from the pelvis can result in major blood loss. The exact site should be identified if at all possible and ligation carried out with clips or sutures. Often this is difficult, and packing with hot pads will be necessary to control small venous hemorrhage. If not, it can help isolate the bleeding, which can then be ligated directly. To put a clip or suture into the area of hemorrhage is usually unsuccessful. The identification of the actual hemorrhage point cannot be overemphasized; identification is important so that control of bleeding may be made complete. Avitene has been shown to be successful in controlling some venous bleeding when packing has not succeeded. Thrombin can be used to control minor oozing but has been unsuccessful for major hemorrhage. We still favor the traditional methods of packing and ligation of major bleeding points, because the amount of clot and foreign material left to be absorbed is minimized.

Intraoperative genitourinary injuries

Injuries to the GU tract may occur immediately as the direct result of surgery or subsequently after radiation therapy. Surgical injuries to the bladder or ureters are more common after treatment of benign pelvic disease than after radical surgery because when the latter is done the ureters and bladder are usually identified and isolated. Identification of the urinary system at all surgery is helpful in preventing injuries. If the ureter cannot be located on the medial leaf of the broad ligament, the bifurcation of the iliac vessels should be sought because the ureter usually crosses the vessel at this point. In many benign cases (pelvic masses, pelvic inflammatory disease, and endometriosis, to name a few) the dissection is usually considerably easier if the retroperitoneal approach is initially undertaken. With distorted anatomy, it is imperative to identify the ureter before the infundibulopelvic ligament is ligated. In such situations a preoperative IVP is important to help identify the patient with duplication of the collecting system. At the time of surgery, if injury to the GU tract occurs, immediate surgical correction can be accomplished with excellent results. Small injuries can be identified by watching for extravasation of urine after coloring it with the intravenous administration of indigo carmine dye. If the lower ureter is involved with tumor and requires resection, or injury occurs during surgery, reimplantation of the ureter into the bladder (ureteroneocystotomy with psoas hitch) can be performed with good results. If there is a question about ureteral occlusion, such as with a suture ligation, the ureter can be opened longitudinally at the pelvic brim and a catheter passed caudally. If the catheter slips into the bladder without difficulty, ligation is unlikely. The

incision made in the ureter can be closed with simple interrupted light suture ligatures placed along the longitudinal incision. Patency can also be established by opening the bladder and passing the catheter retrograde into the ureter. A retroperitoneal drain placed at the site of surgery to the ureter is recommended. Lacerations to the bladder can usually be managed by simple closure of the bladder (two-layer closure is recommended), with a Foley catheter left in place for 5-7 days.

Postoperative genitourinary injuries

Anuria or severe oliguria in the immediate postoperative period should alert the physician to the possibility of bilateral ureteral injuries. In most instances the findings can be explained by a prerenal process, and forced diuresis will resolve the differential diagnoses. On the other hand, unilateral injury may not be recognized until several days postoperatively. The volume of urinary output is usually not noticeably affected. The patient may develop chills, fevers, flank pain, and subsequently urinary leakage usually through the vagina, particularly if a hysterectomy has been performed. Once it is obvious that a fistula has developed, determining the site is the next priority. Placing dye-colored saline into the bladder via a Foley catheter and observing for leakage into the vagina will confirm a vesicovaginal fistula. If a vesicovaginal fistula is present, the colored fluid is usually observed in the vagina immediately. Occasionally, when a fistula is not readily identified, placing a tampon in the vagina and having the patient ambulate will allow a small opening to be identified. If no dye is present on the tampon in the vagina, a vesicovaginal fistula has been ruled out. Intravenous dye (i.e., indigo carmine) should then be injected, and if stained urine is present on the tampon, it is reasonable to assume a ureterovaginal fistula is the source of the urinary leakage. It is then important to determine which ureter has the fistula. An IVP may be of help here, since extravasation along with other findings such as hydronephrosis, delayed excretion, or ureteral stricture can be identified. Occasionally, cystoscopy with retrograde catheterization will be needed for final diagnosis. The fistula opening may be very difficult to identify with the patient in the lithotomy position. Placing her in the knee chest position facilitates the identification of a fistula, particularly if the opening is high.

Subsequent management depends on the extent of the ureteral injury. If a simple ureteral fistula is present, a retrograde or antegrade catheter is placed in the affected ureter and left for several days or weeks. In some instances the fistula will spontaneously close. If a complete transection or considerable necrosis of the ureter has occurred, placement of a catheter may be impossible. The use of percutaneous nephrostomy with diversion of urine may be of help but rarely keeps the patient dry. Because of edema and infection at the future operative site, some recommend that drainage be established in the retroperitoneal area without attempted correction of the fistula for several months. If the fistula is within 4-5 cm of the bladder, actual repair of the fistula even without edema or infection is difficult. As a result, reimplantation of the ureter can usually be done initially because the implantation is out of the affected field. This will save the patient another surgical procedure and is usually successful.

If the fistula is higher (toward the pelvic brim) a ureteroureteral anastomosis is usually recommended. Others have used a ureteroileoneocystotomy to reach the bladder with these high injuries. Seldom will permanent diversion procedures be necessary.

Fortunately, the occurrence of GU fistulae has decreased considerably over the last two decades, particularly after radical hysterectomy. Previous reports suggested that as many as 10% of patients treated with radical hysterectomy and pelvic lymphadenectomy developed a vesicovaginal or ureterovaginal fistula. Current studies suggest that this incidence has dropped to approximately 1%-2%.

Hatch et al. reported on 300 patients who had undergone radical hysterectomies and pelvic node dissections and noted that ureterovaginal fistulae occurred in 4 patients (1.3%). None of these were associated with recurrent cancer. Two occurred because of intraoperative trauma, and two were unexplained. There were ureteral strictures in 13 (4.3%). Ten of these were late and were caused by recurrent cancer. It is interesting that 32 patients received whole-pelvis irradiation for positive nodes or positive margins postoperatively and none developed ureterovaginal fistulae. The GU injuries are similar whether radical or simple hysterectomy is done. Reduction in fistulae after radical surgery has been credited to changes in the surgical procedure. These changes include suspending the ureter to the obliterate hypogastric, encasing the ureter in peritoneum, and providing prolonged bladder drainage. Most would agree that suction drainage to the retroperitoneal space has been responsible for the lower complication rate. The routine of not reperitonealizing the retroperitoneal space may have also contributed to this reduction of fistula.

Both ureterovaginal fistulae and vesicovaginal fistulae manifest within a week to 10 days after surgery. Once a vesicovaginal fistula has been identified, an attempt is made to keep the patient dry by use of a Foley catheter. Most authorities suggest waiting 3-6 months before repair is attempted. If the fistula is small and high, an immediate repair with the Lazko technique may be successful. Before surgical repair, cystoscopy and IVP should be repeated so that the relationship of the fistula to the urethral orifices can be established. With long-term Foley catheter drainage, there can be a tendency to develop calculi in the bladder around the catheter. In this event the catheter must be removed and a period of time must elapse before repair is attempted. Surgery is contraindi-

cated in the presence of chronic infection and calculi formation. In most instances the repair of vesicovaginal fistulae can be done successfully through the vagina even when the fistula is high in the vagina and small. Tedious dissection is required, and mobilization of all tissues is mandatory for a successful repair. Appropriate instruments, particularly proper retractors, are of tremendous value when attempting a repair. In these fistula repairs it is usually unnecessary in an unirradiated patient to interpose a source of neovascularization. However, several techniques have been described if this is indicated, such as transposition of the gracilis muscle or the bulbocavernosus labial fat pad to the operative site. Postoperatively a Foley catheter or suprapubic catheter should be used to drain the bladder until adequate healing has occurred (usually 2-3 weeks in the unirradiated patient and 4-6 weeks in the irradiated patient). It has been suggested that the combined use of radiation therapy and radical hysterectomy would have an increased complication rate. Jacobs et al. reported on 102 patients so treated. There were five major complications, and four of the five involved the GU tract. The one sigmoid stricture required a diverting colostomy with resection and reanastomosis. Ureteral obstruction and fistulae were the other complications. Complications were more likely if the dose at point A was greater than 7000 cGy or the dose to point B was greater than 4000 cGy. No complications were seen if the bladder dose was less than 5000 cGy. The rate rose significantly if more than 6000 cGy was delivered to the rectum or to the bladder. Stern et al. reported two patients who developed postoperative conduit fistulae after total pelvic exenteration. The antegrade ureteral stent catheter was placed via percutaneous nephrostomy, and both fistulae spontaneously closed. This technique prevented surgical revision of the conduit.

Bladder dysfunction after radical surgery

The pathophysiology of voiding dysfunction after radical hysterectomy is still not clearly understood. Roman-Lopez felt that incomplete innervation of the bladder produced a temporary parasympathometic predominance that usually resolved with nerve regeneration. The use of parasympatholytic drugs, however, have been ineffective in altering the detrusor muscle. Forney suggested that disruption of the sympathetic fibers that travel through the paracervical web result in loss of inhibition for the detrusor and trigone, leaving an uncoordinated parasympathetic dominance. This is supported by the observation that incomplete division of the cardinal ligament resulted in decreased postoperative detrusor hypertonia compared with complete division. Kader found significantly fewer long-term bladder symptoms, especially incontinence and sensory loss, in patients with incomplete division of the cardinal ligament. Recent serial cystometric studies of patients undergoing radical hysterectomy have defined the natural history of bladder function in the perioperative period. There is a near uniform development of detrusor hypertonia characterized by low capacity, high resting tone, and high filling pressure in the immediate postoperative phase. Bladder insensitivity to filling is also present. The patient often has difficulty initiating her stream and may have overflow incontinence when the capacity is exceeded. Hypertonia generally subsides within 3-6 months but other abnormalities often persist for years. Older series that studied patients many years after surgery described a high incidence of detrusor hypotonia. This is manifested by retention, overflow incontinence, recurrent infections, and the need for cholinergic drugs and catheterization. More recent studies indicate that overdistention of the bladder may be casually related to this complication. In a study of 40 patients treated with radical hysterectomy, Ralph performed urologic evaluation and urodynamic studies before and 2 weeks, 6 months, and 12 months after surgery. Two weeks postoperation, all patients had small, spastic bladders and 68% had residual urine. Bladder sensation was impaired in all patients at 2 weeks and in 63% at 1 year. At 1 year, almost two thirds had abnormal compliance and 85% used abdominal straining to initiate voiding. Three developed overflow incontinence and 8 had stress incontinence.

Various types and durations of postoperative bladder drainage have been used to correct these complications. Whether the type of bladder drainage is transurethral for a short or long period of time, suprapubic for varying lengths of time, or self-catheterization, all have their proponents and varying degrees of success. It has been our practice to use a suprapubic catheter, and after a week of continuous drainage, voiding is attempted. When spontaneous voiding has resumed in the 200-300 ml range with residuals less than 100 ml, the catheter is removed. The patients are then trained to void "by the clock" for several weeks after surgery. Our experience with 61 patients with stage Ib carcinomas of the cervix who were treated with radical hysterectomy has been reported by Bandy et al. All underwent water cystometry 6 months or longer after surgery. Adjunctive pelvic irradiation in 10 patients was associated with significantly more contracted and unstable bladders than in those patients who had only surgery. The necessity for bladder drainage 30 days or longer after surgery alone in 17 patients was associated with significantly worse long-term postvoid residual and total bladder capacity as well as volume for the first urge to void compared with 34 patients treated only with surgery who required short-term drainage. Photopulos and others suggest that a less radical operation (type II rather than type III) would decrease the morbidity, including bladder dysfunction. In a comparison of 21 type II cases with 81 class III cases (the traditional radical hysterectomy), he noted no GU fistulas in the former group, but there were 3 in the latter group. Those patients with class II had a mean time to voiding of 16.5 days, compared to 32.7 days with a class III hysterectomy. It is probably the degree of radicality of the surgery, not the method of drainage, that is important relative to bladder function after radical hysterectomy.

Gastrointestinal injuries (intraoperative)

Surgical injuries to the gastrointestinal tract can occur at any time during the operative procedure but may be common at the time that the peritoneal cavity is entered, particularly if the patient has had previous surgery or radiation and adhesions are present to the anterior abdominal wall. These are usually recognized immediately and can be repaired with a high degree of success. We have found it advantageous to have performed a mechanical bowel preparation on all patients undergoing abdominal surgery. This can be easily accomplished with 240 ml of magnesium citrate or other saline cathartic 36 hours before surgery with the simultaneous commencement of a clear liquid diet and continuing until surgery. Some recommend Co-Lyte liquid, which is very successful but usually requires the patient to drink a gallon of fluid, which many times is impossible. A good alternative is 30 cc of milk of magnesia, given the two nights before admission, along with a clear liquid diet. An antibiotic bowel prep (neomycin and erythromycin are commonly used) is usually unnecessary unless one is planning bowel surgery. This not only allows the bowel to be relatively empty of any contents but also insures that if an injury to the GI tract occurs, contamination of the peritoneal cavity is relatively minor compared with an unprepared bowel. If the mucosa of the GI tract is entered, a two-layer closure is usually performed using a polyglycolic acid suture on the mucosal layer with the knot tied intralumenally, followed by a serosal suture layer usually of a permanent-type material. The closure should always be accomplished in a manner in which the lumen is largest after the repair. If only the serosa has been incised, interrupted polyglycolic acid suture is usually all that is necessary. Primary repair of the stomach and small bowel usually poses no problems, and healing is rapid.

If the large bowel is injured, particularly in the pelvic area, the question arises as to whether a temporary diverting colostomy should be done to protect the operative site. If the bowel has been prepared as previously noted, it is usually unnecessary to do a diverting colostomy unless the bowel has been transected completely, there is considerable tissue trauma in the area, or the patient has had heavy irradiation to the involved area.

Postoperative gastrointestinal problems.. Patients who have had extensive pelvic dissection, particularly with extensive tumor or with a history of irradiation, are at risk for developing enteric fistulae, which at times will become apparent by vaginal drainage of GI content. On other occasions, particularly if a bowel anastomosis has been done at the time of surgery and there is subsequent leakage at the anastomosis site, an enterocutaneous fistula to the anterior abdominal wall, often through the incision, will result. It is important to determine whether the fistula is from the large or small bowel. Drainage of small bowel contents through the fistula to the skin creates a serious nursing problem because the tissue is vulnerable to the irritation caused by the digestive enzymes. A similar process will occur in the vulvar area if there is an enterovaginal fistula. The patient who has an enterovaginal fistula that is not complicated by active tumor, previous high-dose irradiation, or leakage from a small bowel anastomosis may occasionally heal spontaneously if the fecal stream can be diverted or stopped. Often this can be accomplished by giving the patient an elemental diet in which there is essentially no stool produced or by administering total parenteral nutrition (TPN). The use of TPN reduces GI secretory capacities by 30%-50% but this could take several weeks. Unfortunately, TPN with its aminoacids and lipids can stimulate gastric or pancreatic secretions. The use of somatostatin in conjunction with TPN has been successful in the spontaneous closure of enteric fistula, both large and small bowel. Somatostatin inhibits the basal exocrine GI secretions and prevents the possibility of exogenous stimuli. There is a synergistic effect of TPN and somatostatin. The GI output decreases rapidly within 1-2 days. Fistulae that close spontaneously do so very quickly, usually within 1 week. Although most experience has been in nonradiated patients this regimen appears to be successful even in those who have had prior radiation. Experience suggests that up to 75% of fistulae will heal with this medical management. It should certainly be tried as the initial treatment. Although both are time consuming and expensive, these techniques may be successful and save the patient a second surgical procedure in many instances. In the patient with a large bowel fistula (usually rectovaginal fistula), it is usually necessary to perform a three-stage procedure. This usually means a diverting colostomy with a subsequent repair of the vesicovaginal fistula a few months later, and after demonstrable healing of the fistula closure, a reanastomosis of the large bowel with closure of the colostomy site. Complex fistulae involving multiple sites from both the GI and GU systems must have exhaustive documentation, and the surgical correction must be highly individualized. Patients undergoing large bowel surgery as part of planned procedures are, by nature of the disease being treated, at high risk for complications. Hatch et al. reported their experience with low rectal anastomosis in conjunction with pelvic exenteration. Their experience with 31 patients noted that only 16 (52%) achieved complete healing. Six (19%) experienced early anastomosis breakdown, and 9 (29%) developed late fistula, although 3 were associated with recurrent cancer. Protective colostomy was used in 12 patients, but it has been discontinued because it has not been shown to decrease the fistula rate. Hatch et al. noted "an omental wrap" around the anastomosis resulted in complete healing in 11 of 13 patients.

Rectal dysfunction has been addressed by Barnes et al. In 15 patients undergoing radical hysterectomy, anorectal pressure profiles were obtained pre- and postoperatively. All patients had normal preoperative profiles, and all were abnormal postoperatively. Twelve patients reported problems with rectal function, mainly relaxation of internal sphincter, increased distention, and decreased rectal sensation, but no patients reported incontinence of stool or gas. It is felt that these problems were probably caused by partial denervation of the rectal plexus during the lateral dissection, much like what occurs with denervation of the hypogastric or ureterovaginal plexus in the cardinal ligament, which leads to well-recognized bladder dysfunction. Studies of bowel dysfunction in patients with type II hysterectomy have not been done.

Diarrhea in any patient may indicate underlying pathology. In a report from UCLA, about 10% of hospitalized gynecologic cancer patients developed diarrhea. This was more common in patients receiving chemotherapy than in the surgical patient. In only 10% of the patients with diarrhea was *Clostridium difficile* identified as the etiology. *C. difficile* colitis can cause severe diarrhea, hypovolemic shock, cecal perforation, hemorrhage, and death. Fortunately, when *C. difficile* is the source of diarrhea in the gynecologic patient, symptoms are usually mild or moderate. This entity is most commonly associated with antibiotic use. Clindamycin has been the most frequently used antibiotic but many different antibiotics may be related. Profuse, watery, foul-smelling, or bloody diarrhea with crampy abdominal pain are the most frequent symptoms. Pseudomembranous colitis may also cause high fever, leukocytosis, and dehydration. Positive cultures usually confirm the diagnosis. The use of ELISA tests for the *C. difficile* toxins are rapid and relatively inexpensive. Treatment is supportive; e.g., fluids and electrolyte replacement. Vancomycin is highly effective against the *C. difficile* organism. In mild or moderate cases, metronidazole is usually active and appears to be as effective as vancomycin, well tolerated, and considerably less expensive. In severe cases, vancomycin is the treatment of choice. Antibiotics are best given orally.

Lymphocysts

Fortunately, lymphocysts occur infrequently after lymphadenectomy; when they do appear, only a small fraction of them require surgical intervention. It has been suggested that prevention may be initiated by ligating the multiple lymphatic branches during a lymphadenectomy, thus diminishing the incidence of lymphocysts. The use of operative site suction drainage, particularly in the patient undergoing radical hysterectomy, appears to be extremely helpful in preventing lymphocysts. Lymphocysts, when they do develop, usually occur anteriorly in the pelvis and are more easily appreciated on abdominal examination than on pelvic examination. Seldom do they become infected, and in most instances they are small and can be treated expectantly, because over time most will slowly resolve. If the lymphocyst is large enough or critically placed, obstruction of the ureter or the pelvic veins can occur, leading to ureteral obstruction or venous thrombosis. When these complications occur, surgical drainage is imperative. This can usually be done simply by approaching the lymphocyst retroperitoneally with a small incision and immediate drainage. Suction drainage is usually placed in the lymphocyst with the hope that the cyst wall will collapse and fluid will not reaccumulate. We routinely leave the pelvic peritoneum open after both lymph node sampling and radical hysterectomy, which allows the fluid to drain directly into the peritoneal cavity. Retroperitoneal suction drainage is no longer used after lymphadenectomy or radical hysterectomy. It is our impression that the incidence of lymphocysts is less with this latter technique, although lymphocysts have not been completely eliminated.

Lymphocysts can occur in the inguinal area after lymphadenectomy. Although suction drainage is used routinely in these cases, from time to time we have seen individuals develop rather large lymphocysts after such removal (usually after hospital discharge). These can be managed with aspiration and pressure dressing, but occasionally suction drainage is again required to prevent recurrence. Repeat aspirations can lead to infected lymphocysts. Small lymphocysts can be managed expectantly, but large ones can cause discomfort and lymphedema.

Sepsis

Infection is a constant problem in patients with gynecologic cancer The fact that the GI and GU tracts may be interrupted increases the possibility for infection, especially anaerobic infections that are a very real concern. Prophylaxis is an area that has been extensively evaluated over the past several years especially with regard to benign gynecologic surgery. It does appear to be of benefit particularly in vaginal and possibly abdominal hysterectomies. Unfortunately, there is little research concerning the use of prophylactic antibiotics in radical gynecologic surgery. If it appears to be of benefit in the patient undergoing benign gynecologic surgery, would it not also be appropriate for patients with gynecologic cancers?

It is generally stated that a simple hysterectomy should not be done after a conization of the cervix even with antibiotic coverage unless it is done within 48 hours or after 6 weeks. This tenet apparently does not apply to radical hysterectomy. A study from the Mayo Clinic has shown that there is no increased infection rate when radical hysterectomy is done after 48 hours and before 6 weeks after conization, presumably because the potentially infected parametrium is removed with a radical hysterectomy.

Only two prospective randomized studies with prophylactic antibiotics in gynecologic cancer patients have been done to date. Both studies showed a decrease of febrile morbidity in the antibiotic group. However, serious pelvic infections were not a common problem in either the antibiotic- or the placebo-treated population. Additional studies are needed to further elucidate the possible advantage of this therapy. Until such studies are performed, many physicians treating gynecologic cancers will continue to use prophylactic antibiotics. A good mechanical and antibiotic prep before bowel surgery certainly deceases the likelihood of postoperative infections.

Other preventive measures appear to have decreased infection in patients with gynecologic cancers. A good example is the patient who is undergoing a pelvic exenteration. Infection has been and remains a real concern in these patients. The pelvic floor may become infected because of the large raw areas that remain exposed. The use of a bilateral myocutaneous graft will form a neovagina and also replace the void left by the exenterative procedure, thus significantly decreasing the possibility of infection in this area. These grafts have also been used in patients undergoing radical vulvectomies and inguinal lymphadenectomies, particularly if an extra large amount of tissue has to be removed.

Necrotizing fasciitis

Necrotizing fasciitis is an uncommon but serious infectious process that can be life threatening and must be aggressively treated. Diabetes is present in about 70% of gynecologic patients with this infectious process. Initially, the infection may be insidious but then becomes rampant. Skin changes are usually the first indications of potential problem. Reddish purple to blue gray color of the skin with skin breakdown and bullae is usually present. Gangrene appears shortly thereafter. The area at this point is usually nontender due to thrombosis of small vessels and destruction of superficial nerves. Most patients are actively ill with fever and leukocytosis. The bacterial flora may be a polymicrobial involving anaerobic and facultative aerobic bacteria or primarily *Streptococcus pyrogenes* (group A) with or without *Staphylococcus aureus*. Necrosis of skin, subcutaneous tissue, and superficial fascia is present without involvement of underlying muscle. Extensive surgical debridement is the hallmark of therapy. All necrotic tissue should be removed. Wide excision to bleeding edges should be done. Nonviable muscle should be removed. The wound is packed. Frequent debridement may be required. Fluid and electrolyte replacement with broad spectrum antibiotic therapy should be started prior to surgery. After infection has resolved, secondary closure or skin grafting may be done

Septic shock

Septic shock is due to an infection with peripheral circulatory failure and inadequate tissue profusion, which ultimately leads to cell death. The underlying septicemia is a systemic disease associated with pathogenic microorganisms or their toxins in the blood. It is the thirteenth leading cause of death in the United States and seems to be increasing in frequency. This may be due to several causes, including HIV infection, organ transplants, and patients undergoing chemotherapy for a malignancy. In obstetrics and gynecology, this is an unusual finding that appears to be more frequently seen in the obstetrical or postpartum patient and accompanying fetal or uterine infection. Septic shock is usually due to a gram-negative organism, but gram-positive bacteria, fungi, and viruses have also been implicated. Gram-negative shock is due to an endotoxin usually found in the gram-negative organism's cell wall. The very complicated cascade that follows appears to involve cytokines that may contribute to the septic shock. Activation of the coagulation cascade may also occur. About three fourths of all septic shock is caused by gram-negative facultative anaerobic organisms for which *Escherichia coli* is the one most frequently seen. Gram-positive infections with streptococci, staphylococci, and obligate anaerobic infections may also be the culprit.

The cardiovascular effect may be the initial clinical change identified. This effect is a continuum that may begin with tachycardia and respiratory alkalosis. Increased cardiac output and diminished systemic vascular resistance can occur with little change in the blood pressure. This state can usually be treated successfully with volume expansion. Marked hypotension with systolic pressures less than 60 mm Hg results from a decrease in systemic vascular resistance with significant increase in cardiac output. This is followed by a decreasing cardiac index because of poor left ventricular performance and an increase in systemic vascular resistance. This results in an anaerobic metabolism with lactic acid accumulation and metabolic acidosis. The patient is usually cold and clammy with hypoxemia and oliguria.

Sepsis can lead to ARDS with a clinical picture of hypoxemia even with increased oxygenization. Bilateral diffuse pulmonary infiltrates are commonly seen suggestive of pulmonary edema without volume overload. Altered renal function is also a continuum ranging from minimal proteinuria to acute tubular necrosis and renal failure. Decreased circulating volume and hypotension contributes to the renal hyperprofusion and possible acute tubular necrosis. Care must be made in prescribing antibiotics that are nephrotoxic, since this can potentiate the already decreased renal function.

As noted earlier, the infectious process can stimulate the coagulation cascade, which can result in a disseminated intervascular coagulopathy (DIC). Consumption of platelets and coagulation factors take place with fibrin deposition within small blood vessels, which in severe cases can lead to death secondary to necrosis from the fibrin deposition. DIC is seen more frequently with gram-negative than gram-positive sepsis.

Management is directed toward the clinical effects of the septic patient with probably the most important point being recognition of the syndrome. Initial adequate oxygenization, fluid replacement, cardiac output monitoring, and administration of broad spectrum antibiotics is extremely important. The placement of a Swan-Ganz catheter certainly aids with the hemodynamic therapy. If ARDS develops, intubation and mechanical respiration is needed. If cardiovascular function is suboptimal, dopamine is usually the drug of choice for improving cardiac function. Inotropic therapy may also be needed, as well as a peripheral vasodilator if vasoconstriction continues to be a problem. Elimination of the infecting organism, of course, is tantamount to successful management. Not only are appropriate antibiotics needed but the infected tissue should be removed, such as the drainage of a pelvic abscess in the postoperative patient. Because of the serious life-threatening condition, these patients require intensive care admission, and consultation with physicians experienced in the management of these patients should be sought.

Neutropenia

Neutropenia, with or without fever, is a common finding after chemotherapy, particularly if multiple agents are used over a protracted period of time, as is the case in patients with ovarian cancer. Short-term neoadjuvant therapy as it is used today by some in carcinoma of the cervix does not seem to place patients at high risk for neutropenia. The febrile neutropenic patient has a very high possibility of being infected. If the neutrophil count is less than 100 cells/ml, almost one quarter of the febrile episodes will have an associated bacteremia. These are usually caused by gram-negative aerobic bacilli, particularly *E. coli*, *Klebsiella pneumoniae*, and *Pseudomonas aeruginosa*, and by gram-positive cocci, particularly coagulase-negative staphylococci, alpha hemolytic streptococci, and *Staphylococcus aureus*. It is suggested that relatively few anatomic sites might be affected and relatively few organisms cause these infections. The alimentary tract, with its mucosal changes induced by chemotherapy, may be a primary site of infection. Invasive procedures can also cause the skin to be a port of infection, especially where the placement or maintenance of a vascular access device is involved. In many instances, if not most, the febrile episodes in the neutropenic patient are of unexplained pathogenesis. The role of multiple site cultures, including blood cultures, appears to have limited clinical usefulness. The reason for this is that no single site is a predictable source. Other less common potential pathogens were usually isolated, and the true pathogen (as noted on a blood culture) was usually known prior to its identification in the blood. As a result, many investigators do not recommend routine cultures in the neutropenic patient. An exception to this might be the individual who has an indwelling intravenous device. If only a catheter is in place, over 90% of the catheter-related bacteremias in the neutropenic patient can be successfully treated with appropriate antibiotics without catheter removal. However, a subcutaneous tunnel infection in a patient with an indwelling intravenous access device (such as a Porta-Cath) will usually not be cleared with antibiotics only, and the device should be removed. It has been suggested that if a central venous catheter is in place cultures should be taken from the device as well as peripherally. If the bacteremia or septicemia is caused by a fungus, the line is usually removed. S. aureus and coagulase-negative staphylococci are the most frequent cause of catheter-induced infection. Only about 5% of septicemic episodes are caused by anaerobic bacteria.

Empiric antibody coverage is given to neutropenic patients when they become febrile. Many patients may have a neutropenia of less than 1000/ml and remain afebrile. Although some people have suggested prophylactic antibiotics in this group, it has been our practice to not use antibiotics unless fever is associated with the neutropenia. It should be remembered that a low-grade fever in the neutropenic patient is as significant as a high-grade fever in the nonneutropenic patient. If fever is present in the neutropenic patient, combination antibiotic therapy is usually recommended. Probably the most common combination is that of an aminoglycoside with an antipseudomonal betalactam. The advantages of combination therapy are potential synergistic effects against some gram-negative bacilli, coverage of anaerobes, and the lessened likelihood that resistance may develop. The disadvantages are the lack of activity against some gram-positive bacteria and toxicity noted with aminoglycosides. Serum levels of aminoglycosides should be monitored and dose adjusted accordingly. The use of aminoglycoside alone is not recommended, even though it may be sensitive against the presumed causative bacteria. Other suggestive combinations have been two betalactam antibiotics. In some studies, these have been shown to be as effective as the previously noted combination. A major disadvantage is the relatively high cost. If a patient is known to have coagulase-negative staphylococci, methicillin-resistant S. aureus, corynebacteria, or alpha hemolytic streptococci, vancomycin may be included in combination therapy of aminoglycoside and antipseudomonal penicillin. This situation is seen more frequently in patients with indwelling central venous catheters. The role of monotherapy with the third generation cephalosporins as a substitute for multiple agents continues to gain support. Meta-analysis notes no significant difference in efficacy and clinical outcome when monotherapy with ceftazidine was compared with ceftazidine or other β-lactam plus an aminoglycoside. Ceftazidine demonstrated a lack of efficacy against gram-positive and anaerobic bacteria. Imipenem monotherapy provides good coverage of gram-negative and anaerobic bacteria. If the patient does not respond promptly, multiple agents should be used. In the past, the length of antibiotic coverage varied. Many investigators have suggested a minimum of 7 days of antibiotics after blood cultures have returned to normal or sites of

infection have cleared. It has been suggested that the neutrophil count should be greater than 500/ml before the antibiotics are stopped. In most instances when no organism is isolated, it is suggested that antibiotics should be continued for a minimum of 7 days, assuming that the patient responds promptly (usually within 3 days) to the antibiotic regimen. Obviously, if the fever and neutropenia continue, consideration for a change in antibiotics along with central line catheter removal should be taken under advisement. We have noted that once the nadir has passed and the neutrophil count begins to return toward normal, the febrile episode usually disappears fairly soon. If the neutrophil count is greater than 500/ml, the likelihood of persistent or recurrent infection is greatly reduced. In patients who remain febrile, the use of antifungal and antiviral agents should be considered. Patients with a history of neutropenia and fever are followed closely, and antibiotics are used liberally in subsequent courses.

Drug Related Leukemias

Several chemotherapeutic agents have been related to the development of subsequent leukemias. The alkylating agents were the first to be noted as a possible leukemia associated malignancy. More recently, studies have reported that patients treated with epipodophyllotoxins (etoposide and teniposide) have had secondary acute myeloid leukemia (AML). Although these numbers are small (1% in germ cell tumors), one must be aware of this relationship. It appears that in patients who developed AML, most, if not all, received a high cumulative dose (>2 g/m^2) weekly or twice weekly and doses were given in combination with other drugs that inhibit DNA repair. There is a relatively short latency period (mean 35 months) and a good response to chemotherapy (CR 50%-60%). In contrast, leukemias seen after alkylating agents develop relatively late (over 5 years) and frequently go through the myelodysplasia or preleukemic stage. The response of the AML to therapy is generally poor. It appears that AML after these two agent families differs either by arising by a different mechanism of action or it effects a different target cell.

Hypercalcemia

Hypercalcemia of malignancy is the most common metabolic complication of cancer. Although seen more frequently in non-gynecologic cancers, hypercalcemia is seen from time to time and should be recognized and aggressively managed. Increased bone reabsorption is the common denominator that takes place at the site of osteolytic metastasis. This is mediated by normal osteoclasts rather than tumor cells. There does not, however, appear to be a relationship between the number of boney metastases and the level of serum calcium. Serum calcium levels greater than 13 mg/dl is considered a medical emergency. Symptoms produced by hypercalcemia include somnolence, nausea, weakness, and personality changes. Immobilization and medications such as thiazide diuretics can contribute to the disease process. Hydration is the cornerstone of management. Patients are usually dehydrated and have impaired renal calcium excretion. Saline infusion to replace blood volume deficit will help to increase urinary output and hopefully calciuresis. Furosemide may enhance calcium excretion by blocking calcium reabsorption. Adequate hydration should take place before furosemide is given. Serum electrolytes need to be monitored and replaced as needed. The use of osteoclast inhibitors appears to be most helpful. The newer bisphosphonates, particularly pamidronate, appear to be the treatment of choice by some investigators. It is given as a single 12-14 hr infusion. A 90 mg infusion is used for a calcium of $\geq$14 and 60 mg if Ca is <14/mg/dl. Its effect takes 3-4 days with maximum effect at 7-10 days.

Chemotherapy-produced Nausea and Vomiting

One of the significant side effects of chemotherapy is its associated nausea and vomiting. One of the drugs that has a high emetogenic potential is cisplatin, which is frequently used in gynecologic cancers. Because of its high frequency of nausea and vomiting, antiemetics are routinely used before and during infusion of the drug. For several years, metoclopramide, usually in combination with dexamethasone, was the standard antiemetic. Its effectiveness was usually present in about one half of cycles. Limiting side effects included sedation, akathisia, and dystonic reactions. As the role of serotonin receptors in the mechanism of emesis was defined, newer specific 5-HT$_3$ receptor antagonists were developed. Several prospective randomized double blind studies have shown the superiority of these antagonists, usually in combination with dexamethasone compared to the antagonist alone or in other combinations. Granisetron (Kytril) 1 mg and dexamethasone 20 mg given before chemotherapy is effective in controlling nausea and vomiting (see box).

Patients over 65

The average life-span of women in the United States is 78 years, and a 75-year-old woman on the average can expect to live another 10 years. The elderly patient is at high risk of developing gynecologic malignancies in that 27% of the cervical, 45% of endometrial, 43% of epithelial ovarian, and 65% of vulvar cancers occur in women over 65. Management of gynecologic cancer in these individuals in many instances poses a therapeutic dilemma. For many years, it was felt that surgery, particularly radical surgery, should be restricted to younger people. As a result, radiation therapy, when appropriate, was almost routinely given to older individuals. Experience has shown that older patients can withstand radical surgery and are not without major complications when radiation therapy is used. Nutritional supplementation, when needed, along with improvement in anesthesia, intraoperative monitoring, blood banking, and postoperative care, has reduced the risk of radical surgery. Lawton and Hacker reviewed their experience in 226 consecutive patients, of whom 72 were over 70 years old and 154 were younger, in regard to their ability to undergo surgery. The older patients presented with more advanced-stage disease and generally had significantly poorer presurgical performance status and more intercurrent medical problems than the younger patients. The planned radical surgical procedure, however, could be carried out in 90% of the elderly patients, with a postoperative mortality of 1.5%. Postoperative minor complications were similar in the two groups, and the mean inpatient stay was the same, except for the vulvectomy patients. It appears from this study that older patients can withstand radical surgery almost as well as younger patients. Lawton and Hacker felt that chronological age alone was not a detriment of surgical risks. The group at the Mayo Clinic reported 38 patients 65 years of age or older who underwent radical hysterectomy as primary treatment for carcinoma of the cervix. There was no perioperative mortality or ureteral fistulae. They compared this group of patients with a group of 320 patients under 65 who were treated in a similar fashion. Transfusion requirements and incidence of postoperative lower-extremity edema were similar between the two groups. Febrile morbidity was less frequent in the older patients, but postoperative small bowel obstruction, bladder dysfunction, and pulmonary emboli were more frequent. The survival estimates for the two groups were identical.

Complications from radiation therapy in the older patient are increased. The thin, hypertensive patient appears to be at greater risk for radiation therapy complications to both the GI and GU tracts. Kennedy reported that 10 of 30 elderly women receiving definitive radiotherapy for gynecologic cancers had to have their treatments modified because of complications. Two patients (7%) had treatment-related mortality, and major complications occurred in 12 patients, 4 of them life threatening. There was a 10% fistula rate. Grant and his associates noted that 10 of 31 elderly patients receiving radiotherapy as primary treatment for their gynecologic malignancies failed to complete the planned therapy and

---

SUGGESTED CHEMOTHERAPY EMESIS PREVENTION

- Acute emesis prevention
  Granisetron (Kytril) 1 mg   } PO or IV 30"
  Dexamethasone (Decadron) 20 mg } before chemo
- Delayed emesis prevention
  Metroclopramide (Reglan) 30 mg t.i.d. × 3 days
  Dexamethasone (Decadron) 8 mg b.i.d. × 3 days

4 (13%) died of treatment-related complications. In those with a poor performance status, 70% failed to complete radiotherapy, and there was a 30% mortality in that group. The argument has been put forth that since ovarian preservation is not a consideration in elderly patients, surgery does not offer any advantage over radiation therapy for the treatment of carcinoma of the cervix. It has been our observation that such patients appear to be extremely vulnerable to vaginal scarring and stenosis from radiation therapy, particularly when brachytherapy is utilized. Sexual dysfunction after radical surgery in these individuals is much less frequent than it is after radiation therapy. It is believed that functional age, not chronological age, is a more important criterion in determining whether a patient is a tolerable surgical risk.

Invasive hemodynamic monitoring

Before the introduction of invasive hemodynamic monitoring, one could rely only on physical signs and symptoms to evaluate cardiopulmonary function and determine proper therapy. Clinical findings, which usually indicated events that had already occurred, were neither a sensitive indicator of current status nor predictive of what might occur. For instance, late findings of left ventricular failure included dyspnea, extended jugular vein, and tachycardia, which usually were secondary to pulmonary edema and right ventricular failure. The lag time between corrective action and resolution of the clinical findings could be several hours, and this could very well be critical in the correct management of patients with significant cardiopulmonary dysfunction. In 1962, central venous pressure (CVP) allowed direct cardiac monitoring and was an indicator of right ventricular filling pressure (preload) if tricuspid valve disease was not present. Unfortunately, accurate evaluation of left ventricular filling pressure is impossible with CVP. Since the left ventricle is a prime mover of blood, an accurate assessment of left ventricular function is necessary in the management of the critically ill patient. In 1970 the development of the Swan-Gantz catheter allowed assessment of the left ventricular function with pulmonary artery wedge pressure. In addition, pulmonary artery, systolic, and diastolic pressures could be measured. It was now possible to distinguish cardiogenic from noncardiogenic pulmonary edema. With the improvement of the original Swan-Gantz catheter, cardiac output, right arterial pressure, calculated pulmonary and systemic vascular resistance, monitored mixed venous oxygen saturation, and the function of the ventricles can now be determined.

The quadruple lumen thermodilution catheter is the most commonly used invasive monitoring device today. One port, which runs the entire length of the catheter and terminates at its tip, is used to measure pulmonary artery pressure and wedge pressure. The balloon inflation port terminates within the balloon. The proximal right atrium port terminates 30 cm from the tip of the catheter, and the opening is in the right atrium when the tip of the catheter is in the pulmonary artery. This port is used to monitor right atrium pressure, obtain blood samples, and administer IV fluid or medication, as well as other solutions for cardiac output studies. The thermistor port contains a temperature-sensitive wire that terminates 4-6 cm from the tip of the catheter. The catheter is inserted through a peripheral or a central vessel. The catheter is advanced into the right atrium. Pressure profiles are obtained with the advancement of the catheter, and location is determined accordingly. The low pressure is usually present in the right atrium; and as it is passed into the right ventricle the pressure is increased from a level of 0-8 mm of mercury to a level of 15-25 mm of mercury. With the passage into the pulmonary artery, normal pressure values are 4-12 mm of mercury. As the catheter is directed into the more peripheral pulmonary circulation, the balloon becomes lodged in a segment of the pulmonary artery and the pulmonary artery wedge pressure can be obtained.

Probably the greatest use for invasive monitoring in gynecologic oncology is to determine the cause of hypotension and low urinary output, particularly during the postoperative period. This may be caused by hypovolemia, congestive heart failure, myocardial infarction, or sepsis, all of which require different treatments. A patient with hypotension secondary to hypovolemia will tend to have a decrease in cardiac index and in pulmonary artery and pulmonary capillary wedge pressure with a rise in the systemic vascular resistance. Systemic vascular resistance—the average or total resistance to blood flow in the entire vascular system—is calculated from measured parameters. Because of the rise in the systemic vascular resistance, the blood pressure may remain within normal range until severe hypovolemia is present. In the postoperative patient, hypovolemia could be caused by dehydration, hemorrhage, or third space fluid loss. This latter situation can be exhibited by an ovarian cancer patient with ascites, and the hypovolemia should be corrected with colloid and crystalloid.

Invasive hemodynamic monitoring can certainly make a difference for critically ill patients, determine the etiology of their impaired cardiovascular status, and aid in directing correct therapy. Obviously, the anticipated benefit must clearly outweigh the risks and expenses. Although general guidelines are available for its use, individual patient circumstances must be considered carefully before the decision is made to use these monitoring techniques. The use of the APACHE II scoring system has been shown to predict mortality in gynecology patients. The APACHE II score reflects chronic health status, age, and 12 health characteristics such as heart rate and mean arterial pressure. The experience at the University of North Carolina was reported in patients admitted to the ICU for various reasons. Only 1 of 37 patients (3%) died if APACHE II score was less then 20; 7 of 8 patients with a score of ≥20 died. Although this score predicts mortality, the authors, as well as others, do not feel that the score should be used to dictate management of the individual patient.

Radiation Therapy

Morbidity resulting from properly conducted radiation therapy in patients with carcinoma of the cervix is usually minimal. Unfortunate misconceptions about the magnitude of this small radiation morbidity have several origins. Many investigators fail to distinguish that unnecessary adverse effects result from bad techniques and should not be extrapolated to the use of proper techniques. In addition, there has been a failure to recognize that a great deal of radiation morbidity is usually related to compromised treatment of patients with extensive tumors in whom surgery is not applicable. Results in these patients cannot be extrapolated to the use of optimal techniques in the treatment of patients with limited malignancy. Also, it often is an unrecognized fact that a great deal of morbidity attributed to irradiation results from an uncontrolled tumor (i.e., rectovaginal and vesicovaginal fistulae). As in the case of surgery, the treatment-related morbidity can be minimized by good application, but it cannot be eliminated.

Because the bladder and rectum are adjacent to the female genital tract, most of the side effects and complications of radiation involve these adjacent organs. Radiation complications are related to the dose, field size, and type of equipment used. The larger the field, the greater the risk of problems if the dose remains constant. Usually as the fields enlarge, the dose must be decreased; conversely, as the fields become smaller, a larger dose can be tolerated.

With the orthovoltage equipment, skin intolerance was a real problem. Multiple ports were used in an attempt to decrease skin irritation. This situation was encountered because 100% of the given dose was absorbed at the skin level. With the newer megavoltage equipment, the 100% absorption isodose level may be several centimeters beneath the skin. With orthovoltage, and even with cobalt-60, hyperemia almost always occurred on the skin. In some instances large areas of the skin ports sloughed with no or very slow healing. Fortunately this situation is rarely seen today.

Gastrointestinal complications

In most patients receiving external radiation to the pelvis, radiation proctitis and/or enteritis is seen with its resultant diarrhea. The extent varies from patient to patient. It usually manifests within a week or two of the commencement of radiation therapy and resolves within a week or 10 days after therapy has been completed. Some of the transitory symptoms are tenesmus and the passage of mucus and even blood per rectum. Diarrhea and abdominal cramping characterize small intestinal irritation. Such morbidity is more common when a portion of intestine is fixed in the pelvis by previous surgical adhesions or other pathologic conditions. The severity (one or two loose stools to many diarrheal stools per day) is variable from patient to patient. Diet and the use of antidiarrheal medication (e.g., diphenoxylate [Lomotil]) usually keep the symptoms tolerable. Anorexia may also be present during treatment. Nausea and vomiting can occur, but they are unusual. If present, they can lead to dehydration with a resultant need for intravenous hydration and electrolyte supplementation in some instances. Patients will usually lose a few pounds during the radiation treatment. Occasionally weight loss may be severe, and nutritional augmentation is required. The most common offending agent in proctitis is vaginal radium, particularly if physical separation (of the radioactive source) from the rectovaginal septum is less than adequate.

Postradiation injuries to the bowel may manifest at any time after therapy. A typical patient with small bowel injury is initially seen with postprandial crampy abdominal pain and anorexia. All too often these patients are classified as having recurrent disease and are allowed to waste away. In the study from the MD Anderson Hospital about one half of small bowel injuries occurred within 1 year after radiation and three fourths occurred within 2 years. Another study from the same institution evaluated small bowel dysfunction in Stage Ib cervical cancer patients. They compared 224 patients who were radiated compared with 100 treated with radical hysterectomy. A significantly greater number of patients treated with radiation experienced weight loss, had more diarrhea, and required medication for diarrhea. Pretreatment lap was a significant predictor of diarrhea requiring medication. About one fifth of patients developed diarrhea and about one half of those required medication. The interval between end of therapy and onset of diarrhea was a median of 26 months. Patients are usually initially seen with partial or complete obstruction with or without perforation or fistulae. Surgical correction depends on the situations encountered at the time of surgery. Many times a long intestinal tube is of help not only in decompressing the bowel but also in identifying proximal segments of the bowel at the time of surgery. The obstruction most often is associated with several segments of small bowel stuck in the pelvis, and many surgeons prefer a simple intestinal bypass procedure. Resection with reanastomosis is an option but, at least in some reports, these patients are at increased risk for further obstructive problems. Perforation or fistulae, if present, must be isolated, and diversion with more extensive surgery must be done only if technically feasible. Any anastomosis, whether for bypass or resection, should be done with nonradiated bowel if at all possible (Figure 17-5). Harris and Wheeless reported their experience with end-to-end anastomosis stapler device in low colorectal anastomosis associated with rectal surgery. This was accomplished in 49 patients with 17 (35%) having had prior radiation. All 5 complications

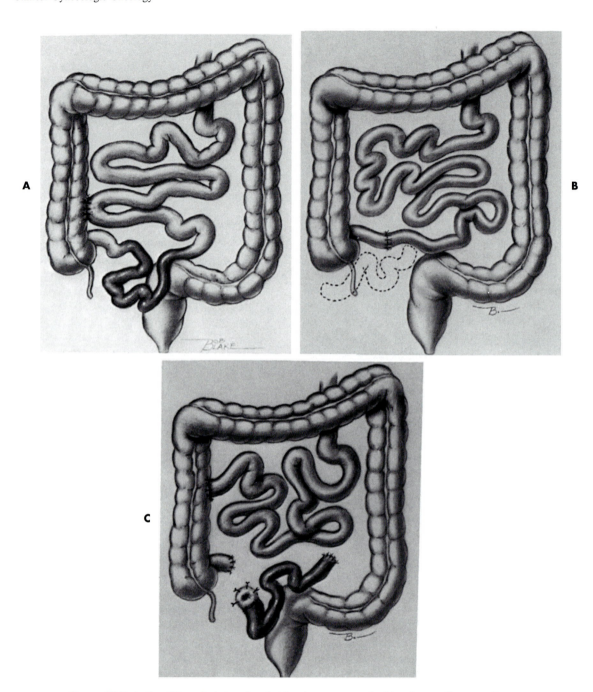

Figure 17-5 A, Small bowel obstruction that has been managed with a bypass ileoascending enteroenterostomy. **B,** Resection of involved bowel has been done with renanastomosis of small bowel. Sufficient terminal ileum must be present for this procedure to be accomplished. **C,** Obstructed bowel has been isolated with formation of mucous fistula. End-to-side anastomosis has also been done.

(2 strictures, 2 anastomosis breakdowns, and 1 fecal incontinence after colostomy closure) occurred in the patients who had prior radiation.

Rectovaginal fistula is the most common significant radiation injury to the large bowel. Sigmoid obstruction and chronic proctosigmoiditis are also frequently encountered. All patients with rectovaginal fistulae should have diverting colostomies performed with subsequent fistula

repair postponed for several months. The problem of poor vascularization in the area of fistula is always present, and the use of neovascularization techniques can improve the success rate (Figure 17-6).

Allen-Mersch et al. have noted that there was a progressive increase in radiation-induced bowel damage (including rectovaginal fistula) after treatment of uterine cancer in their patients treated over the last 20 years. They

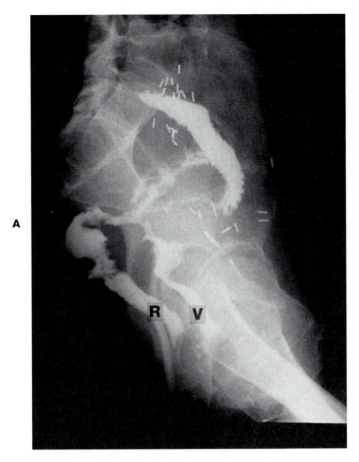

Figure 17-6 A, Barium enema demonstrating rectovaginal fistula after irradiation.

Continued.

treated 1418 cervical and uterine cancer patients and 4.3% had radiation-induced bowel injury. Radiation-induced complications were significantly higher in cervix cancer compared with uterine cancer, which they felt were caused by high rectal doses from intercavitary sources. Most complications were to the rectum or sigmoid colon. Radiation-induced rectovaginal fistulae occurred at a median of 13 months posttreatment and rectal strictures at 24 months. Only after complete healing of the fistulae and absence of obstruction of the bowel have been documented should the colostomy be closed.

Fistulae from the small bowel to the large bowel, bladder, vagina, or skin can occur. These complex fistulae may be difficult to repair and evaluation of their exact nature is a must. Patients are usually malnourished and TPN is important not only to replenish their stores but also to allow optimal healing to take place. The use of TPN is often needed for several weeks before anticipated surgery. If a fistula can be resected, it should be, but at the very least it must be isolated and the intestinal stream diverted around the lesion.

Large bowel obstruction can lead to a surgical emergency with a required colostomy. Fortunately, the radiated patient has usually manifested symptoms that make the physician aware of the possibility, and seeing a patient for the first time with a markedly dilated cecum requiring an emergency colostomy is unusual. When a colostomy is done for radiation-induced obstruction, it is usually permanent.

The symptoms of radiation proctitis may follow an asymptomatic interval of many months to years after treatment. Diarrhea with or without rectal bleeding is the most common finding. Cramping abdominal pain may be associated with the diarrhea. The changes most often are localized to the anterior rectal wall at the site of maximal dosage from radium and range from thickened, fragile mucosa to thin, atrophic mucosa or mucosal ulceration. These changes usually heal with conservative management, including low-residue diet, anticholinergic drugs, stool softeners, and steroid enemas. On occasion a diverting colostomy is necessary for either marked fibrosis of the rectal wall or excessive bleeding from the lower bowel. It is important that these stages be recognized and not be confused with tumor, since diverting procedures are curative and result in the patient returning to a state of well-being.

Occasionally a postirradiated patient may be seen with severe anemia and without a history of melena or active

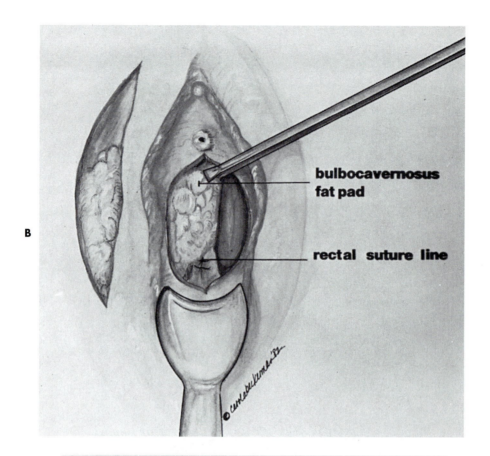

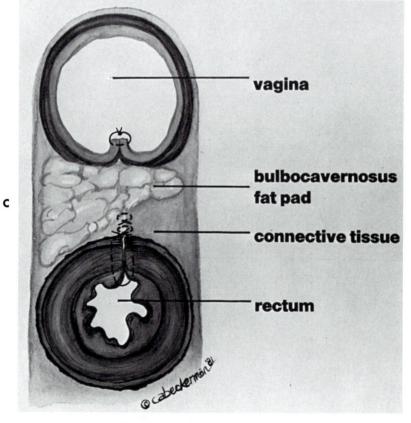

Figure 17-6, cont'd. B, Repair of rectovaginal fistula has been strengthened by interposition of bulbocarvernosus fat pad. **C,** Cross-section shows placement of neovascular fat pad.

rectal bleeding. This may be the result of significant small bowel irradiation (many times in patients previously operated on) that has caused extensive damage to the ileum and eventually vitamin B_{12} deficiency. A Schilling test can differentiate between the vitamin B_{12} and folic acid deficiency. Because vitamin B_{12} is normally absorbed in the distal ileum, radiation and/or surgery to this area may lead to anemia. The use of weekly vitamin B_{12} injections until the hemoglobin returns to a normal level (usually 4-6 weeks) and then monthly injections will prevent recurrence of this type of anemia.

Genitourinary complications

Acute radiation cystitis is occasionally encountered during or in the immediate post-therapy period. Typical symptoms of cystitis are present, but the cultures are usually returned as showing no growth. Increased oral liquid intake and the use of a urinary analgesic will relieve the symptoms, and resolution of symptoms usually occurs within a short time. Chronic radiation cystitis with hematuria is a much different problem. Hemorrhage may be controlled with continuous bladder irrigation using either 0.5% or 1% acetic acid or 1:1000 potassium permanganate solution. Occasionally cystoscopy will be necessary to remove blood clots or fulgurate specific bleeding points; unfortunately, the hemorrhage is often from multiple sites and complete fulguration is not possible. Formaldehyde irrigation can be used if control

of hemorrhage has not been successful with other methods.

Fistulae of both the GU and GI tracts in the irradiated patient usually develop when there is initial extensive disease in the region of the cervix and/or upper vagina. The tumor dose of radiation may have been greater than normal because of the extent of disease. The addition of central surgery (hysterectomy) to irradiation will usually increase the fistula rate. Boronow and Rutledge, in reviewing the MD Anderson Hospital material, noted a 4.1% vesicovaginal fistula rate if radiation and surgery both were used in comparison with 1.4% if radiation alone was used (Table 17-4). In many instances local (vaginal

Table 17-4   Vesicovaginal fistulae after treatment for cervical cancer

	Fistulae	
	Radiation only	**Radiation and surgery**
Stage I	6/562 (1%)	3/60 (5%)
Stage II	6/1080 (0.5%)	5/127 (3.9%)
Stage III	25/971 (2.5%)	2/50 (4%)
Stage IV	2/116 (1.7%)	0/4 (0%)
TOTAL	39/2729 (1.4%)	10/241 (4.1%)

Modified from Boronow RC, Rutledge F: *Am J Obstet Gynecol* 111:85, 1971.

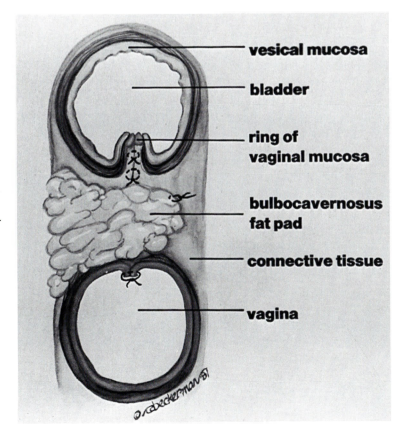

Figure 17-7 Cross section of vesicovaginal repair using bulbocavernosus fat pad as a source of neovascularization.

and cervix) necrosis may precede the fistula by weeks or months. In this type of situation the bladder and rectum both may be involved with the fistula, but they may become apparent at different times. One fistula may be diverted, with the other being manifest a few weeks or months later. Local care, including hydrogen peroxide or zinc peroxide douches and estrogen to the upper vagina, may help remove necrotic material and avoid impending fistulae. If the necrosis is extensive, it is not unusual to have the upper tracts of the GU system involved also, and a ureteral stricture with resultant hydronephrosis may also

be present. Many fistulae occur within 6-12 months after completion of radiation therapy, but others occur years later. If central surgery (hysterectomy) is performed in connection with radiation therapy, the fistula is usually evident within a few weeks of surgery.

Repair of the fistula in irradiated areas is difficult and less successful than fistula repair in nonirradiated areas. A full GU system workup is needed to make sure the ureters are not involved with the process. If only a vesicovaginal fistula is present, several techniques are available. Partial or complete colpocleisis has been used in the past but with

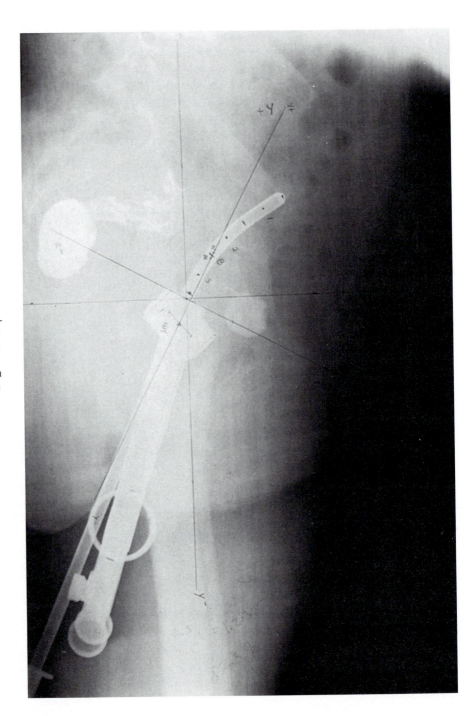

Figure 17-8 Radium placement film (lateral). Fletcher-Suit applicator, Hypaque in Foley catheter balloon, and contrast material in rectum allow estimation of dose to these structures. This is a good application with reasonable distances between radium system (tandem and ovoids) and bladder anteriorly and rectum posteriorly.

a definite loss of sexual function. In all of these patients the problem of adequate blood supply in the irradiated area is a major consideration. The use of the bulbocavernosus labial fat pad mobilized to a position between the bladder and vagina has proved very successful (Figure 17-7). Surgeons repairing this type of fistula are advised to use this or some other type of neovascularization to help ensure success. When repairing this type of fistula abdominally with an intravesical approach, the omentum with its attached blood supply lends itself nicely as the neovascular contributor. If the ureter is involved, an abdominal approach is mandatory. Repair of the vesicovaginal fistula can be done, with reimplantation of the ureter into the dome of the bladder accomplished at the same time.

If both ureters are involved and reimplantation is not feasible, a conduit may be the only option. A piece of unirradiated bowel must be selected for the conduit, and the use of the transverse colon as advocated by Nelson has become popular. If the bladder is not involved, an ilioneoureterocystotomy may be considered. Subsequent renal embarrassment can occur with either of these approaches.

Kagan et al. have proposed a staging system for irradiation injuries after treatment for cancer of the cervix uteri that we find particularly useful:

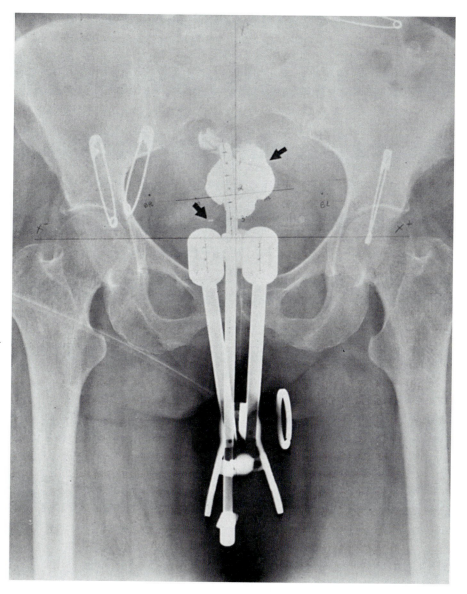

Figure 17-9 Anteroposterior view of system in Figure 17-8. Arrows point to contrast material in rectum and stainless steel seeds placed 1 cm into cervical tissue to identify that organ. Risk of injury from such an application would be low with average doses because of good central positioning.

R[1]   Type of injury that results in complete recovery from all acute symptoms such as dysuria and hematuria, diarrhea and cramps, rectal bleeding, and hydroureter.

R[2]   Type of injury in which there is incomplete recovery from urinary bleeding, edematous bladder mucosa, diarrhea, colicky pain, weight loss, persistent hydroureter, or colonic stenosis. Continuous medications and frequent examinations are required.

S[1]   Type of injury that requires surgical intervention from a single-organ injury. This may require total cystectomy, urinary diversion, resection of an obstructed bowel segment, colostomy, or ureteral reimplantation.

S[2]   Type of injury that requires more extensive surgery for injury to two or more organs.

Using this staging system, we, like Kagan et al., have found a positive correlation between increasing dose and severe S[1] and S[2] injuries. There is also a definite correlation between all bladder irradiation injuries (R[1], R[2], S[1], S[2]) and calculated increased bladder dose (Figures 17-8 and 17-9).

The overall complication rate varies considerably, depending on the total dose of radiation used. In general the serious morbidity of pelvic irradiation is less than 5% if the external irradiation is below 5000 cGy. Patients who receive more than 5000 cGy of external irradiation are usually those with advanced disease in whom radical irradiation is a necessity. In these patients the serious complication rate approaches 10%-20%.

BIBLIOGRAPHY

Genitourinary tract

Boronow RC, Rutledge FN: Vesicovaginal fistula, radiation, and gynecologic cancer, *Am J Obstet Gynecol* 111:85, 1971.

Bricker EM: Current status of urinary diversion, *Cancer* 45:2986, 1980.

Carter J, Ramirenz C, Waugh R et al: Percutaneous urinary diversion in gynecologic oncology, *Gynecol Oncol* 40:248, 1991.

Creasman WT, Weed JC Jr: Radical hysterectomy. In Schaefer G, Graber E, editors: *Complications in obstetrics and gynecologic surgery*, New York, 1981, Harper & Row.

Dudley VJ et al: Percutaneous nephrostomy catheter use in gynecological malignancy, *Gynecol Oncol* 24:273, 1986.

Feuer GA, Frauchter R, Souri E et al. Selection for percutaneous nephrostomy in gynecologic cancer patients, *Gynecol Oncol* 42:60, 1991.

Forney, JP: The effects of radical hysterectomy on bladder physiology, *Am J Obstet Gynecol* 138:374, 1980.

Forney JP et al: Long-term effects on bladder function following radical hysterectomy with and without post-operative radiation, *Gynecol Oncol* 26:160, 1987.

Hatch KD, Parham G, Shingleton HM: Ureteral stricture and fistula following radical hysterectomy, *Gynecol Oncol* 19:17, 1984.

Jacobs AL et al: Complications of patients receiving both irradiation and radical hysterectomy for carcinoma of the uterine cervix, *Gynecol Oncol* 22:273, 1985.

Kadar M, Slaliba N, Nelson JH: The frequent causes and prevention of severe urinary dysfunction after radical hysterectomy, *Br J Obstet Gynaecol* 90:859, 1983.

Lee RA, Symmonds RE: Ureterovaginal fistula, *Am J Obstet Gynecol* 109:1032, 1971.

Photopulos EJ, Zwaag RV: Class II radical hysterectomy shows less morbidity and good treatment efficacy compared to class III, *Gynecol Oncol* 40:21, 1991.

Ralph G, Tamussino K, Lictenegger W: Urodynamics following radical abdominal hysterectomy for cervical cancer, *Arch Gynecol Onstet* 243:215, 1988.

Roman-Lopez JJ, Barkley DL: Bladder dysfunction following Schanta hysterectomy, *Am J Obstet Gynecol* 115:81, 1973.

Seski JC, Diokno AC: Bladder dysfunction after radical abdominal hysterectomy, *Am J Obstet Gynecol* 128:643, 1977.

Stern JL, Maroney TP, Lace C: Treatment of urinary conduit fistula by antegrade ureteral stent catheter, *Obstet Gynecol* 70:276, 1987.

Swan RW, Rutledge FN: Urinary conduit in pelvic cancer patients: a report of sixteen years' experience, *Am J Obstet Gynecol* 119:6, 1974.

Symmonds RE: Urological injuries: ureter. In Schaefer G, Graber E, editors: *Complications in obstetrics and gynecologic surgery*, New York, 1981, Harper & Row.

Underwood RB, Lutz MH, Smoak DL: Ureteral injury following irradiation therapy for carcinoma of the cervix, *Obstet Gynecol* 49:663, 1977.

Gastrointestinal tract

Adelson MD, Kasowitz MH: Percutaneous endoscopic drainage gastrostomy in the treatment of gastrointestinal obstruction from intraperitoneal malignancy, *Obstet Gynecol* 81:467, 1993.

Allen-Mersch TG et al: Has the incidence of radiation-induced bowel damage following treatment of uterine carcinoma changed in the last 20 years? *J Soc Med* 79:387, 1986.

Barnes W, Waggoner S, Delgado G et al: Mamometric characterization of rectal dysfunction following radical hysterectomy, *Gynecol Oncol* 42:116, 1991.

Barnhill D, Doering D, Remmenga S et al: Intestinal surgery performed on gynecologic cancer patients, *Gynecol Oncol* 40:38, 1991.

Boike GM, Sightler SE, Averett HE: Treatment of small intestinal fistulas with octreotide, a somatostatin analog, *J Surg Oncol* 49:63. 1992.

Borison DI, Bloom AD, Pritchard TJ: Treatment of enterocutaneous and colocutaneous fistulas with early surgery or somatostatin analog, *Dis Colon Rectum* 35:635, 1992.

Bricker EM, Johnston WD: Repair of post-irradiation rectovaginal fistula and stricture, *Surg Gynecol Obstet* 148:499, 1979.

Cirisano FD, Greenspoon JS, Stenson et al: The etiology and management of diarrhea in the gynecologic oncology patient, *Gynecol Oncol* 50-45, 1993.

Clarke-Pearson DL et al: Surgical management of intestinal obstruction in ovarian cancer, *Gynecol Oncol* 26:11, 1987.

DiCostanzo J, Cano N, Martin J et al: Treatment of external gastrointestinal fistulas by a combination of total parenteral nutrition and somatostatin, *J Paternal Enteral Nutrition* 11:465, 1987.

Harris WJ, Wheeless CR: Use of the end in anastomosis stapling device in low colorectal anastomosis associated with radical gynecologic surgery, *Gynecol Oncol* 23:350, 1986.

Hatch KD, Gelder MS, Soong SJ et al: Pelvic exenteration with low rectal anastomosis: survival complications and prognostic factors, *Gynecol Oncol* 38:462, 1990.

Kagan AR et al: A new staging system for irradiation injuries following treatment for cancer of the cervix uteri, *Gynecol Oncol* 7:166, 1979.

Mangili G, Franchi M, Mariani A et al: Octreotide in the management of bowel obstruction in terminal ovarian cancer, *Gynecol Oncol* 345, 1996.

Marchant DJ: Special problems of the intestinal tract. In Schaefer G, Graber E, editors: *Complications in obstetrics and gynecologic surgery,* New York, 1981, Harper & Row.

Patton TJ, Mitchel MF, Atkinson EN et al: Parameters of small bowel dysfunction in cervical cancer patients undergoing radiotherapy, *Int J Gynecol Cancer* 3:175, 1993.

Photopulos JC et al: Intestinal anastomosis after radiation therapy by surgical stapling instruments, *Obstet Gynecol* 54:515, 1979.

Smith JP, Golden PE, Rutledge FN: The surgical management of intestinal injuries following radiation for carcinoma of the cervix. In University of Texas MD Anderson Hospital and Tumor Institute: *Cancer of the uterus and ovary*, Chicago, 1969, Year Book Medical.

Stockbine MF, Hancock JC, Fletcher GH: Complications in 831 patients with squamous cell carcinoma of the intact cervix treated with 3000 rad or more whole pelvic irradiation, *Am J Roent Radium Ther Nuc Med* 108:293, 1970.

Swan RW, Fowler WC, Boronow RC: Surgical management of radiation injury to the small intestine, *Surg Gynecol Obstet* 142:325, 1976.

Symmonds RE: Ureteral injuries associated with gynecologic surgery: prevention and management, *Clin Obstet Gynecol* 19:623, 1976.

Thromboembolism

Clarke-Pearson DL, Creasman WT: Diagnosis of deep venous thrombosis in obstetrics and gynecology by impedence phlebography, *Obstet Gynecol* 58:52, 1981.

Clarke-Pearson DL, Jelovsek FR, Creasman WT: Thromboembolism complicating surgery for cervical and uterine malignancy: incidence, risk factors, and prophylaxis, *Obstet Gynecol* 61:87, 1983.

Clarke-Pearson DL et al: Venous thromboembolism prophylaxis in gynecologic oncology: a prospective controlled trial of low-dose heparin, *Am J Obstet Gynecol* 145:606, 1983.

Clarke-Pearson DL et al: Variables associated with post-operative deep venous thrombosis: a prospective study of 411 gynecologic patients and the creation of a prognostic model, *Obstet Gynecol* 69:146, 1987.

Metz SA: Thromboembolism in gynecologic surgery, *The Female Patient* 20:15, 1995.

Moser KM, Fedullo PF, LittleJohn JK et al: Frequent asymptomatic pulmonary embolism in patients with deep vein thrombosis, *JAMA* 271:223, 1994.

The multicenter trial committee: Dihydroergotamine-heparin prophylaxis of postoperative deep venous thrombosis, *JAMA* 251:2960, 1984.

Myhand RC, Weiss RB: Causes and management of treatment-related thrombosis, *Contemporary Oncol*, August, pp 37-45, 1994.

Prandoni P, Lensing AWA, Buller HR et al: Comparison of subcutaneous low-molecular-weight heparin with intravenous standard heparin in proximal deep-vein thrombosis, *Lancet* 339:441, 1992.

Others

ACOG Technical Bulletin, 204, 1995.

Bajorunas DR: Clinical manifestations of cancer-related hypercalcemia, *Seminars in Oncology* 17:16, 1990.

Bandy LC, Clarke-Pearson DL, Creasman WT: Vitamin B-12 deficiency following therapy in gynecologic oncology, *Gynecol Oncol* 17:370, 1984.

Bergan JJ, Dean RH, Yao JST: Vascular injury in pelvic cancer surgery, *Am J Obstet Gynecol* 124:562, 1976.

Bone RC, Balk RA, Cerra FR et al: ACCP/SCCM consensus conference, *Chest* 101:1646, 1992.

Boronow RC: Management of radiation-induced vaginal fistulae, *Am J Obstet Gynecol* 110:1, 1971.

Delgado G, Smith PJ: *Management of complications in gynecologic oncology*, New York, 1982, John Wiley & Sons.

Editorial: *Seminars in Oncology* 17:1, 1990.

Escalante CP: Causes and management of superior vena cava syndrome, *Oncol* 7:61, 1993.

Fekety R, Shah AB: Diagnosis and treatment of *Clostridium difficile* colitis, *JAMA* 269:71, 1993.

Fox SM, Einhorn LH, Cox E et al: Ondansetron versus ondansetron, dexamethasone and chlorpromazine in the prevention of nausea and vomiting associated with multiple-day cisplatin chemotherapy, *J Clin Oncol* 11:2391, 1993.

Grant JP: *Handbook of total parenteral nutrition*, Philadelphia, 1980, WB Saunders.

Grant PT, Jeffrey JF, Frazier RC et al: Pelvic radiation therapy for gynecologic malignancy in geriatric patients, *Gynecol Oncol* 33:185, 1989.

Gurney H, Grill V, Martin TJ: Parathyroid hormone-related protein and response to pamidronate in tumour-induced hypercalcaemia, *Lancet* 341:1611, 1993.

Heath D, Baron R: *Nutrition handbook of medical treatment*, Skach W, Daly CL, Foramark CE, and Jones Medical Publication, California, 1988.

Hughes WT, Armstrong D, Bodez GP, et al: Guidelines for the use of antimicrobial agents in neutropenic patients with unexplained fever, *J Infect Dis* 161:381, 1990.

Italian Group for Antiemetic Research: Ondansetron + dexamethasone vs metoclopramide + dexamethasone + diphenhydramine in prevention of cisplatin-induced emesis, *Lancet* 340:96, 1992.

Italian Group for Antiemetic Research: Dexamethasone, granisetron, or both for the prevention of nausea and vomiting during chemotherapy for cancer, *N Eng J Med* 332:1, 1995.

Karp JE, Merz WG, Dick JD: Management of infections in neutropenic patients: advances in therapy and prevention, *Current Opinion in Infectious Diseases* 6:405, 1993.

Kinney WK, Egorshin EVB, Podratz KC: Wertheim hysterectomy in the geriatric population, *Gynecol Oncol* 31:227, 1988.

Kumar L: Epipodophyllotoxins and secondary leukaemia, *Lancet* 342:819, 1993.

Lawton FR, Hacker N: Surgery for invasive gynecologic cancer in the elderly female population, *Obstet Gynecol* 76:287, 1990.

McCraw JB et al: Vaginal reconstruction with gracilis myocutaneous flaps, *Plast Reconstr Surg* 58:176, 1976.

McDonald PT et al: Vascular trauma secondary to diagnostic and therapeutic procedures: laparoscopy, *Am J Surg* 135:651, 1978.

Muggia FM: Overview of cancer-related hypercalcemia: epidemiology and etiology, *Seminars in Oncology* 17:3, 1990.

Mundy GR: Pathophysiology of cancer-associated hypercalcemia, *Seminars in Oncology* 17:10, 1990.

Myhand RC, Weiss RB: Causes and management of treatment-related thrombosis, *Contemporary Oncol*, August, pp 37-45, 1994.

Nelson JH: *Atlas of radical pelvic surgery*, New York, 1977, Appleton-Century-Croft.

O'Quinn AG, Fletcher GH, Wharton JT: Guidelines for conservative hysterectomy after irradiation, *Gynecol Oncol* 9:68, 1978.

Parnes HL, How to manage metabolic emergencies, *Contemp Oncol* 1993, September, pp. 54-67.

Pearlman MD, Faro AE: Obstetrical septic shock: a pathophysiological basis for management, *Clin Obstet Gynecol 33:485, 1990.*

Perez EA, Hallstrom AE: Chemotherapy-induced emesis: prevention and management, *Contem Oncol* 1992, December, pp. 33-43.

Pizzo PA: Management of fever in patients with cancer and treatment-induced neutropenia, *N Engl J Med* 328:1323, 1993.

Rich NM, Spencer FC: *Management of acute injuries in vascular trauma*, Philadelphia, 1978, WB Saunders.

Ritch PS: Treatment of cancer-related hypercalcemia, *Seminars in Oncology* 17:26, 1990.

Rosenthal DM, Colapinto R: Angiographic arterial embolization in the management of postoperative vaginal hemorrhage, *Am J Obstet Gynecol* 151:227, 1985.

Soper DE: Necrotizing fasciitis and related entities. In Postosk JG, III, editor: *Obstetric and Gynecologic Infectious Diseases*, Raven Press, Ltd, New York, 1994.

Swartz PE et al: Control of arterial hemorrhage using percutaneous arterial catheter technique in patients with gynecologic malignancies, *Gynecol Oncol* 3:276, 1975.

Van Le L, Fakhry S, Walton LA et al: Use of the APACHE II scoring system to determine mortality of gynecologic oncology patients in the intensive care unit, *Obstet Gynecol* 85:53, 1995.

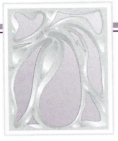

Basic Principles of Chemotherapy

All living things have an inherent capacity to multiply, and they cease multiplication for a variety of reasons. Control appears to be mediated by an unknown feedback mechanism, probably resulting from contact phenomena when cells are crowded together. In the malignant growth, cells do not cease multiplying when they reach a critical mass, and the uncontrolled growth leads to the death of the host. In the early phases of growth, tumor cells appear to grow exponentially, but as tumor mass increases, the time that a particular tumor requires to double its volume appears to increase. Three explanations have been given for this prolonged volume-doubling time: (1) an increase in cell cycle time (the time from one mitosis to the next), (2) a decrease in the growth fraction (cells participating in cell division in the tumor), and (3) an increase in cell loss from tumor cells with insufficient nutrients and vascular supply.

The outcome of cancer chemotherapy is not fully predictable, but the chances of remission can be improved by judicious selection of patients, careful assessment of the tumor's growth pattern, and treatment of the neoplasm with the drug or drugs most likely to be effective. The clinical response to chemotherapy is assessed utilizing standard criteria (Table 18-1)

Not all cancer patients can be treated with drugs. The suitability of a patient for chemotherapy depends on at least three critical criteria: (1) the nature of the neoplasm, (2) its extent of spread or stage, and (3) the patient's clinical condition. Not all cancers are equally sensitive to drugs. Factors that determine a tumor's susceptibility include how the drug is distributed to the tumor, drug transport into the cell, whether a drug-sensitive biochemical pathway is present in the tumor cell, and the relative rates of intracellular activation and inactivation of the drug. In many instances some of these factors are unknown for the drug and the tumor type. Investigational trials are being conducted with multiple agents to give us a better understanding of these parameters.

At present, only disseminated neoplasia is regularly treated with chemotherapy; surgery, radiotherapy, or both are the current treatment choices for localized disease. These concepts are rapidly changing, however, and the use of adjuvant chemotherapy soon after eradicating surgery is increasing, especially in the treatment of ovarian and uterine cancer. Treatment of a patient with metastatic disease should not mean waiting until the patient is cachectic or moribund. The patient should be treated as soon as she has symptoms attributable to the tumor, not only symptoms as obvious as pain caused by nerve route compression or dyspnea from lymphangitic pulmonary metastases but also anorexia and general weakness. Even asymptomatic patients who have diseases in which long remissions or cures can be achieved (such as choriocarcinoma or childhood acute leukemia) must be treated as early as possible. In most instances chemotherapy is palliative rather than curative; for this reason,

Table 18-1   Definitions of response

Type	Definition	Subtype
Complete Response (CR)	Complete resolution of all evidence of disease lasting at least 1 month	■ Complete Clinical Response (CCR) ■ Complete Pathologic Response: surgically documented (CPR) ■ Partial Clinical Response (PCR) ■ Partial Pathologic Response: surgically documented (PPR)
Partial Response (PR)	A decrease of ≥50% in the product of the diameters (maximal and minimal) of all measurable lesions lasting at least 1 month without the development of new lesions	
Stable Disease (SD)	A decrease of <50% or an increase of <25% in the product of the diameters of all measurable disease	
Progression	An increase of ≥25% in the measurable lesions as described above or the identification of new lesions	

side effects produced by these potent agents can be justified only by the more persistent removal of symptoms caused by the tumor or by a reasonable expectation of improved survival even in the absence of symptoms. Chemotherapy in a severely debilitated patient is usually futile and often dangerous and thus should be avoided.

The rationale for the use of drugs in the treatment of cancer is to achieve the selective killing of tumor cells. Underlying this rationale are the basic principles of the "cell kill" hypothesis first described by Skipper et al. The following principles were worked out in the L1210 leukemia model:

1. The survival of an animal with cancer is inversely related to the number of cancer cells
2. A single cell is capable of multiplying and eventually killing the host
3. For most drugs, a clear relationship exists between the dose of drug and its ability to eradicate tumor cells
4. A given dose of a drug kills a constant fraction of cells, not a constant number, regardless of the cell numbers present

This fourth and most important principle implies that cell destruction by drugs follows first-order kinetics. For example, treatment reducing a population from 1 million to 10^3 cells should reduce a population of 1000 to 1 cell. Implication for the clinician of this first-order cell destruction is that to eradicate a tumor population effectively, it is necessary to increase the total dose of drug or drugs to the maximal limits tolerated by the host or to start treatment when the number of cells is small enough to allow the destruction of tumor at total doses of drug that are reasonably tolerated. The logical conclusion derived from this hypothesis is that the maximal opportunity for achieving cure exists during the early stage of disease. It is more difficult to eradicate disseminated

disease than localized cancer, and it is much easier to control small tumors than large ones.

GOMPERTZIAN GROWTH

The experimental model (Figure 18-1) view of the growth curve of a cancer is that it follows a Gompertzian process whereby, as tumor mass increases in size, its mass-doubling time becomes progressively longer. The Gompertzian aspect of tumor growth is recognizable only when a tumor is measured in its clinically palpable range. In the subclinical period the growth is assumed to be exponential. Although all this is true in the rodent model, no data prove that it is applicable to humans. The Gompertzian model has significant clinical implications that have guided a good deal of clinical chemotherapy research over the past two decades. As a mass responds to treatment (i.e., gets smaller), the doubling time has been assumed to decrease as a consequence of a greater number of cells moving into cycle. This larger percentage of metabolically active cells would, therefore, increase the sensitivity of the neoplastic population of cell cycle-specific agents. This has led to the sequential use of cell cycle-nonspecific agents, such as cyclophosphamide, to bring down the mass, to be followed by cell cycle-specific agents such as methotrexate. Although these sequential combinations have been theoretically attractive, none has shown clear superiority in clinical trials. Another implication of the Gompertzian growth concept is that metastases can be expected to be more sensitive to chemotherapy in general, and to cell cycle-specific agents in particular, than the primary tumor from which they arise. The smaller the size of the metastatic focus, the greater the differential sensitivity will be. Therefore, the insensitivity of a primary tumor to a given drug regimen might not necessarily predict the response of metastasis to the same

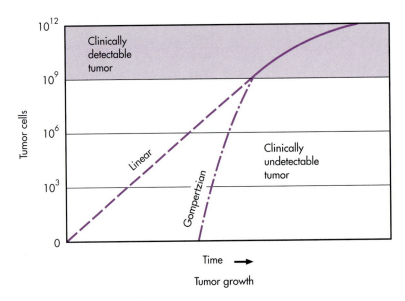

Figure 18-1 Tumor growth.

regimen. This theory has made adjuvant chemotherapy highly attractive.

A basic principle of the cell kill hypothesis and the Gompertzian growth concept is an inverse relationship between the sensitivity to chemotherapy and the tumor burden. This is based on pure kinetic construct and also on biochemical resistance. It means that the larger the total malignant mass, the higher the proportion of the permanently drug-resistant variance to any given compound or regimen. Another factor besides kinetics and resistance that can explain why clinical results differ from experimental models is pharmacology. The higher the cell number, the greater the chances for the existence of sites, either within the tumor or in selected organs, where tumor cells will be protected from efficient exposure to cytotoxic drugs.

DOUBLING TIME

The doubling time of the human tumor is the time it takes for the mass to double its size. There is considerable variation in human doubling times. For example, embryonal tumors and some lymphomas have relatively short doubling times (20-40 days), whereas, adenocarcinomas and squamous cell carcinomas have relatively long doubling times (50-150 days). Metastasis will generally have a shorter doubling time than the primary lesion. If it is assumed that an exponential growth occurs early in the malignancies' history and that the malignancy starts from a single cell, then a 1 mm mass will have undergone approximately 20 tumor doublings. A 5 mm mass (a size first recognizable on an x-ray) may have undergone 27 doublings. It follows, then, that a 1 cm mass will have undergone 30 doublings, and a clinician will be pleased to have detected such an "early" lesion. Unfortunately, this "early" lesion has already undergone 30 doublings

with significant DNA change being possible. Utilizing this rationale, clinical techniques currently available tend to recognize malignancies late in their growth, and metastatic disease may well have occurred long before there was obvious clinical manifestation of the primary lesion. Another implication from this kinetic information is that in late stages of tumor growth a very few doublings in tumor mass make a dramatic impact on the size of the tumor and the status of the patient. Once a tumor becomes palpable (1 cm in diameter), only three more doublings will produce a very large tumor mass (8 cm in diameter). It is obvious that therapeutic modalities such as chemotherapy, hormones, and x-ray therapy may all alter tumor growth; however, tumor growth can also alter the host defense mechanisms, oxygen tension, and vascular supply. Two basic factors regulating the speed with which tumors grow are the growth fraction and cell death. The growth fraction is the number of cells in the tumor mass that are actively involved in cell division. There is marked variation in the growth fraction of humans, ranging from 25% to almost 95%. In the past, it was believed that human tumors contained billions of cells, all growing slowly. In actuality, there is only a small fraction of rapidly proliferating cells within a tumor mass; the majority of cells are often out of the cell cycle and resting.

CELL KINETICS

Skipper et al. believed that for almost all antitumor agents, high-dose intermittent drug treatment was substantially more effective antitumor treatment than low-dose daily treatment. As a result, in the United States most cytotoxic drug treatment follows high-dose intermittent scheduling. It should be noted, however, that the superiority of this high-dose intermittent schedule is not clearly established by review of existing clinical data. Chemo-

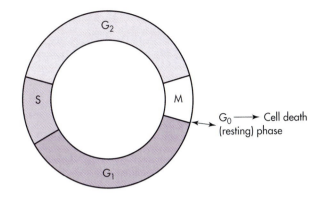

Gap 1 (G₁)	Postmitotic	4-24 hours (variable)
DNA synthesis (S)		10-20 hours
Gap 2 (G₂)		2-10 hours
Mitosis (M)		0.5-1 hour

Figure 18-2 Cell generation time and sequence are similar for all mammalian cells.

therapeutic agents appear to work by first-order kinetics. That is, they kill a constant fraction of cells rather than a constant number. This concept has important implications in cancer treatment. A single exposure of tumor cells to an antineoplastic drug may be capable of producing two to four logs of cell kill. With a common tumor burden 10^{12} cells (1 Kg), a single dose of chemotherapy will destroy a large number of cells but not be curative. Thus there is a need for intermittent courses of chemotherapy to achieve the magnitude of cell kill necessary to produce eradication of the lesion. This concept of "log kill hypothesis" also provides a rationale for multiple drug or combination chemotherapy, as well as for the philosophy of adjuvant chemotherapy. Adjuvant chemotherapy assumes subclinical cell masses of 10^1-10^4 cells that can produce failure but are undetectable following initial surgical therapy. This small tumor burden is particularly vulnerable to effective chemotherapy.

Chemotherapeutic agents are a crucial part of the physician's armamentarium in the ever broadening fight against cancer. With them he or she can ameliorate and, in a few instances, even cure diseases that were usually fatal in the past. Until recently, in most cases, chemotherapy has been reserved for relatively late stages of the disease, but its increasingly successful use, particularly in the treatment of hematologic malignancies, suggests that chemotherapy should be administered earlier. All physicians and surgeons must understand the nature and use of cancer chemotherapy so they can make rational decisions about when it may be indicated.

There are quasi-scientific rationales for modern treatment regimens. Unfortunately, data on solid tumor response are nevertheless still based on empiric observations. To understand the current literature on cell kinetics, it is imperative to visualize cell cycling. All dividing cells follow a predictable pattern for replication called generation time. There are five basic phases (Figure 18-2). G_1 phase (G stands for gap and uncertainty as to purpose) lasts a variable amount of time, usually between 4 and 24 hours. If this phase is prolonged, the cell is usually referred to as being in the G_0, or resting, phase. The S

phase is the phase of DNA synthesis and usually lasts between 10 and 20 hours. The G_2 phase is a premitotic phase lasting from 2 to 10 hours, and the M phase, when actual mitosis takes place, lasts between 0.5 and 1 hour. Tumors do not have faster generation times but have more cells in the active phases of replication than normal tissues. Normal tissues have a large number of cells in the G_0 phase, wherein the cell is not actively committed to division or is "out of cycle."

Some chemotherapeutic agents appear to act at several phases of the cell cycle (Figure 18-3). Alkylating agents appear to act in all phases from G_0 to mitosis. They are termed *cycle-nonspecific agents*. Drugs such as hydroxyurea, doxorubicin (Adriamycin), and methotrexate appear to act primarily in the S phase. Bleomycin appears to act in the G_2 phase, and vincristine appears to act in the M phase. These drugs are termed *cycle-specific agents* (Table 18-2) because they act chemotherapeutically only on cells that are in a specific phase of a cell generation cycle. Steroids, 5-fluorouracil, and cisplatin have rather

Table 18-2   Cell cycle (phase)—specific drugs

Phase	Type	Drugs
S Phase dependent	Antimetabolite	Cytarabine Doxorubicin 5-Fluorouracil 6-Mercaptopurine Methotrexate Hydroxyurea Prednisone
M Phase dependent	Vinca alkaloids	Vincristine Vinblastine Paclitaxel
	Podophyllotoxins	Etoposide Teniposide
G₂ Phase dependent		Bleomycin
G₁ Phase dependent		Corticosteroids

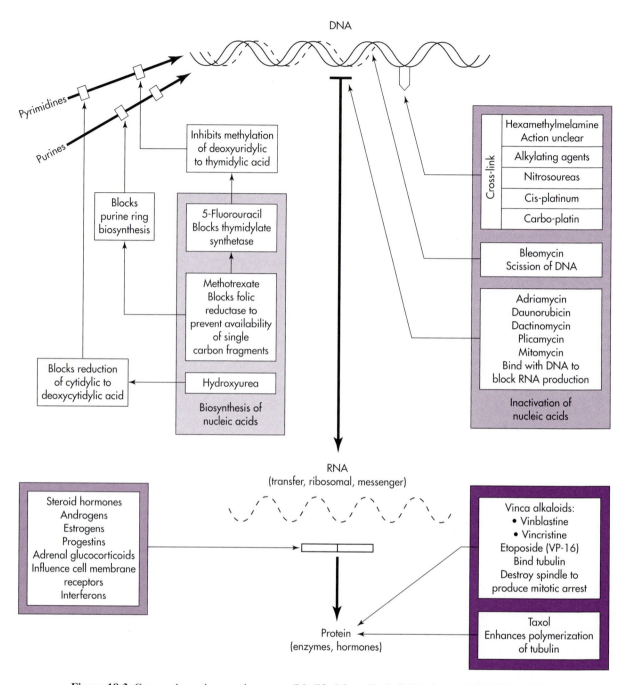

Figure 18-3 Cancer chemotherapeutic agents. (Modified from Krakoff IH: *Cancer* 37:93-105, 1987.)

uniform activity around the cell generation cycle. In theory, if certain cancer therapeutic agents attack only cells that are dividing and more tumor cells are dividing than normal tissue cells, then by properly spacing the chemotherapeutic agent and combining agents that act in different phases of the cell cycle, one should be able to kill tumor cells in far greater numbers than normal cells. Kinetic studies in humans and animals suggest that tumors that have been cured by chemotherapy are those with large fractions of cells in the proliferative phase (e.g., gestational choriocarcinoma and Burkitt lymphoma). The extent of the disease rather than the total mass of tumor

is the most important factor in considering curative radiation or surgery, but in using chemotherapy the total mass is most important. When tumor volume is reduced, the remaining tumor cells can begin to divide actively (they are propelled from the G_0 phase into the more vulnerable cell generation cycle), thereby rendering them susceptible to chemotherapy. These chemotherapeutic agents, as in radiation therapy, kill by first-order kinetics: that is, there is a reduction of the tumor population by a characteristic percentage, regardless of the actual number of tumor cells initially present (Figure 18-4). If the tumor burden is small, fewer cycles of chemotherapy may be

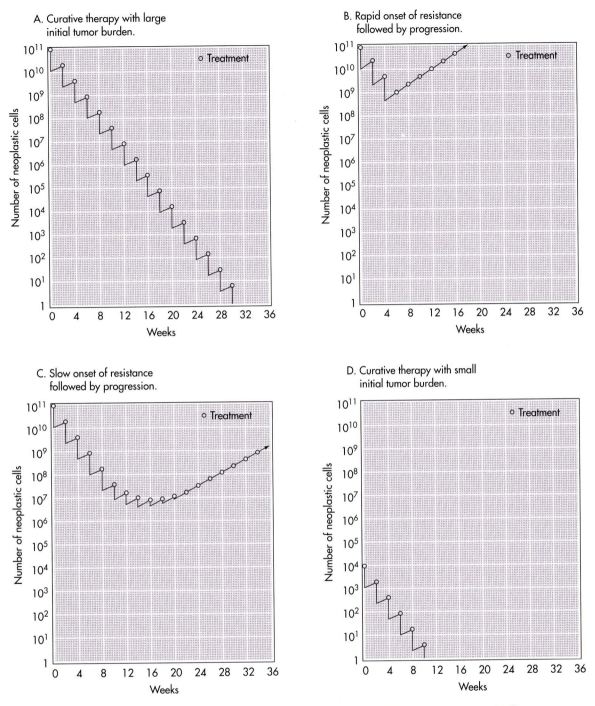

Figure 18-4 Efficacy of chemotherapy related to tumor kinetics. (Modified from Bodye GB Sr, Frei E III, Luce JK: The systematic approach to cancer therapy, *Hosp Pract* 2(10):42, 1967.)

necessary. One milligram of tumor usually consists of 10^6 cells. One cubic centimeter of tumor usually consists of 10^9 cells. Patient death usually occurs at 10^{12} cells.

DYNAMICS OF CHEMOTHERAPY

The time it takes a cell to complete one cycle of growth and division is its generation time. However, the time a

tumor takes to double in size (doubling time) depends on generation time and cell death rate (Figure 18-5). One cannot assume a long generation time simply because a tumor enlarges slowly. Slow tumor growth can result from rapid generation time combined with a high cell death rate. For similar reasons, a small tumor discovered on radiographic or physical examination is not necessarily an early tumor; only serial studies to judge its growth rate will help establish its age. Bulky tumors (diameters >2-3 cm) enlarge more slowly than small ones because their cells, especially those of the inner core (farthest from the blood supply) have a long generation time. Competition for nutrients and other less-defined competitive pressures reduce the activity of the entire mass.

Chemotherapy of cancer requires an edge, a physiologic mechanism that can be exploited to differentially kill cancer cells but spare normal cells as much as possible. Tumor tissues have a more rapid growth rate than normal tissues, and this can be used against them. This is especially true because the growth of tumor cells is characteristically more synchronized than that of normal cells. At any given time, therefore, comparatively large numbers of cancer cells will be in the DNA synthesis phase (S phase) of the cell cycle, the only time during which cycle-dependent agents (those inhibiting DNA synthesis) can act. Thus short-term high-dose chemotherapy with agents affecting DNA synthesis, such as methotrexate, is most effective in killing rapidly dividing tumor cells with relative sparing of normal bone marrow elements. Unfortunately, bone marrow cells, the epithelial cells that line the gastrointestinal tract, and hair follicles all have generation times comparable to those of tumors and are therefore vulnerable to compounds that inhibit DNA synthesis (Table 18-3). However, compared with the more synchronously growing tumor cell population, only a small portion of the bone marrow cells are in their S phase at any given time, and this accounts for the selective toxicity of phase-dependent compounds. A course of therapy extending over a period of several days, or even weeks, may be required to kill a slow-growing tumor in which only a few cells are in the stage of DNA synthesis at any one time. Agents that do not depend on DNA synthesis for their effects (cycle-nonspecific agents), such as alkylating agents, are most effective against bulky, slow-growing tumors. The cells remaining after treatment tend to divide more rapidly and are more susceptible to attack by cycle-specific agents. Thus there is some flexibility in the interplay of chemotherapeutic agents.

The phenomenon of increased susceptibility of tumor cells during recovery from alkylating agents is the rationale for sequentially combining cycle-nonspecific and cycle-specific agents in many new regimens. If, in addition, drugs with different mechanisms of toxicity are combined, each drug can be given safely in the dose used when it is given alone. Each drug chosen for combination therapy should have antitumor activity when used alone.

Whenever possible, intermittent courses of chemotherapy are used to allow restoration of normal cells if they were reduced in number by treatment. In instances in which an antidote to the chemotherapeutic agent is known, for example, leucovorin (citrovorum factor-folinic acid) for methotrexate, this antidote can also be given to hasten normal cell recovery. Of course, the danger of revitalizing sublethally injured tumor cells also

exists and must be evaluated with each new treatment regimen. Although careful studies are needed to compare each new combination with the single agents concerned, the trend in chemotherapy is unquestionably toward exploitation of drug combinations used simultaneously and sequentially (Table 18-4).

Drug Resistance

The effectiveness of any cancer treatment is limited by the development of acquired drug resistance. The development of resistance to individual drugs is frequently associated with a broad cross-resistance to structurally dissimilar drugs. This probably explains the 6%-10% response rate to salvage therapy seen in many diseases. The mechanisms responsible for the development of resistance and multiple-drug resistance that frequently accompanies primary resistance remain to be established (Table 18-5). Some experimental evidence in murine tumors suggests that one form of multiple-drug resistance relates to the ability of drug-resistant tumor cells to limit drug accumulation of structurally unrelated agents. This cross-resistance is most frequently seen with natural products (i.e., doxorubicin, VP-16, and vinca alkaloids). Another mechanism for the multiple-drug resistance phenotype is seen in the cross-resistance present between alkylating agents, cisplatin, and irradiation. Primary resistance and cross-resistance in this group of agents have been linked to elevations in intracellular glutathione levels and are not associated with an overall measurable decrease in drug accumulation. The relative importance of these two separate mechanisms in ovarian cancer remains to be established. However, both mechanisms of resistance may have clinical relevance because there exist pharmacologic ways to reverse the multiple-drug resistance phenotype associated with either an increase of glutathione levels or with a decrease in drug accumulation. Resistant tumor cells may display increased deactivation or decreased activation of drugs. Other suggestions for the development of drug-resistant tumor cells are altered specificity to inhibiting enzymes or increased production of the target enzyme providing the cell with immunity to the chemotherapeutic agent.

It has been suggested that spontaneous mutation is a basis for drug resistance. This spontaneous mutation occurs rapidly in malignant tumors. This concept, the "Goldie-Coldman" hypothesis, has been applied to the growth of malignant tumors and has important clinical implications. The theory suggests that most malignant cells begin with intrinsic sensitivity to chemotherapeutic agents but develop spontaneous resistance at variable rates. Goldie and Coldman have developed a mathematical model relating curability to the time of recurrence of the singly or doubly resistant cells. Assuming a natural mutation rate, the model predicts a variation in the size of the resistant fraction in tumors of the same size and type, depending on the mutation rate and the point at which the mutation develops. During these assumptions, the proportion of resistant cells in any untreated tumor is likely to be small, and the initial response to treatment would not be influenced by the number of resistant cells. In clinical practice, this means that a complete remission could be obtained even if the resistant cell line were present. The failure to cure such a patient, however, would directly depend on the presence of these resistant cells. This model of spontaneous drug resistance implies that minimizing the emergence of drug resistant clones requires that multiple effective drugs or therapies be applied as early as possible in the course of the patient's malignant disease process.

The model described above focuses attention on the mechanisms of drug resistance. If, as stated, failure of drug treatment depends on the spontaneous appearance of resistant cells, the understanding of drug resistance is key to the therapeutic success of most chemotherapeutic regimens. A wide variety of mechanisms for drug resistance had been described but these mechanisms usually account for resistance in a particular drug or drug family. The phenomenon of pleiotropic drug resistance occurs when certain drug resistance mechanisms confer a cross resistance to structurally dissimilar drugs with different mechanisms of action. In pleiotropic resistant cells, Ling's coworkers demonstrated the appearance of a P-glycoprotein with a molecular weight of 170 kilodaltons on the cell membrane. The appearance of pleiotropic drug resistance is associated with permeability of the cell to accumulate and retain antineoplastic drugs. It has been demonstrated that this P-glycoprotein is directly related to the expression of resistance, and cells that revert to the drug sensitive state lose this membrane glycoprotein. DNA can be transferred from resistant cells to the sensitive cells, producing a transfer of pleiotropic resistance to unexposed cells. The gene responsible for the expression of this multidrug resistance has been recently isolated from certain cell populations.

Genetic changes underlying drug resistance can be based on point mutation or gene amplification. Resistance based on an altered gene product resulting from a point mutation would be expected to occur in single cells at a single step. The frequency of resistant cells could be expected to be independent of the concentration of the drug used for selection, and once selected, the mutation

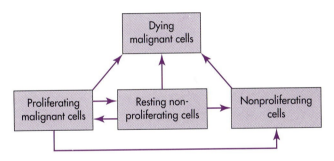

Functional kill table

Figure 18-5 Dynamics of tumor growth showing interrelationship of cell compartments contributing to clinical presence of tumor.

Table 18-3   Classification of normal tissues by rate of proliferation

Rapid proliferation	Slow proliferation	No proliferation
Bone marrow	Lung	Muscle
GI mucosa	Liver	Bone
Ovary	Kidney	Cartilage
Testis	Endocrine glands	Nerve
Hair follicles	Vascular endothelium	

Table 18-4   Chemotherapy in epithelial ovarian cancer*

	CR (%)	PR (%)	Median survival (mo)
Melphalan (n = 104)	19	7	18.6
5-Fluorouracil (n = 21)	19	5	14.3
Hexamethylmelamine (n = 54)	15	17	15.0
Doxorubicin (n = 32)	3	19	16.0
Hexamethylmelamine + cyclophosphamide (n = 48)	19	10	16.2
Cisplatin (n = 22)	27	23	21.2
Hexamethylmelamine + doxorubicin + cyclophosphamide (n = 72)	29	3	26.4
Melphalan + cisplatin (n = 81)	32	5	29.6

Modified from Gershenson DN: Cancer of the ovary—chances for improving therapy results. Paper presented at GBK symposium, Dusseldorf, Germany, June 26, 1982; and Edwards CL et al: *Gynecol Oncol* 15:261, 1983.
*Data collected from several progressive randomized studies frm the MD Anderson Hospital and Tumor Institute in stage III + 10 epithelial carcinoma of the ovary.

Table 18-5 Probable mechanisms associated with resistance to some commonly used anticancer drugs

Mechanism	Drugs
Increase in proficiency of repair of DNA	Alkylating agents, cisplatin
Decrease in cellular uptake or increase in efflux of drugs	Cisplatin, doxorubicin, etoposide melphalan, 6-mercaptopurine, methotrexate, nitrogen mustard, vinblastine, vincristine
Increase in levels of "target" enzyme	Methotrexate
Alterations in "target" enzyme	5-Fluorouracil, 6-mercaptopurine, methotrexate, 6-thioguanine
Decrease in drug activation	Cytosine arabinoside, doxorubicin, 5-fluorouracil, 6-mercaptopurine, 6-thioguanine
Increase in drug degradation	Bleomycin, cytosine arabinoside, 6-mercaptopurine
Alternative biochemical pathways	Cytosine arabinoside
Inactivation of active metabolites by binding to sulfhydryl compounds	Alkylating agents, cisplatin, doxorubicin
Decrease activity of topoisomerase	Amsacrine, doxorubicin, etoposide

From Tannock IF, Hill RT, eds: *The basic science of oncology,* ed 2, New York, 1992, McGraw Hill.

should be stable. Although such mechanisms are common in tissue culture cell circumstances, the significance for human tumor responses to therapy are not clear. In contrast to point mutation, gene amplification appears to occur in a stepwise manner and is influenced by the concentration of the selected drug. Evidence suggests that gene amplification may play a role in clinical drug resistance. There is wide speculation that conditions of chemotherapy treatment may facilitate gene amplification through mutational effects or cell cycle progression delay.

Categories of Drugs in Current Use (Table 18-6)
Cycle-nonspecific agents

Alkylating agents. Alkylating agents prevent cell division primarily by cross-linking strands of DNA. Because of continued synthesis of other cell constituents, such as RNA and protein, growth is unbalanced and the cell dies. Activity of alkylating agents does not depend on DNA synthesis in the target cells. Cyclophosphamide, however, also inhibits DNA synthesis, which makes it distinctive among the alkylating agents in its mode and spectrum of activity. Alkylating agents now used in gynecologic oncology are :

Cyclophosphamide (Cytoxan)
Chlorambucil (Leukeran)
Melphalan (Alkeran)
Triethylenethiophosphoramide (Thiotepa)
Ifosfamide (Ifex)

Cycle-specific agents

Antimetabolites. Antimetabolites act by inhibiting essential metabolic processes that are required for DNA and/or RNA synthesis. The currently used drugs in this category are:

5-Fluorouracil (5-FU)
Methotrexate (MTX, Amethopterin)
Cytarabine (Cytosar-U)

Antibiotics. A number of cytotoxic antibiotics have come into use for chemotherapy of certain neoplasms. Those used in gynecologic oncology are:

Dactinomycin (actinomycin D)
Bleomycin (Blenoxane)
Doxorubicin (Adriamycin)

Plant alkaloids. The two principal vinca alkaloids are similar in structure, mode of action, and metabolism (mainly in the liver) but are different in regard to dose, toxicity, and antitumor spectrum. They arrest cells in metaphase by binding the microtubular protein used in the formation of the mitotic spindle. These drugs are:

Vinblastine (Velban)   Taxol
Vincristine (Onvocin)   Navelbine
Etoposide (VP-16)

Miscellaneous. A number of antineoplastic agents are available that do not clearly fit into any of the above categories. These drugs are:

Dacarbazine (DTIC)
Nitrosoureas (carmustine or lomustine)
Hydroxyurea (Hydrea)
Cis-diamminedichloroplatinum (Cisplatin or Platinol)
Carboplatin (Paraplatin)
Hexamethylmelamine (Hexalen)

Drug Toxicity

Chemotherapeutic agents have been called "poisons." I think this statement is accurate; hopefully they poison the malignancy more than the normal tissue. However, many of the side effects, particularly those to organ systems with rapidly proliferating cell populations, are inevitable. Usually, the mechanism of toxicity is similar to producing the desired cytotoxic effect. Even organs with limited cell proliferation can be damaged by chemotherapeutic agents, especially if the agents are utilized at high doses. Chemotherapeutic agents must be used at doses that produce some degree of toxicity to normal tissue in order to be effective. The incidence of severe side effects of chemotherapeutic agents is greatly influenced by states

Text continued on p. 524.

Table 18-6   Chemotherapy agents used in treatment of gynecologic cancer

Drug	Dosage and route of administration	Acute side effects	Toxicity	Precautions*	Major indications
Alkylating agents					
Cyclophosphamide (Cytoxan)	50-1500 mg/m² as a single dose IV or 60-120 mg/m² day PO; dose decreased if severe leukopenia develops	Nausea and vomiting	Bone marrow depression, alopecia, cystitis	Maintain adequate fluid intake to avoid cystitis	Carcinoma of the cervix, ovary, endometrium, and fallopian tube
Chlorambucil (Leukeran)	0.1-0.2 mg/kg/day PO; dose decreased if severe bone marrow depression develops	Nausea, vomiting (with high doses)	Bone marrow depression	None	
Melphalan (Alkeran)	0.2 mg/kg/day PO for 4 days every 4-6 weeks	Nausea, vomiting (with high doses)	Bone marrow depression	None	
Triethylenethio-phosphoramide (Thiotepa)	0.2 mg/kg/day IV for 5 days	None	Bone marrow depression	None	
Ifosfamide (IFEX)	7-10 gm/m² IV over 3-5 days every 3-4 weeks	Nausea, vomiting	Bone marrow depression, alopecia cystitis	Uroprotector to prevent hermorrhagic cystitis	Carcinoma and sarcoma of ovary, cervix, and endometrium Germ cell tumors
Cycle-specific antimetabolites					
5-Fluorouracil (5-FU, fluorouracil)	12 mg/kg/day IV for 4 days, then alternate days at 6 mg/kg for 4 days or until toxicity; repeat course monthly or give weekly IV dose of 12-15 mg/kg; maximal dose 1 g for either regimen; often used as one drug in combination regimens at a dose of 500 mg/m² IV	Occasional nausea and vomiting	Bone marrow depression, diarrhea, stomatitis, alopecia	Decrease dose in patients with diminished liver, renal, or bone marrow function or after adrenalectomy	Carcinoma of the ovary and endometrium
Methotrexate (MTX, Amethopterin)	Choriocarcinoma: 10-30 mg/day IV for 5 days Ovarian or cervical carcinoma: 200-2000 mg/m² IV with concomitant and/or sequential systematic antidote leucovorin ("leucovorin rescue")	None	Bone marrow depression, megaloblastic anemia, diarrhea, stomatitis, vomiting; alopecia less common; occasional hepatic fibrosis, vasculitis, pulmonary fibrosis	Adequate renal function must be present, and urine output must be maintained	Choriocarcinoma, carcinoma of the ovary and cervix

*All alkylating agents and many other antineoplastic drugs should be used only if absolutely necessary in pregnant women, since they may be abortifacient or teratogenic.

Continued.

Table 18-6   Chemotherapy agents used in treatment of gynecologic cancer—cont'd

Drug	Dosage and route of administration	Acute side effects	Toxicity	Precautions*	Major indications
Cycle-specific antimetabolites—cont'd					
Cytarabine (Ara-C, Cytosar-U)	200 mg/m² daily for 5 days by continuous infusion	Nausea and vomiting	Bone marrow depression, megaloblastosis, leukopenia, thrombocytopenia	None	Carcinoma of the ovary (intraperitoneal use)
Gemcitabine (Gemzar) (2',2'-difluorodeoxy cytabidine)	800-1000 mg/m²IV weekly every 3 weeks	Mild nausea, vomiting, malaise (usually mild), transient febrile episodes, maculopapular rash	Bone marrow suppression	None	Carcinoma of breast and ovary
Antibiotics					
Dactinomycin (actinomycin D, Cosmegen)	15 μg/kg/day IV or 0.5 mg/day for 5 days	Pain on local infiltration with skin necrosis; nausea and vomiting in many patients 2 hours after dose; occasional cramps and diarrhea	Bone marrow depression, stomatitis, diarrhea, erythema, hyperpigmentation with occasional desquamation in areas of previous irradiation	Administer through running IV infusion; use with care in liver disease and in presence of inadequate marrow function; prophylactic antiemetics are helpful	Embryonal rhabdomyosarcoma, choriocarcinoma, ovarian germ cell tumors
Mitomycin C (Mutamycin)	0.05 mg/kg/day IV for 6 days, then alternate days until 50 mg total dose	Nausea, vomiting, local inflammation and ulceration if extravasated	Neutropenia, thrombocytopenia, oral ulceration, nausea, vomiting, diarrhea	Administer through running IV infusion or inject with great care to prevent extravasation	Carcinoma of the cervix
Bleomycin (Bleonoxane)	10-20 mg/m² IV or IM 1-2 times a week; start with 5 mg for first 2 doses in lymphoma	Fever, chills, nausea, vomiting; local pain and phlebitis less frequent	Skin: hyperpigmentation, thickening, nail changes, ulceration, rash, peeling, alopecia Pulmonary: pneumonitis with dyspnea, rales, infiltrate can progress to fibrosis; more common in patients over 70 and with more than 400 mg total dose, but unpredictable	Watch for hypersensitivity in lymphoma with first 1-2 doses; use with extreme caution in presence of renal or pulmonary disease; start in hospital under observation; do not exceed total dose of 400 mg	Squamous cell carcinoma of the skin, vulva, and cervix; choriocarcinoma
Doxorubicin (Adriamycin)	60-100 mg/m² IV every 3 weeks	Nausea, vomiting, fever, local phlebitis, necrosis if extravasated, red urine (not blood)	Bone marrow depression, alopecia, cardiac toxicity related to cumulative dose, stomatitis; atrophy of the myocardia can occur, especially if a total dose of 450-500 mg/m² is exceeded	Administer through running IV infusion; avoid giving to patients with significant heart disease; follow for ECG abnormalities and signs of heart failure	Adenocarcinoma of the endometrium, fallopian tube, ovary, and vagina; uterine sarcoma

Plant alkaloids

Drug	Dose	Acute toxicity	Delayed or chronic toxicity	Comments	Indications
Vinblastine (Velban)	0.10-0.15 mg/kg/week IV	Severe, prolonged inflammation if extravasated; occasional nausea, vomiting, headache, and paresthesias	Bone marrow depression, particularly neutropenia; alopecia, muscle weakness, occasional mild peripheral neuropathy, mental depression 2-3 days after treatment, rarely stomatitis	Administer through running IV infusion or inject with great care to prevent extravasation; decrease dose in liver disease	Choriocarcinoma
Vincristine (Oncovin)	0.4-1.4 mg/m² IV weekly in adults; 2 mg/m² weekly in children	Local inflammation if extravasated	Paresthesias, weakness, loss of reflexes; constipation; abdominal, chest, and jaw pain; hoarseness, foot-drop; mental depression; marrow toxicity generally mild, anemia and reticulocytopenia most prominent; alopecia	Administer through running IV infusion or inject with great care to prevent extravasation; decrease dose in liver disease; patients with underlying neurologic problems may be more susceptible to neurotoxicity; alopecia may be prevented by use of a scalp tourniquet for 5 minutes during and after administration	Uterine sarcoma, germ cell tumor of the ovary
Etoposide (VP-16) (4-demethyl-epipodophyllotoxin)	100 mg/m² IV days 1, 3, and 5; repeat in 4 weeks	Nausea and vomiting	Leukopenia, thrombocytopenia, alopecia, headache, fever, occasional hypotension	Reduce dose by 25%-50% for hematologic toxicity	Trophoblastic disease, germ cell tumors
Paclitaxel (Taxol)	170-250 mg/m² IV every 3-4 weeks	Allergic reaction, nausea, vomiting	Bone marrow depression, severe allergic-like reactions with facial erythema, dyspnea, tachycardia, and hypotension cardiotoxicity with bradycardia, alopecia, stomatitis, fatigue	Cardiac monitoring may be necessary	Ovarian carcinoma
Vinorelbine tartrate (Navelbine)	30 mg/m² weekly IV	Mild nausea, 10% alopecia	Bone marrow depression, mild to moderate peripheral neuropathy	Local irritant, dose modification with hepatic dysfunction	Ovarian carcinoma

Continued.

Table 18-6 Chemotherapy agents used in treatment of gynecologic cancer—cont'd

Drug	Dosage and route of administration	Acute side effects	Toxicity	Precautions*	Major indications
Miscellaneous					
Hydroxyurea (Hydrea)	80 mg/kg PO every 3 days or 20-30 mg/kg/day	Anorexia and nausea	Bone marrow depression, megaloblastic anemia; stomatitis, diarrhea, and alopecia less common	Decrease dose in patients with marrow and renal dysfunction	Carcinoma of the cervix (with radiotherapy)
Cis-diamminedichloroplatinum (Cisplatin or Platinol)	50-100 mg/m^2 IV every 3 weeks	Nausea and vomiting, often severe	Renal damage, moderate myelosuppression, neurotoxicity; severe renal damage can be minimized by not exceeding a total dose of 500 mg/m^2 in any treatment course	Infuse at a rate not to exceed 1 mg/min and only after 10-12 hours of hydration; avoid nephrotoxic antibodies; watch renal function and discontinue if BUN exceeds 30 or creatinine exceeds 2	Carcinoma of the ovary, endometrium, or cervix
Carboplatin (Paraplatin)	250-400 mg/m^2 IV bolus or by 24-hr continuous infusion every 2-4 weeks	Mild nausea and vomiting	Bone marrow suppression, especially thrombocytopenia	Decreased dose in patients who have had previous chemotherapy	Carcinoma of the cervix, ovary, and endometrium
Hexymethylmelamine (Hexalen)	4-12 mg/kg/day, PO in divided doses for 14-21 days, repeated every 6 weeks	Nausea and vomiting	Bone marrow depression, neurotoxicity, both central and peripheral	None	Ovarian carcinoma
Dacarbazine (DTIC-Dome)	80/160 mg/m^2 daily for 10 days	Nausea and vomiting	Bone marrow depression	Patients may develop severe dehydration from nausea and vomiting	Uterine sarcoma
Hycomptamine (Topotecan)	1.5 mg/m^2 daily for 5 days	Maculopapular pruritic exanthema	Bone marrow depression	Watch for neutropenic fever	Ovarian carcinoma

Hycomptamine (Topotecan)	1.5 mg/m² daily for 5 days	Maculopapular pruritic exanthema	Bone marrow depression	Watch for neutropenic fever	Ovarian carcinoma
Progestational agents					
Medroxyprogesterone acetate	400-800 mg/week IM or PO	None	Occasional liver function abnormalities, occasional alopecia and hypersensitivity reactions	Use with care in presence of liver dysfunction	Carcinoma of the endometrium
Hydroxyprogesterone caproate	1000 mg IM twice weekly				
Megestrol acetate (Megace)	20-80 mg PO twice a day				
"Antiestrogenic" agents					
Tamoxifen	10-20 mg PO twice daily	Nausea, usually mild	Caused by antiestrogenic action (e.g., hot flashes, pruritus vulvae, and occasionally vaginal bleeding)	None	Breast cancer, possibly useful in endometrial carcinoma (metastatic)
Leuprolide (Lupron)	1 mg daily subcutaneously or PO	Nausea and vomiting	Hot flashes	None	Well-differentiated ovarian epithelial lesions, possibly breast cancer and endometrial cancer

Table 18-7 Drug dose modification (sliding scale)

Count before next course (mm³)	Dose modification*
Leukocytes	
>4,000	100% of dose
3999-3000	100% of nonmyelotoxic agents
	50% of myelotoxic agents
2999-2000	100% of nonmyelotoxic agents
	25% of myelotoxic agents
1999-1000	25% of myelotoxic agents
≤999	No drug
Platelets	
>100,000	100% of dose
50,000-100,000	100% of nonmyelotoxic agents
<50,000	No drug

*Based on myelosuppression.

such as severe disability, advancing age, poor nutrition and/or direct organ involvement by primary or metastatic lesions. The physician must monitor these patients with extreme care and appropriate dose modifications must be made (Table 18-7).

Hematologic toxicity

Hematologic toxicity is the most frequently seen side effect. Acute granulocytopenia occurs 6-12 days after administration of most myelosuppressive chemotherapeutic agents. Recovery occurs in 10-14 days. The Megakarocyte series is affected later such that platelet suppression usually occurs four or five days following granulocytopenia and recovers several days after the white count. Mitomycin-C and Nitrosourea are particularly unique in their ability to produce delayed bone marrow suppression. Myelosuppression with these two drugs commonly occurs 28-42 days with recovery 40-60 days after treatment.

Most clinicians consider patients with absolute granulocyte counts greater than 500/mm³ for 5 days or longer to be at a higher risk for sepsis. The practice of utilizing prophylactic broad spectrum antibiotics in febrile granulocytopenic cancer patients has significantly decreased the incidence of life threatening infections in this group of patients. Granulocytopenic patients should have their temperature checked every four hours, and they should be examined frequently for evidences of infection. Thrombocytopenic patients with platelet counts less than 20,000/mm³ are at increased risk for spontaneous hemorrhage, particularly from the gastrointestinal tract. Routine platelet transfusions for platelets under 20,000/mm³ have been utilized by some clinicians. It is common to transfuse six to ten units of random donor platelets to such patients. Others wait and watch until patients manifest some evidence of bleeding. Repeat transfusions of platelets at 2 to 3-day intervals may be necessary in patients with severe thrombocytopenia. Patients with active peptic ulcer disease and patients needing surgical procedures need to be transfused with counts lower than 50,000/mm³.

Gastrointestinal toxicity

Gastrointestinal toxicity is another frequent manifestation of chemotherapeutic agents. Mucositis could be caused by direct effect on the rapidly dividing epithelial mucosa. Concomitant granulocytopenia allows the injured mucosa to become infected and serve as a portal of entry for bacteria and fungi. The onset of mucositis is frequently 3-5 days earlier than myelosuppression. The nasopharyngeal lesions are difficult to distinguish from viral lesions. Candidiasis is frequently seen and is difficult to distinguish from stomatitis secondary to chemotherapy; antifungal agents have been very effective in treating this condition.

Necrotizing enterocolitis is another condition seen in patients on chemotherapy. Symptoms of this condition are watery or bloody diarrhea, abdominal pain, nausea, vomiting, and fever. Patients usually have abdominal tenderness and distention. They also have a history of broad spectrum antibiotic use. Most necrotizing enterocolitis is caused by anaerobic bacteria such as *Clostridium difficile*. The treatment of choice for *C. difficile* infection is oral Vancomycin, 125 mg four times daily for 10-14 days.

Skin reactions

Skin reactions, including alopecia and allergic hypersensitivity reactions, are also frequently seen with chemotherapeutic agents. Skin necrosis and sloughing at the site of intravenous extravasation is associated particularly with agents such as Adriamycin, actinomycin D, mitomycin C, vinblastine, vincristine, and nitrogen mustard. The extent of the necrosis is determined by the amount of extravasated drug. Management includes removal of the intravenous line and local infiltration of the area with corticosteroids, as well as ice pack therapy 4-5 times a day for 3 days. Long term monitoring of these patients is essential. Alopecia is a common side effect of many chemotherapeutic agents. Therapies designed to reduce alopecia have not been successful. Hair growth will resume 10-20 days after treatment is completed. Generalized allergic skin reactions occur primarily with drugs such as Adriamycin, actinomycin D, methotrexate, and Taxol. Taxol administration can be associated with severe hypersensitivity reactions and prophylaxis has become a routine (Table 18-8).

Hepatic toxicity

Hepatic toxicity is uncommon. Mild elevations in transaminase, alkaline phosphatase, and bilirubin are seen with

Table 18-8   Taxol hypersensitivity management

Taxol prophylactic pretreatment	
Drug	Dose, route, time
Dexamethasone	20 mg PO or IV, 14 and 7 hours prior to treatment
Diphenhydramine	50 mg IV, 30 minutes prior to treatment
Cimetidine or ranitidine	300 or 50 mg, respectively, 30 minutes prior to treatment

many agents, but rarely is the condition severe. Psoriases and drug-induced hepatitis can affect the amount of the chemotherapeutic agent given, as can pre-existing liver disease or exposure to other hepatic toxins.

Interstitial pneumonitis

Interstitial pneumonitis with pulmonary fibrosis is seen with certain chemotherapeutic agents. The agents most likely to produce this are Adriamycin, alkylating agents, and nitrosoureas. Management of patients with drug-induced interstitial pneumonitis involves discontinuation of the cytotoxic agent and supportive care. Steroids may be of some benefit.

Cardiac toxicity

The risk of cardiac toxicity is seen primarily with Adriamycin. The risk increases dramatically when the cumulative dose exceeds 500 mg/m^2 of ideal body surface area. In recent years, this limit has rarely been exceeded, so cardiomyopathy has diminished greatly in incidence. Acute arrhythmias frequently may be seen but these disappear with a few days of supportive care. On rare occasions, cyclophosphamide has been reported to produce cardiotoxicity, particularly when it is used in massive doses. Mitomycin C has been reported to cause endocardial fibrosis and myocardial fibrosis, but again these are rare events.

Genitourinary toxicity

Metabolites of cyclophosphamide are irritants to the bladder mucosa and can cause a chronic hemorrhagic cystitis. The toxic metabolite of cyclophosphamide that causes bladder toxicity is known as acroleim. Vigorous hydration and diuresis during administration of cyclophosphamide is essential. Cisplatin produces renal tubular toxicity associated with azotemia and magnesium wasting. Again, this complication can be minimized with diuresis during administration of cisplatin. Other agents known to cause genitourinary toxicity are methotrexate, nitrosoureas, and mitomycin C. Mesna or n-acetyl-cysteine has been used in recent times in conjunction with cyclophosphamide to prevent bladder toxicity. This agent acts by inactivating the toxic metabolite acroleim.

Neurologic toxicity

In general, most antineoplastic drugs are associated with mild neurologic side effects. There are some exceptions, however. Vinca alkaloids are commonly associated with peripheral motor sensory and autonomic neuropathies. Agents such as vincristine, vinblastine, Taxol, and Navelbine can produce loss of deep tendon reflexes with distal paraesthesias. In almost all instances, these neurologic toxicities are reversible following cessation of the drug. Cisplatin produces ototoxicity and peripheral neuropathy and occasional retrobulbar neuritis. High doses of cisplatin, often used in ovarian cancer therapy, are particularly likely to produce progressive and somewhat delayed peripheral neuropathy. 5-Fluorouracil (5-FU) has been associated with acute cerebellar toxicity. Hexamethylmelamine is reported to produce peripheral neuropathy and encephalopathy. Ifosfamide has also been associated with encephalopathy.

Gonadal dysfunction

Many chemotherapeutic agents have lasting effects on testicular and ovarian functions. This is particularly true of alkylating agents which can cause azoospermia and amenorrhea. The onset of amenorrhea and ovarian failure is accompanied by an elevation of the serum FSH and a fall in serum estradiol. Indeed, these patients often end up with premature menopause. The younger the patient at the onset of therapy, the less likely it is that chemotherapy would eventuate in permanent gonadal dysfunction. In women over the age of thirty, most chemotherapeutic regimens would be associated with a high incidence of premature ovarian failure.

Evaluation of New Agents

A number of trials will be necessary to demonstrate that a newly developed agent should be allowed in regular medical practice. Such trials have been defined as follows:

- **Phase I:** These initial trials are designed to test new drugs at various doses to evaluate toxicity and determine the tolerance to a particular agent. Some therapeutic effects may be observed, even though the intent of these trials is not response measurement.
- **Phase II:** Phase II studies attempt to determine the therapeutic effectiveness as well as the extent of toxicity of the particular agent at doses expected to be effective against specific tumor types. Phase II trials are often conducted for multiple disease sites.
- **Phase III:** Phase III trials are designed to compare the drug to treatment currently in use. Commonly, a new drug will be tested against the accepted "gold

standard" drug therapy for a particular disease site and histology.

Chemosensitivity Testing

The diversity of pathologic processes in the malignancy and the resistance mechanisms that may develop at any time make it difficult for the clinician to select the most appropriate therapy for an individual patient. Clinical trials indicate which therapeutic options are best for most cases. However, the individual patient's response can be determined only after administration of at least two courses of chemotherapy. This has given rise to the premise of in vitro drug response testing that might provide knowledge of the efficacy for various agents. The majority of ovarian cancers are resistant to some chemotherapy, and there is an ever increasing need to be precise with salvage drugs.

The origin of in vitro drug-response testing stems from the work of Ehrlich and Pasteur, who evaluated agents of microbial and synthetic origin on the growth of cultured microbes in the late nineteenth century.

Flemming's discovery of penicillin in 1929 introduced the modern era of culture and sensitivity testing. The subsequent discoveries of bacterial antibiotic resistance mechanisms and improvements in tissue culture technology paved the way for translating this approach to the evaluation of the cancer patient.

A clonogenic assay was developed in the mid 1950s by Puck and Marcus in their attempts to assess the impact of radiation on tumor cell growth. Several hurdles were encountered in the substantiation of their early studies. The cellular heterogeneity of malignancies makes it necessary to show that a given assay has an end point that is generated by the tumor cells, with minimal contribution by nonmalignant fibroblast or endothelial cells. In vitro drug-response testing must be validated clinically by correlations with patient outcome. A method should be reliable enough to provide information for a variety of chemo responsive tumor types. The turn around time of the procedure should make results available in a clinically relevant period of time. In vitro drug sensitivity assays essentially require four procedures:

1. Isolation of cells: In solid tumors, liberation of tumor cells is accomplished by various mechanical and enzymatic techniques.
2. Incubation of cells: The cells must be incubated with drugs for a specific period of time.
3. Assessment of cell survival
4. Interpretation of the results: An individual who understands what the clinician needs to report should interpret results in a clinically relevant fashion.

Currently, there are at least seven different types of assays. A discussion of each of these assays is beyond the scope of this text. Good clinical correlations are not available for most assays. The clinical utility of any test must be judged by how a test influences a patient's care. For a particular assay to be useful, its results should modify patient care in a significant portion of cases. The greatest value to date of chemosensitivity testing is to predict resistance to specific drugs. However, drug resistance is not usually an all or none phenomenon. Therefore, many assays state resistance and sensitivity as a percent probability. The clinician may then utilize this information in selecting the drug therapy.

Supportive Care

Because severe bone marrow depression can occur, facilities for supportive care should always be available. Platelet and erythrocyte transfusions, and, where possible, leukocyte transfusions, are often required until a patient's own normal bone marrow elements recover, a process that can take days or several weeks. The need for such support has increased with the widespread use of combination chemotherapy.

In addition, the performance status of the patient should be watched carefully (Table 18-9).

Supportive social workers, chaplains, and psychiatrists in a concentrated total care setting are of great value in enabling a patient to cope with the emotionally and financially shattering experience of having cancer. Home health care services have improved in most areas of the country, so that intravenous fluids, antibiotics, intravenous alimentation, and even chemotherapy can be administered in the home if the situation allows. Although treatment of many patients must be conducted at large medical centers where new agents and multidisciplinary facilities are available, continuing collaboration between the medical center and the patient's primary physician is

Table 18-9 Performance status

GOG* score	ECOG† score	Karnofsky score	Activity level
0	0	90-100	Fully active; unrestricted activities of daily living
1	1	70-80	Ambulatory but restricted in strenuous activity
2	2	50-60	Ambulatory but capable of self-care; unable to work; out of bed greater than 50% of working hours
3	3	30-40	Limited self-care or confined to bed or chair 50% of waking hours; needs special assistance
4	4	10-20	Completely disabled and no self-care
5	5	0	Dead

*GOG, Gynecologic Oncology Group.
†ECOG, Eastern Cooperative Oncology Group.

essential. Problems caused by the disease or its treatment often arise when the patient returns to her community. An informed local physician can rapidly evaluate these crises and take appropriate action.

Growth Factors

The application of hematopoietic drug factors to supportive care has been dramatic. Rapid advances in unraveling the molecular biology and biochemistry of these glycoprotein hormones that regulate hematopoiesis has led to their routine clinical use. Their emergence in 1989 allowed:

1. Amelioration of therapy related myelosuppression
2. Modulation of disease related myelosuppression
3. An enhanced host defense to infection

This class of agents includes molecules such as granulocyte colony-stimulating factor (G-CSF) and granulocyte-macrophage colony-stimulating factor (GM-CSF). The biologic activities of these proteins are complex and multifunctional, stimulating potent changes in the growth, differentiation, distribution and functional status of mature cells as well as their precursors (Table 18-10).

One of the more interesting and poorly understood activities of certain hemopoietic growth factors, such as G-CSF and GM-CSF, is the ability of these molecules to induce large numbers of hemopoietic stem and progenitor cells to leave their normal havens within the intermedullary compartment of the bone marrow and to circulate in the peripheral blood. This mobilizing activity of hemopoietic growth factors and the biological properties of peripheral blood progenitor cells (PBPCs) allows for easy access to cells that were formally obtainable by bone marrow aspiration.

G-CSF and GM-CSF. Initial studies with G-CSF and GM-CSF focused on their administration via the intravenous route. Since then, numerous studies have shown that subcutaneous administration once or twice a day is even more myelostimulatory than two to four hour intravenous infusions. There also appears to be less GM-CSF required when the drug is given subcutaneously. The recommended dose of GM-CSF is 250 micrograms per m^2 or 3-5 micrograms per kilogram. Interestingly, at least in some cases, a fairly low dose of GM-CSF may be more myelostimulatory than higher doses. The enhancement of neutrophil function in terms of adherence, phagocytosis, and chemotaxis have also been noted in clinical studies. GM-CSF can activate lymphocytes. The recommended dose of G-CSF is 5 micrograms per kilogram but unlike GM-CSF there does not appear to be any definitive dose limit. Bone pain often develops at higher doses of G-CSF. The adverse effects that are seen following administration of both of these agents are as follows:

A cutaneous eruption of macules and papules

Exacerbation of underlying autoimmune disease

Stomach distension and, on rare occasions, rupture

Anaphylaxis, which is rare

Mild increased risk of thrombosis

A theoretical possibility of the exacerbation of the underlying malignancy

Unquestionably, the administration of G-CSF or GM-CSF would accelerate neutrophil recovery to a significant degree following standard dose chemotherapy. Less dramatic but still significant is the beneficial effect on secondary end points such as the incidence of fever, antibiotic usage, and days in the hospital. Cost analysis of the use of growth factors are not complete but any randomized study of these agents should include such an analysis. Randomized trials comparing the prophylactic use of growth factors with prophylactic oral antibiotics are of interest and are contemplated. The more conservative approach currently being explored calls for reserving the use of growth factors until the onset of

Table 18-10 Characteristics of the hematopoietic growth factor family of cytokines		
Cytokine	**Source**	**Function**
GM-CSF	T cells, endothelial cells, stromal cells	Stimulates hematopoiesis of granulocyte and macrophage lineage; activates granulocytes and macrophages
G-CSF	Endothelial cells, monocytes, stromal cell	Stimulates hematopoiesis of granulocyte lineage; activates granulocytes
Erythropoietin	Kidney	Stimulates erythroid growth and development
IL-1	Monocytes/macrophages, B and T cells, endothelial cells	Co-stimulates early stages of hematopoiesis; T and B cell activation
IL-3	T cells	Stimulates early stages of hematopoiesis
IL-6	T cells, monocytes/macrophages, fibroblasts	Co-stimulates early stages of hematopoiesis; T and B cell activation

Modified from Kouides PA: The hematopoietic growth factors: In Charles M. Haskell, ed. *Principles of cancer treatment,* ed 4, Philadelphia, WB Saunders Co., 1995.

neutropenia fever when systemic antibiotic therapy is initiated. This approach is certainly more cost effective.

Erythropoietin. The existence of a hormone that regulates erythropoiesis has been proposed for a hundred years. In 1985, two independent groups cloned the gene responsible for this growth factor. This gene was labeled the Epo gene. The kidney appears to be the major site of production of erythropoiesis growth factor (Epo). Apparently, the site of production in the fetus is the liver, and in the last third of the gestational period, the responsibility is gradually transferred to the kidney. Tissue hypoxia is the chief stimulus for the production of Epo. Relatively small blood losses such as one unit of blood only modestly stimulates Epo production. The majority of patients on chemotherapy develop anemia at some point during the course of their illness, the hemoglobin concentration of these patients usually ranges from 7-12 g/dL, and the hematocrit is somewhere between 25%-38%. This is sufficient to stimulate the production of Epo endogenously. However, there appears to be a large blunting of response to Epo in patients who have undergone chemotherapy. A dose of 150 units/kilogram subcutaneously three times a week for 12 weeks has been used by many clinicians. Others utilize a daily dose of 60 units/kilogram progressing to a maximum dose of 90 units/kilogram/day. Adverse effects are extremely uncommon.

Other growth factors. Interleukin 3 (IL-3) and Interleukin 6 (IL-6) are currently are under investigation as growth factors. With IL-3, there is a moderate, dose dependent increase in neutrophils, platelets, and total white blood cells after continuous intravenous infusion or subcutaneous infusion. The leukocytosis mostly consists of neutrophils, eosinophils, and lymphocytes. Flu-like symptoms have been reported but are uncommon; headaches are relatively frequent. IL-6 shows a dose dependent 2-3 increase in platelet count. Hepatotoxicity and cardiac arrhythmias have been seen with the use of this agent.

IL-1 has demonstrated significant effects on platelet recovery after high dose carboplatin. Pretreating patients with IL-1 before carboplatin administration does not seem to be effective in preventing thrombocytopenia.

Minimizing the Most Common Side Effects

Nausea and vomiting are common acute side effects of many antineoplastic drugs (Table 18-11). Administration of the drug at night, preceded by a sedative and phenothiazine when possible, often minimizes these symptoms. Administration through an established intravenous line sometimes prevents drug extravasation and consequent pain and necrosis, which can occur with many of the agents. Phlebitis can often be prevented by administering the most irritating agents (such as dactinomycin and doxorubicin) through a running infusion. Continuation of the infusion will prevent dehydration.

Rich and DiSaia reported data that suggested short-term high-dose steroid therapy (methylprednisolone, 250-1000 mg every 6 hours for four doses beginning 2 hours before administration of intravenous chemotherapy) can significantly reduce the nausea and vomiting caused by chemotherapy. One of the mechanisms of action proposed is associated with the inhibitory effect of steroids on prostaglandin synthesis. Other prostaglandin inhibitors may have a similar action. Steroid therapy appears to be inadequate in controlling nausea if cisplatin chemotherapy is given. For control of gastrointestinal toxicity from this latter agent, drugs such as delta-9-tetrahydrocannabinol (THC), 5 mg/m^2 every 3 hours for four doses; droperidol, 1 mg hourly up to 12 hours beginning 1 hour before administration of chemotherapy; metoclopramide (Reglan), 80-120 mg every 3-4 hours for a maximum of five doses; and lorazepam (Ativan), 2 mg beginning 1 hour before chemotherapy and continuing every 4 hours for a total of three doses may be more effective. The newest drug is Ondansetron (Zofran), a selective serotonin, subtype-3, receptor antagonist. Given intravenously at 4-hour intervals at a dose of 0.15 mg/kg, the drug is very effective at reducing and eliminating the nausea produced by cisplatin chemotherapy. Control of nausea with mild antiemetics, such as prochlorperazine used as a single agent, is often adequate for drugs with low potential for inducing emesis. Moderately emetogenic chemotherapy commonly requires more intensive prevention techniques, usually with dexamethasone or ondansetron. The dose of dexamethasone is 10-20 mg IV before chemotherapy; the dose of ondansetron is 8 mg by mouth or 10 mg IV. Combinations of antiemetics are almost always required for drugs, such as cisplatin,

Table 18-11 Emetogenic potential of cancer chemotherapeutic agents used in gynecologic oncology

Emetogenic potential	Agent
High	Cisplatin
	Dacarbazine
	Dactinomycin
Moderate	Cyclophosphamide
	Doxorubicin
	Carboplatin
	Mitomycin
Low	Fluorouracil
	Methotrexate
	Etoposide
	Vincristine
	Bleomycin
	Topotecan,
	Navelbine

Table 18-12   Combination antiemetic regimens for highly emetogenic chemotherapy

Drug combination	Doses
Dexamethasone	20 mg IV
Ondansetron	32 mg IV (may be given in divided doses)
Dexamethasone	20 mg IV
Metoclopramide	3 mg/kg IV (repeat q 2 hr prn)
Diphenhydramine	25-50 mg IV (repeat q 2 hr prn)
Lorazepam	1-2 mg IV

nitrosoureas and cyclophosphamide, as well as dacarbazine, that cause severe nausea and vomiting when used in high doses (Table 18-12).

Alopecia is a common consequence of therapy. The use of a scalp tourniquet during administration of such drugs as vincristine, dactinomycin, and doxorubicin is reported to be helpful in preventing hair loss. These reports have not been confirmed widely. The scalp tourniquet can be effective only when a large percentage of the drug administered is inactivated during the period (usually 20-25 minutes) of its application. Thus it is rarely effective when slowly deactivated drugs such as cyclophosphamide are employed. Patients should be encouraged to explore the use of artifical hair pieces and wigs. Many communities have support groups consisting of patients who have experienced total alopecia and accommodated this often perceived demoralizing side effect of many chemotherapeutic agents. Patients seem to gain strength from association with others who have tolerated and overcome this disability.

Renal toxicity with drugs such as cisplatin is reduced with adequate intravenous hydration and mannitol- induced diuresis. Antibiotic therapy with aminoglycosides potentiates the nephrotoxicity of drugs such as cisplatin and should be avoided if possible.

Peripheral neuropathy is regularly produced by vincristine, hexamethylmelamine, cisplatin, and, occasionally, by vinblastine. Several clinicians are convinced that these side effects can be minimized by the administration of pyridoxine but this issue is unclear, except that no direct effect or antitumor properties can be attributed to pyridoxine. Patients should be encouraged that much of the peripheral neuropathy will slowly recede following cessation of chemotherapy.

Calculation of Dosage

Dosages of chemotherapeutic agents are usually discussed as milligrams per kilogram of body weight or milligrams per square meter of total body surface area (BSA) (Table 18-13). Dosage based on surface area is preferable to that based on weight because surface area

changes much less during the course of the a more consistent absolute amount of dru throughout therapy. Dosages per unit a comparable in adults and children (Figu

Table 18-13   Body Surface Area (BSA)

Mostellar equation (m^2): $\sqrt{\text{wt} \times \text{ht}/3600}$
DuBois and DuBois (m^2): $(\text{wt}^{0.425}) \times (\text{ht}^{0.725}) \times 71.84$
Haycock (m^2): $(\text{wt}^{0.5378}) \times (\text{ht}^{0.3964}) \times 0.024265$

m^2, Meters squared; wt, weight in kilograms; ht, height in centimeters.

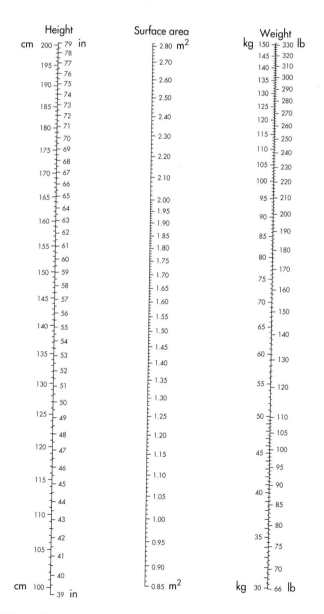

Figure 18-6 Nomogram for calculating body surface area of adults.

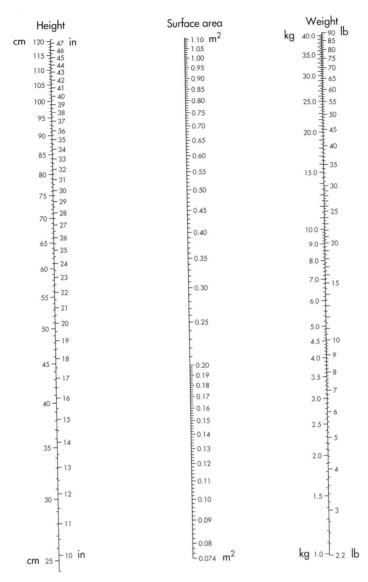

Figure 18-7 Nomogram for calculating body surface area of children.

18-7), and the variation in total dose between very obese and very thin people is minimized. Dosage in experimental animals expressed as milligrams per square meter is more easily related to that in humans. In adults, milligrams per kilogram can be converted with reasonable accuracy to milligrams per square meter by multiplying by 40.

Dose adjustments should be made for patients who are likely to have a compromised bone marrow reserve, that is, those over 70 years of age, those who have received previous pelvic or abdominal irradiation, and those who have had previous chemotherapy. In these subsets of patients, the physician should consider beginning with a dose reduced by 35%-50% and escalate up to full dose with subsequent courses if initial doses are well tolerated. In a similar manner, any moderate to severe toxicity during the patient's course of therapy should direct a reduction in future doses. Many clinicians favor limiting surface area to 2.0 milligrams per square meter in calculation of dosage. The adverse effects criteria table used by the GOG is included as Appendix B.

Dose adjustments are often required in patients receiving anticancer agents that are eliminated by the kidneys. These adjustments lessen the likelihood of overly high plasma drug concentrations and the attendant risk of serious renal toxicity. A number of techniques have been used to assess renal function (glomerular filtration rate [GFR]) in individuals with cancer. The calculated creatinine clearance (Cr Cl) using serum creatinine is the most commonly used. The elimination of creatine is primarily via glomerular filtration, although a small fraction may be secreted in the renal tubules. A number of studies have compared the different methods of estimating Cr Cl using a serum creatinine value. These methods are based on correlations of Cr Cl with age, body weight, serum creatinine (Scr), and creatinine metabolism. The most utilized methods are as follows:

Jelliffe Method: The Jelliffe Method was originally used as a simple estimate of Cr Cl using serum creatinine, making minor adjustments in the calculation for females. The current Jelliffe formula takes into consideration age and renal function and is as follows:

$$\text{Cr Cl (mL/min/1.73 m}^2) = \frac{98 - 0.8 \, (\text{Age} - 20)}{\text{SCR}}$$

(For females, use 90% of predicted Cr Cl)

Cockroft-Gault Method: This equation includes factors for lean body weight, which is especially important for obese patients, and correlation for females wherein Cr Cl is reduced from the value calculated for the male by 15%. This method is similar to the Jelliffe calculation and is as follows:

$$\text{Cr Cl} = \frac{(140 - \text{Age}) \, (\text{Wt kg})}{27 \times \text{Scr (gm/100 mL)}}$$

(15% less in females)

The use of the Cr Cl has also been incorporated into the so-called Calvert formula. Based on good data, there is evidence showing that there is an inverse linear correlation between the GFR and the area under the curve (AUC) of drugs such as carboplatin (Table 18-14). This finding suggests that in order to obtain the desired AUC the dose not only must be decreased in patients with low renal function, but higher than standard doses may be required for patients with high renal clearance values. The Calvert formula is as follows:

$$\text{Dose (mg)} = \text{AUC} \times (\text{GFR} + 25)$$

Carcinogenicity of Anticancer Drugs

Many antineoplastic agents in current use are mutagenic and teratogenic. Alkylating agents, procarbazine, and the nitrosoureas are major offenders. Antimetabolites, in contrast, seem less risky. Long-term studies in Hodgkin's disease suggest a major risk with the combination of chemotherapy and radiation therapy. The second malignancy commonly occurs 4-7 years after successful therapy. After 11 years, the risk of leukemia in patients treated for Hodgkin's disease decreases to that of the normal population. The long-term follow-up of women treated for choriocarcinoma shows no increase in risk of a second malignancy (most were treated with an antimetabolite). There is clear evidence from several reports that the incidence of acute leukemia is increased in patients who have been treated with alkylating cytotoxic agents for ovarian epithelial cancer. In 1976, Sotrel et al. reported two cases of advanced ovarian carcinoma treated with chlorambucil that eventually succumbed to acute leukemia. The patients were treated for 7 and 5 years,

Table 18-14   Recommended individualized dosing of carboplatin

Carboplatin dose (mg) = target AUC × (GFR + 25)

AUC is selected for appropriate clinical situation:
   AUC, 5 in untreated patients, when used in combination chemotherapy
   AUC, 5 in previously treated patients
   AUC, 7 in previously untreated patients
GFR is equivalent to Cr Cl, which can be measured or can be estimated from patient's age, weight, and serum creatinine.

AUC, Area under the curve; GFR, glomerular filtration value; Cr Cl, creatinine clearance.

Table 18-15   Alkylating agents—leukemia

Drug	Median (total dose)		Cumulative risk (10 years)
Cyclophos-phamide	Low dose	(7600 mg)	0
	Medium dose	(19,500 mg)	0
	High dose	(46,300 mg)	11.1
Melphalan	Low dose	(251 mg)	1.1
	Medium dose	(600 mg)	5.0
	High dose	(965 mg)	19.5

respectively, with continuous maintenance doses of chlorambucil. Other reviews of ovarian cancer patients surviving 3 years or more point to similar increased incidences of acute leukemia in patients treated with melphalan pulse therapy. Long-term follow-up of this same group of patients has revealed increased risk with high-dose (cumulative dose) therapy (Table 18-15). Much of the data on the occurrence of acute leukemia in patients treated with alkylating agents are clouded by detection bias. Obviously, the patients who survive 3 years or more are a very small portion of the total group treated, since the disease claims the lives of most patients in less than 3 years. In addition, a significant number of patients have received concomitant radiotherapy, and other patients have received additional chemotherapeutic agents. However, retrospective data strongly suggest that alkylating agent therapy results in a significant increase in the occurrence of acute leukemia in patients with ovarian cancer who survive after therapy.

Reimer et al. reported the results of a national survey of 70 institutions using alkylating agents in the treatment of ovarian carcinoma. Patients with advanced ovarian carcinoma who had survived 2 years had a relative risk for subsequent acute nonlymphocytic leukemia of more than 170%. Review of a historical control group of more than 13,000 patients with ovarian carcinoma who had surgery, radiation therapy, or both suggested that this excess risk was not related to an underlying predisposition to develop leukemia. On the basis of this survey, Reimer et al. predicted that as many as 5%-10% of a hypothetical group of 10-year survivors might develop acute leukemia. Kaldor reported that chemotherapy alone was associated with a relative risk of 12, compared to surgery alone. Patients treated with chemotherapy and radiotherapy had a relative risk of 10. Radiotherapy alone did not produce a significant increase in risk compared to surgery alone. The risk of leukemia was greatest 4 to 5 years after chemotherapy began, and the risk was elevated for at least 8 years after cessation of chemotherapy. Chlorambucil and melphalan were the most leukemogenic drugs, followed by thiotepa, cyclophosphamide, and busulfan, which were the weakest leukemogens.

This matter is of particular concern for patients receiving adjuvant chemotherapy when the risk of recurrence is not great. Such a category would include individuals with stage I, grade 1, epithelial cancer of the ovary. In this category of patients and in similar groups where a reasonably high survival rate is anticipated, the risks of adjuvant therapy in the form of the traditional single-drug alkylating agent must be weighed against the possible benefits. Since the benefits of adjuvant chemotherapy are unclear in this low-risk category, it appears that therapy should be withheld until better evidence is available.

The carcinogenic potential of many chemotherapeutic agents could pose significant safety problems for health care professionals as well as patients. In the past, these drugs were commonly prepared by physicians and nurses without sufficient precautions. This is no longer accepted in most institutions, largely because of evidence that unprotected individuals preparing these drugs appear to have higher than normal levels of agents in their urine. In addition, patients who become pregnant during the presence of such agents appear to have a high rate of fetal loss. It is now standard for cancer chemotherapeutic agents to be solely prepared by trained individuals (usually pharmacists) inside a biohazard safety hood where protective clothing and disposable gloves made of latex or polyvinyl can be utilized. Subsequent administration of drugs to the patient is done with care to avoid aerosols or gross spills, and the empty syringe and tubing are disposed of as toxic wastes. Special kits should be readily available in case of accidental contamination of the environment around the patient.

BIBLIOGRAPHY

Bradley G, Juranka PF, Ling V: Mechanisms of multidrug resistance, *Biochem Biophysi Acta* 948:87, 1988.

Charbit A, Malaise EP, Tubiana M: Relation between the pathological nature and the growth rate of human tumors, *Eur J Cancer* 7:307, 1971.

DeVita VT: The influence of information on drug resistance on protocol design: the Harry Kaplan Memorial Lecture given at the Fourth International Conference on malignant lymphoma, June 6-9, 1990, Lugnao, Switzerland, *Ann Oncol* 2:93, 1991.

DeVita VT, Hellman S, Rosenberg SA: *Cancer Principles and Practice of Oncology*, ed 4, Philadelphia, J.B. Lippincott Company, 1993.

Endicott JA, Ling V: The biochemistry of P-glycoprotein-mediated drug resistance, *Annu Rev Biochem*, Berlin: Sprinter-Verlag, 1984.

Epstein RA: Drug-induced DNA damage and tumor chemosensitivity, *J Clin Oncol* 8:2062, 1990.

Goldie JH: Scientific basis for adjuvant and primary (neoadjuvant) chemotherapy, *Semin Oncol* 14:1, 1987.

Goldie JH, Coldman AJ: A mathematical model for relating the drug sensitivity of tumors to spontaneous mutation rate, *Cancer Treat Rep* 63:1727, 1979.

Goldstein U et al: Expression of a multidrug resistant gene in human cancers, *JNCL* 81:116, 1989.

Ling V: Drug resistance and membrane mutase of mammalian cells, *Cancer J Genet Cytol*, 17:503, 1975.

Reimer RR, Hoover R, Fraumeni JF, Young RC: Acute leukemia after alkylating agent therapy, *NEJM* 297:117, 1977.

Rich WM, Abdulham G, DiSaia PJ: Methylprednisolone as an antiemetic during cancer chemotherapy: a pilot study, *Gynecol Oncol* 9(2):193, 1980.

Rowinsky EK, McGuire WP, Donehower RC: The current status of Taxol. In *Principles and Practice of Gynecologic Oncology Updates*, ed Hoskins WJ et al, Philadelphia: J.B. Lippincott Company, 1993.

Shoemaker RH et al: Potentials and drawbacks of the tumor stem cell assay, *Behring Inst Mitt* 74:262, 1984.

Skipper HE, Schabel FM, Jr, Wilcox WS: Experimental evaluation of potential anticancer agents: XII. On the criteria and kinetics associated with "curability" of experimental leukemia, *Cancer Chemother Rep* 35:1, 1964.

Sotrel G et al: Acute leukemia in advanced ovarian carcinoma after treatment with alkylating agents, *Obstet Gynecol* 47:675, 1976.

Skipper HE et al: Implications of biochemical, cytokinetic, pharmacologic, and toxicologic relationships in the design of optimal therapeutic schedules, *Cancer Chemother Rep* 54:431, 1950.

Stierle A, Strobel G, Stierle D: Taxol and Taxane production by *Taxomyces andreane*, an endophytic fungus of pacific yew, *Science* 260:214, 1993.

Chemosensitivity testing

Hamburger AW, Salmon SE: Primary bioassay of human tumor stem cells, *Science* 197:461, 1977.

Kern DH, Weisenthal LM: Highly specific prediction of antineoplastic drug resistance with in vitro assay using suprapharmacologic drug doses, *J Natl Cancer Inst* 82:582, 1990.

Puck TT, Marcus PI: Action of x-rays on mammalian cells, *J Exp Med* 103:653, 1956.

Sevin B-U et al: Chemosensitivity testing in ovarian cancer, *Cancer* 71:1613, 1993.

Weisenthal LM: Predictive assays for drug resistance and radiation resistance. In Masters J, ed: *Human Cancer in Primary Culture: A Handbook*, p103. Dordrecht, Wolters Kluwwe, 1991.

Growth factors

Demetri GD: Hematopoietic growth factors: current knowledge, future prospects, *Curr Probl Cancer* 16:179, 1992.

Kouides PA, Dipersio JF: The hematopoietic growth factors. In *Principles of Cancer Treatment*, ed 4, Charles M. Haskell, ed, WB Saunders Co, Philadelphia 1995.

Lieschke GJ, Burgess AW: Granulocyte colony stimulating factor and granulocyte-macrophage colony-stimulating factor, *N Engl J Med* 327(1):28, 1992.

Lieschke GJ, Burgess Aw: Granulocyte colony stimulating factor and granulocyte-macrophage colony-stimulating factor, *N Engl J Med* 327(2):99, 1992.

Miller CB et al: Decreased erythropoietin response in patients with the anemia of cancer, *N Engl J Med* 322:1689-1692, 1990.

Neidhart JA: Hematopoietic colony-stimulating factors, *Cancer* 70:913, 1992.

Piroso E, Erslev AJ, Caro J: Inappropriate increase in erythropoietin titers during chemotherapy, *Am J Hematol* 32:248, 1989.

Schapira L et al: Serum erythropoietin levels in patients receiving intensive chemotherapy and radiotherapy, *Blood* 76:2354, 1990.

Tepler I et al: Use of peripheral blood progenitor cells abrogates the myelotoxicity of repetitive outpatient high-dose carboplatin and cyclophosphamide chemotherapy, *J Clin Oncol* 11:1583, 1993.

Zucker S: Anemia in cancer, *Cancer Invest* 3:249, 1985.

Calculation of dosage

Calvert AH et al: Carboplatin dosage: prospective evaluation of a simple formula based on renal function, *J Clin Oncol* 7:1748, 1989.

Cockroft DW, Gault MH: Prediction of creatinine clearance from serum creatinine, *Nephron* 16:31, 1976.

Jelliffe RW, Jelliffe SM: A computer program for estimation of creatinine clearance from unstable serum creatinine levels, age, sex, and weight, *Math Biosci* 14:17, 1972.

Safe handling of cytotoxic drugs

American Society of hospital pharmacists technical assistance bulletin on handling cytotoxic and hazardous drugs, *Am J Hosp Pharm* 47:1033, 1990.

Jones RB et al: Safe handling of chemotherapeutic agents: a report from the Mount Sinai Medical Center, *CA-A Cancer J Clinic*, Sep/Oct:258, 1983.

OSHA Work-Practice guidelines for personnel dealing with cytotoxic (antineoplastic) drugs. *Am J Hosp Pharm* 43:1193, 1986.

Recommendations for the safe handling of parenteral antineoplastic drugs. NIH publication No. 83-2621. For sale by the superintendent of documents. US Government Printing Office. Washington, DC 20402.

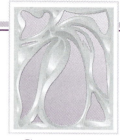

CHAPTER

19

Tumor Immunology, Host Defense Mechanisms, and Biologic Therapy

I am convinced that during development and growth, malignant cells arise frequently, but that in the majority of individuals they remain latent due to the protective action of the host. I am convinced that this natural immunity is not due to the presence of antimicrobial bodies, but is determined purely by cellular factors. These may be weakened in older age groups in which cancer is more prevalent.

Paul Ehrlich (1909)

HISTORICAL REVIEW

The word *immunity* means freedom from burden, and in its original application the burden was that of invasion by microorganisms. In modern times the burden is much larger and also encompasses the reaction of the body to foreign tissue, such as organ transplants, and to altered tissue, such as neoplastic growths. The nineteenth century saw the emergence of microbiology and immunology and witnessed the beginnings of vaccination in the prevention of disease. Edward Jenner successfully inoculated cowpox into humans and was able to offer protection against smallpox. The practices of Jenner were extended by Pasteur, who established the value of preventive inoculation against a variety of animal and human diseases. It was because of Pasteur that the skepticism about the "germ theory" finally was dispelled, and Koch was able to lay down the fundamental laws regarding infectious agents with the "Koch postulates." The field of immunology became a firm scientific foundation around the turn of the twentieth century with the recognition of immunolysis of foreign red cells by Bordet in 1898 and the description of the ABO blood groups by Landsteiner in 1904. In the early part of the twentieth century, the relative importance of phagocytosis and antibody production to host defense caused a sharp division of scientific opinion. One group of scientists led by a Russian, Elie Metchnikoff, held phagocytosis to be more crucial. Paul Ehrlich and his followers attributed greater importance to antibody attack on the parasite. Ehrlich developed the theory of antigenic specificity, which depended, according to him, on chemical union between the antigen and side chains on the corresponding antibody. In 1908 the Nobel Prize was awarded to Ehrlich and Metchnikoff for their work on immunity.

Tumor immunology developed as an offshoot of transplantation immunology. The roots of transplantation immunology are found in the work of a Hungarian-born Viennese surgeon, Emerich Ullman, who successfully transplanted a kidney into a dog. His technique was perfected by Alexis Carrel, a graduate of the University of Lyon, who was working in Chicago between 1902 and 1904. Carrel applied the principles of vascular anastomosis to transplantation of various organs. The techniques described by Carrel for developing vascular suture substances and his technique of vascular surgery have persisted to modern times. Carrel won the Nobel Prize in medicine for his work.

In 1923 and 1924 the pathology of transplantation rejection was described by Carol S. Williamson of the Mayo Clinic, and the phenomenon of first and second set rejection was documented by Holman, who worked with skin allografts on a burn victim. These findings laid the foundation for the classic work of Peter Gorer leading to the formulation of the theory of antigenic specificity of tissues from different individuals. The first clinical attempt at human kidney transplantation was at the Peter Bent Brigham Hospital in Boston by Charles A. Hufnagel, David A. Hume, and Ernest Landsteiner in 1947.

About the same time an interesting observation made in 1945 by R. Owen, a veterinary surgeon from Wisconsin, began to be widely appreciated by the scientific community. Owen noted that in utero mixing of the circulation of monoplacental cattle led to the coexistence in the adult animal of two different blood groups, a condition called chimerism. In 1955, Billingham et al. published their landmark paper on actively acquired tolerance of foreign cells in which they showed that when fetal mice were exposed to foreign cells in utero, those mice, on attaining adult age, would become tolerant to tissues from the original donor of the cells. In 1959, Macfarlane Burnet refined this concept and detailed the clonal selection theory of immunity. By 1960 teams of surgeons in the United States, France, and Britain were successfully transplanting kidneys, and their techniques have continued. Burnet and Medawar were awarded the Nobel Prize in medicine in 1960 for their monumental work. The importance of cell surface antigens in transplantation immunity became well recognized and led to advances such as those of Paul Terasaki, who developed and popularized a method for matching tissues of organ donors and recipients to prolong transplantation survival.

As transplantation immunology (Table 19-1) became more thoroughly understood, some scientists referred to the hypothesis of Paul Ehrlich, which stated that malignant neoplasms were antigenic and, as such, could be recognized by the host as foreign in much the same manner as allogenic tissue. Indeed, in 1908 Ehrlich indirectly suggested the theory of immunologic surveillance. Cancer-specific antigens were identified for the first time in experiments by Gross in 1943. He described the failure of mice to accept a transplant of a specific cancer after they had been immunized with material from the same cancer growing in pedigreed mice. Gross immunized mice by intradermal inoculation of tumor cells. The immunized animals rejected a subcutaneous transplant of the same tumor, but **nonimmunized** animals did not. His work was all but **ignored** until 1957, when Prehn and Main reported **their** experiments using syngeneic methylcholanthrene-induced fibrosarcomas. They observed that mice immunized against these fibrosarcomas by inoculation of living sarcoma tissue, after surgical removal of the growing tumor, were resistant to subsequent grafts of the same tumor. In addition, immunization with normal tissue did not confer resistance to the tumor graft. The mice that had become resistant to the tumors still accepted skin grafts from the primary host of these tumors. The rejection of the tumor tissue with simultaneous acceptance of normal tissue from the same donor to the same recipient proved Ehrlich's hypothesis correct. The malignant neoplasm appeared to have acquired an antigenic moiety during the malignant transformation of the mouse tissue that allowed that malignant tissue now to be recognized as "non-self," whereas corresponding normal tissue was still accepted as "self."

The experiments of Prehn and Main were repeated by many others in different tumor systems, and the following conclusions have been reached. Antigenic differences exist between cancer cells and their normal counterparts, and these differences are equivalent to weak transplantation antigens. It appears that malignant tissues evoke a measurable immunologic response in most organisms in which they appear, including the human. The specificity

Table 19-1   Tumor immunology is a form of transplantation immunology and the same terminology applies

Genetic relationship	Antibody	Transplant	
		Old term	New term
Identical, same individual	Auto	Auto	Autologous
Identical twin (same inbred strain)	Iso	Iso	Syngeneic
Different individual, same species	Iso	Homo	Allogeneic
Different species	Hetero	Hetero	Xenogeneic

From DiSaia PJ: Tumor immunology: general aspects, *Contemporary Ob/Gyn* 4:91, 1974, Medical Economics Co.

of the cell surface tumor antigens is in doubt, and therefore they have been termed *tumor-associated antigens*.

In the late 1950s, the term *immunological surveillance* was coined by Burnet, who postulated that cell-mediated immunity evolved to recognize and destroy cells that had non-self markers, such as tumor cells bearing tumor antigens. The theory of immune surveillance, then, hypothesizes that immune mechanisms may eliminate newly appearing tumor cells and thus serve as a surveillance system for cancer. This theory continues to be investigated from many aspects, especially with regard to the role of cell mediated and cytokine mediated mechanisms.

In 1959, Macfarlane Burnet conceived the clonal selection theory, which states in essence that immunocompetent cells are already endowed with the genetic ability to make a certain antibody. Through combination with its specific cell via antigen-specific receptors on the surface membrane, an antigen causes that specific cell to proliferate, an activity that results in observable antibody formation. In addition, each lymphocyte carries on its surface receptor molecules of only a single specificity.

An attractive portion of the clonal selection theory is its application to specific immunological tolerance: the failure to make an antibody to a normally antigenic material because of a previous exposure to the antigen. Burnet suggested that self-recognition occurs in neonatal life by contact of the antibody-forming cells with new antigens as the fetus first forms them. The result in utero is a functional shutdown of such a cell, so that one does not make antibodies to one's own antigens. Peter Medawar tested this hypothesis with fetal exposure to non-self antigens and measured the results. As the theory predicted, the animal, when grown to adulthood, did not respond to the antigen.

In the mid-1970s, research conducted primarily by Milstein and Kohler led to the description of immunoglobulin-sensitizing hybridomas and the discovery and development of hybridoma technology (Figure 19-14). Kohler and Milstein received a Nobel prize in physiology and medicine in 1984. In 1987, the Nobel Prize in medicine and physiology was awarded to the Japanese-American Susumu Tonegawa for his important discoveries based on the analysis of immunoglobulin genes. He clearly demonstrated that more than one gene was involved in the synthesis of a single peptide or immunoglobulin.

In the last three decades, various methods to stimulate a patient's immune system non-specifically have been tried with minimal success (e.g., BCG, *Corynebacterium parvum*, etc.). Other approaches have used monoclonal antibodies or various lymphokines and other immune system stimulatory factors (so-called "biological response modifiers"). All will be discussed in the pages that follow.

ANATOMY OF THE IMMUNE SYSTEM
Antigens

Tumor cells express most of the same cell surface antigens (e.g., transplantation or HLA antigens) as normal cells (Figure 19-1). In addition, many tumor cells express specific antigens not found in similar normal cells. An antigen announces its foreignness by means of intricate and characteristic shapes called epitopes or antigen determinants, which protrude from its surface. Most antigens carry several different kinds of epitopes on their surface: some may carry several hundred epitopes, and some will be more effective at stimulating an immune response (Figure 19-2). These antigens (often rare and weak) are termed *tumor-specific antigens* (TSAs) in animal studies and *tumor-associated antigens* (TAAs) in human malignancies. Experiments to demonstrate tumor-specific antigens involve a demonstration that pretreatment with a

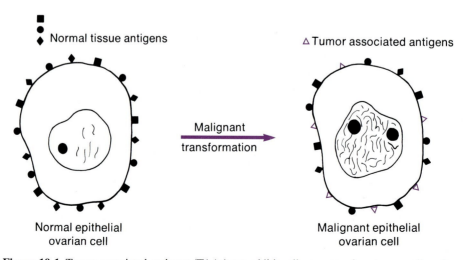

Figure 19-1 Tumor-associated antigens (TAAs) are additionally expressed on tumor cell surface.

syngeneic tumor will influence the growth of a subsequent challenge with the same tumor. In animals this was possible after introduction of syngeneic inbred mouse strains, and in 1953 Foley produced the first such evidence. This was followed by the studies of Prehn and Main (described previously). Such studies are not possible in humans; however, there are in vitro techniques for detection of tumor antigens and these have been liberally applied to human tumors. Tumors vary widely in their immunogenicity. In general, neoplasms induced experimentally in vivo with chemical or viral agents are highly immunogenic; tumors arising spontaneously in vivo (e.g., human malignancies) are poorly immunogenic.

Oncofetal antigens have also been described; these are antigens that are found in fetal and malignant tissue and tend to occur more commonly than TAAs. These normal antigens in the fetus are repressed as the process of intrauterine development proceeds toward birth and then derepressed during the malignant transformation process. Their existence supports the concept that cancer represents a dedifferentiation to a more primitive cell type. The relationship between malignant neoplasms, specific tumor antigens, and fetal antigens is not clear. The most carefully studied oncofetal antigens in gynecologic cancer are carcinoembryonic antigen (CEA) and alphafetoprotein (AFP). The most apparent importance of these antigens is not in their possible protective value but in their ability to serve as tumor markers for various cancers. CEA initially stimulated great interest as a possible accurate diagnostic assay for gastrointestinal tract malignancies. However, with further study, elevated levels were found in patients with benign disease (e.g., colonic polyps, severe cirrhosis, uremia, and inflammatory disease of the bowel). Indeed, CEA can be found in many nongastrointestinal tract cancers, including several gynecologic malignancies, and its value as a clinically usable tumor marker is limited. AFP is detectable immunologically in serum from human fetuses. In the adult, it is found in patients with malignancies of endodermal origin, for example, liver tumors and gonadal tumors such as endodermal sinus tumor of the ovary. As with CEA, there does not appear to be a clear correlation between the level of AFP and the prognosis for the patient, and, also like CEA, it is not disease specific. The presence of AFP with an ovarian neoplasm strongly suggests a diagnosis of endodermal sinus tumor, and the reappearance of detectable serum levels after a period of negative titers strongly suggests recurrent disease.

With very few exceptions, it has not been possible to demonstrate antigens in human neoplasms that have as high degree of tumor specificity as that reported for most TSAs in animals. Rather, the great majority of human tumor antigens known today are tumor-associated antigens. Some have described these as tumor-associated differentiation antigens (TADAs). These antigens (TAAs or TADAs) are sometimes referred to as fetal antigens that have relative rather than absolute specificity for cancer cells. If highly specific antigens could be found in human cancer similar to those encoded by certain tumor viruses, they would provide excellent targets for active and passive immunotherapy. However, even the weak TAAs known today offer some promise for clinical applications in that they provide markers for diagnosis, both by histologic and cytologic techniques and through the assays of sera. They can be used to detect how cancer patients respond to therapy, and they can be used in vivo for detection of tumors via nuclear imaging.

Each human tumor may express many TAAs. For example, melanomas, which are among the neoplasms most thoroughly studied, express different proteins as well as glycolipid antigens. There is considerable heterogenicity in the expression of many TAAs, both between different tumors of the same type and between different cells of the same tumor. Heterogeneity is reflected even in

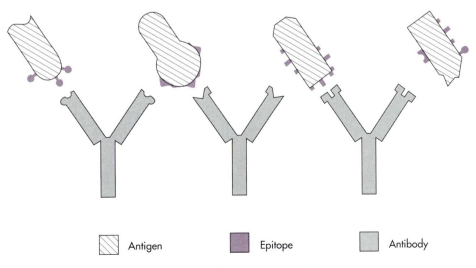

Antigen   Epitope   Antibody

Figure 19-2 Antigens and antibodies.

a different expression of a TAA in a primary tumor and its metastases. Antigens that are expressed more in some tumor types than in others do exist but most TAAs are shared by neoplasms of many different types.

With the development of the monoclonal technology, it is possible to identify several novel serum markers for different human tumors. One of these markers, CA-125, has been used to monitor patients who have epithelial ovarian cancer. CA-125 is recognized by a murine monoclonal IgGl immunoglobulin OC-125. The antibody was developed using the technique of Kohler and Milstein. Murine myeloma cells were hybridized with spleen cells from a mouse that had been immunized with a human serous cystadenocarcinoma cell line. Stable hybrid clones were screened for reactivity against the ovarian tumor cell line used for immunization and for lack of reactivity with a B lymphocyte line established from the tumor donor using Epstein-Barr virus transformation. Clones were also screened for a lack of reactivity with allogeneic human ovary. CA-125 determinants are associated with the derivatives of the coelomic epithelium in the embryo and adult, including the pleura, pericardium, peritoneum, fallopian tube, endometrium, and endocervix. Outside of this lineage, CA-125 has also been detected in tracheobronchial epithelium and glands, amnion, amniotic fluid, milk, cervical mucus, and seminal fluid. Interestingly, CA-125 has not been found in sections of normal ovary, either in the fetus or the adult. The antigen is present at the cell surface in more than 80% of nonmucinous epithelial ovarian cancers, as well as in a smaller fraction of carcinomas that arise from the endometrium, fallopian tube, endocervix, pancreas, colon, breast, and lung.

An immunoradiometric assay has been developed to measure CA-125 determinants in serum or ascites fluid. In this assay, CA-125 antigen is bound to OC-125 antibody on a solid phase immunoabsorbent. Because there are multiple CA-125 determinants on each antigen molecule or complex, I-125-labeled OC-125 can be used as a probe to detect bound antigen in a double determinant simultaneous "sandwich" assay. Antigen in body fluids is compared with a standard prepared from culture supernatants of an ovarian tumor cell line. Antigen activity has been expressed on an arbitrary scale from 1 to 20,000 U/ml. The day-to-day coefficient of variation for the assay is 12%-15%, and a doubling or halving of antigen levels has been considered significant.

A number of additional monoclonal antibodies that react with ovarian cancers have been generated; e.g., NB/70K, CA 19-9, etc. CA 19-9 monoclonal antibody can be co-expressed with the CA-125 determinant, CA 19-9 is found in the serum of about 25% of ovarian cancer patients. Requirements for a successful tumor marker include sensitivity, specificity, and the availability of effective treatment. Sensitivity is defined as the proportion of assay positives to true positives; specificity is defined as a proportion of assay negatives to true

negatives. Even when it is highly specific and sensitive, the utility of a tumor marker depends ultimately on its ability to influence decisions between alternative plans for patient management. Consequently, requirements for a useful gynecologic tumor marker must depend on the particular clinical problems for which it is applied. One of the most useful applications for a tumor marker is the detection of early disease at a time when it can be cured. In gynecologic practice, cytologic analysis has provided an appropriate screening technique for the detection of cervical carcinomas, but there has been no comparable strategy to detect neoplasms of the ovary and fallopian tube. High sensitivity is needed to detect disease at an early stage. Specificity must be sufficient to discriminate malignant disease from a broad spectrum of intercurrent benign conditions. If additional noninvasive tests could localize the site of primary tumor growth, an effective screening test might not need to distinguish different primary sites of malignancy. If a test was sufficiently specific to identify sites of primary tumor growth, it might prove useful in evaluating patients who have malignant ascites. In this setting, tumor burden is often substantial, and high sensitivity would not be as critical as in the detection of early stage disease.

In gynecologic practice, discrimination of benign from malignant pelvic masses would be of great value, particularly in patients who might be referred to tertiary centers for cytoreductive surgery. Because gross disease is often present, requirements for sensitivity are reduced. Specificity is still important in that the test must effectively distinguish malignant from benign conditions. Tumor markers have been used most often to monitor response to therapy in patients known to have cancer. For this application, antigen levels must parallel tumor burden. Ideally, the range of assay values should be broad relative to the precision of the assay, permitting measurement of tumor burden over several orders of magnitude. Markers with a short half-life in serum would reflect decreases in tumor burden more promptly than markers with slow clearance. For effective monitoring, the degree of specificity is somewhat less critical than that of sensitivity. The assay should not be affected by benign conditions that occur during treatment, but these conditions would include only a small subset of the broad spectrum of benign conditions that could be encountered during screening of an apparently healthy population. Assays for persistent or recurrent disease are of greatest value in settings where there is an effective salvage therapy. If, however, treatment with cytotoxic drugs is sufficiently morbid, progressive elevation of a marker might prompt discontinuation of ineffective chemotherapy in selected patients.

Humoral Factors

Some immunoblasts differentiate into plasma cells, which are largely responsible for humoral immunity. Antibodies are secreted by plasma cells into the vicinity of the antigenic stimulus, and there binding takes place with the inciting antigen. A given antibody matches an antigen much as a key matches a lock. The fit varies: some times it is very precise; at other times it is imprecise. To some degree, however, the antibody interlocks with the antigen. The basic unit of all antibodies is composed of four polypeptides, two light chains, and two heavy chains linked to each other by several disulfide bridges. The sections that make up the tips of the Y's arms vary greatly from one antibody to another, creating a pocket uniquely shaped to lock in a specific antigen. This is called the variable region. The stem of the Y serves to link the antibody to other participants in the immune system (e.g., a T cell). This area is identical in all antibodies of the same class and is called the constant region (Figure 19-3). The unique variable region of an antibody can itself act as an antigen. The variable region contains a number of antigen-like segments and these are known collectively as an idiotype. Like any other antigen, an idiotype can trigger complementary antibody. This second-rowed antibody is known as an anti-idiotype.

There are five classes of antibodies: IgG, IgM, IgA, IgE, and IgD. It is estimated that 100,000 different antibodies can be produced by a human; specificity is a basic property of this system. An antibody directed toward a particular antigen will not confer protection against other antigens. This concept is termed the *clonal selection theory*, which states that each antibody- producing cell is committed to one particular antibody in production.

Antibodies have been demonstrated in the serum of many animals bearing a variety of experimentally induced tumors. Although these antibodies have been useful in serologic characterization and in isolation of tumor-associated antigens, the presence of a humoral response is not consistently correlated with increased tumor resistance in the host. Nonetheless, there are several ways in which tumor-specific antibodies could theoretically mediate antitumor activity. If tumor-associated antigens induce a humoral response, it is likely that the interaction of the tumor cell with some of the antibodies will activate the complement system, leading to lesions in the cell membrane and eventually lysis. Lysis by complement has been shown to be effective in vitro against certain cells in suspension; however, cell death is not usually evident when treating target cells of solid tumor tissue. Opsonization is the binding of specific antibody and complement components with particulate antigen to facilitate its phagocytosis. In vitro studies demonstrated the ability of macrophages to exert cytotoxic activity against some tumor cells by cytophagocytosis in the presence of immune serum. The relevance of this activity in vivo is difficult to assess. The ability of antibodies to bind to the surface of tumor cells in vivo may be important in antitumor activities other than those mediated by complement-dependent lysis or phagocytosis by macrophages. Antibodies bound to the membranes of malignant cells may modulate surface structures and thereby interfere with cell adhesive properties. This could have a deleterious effect on certain types of tumors because the ability to adhere to each other and to surrounding host tissue may be essential for successful establishment of the malignant clone by providing cellular organization and support. Furthermore, adherence of circulating tumor cells to the endothelium of blood vessels appears to precede metastatic spread. Antibodies specifically bound to the membranes of tumor cells may result in loss of the adhesive properties important to the establishment of bloodborne metastatic foci.

T Lymphocytes (Thymus Dependent)

Thymus-dependent (T) lymphocytes recognize and destroy foreign cells and regulate immune reactions. T lymphocytes carry out these functions directly by cell-to-cell contact or indirectly by using factors they produce and secrete. T cells regulate the activity of other T cells, macrophages, B cells, neutrophils, eosinophils, and basophils. T lymphocytes mature in the thymus because lymphoid cells differentiate in the thymus, they require specialized functions, and their cell membranes display distinguishing profiles or differentiation antigens. The biological function of many of the differentiating antigens is not yet understood but these cell surface markers are extremely useful for identifying lymphoid T cell subsets in normal and lymphoproliferate disease states. T lymphocytes, after leaving the thymus, are mainly found in the blood and thymic-dependent areas of the lymphoid tissues (e.g., spleen, lymph nodes, and Peyer's patches). In the circulation, they make up 80%-90% of the total lymphocytes. Utilizing the differ-

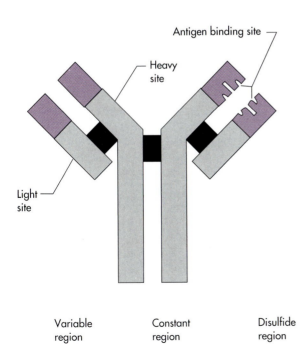

Figure 19-3 Antibody structure with antigen-binding site.

Table 19-2   Cytokines

Cytokine	Biologic activity
Interferon (IFN), alpha or beta	Antiviral, augments NK cell activity, antiproliferative properties
Interferon (IFN), gamma	Activates macrophages, augments NK cell activity, augments or inhibits other cytokine activities
Interleukin-1 (IL-1), alpha or beta	Activates resting T cells, induces CSF production, stimulates synthesis of other cytokines
Interleukin-2 (IL-2)	Augments lymphocyte killer activity, induces production of other cytokines
Interleukin-3 (IL-3)	Stimulates early growth of monocyte, granulocyte, erythrocyte, and megakaryocyte progenitor cells
Interleukin-4 (IL-4)	Growth factor for activated B cells, enhances growth of most cell lines
Interleukin-5 (IL-5)	Induces proliferation and differentiation of eosinophil progenitors
Interleukin-6 (IL-6)	Induces differentiation of B cells; enhances I_g secretion by B cells
Interleukin-7 (IL-7)	Supports growth of pre-B cells
Interleukin-8 (IL-8)	Activates neutrophils; attenuates inflammatory events at blood vessel endothelium
Tumor necrosis factor (TNF), alpha or beta	Cytotoxic for some tumor cells, activates macrophages, stimulates synthesis of other cytokines
Granulocyte colony-stimulating factor (G-CSF)	Stimulates growth of granulocyte to colonies and activates mature granulocytes
Granulocyte macrophage colony-stimulating factor (GM-CSF)	Stimulates growth of granulocyte, monocyte, and early erythrocyte progenitors; less megakaryocyte progenitors
Macrophage colony-stimulating factor (M-CSF)	Stimulates growth of monocyte colonies, enhances antibody-dependent, monocyte-mediated cytotoxicity

entiating antigens, human T cells have been characterized by monoclonal antibody techniques and are divided into three functional subgroups: helper, suppressor, and cytotoxic lymphocytes. T helper lymphocytes, which constitute about one third of the mature cell population, are programmed to produce factors that amplify the functions of other cells (B lymphocytes and other T lymphocytes). Suppressor lymphocytes also have characteristic functions and can suppress effector lymphocytes by direct interaction or by the release of soluble suppressor factors. Cytotoxic T cells also express antigens, which can be detected by monoclonal antibodies.

T lymphocytes primarily recognize cell-associated antigens. Specifically, T cells simultaneously recognize both the antigen and a portion of one of the self class I or class II major histocompatibility complex (MHC) gene products. It is not clear whether T cells have distinct receptors for this MHC and the antigenic determinant or single receptors that have both specificities combined. Activated lymphocytes can produce a variety of soluble effector substances. They participate in the complicated process called the immune response. These substances are called cytokines and include, among others, those listed in Table 19-2.

T lymphocytes are required for several types of reactions such as regulating immunoglobulin production, mediating delayed hypersensitivity, and lysing early virus-infected cells. An important advance in understanding how T cells develop into functionally mature populations and how they mediate these functions was the demonstration that distinct stages of T cell differentiation and function correlate with the expression of specific surface molecules. These molecules are designated by the letter "T" followed by a number (T1 through T11) and can be detected by monoclonal antibodies.

All lymphocytes are relatively indistinguishable by light microscopy but various markers have been found that serve to identify their phenotypes. Most useful among these markers are those on the surface of the cell (Table 19-3) and, although their function in many instances is unknown, their presence can be exploited for purification as well as identification of these cells. The development of monoclonal antibodies has assisted greatly in the mapping of these cell surface molecules. Initially, these monoclonal antibodies to lymphocyte markers were developed in many laboratories and given different designations. Indeed, the same antibody ended up having several designations, each applied by a laboratory involved with research utilizing that antibody. To overcome this confusion, a uniform system of nomenclature has been adopted in which all surface markers are called CD followed by a number indicating the sequence of their acceptance. The list extends to at least CD 80. This term, CD (cluster determinant), describes the cluster of antigens with which antibodies react, and the number indicates its order of discovery. Thus, anti-CD 4 designates antibodies

Table 19-3   Surface antigens useful for exploring human T cell differentiation and function

Antigens	Molecular weight	Monoclonal antibody	Comments
CD 1	67,000	OKT 1	Equivalent to murine Thy 1 antigen
		Leu 1	
CD 3	20,000	OKT 3	Associated with T cell receptor for antigen
	23,000	Leu 4	
CD 4	60,000	OKT 4	Present on helper/inducer T cells
		Leu 3	
4B4			Helper/inducer
4H4			Suppressor/inducer
CD 6	44,000	OKT 6	Equivalent to murine T1 antigens
		Leu 6	
CD 8	32,000	OKT	Present on cytotoxic/suppressor cells
	43,000	Leu 2a	
		Leu 2b	
CD 9	190,000	OKT 9	Transferrin receptor, present on activated T cells
CD 10	37,000	OKT 10	Present on early stem cells, some B cells, activated peripheral T cells
CD 11	55,000	OKT	Associated with SRBC rosette receptor
		Leu	

that would react with a particular cell surface protein called CD 4, regardless of the epitope on the CD 4 they recognize. Many of these cell surface molecules have been detected by appropriate antibodies, and a list of at least 80 exists at this time. However, the functions of only a few have been adequately elaborated. Utilizing the current nomenclature, similar molecules in any species bear the same designation.

B Lymphocytes

The most salient characteristics of the B lymphocyte is the production of immunoglobulins upon activation (Figure 19-4). B lymphocytes are derived from the hematopoietic stem cells, and they receive their name from the discovery of their dependency on the bursa of Fabricius in birds. Studies have revealed the existence of at least five different cell types in the B lymphocyte differentiation pathway: pre-B cells, immature B cells, mature B cells, memory cells, and effector cells. There are also five immunoglobulin classes: IgM, IgG, IgA, IgE, IgD. The pre-B cell is the earliest cell identifiable as belonging to the B lymphocyte lineage. Conversion of the pre-B cell to an immature B cell begins near the end of the first trimester and persists through the second trimester of pregnancy. As pregnancy progresses, the stem cell pool shifts from the liver to the bone marrow, where differentiation continues throughout life. The expression of membrane-bound immunoglobulins is the common feature of all immature B cells; this feature allows clonal selection by antigen. When stimulated by antigen, B cells undergo a series of changes in cell surface structures and

in functional capabilities and differentiate into plasma cells. Plasma cells, the final stage in B cell differentiation, secrete large amounts of immunoglobulin. An individual plasma cell initially secretes antibodies of the IgM class but can switch to producing antibodies of other subclasses with the same antigen specificity.

Natural Killer Cells

Natural killer (NK) cells are a subpopulation of lymphoid cells present in most normal individuals and in a variety of mammalian and avian species. They do not result from a classic cellular immune response. They are cytolytically active in a nonspecific fashion when taken from an unimmunized host. NK cells do not depend on the thymus for maturation. There is no memory response by NK cells following re-exposure of the host to a reactive target. NK cells have spontaneous cytolytic activity against a variety of tumor cells and some normal cells, and their reactivity can be rapidly augmented by interferon. They have characteristics distinct from other types of lymphoid cells and are closely associated with large granular lymphocytes, which comprise about 5% of blood or splenic leukocytes. There is increasing evidence that NK cells, with the ability to mediate natural resistance against tumors in vivo, certain viruses and other microbial diseases, and bone marrow transplants may play an important role in the immune surveillance. NK cells share several features with macrophages and polymorphonuclear leukocytes (PMNs). NK cells have spontaneous activity in normal individuals, and this activity appears to be well regulated, subject to various inhibitory cells and

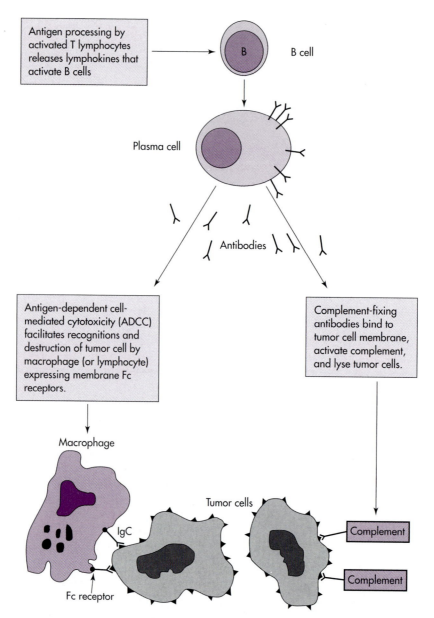

Figure 19-4 Role of the B cell in the immune response to malignancy.

factors. The nature of target cell recognition by NK cells seems to be intermediate between the exquisite specificity of T cells and the ill-defined or absent specificity of macrophages or PMNs. NK cells can react against a wide variety of syngeneic, allogeneic, and xenogeneic cells. Susceptibility to cytotoxic activity is not restricted to malignant cells; fetal cells, virus-infected cells, and some subpopulations of thymus cells, bone marrow cells, and macrophages are also sensitive to lysis. It appears that NK cells can recognize at least several widely distributed antigenic specificities and that such recognition is clonally distributed. The nature of the recognition for interferon production and for cytotoxic interactions of NK cells with target cells is not clear. The mechanism of killing by NK cells is also unclear, but, as with T cells,

binding to target cells is first required, followed by the lytic event. The actual lysis may be mediated by neutral serine proteases, phospholipases, or both.

NK cells represent an interesting and unusual type of effector cell. Research to date has led to a good understanding of the nature and characteristics of these cells but has also raised a number of questions. For example, it would be of interest to determine more clearly the lineage of NK cells and their relation to the T cell and the myelomonocytic lineages: the nature of the recognition receptors on NK cells and of the antigens on the target cells, the detailed mechanisms for regulation of their activities, and the biochemical sequence of events that led to their lysis of target cells. Data on the roles of NK cells in vivo suggest that these cells may be important in the first line of defense against tumor growth and against infection by some microbial agents. It is now necessary to determine more directly the role of NK cells in immunosurveillance. Ideally, one would like to show increased tumorigenesis when NK activity is selectively depressed and reduced tumor formation when such deficiencies are selectively reconstituted or normal levels of reactivity are selectively augmented. However, there are several practical problems in conducting such experiments. In addition to the long time needed for such studies and the difficulties in identifying the most relevant experimental carcinogenesis models, completely selective and sustained alterations of NK activity are not easily found or produced. If a major role for NK cells in resistance against tumor growth or other diseases can be sustained, this might lead to alternative strategies for immunoprevention or immunotherapy.

Lymphokine-activated killer (LAK) cells result from culturing lymphocytes with relatively high doses of IL-2. The fundamental characteristic of LAK cells is that they selectively lyse a broad spectrum of fresh autologous, syngeneic, or allogeneic cells in an independent fashion. They are activated cells, derived largely from two sources: NK cells and T cells. The NK cells are the primary source of LAK activity generated in response to high doses of IL-2. After exposure to IL-2 for a day or more, these cells are cytotoxic for tumor cells relatively insensitive to normal NK-mediated cytotoxicity. The T cells also generate LAK activity. Peripheral blood T cells or IL-2-dependent T-cell lines exhibit LAK activity after exposure to relatively high doses of IL-2. The cytotoxic mechanisms of LAK cells appear to be similar to those of NK cells and cytotoxic T lymphocytes.

Macrophage and Antigen-presenting Cells (APCs)

For cells involved in the immune response to react to foreign antigens, these antigens must be presented in a manner that the immune cells can recognize them. This requires that the foreign antigens be processed into smaller bits of information and be presented to immune cells or a part of an immune complex with cell surface MHC molecules. There are two types of MHC molecules: Class I, expressed on all cells, and class II, expressed on macrophages, dendritic cells, and B cells. All three of these cell types can present antigens to CD-4 bearing T cells (see Figure 19-8).

The macrophage is emerging as a major player in the host reaction to a tumor. Recent evidence has illustrated that the macrophage can be activated by lymphocytes and exert a killing effect on tumor cells. The mechanism of this killing is unclear but it appears that direct contact with the target cell is necessary. The macrophage is derived from the bone marrow. Widely distributed throughout the body (blood, bone marrow, lymphoid tissue, liver, connective tissue), macrophage cells form a critical part of the immune defense system. These cells serve at least three distinct but interrelated functions in host defense (Figure 19-5):

1. Secretion of biologically active molecules
2. Antigen clearance
3. Antigen presentation to lymphocytes (induction of the immune response)

The antigen-activated macrophage secretes a wide range of biologically active molecules that can have regulatory influences on surrounding cells in the process of tissue repair, inflammation, infection, and the immune response. Secretory products of the macrophage include enzymes, complement products, growth and differentiation factors (i.e., interleukin-1), cytotoxins for tumor and infectious agents, and other substances such as prostaglandins. In the immune system, prostaglandin E_2 can induce immature thymocytes, B lymphocytes, and hematopoietic cell precursors to differentiate and acquire the functional and immunologic characteristics of mature lymphocytes. Perhaps the most important role of the macrophage in the immune response is the processing and presentation of antigen to T cells to generate an immune response.

Although many in vitro studies have demonstrated the cytotoxicity of appropriately stimulated macrophages, evidence that they play a crucial role in the natural defense of the host against malignant disease has been difficult to assess directly. Nonetheless, activated macrophages isolated from donors infected with certain intracellular microorganisms or exposed to general immunopotentiating agents such as endotoxin express nonspecific cytotoxicity for a wide range of tumor types but not for normal cells. Several mechanisms may be involved in generating these cytotoxic macrophages. Agents that consist of endotoxin and other stimulants may activate macrophages directly. In general, however, many agents indirectly lead to macrophage activation by functioning as specific antigen stimuli for immune lymphocytes that release a variety of lymphokines. Some of these lymphokines attract macrophages to the site of the immunologic reaction and prevent their migration away (migration inhibitory factor [MIF]) as well as stimulate them with macrophage activating factor to undergo morphologic changes resulting in enhanced killing capabilities. Because the enhanced killing mediated by these mechanisms can be demonstrated against a variety of tumor target cells, the macrophage appears to be an important nonspecific effector of an antigen-specific cell-mediated response.

Mechanisms of Immunity

The immune mechanism consists basically of initial recognition and processing of foreign matter, an afferent mechanism leading to activation of the central immune system, and an efferent mechanism leading to the elimination of the offending material. The basic study of immunology concerns the reactions of the body to certain

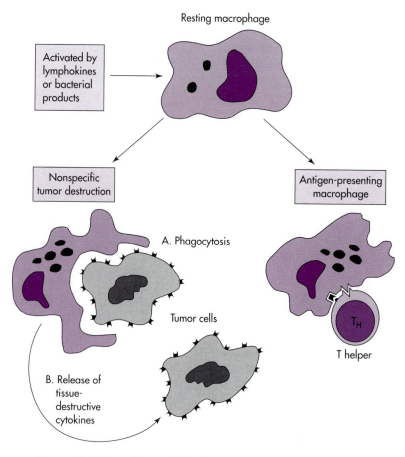

Figure 19-5 Macrophage role in the immune response to malignancy.

foreign materials presented to it, both living and nonliving. The immune reaction can be defined as an interaction between the invading foreign material and the defending host tissue. The cells of the afferent arm process the antigenic information and convey it to the central immune mechanism capable of reacting specifically to this information. The cells of the central mechanism are termed *immunologically competent* and are of the lymphoid series. This lymphoid tissue is present in peripheral lymph nodes, bone marrow, spleen, thymus, Peyer's patches of the intestine, thoracic duct, and the bloodstream itself. All antigens are recognized as "self" or "non-self." It is known, however, that when recognition occurs, it is very specific and precisely directed against certain molecular configurations on the antigen. In addition, antigen and immunocompetent cells apparently have physical contact to evoke a response.

Specific immune responses are mediated by two categories of effectors, with considerable interaction between the two. One category of response can be transferred from one individual to another only by transferring living immunologically competent cells or cultured products of these cells. This type of response is termed *cell-mediated immunity* (CMI). The second type

of response can be transferred by cell-free serum and therefore is called *humoral immunity* (Figure 19-6). The key to both these responses is the small lymphocyte, which until recently was relegated to a position of relative obscurity in textbooks of physiology and hematology. The small lymphocyte is formed in the bone marrow from precursor stem cells and then released into the circulation, eventually coming to rest in the lymphoid organs. The small lymphocytes specialize early in their life by passing through the thymus gland and differentiating into cells that will participate in CMI (T cells) or bypassing the thymus and undergoing differentiation into cells that will mediate humoral immunity (B cells). Despite the crucial differences between these two types of cells, they are morphologically indistinguishable by light microscopy.

Cell-mediated Immunity

Cell-mediated immunity (CMI, cellular immunity, transplantation immunity, or delayed hypersensitivity) is mediated by the lymphocyte that has passed through the thymus in its development. The exact mechanism of the thymic influence is not well understood in the human organism but is suspected of being hormonal. After the lymphocyte passes through the thymus in its develop-

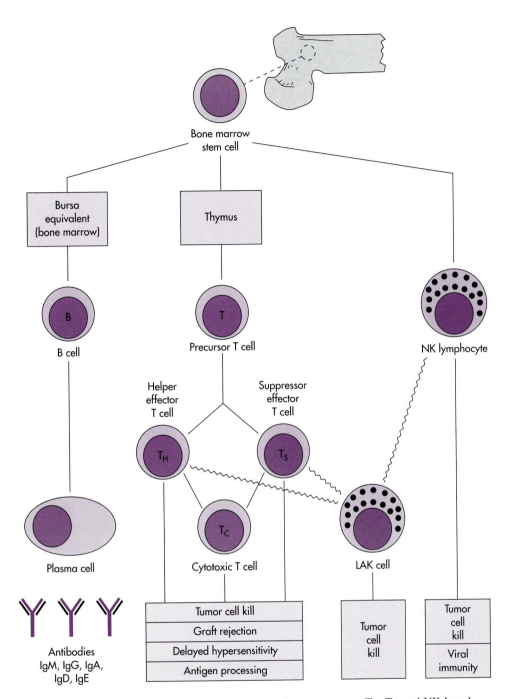

Figure 19-6 Development of effector cells within the immune system. T_H, T_S, and NK lympho-cytes require cytokine activation to differentiate into LAK cells.

ment, it remains under the influence of the thymus and is variously termed the *thymic-dependent lymphocyte, T lymphocyte*, or, simply, *T cell* (Figure 19-7).

Many studies, both in vivo and in vitro indicate that, in addition to that of T cells and B cells, a central role in the inductive phase of the immune response is played by "accessory cells" of the monocyte-macrophage series. After the injection of antigen, macrophages, in draining lymph nodes and in the spleen, trap and concentrate the antigen. Studies in vitro have shown that the production of antibodies involves the formation of clusters of lymphocytes around central macrophages or other dendritic cells with subsequent intimate contact of these accessory cells with B and T lymphocytes. Furthermore, if accessory cells are removed from cultures of lymphocytes, the immune response is, in large part, abrogated.

We now have a widely accepted mechanism that follows the injection of an immunogen that elucidates the

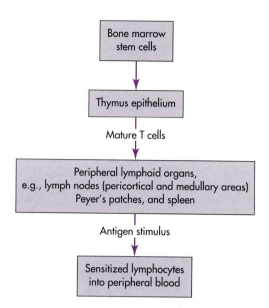

Figure 19-7 Progress of T cell lymphocyte maturation.

role of accessory cells in immune induction. By far the great majority of antigens involved in immune responses are proteins, and these responses depend on the presence of T cells. These antigens are therefore commonly referred to as T-dependent antigens and are to be distinguished from another major category of antigen, polysaccharides, which generally induce antibody in the absence of T cells and are thereby termed *thymus-independent responses*. Unlike B cells, T cells are not activated by free antigen. The antigen involved in T cell activation must be presented by other cells, such as macrophages or even B cells. These accessory, or antigen-presenting, cells play a crucial role in the processing of a polypeptide. The accessory cells break the polypeptide down intracellularly into smaller peptide fragments. Some of these peptide fragments become associated with glycoprotein molecules, which are coated by genes located in the major histocompatibility complex. These complexes of peptides and MHC molecules are somehow transported to the surface of the cell where they are recognized by the T cell receptor.

The key functions of the molecules coded for by the MHC and the T cell responses to such underlie the mechanism of the immunity response (Figure 19-8). These key functions are as follows: (1) establishing a T cell repertoire, as a consequence of the positive and negative selection events that occur when T lymphocyte precursors interact with MHC molecules expressed on the surface of accessory cells, and (2) activating mature T cells. The activation of mature T cells is the result of the antigen-specific T cell receptor interacting with antigen only when the polypeptide antigen is bound to the MHC molecule of an accessory cell. These polypeptide antigens are processed within an accessory cell, where smaller peptides between 10 and 20 amino acids in length are

produced. When these smaller peptides become associated with MHC molecules inside the cell, the complex can then be transported to the cell surface where it can be recognized by the T cell receptor (TcR). The combination of antigen-recognizing T and signal transducer CD 3 comprises the T cell receptor (TcR). The engagement of the T cell receptor (Ti-CD 3) by the antigen-class II complex is still insufficient to activate the T cells. This may be due to a low affinity of such reactions. This interaction of the Ti-CD 3 with the peptide-MHC class II is enhanced by yet another molecule, CD 4 (see Figure 19-8), found on the surface of yet another set of T cells, the CD 4 T cells. The function of the CD 4 seems to be to bind to a portion of the MHC class II molecule. In summary, the sequence of events leading to the activation of CD 4 T cells starts with the engagement of the Ti-CD 3 receptors that recognize the specific antigen in association with the class II molecule on an accessory cell, followed by the further stabilization of this molecular interaction through CD 4 class II association and through the cellular interaction of adhesion molecules. Thus, by a combination of antigen-specific and nonspecific interactions, sufficient receptors are engaged with sufficient energy to start the T cell on its activation route. The way in which T cells bind antigen provides a useful mechanism for avoiding engagement of T cells by free antigen. The interaction with free antigen is a role left to antibodies.

T cell activation results in the secretion of a number of antigen-nonspecific soluble factors known as lymphokines. Each lymphokine has a specific cell surface receptor, expressed on various different cell types. Soluble products released by lymphocytes, lymphokines belong to the general category of substances known as cytokines. Cytokines are soluble substances, produced by cells, that have various effects on other cells (see Table 19-2). The soluble products of monocytes are known as monokines. Substances produced by one of the leukocytes, which can in turn effect other leukocytes, are known as interleukins. As a consequence of T cell activation, many different cytokines are produced. These cytokines have profound effects, not only on the proliferation and differentiation of T cells but also on the activation and growth of many different cell types.

The thymus manufactures a large number of T lymphocytes. These T cells leave the thymus to enter the bloodstream, where they comprise about 60% of the peripheral blood lymphocytes. They then enter a unique pattern of recirculation, with many moving from blood to lymph node to thoracic duct; from there they return to the blood. In the lymph node most T cells reside in the deep cortex in areas in and between germinal centers. This pool of mature T lymphocytes is often called the recirculating pool of long-lived T lymphocytes (some undoubtedly memory cells), and some of these resting cells have been shown to live longer than 20 years without dividing. It is

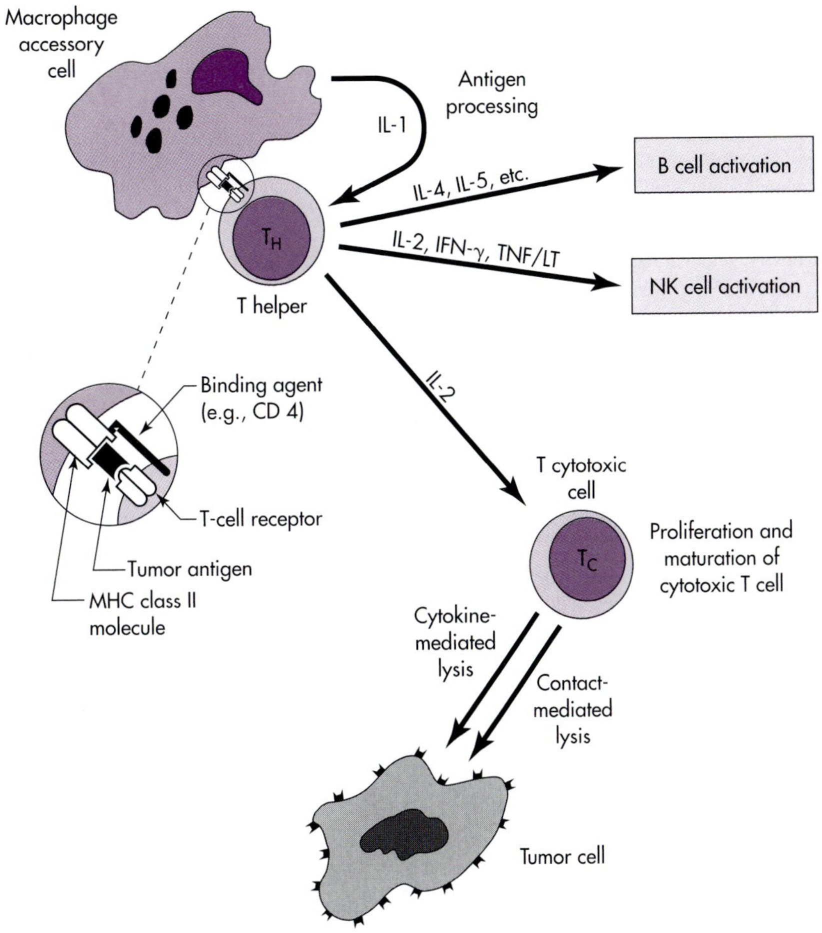

Figure 19-8 T cell activity in the immune response to malignancy. T helper cells (T_HMHC class II restricted) mediate effects by secretion of cytokines to activate other cells. T cytotoxic cells (T_CMHC class I restricted) mediate effects by direct lysis of tumor cells. The complex formed by the immunogenic peptide (antigen) bound in the cleft of a class II molecule is recognized by the antigen receptor on a specific helper T cell. A binding agent such as CD 4 is necessary to finally activate the T cell.

important to note that the path of recirculation does not involve the thymus; for unknown reasons, after a T cell leaves the thymus, it does not appear to return to it.

Subpopulations of T Cells

There are several subpopulations of T cells, each with a different function. There is substantial evidence for separate categories of functional T lymphocytes, such as the "helper" cell or "cytotoxic" or even "suppressor" cells (see Figure 19-6) but it is unclear whether these categories represent different functional states in the common differentiation pathway or have quite separate pathways of maturation. Normal T cells do not produce conventional immunoglobulin as is characteristic of B cells. However, T cells do have a crucial role in the regulation of immune responses by acting as potentiators or inhibitors of the B cell transition into immunoglobulin-secreting plasma cells. The cells that potentiate this B cell transition are classified as helper cells; those that inhibit

it are classified as suppressor cells. Suppressor cells have been identified in humans through a variety of circumstances. There is compelling evidence in mice and corroborating evidence in humans that help and suppression are mediated by distinct subsets of T cells, each genetically committed to mediate only one of these two functions. Other evidence suggests that immunoregulatory T cells may have an interim existence as inactive precursors, which might be referred to as pro-helper cells and pro-suppressor cells, that must react with a different set of activated T cells before maturing into fully functional helper effector cells or suppressor effector cells. Physiologically, suppressor cells may terminate excessive immune responses after antigenic exposure, and they probably provide a safeguard against autoimmune reactions. It is not surprising, therefore, that recent evidence from a number of animal models of autoimmunity suggests that impaired suppressor T cell function can lead to overt autoimmune disease.

An understanding of suppressor cell function in human neoplasia may alter the perspective and direction of oncologic researchers and clinicians. There is a real possibility that chemotherapy, radiation, and surgery might, in certain cases, benefit cancer patients by an indirect effect on suppressor cells, as well as the obvious effect on the neoplasm itself. New immunotherapeutic strategies that incorporate recent insight regarding the suppressor cell network are nullifying suppressor cell systems that oppose tumoricidal immune effector mechanisms. In addition to switching off antibody production by B cells, suppressor T cells apparently are also capable of preventing lymphokine production by other T cells.

Humoral Immunity

As the term suggests, *humoral immunity* is mediated by factors present in, and transferable by, serum; these include the classical antibody globulins. The cell responsible for the production of these antibodies is the second type of small lymphocyte, the B cell (Figure 19-9). In the chicken these lymphocytes aggregate in a small organ called the bursa of Fabricius. Removal of the bursa was noted to render the chicken unable to produce antibodies; the B cells have thus come to be known as bursa-dependent cells. In humans there was a great deal of controversy as to the origin of these cells but recent evidence has made it clear that these cells originate from the bone marrow and do not undergo maturation in the thymus. In humans (who have no bursa of Fabricius) no one organ appears to have control of the B cell production. Rather, B cells are distributed in all areas of lymphoid tissue, including the spleen, lymph nodes, tonsils, appendix, and Peyer's patches of the small intestine. With suitable stimulation, B cells become metabolically active and begin to synthesize antibodies with great facility. The antibodies soon become detectable in the cytoplasm and then are secreted into the surrounding medium. It is at this point that the B cell has undergone transformation into a plasma cell, which is the actual antibody producer. In a typical peripheral lymph node, B cells occupy the germinal centers and T cells occupy the cortical areas; these areas are referred to, respectively, as the bursa-dependent and thymus-dependent areas of the node. Although the bone marrow appears to be the source of cells destined to make antibodies, the bone marrow itself is not the locus of large-scale antibody formation. Rather, it is the site of intense lymphocyte proliferation leading to the production of mature B lymphocytes, which quickly leave the marrow and travel to peripheral lymphoid tissues. There they may meet the appropriate antigen, become stimulated to divide and differentiate into large lymphocytes and plasma cells, and actively manufacture antibodies. Resting B lymphocytes are the typical small lymphocytes of the peripheral blood and, in fact, cannot be distinguished from resting T lymphocytes under the usual light microscope (Table 19-4). Under the scanning

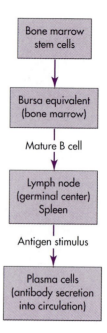

Figure 19-9 Progress of B cell lymphocyte maturation.

electron microscope, typical B cells have a hairy appearance with many small hairlike projections, whereas typical T cells are smoother (Figure 19-10). B lymphocytes are particularly plentiful in areas where antibody production occurs, for example, in the germinal centers of the lymph nodes and in the diffuse lymphoid tissue of the gastrointestinal and respiratory tracts. They are less common in the blood, rare in the lymphatics and thoracic duct, and virtually absent from the thymus.

There is clear evidence that the functional separation of T cells and B cells into two systems is not as clear-cut as formerly thought. An increasing number of biologically important responses are being discovered for which interplay of two systems is essential. This has been termed *T-B cooperation*. The presence of healthy T cells is necessary for production by B cells or many antibodies in response to antigenic stimulation and probably for the maintenance of immunologic memory for most antigens. The precise mechanism of this T-B cooperation is unknown; it may take the form of some messenger protein or actual physical contact and cytoplasmic bridging. Under suitable circumstances, B cells are capable of secreting some of the nonimmunoglobulin-soluble products (lymphokines) that were formerly thought to be characteristic of T cells. The biologic role of T-B cooperation is one of the most important areas for future research. There is much controversy regarding the order of production of immunoglobulins by the B cell. Currently it is thought that IgM is the first antibody produced, and then a switch to IgG production follows a signal possibly initiated by helper T cells. It has been theorized that IgD antedates the secretion of both IgM and IgG in embryonic life, as well as in the adult. This is one of many

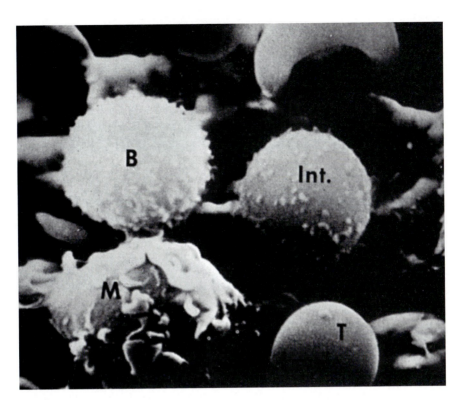

Figure 19-10 Scanning electron microscopic view of peripheral blood leukocytes. (*B*, B cell; *M*, macrophage; *T*, T cell; *Int.*, intermediate form, which may be of the "double cell" variety.)

Table 19-4   Comparison of T and B cells

T cells (thymus dependent)	B cells (thymus independent)
Bone marrow origin	**Bone marrow origin**
Mature in thymus	Mature in lymph node
Concentrated in paracortical areas of the lymph node	Concentrated in germinal centers of the lymph node
Long-lived (months to years)	Short-lived (days to weeks)
Circulate widely	Less mobile, concentrated in lymph nodes and spleen
Sensitive to phytohemagglutinin	Insensitive to phytohemagglutinin
Sensitive to pokeweed mitogen	Sensitive to pokeweed mitogen
No immunoglobulins	Synthesize immunoglobulins
Cell-mediated immunity	Humoral immunity
Delayed hypersensitivity	Antibody production
Produce lymphokines	Do not usually produce lymphokines

unanswered questions. Deficiencies of either or both of the thymic-dependent and bursa-dependent systems occur in various congenital and acquired diseases. A list of the primary immunodeficiency syndromes includes chronic granulomatous disease, Chediak-Higashi disease, Bruton syndrome, DiGeorge syndrome, ataxia-telangiectasia (Louis-Bar syndrome), and Wiskott-Aldrich syndrome. The incidence of spontaneously occurring malignancy is increased appreciably in most of these conditions.

Suppression of the immunologic responses is a natural result of certain biologic processes such as pregnancy and aging. It also occurs in several systemic diseases, as a result of radiation or drug therapy, and following severe injuries. In most instances CMI is suppressed more rapidly or profoundly than humoral immunity. With modern advances in immunologic techniques, the precise nature of the defect may be uncovered but is not known at present for many of these conditions. This kind of knowledge is essential if one is to treat these disorders effectively by immunologic means. Immunotherapy will be available in the near future but its effectiveness will depend on the accurate diagnosis of the relevant immunologic defect and selective reversal. Conditions such as malnutrition, surgical trauma, burns, and accidental injuries will result in suppression of the host defense mechanism. This should be kept in mind in the design of an overall treatment plan for any patient.

Interactions that Regulate Immune Responses

The discovery of a complex series of regulatory interactions among components of the immune system has proved to be a major advance in our understanding of the system. In the 1960s it was demonstrated that the development of the antibody responses depended on T cell–B cell interactions, and our perspective has now widened to reveal the workings of various genes, molecules, and cells in regulation of this immune system. It is known that genes of the system produce (1) antigen-specific receptors on lymphocyte surface membranes, (2) circulating antibodies that perform effective functions and exert feedback regulation, (3) crucial regulatory effects on various cell-cell interactions necessary for normal immunologic homeostasis, and (4) biologically active molecules capable of enhancing or suppressing T cell or B cell activity. The cells of the system are interdependent. The development of cell-mediated or humoral immunity, therefore, is regulated by a series of essential interactions between macrophages, T cells, and B cells. Regulatory interactions between constituents of the immune system may enhance or suppress the immune responses. The qualitative or quantitative response occurring in any given time,

however, will reflect the net effect of the extremely dynamic interplay among the system's components.

Immunosurveillance

The mechanisms used by the host to mount a response against any antigens that are expressed by a neoplasm are called immunosurveillance. The primary function of the immune system is to recognize and degrade foreign (non-self) antigens in the body that arise de novo or are inflicted on the host. In tumor surveillance the assumption is made that the mutant cell will express one or more antigens that can be recognized as non-self. A popular concept holds that mutant cells develop frequently in the human and are rapidly victimized by the ubiquitous and ideally competent immunologic mechanisms. Mice deprived of CMI and exposed to an oncogenic agent will spontaneously develop more tumors. This is regarded as evidence of an immunosurveillance mechanism. Patients with advanced disease are often more immunosuppressed than patients with early disease (Figure 19-11). Patients taking immunosuppressive drugs after renal transplantation have an increased incidence of malignancies (100 times greater than matched controls). Nearly 50% of these tumors in immunosuppressed individuals are of mesenchymal origin, for example, reticulum cell sarcomas, but a higher incidence of epithelial neoplasia, especially cervical intraepithelial neoplasia, has also been reported. Complementary evidence for the importance of tumor surveillance comes from the relationship between congenital or acquired immunodeficiency disease and tumor

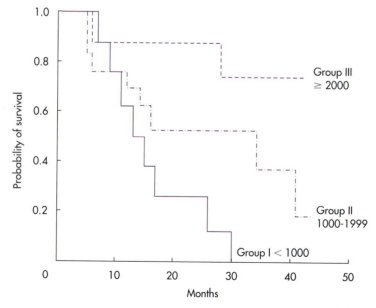

Figure 19-11 Patients with stage III cervical cancer who received optimal radiation therapy. Survival (months) is correlated with initial peripheral blood lymphocyte counts. (Reprinted with permission from DiSaia PJ, Morrow CP, Hill A et al: Immune competence and survival in patients with advanced cervical cancer; peripheral lymphocyte counts, *J Radiat Oncol* 4:449, 1978, Copyright 1978, Pergamon Press.)

development; these patients also demonstrate an incidence of malignancy far in excess of matched controls.

Although there are explanations of how immune surveillance may be circumvented by cancer, there is much less evidence that there is an immune mechanism for limiting tumor growth. Examples of tumor immunity have been demonstrated in experimental animals, particularly for early induced tumors and tumors induced by "strong" chemical carcinogens. However, other evidence indicates that tumors induced by "weak" carcinogens or those arising "spontaneously" are weakly antigenic or not antigenic at all. Evidence of tumor-limiting factors in humans is only circumstantial, and this is listed in the box below. Although this list is impressive at first glance, the number of patients exhibiting tumor immunity is relatively low. Most untreated human tumors grow without evidence of tumor immunity. Documented spontaneous regressions are rare and occur most often in tumors of embryonal tissue such as choriocarcinomas, hypernephromas, and neuroblastomas, suggesting developmental controlling factors rather than immunity. Regression of metastases without chemotherapy or radiation is extremely rare. Reappearance of metastases after long latent periods may be explained by several factors controlling dormancy other than immunity. Although infiltration of tumors by mononuclear cells is often used to support some role of the immune response in the fate of the tumor, there is limited evidence that such infiltration actually affects the growth of the tumor. The tumors found in immunosuppressed or immunodeficient patients are frequently of lymphoid elements, suggesting an abnormality in lymphocyte-controlling mechanism rather than specific tumor immunity. Finally, a number of immune abnormalities occur in the elderly, including loss of the thymic cortex and the appearance of a variety of autoantibodies. However, there is no directly demonstrable cause-and-effect relationship between abnormality of the immune response associated with aging and the increased incidence of cancer associated with aging. In summary, the role of immunity in immunosurveillance against newly arising tumors remains controversial.

Takasugi, Mickey, and Terasaki call attention to the role of NK lymphocytes in the immunosurveillance of tumors. NK cells from several species preferentially destroy malignant target cells in vitro and appear to need no prior sensitization. Indeed, NK cells may be the effectors of tumor surveillance.

One of the major predictions of the immunosurveillance theory is that tumor development should be associated with, in fact be preceded by, depressed immunity. Several observations fit this prediction, including the fact that kidney allograft recipients who have received immunosuppressive drugs and have a high risk of developing lymphoproliferative and other tumors also have severely depressed NK activity. Many other observations of the animal system support the possibility that one of the requisites for tumor induction by carcinogenic agents may be interference with host defenses, including those mediated by NK cells.

Doubt is cast on the validity of the theory of immune surveillance by the finding that the incidence of tumors in athymic mice, which have no T cell-mediated response, is no higher than incidence in their normal counterparts. However, such athymic mice have normal or, in some instances, increased numbers of NK cells.

Escape from Surveillance (Figure 19-12)

There are several postulated mechanisms by which mutant cells might avoid an interaction with a potentially damaging immune system.

Lowered tumor antigenicity (antigenic modulation)

Neoplasms that arise spontaneously are noted to be considerably less antigenic than those induced experimentally. Many human tumors may be weakly antigenic or nonantigenic. In addition, antigenic modulation may occur. Antigenic modulation is a loss of antigenicity or a change in the antigenic markers by which tumor cells may avoid immunologic destruction. Antigenic modulation has been demonstrated with murine leukemia cells expressing thymic lymphocyte (TL) antigens. When these tumor cells are grown in the presence of cytotoxic serum that contains anti-TL antibodies, certain cells lose their TL antigens, perhaps by shedding or internalization of membrane receptors. These variants become predominant in the culture. However, removal of the antiserum leads to the reappearance of the TL antigens. This indicates that the antigenic selection has not taken place but that specific antibodies suppress the production of the corresponding antigen.

CIRCUMSTANTIAL EVIDENCES FOR TUMOR-LIMITING FACTORS IN HUMANS

1. Spontaneous regression
2. Self-healing melanomas
3. Regression of metastases after resection of primary neoplasms
4. Regression of tumor after "noncytotoxic" doses of chemotherapy
5. Reappearance of metastasis after long latent periods
6. Frequent failure of circulating tumor cells to form metastases
7. Infiltration of tumors by mononuclear cells
8. Higher incidence of tumors after clinical immunosuppression
9. High incidence of tumors in immune deficiency diseases
10. Increased incidence of malignancy with aging

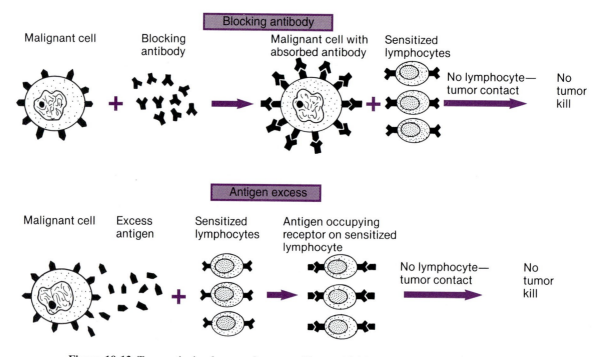

Figure 19-12 Two methods of escape from surveillance: (1) blocking antibody absorbed onto antigen sites on tumor cell surface, and (2) excess antigen flooding the tumor cell environment, preventing lymphocyte attack.

Sneaking through

Old et al. report neoplastic systems in which large inocula of immunogenic tumor cells fail to grow in a syngeneic recipient but smaller doses will grow and eventually overwhelm the host. The mechanism of "sneaking through" is unknown but it may be related to the time of vascularization of the neoplasm.

Immunoresistance

Diminished sensitivity to rejection may develop in the same way that bacteria develop resistance to antibodies after repeated exposure. The cells may develop a decrease in cell surface antigenic sites (antigenic modulation) or relevant antibody-binding sites. Another mechanism that is easy to conceive calls for antigenic molecules or receptors for cytokines on the surface of the tumor cell to be shed in large amounts into the surrounding extracellular fluid. The cell surface will then be rendered relatively immunoresistant as its locality becomes flooded with excess antigens or receptors. This may be classified then as a "blocking factor." Some suggest that tumors that shed antigen rapidly are those of low immunogenicity and metastasize most rapidly.

Vascularization

Tumors probably reach 1-2 mm in diameter before vascularization takes place. Folkman and Hochberg suggested that the vessels result from ingrowth of host cells, and thus the endothelium of the tumor vessels may be recognized as "self" and not rejected. Therefore some neoplasms may proliferate with their antigens locked away behind a wall of "normal" endothelial cells unpenetrated by attack lymphocytes.

Immunosuppression

It has been well established that the presence of a cancer can significantly reduce an individual's capacity to mount a response to a great variety of antigens. Immunosuppressive factors have been described in the serum of cancer patients and confirmed in vitro. The mechanism by which these factors cause immunosuppression is not understood, but some authors have suggested that they suppress macrophage function. Some degree of immunosuppression has been found in almost all cancer patients studied. DNCB, DNFB, and a variety of skin test antigens have been used on patients with gynecologic malignancies. An increase in tumor burden is associated with a decreased percentage of patients responding to these tests, and both are associated with poorer prognoses.

Certain types of tumors synthesize compounds, such as prostaglandins, that reduce many aspects of the immune responsiveness. The role of prostaglandins in the mechanism whereby tumors escape destruction by the immune system is unclear.

Although the mechanism suggested in the preceding paragraph is nonspecific suppression, antigen-specific suppressor T cells may also play an important role in the regulation of the immune response to an antigen. An increase in tumor-specific suppressor T cells has been demonstrated in many experimental systems, especially in patients with advanced malignancy. Whether this increase can be attributed to immunologically specific suppressor mechanisms or to a more generalized suppression mediated by tumor cells is unknown at this time.

Blocking factors

Neoplasms may escape the immune mechanism by the development of systemic factors that abrogate the usual interaction with host defense capabilities. Several serum factors have been identified in vitro: blocking antibodies, antigen-antibody complexes, and soluble antigen excess. When these blocking factors are operational, the state of the tumor-host relationship is one of tumor enhancement. The mechanisms involved may be quite similar to those described under immunoresistance. Excess free antibody may saturate antigenic sites on the cell surface, or conversely, excess free antigen may paralyze lymphocyte activity. In addition, recent studies suggest that the cellular factors of the immune system may be capable of causing tumor enhancement. In some animal and in vivo systems, small numbers of sensitized (tumor specific) lymphocytes can enhance tumor growth, whereas larger numbers of the same cells will retard growth. This phenomenon has been referred to as immunostimulation, and if valid it will help to explain the emergence of neoplasms beyond the subclinical stage where tumor cell numbers are small and vulnerable. The puzzle is made more difficult because "deblocking" factors have also been described in the serum of cancer patients undergoing remission or following surgical debulking procedures. The mechanism involved in deblocking is unknown.

IMMUNOPROPHYLAXIS

Immunoprophylaxis is the induction of resistance to a tumor before its origination and should be clearly separated from immunotherapy, which is the treatment of established neoplasms and is a more difficult problem. Everyone interested in tumor immunology dreams of successes with immunoprophylaxis similar to those achieved with bacterial and viral illnesses. Immunoprophylaxis theoretically may be achieved by immunization either against the etiologic agent of the cancer, for example, an oncogenic virus, or against the tumor-specific cell surface antigens of the neoplasm. However, the oncogenic viruses of human cancer (if they exist) have not as yet been clearly identified, and even if they exist there is uncertainty whether transmission is vertical or horizontal. The tumor-specific cell surface antigens needed for the other approach have not as yet been adequately purified. Both pathways can be made to work in animal systems but have not been truly tested in humans. Some indirect confirmation comes from studies such as that of Rosenthal et al., who reported a retrospective analysis of the leukemia death rate in an infant population from Chicago who received Bacillus

Calmette-Guérin (BCG) vaccine compared with a similar population who had not received the vaccine. During the period 1964 to 1969, the death rate in the infants who were not vaccinated was 6-7 times greater than the vaccinated group. At least one other study from Canada confirms the Rosenthal et al. study, but others have not.

Prophylaxis against tumors by vaccination depends on immunologic reactivity between the immunogen and the tumor. Thus, at least theoretically, it should be feasible to immunize against only virally induced tumors and other tumors that exhibit immunologic reactivity. For example, positive reactivity has been demonstrated among patients who have Burkitt's lymphoma, nasopharyngeal carcinoma, melanoma, and neuroblastoma, suggesting the possibility of preparing tumor vaccines for prophylactic purposes. However, it should be remembered that immunization would not necessarily result in protection against the tumor. It may lead to induction of immune complexes (such as blocking antibodies) that will enhance rather than impede tumor growth and metastasis. Such considerations must be taken into account before any trial of immunization.

PRINCIPLES OF IMMUNOTHERAPY

It is obvious that the ultimate goal of immunotherapy is the complete destruction of all neoplastic cells. Short of obtaining that, the suppression of growth of tumor cells is desired. An expression of this therapeutic effect would be the prolongation of remission and the prevention of the appearance of metastatic disease. More often than not, the immunotherapist must be satisfied with evidence that the approach has achieved at least a reduction in the mass of tumor cells. Before the institution of immunotherapy, it is crucial to reduce tumor mass to a minimum, preferably less than 10^8 cells, by whatever means at hand—radical surgical procedures, chemotherapy, or irradiation therapy. It has been shown that immunotherapy can achieve little against an overwhelming tumor burden, and single-agent immunotherapy by itself appears to be relatively ineffectual. At present it is always used with other cancericidal modalities, which are depended on to significantly reduce the tumor burden. As one would expect, immunotherapy has shown more effectiveness in neoplasms that are highly antigenic, such as Burkitt's lymphoma, malignant melanoma, and neuroblastoma.

Most clinical trials to date have utilized single immunoactive agents ineffectively. In fact, several elements of the immune system are probably necessary and should be orchestrated in as yet an unknown manner to achieve the desired effect. Immunotherapeutic approaches can be classified into two broad categories: (1) active, those that attempt to induce in the host a state of immune responsiveness to the tumor; or (2) passive, those that transfer directly to the host immunologically active substances that mediate an antitumor response themselves. There is overlap, such as monoclonal antibodies (passive), that induce a host-specific antitumor response (active). In general, however, the classification is appropriate; and both active and passive can be further subdivided into specific and nonspecific. Most important, the reader should fully comprehend the embryonic nature of immunotherapy, and an attitude of cautious optimism must be maintained as this fetal area of research is brought to full term.

Active Immunotherapy (box below)
Nonspecific

Central to tumor immunology and especially to active immunotherapy is the question of whether antigens recognizable by the host exist on the surface of the tumor cell. One of the theoretical concerns about active immunotherapy as a proposed modality is the apparent lack of a response in the host observed in the setting of a progressively growing tumor. Recognition of this fact has led to several approaches designed to increase the immunogenicity of these human tumors. These have included co-stimulation with biological immunostimulants, including BCG, MER, *C. parvum*, and other products.

A substance that increases response to an antigen is an adjuvant. Adjuvants may be effective by altering the antigen itself or the immunologic reaction to the antigen. In the former instance one can postulate a mechanism whereby the adjuvant would increase the release of antigen. Nonspecific immunotherapy directed toward the reaction to the antigen has focused on the cellular response. Later studies suggest, however, at least two cellular cytotoxic mechanisms. One involves thymus-processed cytotoxic cells (T cells), which recognize target antigens, and the other is controlled by a thymus-independent effector cell system, which is independent of the target antigen. The latter system is triggered to kill by recognition of antibody bound to the target, and it refutes our previously held simplistic view that stimulation of the cellular mechanism is beneficial whereas humoral immunity is of no aid.

The most widely used nonspecific immunotherapy has employed adjuvants such as BCG, *Corynebacterium parvum* (*C. parvum*), levamisole, and MER. BCG is a live, attenuated strain of *Mycobacterium bovis*. *C. parvum* is a gram-negative anaerobe given in a nonviable form. Levamisole is a synthetic antihelminthic drug that has been found to have significant effects on tumor immunity. MER is a methanol extraction of killed tuberculin bacilli (BCG).

The current era of experimentation with bacterial products began in 1959, when Old et al. demonstrated that injection of BCG was capable of inhibiting growth of tumors in mice. BCG had been introduced into clinical medicine in 1921 with its use as a vaccine against tuberculosis. Since 1921, many effects of BCG stimulating nonspecific immune responses in animals and humans have been demonstrated. Both humoral antibody synthesis and CMI are stimulated by BCG treatment. Mice injected with BCG show an increased resistance to infection with bacteria and are capable of clearing endotoxin and injected carbon particles far more rapidly than untreated mice. BCG injection leads to activation of macrophages as manifested by enhanced phagocytosis, increased microbicidal activity, increased macrophage metabolism, and increased ability of macrophages to kill tumor cell monolayer cultures. The most dramatic work with BCG was that of Rapp et al. with transplantable hepatoma in guinea pigs. They demonstrated that injection of BCG in growing intradermal tumor nodules was capable of eliminating the local nodule and eradicating tumor cells in draining lymph nodes. The dramatic response seen with guinea pig hepatoma may be caused by cross-reactive antigens between BCG and this animal tumor. Recent evidence has shown that BCG may cross-react with antigens on human melanoma cells. In humans, BCG has been used primarily in three ways: (1) intralesional injection; (2) systemic administration, generally by scarification or intradermal injection; and (3) mixed with cells and administered as a vaccine.

Intralesional use of BCG has largely been confined to treatment of cutaneous recurrences of malignant melanoma. In one series, approximately 90% of over 700 intracutaneously injected lesions in 36 patients could be made to undergo complete regression by BCG injection. Subcutaneous and visceral deposits of melanoma, however, are far more resistant to BCG treatment. Uninjected nodules surrounding the injected lesion that also undergo regression are always in the drainage area of the injected nodule. It appears that direct contact between BCG and the tumor is essential for the therapeutic effect.

ACTIVE IMMUNOTHERAPY

Nonspecific

Biological immunostimulants—BCG, MER, *C. parvum*, OK 432, etc.

Chemical immunostimulants—levamisole, cimetidine, lysosomes containing macrophage-activating substances

Chemotherapeutic agents—Cyclophosphamide, doxorubicin, vinca alkaloids, cisplatin

Cytokines—interferon, IL-2, TNF

Specific

Inactivated tumor vaccines (autologous, allogeneic) Monoclonal tumor autoidiotypic antibodies Human tumor hybrids (with xenogeneic antigen-bearing fusion partners)

BCG administered intradermally by direct injection or by scarification techniques has been used in patients who have leukemia or one of a variety of solid tumors. Most of the evidence for antitumor activity of BCG used systemically is derived from experiments involving pretreatment of animals. As immunotherapy in the treatment of established experimental tumors, it is remarkably ineffective.

Corynebacterium parvum, like BCG, belongs to a group of bacterial agents that have stimulatory effects on the reticuloendothelial system, increase the phagocytic capacity of macrophages, and increase the resistance of animals to both infections and subsequent implantation or induction of experimental tumors. *C. parvum* is also active by direct intralesional injection. In animal systems, *C. parvum* given intravenously can induce regression of established local and pulmonary metastasis. *C. parvum* was originally administered subcutaneously in combination with chemotherapy, and now several trials are under way using this immunopotentiator intravenously. When used intravenously, the drug produces high fever and shaking chills, and some patients have experienced thrombotic thrombocytopenic purpura. Some investigators suggest that its action may be to cause release of TNF. Unlike BCG, *C. parvum* seems to act primarily by stimulating macrophage function; its effect on T cell immunity is less clear. Trials have been conducted in solid tumor therapy without notable success.

A second group of substances includes a variety of synthetic compounds that are believed to be immunostimulants (e.g., levamisole, cimetidine, and others). These substances have demonstrated some effects on the immune system, including increases in delayed-type hypersensitivity response, total number of T cells, increased lymphocyte proliferation, and mitogenic response. Firm evidence that these changes in immune parameters translate to improved tumor control is not available.

Levamisole has been studied in animal systems, where it has shown to potentiate the antibody and delayed hypersensitivity responses to a variety of antigens. It appears that levamisole can potentiate or permit expression of established delayed-type hypersensitivity reactions in previously immunocompetent individuals. One mechanism of levamisole action may be by causing maturation of thymus-derived immature lymphocyte precursors. It has been termed by some an *immunomodulator* in that it seems to reconstitute immunologic competence in patients who are immunosuppressed. Administration of levamisole before or concurrent with a bacterial adjuvant may augment the activity of the latter.

MER is the methanol extraction residue of BCG and was devised to overcome the problems associated with viable BCG preparations, including systemic BCG infection. This material, which is supplied as a particulate aqueous suspension has shown both immunoprophylactic and immunotherapeutic activity comparable to that of BCG in a variety of animal models. It is administered intradermally or subcutaneously to humans. It produces severe local reactions characterized by inflammatory ulceration and/or sterile abscess formation. MER appears to be more immunopotentiating than BCG in humans and can restore established delayed hypersensitivity in approximately 20% of patients with widely metastatic solid tumors. A number of clinical trials with MER have been completed with little success.

A third class of drugs includes chemotherapeutic agents such as cyclophosphamide, doxorubicin, and others. These agents are presumed to work by inhibiting suppressor mechanisms.

Active nonspecific immune mechanisms can also be evoked by a variety of natural and recombinant cytokines. The three major species of interferons (alpha, beta, and gamma) have in vitro and in vivo antitumor effects. IL-2 is a glycoprotein acting to cause T cell proliferation after an initial antigen recognition and presentation. Another directly cytotoxic and/or cytostatic cytokine is TNF.

Specific

Tumor immunotherapy has been under study with extensive clinical trials, but less has been attempted using specific immunotherapy as compared with nonspecific modes. Specific immunotherapy can be active, passive, or adoptive.

Active specific immunotherapy calls for administration to the cancer patient of tumor cells (vaccines) or their equivalent, bearing antigens that will cross-react with the neoplasm. Tumor antigens are usually weakly antigenic, so that often immunostimulants (e.g., BCG) are administered jointly. Other attempts to heighten the immunogenicity of the tumor cells have been studied, such as surface changes by enzymes, viral incorporation, physical treatments, and chemical modifications. Although this remains an exciting field for future research, trials to date in humans have been disappointing.

Several cancer vaccines are under development and some of these have reached the point of clinical trials. Various approaches include:

1. Use of synthetic peptides representing the immunoglobulin epitope of B-cell malignancies
2. Fusion of cancer cells with activated B lymphocytes to increase cytotoxic T-lymphocyte recognition of tumor cells
3. Injections of gene complexes into tumor cell nuclei, which render the transformed cells capable of secreting large amounts of cytokine into the surrounding area

Some studies suggest that antibodies to murine monoclonal antitumor antibodies (so-called anti-idiotype) might resemble antigen and evoke a specific host antitumor response. Other modifications of the tumor cell potentially to increase antigenicity involve chemical treatment of the cell surface, including stripping off sialic acid residues. All these approaches have yet to demonstrate effectiveness in humans.

Passive Adoptive Immunotherapy (box below)

The use of immunological reagents like monoclonal antibodies or the adoptive transfer of cells to mediate direct antitumor response (without requiring a host response) has been a subject of much study. The earliest studies used heterologous sera obtained from immunized humans or animals. These did not have convincing efficacy and have largely been abandoned. The development of monoclonal antibodies allowed the evolution of potentially powerful new serologic reagents for the diagnosis and treatment of patients with cancer. The development of the lymphokine interleukin-2 made possible the in vitro propagation of T lymphocytes taken from the peripheral blood or directly from tumors, which allowed their use in human therapeutic protocols. The demonstration that IL-2 could also induce a subset of normal lymphoid cells to lyse tumor, a phenomenon we have termed *lymphokine-activated killing* (LAK), has also been exploited in immunotherapy trials.

Nonspecific

Nonspecific immunotherapies include the use of LAK cells, activated macrophages, and the directly cytotoxic or cytostatic cytokines such as interferon (alpha, beta, and gamma) and TNF.

In the mid-1980s passive immunotherapy with sensitized cells, referred to as adoptive immunotherapy, received a resurgence of interest because of the work of

---

PASSIVE ADOPTIVE IMMUNOTHERAPY

Nonspecific

LAK cells—generated by IL-2
Activated macrophages—interferon
Cytostatic or cytotoxic cytokines—interferon and TNF

Specific

Heterologous antiserum from an immunized human
Monoclonal antibodies—murine or human
Radiotherapeutic coupled to alpha- or beta-emitting radionuclides
Chemotherapeutic—Adriamycin, methotrexate, or ricin conjugates
Biologic—complement fixation or antibody dependent and cellular cytotoxic mechanisms
T lymphocytes—autologous, allogeneic, or xenogeneic from in vitro sensitization or tumor-draining lymph nodes
Allogeneic bone marrow transplants with ablative chemotherapy or radiation therapy (graft vs tumor)

Steven Rosenberg using activated lymphocytes. Leukopheresis machines were used to remove circulating lymphocytes from patients. These lymphocytes were then treated with a lymphokine called Interleukin-2 (IL-2). This converted the lymphocytes into lymphokine-activated killer (LAK) cells that were capable of destroying cancer cells but not normal cells. These LAK cells were infused along with IL-2 back into the patient. The IL-2 induced the LAK cells to multiply for a short time in the body, thus enhancing their ability to destroy cancer cells. The development of the genetically engineered or recombinant form of IL-2 in 1984 made available to scientists a large amount of this substance, which was necessary for treating patients in clinical trials. Rosenberg noted that the adoptive transfer of LAK cells plus additional IL-2 administration was capable of mediating regression of established pulmonary and hepatic metastasis in a variety of human neoplasms. The dose-limiting toxicity for IL-2 was noted at 100,000 units per kilogram by intravenous bolus every 8 hours, and that toxicity consisted primarily of capillary permeability leak, which can lead to intravascular fluid leaking into subcutaneous tissue. In October 1987 Rosenberg reported on 104 patients treated in this manner. A total of seven complete regressions were noted in patients who had renal cell carcinoma, melanoma, colorectal cancer, or non-Hodgkin's lymphoma in a very advanced state. The longest response was 36 months in a patient with widespread melanoma who received a single treatment. The mechanism by which adoptive transfer of LAK cells in conjunction with IL-2 (Figure 19-13) is effective in humans is as yet unclear, and the role of IL-2 and the LAK cell remains to be defined. Murine studies suggest that IL-2 leads to the general proliferation of LAK cells in vivo when given alone and that responsiveness is in part dictated by the immunogenicity of the tumor. Refinement of the technique for improved effectiveness was anticipated.

West and his colleagues reported another series of patients using adoptive immunotherapy involving constant infusion rather than bolus-dose recombinant Interleukin-2 as well as LAK cells. Forty patients were reported in 1987, and there were 13 partial responses in a variety of neoplasms. The authors concluded that administering IL-2 by constant infusion rather than by bolus-dose was less toxic.

Studies of tumor-infiltrating lymphocytes (TILs) in mice suggested to Rosenberg et al. that other populations of IL-2-stimulated cytotoxic cells might provide more effective antitumor activity than LAK cells. Both human and murine tumors are known to be infiltrated by a variety of host immune cells, including significant numbers of T cells or TILs. Because tumor growth occurs despite the presence of these cells, freshly extracted TILs would not be expected to have significant antitumor activity. A method for activating and expanding these cells was

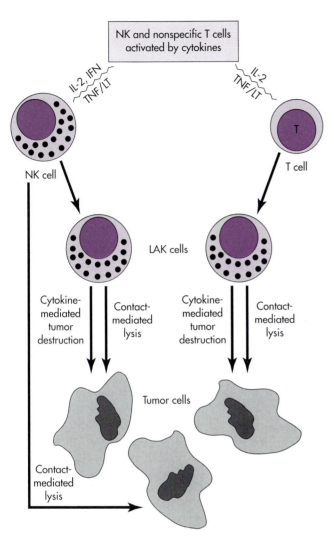

Figure 19-13 Role of the NK and LAK cells in the immune response to malignancy. NK (natural killer) cells are the first line of defense against growth of transformed cells. LAK (lymphokine activated killer) cells are IL-2 dependent and are nongenetically restricted killer cells.

required, and again IL-2 proved to be crucial. Initial experience with murine TIL therapy revealed two significant remaining limitations on adapting this therapy to patient protocols. Tumor-infiltrating lymphocytes could not be generated from nonimmunogenic tumors and were not effective against large, advanced tumor burdens in mice. Subsequent modifications of the techniques for TIL culture, as well as adjuvant therapies directed at the TIL recipient, have partially addressed these limitations. In searching for sources of lymphocytes with antitumor activity in the tumor-bearing hosts, a second site outside the tumor itself was found where T cells demonstrated this activity. Within the lymph nodes that drain the tumor site are lymphocytes with many features similar to TILs. These lymphocytes have the opportunity to be tumor sensitized, and with the proper stimulation and expansion

in culture, they can be shown to have activity against established murine tumors.

The concept of generating and augmenting antitumor activity in an immune-cell population, expanding these cells in vitro, and readministering them in the treatment of cancer has considerable appeal. Evidence to suggest that this can be done effectively has existed in preclinical animal systems for some time. More recently, preliminary data suggest that it can be applied successfully to the treatment of some human tumors. Models demonstrating the effectiveness of LAK cells, TILs, and tumor-draining lymph node lymphocytes have provided the technology to obtain cells for some early trials. Areas for research are related to the survival and localization of adoptively transferred cells in the tumor-bearing host and the precise mechanism and effectors of tumor regression. Ongoing investigation should be watched carefully but the data to date suggest that this costly approach may be associated with morbidity that far outweighs the limited success.

Specific

An example of passive specific immunotherapy would be producing antisera to a patient's cancer in an animal (a great deal of absorption of foreign antigens would be necessary before use) or another cancer patient and then injecting the antisera into the patient. Passive transfer of antibodies has been attempted with no significant results. With further knowledge of the precarious role of antibodies, much less enthusiasm has recently been noted, except in the area of "deblocking antibodies." Monoclonal antibodies are produced by hybridoma techniques. This involves immunizing an animal with antigen and fusing its spleen cells with a long-lived malignant B cell line (Figure 19-14). Subsequently, antibodies produced by the fused, normal, and malignant B cells are selected for their ability to recognize an antigen of interest. To tumor cells, this would represent a tumor-differentiation antigen or a tumor-associated antigen. The advantage of this approach is that large quantities of antibodies, specific only for antigens on tumors and not antigens present on normal cells, can be produced. Similar strategies have been used in humans to produce human monoclonal antibodies from human splenocytes but with much less success. The majority of currently available monoclonal antibodies come from murine sources. However, recombinant biologic techniques have also been applied to obtain monoclonal antibodies and this technology should be helpful in promoting the development of human products. The potential use of monoclonal antibodies (Mabs) that recognize tumor associated antigens is far reaching. While monoclonal antibodies directed against tumor cell surface determinants can inhibit tumor cell proliferation in culture and in animals, direct administration to patients has found limited success to date. Monoclonal antibodies could be of benefit in clearing tumor cells from the blood and in diminishing the amount

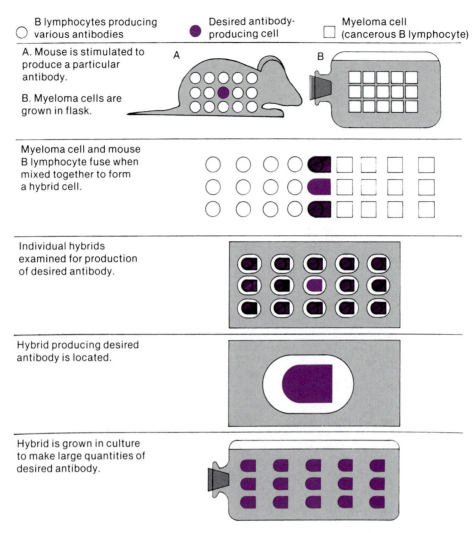

○ B lymphocytes producing various antibodies   ● Desired antibody-producing cell   ☐ Myeloma cell (cancerous B lymphocyte)

A. Mouse is stimulated to produce a particular antibody.

B. Myeloma cells are grown in flask.

Myeloma cell and mouse B lymphocyte fuse when mixed together to form a hybrid cell.

Individual hybrids examined for production of desired antibody.

Hybrid producing desired antibody is located.

Hybrid is grown in culture to make large quantities of desired antibody.

Figure 19-14 Hybridoma technique for production of monoclonal antibodies.

of circulating tumor antigen that could have a blocking effect on subsequent immunotherapy. Monoclonal antibodies can also be attached to antitumor drugs, toxins, or radionuclides. The rationale of this latter approach would be to target toxic substances directly to the tumor cells and spare normal cells. This approach has been piloted with some success.

IMMUNODIAGNOSIS

Immunodiagnosis is a field of investigative medicine largely based on the science of radioimmunoassay. Substances that are antigenic in animals or that can be bound to antigens can be measured in body fluids in very low concentrations. Tumor immunodiagnosis depends on the liberation by tumors of such substances into the bloodstream or other body fluids in a form or concentra-

tion not commonly found in healthy individuals. These substances, usually called tumor markers, are sometimes referred to as antigens, although they may not necessarily produce an immune response in the tumor-bearing host. Other substances may actually play a role in immunodiagnosis, such as hormones or the pregnancy-associated proteins. Tumor-associated antigens and oncofetal antigens have been the major interest of tumor immunologists. In humans, evidence for the liberation of specific neoantigens is scanty, and in ovarian cancer early claims of the specificity of tumor extract antigenicity by Levi and Barber have awaited confirmation. Tumor-associated antigens have been roughly identified and characterized by Gall, Walling, and Pearl and DiSaia. However, these antigens appear to have a unique ability to camouflage themselves among the normal proteins of the cell, defying attempts at refined isolation. Since the foundation of modern immunodiagnosis is the radioimmunoassay, one must have an absolutely pure antigen to begin the process that will lead to a clinically useful tool.

Secreted products released into the bloodstream provide the best diagnostic markers to date. The most useful of these are myeloma proteins produced by plasma cell myelomas, alpha-fetoprotein produced by hepatocellular carcinomas, and teratocarcinoma containing yolk sac elements, and carcinoembryonic antigen, produced by tumors of the gastrointestinal tract. Human chorionic gonadotropin is another example of an excellent tumor marker for gestational trophoblastic disease.

Monoclonal antibodies using the hybridoma technique (Figure 19-14) are being employed by investigators in many scientific disciplines and have led to a revolution in diagnostic immunology. With respect to cancer immunodiagnosis, monoclonal antibodies have aided in the recognition and identification of tumor-associated antigens (differentiation antigens and other marker molecules) with heretofore unobtainable specificity. Such antigenic determinants have been described on or in tumor cells from patients with leukemia and malignant lymphoma, as well as a variety of solid tumors including melanoma and carcinomas of the lung, breast, prostate, and gastrointestinal tract. In addition to their role in detection, monoclonal agents can be used as immunoadsorbents to purify and characterize tumor-associated antigens. Although truly "tumor-specific" antigens do not exist, the exquisite resolving power of monoclonal antibodies provides a means to detect antigens present on tumor cells that are not commonly found on normal adult tissue cells. These antigenic differences can conceivably be exploited in several ways relating to diagnosis, staging, and the treatment of cancer patients. Circulating antigens secreted or shed by tumor cells can be detected by monoclonal antibodies employed as serologic reagents. Detection of circulating tumor antigen in this way would be helpful both in initial diagnosis and serially monitoring the results of therapy. Monoclonal antibodies to tumor and to normal tissue antigens appear valuable as immunohistologic reagents for the analysis of lymphoid infiltrates in lymph nodes, improved taxonomy of lymphomas and leukemias, and primary identification of undifferentiated carcinomas or adenocarcinomas of an unknown origin. These examples illustrate how monoclonal antibodies seem certain to lead to earlier diagnosis and more accurate classification of malignant neoplasms.

With regard to staging, monoclonal antibodies directed to tumor antigens or markers also offer a promising approach. Photoscanning after injection of radiolabeled monoclonal antibodies can be used to identify sites of tumor involvement that might otherwise go unrecognized. This will reduce the likelihood of understaging patients and of administering inadequate therapy. Although a number of problems remain, studies in animals and preliminary data in patients suggest that staging with radiolabeled monoclonal antibodies is likely to become available for clinical use in the near future.

BIOLOGIC RESPONSE MODIFIERS

Biologic response modifier (BRM) is a term that includes the many agents and approaches to the treatment of cancer with mechanism of action that involve modulation of the individual's own biologic responses. BRMs are molecules produced by the body to regulate cellular response. Activation of host responses, particularly the host immune response, has been the ideal of therapists for many generations, but recent technologic advances have improved our understanding and made manipulation of biologic responses a practical goal in therapy. Because of these recent advantages, biologic response-modifying therapy is now a reality, and BRMs are likely to be valuable in increasing our understanding of cancer biology and improving cancer therapeutics in this decade. Indeed, the Biological Response Modifiers Program is a comprehensive program of the Division of Cancer Treatment, National Cancer Institute, intended to investigate, develop, and bring to clinical trials potentially therapeutic agents that may alter biologic responses important in cancer growth and metastasis.

Cytokines (see Table 19-2)

The term *cytokines* defines a large group of secreted polypeptides released by living cells that act nonenzymatically to regulate cellular functions. These cellular functions include regulation of immune cell activity (interferons and interleukins), hematopoiesis (colony stimulating factor) and regulation of proliferation and differentiation (e.g., TGFa, EGF). This chapter will discuss only those that affect the immune system. Lymphokines and other cytokines have a specific ability to regulate certain components of the immune response, which may be useful in altering the growth of cancer in humans. There are early indications of a specific ability of these substances to alter immune responses in ways that may be beneficial in the host-tumor interaction. For example, it is possible that certain cytokines or lymphokines may augment the ability of T cells to respond to tumor-associated antigens, and others may induce higher responsiveness with respect to B cell activity in cancer patients. Lymphokines also decrease suppressive functions of the immune system and may be useful in enhancing immune responses by lessening the suppressive effects of suppressive factors or suppressive cells in cancer patients. Another specific use of lymphokines may be in the pharmacologic regulation of tumors of the lymphoid system. Although many of these malignant tissues are considered to be unresponsive to normal growth-controlling mechanisms mediated by lymphokines, it is possible that the large quantities of pure lymphokines, administered pharmacologically, or the use of certain molecular analogues of these naturally occurring lymphokines, may be useful in the treatment of lymphoid malignancies. A further use of lymphokines may be the manipulation of the immune response in vitro to produce products that may subsequently be used therapeutically in vivo. Interleukin-1 alpha or beta activates resting T cells and makes early hematopoietic progenitors more sensitive to other factors. It also stimulates the synthesis of other cytokines, including possibly IL-2. IL-2 is also known as T cell growth factor. Pharmacologic doses of these lymphokines can conceivably be used to alter the maturation and kinetic capabilities of various T cell malignancies. Cloning of IL-1 and IL-2 has made large quantities of highly purified materials available for clinical trials. Some of these trials with LAK cells have been discussed in the section on Specific Immunotherapy.

Interferons (IFN)

The interferons are a family of glycoproteins produced by several different cell types. Type 1 (alpha and beta) interferons, which are produced, respectively, by induced leukocytes and fibroblasts, show about 30% homology of amino acids. Type 2 (gamma) interferon, which is produced by lymphocytes and monocytes in response to antigenic or mitogenic stimulation, differs significantly in amino acid composition. The interferons were thought at first to have only antiviral activity, but multiple other functions (previously postulated to have been related to impurities in the preparations) have been documented. Further documentation of these multiple functions as definite interferon effects is now possible since highly purified products have become available to study in clinical use. In addition to antiviral activity, the interferons have profound effects on the immune system. Relatively low doses will enhance antibody formation and lymphocyte blastogenesis, whereas higher doses will inhibit both of these functions. Moderate to high doses may inhibit delayed hypersensitivity while enhancing macrophage phagocytosis and cytotoxicity, sensitized lymphocyte cytotoxicity, NK activity, and surface antigenic expression. Interferons also prolong and inhibit cell division, having this effect on almost every cell system studied, whether transformed or not. Interferons also stimulate the induction of several intracellular enzyme systems, with resultant profound effects on macromolecular activities and protein synthesis.

Antitumor effects of interferon were first demonstrated in tumors considered to be induced by oncogenic viruses. Late appearance of tumors and increased animal survival have been reported with many animal tumors induced by viruses. The antitumor immune modulating effect of IFN in vivo and the relatively low host toxicity has led to a number of clinical trials. The greatest therapeutic usefulness of IFN has been in a rare form of leukemia: hairy cell leukemia. Early trials used IFNa purified from human leukocytes and later obtained by recombinant DNA techniques. Various recombinant forms of IFN are now in clinical trials for various malignancies.

Interleukins

The interleukins belong to a family of polypeptide growth and differentiation factors called lymphokines. These are factors, produced by lymphocytes or macrophages, that stimulate the proliferation, differentiation, and function of T lymphocytes, B lymphocytes, and certain other cells involved in the immune response (see Table 19-2). Initially discovered as soluble factors present in the growth medium of cultured lymphocytes, several activities have now been identified for these substances. These substances are usually defined by their role in stimulating an in vitro immune reaction such as promoting the activation and/or proliferation of immune system cells. However, it has become clear that several of the activities previously described could be attributed to two distinct polypeptides. One of these polypeptides is Interleukin-1 (IL-1), and the other is interleukin-2 (IL-2). The term *interleukin* was chosen because it indicates the basic property of these secreted mediators to serve as intercellular signals between leukocytes. Several additional interleukins have now been identified (see Table 19-2); IL-1, 2, 3, and 4 have been introduced into clinical trials for various malignant diseases. IL-2 has been used in adoptive immunotherapy to stimulate colonal expansion of lymphokine activated killer (LAK) cells and tumor-infiltrated lymphocytes (TIL). IL-3 has been utilized to stimulate bone marrow recovery in bone marrow or peripheral stem cell transplantation. IL-4 has been introduced as an immune system stimulator in various cancer treatment regimens. Macrophages produce interleukin-1 when the T cell antigen receptor interacts with antigen class II MHC complexes on the macrophage surface. The IL-1 molecule released by the macrophage induces the T-lymphocyte to express a cell surface receptor for interleukin-2. These events lead to the synthesis of IL-2, a growth factor produced by T cells that drives the proliferation of T cells bearing IL-2 receptors, resulting in clonal expansion of the responding T cells. In addition to the IL-2 receptor, activated T cells express other cell surface markers not found on resting T cells, including class II MHC molecules, transferrin receptors, and several antigens restricted to activated T cells. After activation, T cells of the helper-inducer subset produce a large number of mediators in addition to IL-2.

Tumor Necrosis Factor

A unique pair of cytokines produced by activated monocytes and lymphocytes are the agents referred to as tumor necrosis factors, alpha and beta. These substances were originally identified by their capacity to induce hemorrhagic necrosis and regression in a mouse tumor model in vivo and by their cytotoxic-cytostatic activity against mouse L cell in vitro. There are two closely related molecules with tumor necrosis factor (TNF) activity: TNF alpha (a monokine) and TNF beta (lymphotoxin), a product of activated lymphocytes. The two molecules, which are structurally related and share about 30% amino acid sequence homology, compete for the same cellular receptors. Both are now being produced by recombinant DNA technology. Currently only the TNF that is a monokine is being evaluated in the clinic. Nonetheless, it seems worthwhile to develop both species of TNF because the two molecules may have different antitumor spectra despite the fact that they share a number of functional attributes. Because TNFs are products of normal cells, they are capable of pleiotropic biologic activities, including cytotoxic-cytostatic activity against tumor cells, immunomodulatory functions, interactions with other BRMs, and modulation of gene expression. TNFs can destroy tumor cells in vitro in the absence of cells of the immune system. Several lines of evidence suggest that TNFs may modulate cell-mediated immune defenses against tumors. TNFs can activate and enhance neutrophil and eosinophil functions and can augment expression of class I and class II histocompatibility antigens. Binding of TNF molecules to specific high-affinity receptors is an initial event in the action of TNFs, and cells that do not possess these receptors appear to be resistant to TNFs. Cytotoxic-cytostatic activity has been documented in a broad spectrum of mouse and human tumor cells in vitro. Hemorrhagic necrosis and regression have been achieved in a comparable spectrum of mouse tumors growing in syngeneic mice and in human tumors growing in the xenogenic nude mouse model. Responsive tumor cell lines have included melanoma, colon cancer, breast cancer, cervical cancer, ovarian cancer, lung cancer, and astrocytoma. However, there is considerable heterogeneity of response within any given tumor type. Responsiveness to TNFs does not depend on tumor type or on any potentially prognostic factor. Clinical toxicities of recombinant TNF are similar to those of recombinant interferons—primarily, fever, chills, headaches, and other constitutional symptoms. A dose-dependent, reversible, local inflammatory response is not uncommon. Hypotension may occur occasionally but can be managed with intravenous hydration. Neurologic symptoms such as confusion may develop in rare instances. Myelosuppression may occur but this is dose-dependent and reversible. These data suggest a tolerance for TNFs used in combination with myelosuppressive chemotherapy. A few patients will require transfusion for anemia but this does not present a major clinical problem. To date, the clinical usefulness of TNF has been very limited becasue the systemic toxicity observed after intravenous infusion limits its utility. Efforts are being made to deliver TNF directly to the tumor, which should lower toxicity.

Retinoids

Vitamin A has a number of important functions in the body. Among others, it is apparently essential for the integrity of epithelial cells. The functional and structural integrity of epithelial cells throughout the body depends on an adequate supply of vitamin A. This vitamin plays a major role in the induction of control in epithelial differentiation in mucus-secreting or keratinizing tissue. In the presence of retinol, basal epithelial cells are stimulated to produce mucus. Excessive retinol will lead to the production of a thick layer of mucin with an array of goblet cells and inhibition of keratinization. In the absence of retinol, atrophy of the epithelium occurs followed by a proliferation of basal cells with an increase of mucous cells. It has been established that epithelial systems need vitamin A for display of a proper morphology and function. In vitro studies support the concept of vitamin A as directly involved in maintaining normal phenotypic expression. This concept, therefore, puts vitamin A in a special position among nutrients if one considers that most solid tumors arise from epithelial tissues. Studies on the protective effect of vitamin A against the development of epithelial tumors has been conducted for many years. Numerous studies have been done, and in general vitamin A either fed to the animal in its diet or applied locally appeared to have a protective and therapeutic effect on chemically produced tumors. One derivative of vitamin A, retinoic acid, has been studied most for human epithelial malignancies. Topically applied retinoic acid has been successful in certain dermatologic disorders such as actinokeratosis, a precancerous condition, and basal cell carcinomas. Studies suggesting activity have also been done with urinary bladder papillomas and intraepithelial neoplasia of the cervix. These substances show great promise for treating the increasing numbers of patients who have intraepithelial neoplasia of the cervix.

In summary BRM therapy and the use of various biologic products of the human genome in the clinical setting are now realities. We can expect to see the induction of partial responses and, ultimately, the induction of complete responses in patients with malignancy that will lead to a new era in treatment. The use of these agents will become the fourth modality of cancer therapy, acting effectively and independently in patients with clinically perceptible disease but perhaps acting optimally in the minimal disease setting, especially when combined with existing treatment modalities.

ADDITIONAL IMMUNOTHERAPY TRIALS

Nonspecific immunotherapy implies the stimulation of the reticuloendothelial system by injection of various substances not related to the malignancy under therapy. BCG, MER, and *C. parvum* have been utilized as nonspecific reticuloendothelial stimulants. Various trials using nonspecific immunotherapy in gynecologic malignancies have been conducted with mostly negative results.

Olkowski et al. reported on the effects of combined immunotherapy with levamisole and BCG on immunocompetence of patients with squamous cell carcinoma of the cervix. Immunologic tests were performed before and immediately after a full course of radiotherapy in 25 patients with squamous cell carcinoma of the cervix, stage Ib through III. The patients were randomized to immunotherapy with oral levamisole and intradermal BCG or no immunotherapy. Lymphocyte responses to phytohemagglutinin and pokeweed mitogen were subnormal before radiotherapy and declined still further after radiotherapy. Both treatment groups showed a gradual recovery from immunosuppression (T and B lymphocyte counts and mitogenic responses) during follow-up, but the immunotherapy group showed a tendency (not significant in the preliminary data) toward slower recovery. Lymphocyte cytotoxicity to allogeneic tumor cells was variably affected by radiotherapy but was generally higher 8 weeks after radiotherapy than in preceding tests.

DiSaia reported the results of a Gynecologic Oncology Group study on the treatment of women with advanced carcinoma of the uterine cervix with radiotherapy alone vs radiotherapy plus immunotherapy with intravenous *C. parvum*. One hundred sixty-seven patients in the preliminary report and 295 patients in the final unpublished study were considered evaluable at the time of analysis. The conclusion reached was the *C. parvum* did not add any therapeutic effect as an adjuvant to radiotherapy in the patient population study.

Alberts has an exciting report in the literature concerning nonspecific immunotherapy of ovarian carcinoma. He studied the effect of adding BCG to doxorubicin (Adriamycin) and cyclophosphamide (A-C) for the treatment of stages III and IV or recurrent epithelial ovarian carcinoma. In his study 131 patients with no prior chemotherapy and measurable disease were randomly assigned to receive A-C or A-C and BCG. Doxorubicin, 40 mg/m^2 on day 1, and cyclophosphamide, 200 mg/m^2/day on days 3 through 6, were given every 3 to 4 weeks for a total doxorubicin dose of 500 mg/m^2. BCG was administered by scarification to alternating upper and lower extremity sites on days 8 and 15. There was a similar distribution between the two study arms of patients with stage IV disease, bulky tumor masses, types of surgical procedures, performance status, prior radiation therapy exposure, and type and grade tumor histology. The complete remission and partial remission rate of 52% for patients receiving A-C and BCG was significantly different ($p <0.05$) from the 30% rate observed in the group receiving A-C. The median duration of responses of 13+ months for the groups receiving A-C plus BCG was not statistically better than the 7⅙ months for the patients receiving A-C. Median survival duration of the patients

receiving A-C plus BCG (21 months) was statistically better than that of patients receiving only A-C (13½ months) ($p <0.005$). Therapy was well tolerated. There were no drug-related deaths and no serious systemic BCG toxicities. The addition of BCG to the standard A-C treatment for far advanced ovarian carcinoma appears to have increased response rates and overall survival duration without markedly adding to drug toxicity.

The Gynecologic Oncology Group (GOG) initiated another prospective randomized trial to test the efficacy of BCG by scarification in patients with advanced ovarian adenocarcinoma. Suboptimal patients with bulky residual disease stages III and IV were randomized between chemotherapy with cisplatin, doxorubicin, and cyclophosphamide (CAP) vs CAP plus BCG given in a manner identical to that reported by Alberts. Although the chemotherapy given in this study by the Gynecologic Oncology Group is at variance with that used by Alberts, the methodology was otherwise identical. It was thought that this study would test the value of BCG in patients with advanced epithelial cancer of the ovary. In 1987, the GOG study in which BCG was used was closed, and analysis did not substantiate the efficacy of BCG as reported by Alberts.

Gall reported a prospective, randomized trial (done under the auspices of the GOG) in patients with stage III optimal epithelial carcinoma of the ovary that utilized melphalan vs melphalan plus *Corynebacterium parvum* (*C. parvum*). There were 185 patients eligible for evaluation, 87 in the melphalan group and 98 in the melphalan plus *C. parvum* group. The comparison of the treatment regimens showed no differences regarding progression-free interval or survival. However, it should be noted that a 3-year survival of 50% was obtained. Both the maximum size of residual tumor and performance status were prognostically significant. In summary, this study demonstrated a lack of efficacy of the addition of *C. parvum* to melphalan for this patient population.

Berek reported the treatment of 21 patients who had recurrent and advanced epithelial ovarian cancer using *Corynebacterium parvum* administered intraperitoneally. Nineteen patients had surgically measurable disease, and two received adjuvant therapy. Surgically confirmed responses were documented in 6 of 19 patients (31.6%), which included 2 complete responses (10.5%) and 4 partial responses (21.1%). Three patients (15.8%) had stable disease, and 10 patients (52.6%) had disease progression. The mean survival of the patients who had complete response was 35½ months; the four patients who had partial response had a median survival of 26⅗ months. Of the non-responders the mean survival was 12⅗ months. Stimulation of cytotoxic lymphocytes resulted from the administration of *C. parvum*, which induced a significant increase of both intraperitoneal natural killer lymphocyte cytotoxicity and antibody-dependent cell-mediated cytotoxicity in 6 of 9 patients tested. Toxicity in 86 courses of therapy included abdominal pain in 78% of cases, fever in 56%, nausea in 40%, and vomiting in 22%.

Active specific immunotherapy in ovarian cancer has been reported by Crowther et al. and Hudson et al. Cryopreserved, desiccated, and irradiated allogeneic tumor cells mixed with BCG were given to patients who had advanced ovarian cancers. These small non- randomized trials suggested activity for active specific immunotherapy.

Ikic et al. studied interferon treatment of uterine cervical precancerous lesions. Human leukocyte interferon (INF) was applied topically on the uterine cervix in 10 patients with persistent cytologic findings of non-dysplastic atypia and dysplastic atypia. Patients were treated 14 to 21 days at a daily dose of 1×10^6 IU. Cytologic findings after treatment were minor inflammations, that is, normalized cytologic findings (IIa according to Papanicolaou nomenclature) in all 10 patients. No relapses were found in the 6-month interval after treatment. A follow-up report in 1981 by Ikic et al. studied groups of patients with cervical intraepithelial neoplasia who were randomly selected for treatment with INF (13 patients with cervical intraepithelial neoplasia, stages I and II) or placebo (18 patients with cervical intraepithelial neoplasia, stages I through III). Follow-up studies at 2 years showed significant differences between the treatment and the placebo groups with regard to cytologic findings and histologic diagnoses. In the controls the pathologically changed epithelium was persistent in 7 of 18 cases, and there were 7 of 18 progressions. Among the controls, no regressions were observed. In the patients treated with INF, abnormal epithelium persisted in 4 of 13 cases, progressed in 1 of 13, and regressed in 8 of 13. The results indicate that INF has an impact on the regression of cervical intraepithelial neoplasia. Therapy with INF may be particularly indicated in women in the reproductive age in whom fertility is to be preserved because it may obviate the need for surgery.

Krusic et al. reported on the application of INF in patients with invasive cervical carcinoma. In his study, 15 patients with invasive squamous cell carcinoma of the uterine cervix were treated with crude INF for 3 weeks before surgical removal of the tumor. Nine patients were given INF topically and intramuscularly and 6 were given INF topically only. In 3 patients the surgical material was free from tumor cells, in 3 it showed a lower grade of carcinoma, and in 9 the findings remained unchanged. In only 1 patient the tumor metastasized to the lymph nodes. Typically a tumor regressed to about one third of its original size. There was a sharp distinction between the tumor mass and the healthy tissue manifested in the formation of a fibrous wall. The overall appraisal of the response caused by INF therapy was as follows:

Number of cases	Response
6	Excellent
5	Very good
1	Moderate
2	Poor
1	No response

It is suggested that INF is suitable for administration before and after surgery in patients with stage I or II cervical cancer. If stroma cannot be induced to respond within 21 days of treatment, INF application should be discontinued.

Einhorn et al. reported on a series of patients treated with INF for advanced ovarian carcinoma. Daily intramuscular injections of 3×10^6 IU of INF were given to 5 patients with advanced ovarian carcinoma, all of whom previously received other forms of treatment. Ascitic fluid production ceased in 2 of 2 patients. According to the criteria specified by Young and DeVita, a partial response was observed in 1 patient, and in 2 other patients the disease was stable for more than 1 year. Side effects of the interferon therapy were relatively mild.

The introduction of interferon therapy was followed by an increase in NK cell activity of peripheral blood lymphocytes in all three patients examined. NK cell activity decreased after cessation of interferon therapy in the one patient in whom this was tested.

Abdulhay reported on 36 patients who had measurable epithelial ovarian cancers who had failed conventional chemotherapy and were treated with lymphoblastoid interferon alone. Twenty-eight patients were evaluable for response: 2 had complete response (7.1%), 3 had partial response (10.8%), 14 had stable disease (50.0%), and 9 had increasing disease (32.2%). Abdulhay concluded that interferon therapy may have cytostatic and possibly cytotoxic effects. This Gynecologic Oncology Group pilot study was followed by another pilot study in patients immediately after surgery who had advanced epithelial ovarian cancers who received interferon in addition to CAP chemotherapy. This study was reported by DiSaia who noted unacceptable toxicity, especially that of cumulative myelotoxicity with prolonged leukopenia.

Berek reported 14 patients who had persistent epithelial ovarian cancers documented at second-look laparotomy after combination chemotherapy who were treated with 146 cycles of alpha-recombinant interferon administered intraperitoneally. The initial dose was 5×10^6 units, which was escalated weekly to 50×10^6 units over 4 weeks and then continued weekly for a total of 16 weeks. Eleven patients underwent surgical reevaluation after therapy that confirmed by pathologic examination complete responses (36%), 1 partial response (9%), and disease progression in 6 patients (55%). Five of 7 patients (71%) who had residual tumor less than 5 mm had a surgically documented response, whereas there was no response in the 4 patients whose tumors were greater than or equal to 5 mm. Significant fever was seen in 58%, vomiting in 37%, abdominal pain in 22%, and 1 patient had infectious peritonitis.

On the basis of a report of Verhaegen et al., who demonstrated a survival advantage in patients with colorectal carcinoma who were adjuvantly treated with levamisole, the North Central Cancer Treatment Group conducted a trial that randomly allocated 401 postoperative patients with Dukes' B or C carcinomas to (1) observation, (2) levamisole alone, or (3) a combination of levamisole and 5-FU. Levamisole was administered at 150 mg daily for 3 consecutive days every 2 weeks. Therapy was continued for 1 year; the median follow-up exceeded 7 years. Therapy with 5-FU and levamisole significantly reduced cancer recurrences, and an improvement in survival was observed in patients with Dukes' C colon cancer (p = 0.03) over that of patients receiving no additional postoperative therapy. Results in the group treated with levamisole alone suggested a reduction in recurrences (p = 0.05) but no influence on survival.

Many pilot studies have been initiated utilizing a host of cytokines, usually as single agents alone and without chemotherapy, in an attempt at active immunotherapy. More and more is being learned about these complex and often pleiotropic molecules and the multiple populations of effector cells under their control. The future promises to allow for selection of cytokines and proper orchestration of those selected to create the desired effect. The biology involved is complex and the therapeutic trials to date have been simplistic. The future promises more rational schedules, sequences, and doses of these agents, with or without chemotherapeutic therapy.

MONOCLONAL ANTIBODY THERAPY

The use of monoclonal antibody and its conjugates in the treatment of cancer is in an early stage. Although it is clear that much needs to be done to clarify many of the issues surrounding the use of antibody alone or conjugates of the antibody with other toxic substances, it has been demonstrated in animal tumor models and in man that antibody alone and antibody conjugated with drugs, toxins, and radioisotopes can have therapeutic effects. The potential for monoclonal antibodies in cancer therapeutics is enormous given the specificity that is inherent in the antibody-antigen reaction. The use of isotope-labeled antibody has enormous potential for the detection and treatment of cancer. There are still significant problems with these conjugates because of potential toxicity from the organ's nonspecific accumulation of radioactivity or toxins from the conjugate or its products. In addition, any nonspecific binding of the isotope-labeled conjugates will represent a significant clinical problem for the use of these conjugates in therapy. The hypothesis that lower levels of drug toxicity and greater antitumor activity may be seen by virtue of increased

specificity of the drug-antibody conjugate remains to be demonstrated in humans.

Most monoclonal antibodies directed at human tumors are of murine or other rodent origin and activate human immune-effector mechanisms poorly. The prospect of developing antitumor antibodies of human origin certainly will improve this situation. However, there are still few human cell lines that are as compatible as fusion partners as the murine myeloma lines, and the technique for immunizing humans to get antitumor antibodies of high affinity and IgG isotype has not yet been perfected. However, the application of recombinant DNA technology to fuse the human heavy chain constant region gene to a rearranged *VDJ* murine gene encoding an antitumor variable region may yield recombinant genes capable of producing high affinity antibody with the capacity to activate the human immune response efficiently (Figure 19-15). Thus, arming the available murine antitumor antibodies with some sort of killer molecule appears to be the most promising lead immediately available. There is considerable discussion, however, as to whether the use of conventional drugs, radionuclides, or bacterial toxins is best for this purpose. Most interest is focused on the latter two.

Radionuclides have many attractive features in their use as lethal moieties on monoclonal antibodies (Figure 19-16). They allow for diagnosis through imaging that might be accomplished with low specific activity conjugates. These results could be used in dosimetry calculations to produce a theoretic therapeutic index for the use of the conjugate at higher specific activity in the individual patient. The use of radionuclides also circumvents the problem of tumor cell antigen heterogeneity, modulation, and the need for internalization of the

NAKED ANTIBODIES

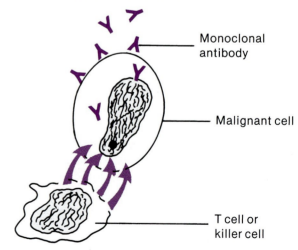

Figure 19-15 Monoclonal antibodies can be made to recognize and attach to unique proteins on the surface of cancer cells. After the cancer cell is coated with antibodies, cells of the immune system recognize and destroy the malignant cell.

complex, because the isotope of interest can have killing distances of many centimeters. These assumed advantages, however, by their nature decrease the specificity of the treatment, and there must be consideration as to whether, for example, a metastatic tumor in the liver with localization of the isotope-antibody complex in that organ could result in marked hepatic toxicity. In addition, there are technical limitations to the use of some of the more preferable isotopes because of incompletely defined practical and stable conjugation chemistry. The ideal isotope is of high specific activity, has a short half-life, has high energy at a short distance, is safe to work with from a radiation standpoint, possesses well-defined and stable conjugation chemistry, and is rapidly cleared from the body. At present, none of the radionuclides fulfill all of these criteria.

The use of natural toxins, for example, *Pseudomonas* exotoxin and the A-chain of ricin (from the castor bean), as the cytotoxic component on a monoclonal antibody also has potential advantages (Figure 19-17). These agents exhibit their cytotoxic effect by irreversible inhibition of protein synthesis. They catalyze the inhibition of elongation factor-2 or inhibit ATP ribosylation, processes essential to protein synthesis. The inhibition is so efficient that as few as one or two molecules of the toxin can kill the cell. The toxins are usually composed of two separate chains, an A-chain that is the active toxic moiety, and the B-chain that is responsible for binding the toxin to the cell and for getting it internalized from receptosomes to the cytoplasm. An isolated A-chain is essentially nontoxic because it has no capability for entering cells. After the toxin binds its target, it is taken up by receptor-mediated endocytosis and enters the cytoplasm. Both binding and internalization into the cytoplasm must take place for toxins to exert their effects. Therefore they are exceedingly specific. The extreme specificity of immunotoxins is a potential liability because of the tumor cell antigen heterogeneity where the use of only one monoclonal antibody would kill only those cells expressing the target antigen. The use of a "cocktail" of toxin conjugates might circumvent this problem and yet allow for retention of the killing specificity dictated by the need for internalization. Another danger relates to the fact that antigens may be shared with some normal cells so that these normal cells will also be targeted.

The need for internalization places potential constraints on some of the antibodies applicable to the production of immunotoxins. Some target antigens are shed and are poorly internalized. Therefore, in addition to the search for appropriate antitumor antibodies, antibodies must be directed against components of an actively growing cell, such as growth factor receptors and the transferrin receptor, which are potential candidates for immunotherapy. These antibodies are efficiently internalized and might quantitatively discriminate between carcinoma cells characterized by their uncontrolled growth and normal cells, which generally are dividing at a less rapid rate. Such a differential in growth rate may be particularly relevant to intraperitoneal therapy in ovarian cancer because the only rapidly dividing cells in the

RADIOACTIVE ANTIBODIES

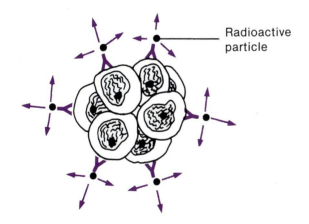

Figure 19-16 Radioactive particles can be attached to monoclonal antibodies. The antibodies carry the particles to cancer cells where the radioactive material is then concentrated to kill the neoplastic cells.

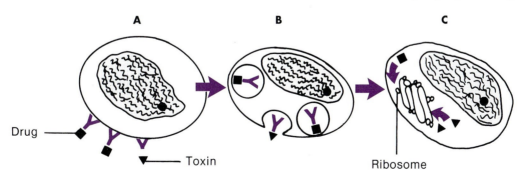

Figure 19-17 A, The drug-laden antibody attaches to the cancer cell's surface. **B,** The drugs of toxins—though not necessarily the antibody—are engulfed by the cell. **C,** When inside the cell, the drugs or toxins poison the cell. One toxin, for example, destroys the ribosomes, which are the cell's protein factories.

peritoneal cavity should be malignant ovarian cancer cells.

Few monoclonal-conjugate clinical studies have been done but preliminary results from one of these in which antiferritin antibody was linked to I-131 suggest some promise for the treatment of hepatocellular carcinoma. Because any monoclonal antibody conjugate is expected to be transported primarily to the liver, it is unclear what, if anything, the specific antibody contributes to the observed responses. Monoclonal antibodies directed against cell-surface antigens in conjunction with immunoconjugates or complement have already proved useful in autologous bone marrow transplantation. They have been used to clear the bone marrow in vitro either of normal T cells, to decrease graft vs host reactions, or of malignant cells. Another useful clinical role of conjugated antibodies is to provide staging information. Such reagents have been useful in cutaneous T cell lymphoma and melanoma. The monoclonal antibody is labeled with a radioisotope such as I-135 or I-131, the conjugate administered intravenously or intralymphatically, and the patient scanned with a gamma camera. This technique may also provide a sensitive and specific way of determining the location of metastases undetectable by other methods.

The rapid development of DNA technology has significant implication for monoclonal antibody research. For example, genetic engineering has made it possible to tailor chimeric antibodies consisting of murine light chains and human heavy chains, resulting in less immunogenicity. Recombinant technology also allows one to make novel bifunctional molecules in which one end contains the antigen-combining site and a second end binds to a drug, toxin, effector cell, or other matter. Future clinical trials may well involve the use of monoclonal antibodies or bifunctional molecules combined with other biologics such as interferon, tumor necrosis factor, or interleukin-2. The rationale for such studies stems from the preclinical data showing enhancement of the antibody-dependent cellular cytotoxicity and other immune functions generated by these cytokines. Genetically engineered monoclonal antibody constructs may eliminate several problems associated with current murine monoclonal antibodies.

Various other factors can also inhibit the efficacy of monoclonal antibody therapy: circulating tumor antigen in the serum can bind most of the antibody and prevent its effective delivery to the site of the tumor, a subset of the tumor cells may not express the tumor antigen or may express it only in low amounts, and modulation of the antigen from the cell surface will remove the antibody's target. The potential of monoclonal antibodies in cancer treatment has not yet been realized. The obvious appeal of monoclonal antibodies is their specificity and their potential for focusing immune mechanisms of the host or cytotoxic agents on the tumor cell. The initial experimental work in clinical trials defined some problems that must

be resolved. They also provided some intriguing results that will certainly be an impetus to further work and to exploration of new approaches to their use in therapy. The authors are more optimistic for the immediate future regarding the potential use of monoclonal antibodies as a tool for imaging and diagnosis.

CONCLUSIONS

The field of tumor immunology and biologic response modifiers has grown significantly in recent years, and it is impossible to address all aspects of this highly evolving area of scientific development in a chapter such as this. The reader is encouraged to obtain some of the references if additional information is desired. The main objective among those interested in clinical gynecologic tumor immunology and the use of biologic response modifiers continues to be determining methods of immunodiagnosis and methods of immunotherapy. Immunodiagnosis is hampered at this point by the weakness of the tumor-associated antigens in gynecologic malignancies and physicochemical and other technical problems associated with isolation of substances from the cell surface that vary only slightly from normal cellular molecules. The presence of tumor-associated antigens in gynecologic malignancies has been demonstrated by a number of indirect methods, and therefore the probability that several immunodiagnostic tools will be developed for the clinician is quite promising. It is hoped that the technology developed around CA-125 testing in epithelial ovarian cancer will be the first of many clinically useful immunodiagnostic methods.

The status of immunotherapy in gynecologic cancer is similar to that in other human malignancies. Immunoprophylaxis awaits identification of viral or other etiologic agents and/or purification of tumor-associated antigens. Both specific and nonspecific immunotherapeutic trials have been performed and are currently under way in various institutions, with mixed results. These less than optimal results are understandable if one considers the following factors. Most trials have used nonspecific immunotherapy, which relies on a generalized stimulation of the reticuloendothelial system with concomitant specific stimulation of clones directed toward the malignancy as a by-product. Specific immunotherapy has not been successful because of the weak immunogenic properties of the antigens involved. In addition, most clinical trials have been conducted in patients with large tumor burdens in whom reduction of those burdens was assigned to surgery, chemotherapy, and/or radiotherapy. These cancericidal modalities are immunosuppressive in and of themselves and may abrogate the effectiveness of the immunopotentiator.

In 1996 the status of most immune monitoring techniques is disappointing. Indeed, most of the immune monitoring techniques that the immunotherapist formerly relied on to demonstrate an effect from immunotherapeutic agents have been demonstrated to be unreliable or inaccurate. Thus the immunotherapist is forced to rely on clinical response as an end point, and clinical response is confused by the multiplicity of other factors involved in the patient's condition, such as other tumoricidal therapies, nutrition, and genetic makeup. In many ways the cards have been stacked against the immunotherapist, and a certain amount of patience is appropriate among clinicians as these complex issues are unraveled.

The therapeutic application of monoclonal antibodies offers perhaps the most exciting potential and the greatest challenge. Although already hailed as "magic bullets" or "guided missiles," the use of monoclonal antibodies in treatment is just beginning to be explored, and their ultimate role is undefined. However, early results in patients with leukemia, lymphoma, and cancer of the gastrointestinal tract have been encouraging. Monoclonal antibodies have themselves been shown to destroy tumor cells in vitro and in vivo using a nude mouse system. The mechanisms for this direct antitumor effect appear to involve antibody-dependent cellular cytotoxicity and macrophages. Other tumor cell agents such as chemotherapy drugs, toxins, radioisotopes, or interferon may be conjugated to carrier monoclonal antibodies for precise delivery to tumor cells.

Several obstacles must be overcome if the potential of monoclonal antibodies as a significant therapeutic modality in cancer is to be realized, including:

1. The problem of circulating tumor antigen, which can activate the antibody and theoretically lead to immune complex disease
2. The appearance in the recipient of human antibody to mouse protein with the same consequence
3. The phenomenon of antigenic modulation (temporary disappearance of target antigen from the tumor cell surface in the presence of antibody)
4. The existence of antigenic heterogeneity of tumor cells
5. The varying affinity in antitumor properties of different classes of antibodies
6. The delineation of optimal methods of conjugating tumor cell compounds to monoclonal antibodies

Solutions to some or all of these obstacles seem likely. The development of methods to produce human hybridomas, the use of mixtures of monoclonal antibodies to enhance the affinity and specificity for tumor cells, the direct linkage of monoclonal antibodies to effector cells, and the generation of monoclonal reagents to tumor stem cell or chemoresistant cell subpopulations are examples that are currently under active investigation in many laboratories.

GLOSSARY

accessible antigens   Antigens of self that are in contact with antibody-forming tissues and to a host that is normally tolerant.

accessory cell   Cell required for, but not actually mediating, a specific immune response. Often used to describe antigen-presenting cells.

active immunization   Direct immunization of the intact individual or of immunocompetent cells derived from the individual and returned to him.

active immunotherapy   May be divided into two groups: specific immunogens and non-specific adjuvants. Active specific immunotherapy is attempted by the immunization of a tumor-bearing patient with autochthonous altered (radiation, chemical) tumor cells. Non-specific immunotherapy attempts to augment antitumor immunologic activity with non-specific stimulants such as BCG or *C. parvum*.

adaptation   A process whereby protection accorded a foreign graft from the immune reaction of the recipient renders it less vulnerable to immunologic attack by the host.

adjuvant   A substance that when mixed with an antigen enhances its antigenicity.

adoptive immunization   The transfer of immunity from one individual to another by means of specifically

immune lymphoid cells or materials derived from such cells that are capable of transferring specific immunologic information to the recipient's lymphocytes.

agglutinin   Any antibody that produces aggregation or agglutination of a particular or insoluble antigen.

allele   An alternative gene acting at the same locus on the chromosome.

allergen   A substance (antigen or hapten) that incites allergy.

allergy   A state of specific increased reactivity to an antigen or hapten such as occurs in hay fever. The term is used to designate states of delayed sensitivity caused by contact allergens.

alloantibody (isoantibody)   Any antibody produced by one individual that reacts specifically with an antigen present in another individual of the same species. The term *isoantibody* is commonly used in hematology; the term *alloantibody* is used in tissue transplantation.

alloantigen (isoantigen)   Any antigen that incites the formation of antibodies in genetically dissimilar members of the same species.

allogeneic   Referring to genetically dissimilar individuals of the same species.

allogeneic disease   Any systemic illness resulting from a graft vs host response when the graft contains immunologically competent cells and the host is immunologically incompetent (e.g., runt disease).

allograft (homograft) A graft derived from an allogeneic donor.

alloimmune Specifically immune to an allogeneic antigen.

alpha-fetoprotein (AFP) Synthesized in the fetus by perivascular hepatic parenchymal cells. It is found in a high percentage of patients with hepatomas and endodermal sinus tumor of the ovary or testes. It is a serum protein present in concentrations up to 400 mg/dl in early fetal life, falling to less than 3 µg/dl in adults. Increased levels may be detected in the serum of adults with hepatoma (80% positive) and endodermal sinus tumor (60%-80% positive) and may be used to observe the disease progression.

anamnestic response (recall phenomenon, memory phenomenon) An accelerated response of antibody production to an antigen that occurs in an animal that has previously responded to the antigen.

anaphylaxis, acute Systemic shock (often fatal) that develops in a matter of minutes after subsequent exposure to a specific foreign antigen to which the host has already reacted.

anergy Absence of a hypersensitivity reaction that would be expected in other similarly sensitized individuals.

antibody (Ab) A substance (usually a gamma globulin) that can be incited in an animal by an antigen or by a hapten combined with a carrier and that reacts specifically with the antigen or hapten. Some antibodies can occur naturally without known antigen stimulation.

antibody reaction site (antigen binding site, antibody combining site) The inverted surface site on antibody that reacts with the antigen determinant site on the antigen.

antibody response The production of antibody in response to stimulation by specific antigen.

antigen (Ag) A substance that can react specifically with antibodies and under certain conditions can incite an animal to form specific antibodies. *Extrinsic:* An antigen that is not a constituent or product of the cell. *Intrinsic:* An antigen that is a constituent or product of the cell.

antigen-presenting cell A specialized type of cell, bearing cell antigen-presenting cell surface class II major histocompatibility complex (MHC) molecules, involved in the processing and presentation of antigen to inducer or helper T cells.

antigen determinant A small, three-dimensional everted surface configuration on the antigen molecule that specifically reacts with the antibody reaction site on the antibody molecule.

antigen receptor The specific antigen-binding receptor on T or B lymphocytes; these receptors are transcribed and translated from rearrangements of *V* genes.

antigenic modulation Loss of antigenicity or change in antigenic markers by which tumor cells may avoid immunologic identification or destruction.

antigenic paralysis See Immunologic tolerance.

Arthus reaction An inflammatory reaction characterized by edema, hemorrhage, and necrosis that follows the administration of antigen to an animal that already possesses precipitating antibody to that antigen.

atopy A hereditary predisposition of various individuals to develop immediate-type hypersensitivity on contact with certain antigens.

auto- Self or same.

autoantibodies Antibodies produced by an animal that react with the animal's own antigens. The stimulus is not known but could be the animal's own antigens or cross-reacting foreign antigens.

autoantigen A "self-antigen" that incites the formation of autoantibodies.

autochthonous (indigenous) Found in the same individual in which it originates, as in the case of a neoplasm; autochthonous tumor is a tumor borne by the host of origin.

autograft A graft derived from the same individual to whom it is transplanted.

autologous Derived from the recipient itself.

B cell or B lymphocyte A bone marrow cell. These cells mediate humoral immunity and are thymus- independent cells. In the avian species these cells are derived from the bursa of Fabricius. In humans they originate in the bone marrow.

binding site A term used for the antibody-combining site and other sites of specific attachment of macromolecules to one another.

biologic response modifier (BRM) The molecule produced by the body to regulate cellular responses.

blocking factor A humoral antibody or an antigen-antibody complex or other factor that coats antigenic sites with a protective covering so that neither complement nor killer lymphocytes can attack the cell.

bursa of Fabricius A cloacal structure in avian species containing immature lymphoid elements (B cells) and presumed to govern the production of humoral antibodies through these B cells.

cell-mediated cytotoxicity (CMC) Killing (lysis) of a target cell by an effector lymphocyte.

cell-mediated immunity (CMI) Immune reaction mediated by T cells; in contrast to humoral immunity, which is antibody mediated. Also referred to as delayed-type hypersensitivity.

chimera An individual composed of genetically dissimilar tissues.

class I, II, and III MHC molecules Proteins encoded by genes in the major histocompatibility complex.

clonal selection theory The prevalent concept that specificity and diversity of an immune response are the result of selection by antigen of specifically reactive clones from a large repertoire of preformed lymphocytes, each with individual specificities.

clone A population of cells derived from a single cell by asexual division.

colony-forming units Hematopoietic progenitors that proliferate and give rise to a colony of hematopoietic cells.

Colony-stimulating factor (CSF) A polypeptide that promotes the growth of hematopoietic progenitors.

committed cell A cell committed to the production of specific antibodies to a given antigen determinant. Committed cells include primed cells, memory cells, and antibody-producing cells.

complement (C') A multifactorial system of one or more normal serum components characterized by their capacity to participate in certain and specific antigen-antibody reactions.

complement activation Promotion of the killing or lytic actions of complement.

complement cascade A precise sequence of events usually triggered by an antigen-antibody complex, in which each component of the complement system is activated in turn.

complement fixation The fixation of C' to an antigen-antibody complex.

conjugates Yoked or coupled substances, that is, immunoconjugates, such as monoclonal antibodies conjugated with drugs, toxins, or radioisotopes.

cytokines Cell-derived regulatory molecules.

cytophilic antibodies Antibodies with an affinity for cells that depend on bonding forces independent of those that bind antigen to antibody.

D cell (double cell) Lymphocytes that appear to have characteristics of both T and B cells.

delayed hypersensitivity A specific sensitive state characterized by a delay of many hours in initiation time and course of reaction. It is transferable with cells but not with serum.

dendritic cells White blood cells found in the spleen and other lymphoid organs. Dendritic cells typically use thread-like tentacles to enmesh antigens, which they present to T cells.

desensitization The procedure of rendering a sensitive individual insensitive to an antigen or hapten by treatment with that specific agent.

determinant group That part of the structure of an antigen molecule that is responsible for specific interaction with antibody molecules evoked by the same or a similar antigen.

enhancement factor See Blocking factor.

enhancing antibodies Antibodies that enhance the survival of a graft or of a tumor.

enzyme-linked immunosorbent assay (ELISA) The assay in which an enzyme is linked to an antibody and a colored substrate is used to measure the activity of bound enzyme and the amount of bound antibody.

epitope An alternative term for antigenic determinant.

Fab (fragment antigen binding) That segment of the IgG antibody molecule, derived by papain treatment and reduction, containing only one antibody reaction site. Under oxidizing conditions, Fab fragments recombine to form the divalent molecule $F(ab)_2$ devoid of the Fe segment of the original molecule.

Forssman antigen An interspecies-specific antigen present in erythrocytes of many species, including some microorganisms, that is capable of inducing in animals devoid of such antigen the formation of lysin for sheep erythrocytes.

Freund adjuvant *Complete*: Freund emulsion of mineral oil, plant waxes, and killed tubercle bacilli used to combine with antigen to stimulate antibody production. *Incomplete*: Freund mixture without tubercle bacilli.

hapten A substance that combines specifically with antibody but does not initiate the formation of antibody unless attached to a high molecular weight carrier.

helper factor Sensitized T lymphocyte subpopulations release a helper factor that enables immunocompetent B cells to respond to antigens that they otherwise are unable to recognize. The stimulated B lymphocytes differentiate into plasma cells that produce antibody. The helper factor can also stimulate the B lymphocyte to produce a variant of the B cell, termed a *killer cell* (K), which is able to attack tumor cells only after the tumor cells have been exposed to specific antibody. Complement is not required for this action. See also Killer cell (K cell).

hemagglutinin An antibody that reacts with (a) surface antigen determinant(s) on red cells to cause agglutination of those red cells.

hemolysin (amboceptor) An anti-red cell antibody that can specifically activate complement (C') to cause lysis of red cells.

hetero- Other or different; often used to mean "of a different species."

heterophil Pertains to antigenic specificity shared between species.

heterophil antigens Antigens common to more than one species.

heterozygosity The presence in a chromosome of dissimilar genes.

histocompatibility antigens (transplantation or HLA antigens) Antigens coded for by "histocompatibility genes" that determine the specific compatibility of grafted tissues and organs.

HLA antigens (human leukocyte antigen) A genetic locus containing two closely linked groups of several alleles (a subloci). They are present on the cell membranes of all nucleated cells and play a major role in determining graft take and rejection.

homologous See Allogeneic.

homologous disease See Allogeneic disease.

horizontal transmission of viruses Transmission of viruses between individual hosts of the same generation. See also Vertical transmission of viruses.

host The organism whose body serves to sustain a graft; interchangeable with the recipient.

humoral antibodies Antibodies present in body fluids.

humoral immunity Pertains to the body fluids in contrast to cellular elements. It is initiated by the thymus-independent B cells. These B lymphocytes proliferate and differentiate into plasma cells that secrete immunoglobulins (IgG, IgM, IgA, IgD, and IgE).

hybridoma A hybrid cell that results from the fusion of an antibody-creating cell with a malignant cell; the progeny secrete antibody without stimulation and proliferate continuously in vivo and in vitro.

idiotypes The unique and characteristic parts of an antibody's variable region, which can themselves serve as antigens.

immune The state of being secure against harmful agents (e.g., bacteria, virus, or other foreign proteins) or influences.

immune clearance Clearance of antigen from the circulation after complexing with antibodies.

immune response A specific response that results in immunity. The total response includes an afferent phase during which responsive cells are "primed" by antigen, a central response during which antibodies or sensitized lymphoid cells are formed, and an efferent or effector response during which immunity is effected by antibodies or immune cells.

immunity The state of being able to resist and/or overcome harmful agents or influences. *Active*: Immunity acquired as the result of experience with an organism or other foreign substance. *Passive*: Immunity resulting from acquisition of antibody or sensitized lymphoid cells.

immunize The act or process of rendering an individual resistant or immune to a harmful agent.

immunocompetent cell (antigen-sensitive cell) Any cell that can be stimulated by antigen to form antibodies or give rise to sensitized lymphoid cells, including inducible cells, primed cells, and memory cells.

immunoconjugate A monoclonal antibody linked to a chemotherapy agent, radioisotope, or natural toxin to increase ability to kill target cells.

immunogen An antigen that incites specific immunity.

immunoglobulins (Ig) Classes of globulins to which all antibodies belong.

immunologic enhancement Enhanced survival of incompatible tissue grafts (tumor or normal tissue) caused by specific humoral or other blocking factors.

immunologic paralysis Absence of normal specific immunologic response to an antigen, resulting from previous contact with the same antigen, administered in a quantity greatly exceeding that required to elicit an immunologic response. The normal capacity to respond to other unrelated antigens is retained.

immunologic surveillance Effective immunologic surveillance relies on the presence of tumor-specific antigenic determinants on the surfaces of neoplastic cells, which enable these altered cells to be recognized as "non-self" and to be destroyed by immunologic reactions.

immunologic tolerance (antigenic paralysis, immunologic suppression, immunologic unresponsiveness, antigen tolerance) Failure of the antibody response to a potential antigen after exposure to that antigen. Tolerance commonly results from prior exposure to antigens.

immunoreaction Reaction between antigen and its antibody.

immunotoxin A monoclonal antibody linked to a natural toxin.

interferon A family of proteins released by cells in response to a virus infection. These substances represent non-specific immunity and appear to have non-specific tumoricidal characteristics.

interleukin-1(IL-1) A macrophage-derived cytokine that is necessary for the initial step in activation of specific T cells and the process of in vivo production of effector T cells.

interleukin-2 (IL-2) A lymphokine with multiple in vitro and in vivo effects. It is an essential factor for the growth of T cells; it augments various T cell functions; it supports the preservation and augmentation of natural killer (NK) cell function; and it is critical for the generation of lymphokine-activated killer (LAK) cells.

interleukins Polypeptides secreted by lymphocytes, monocytes, or other accessory cells, which function in the regulation of the hematopoietic and/or immune system; these molecules have an important role in cell-to-cell communication.

iso- Identical.

isoantibody The term used in blood grouping studies to designate an antibody formed by one individual that reacts with antigens of another individual of the same species. See also Alloantibody.

isoantigen See Alloantigen. The term *isoantigen* is commonly used in hematology.

isogeneic See Syngeneic.

isograft See Syngraft.

isoimmune See Alloimmune.

isologous See Syngeneic.

killer cell (K cell) Sensitized T lymphocytes produce a helper factor that acts on the immunocompetent lymphoid cell to produce a population of cells, probably variants of the B cell, termed *killer cells* (K cells), which are able to attack tumor cells that have been exposed to a specific sensitizing antibody. Unlike the usual humoral antibody (immunoglobulin) response, complement is not needed.

killer T cell A T cell with a particular immune specificity and an endogenously produced receptor for antigen, capable of specifically killing its target cell after attachment to the target cell by this receptor. Also called cytotoxic T cell.

locus   The precise location of a gene on a chromosome. Different forms of the gene (alleles) are always found at the same location on the chromosome.

lymphocyte   A round cell with scanty cytoplasm and a diameter of 7-12 μm. The nucleus is round, sometimes indented, with chromatin arranged in coarse masses and without visible nucleoli. Lymphocytes may be actively mobile.

lymphoid cell(s)   Any or all cells of the lymphocytic and plasmacytic series.

lymphokine   Substances released by sensitized lymphocytes when they come in contact with the antigen to which they are sensitized; examples include transfer factor (TF), lymphocyte-transforming activity (LTA), migration- inhibition factor (MIF), and lymphotoxin (LT).

macrophage   Large mononuclear phagocyte; in the tissues this cell may be called a histiocyte and in the blood it is called a monocyte. An antigen must come in contact with or pass through a macrophage before it can become a processed antigen with the ability to encounter and then sensitize a small lymphocyte.

macrophage-activating factor (MAF)   Sensitized T lymphocytes can release a non-specific macrophage-activating factor that creates a cytotoxic population of macrophages that appears to distinguish malignant from normal cells, killing only malignant ones.

major histocompatibility complex (MHC)   A cluster of genes encoding cell surface molecules that are polymorphic within a species and that code for antigens, which leads to rapid graft rejection between members of a single species that differ at these loci. Several classes of protein such as MHC class I and II proteins are encoded in this region.

memory cells   Cells that can mount an accelerated antibody response to antigen.

migration-inhibition factor (MIF)   A lymphokine produced when a sensitized lymphocyte is exposed to an antigen to which it is sensitized. MIF inhibits the migration of these lymphocytes.

minor histocompatibility antigens   These antigens, encoded outside the MHC, are numerous but do not generate rapid graft rejection or primary responses of T cells in vitro. They do not serve as restricting elements in cell interactions.

mitogen   A substance that induces immunocompetent lymphocytes to undergo blast transformation, mitosis, and cell division (causing mitosis or cell division).

monoclonal antibody   Antibodies with such high intrinsic specificity that only one or two antigenic determinants are recognized.

monokines   Soluble substances, secreted by monocytes, which have a variety of effects on other cells.

mosaic   An individual composed of two or more genetically dissimilar cell lines but from the same species. This can come about by somatic mutation or by grafting cells between individuals of very close genetic constitution, such as dizygotic twins.

natural antibodies   Antibodies that occur naturally without deliberate antigen stimulation.

natural killer lymphocytes (NK cells)   Lymphocytes that are active in the immune surveillance of tumor. NK cells can lyse malignant target cells in vitro and appear to need no prior sensitization.

non-specific immunization   Refers to stimulation of the general immune response by the use of materials (e.g., BCG or PHA) that are not antigenetically related to the specific tumor.

nude mice   Mice born with a congenital absence of the thymus. The blood and thymus-dependent areas of the lymph nodes and spleen are depleted of lymphocytes.

oncogenic   An agent capable of causing normal cells to acquire neoplastic characteristics. The term is often applied to viruses, such as adenoviruses.

passive transfer of immunity   The transfer of specific antibody from one individual to another.

phytohemagglutinins   Lectins extracted from the red kidney bean, *Phaseolus vulgaris* or *P. communis*; the extract can be purified to yield a glycoprotein mitogen that stimulates lymphocyte transformation and causes agglutination of certain red cells; provides a method for calculating the pool of thymus-dependent lymphocytes (T cells).

pokeweed mitogen (PWM)   A mitogen extracted from the pokeweed plant; it can be purified to yield a specific glycoprotein. PWM stimulates blast formation of both B and T cells.

plasma cell   End-stage differentiation of a B cell to an antibody-producing cell.

precipitin   An antibody that reacts specifically with soluble antigen to form a precipitate.

prophylactic immunization   Represents pre-immunization of an individual against a causative agent (e.g., oncogenic virus) or tumor-specific antigen, in advance of any natural encounter with the agent or tumor.

recombinant   A gene that has been isolated and recombined with other sequences responsible for gene expression.

runt disease   A condition of dwarfing that follows the injection of mature allogeneic immunologically competent cells into immunologically immature recipients. It is characterized by failure to thrive, lymph node atrophy, hepatomegaly and splenomegaly, anemia, and diarrhea.

sensitize   The process of increasing the specific reactivity of a subject or cell to an agent. Commonly used to designate the process of increasing reactivity caused by specific antibodies or "immune cells."

Shwartzman reaction A local non-immunologic inflammatory reaction with hemorrhage and necrosis produced by the injection of a bacterial endotoxin.

suppression A mechanism for producing a specific state of immunological unresponsiveness by the induction of suppressor T cells. This type of unresponsiveness is passively transferable by suppressor T cells or their soluble products.

suppressor T cells Represent an important set of feedback controls, centered around sensitized T lymphocytes, through which inhibitory populations of these T cells suppress the production of sensitized lymphocytes and antibody-forming cells.

syngeneic (isogeneic) Pertaining to genetically identical or nearly identical animals, such as identical twins or highly inbred animals.

syngraft (isograft) A graft derived from a syngeneic donor.

T lymphocyte (T cell) Lymphocytes that have matured and differentiated under thymic influence, termed *thymic-dependent lymphocytes*. These cells are primarily involved in the mediation of cellular immunity, as well as tissue and organ graft rejection.

topoisomerase An enzyme that controls conformational changes in DNA and aids in orderly progression of DNA replication, gene transcription, and separation of daughter chromosomes by cell division.

transfer factor A heat-labile, dialyzable extract of human lymphocytes (a lymphokine) that is capable of conferring specific antigen reactivity to the donor.

tumor angiogenesis factor (TAF) Represents the induction of the growth of blood vessels caused by this stimulant released by tumor cells. The growth of a tumor appears to parallel the development of new blood vessels.

tumor necrosis factor (TNF) A family of cytokines produced by activated monocytes and lymphocytes that can induce hemorrhagic necrosis and regression of tumors.

vaccination Injection or ingestion of an immunogenic antigen(s) for the purpose of producing active immunity.

vaccine A suspension of dead or living microorganisms that is injected or ingested for the purpose of producing active immunity.

vertical transmission of viruses Transmission from one generation to another. Can include transmission from one generation to the next via milk or through the placenta.

xenogeneic (heterologous) Pertaining to individuals of different species.

xenograft (heterograft) A graft derived from an animal of a different species than that of the one receiving the graft.

BIBLIOGRAPHY

Mechanisms of immunity

Billingham RE, Brent L, Medawar PB: Acquired tolerance of skin homografts, *Ann NY Acad Sci* 59:409, 1955.

Broder S, Waldmann TA: The suppressor-cell network in cancer, *N Engl J Med* 229:1281, 1978.

Currie GA: *Cancer and the immune response*, London, 1974, Edward Arnold.

Currie GA, Alexander P: Spontaneous shedding of TSTA by viable sarcoma cells: its possible role in facilitating metastatic spread, *Br J Cancer* 29:72, 1974.

DiSaia PJ: Studies in cell-mediated immunity in two gynecologic malignancies, *Cancer Bull* 23:65, 1971.

DiSaia PJ: Overview of tumor immunology in gynecologic oncology, *Cancer* 38:566, 1976.

DiSaia PJ, Morrow CP, Townsend DE: *Synopsis of gynecologic oncology*, New York, 1975, John Wiley & Sons.

DiSaia PJ et al: Immune competence and survival in patients with advanced cervical cancer: peripheral lymphocyte counts, *J Radiat Oncol* 4:449, 1978.

Germain RN: MHC-dependent antigen processing and peptide presentation: providing ligands for T lymphocyte activation, *Cell* 76:287, 1994.

Hanna N: The role of natural killer cells in the control of tumor growth and metastasis, *Biochem Biophys Acta* 780:213, 1985.

Herberman RB: Animal tumor models and their relevance to tumor immunology, *J Biol Resp Mod* 2:39, 1983.

Janeway, Jr. CA, Bottomly K: Signals and signs for lymphocyte responses, *Cell* 76:275, 1994.

Oldham RK: Natural killer cells: history and significance, *J Biol Resp Mod* 1:217, 1982.

Paul WE, Seder RA: Lymphocyte responses and cytokines, *Cell* 76:241, 1994.

Rapp HJ et al: Antigenicity of new diethylnitrosamine-induced transplantable guinea pig hepatoma, *J Natl Ca Inst* 41:1, 1968.

Schnipper LE: Clinical implications of tumor-cell heterogeneity, *N Engl J Med* 314:1423, 1986.

Sinkovics JG, DiSaia PJ, Rutledge FN: Tumour immunology and evolution of the placenta, *Lancet* 2:1190, 1970.

Sjogren HO: Blocking and unblocking of cell-mediated tumour immunity. In Busch H, editor: *Methods in cancer research*, New York, 1973, Academic Press.

Takasugi M, Mickey MR, Terasaki PI: Reactivity of lymphocytes from normal persons on cultured tumor cells, *Cancer Res* 33:2898, 1973.

Weiss A, Littman DR: Signal transduction by lymphocyte antigen receptors, *Cell* 76:263, 1994.

Weissman IL: Developmental switches in the immune system, *Cell* 76:207, 1994.

Welch WR, Niloff JM, Anderson D et al: Antigenic heterogeneity ovarian cancer, *Gynecol Oncol* 38:12, 1990.

Immunoprophylaxis

Barber HR: *Immunobiology for the clinician*, New York, 1977, John Wiley & Sons.

Nalick RH et al: Immunologic response in gynecologic malignancy as demonstrated by the delayed hypersensitivity reaction: clinical correlations, *Am J Obstet Gynecol* 118:393, 1974.

Old LJ et al: The role of the reticuloendothelial system in the host reaction to neoplasia, *Cancer Res* 21:1281, 1961.

Old LJ et al: Antigenic properties of chemically-induced tumors, *Ann NY Acad Sci* 101:80, 1962.

Romney FL et al: Retinoids and the prevention of cervical dysplasias, *Am J Obstet Gynecol* 1411:890, 1981.

Rosenthal SR et al: BCG vaccination and leukemia mortality, *JAMA* 222:1543, 1972.

Springer TA: Traffic signals for lymphocyte recirculation and leukocyte emigration: the multistep paradigm, *Cell* 76:301, 1994.

Surwit EA et al: Evaluation of topically applied transretinoic acid in the treatment of cervical intraepithelial lesions, *Am J Obstet Gynecol* 143:821, 1982.

Immunotherapy

Alberts DS: BCG as an adjuvant to Adriamycin-Cytoxan for advanced ovarian cancer: a Southwest Oncology Group study (meeting abstract). Program and abstracts of the second International Conference on the Adjuvant Therapy of Cancer, University of Arizona Cancer Center, Tucson, Ariz, March 28-31, 1979.

Arca MJ, Mulé JJ, Change AE: Genetic approaches to adoptive cellular therapy of malignancy, *Semin Oncol* 23(1):108, 1996.

Berek JS, Welander C, Schink JC et al: A phase I-II trial of intraperitoneal cisplatin and alpha-interferon in patients with persistent epithelial ovarian cancer, *Gynecol Oncol* 40(3):237, 1991.

Campo MS: Prophylactic and therapeutic vaccination against a mucosal papillomavirus, *J Gen Virol* 74:945, 1993.

Creasman WT et al: Chemoimmunotherapy in the management of primary stage III carcinoma of the ovary, *Cancer Treat Rep* 63:319, 1979.

Crowther ME, Hudson C: Experience with a pilot study of active specific immunotherapy in advanced ovarian cancer (meeting abstract), *Clin Oncol* 3:397, 1977.

Crowther ME, Hudson C: Experience with a pilot study of active specific intralymphatic immunotherapy, *Cancer* 41:2215, 1978.

Crowther ME et al: Active specific immunotherapy in ovarian cancer, *Recent Results Cancer Res* 68:166, 1979.

Currie GA: Eighty years of immunotherapy: a review of immunological methods used for the treatment of human cancer, *Br J Cancer* 26:141, 1972.

Debois JM: Five-year experience with levamisole in cancer patients. Third interim report. Clinical Research Report on R 12564/69, 1978, Janssen Research Productive Information Service.

DiSaia PJ, Nalick RH, Townsend DE: Antibody cryotoxicity studies in ovarian and cervical malignancies, *Obstet Gynecol* 1:314, 1973.

DiSaia PJ et al: Preliminary report on the treatment of women with cervical cancer, stages IIB, IIIB, IVA (confined to the pelvis and/or periaortic nodes), with radiotherapy plus immunotherapy with intravenous *Corynebacterium parvum*, phase II. In Terry WD, Rosenberg SA, editors: *Immunotherapy of human cancer*, New York, 1982, Elsevier North-Holland.

Eilber FR et al: Immunotherapy as a adjunct to surgery in the treatment of cancer, *World J Surg* 1:547, 1977.

Flander AN et al: Immunocompetent for immunotherapy? A study of the immunocompetence of cervical cancer patients, *Int J Gynecol Cancer* 5:438, 1995.

Folkman J, Hochberg M: Self-regulation of growth in three dimensions, *J Exp Med* 138:745, 1973.

Foon KA, Bernard M, Oldham RK: Monoclonal antibody therapy, *J Biol Resp Mod* 1:277, 1982.

Freedman RS et al: Novel immunologic strategies in ovarian carcinoma, *Am J Obstet Gynecol* 167:1470, 1992.

Gall S, Bundy B, Beecham J et al: Therapy of stage III (optimal) epithelial carcinoma of the ovary with melphalan or melphalan plus *Corynebacterium parvum* (a Gynecologic Oncology Group study), *Gynecol Oncol* 25:26, 1986.

Guo Y et al: Effective tumor vaccine generated by fusion of hepatoma cells with activated B cells, *Science* 263:518, 1994.

Hawkins MJ: PPO updates IL-2/LAK, *Prin Prac Oncol* 3(8):1, 1989.

Herberman RB, Oldham RK: Cell-mediated cytotoxicity against human tumors: lessons learned and future prospects, *J Biol Resp Mod* 2:111, 1983.

Herberman RB, Ortaldo JR: Natural killer cells: their role in defenses against disease, *Science* 214:24, 1981.

Hewitt HB: Animal tumor models and their relevance to human tumor immunology, *J Biol Resp Mod* 1:107, 1982.

Hudson CN et al: Experience of a pilot study of active specific immunotherapy in advanced ovarian cancer. In Davis W, Harrap KR, editors: *Characterization and treatment of human tumours.* Proceedings of the Seventh International Symposium on the Biological Characterization of Human Tumours, Amsterdam, Excerpta Medica Foundation, *Advances in Tumour Prevention, Detection and Characterization* 4:332, 1978.

Juillard GJ, Boyer PJ, Yamashiro CH: A phase I study of active specific intralymphatic immunotherapy, *Cancer* 41:2215, 1978.

Kamada M, Sakamoto Y, Furumoto H et al: Treatment of malignant ascites with allogeneic and autologous lymphokine-activated killer cells, *Gynecol Oncol* 34:34, 1989.

Kohler G, Milstein C: Continuous cultures of fused cells secreting antibody of predefined specificity, *Nature* 256:495, 1975.

Lanzavecchia A: Identifying strategies for immune intervention, *Science* 260:937, 1993.

Levy R: Biological forecaster treatment: monoclonal antibodies, *Hosp Pract* 20:67, 1985.

Maiman M et al: Human immunodeficiency virus infection and invasive cervical carcinoma, *Cancer* 71:402, 1993.

Mastrangelo MJ, Beard D, Maguire HC Jr: Current condition and prognosis of tumor immunotherapy: a second opinion, *Cancer Treat Rep* 68:207, 1984.

Meeker TC et al: A clinical trial of anti-idiotype therapy for B cell malignancy, *Blood* 65:1349, 1985.

Melchert F et al: Influencing the immune system of carcinoma patients with oral BCG treatment, *Arch Gynaekol* 224:476, 1977.

Morton D, Eilber FR, Malmgren RA: Immunological factors which influence response to immunotherapy in malignant melanoma, *Surgery* 68:158, 1970.

Morton DL, Goodnight JE: Clinical trials of immunotherapy, *Cancer* 42:2224, 1978.

Oldham RK, Smalley RV: Immunotherapy: the old and the new, *J Biol Resp Mod* 2:1, 1983.

Olkowski ZL, McLaren JR, Skeen MJ: Effects of combined immunotherapy with levamisole and bacillus Calmette-Guérin on immunocompetence of patients with squamous cell carcinoma of the cervix, head and neck, and lung undergoing radiation therapy, *Cancer Treat Rep* 62:1651, 1978.

Onsrud M, Thorsby E: Long-term changes in natural killer activity after external pelvic radiotherapy, *Int J Radiat Oncol Biol Phys* 7:609, 1981.

Rao B et al: Intravenous *Corynebacterium parvum*: an adjunct to chemotherapy for resistant advanced ovarian cancer, *Cancer* 39:514, 1977.

Rosenberg SA: Adoptive immunotherapy of cancer: accomplishments and prospectives, *Cancer Treat Rep* 68:233, 1984.

Rosenberg SA: The development of new immunotherapies for the treatment of cancer using interleukin-2, *Ann Surg* 208(2):121, 1988.

Rosenberg SA: The immunotherapy and gene therapy of cancer, *J Clin Oncol* 10:180, 1992.

Rosenberg SA, Lotze MT, Yang JC et al: Experience with the use of high-dose interleukin-2 in the treatment of 652 cancer patients, *Ann Surg* 210(4):474, 1989.

Schafer A et al: The increased frequency of cervical dysplasia-neoplasia in women infected with the human immunodeficiency virus is related to the degree of immunosuppression, *Am J Obstet Gynecol* 164:593, 1991.

Smith RT: Possibilities and problems of immunologic intervention in cancer, *N Engl J Med* 287:439, 1972.

Spirtos NM, Smith LH, Teng NNH: Prospective randomized trial of topical x-interferon (x-interferon gels) for the treatment of vulvar intraepithelial neoplasia III, *Gynecol Oncol* 37:34, 1990.

Streilein JW: Immunotherapy of cancer, *Surg Gynecol Obstet* 147:769, 1978.

Yannelli JR et al: An improved method for the generation of human lymphokine-activated killer cells, *J Immunol Methods* 100:137, 1987.

Immunodiagnosis

Barlow JJ, Bhattacharya M: Tumor markers in ovarian cancer: tumor associated antigens, *Sem Oncol* 11:203, 1975.

Bast RC Jr et al: A radioimmune assay using a monoclonal antibody to monitor the course of epithelial ovarian cancer, *N Eng J Med* 309:883, 1983.

Bast RC Jr et al: Monitoring ovarian carcinoma with a combination of CA-125, CA-19-9, and carcinoembryonic antigen, *Am J Obstet Gynecol* 149:553, 1984.

Berchuck A et al: Heterogeneity of antigen expression in advanced epithelial ovarian cancer, *Am J Obstet Gynecol* 162:883, 1990.

Cole LA et al: Urinary human chorionic gonadotropin free b-Subunit and b-Core fragment; a new marker of gynecological cancers, *Cancer Res* 48:1356, 1988.

Dini MM, Faiferman I: Sequential in vitro reactivity of lymphocytes from patients with cervical squamous malignancy in a cytotoxicity assay, *Am J Obstet Gynecol* 144:341, 1982.

DiSaia PJ, Rich WM: Value of immune monitoring in gynecologic cancer patients receiving immunotherapy, *Am J Obstet Gynecol* 135:907, 1979.

DiSaia PJ et al: Carcinoembryonic antigen in patients with gynecologic malignancies, *Am J Obstet Gynecol* 121:159, 1975.

DiSaia PJ et al: Carcinoembryonic antigen in cancer of the female reproductive system: serial plasma values correlated with disease state, *Cancer* 39:1265, 1977.

Gall SA, Walling J, Pearl J: Demonstration of tumor-associated antigens in human gynecologic malignancies, *Am J Obstet Gynecol* 115:387, 1973.

Goldenberg DM, DeLand FH: History and status of tumor imaging with radio-labeled antibodies, *J Biol Resp Mod* 1:121, 1982.

Kato H et al: Value of tumor-antigens (TA-4) of squamous cell carcinoma in predicting the extent of cervical cancer, *Cancer* 50:1294, 1982.

Levi MM: Antigenicity of ovarian and cervical malignancy in a view toward possible immunodiagnosis, *Am J Obstet Gynecol* 109:689, 1971.

Maserang VL et al: Immunodiagnosis of human malignancy, *South Med J* 70:222, 1977.

Mills GB et al: Ascitic fluid from human ovarian cancer patients contains growth factors necessary for intraperitoneal growth of human ovarian adenocarcinoma cells, *J Clin Invest* 86:851, 1990.

Molthoff CFM et al: Human ovarian cancer xenografts in nude mice: characterization and analysis of antigen expression, *Int J Cancer* 43:55, 1989.

Nam JH et al: Urinary gonadotropin fragment, a new tumor marker, *Gynecol Oncol* 36:383, 1990.

Biological response modifiers

Abdulhay GA et al: Human lymphoblastoid interferon in the treatment of advanced epithelial ovarian malignancies: a GOG study, *Am J Obstet Gynecol* 152:418, 1985.

Antman KS, Griffin JD, Elias A et al: Effect of recombinant human granulocyte-macrophage colony stimulating factor on chemotherapy-induced myelosuppression, *N Engl J Med* 319:1, 1988.

Balkwill F; Tumor necrosis factor: improving on the formula, *Nature* 361:206, 1993.

Berchuck A, Olt GJ, Everitt L et al: The role of peptide growth factors in epithelial ovarian cancer, *Obstet Gynecol* 75:1, 1990.

Berek JS et al: Intraperitoneal immunotherapy of epithelial ovarian carcinoma with *Corynebacterium parvum, Am J Obstet Gynecol* 152:1984.

Berek JS et al: Intraperitoneal recombinant alpha-interferon for "salvage" immunotherapy in stage III epithelial ovarian cancer: a GOG study, *Cancer Res* 45:4447, 1985.

Berek JS et al: Serum interleukin-6 levels correlate with disease status in patients with epithelial ovarian cancer, *Am J Obstet Gynecol* 164:1038, 1991.

Borden EC, Sondel PM: Lymphokines and cytokines as cancer treatment: immunotherapy realized, *Cancer* 65:800, 1990.

Champlin RE: Peripheral blood progenitor cells: a replacement for marrow transplantation? *Semin Oncol* 23(2):15, 1996.

Dinarello CA: Biology of interleukin 1, *FASEB J* 2:108, 1988.

Einhorn N et al: Human leukocyte interferon therapy for advanced ovarian carcinoma, *Am J Clin Oncol* 5:167, 1982.

Fraser JK, Lill MCC, Figlin RA: The biology of the cytokine sequence cascade, *Semin Oncol* 23(2), 1996.

Freedman RS, Ioannides CG: Biologic response modifiers in the treatment of gynecologic malignancies, *Cancer Bull* 42:98, 1990.

Freedman RS et al: Leukocyte interferon in patients with epithelial ovarian cancer, *J Biol Resp Mod* 2:133, 1983.

Gabrilove JL, Jakubowski A, Scher H et al: Effect of granulocyte colony-stimulating factor on neutropenia and associated morbidity due to chemotherapy for transitional-cell carcinoma of the urothelium, *N Engl J Med* 318:1414, 1988.

Gadducci A et al: Serum levels of tumor necrosis factor (TNF), soluble receptors for TNF (55- and 75-kDa sTNFr), and soluble CD14 (sCD14) in epithelial ovarian cancer, *Gynecol Oncol* 58:184, 1995.

Grosen EA et al: Blocking factors (Soluble Membrane Receptors) for tumor necrosis factor and lymphotoxin detected in ascites and released in short-term cultures obtained from ascites and solid tumors in women with gynecologic malignancy, *Lymphokine Cytokine Res* 11(6):347, 1992.

Grosen EA et al: Measurement of the soluble membrane receptors for tumor necrosis factor and lymphotoxin in the sera of patients with gynecologic malignancy, *Gynecol Oncol* 50:68, 1993.

Heo DS, Whiteside TL, Kanbour A et al: Lymphocytes infiltrating human ovarian tumors. I. Role of Leu-19 (NKH1)-positive recombinant IL-2 activated cultures of lymphocytes infiltrating human ovarian tumors, *J Immunol* 140:4042, 1988.

Hoover HC Jr, Surdyke MG, Dangel RB et al: Prospectively randomized trial of adjuvant active-specific immunotherapy for human colorectal cancer, *Cancer* 55:1236, 1985.

Horning SJ et al: Phase I study of human leukocyte interferon in patients with advanced cancer, *J Biol Resp Mod* 2:47, 1983.

Ikic D et al: Interferon treatment of uterine cervical precancerosis, *J Cancer Res Clin Oncol* 101:303, 1981.

Itri LM: The interferons, *Cancer* 70(4):940, 1992.

Krusic J et al: Influence of human leukocyte interferon on squamous cell carcinoma of the uterine cervix: clinical, histological, and histochemical observations. III. Communication, *J Cancer Res Clin Oncol* 101:309, 1981.

Le J, Vilcek J: Tumour necrosis factor and interleukin 1: cytokines with multiple overlapping biological activities, *Lab Invest* 56:234, 1987.

Lotzova E, Savary CA, Freedman RS et al: Recombinant IL-2 activated NK cells mediate LAK activity against ovarian cancer, *Int J Cancer* 42:225, 1988.

Manetta A, Lucci J, Soopikian J et al: In vitro cytotoxicity of human recombinant tumor necrosis factor x in association with radiotherapy in a human ovarian carcinoma cell line, *Gynecol Oncol* 38:200, 1990.

Mills GB, May C, McGill M et al: A putative new growth factor in ascitic fluid from ovarian cancer patients: identification, characterization, and mechanism of action, *Cancer Res* 48:1066, 1988.

Mills GB, Paetkau V: Generation of cytotoxic lymphocytes to syngeneic tumor by using co-stimulator (interleukin 2), *J Immunol* 125:1897, 1980.

Mutch DG, Powell CB, Kao MS et al: In vitro analysis of the anticancer potential of tumor necrosis factor in combination with cisplatin, *Gynecol Oncol* 34:328, 1989.

Neumaitis J: Cytokine-mobilized peripheral blood progenitor cells, *Sem Oncol* 23(2), 1996.

Oldham RK: Biological and biological response modifiers: 4th modality of cancer treatment. *Cancer Treat Rep* 68:1, 1984.

Oldham RK: Biological and biological response modifiers: new approaches to cancer treatment, *Cancer Invest* 3:53, 1985.

Rosenberg SA, Schwarz SL, Spiess PJ: Combination immunotherapy for cancer: synergistic antitumor interactions of interleukin-2, alfa interferon, and tumor-infiltrating lymphocytes, *J Natl Ca Inst* 80:1393, 1988.

Rosenberg SA, Lotze MT, Yang JC et al: Experience with the use of high dose interleukin-2 in the treatment of 652 cancer patients, *Ann Surg* 210:474, 1989.

Rosenberg SA, Packard BS, Aebersold PM et al: Use of tumor-infiltrating lymphocytes and interleukin-2 in the immunotherapy of patients with metastatic melanoma: a preliminary report, *N Engl J Med* 319:1676, 1988.

Smith CA et al: The TNF receptor superfamily of cellular and viral proteins: Activation, costimualtion, and death, *Cell* 76:959, 1994.

Topolian SL, Soloman D, Avis FP et al: Immunotherapy of patients with advanced cancer using tumor-infiltrating lymphocytes and recombinant interleukin-2: a pilot study, *J Clin Oncol* 6:839, 1988.

Verhaegen H, DeCree J, DeCock W et al: Levamisole therapy in patients with colorectal cancer. In Terry WD, Rosenberg SA, editors: *Immunotherapy of Human Cancer,* New York, 1982, Elsevier Press.

Wadler S. The role of interferons in the treatment of solid tumors, *Cancer* 70(4):949, 1992.

West WH et al: Constant-infusion recombinant Interleukin-2 in adoptive immunotherapy of advanced cancers, *N Engl J Med* 316:898, 1987.

Zimmerman RJ, Gauny S, Chan A et al: Sequence dependence of murine tumor therapy with human recombinant tumor necrosis factor and interleukin-2, *J Natl Ca Inst* 981:227, 1989.

Monoclonal antibodies

Bast R, Klug T, St John E et al: A radioimmunoassay using a monoclonal antibody to monitor the course of epithelial ovarian cancer, *N Engl J Med* 309:883, 1983.

Colcher D, Esteban J, Carrasquillo JA et al: Complementation of intracavitary and intravenous administration of a monoclonal antibody (B72.3) in patients with carcinoma, *Cancer Res* 47:4218, 1987.

Dillman RO: Monoclonal antibodies for treating cancer, *Ann Intern Med* 111:592, 1989.

Fitzgerald D, Pastan I: Targeted toxin therapy for the treatment of cancer, *J Natl Ca Inst* 81:1455, 1989.

Goldenberg DM: New developments in monoclonal antibodies for cancer detection and therapy, *CA* 44:43, 1994.

Junghans RP, Waldmann TA, Landolfi NF et al: Anti-Tac-H, a humanized antibody to the interleukin 2 receptor with new features for immunotherapy in malignant and immune disorders, *Cancer Res* 50:1495, 1990.

Kawase I, Komuta K, Hara H et al: Combined therapy of mice bearing a lymphokine-activated killer-resistant tumor with recombinant interleukin-2 and an antitumor monoclonal antibody capable of inducing anti-dependent cellular cytotoxicity, *Cancer Res* 48:1173, 1988.

Kohler G, Milstein G: Continuous culture of fused cells secreting antibody of predefined specificity, *Nature* 256:495, 1975.

Lamki LM, Zukiwski AA, Shanken LJ et al: Radioimaging of melanoma using Tc-labeled Mab fragment reactive with a high molecular weight melanoma antigen, *Cancer Res* 50(suppl):904s, 1990.

Murray JL, Unger MW: Radioimmuno-detection of cancer with monoclonal antibodies: current status, problems, and future directions, *Crit Rev Oncol Hematol* 8:227, 1988.

Murray JL, Zukiwski AA, Mujoo K et al: Recombinant alpha interferon enhances tumor targeting of an anti-melanoma monoclonal antibody in vivo, *J Biol Resp Mod* 9:556, 1990.

Oldham RK, Lewis M, Orr DW et al: Adriamycin custom-tailored immuno-conjugate in the treatment of human malignancies, *Mol Biother* 1:103, 1988.

Smith LH et al: Human monoclonal antibody recognizing an antigen associated with ovarian and other adenocarcinomas, *Am J Obstet Gynecol* 166(2):634, 1992.

Waldmann TA: Monoclonal antibodies in diagnosis and therapy, *Science* 252, 1657, 1991.

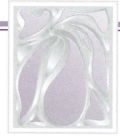

Genes and Cancer

Most investigators support the concept that carcinogenesis is a multistep and mutlifunctional process. The process of carcinognenesis can be divided into three phases of tumor (initiation, promotion, and progression) (Figure 20-1) and can most easily be defined with some human lesions such as skin, liver, breast, colon, and prostate. The tumor initiation stage appears to be an irreversible step that probably involves a somatic mutation caused by DNA damage. The tumor progression stage is characterized by an expansion of initiated stem cells in the benign lesion with production and maintenance of chronic cell proliferation. Also characteristic of this stage is the development of benign outgrowth (e.g., papillomas) and altered patterns of differentiation with a diploid stem line. The final step of progression can be divided into a preinvasive phase where additional genetic events occur and aneuploidy develops followed by loss of heterozygosity and further alteration in patterns of differentiation. This phase is followed by invasion, metastasis, loss of tumor suppressor activity (e.g., *p53* mutation), and gene amplification.

The past 20 years have seen a veritable explosion in biotechnology that has had a dramatic and direct impact on our knowledge of human disease and disease processes. A major beneficiary of this new technology has been the field of cancer biology. Cancer researchers have had an increasing armamentarium of techniques that have allowed them, for the first time, to critically evaluate specific genes and gene products, various aspects of the cell cycle, signal transduction and regulatory pathways within cells, cell-cell as well as cell-matrix interactions that facilitate cell migration and metastasis, and the molecular and cellular aspects of the host immune response to malignant cells. Several of the insights gained from these fundamental studies of cancer biology have already been put into clinical practice, and many more are likely to be clinically applicable in the near future.

The hypothesis that specific genes might be responsible for the induction or maintenance of malignancy is by no means new. It was the molecular characterization of the genomic structure of acutely transforming retroviruses that first provided direct evidence for the existence of such sequences. These viruses are known to be causative agents of cancer in both laboratory animals and animals in the wild. The types of cancer caused in various vertebrate species span the same clinical spectrum of malignancy seen in humans, including sarcomas, carcinomas, lymphomas, and leukemias. Cloning and sequenc-

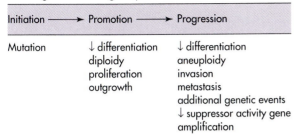

Figure 20-1 Carcinogenesis multi-stage sequence.

ing the genomes of the viruses comprising this group led to identification of the individual genes encoding their transforming capability. Each member of the group was found to contain a unique transforming gene. Collectively, these sequences are known as the *viral oncogenes* (*v-onc*).

Given the relatively unique life cycle of these retroviruses, it was then postulated that the viral oncogenic sequences might actually have arisen from genes contained in the host cell. Formal proof of this came with the discovery that normal, uninfected vertebrate DNA contained homologues to the viral oncogenes and that these homologues were transduced by recombination-type events occurring between viral and cellular sequences. The cellular homologues to the viral oncogenes are collectively known as *proto-oncogenes*, and their nomenclature is similar to that of their viral counterparts: *c-src*, *c-abl*, and *c-myc*. Several of these proto-oncogenes are now known to be important in normal cellular growth, differentiation, and proliferation. Indeed, at least five members of the group have been shown to be identical or closely related to known growth factors, growth factor receptors, or transcriptional factors. It is very likely that this list will grow as more is learned about the normal physiologic function of proto-oncogenes.

A second group of genes, known as tumor suppressor genes, has been identified by virtue of their inactivation or deletion in human tumor cells. These genes also appear to play a critical role in the control of cellular growth, proliferation, and, perhaps, differentiation. The key role of tumor suppressor genes in the growth process is inhibitory in nature, and their inactivation or deletion is believed to promote growth by the resultant absence of critical controls to check proliferation. The prototype of this family is the retinoblastoma (*RB*) gene.

There is clear evidence that members of these two gene groups are important in normal physiologic processes related to cell and tissue growth. There is also considerable circumstantial evidence that alterations in these genes may play a role in the induction or maintenance of malignancies. This circumstantial evidence is as follows:

1. The viral oncogenes, which are oncogenic, are derived from proto-oncogenes, and, as a result, one can envision that proto-oncogenes might also encode oncogenic potential independent of viruses.

2. At least some proto-oncogenes, when coupled with the appropriate control or promoter elements and transfected into normal cells, induce transformation in vitro and tumorigenesis in vivo. Transfection assays using DNA from tumor cell lines or, in some cases, tumor tissues have resulted in identification of dominant transforming oncogenes. Many, although not all, of these dominant transforming genes have been found to be related or identical to known proto-oncogenes. Similarly, transfection studies performed with intact and functional tumor suppressor genes placed into cells that have an inactivated or deleted gene can reverse the transformed phenotype and tumorigenicity of these cells.

3. Direct evidence that a proto-oncogene can be involved in the pathogenesis of an animal tumor again came from studies with transforming retroviruses—in this case, the long-latency transforming viruses. These viruses do not contain a viral oncogene but insert themselves at or near the site of a proto-oncogene, resulting in the presumed activation of these cellular sequences. It is believed that the activation of proto-oncogene sequences is important in the pathogenesis of the tumors caused by these viruses.

4. Many of these studies, including the original one, demonstrated proto-oncogene expression patterns altered in malignant tissue as compared to normal tissue. More recently, the same approach has been taken with tumor suppressor genes, and the results are similar—altered expression exists in many malignant tissues.

5. Classic cytogenetic studies demonstrated an association between specific chromosomal abnormalities and certain human malignancies. Subsequently, the technique of gene mapping using in situ hybridization allowed for exact localization of genes of interest on an individual chromosome. Combining these two techniques led to the observation that many (although, again, not all) specific chromosomal translocations found in human malignancies occurred at or near the site of proto-oncogenes.

   In addition, identification of the sites of tumor suppressor genes came about in the overexpression of a normal proto-oncogene product or in production of a novel, structurally altered gene product.

6. Finally, studies examining human tumor cell lines and fresh tumors for evidence of gene amplification demonstrated that the sequences most frequently amplified are proto-oncogenes. The first proto-oncogene found to be amplified in a human malignant cell line was the *c-myc* gene in I IL-60 leukemia cells. Subsequent studies identified am-

plification of *c-myc* in human small cell carcinoma cell lines.

This approach was used to identify potentially important alterations in two other human malignancies, breast and ovarian cancers. Studies identified alterations in the *HER-2/neu* gene and showed a similar association: women whose tumors contained amplification or overexpression of the gene were more likely to develop recurrence and had shortened overall survival. Analysis of this gene and gene product is now being used by some physicians to aid in prognostic evaluation of these diseases. Similar approaches have been, and continue to be, used to identify both tumor suppressor genes and their alteration in human malignancies.

For a long time, cancer was conceived as a genetic disease at the level of the somatic cell. Advances in understanding cancer at the molecular level have led to the identification of several genes whose somatic alterations are involved in the complex multiple steps in carcinogenesis. As stated above, in addition to the oncogenes first discovered, a second category of tumor-associated genes, the tumor suppressor genes, has been identified, and some of them have been molecularly cloned. The analysis of tumor suppressor genes and of their loss-of-function mutations lends support to the idea that cancer is a genetic disease also at the germline level.

Cellular oncogenes comprise a very small family of genes, highly conserved throughout vertebrate evolution, that code for proteins with diverse functions, including DNA binding, as well as protein kinase and cellular growth factor activities. Cellular oncogenes are more important in certain aspects of the proliferation and differentiation of normal cells. Various mechanisms must underlie their development in carcinogenesis. Several viral oncogenes encode proteins that act as enzymes, which add phosphate groups to amino acid residues in proteins, a process known as phosphorylation.

Cellular proto-oncogenes are deoxyribonucleic acid (DNA) sequences homologous to the transforming genes of ribonucleic acid (RNA) tumor viruses. Because of their high degree of sequence conservation and the high levels of expression in embryonic and rapidly dividing tissues, many have speculated that these genes play a role in the regulation of normal cell growth and differentiation. Studies have shown that oncogene activation, resulting in increased gene expression (amplification) or the synthesis of an altered gene product (mutation), plays a role in the process of malignant transformation. Expression of the *c-myc* proto-oncogene correlates with the proliferative capacity of a number of malignant and nonmalignant cell types. Decreased *c-myc* expression is associated with cellular differentiation and entry into the G_0 phase of the cell cycle. Expression of this gene appears to be regulated at both the transcriptional and post-transcriptional levels. Abnormal expression and structural alterations of the *c-myc* gene have been observed in numerous hematopoi-

etic and solid cancers, including B and T cell malignancies.

Zheng et al. studied another oncogene, called *HER-2/neu*, in ovarian carcinoma. Their group showed application of this gene in approximately one third of such tumors. Examination for the presence of another oncogene, called *H-ras*, was negative. Their studies also suggested that the more aggressive lesions were more likely to contain the *Her-2/neu* amplification. A relationship between *Her-2/neu* amplification and poor prognosis was demonstrated by Slamon for both ovarian and breast carcinomas. It is therefore possible that tumors with such amplifications behave more aggressively than other tumors of similar histological grades. The relevance of this to therapy is only speculative at this time. With more than 20 oncogenes currently known in human malignancies, only very preliminary work in gynecologic malignancies has been done. Details on this exciting area of investigation must await future editions.

GENETIC ALTERATIONS IN CANCER

All cancer cells have some alteration of gene expression. Much of the data about genetic alterations in cancer has come from studies of leukemia and lymphoma where it is easier to obtain relatively pure single-cell dispersions of malignant cells from peripheral blood or bone marrow aspirates. More recently, some similar information has been obtained in solid tumors.

Translocations and Inversions

More than 100 commonly occurring translocations have been observed in malignant cells. Many of these occur consistently in certain specific cancer types, which argues strongly that they are involved in the malignant process of the cell. Some of the translocations may occur as secondary events in the evolution of more aggressive phenotypic changes. The inherent genetic instability of malignant cells leads to further karyotypic abnormalities as the disease progresses, reflecting additional genetic alterations that increase growth potential. Evidence that malignant transformation of cells does not usually result from single translocation event comes from study of patients suffering from telangiectasia ataxia who are at high risk for leukemia. These patients have lymphocytes with a characteristic translocation present for many years before developing leukemia, so additional genetic events are necessary before a malignancy develops in the patient. Table 20-1 lists the translocations found in some common solid tumors encountered by the gynecologist.

Chromosomal Deletions

The application of the techniques of molecular biology, e.g., gene cloning, in situ hybridization, restriction endonuclease mapping of gene sequences, and polymerase chain reaction (PCR) analysis of gene transcrip-

Table 20-1   Translocations in solid tumors

Tumor	Translocation
Breast adenocarcinoma	t(1)(q21-23)
Leiomyoma (uterus)	t(12; 14) (q13-15; q23-24)
Melanoma	t(1) (q11-q12)
	t(1; 6) (q11-12; q15-21)
	t(1;19) (q12; p13)
	t(6) (p11-q11)
	t(7) (q11)
Ovarian adenocarcinoma	t(6;14) (q21; q24)
Rhabdo myosarcoma	t(2; 13) (q35-37; q14)

Modified from Solomon E, Borrow J, Goddard AD: Chromosome aberrations and cancer, *Science* 254:1153, 1991.

Table 20-2   Deletion and loss of heterozygosity in solid tumors

Tumor	Chromosomal deletion	Allele loss
Uterine adenocarcinoma	1q 21-23	3p
Ovarian adenocarcinoma	3p 13-21	3p;6q;11p;17q
	6q 15-23	
Melanoma	1p 11-12	1p
	6q 11-27	
Leiomyoma (uterus)	6p 21	Not tested
	7q 21-31	
Breast adenocarcinoma	1p 11-13	1p;1q;3p;11p
	3p 11-13	13q;16q;17p
	3q 11-13	17q;18q
Bladder adenocarcinoma	1q 21-23	9q;11p;17q
Colorectal adenocarcinoma	17p	5q;17p;18q
	18q	

Modified from Solomon E, Borrow J, Goddard AD: Chromosome aberrations and cancer, *Science* 254; 1153, 1991.

tion, has led to the conclusion that a given chromosomal abnormality may be associated with a variety of neoplasms and that a given oncogene may be activated in a variety of human cancers. The most common defects obscured in solid tumors are deletions in specific gene sequences, observed as loss of a part of a banding region or the loss of heterozygosity of a specific genetic allele. Deletion of genetic material in a cancer cell suggests loss of function that regulates cell proliferation and differentiation. More than 20 human solid tumors have been shown to have some type of chromosomal deletion. Table 20-2 lists some solid tumors of interest to the gynecologist. The *p53* tumor suppressor gene-containing region of chromosome 17p is deleted or mutated in a wide variety of human cancers. The fact that there is such commonality among cancer cell types in the loss of chromosomal material suggests that these regions contain genes coding for regulating functions of a wide variety of cell types. Induction of the malignant neoplastic process must involve at least two genetic "hits." This "two hits" theory introduced by Alfred G. Knudson Jr. answered several questions. Why did patients with inherited disease typically acquire only one or a few cancers? Did the existence of familial cancers mean that sporadic (nonfamilial) disease also had a genetic basis? Did sporadic cancer arise by a completely different process? In a genetically predisposed individual the first genetic alteration may be inherited but the second, third, etc. occur after birth. In a genetically predisposed cell, the remaining single normal allele may be sufficient to maintain normal growth regulation and a second deletion or mutation is required to inactivate the remaining normal allele.

Point Mutations

Point mutations can lead to single changes in a DNA sequence. If this mutation is in a regulatory element of a gene, loss or alteration of regulation of gene expression can occur. If the mutation is in a coding region of a gene, an altered protein may be formed.

Gene Amplification

Gene amplification can occur in many ways. A gene that is usually present in a single copy in the normal cell may be duplicated or may undergo a small increase in the copy number. Another type of amplification may involve 10-100–fold increase in copies of a genetic locus containing key genes. A third method of amplification can result from the duplication of whole chromosomes leading to trisomy or polyploidy. Examples of amplification in human cancers include amplification of the *her-2/neu* gene in advanced breast and ovarian cancer.

Aneuploidy

Although subtle changes in the genome such as point mutations, gene deletion, and gene rearrangements may be associated with the initiation of the malignant transformation, gross changes in the number of chromosomes occur as tumors progress in the malignant process. Chromosomal deletions, translocations, and trisomies are precise non-random chromosomal alterations to be contrasted with changes in cell ploidy occurring later in the malignant progression, which is random without a definitive pattern of chromosomal number. In general, tumors that remain localized without metastases have a much lower incidence of aneuploidy.

Comment

Several similarities to chromosomal alterations in other human solid tumors have been observed in human ovarian carcinoma. In one study of 14 cases, 64% had allelic loss at the estrogen receptor locus of chromosome 6q; 75% had loss of heterozygosity (LOH) at the 17p locus; and 46% had LOH at the H-ras-1 locus of chromosome 11p.

Some of the tumor suppressor genes are also lost or inactivated in ovarian carcinoma. Allelic loss of the *p53* gene was observed in 16 of 20 ovarian carcinomas reported by Carter. Allelic loss of the RB gene has also been observed in 30% of ovarian cancers.

The fact that multiple genetic lesions are associated with individual human cancers and that many of these same defects occur consistently in a variety of tumors leads to the conclusion that there are families of tumor suppressor genes and also oncogenes located on different chromosomes and activated in different cell types at different stages of development. Thus, in one tissue type, the *p53* gene may be an important early step of stem cell proliferation and differentiation, whereas in other tissues, it may be more important at a later step. In addition, oncogene activation is also a frequent finding in human cancer and produces the other side of the coin in uncontrolled cell proliferation and loss of ability of cells to differentiate. To all of this, one must add hereditary susceptibility genes. Thus, it is likely that a cascade of events involving several gene types leads to loss of the cellular control that results in cancer.

ONCOGENES

It has been known for many years that viruses can cause malignant tumors in animals. The link noted in animals spurred a great deal of research aimed at identifying the cancer-causing genes carried by the viruses and finding those host genes that were affected. These investigations surprisingly revealed that the genes implicated in malignant diseases were often altered forms of human genes that viruses picked up during their travels. Other times the viruses activated host genes that were normally quiescent. The normal versions of these pirated and activated genes, now termed *proto-oncogenes*, carried codes specifying the composition of proteins that encourage and stimulate cell replication. These growth-promoting genes come in various forms. Some specify the amino acid sequences of receptors that are found on the cell surface and bind to molecules known as growth factors. When bound by such factors, receptors issue an intracellular signal that ultimately causes cells to replicate. Other growth-promoting genes code for proteins that lie inside the cell and govern the propagation of intracellular growth signal. A third group encode proteins that control cell division.

The discovery that viral genes had human counterparts introduced the intriguing possibility that human cancers, including the majority not caused by viruses, might originate from mutations that convert useful proto-oncogenes into carcinogenic forms or oncogenes. Consistent with this notion, studies indicated that alterations of just one copy, or allele, of these proto-oncogenes was enough to transform and render cancerous some types of cells growing in culture. Such dominant mutations cause

cells to overproduce a normal protein or make an aberrant form that is overactive. In either case, the result is that stimulatory signals increase within the cell even when no such signals come from the outside.

It is ironic that research on animal RNA tumor viruses (retroviruses) having no ability to cause human cancer provided the first key to uncovering the identity of oncogenes. These retroviruses, which infect chickens, rodents, cats, and monkeys, were extremely tumorigenic in that infected animals often showed tumors within weeks of initial exposure to the virus. One of these viruses, the Rous sarcoma virus of chicken, was found to carry a specific gene that it used to transform infected cells from a normal to a malignant state. This type of transforming gene was termed a *viral oncogene*. A single oncogene carried into a chicken cell by a Rous sarcoma virus was able to derail and redirect the entire metabolism of the cell, forcing it to grow in a malignant fashion.

In 1976, Varmus and Bishop found that the oncogene in the Rous sarcoma virus was not a viral gene at all; instead, it rose directly from a pre-existing cellular gene that had been captured by an ancestor of the Rous sarcoma virus. Once captured, this gene was used by the virus to transform cells. The early ancestry of the Rous sarcoma virus was capable of replicating in infected cells but was unable to transform them; it instantly gained tumorigenic potency by kidnapping this normal cellular gene, called the proto-oncogene. In the end this work by Varmus and Bishop revealed much more about the cell than it did about the Rous sarcoma virus, since it pointed to the existence of a gene residing in a normal cellular genome that possesses potent transforming ability when appropriately activated, in this case by a retrovirus. *Here* was clear proof of the presence of at least one gene in the normal cellular DNA that might serve as one of the target genes activated by non-viral carcinogens such as mutagenic chemicals and x-rays. By mimicking the effects of the retrovirus, such non-viral agents might also activate this proto-oncogene, converting it to a powerful oncogene. A cell carrying such a mutant gene might, in turn, respond to this damaged gene by launching a program of deregulated growth, and in this way become a cancer cell.

The information uncovered concerning retroviruses and oncogenes provided little immediate comfort to investigators interested in the origins of human cancer. Retroviruses like Rous sarcoma virus never infected humans and therefore could not act to mobilize human proto-oncogenes. The possible connection came from a notion that many such proto-oncogenes could also be activated through an alternative route. Changes in the DNA sequence created by chemical or physical mutants might substitute for the virus. Mutations induced by these chemical or physical mutants in the genomes of target cells in one or another tissue might be as effective as retroviruses in activating the latent carcinogenic potential of proto-oncogenes. By the early 1980s, these suspicions were validated: mutant proto-oncogenes were found in human tumor genomes. In each case, a change in the sequence structure of a gene was identified as being responsible for converting a proto-oncogene into an active oncogene. For example, a *RAS* oncogene in one human bladder carcinoma was found to have arisen through a single base change that altered the DNA sequence of a precursor proto-oncogene (Table 20-2). *MYC* oncogenes arose through gene amplification in various malignancies.

Next researchers tried to ascertain how these genes succeeded in transforming cells. A simple theme emerged that makes it possible to understand and explain the mechanism of action of most, if not all, oncogenes. The concept derives from an understanding of how normal cells regulate their growth. The growth and division of a normal cell residing within a tissue is controlled largely if not exclusively by its surroundings. A normal cell rarely, if ever, decides on its own to proliferate; rather, it listens to and obeys messages that originate from its neighbors in the tissue. These messages may carry growth-stimulatory or growth-inhibitory information and are conveyed largely by growth factors that are released by some cells, traverse the intercellular space, and then impinge on the surfaces of other cells. These latter cells may respond to growth-stimulatory signals by activating their synthetic machinery, copying their DNA, and dividing. A normal cell will never commit itself to such a growth program without having been stimulated by these external signals. Each cell possesses a complex machinery that enables it to receive these signals, process them, and launch a growth program. The machinery consists of an array of proteins that functions to acquire growth-activating signals and transmit them throughout the cell. These proteins include (1) cell surface receptors that recognize the presence of growth factors in the extracellular space and transmits signals into the cell's interior, informing the cell of these encounters, (2) cytoplasmic signal transducers that become activated by these receptors and then pass signals further into the cell, and (3) nuclear transcription factors that are energized by the cytoplasmic signal transducers and, in turn, respond by activating entire banks of cellular genes. These activated gene banks together orchestrate the cell's growth program, they detail events that, acting in concert, enable the cell to grow and divide. Proto-oncogenes encode many of the proteins in this complex signaling circuitry that enables a normal cell to respond to exogenous growth factors. Oncogenes participate in this signaling circuitry by specifying aberrantly functioning versions of the components of this circuitry. Oncogene proteins succeed in activating these signal circuits even in the absence of stimulation by extra-cellular growth factors. In doing so, they force a cell to grow, even when

its surroundings contain none of the clues that are normally required to provoke growth.

Other researchers suggest that mutations in at least two proto-oncogenes have to be present and that only certain combinations of mutations lead to malignancies. These findings suggest that individual oncogenes, although potentially quite powerful, are not capable of causing malignancies by themselves. Thus, oncogenes cannot explain most cancers by themselves. This view was strengthened by the discovery of more than a dozen different oncogenes in human tumors. The results were ultimately disappointing: a mere 20% of human tumors turned out to carry the expected alterations. None of the tumors had pairs of cooperative alterations sometimes found in cultured cells. It also appeared that the inherited mutations responsible for predisposing people to familial cancers were not oncogenes. All of this indicates a need for further study. It became obvious that activated oncogenes were only part of the picture; another class of mutant genes seemed to be equally important. These other genes have been called *anti-oncogene*; however, the term *tumor suppressor genes* is now more widely used.

TUMOR SUPPRESSOR GENES

The first tumor suppressor gene cloned was the *RB* gene; it is the defective gene in retinoblastoma. Several other tumor suppressor genes or likely tumor suppressor genes have been cloned (Table 20-3). This is almost certainly only the tip of the iceberg, and many more tumor suppressor genes will likely be discovered as investigators learn about cancer cell genetics and the map of human genomes. Several generalizations can be made, and a comparison with the activation of oncogenes is instructive. Mutations in oncogenes are gain of function events and lead to increased cell proliferation and decreased cell differentiation. Oncogene mutations do not appear to be inherited through the germ line. Oncogenes are mutated in a wide variety of human cancers (Table 20-4). In contrast, tumor suppressor gene inactivations are loss of function events, usually requiring a mutational event in one allele followed by a loss or inactivation of the other allele. They are recessive in nature, and the resulting mutations may be inherited through the germ line. One point of similarity is that somatic mutational events can occur in oncogenes and in tumor suppressor genes, and they may accumulate over a lifetime (Table 20-5).

Comment

Each cell type in the body follows a slightly different path on its way toward malignancy. Each of these paths is rather long, involving multiple distinct changes in cell genotype and phenotype. These intermediate steps (stages) have long been recognized by pathologist who classify tissues at various stages, including fully normal,

Table 20-3   Tumor suppressor genes

Gene	Gene product	Tumor associations
RBI (13q)*	110-kDa nuclear hypophosphorylated protein, negative cell cycle regulator	Retinoblastoma Osteosarcoma Small cell lung cancer Soft tissue sarcoma Breast cancer Bladder cancer
p53 (17p)	53-kDa sequence-specific DNA-binding protein and transcriptional activator	Li-Fraumeni syndrome Most common alteration in human cancer
DCC (18q)	1447 amino acid transmembrane protein with homology to known adhesion molecules; role in terminal cell differentiation	Colorectal cancer
APC (5q21)	2843 amino acid protein that interacts with membrane-associated cadherin catenin complexes and with microtubules	Familial adenomatous polyposis Garrner's syndrome
MTSI (9q21)	148 amino acid protein inhibitor of cyclin dependent kinase-4	Familial melanoma Bladder cancer Various others
BRCA1 (17q)	1863 amino acid protein with zinc finger-like domains suggesting function as a transcriptional factor	Breast cancer Ovarian cancer
BRCA2 (13q)	Possibly BRUSH I	Familial breast cancer
VHL (3p)	Protein with short homology to a glycan-anchored membrane protein of *Trypanosoma brucei,* no function assigned	Pheochromocytoma Renal cell cancer Pancreatic cancer Hemangioblastomas of CNS and retina
WT-1 (11q)	50-kDa gene, related to the early growth response gene, encodes four 46- to 49-kDa proteins, which appear to function as DNA binding transcriptional repressors	Wilm tumor
NF-1 (17q11.2)	Neurofibromin (about 2500 amino acids), probably negative regulator for p21 *ras*	Von Recklinghausen neurofibromatosis
NF-2 (22q12)	Schwannomin (about 600 amino acids), regulator of cellular response to external environment	Neurofibromatosis type 2

*Chromosomal location.

Mastrangelo MJ et al: Gene therapy for human cancer: an essay for clinicians, *Sem Oncol* 23(1):4, 1996.

hyperplastic, metaplastic, frankly invasive, and metastatic. These discrete stages in tumor development correlate well with the underlying genetic changes in the evolving tumor cell genome. The single altered gene may be able to advance toward full malignancy but the entire process can be completed only when multiple successive changes occur in distinct cellular genes. This requirement for multiple changes creates an important protective mechanism against cancer. If a small number of genetic changes suffice to transform a normal cell into a malignant one, our bodies will be riddled with tumors. By erecting multiple barriers, the circuitry inside ourselves ensures that only the rare cell can sustain the requisite number of changes for making a cancer cell.

GENE THERAPY

One approach to gene therapy for cancer involves the abrogation of oncogene activity and/or the restoration of tumor suppressor gene function. The defective gene could be replaced with a normal gene, a process termed *hemologous recombination*, but progress to date has made this process too inefficient for clinical use. Available vectors can insert a gene into the genome of replicating cells on a random basis but the faulty genes are not removed. The tumor suppressor gene *p53* seems a likely target for gene therapy in that defects in the function of this gene are the most common alteration in human cancer. Mice genetically engineered to be without *p53* look normal at birth but at 6 months all have tumors or are dead. Transfer of the wild-type *p53* gene to deficient cells in vitro will prevent emergence of the neoplastic phenotype, even in tumor cells bearing multiple genetic abnormalities. At this point, the impact of pharmacologic doses of tumor suppressor gene protein on malignant cells is a matter of conjecture because human trials are limited.

Transforming the effects of oncogene function can take one of two approaches. One can attempt to remove the

Table 20-4   Functional classification of selected oncogenes and associated human tumors

Function	Oncogene	Associated tumors
Growth factor	hst	Gastric cancer
	KS3	Kaposi sarcoma
Growth factor receptor	Neu-erB-B2	Breast, ovary, gastric cancers
	erb-B	Breast cancer, glioblastoma
	trk	Papillary thyroid, colon cancers
Signal transducing (GTP-binding) proteins	Ha-ras	Bladder cancer
	Ki-ras	Lung, colon cancers
	N-ras	Leukemias
	gsp	Pituitary tumors
Protein kinases	raf	Gastric cancer
	met	Osteosarcoma
	abl	Leukemia/lymphoma
Nuclear transcription factor	myc	Lymphomas, carcinomas
	N-myc	Neuroblastoma
	L-myc	Small cell lung cancer
Membrane proteins	bcl-2	Follicular, undifferentiated lymphoma
	mas	Breast cancer
	ret	Papillary thyroid cancer

Mastrangelo MJ et al: Gene therapy for human cancer: an essay for clinicians, *Sem Oncol* 23(1):4, 1996.

Table 20-5   Comparison of oncogenes and tumor suppressor genes

Characteristic	Oncogene	Tumor suppressor genes
Number of mutational events in cancer	One	Two
Role of mutation	Gain of function ("Dominant")	Loss of function ("Recessive")
Germ-line inheritance	No	Yes
Somatic mutations	Yes	Yes
Genetic alterations	Point mutations, amplifications, gene rearrangements	Point mutations, deletions
Effect on growth control	Activate cell proliferation	Negatively regulate growth promoting genes
Result of gene transfection	Transforms cells to a partly malignant behavior	Suppress malignant phenotype

oncogene product or block its function. Alternatively, one could use exogenous or intracellular generated antisense oligonucleotides in an attempt to block production of the oncogene product by preventing the transcription of the chromosomal DNA code to RNA message. Antisense oligonucleotides can be administered systemically. Growth suppression has been achieved in vitro with exogenous antisense oligonucleotides. Several human trials are underway using exogenous antisense oligonucleotides, especially in the study of gene therapy for leukemia.

Major successes with gene therapy for cancer have been limited to in vitro systems where tumor cells with well defined genetic defects are easily targeted. Some success has been achieved with systemically administered antisense in preclinical models. Our own research revolved around cytokine gene transfer to tumor cells to enhance the development of immunity. Cytokines provide stimulatory signals important for T cell activation, and enrichment of the cytokine milieu by local injection at the site of immunization can promote the acquisition of cellular immunity. Reasoning that higher and perhaps more effective cytokine levels could be sustained at the immunization site by local production rather than local injection, tumor cells can be genetically engineered to produce the molecule of interest where included in vaccine preparations. Clinical trials are in progress in patients with squamous cell carcinoma, neuroblastoma, glioblastoma, colon cancer, small cell lung cancer, and ovarian epithelial cancer utilizing this technology. Cells are engineered to produce one of several cytokines, including interleukin 2, 4, 5, and 6, as well as macrophage colony stimulating factor, tumor necrosis factor, and the intracellular adhesion molecule.

APOPTOSIS

There has been an extraordinary increase in the interest in the mode of cell deletion known as programmed cell death, or apoptosis. Although apoptosis was described in the 1970s, scientists have only recently recognized its importance in numerous biologic processes such as organism development and metamorphosis and in human diseases such as autoimmunity and cancer. Excitement over research in this area has been driven by discoveries that apoptosis is highly regulated at the molecular level by oncogens and anti-oncogenes. It is also clear that many of these same controlling elements and pathways are also active during development. Thus many now believe that understanding the biochemical and molecular pathways that control apoptosis is essential to understanding the cancer problem.

Apoptosis is a distinct mode of cell death that is responsible for deletions of cells in normal tissues; it also occurs in specific pathologic contexts. Morphologically, it involves rapid condensation and budding of the cell with formation of membrane-enclosed apoptotic bodies containing well-preserved organelles, which are phagocytosed and digested by nearby resident cells. There is no associated inflammation. Apoptosis occurs spontaneously in malignant tumors, often markedly retarding their growth, and it is increased in tumors responding to radiation, cytotoxic chemotherapy, heating, and hormone ablation. In cancer, programmed cell death appears to be a mechanism for deleting cells from the population that has sustained carcinogen-induced DNA damage. When apoptosis of such cells is blocked or inhibited by mutations in oncogenes or anti-oncogenes, such as *bcl-2* or *p53*, these cells are free to propagate their genetic abnormalities through further divisions. This mechanism of genomic instability may be an early step in the development of a cancer cell. After a tumor has formed, many of the current cancer treatments such as radiotherapy and chemotherapy kill cells via the production of DNA damage, and these same mutations in *bcl-2* and *p53* may then influence the effectiveness of these therapies because of their ability to inhibit the apoptotic mode of cell death.

The primary importance of the apoptosis concept for oncology lies in its being a regulated phenomenon subject to stimulation and inhibition. Although little is known about how established therapeutic agents for cancer affect its initiation, it seems reasonable to suggest that greater understanding of the process of involvement might lead to the development of improved treatment regimens. Inhibitory mechanisms such as *bcl-2* proto-oncogene expression may be implicated in the development of resistance of tumors to therapeutic agents and may contribute to tumor growth and perhaps to oncogenesis by allowing the inappropriate survival of cells with DNA abnormalities. It is likely that additional inhibitory mechanisms will be defined. Finally, the discovery that mononuclear antibodies can induced the apoptosis of lymphoid tumor cells may have implications for the development of novel approaches toward therapy. The study of the molecular basis of apoptosis is still in the early stages, and only a limited number of the "central players" have been identified. Most investigators are cautiously optimistic that this area of research will yield important principles to understanding and manipulating cellular behavior in health and disease. Apoptosis is not simply a description of cell death, nor is it a spurious trend in the biology literature; it is a fundamental process and is controlled at the genetic and molecular levels: as such it can be analyzed, understood, and manipulated.

GENETIC TECHNOLOGIES

Through the elucidation of DNA structure by molecular techniques, one can study human genes. Molecular biology is now applied to most branches of clinical medicine. Awareness of the techniques integral to molecular biology is based on an understanding of DNA structure and genes. DNA is a double-helical structure composed of two coils of nucleotide chains connected by nitrogenous bases. The precise complimentary nature of nitrogenous bases provides the basis for the molecular analysis of DNA structure. A gene is a strand of DNA that is transcribed into messenger RNA in the cell's nucleus, then translated into protein in the ribosomes. The amino acid sequence of the protein is determined by the RNA sequence and ultimately the DNA sequence, specifically by groups of three base pairs of nucleotides, termed *codons*. This is referred to as the "genetic code." Individual genes make up only a small percentage of the 3×10^9 base pairs of nucleotides per haploid genome in humans. The function of the remainder of the DNA is speculative but it should be more fully understood with the completion of the human genome mapping project. Characterization of the estimated 50,000-100,000 human genes should be beneficial to the understanding and treatment of genetic disease. It is estimated that the mapping initiative begun in August 1989 should be completed around the year 2005.

Restriction Enzymes

Since human genomic DNA is very large, but specific genes are small, cutting DNA into smaller pieces greatly facilitates its study. Enzymes and bacteria, called restriction enzymes or restriction endonucleases, enable digestion of DNA into smaller pieces. These restriction enzymes are native to the organism and protect against its

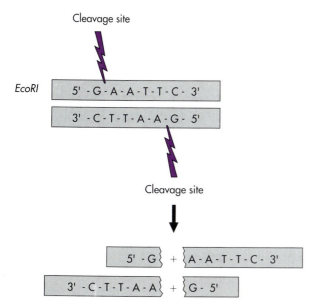

Figure 20-2 Restriction enzymes (endonucleases) recognize specific sequences and cut every time this particular array is encountered. *EcoRI* recognizes the sequence G-A-A-T-T-C, and the enzyme cuts between the G and the A.

destruction by foreign DNA, such as viruses. The restriction enzymes recognize specific sequences and cut every time this particular array of bases is encountered. They are named for the organism in which they are identified, as well as the strain. For example, EcoRI was isolated from *Escherichia coli*, strain R, and was the first such enzyme obtained from this organism. This enzyme recognizes the sequence GAATTC and cuts between the G and the A (Figure 20-2).

Southern Blot Analysis

Southern blot analysis provides a basis for studying genetic disorders at the DNA level. When a normal gene is identified, it can be used as a probe (i.e., a DNA probe to study a gene's structure in an individual's DNA). If the subject's DNA and the DNA probe are each rendered single stranded and then hybridized, complimentary pairing should occur between the DNA probe and the sample DNA. If the pairing does not occur, the subject's DNA does not contain the gene structures present in the probe. For convenience, subject DNA is commonly placed on some type of manageable substance, usually a nylon membrane. This is the Southern blot, named for EM Southern, not for a particular geographic region. A Northern blot, which identifies a particular sequence of RNA, consists of a membrane containing immobilized RNA; a Western blot contains proteins.

A series of steps is required to create a Southern blot (Figure 20-3). DNA is first extracted from nucleated cells, such as leukocytes, trophoblasts, etc. The DNA is then digested with a restriction enzyme into innumerable small pieces. The gene of interest is among these many

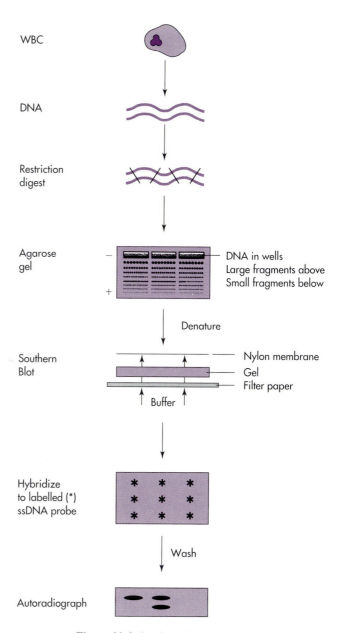

Figure 20-3 Southern Blot preparation.

fragments, but its precise identification and size cannot be determined at this point. The DNA is loaded into an agarose gel and electric current is applied. During this gel electrophoresis, the current causes small DNA fragments to migrate faster and farther than larger fragments (Figure 20-4). The gel is then stained with ethidium bromide, which intercalates between the base pairs and allows visualization of the DNA when it is exposed to ultraviolet light. Because human genomic DNA is so large, the DNA in the lanes appears as a smear but is actually composed of many discrete fragments of varying size. Correct identification of the gene being studied is not yet possible at this point in the procedure.

The DNA contained within the agarose gel is still double stranded at this point. If the gel is exposed to

Step 1. Denaturation. The double-stranded DNA containing the gene of interest is heated to render it single stranded (denatured).

Step 2. Primer annealing. Short pieces of DNA that are complementary to the ends of the double-stranded DNA to be amplified (primers P1, 2) stick (anneal) to their complementary regions of DNA.

Step 3. Extension. In the presence of DNA polymerase and deoxynucleotide triphosphates (dNTPs), the synthesis of the second complementary strand of DNA is completed (extension). The DNA content has been doubled.

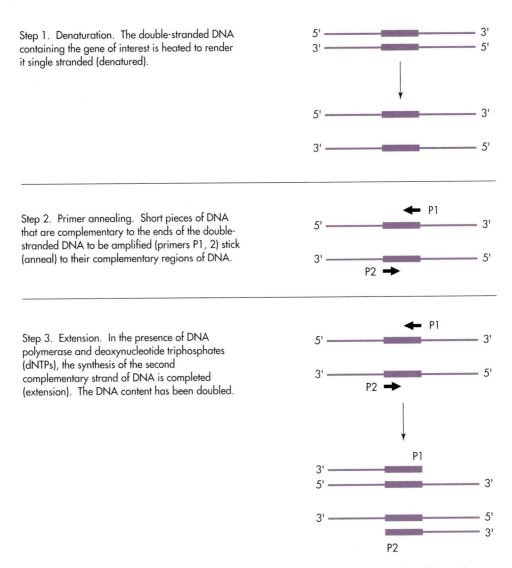

Figure 20-4 Diagram of the polymerase chain reaction. One cycle is shown. The thickened region represents the sequence to be amplified.

alkali, the DNA will denature into single-stranded pieces. The gel now could be studied by hybridization to a single-stranded DNA probe but, because of the fragility of the gel, the DNA is usually transferred to a nylon membrane (the Southern blot). The gel is placed on a platform in a container with buffer. The nylon membrane is positioned directly above the gel, followed by paper towels on top of the membrane. The buffer passes up through the gel by capillary action, causing a single stranded-DNA to migrate to the nylon membrane. The membrane is then baked in a vacuum oven to permanently fix the DNA to the nylon blot. Transfer time may be shortened by using electro blotting or vacuum blotting.

The blot, containing a number of distinct specimens from subjects and control(s), can now be hybridized to a DNA probe. For example, if congenital adrenal hyperplasia due to a deletion in the 21-hydroxylase gene is suspected, the blot could be hybridized to a DNA probe

for 21-hydroxylase. For hybridization, a DNA probe is labeled with some type of marker, usually a radionucleotide such as ^{32}P, although nonradioactive substances such as biotin-avidin may be used. After the probe is labeled, if it is double stranded, it is denatured by boiling or by using an alkaline and placed into a bag or tube with solution and the membrane for hybridization. When hybridization is complete, the unbound, labeled DNA probe is removed by washing. Washes are performed to remove as much of the non-specific material as possible. By washing at high temperatures and low cell concentrations, only sequences that are exactly complimentary remain hybridized. When washing is complete, the blot is placed in a plastic wrap inside a cassette containing film at -70° C. The film is then developed and the presence or absence of bands can be determined. If the same number and size of bands are present in the affected individuals and in the controls, the gene is present and no obvious large rearrangements of the gene are present. This does not preclude the possibility of the presence of smaller mutations, such as a 2-bp deletions or point mutations. Southern blot analyses are not capable of detecting changes this small unless the mutation alters a restriction enzyme's cut site.

Polymerase Chain Reaction (PCR)

Southern blot analysis is labor intensive and generally requires 5-10 µg of DNA for analysis. The development of polymerase chain reaction (PCR) has greatly simplified DNA analysis and shortened laboratory time. As mentioned above, the target gene makes up a minority of the sequences in total chromosomal DNA. Rather than trying to identify a single gene among the many genes per haploid genome with a labeled probe such as in Southern analysis, the PCR allows the exponential amplification of the targeted gene so that its structure can be studied without the need for DNA probes, Only minute quantities of DNA, typically 0.1-1 µg are necessary for PCR. One important prerequisite of PCR not required for the Southern blot analysis is that the sequence of the gene, or at least the borders of the region of DNA to be amplified, must be known.

The PCR procedure has three steps (Figure 20-4). First, DNA is heated to 94°-95° C to render it single stranded or denatured. Second, the temperature is lowered to 37°-55° C, which results in DNA annealing. The reaction solution contains primers, which are short pieces of DNA usually about 20-30 base pairs in length. They are exactly complimentary to the ends of each piece of the double-stranded DNA to be amplified. When the temperature is lowered, these primers will stick, or anneal, to their complimentary regions of DNA. This is the reason the sequence part of the DNA template must be known. The primers are present in such excess that the DNA template is more likely to anneal to the primer rather than to itself. Third, the temperature is raised to about 72° C in the presence of an enzyme (a heat-stable DNA polymerase such as Taq polymerase) and the deoxy nucleotide triphosphates (dNTPs) so that the synthesis of the second complementary strand of DNA will be completed. In practice, the primers, buffer, dNTPs, enzyme, and DNA are mixed together in a tube to a total volume of 25-100 µg and placed in a thermal cycler, an incubator that changes temperature rapidly. The exact cycling parameters and conditions for PCR must be determined empirically for each set of primers.

After one cycle of denaturation, annealing, and primer extension, the DNA content is doubled; one piece of double-stranded DNA becomes two double-stranded pieces of DNA. After two cycles, there are four copies; after three cycles there are eight, and so on. The amount of DNA being amplified increases exponential with each cycle so that the final amount of amplified DNA will be 2^n where n equals the number of cycles. After 30 cycles, which is the typical number of cycles used, the gene of interest may be amplified over 2^{30} or well over one million times. If agarose gel electrophoresis is performed on the amplified product of PCR, the product will migrate to a specific point in the gel and appear as a distinct band. Typically, fragments several kilobases in size can be amplified but sequences up to 10 kb have been successfully amplified.

GENETICS OF COLON CANCER

The colon cancer model developed by Vogelstein and others illustrates in a clear and concise manner some of the concepts discussed above (Figure 20-5). The Adenomatous Polyposis Coli (*APC*) suppressor gene, when present in mutant form, appears to permit the outgrowth of early colonic polyps. In colon disease, samples are easily obtained. As a polyp becomes larger and more irregular, it becomes more readily accessible to the gastroenterologist, and serial studies can be performed. Colon cancer is also convenient to study because certain families are genetically prone to a rare disease called familial adenomatous polyposis. In affected individuals the colon becomes carpeted with hundreds or thousands of polyps, one or more of which is likely to become malignant in mid-life. It was in these patients that the defect in the *APC* gene was first recognized. In most human colonic tumors, the *APC* gene is altered by somatic mutations occurring randomly in colonic epithelial cells. In the rarer situation of familial tumors, the mutant *APC* gene is acquired from a parent and is thus implanted in all cells of the colon, predisposing the recipient to hundreds if not thousands of polyps. The *APC* somatic mutation may later activate a *ras* oncogene, creating a more advanced polyp that is, however, still benign. Over a period of years, this polyp may sustain mutations in its *DCC* and *p53* suppressor genes. These mutations in turn appear to lead to more autonomous uncontrolled growth of colon carcinoma cells.

This work on colon cancer illustrated nicely the multi-step nature of tumorigenesis and the interplay of oncogenes and tumor suppressor genes but unfortunately provides no clues into the later stages of tumorigenesis, including invasiveness and metastasis. These later phenotypes may be governed by yet other mutant genes that remain to be yet discovered. However, the research on colon carcinoma provides a model for researchers working on a number of other tumor types. The hope is to describe the life history of a tumor in terms of a succession of genetic lesions that are sustained in a distinct, relatively small cohort of target genes. Such genetic histories promise to provide a clear view of all the molecular changes required to make a tumor cell and in turn the identities of the molecular targets for future generations of diagnostic and therapeutic techniques.

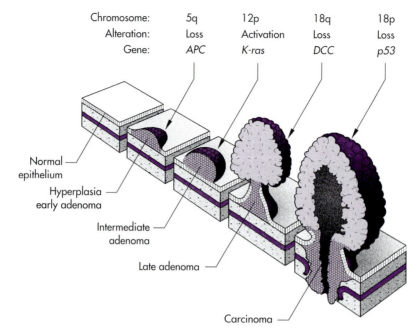

Figure 20-5 A model for colorectal tumorigenesis.

GENETIC STUDIES IN GYNECOLOGIC MALIGNANCIES
Ovarian Cancer

Two neoplasms with the same histology often have divergent clinical behavior, suggesting that the genetic alterations underlying the development and progression of these lesions may not be comparable. Studies are needed correlating specific molecular markers with histologic subtype and appropriate clinical parameters. A few such studies have been reported. There has been controversy for decades as to whether the patterns of ovarian carcinoma with involvement of multiple sites of peritoneal surface reflects a multifocal origin ("field effect") or a unifocal origin with widespread metastatic sites. Well-documented cases of extra-ovarian papillary carcinoma with synchronous uterus endometrial carcinoma support the multifocal concept. Mok reported nine cases with widespread abdominal carcinomatosis in which the pattern of *p53* gene expression was identical in cancer cells from different sites in the same patient, suggesting a unifocal origin. Tsao used X-chromosome inactivation as a molecular marker and showed similar results.

There have been numerous other reports identifying activation of different oncogenes in ovarian cancer. Overexpression of *erb B-2* (*her-2neu*) with and without gene amplification has been reported. Using Southern blot type analysis, Slamon found *erb B-2* amplification in 26% of 120 primary ovarian malignancies. Twelve percent of cases showed *erb B-2* expression without evidence of gene amplification. Over expression of *erb B-2* correlates with poor clinical outcome, suggesting possible clinical use for this molecular marker in future treatment plans.

Baker reported *c-myc* amplification in 29% of ovarian carcinomas. In another study, *c-myc* amplification was reported in 50% of ovarian carcinomas. *C-myc* amplification can not be detected in normal ovarian tissue, benign adenomas, or LMP tumors. This latter observation supports the theory that different genetic alterations account for the development of benign vs malignant ovarian neoplasms. Abnormalities of other oncogenes, such as *ras* gene deletions, amplification, and point mutation, and *fos* gene overexpression also have been reported.

This carcinogenesis of ovarian cancer likely involves inactivation of tumor suppressor genes as well. Sato reported 37 ovarian neoplasms studied with several DNA probes and found allelic losses on 6q, 13q, and 19q in serous carcinomas. They found fewer allelic losses in mucinous type tumors. Sasano found homogenous deletions of the *RB* gene in 1 of 24 ovarian carcinomas. Mazars found *p53* gene mutations in 36% of 34 ovarian carcinomas with most mutations clustered in exons 5 and 7. Marks examined *p53* gene expression in more than 100 ovarian carcinomas and found high levels of mutant p53 protein in more than 50% of the tumors, whereas p53 was undetectable in several benign gynecologic tissue samples. Overexpression of p53 protein was found to correlate closely with the presence of *p53* gene mutation in the tumors. Such studies suggest that the *p53* gene through deletion and/or point mutation plays a role in the development and/or progression of some ovarian cancers.

Most of the above text applies to genetic alterations occurring in somatic cells during cancer development and progression. Primary genetic factors are thought to account for about 5% of ovarian cancer cases. A great deal of research is currently underway to identify and clone the target genes. *BRCA1* is the designation given a gene located in the cells of all humans. Mutant forms of the *BRCA1* has been shown to be associated with disease in some families with multiple cases of ovarian cancer only. In 1995, a combined report from research centers throughout the world reported that |Lf6% of 145 families with multiple cases of ovarian/breast cancer demonstrated the presence of the *BRCA1* gene.

This suggests but does not prove that an altered or mutant form (currently 50 mutants have been identified) of the normal *BRCA1* gene may be passed from generation to generation in these families and that an altered *BRCA1* may predispose a female to develop breast and/or ovarian cancer. The data also suggest that in families in which disease is not linked to *BRCA1*, there may be other, as-yet-unknown, genes responsible for ovarian cancer. In September 1994, the *BRCA1* gene was isolated. This made it possible to identify specific changes in BRCA1 that are associated with disease in cancer cases of *BRCA1*-linked families. It also opens the possibility of identifying individuals in these families who have changes in *BRCAq* but no disease. Such individuals are considered to have a high risk for developing breast and/or ovarian cancer. On the other hand, individuals in these families who have not inherited an altered *BRCA1* gene are not known to be at high risk for developing these diseases. Thus testing for altered *BRCA1* in these families may allow for better evaluation of disease risk for individual members. Because experience with genetic testing for cancer is limited and is an extremely sensitive issue, the American Society of Human Genetics has made recommendations concerning genetic testing for ovarian and breast cancer predisposition. The organization recommends that genetic testing be limited to members of families with a strong ovarian/breast cancer history and that testing should be performed in conjunction with established research programs by trained professionals. These trained professionals are aware of genetic, clinical, and psychologic implications of the testing and of the technical limitations of the testing methods.

Cervical Cancer

Although the association of HPV infection with cervical cancer suggests HPV as a causative agent, several other facts suggest that HPV infection alone is insufficient to bring about the neoplasm. The viral genome contains several open frames (ORFs) encoding many proteins and is stably integrated into the host DNA. Although a common point of integration has not been found, HPV sequences have been found integrated near cellular oncogenes *c-myc* and *n-myc* in at least a few cervical cancer cell lines. In most cases, integration interrupts the E1 and E2 open reading frames but leaves E6 and E7

ORFs intact. The proteins encoded by E6 and E7 of oncogenesis HPV strains can effectively immortalize primary keratinocytes; this was demonstrated by Barbosa in a report in 1989.

The molecular basis for differences in the oncogenic potential between various strains of HPV remains unclear. Münger has shown some biochemical and biologic differences between E7 proteins of low-risk viruses such as HPV-6 and high-risk viruses such as HPV 16.

Kastan suggested that *p53* may function as an "emergency brake" in cells that have sustained DNA damage. Cells damaged by irradiation or drugs often arrest in the G_1-S phase of the cell cycle, presumably allowing for DNA repair. This cell cycle arrest is associated with transient increases in wild-type *p53* and is not seen in cells containing mutant *p53* genes. Kessis suggested that oncogenic HPV E6 expression may also disrupt the *p53*-mediated cellular response to DNA damage. When HPV 16 E6 is transfected into cells exhibiting normal DNA damage response, p53 protein levels are essentially undetectable and cell cycle arrest after DNA damage is abolished. Thus genomic instability is achieved, possibly leading to further genetic alterations and tumorigenesis.

Vulvar Cancer

Like cervical cancer, a sexually transmitted agent is suspected to play a role in the pathogenesis of vulvar cancer. HPV 16 and 18 have been identified in VIN and invasive squamous carcinoma. Worsham found that vulvar cancers tend to contain certain consistent chromosomal abnormalities, including losses of chromosomes 3p, 8p, 22q, and gains of 3q and 11q. Losses of 10q and 18q were found only in cases that exhibited biologically aggressive behavior. As with cervical malignancies, HPV infection may play a role in the occurrence of molecular alterations that lead to tumor development and progression.

Endometrial Cancer

Like cervical and vulvar cancer, endometrial carcinogenesis has an established preinvasive state (hyperplasia) that is available for study and comparison with more advanced invasive lesions. Several small studies have identified alterations of oncogenes such as the *ras* group, *k-ras*, *c-fms*, and *c-erb-1* that may play a role in the development and progression of endometrial carcinomas. Okamoto studied 24 endometrial adenocarcinomas for allelic losses and found loss of heterozygosity in 7 cases, 5 of which lost loci on 17p, which harbors the *p53* gene. Risinger reported 21 endometrial carcinomas where *p53* gene point mutations were found in 3 cases (14%). Endometrial carcinoma frequently occurs in patients with hereditary non-polyposis colorectal cancer (lynch syndrome II), suggesting that inactivation of the same gene may participate in the development of both cancers.

GLOSSARY

allele Alternative forms of the same gene. Because of the paired nature of chromosomes, every gene exists in two copies. Each copy is an allele.

anti-oncogene See tumor suppressor gene.

c-erb-B-2 proto-oncogene Also referred to as *HER-2* or *neu*, this gene encodes a protein that is structurally similar to the receptor for epidermal growth factor. When it is amplified, the gene is of prognostic significance in breast and ovarian neoplasms.

capping The addition of 7-methylguanosine residues to the 5′ end of most eukaryotic mRNA.

chromosome translocation Exchange of genes or portions of genes between different chromosomes. It is one mechanism for activating oncogenes.

cloning An in vivo method to produce unlimited quantities of specific DNA fragments from as little as a single DNA molecule.

codons A group of three nucleotides forming a base coding message in the gene sequence. In *ras* genes, for example, the 12th, 13th, or 61st codon is often mutated, leading to oncogene activation.

complementary DNA (cDNA) DNA synthesized from a mRNA template such that the DNA sequence is complementary to the mRNA.

cytoplasmic signal transduction molecules Proteins within the cytoplasm of cells responsible for transmitting signals from one event to the next event.

DNA probe A short segment of DNA in which the base sequence is specifically complementary to a particular gene segment. The probe is used, for example, on the Southern blot assay to determine if a certain gene is present in a tumor sample undergoing DNA analysis.

exons The coding portion of genes.

gel electrophoresis A molecular biology laboratory technique in which DNA, RNA, or proteins are separated according to molecular weight, charge, and spatial characteristics in an electric field applied to a gel. For example, because DNA is negatively charged, it migrates toward the positively charged electrode.

gene amplification The presence of multiple copies of a gene within a cell that is normally present in only two copies per somatic cell. An increased number of copies of an individual gene, usually a proto-oncogene, per cell.

gene deletion The deletion of part or all of a gene through removal of DNA sequences by any of several mechanisms.

gene expression The active transcription of a gene into an RNA molecule followed by translation of the protein product.

gene rearrangements The process by which part or all of a gene is moved from its normal location in the genome to another site within the genome.

growth factor Protein that acts on cells to promote cell growth.

growth factor receptors Proteins that interact with growth factors and transmit the growth signal to the cell.

HER-2 See *c-erb-B-2* proto-oncogene.

heteronuclear RNA A form of RNA, a pre-mRNA, that exists before splicing and consists of both introns and exons.

heterozygosity Two different forms of the same gene in a cell. An oncogene is generally heterozygous. For example, one allele may be mutated while the other copy remains normal. In addition, different forms of a gene may be normal variants. Variations in the exact base sequence within DNA are common in the genome among humans. These are called polymorphisms and are often responsible for the heterozygous state.

informative A term used to describe the situation when the two homologous chromosomes from an individual can be distinguished from one another at a given locus; *heterozygous* is an alternative term.

insertions The addition of DNA sequence into the genome.

introns Portions of genomic DNA that are interspersed between exons and are transcribed along with the exons into heteronuclear RNA.

locus A general term to describe a defined chromosomal region.

loss of heterozygosity Losses of specific regions of DNA from one copy of a given chromosome that can be distinguished from the region retained on the other chromosome.

messenger RNA (mRNA) The mature form of processed RNA used as a template for directing translation of proteins.

myc proto-oncogenes The proto-oncogene family that includes *C-myc, N-myc, L-myc,* and *R-myc*. They encode for nuclear-associated DNA-binding proteins that affect DNA replication and transcription.

neu See *c-erb-B-2* proto-oncogene.

nonsense mutations A nucleotide substitution that results in a truncated protein product by generating a stop codon specifying premature cessation of translation within an open reading frame.

nuclear transcription factors Proteins involved in regulating the expression of genes by controlling transcription. Some factors enhance and others repress gene expression and others do both, depending on the intracellular environment.

oncogenes Genes that regulate cell growth in a positive fashion, i.e., to promote cell growth. Oncogenes include transforming genes of viruses and normal cellular genes (proto-oncogenes) that are activated by mutations to promote cell growth.

open reading frame A sequence of DNA representing at least some of the coding portion of a gene that is transcribed and subsequently translated into a protein because it does not contain any internal translation termination codons.

PCR   Polymerase chain reaction. A technique by which genes or portions of genes are multiplied in vitro if the sequence of the gene is known or partially known. A heat-stable enzyme known as polymerase is used to create DNA in the test tube. PCR revolutionized molecular biology by opening genes from very small, even degraded, samples of tissue or tumor to study. Analysis of certain genes is possible from archival paraffin-embedded tissue samples or small quantities of cells.

point mutation   The replacement of one nucleotide in the DNA sequence of the wild-type gene with another nucleotide.

polymorphism   Variation in the exact base sequence of DNA that makes up the genome. These occurrences are normal, and common in humans. Polymorphisms are used in the a study of molecular genetics because they are inherited. Ones found near or within disease genes can be used to study linkage in genetics.

primers   Short DNA sequences that are complimentary to portions of specific DNA sequences.

promoter   The DNA sequence of a gene to which RNA polymerase binds and initiates transcription.

proto-oncogenes   Any of a number of genes that encode for various proteins involved in normal cell growth and proliferation, including growth factors, growth factor receptors, regulators of DNA synthesis, and phosphorylating modifiers of protein function. These are cellular genes that are the normal counterparts of transforming viral oncogenes.

p53 **gene**   A tumor suppressor gene that encodes a nuclear phosphoprotein that arrests cells from entering the S-phase of the cell cycle. Located on chromosome 17(p13), *p53* is postulated to contribute to diverse tumorigenesis.

ras **gene**   A family of genes that encode for similar cell membrane-bound protein involved in signal transduction. Three types, *K-ras*, *N-ras*, and *H-ras*, are the widely studied *ras* genes in human tumors. Their proto-oncogene becomes activated by point mutations, most often in specific codons of the gene sequence.

RB   The first tumor suppressor gene to be discovered. It is a 4.7 kilobase gene, located on chromosome 13q14, and encodes a 110,000 kilodalton nuclear phosphoprotein that suppresses the cell cycle. Absence of *RB* is the cause of retinoblastoma, and research is revealing that it is involved in the pathogenesis of many other neoplasms.

restriction endonucleases   Enzymes that cleave DNA at specific DNA sequences.

restriction fragment length polymorphism (RFLP)   Variations in the DNA of different individuals that create or destroy cleavage sites for a given restriction endonuclease.

reverse transcriptase   An enzyme, discovered in retroviruses, that has the unique ability to transcribe DNA from an RNA template. This is the reverse of the normal physiologic process.

Southern blot analysis   A molecular biology technique in which DNA is transferred to and fixed on a nylon or nitrocellulose membrane and studied with DNA probes that can then detect, for example, the presence of an oncogene.

splice site mutations   Nucleotide substitutions that occur in the sequence adjacent to intron-exon boundaries of genes.

splicing   The process by which introns are removed from heteronuclear RNA and the exons are joined together to maintain the open reading frame of the mRNA.

transcription   The process of converting the DNA code into a complementary messenger RNA segment.

translation   The process by which specific amino acids are incorporated into a protein as dictated by the sequence of the mRNA template.

translocation   Nonhomologous recombination.

tumor suppressor gene   A gene that suppresses cellular growth and proliferation. Therefore, when its protein products are absent, it contributes to tumor development or progression. Also known as anti-oncogene, these normal cellular genes encode proteins that are thought to normally regulate growth in a negative fashion.

uninformative   The term used to describe the situation when the two homologous chromosomes from an individual cannot be distinguished from one another at a given locus; *homozygous* is an alternative term.

vectors   A DNA vehicle that can be propagated in living cells (e.g., bacteria and yeast) into which foreign DNA can be inserted and propagated with the vector DNA. Examples of vectors include bacterial plasmids, cosmids, bacteriophage, and, most recently, yeast artifical chromosomes.

wild-type   The term used to describe the normal gene or gene product. In contrast, a gene that has had its DNA sequence altered is referred to as a mutant gene and its resultant product is a mutant protein. A gene that encodes for a proto-oncogene, for example, is a wild-type gene because it is unaltered.

BIBLIOGRAPHY

Genetic alterations in cancer

Callahan R, Campbell G: Mutations in human breast cancer: an overview, *JNCI* 81:1780, 1989.

Cohen D, Chumakov I, Weissenbach J: A first generation physical map of the human genome, *Nature* 366:698, 1993.

Coles C et al: *P53* mutations in breast cancer, *Cancer Res* 52:5291, 1992.

Fearon ER, Vogelstein B: A genetic model for colorectal tumorigenesis, *Cell* 61:759, 1990.

Fujiwara Y et al: Evidence for the presence of two tumor suppressor genes on chromosome 8p for colorectal carcinoma, *Cancer Res* 53:1172, 1993.

Goldgar DE et al: A large kindred with 17q-linked breast and ovarian cancer: genetic, phenotypic, and genealogical analysis, *JNCI* 86:200, 1994.

Haas OA, Argyriou-Tirita A, Lion T: Parental origin of chromosomes involved in the translocation t(9;22), *Nature* 359:414, 1992.

Houlsworth J et al: Gene amplification in gastric and esophageal adenocarcinomas, *Cancer Res* 50:6417, 1990.

Miki Y et al: A strong candidate for the breast and ovarian cancer susceptibility gene *BRCA1*, *Science* 266:66, 1994.

Mitelman F: *Catalog of Chromosome Aberrations in Cancer*, ed. 3, New York: Alan R Liss, Inc. 1988.

Moul JW: New medicine emerging from genes that control cancer, *Contemp OB/GYN*, Feb 1995.

Rainier S et al: Relaxation of imprinted genes in human cancer, *Nature* 362:747, 1993.

Sato T et al: Accumulation of genetic alterations and progression of primary breast cancer, *Cancer Res* 51:5794, 1991.

Sidransky D et al: Inherited p53 gene mutations in breast cancer, *Cancer Res* 52:2984, 1992.

Solomon E, Borrow J, Goddard AD: Chromosome aberrations and cancer, *Science* 254:1153, 1991.

Oncogenes research

Baker VV, Shingleton HM, Hatch KD et al: Selective inhibition of *C-myc* expression by the ribonucleic acid synthesis inhibitor mithramycin, *Am J Obstet Gynecol* 158:762, 1988.

Buckley I: Oncogenes and the nature of malignancy, *Adv Cancer Res* 50:71, 1988.

Cline MJ, Slamon DJ, Lipsick JS: Oncogenes: implications for the diagnosis and treatment of cancer, *Ann Intern Med* 101:223, 1984.

Karlan BY, Amin W, Casper SE et al: Hormonal regulation of CA 125 tumor marker expression in human ovarian carcinoma cells: inhibition by glucocorticoids, *Cancer Res* 48:3502, 1988.

Lee JH, Kavanagh JJ, Wildrick JJ et al: Frequent loss of heterozygosity on chromosome 6q, 11, and 17 in human ovarian carcinomas, *Cancer Res* 50:2724, 1990.

Marks JR, Davidoff AM, Kerns BJ et al: Overexpression and mutation of p53 in epithelial ovarian cancer, *Cancer Res* 51:2979, 1991.

Nemunaitis J: Cytokine-mobilized peripheral blood progenitor cells, *Semin Oncol* 23(2):9, 1996.

Sagusa M et al: The possible role of bcl-2 expression in the progression of tumors of the uterine cervix, *Cancer* 76, No 11:2297, 1995.

Schreiber G, Dubeau L: C-myc proto-oncogene amplification detected by polymerase chain reaction in archival human ovarian carcinomas, *Am J Pathol* 137:653, 1990.

Scrable HJ, Sapienza C, and Cavenee WK: Genetic and epigenetic losses of heterozygosity in cancer predisposition and progression, *Advances Cancer Res* 54:25, 1990.

Tonkin KS, Berger M, Ormerod M: Epidermal growth factor receptor status in four carcinoma of the cervix cell lines, *Int J Gynecol Cancer* 1:185, 1991.

Weinberg RA: Tumor suppressor genes, *Science* 254:1138, 1991.

Zheng J, Robinson WR, Ehlen T et al: Distinction of low grade from high grade human ovarian carcinomas on the basis of losses of heterozygosity on chromosomes 3, 6, and 11 and HER-2/neu gene amplification, *Cancer Res* 51:4045, 1991.

Tumor suppressor genes

Bertelsen AH et al: Tumor suppressor genes: prospects for cancer therapies, *Biotechnology* 13:127, 1995.

Chen TM et al: The state of p53 in primary human cervical carcinomas and its effects in human papillomavirus-immortalized human cervical cells, *Oncogene* 8(6):1511, 1993.

Gu Z et al: DNA damage induced *p53* transcription is inhibited by human papillomavirus type 18 E6, *Oncogene* 9(2):629, 1994.

Kurvinen K et al: The state of the p53 gene in human papillomavirus (HPV)-positive and HPV negative genital precancer lesions and carcinoma as determined by single-strand conformation polymorphism analysis and sequencing, *Anticancer Res* 14:177, 1994.

Levin AJ, Jamil M, Finlay CA: The p53 tumor suppressor gene, *Nature* 351:453, 1991.

Park D et al: P53 mutations in HPV-negative cervical carcinoma, Oncogene 9(1):205, 1994.

Schneider J et al: Identification of p53 mutations by means of single strand conformation polymorphism analysis in gynecological tumors: comparison with the results of immunohistochemistry, *Eur J Cancer* 30A(4):504, 1994.

Street D, Delgado G: Editorial: the role of p53 and HPV in cervical cancer, *Gynecol Oncol* 58:287, 1995.

Gene therapy

Brenner MK: Human somatic gene therapy: progress and problems, *J Intern Med* 237:229, 1995.

Champlin RE: Peripheral blood progenitor cells: a replacement for marrow transplantation? *Semin Oncol* 23(2):15, 1996.

Fraser JK, Michael CC Lill, Figlin RA: The biology of the cytokine sequence cascade, *Semin Oncol* 23(2):2:1996.

Holzman D: New cancer genes crowd the horizon, create possibilities, *J Natl Cancer Inst* 87:1108, 1996.

Hwu P: The gene therapy of cancer, *PPO Updates* 9:1, 1995.

Jolly D: Viral vector systems for gene therapy, *Cancer Gene Ther* 1:51, 1994.

Krotiris TG: Oncogenes, *N Engl J Med* 333:303, 1995.

Mastrangelo MJ et al: A pilot study demonstrating the feasibility of using intratumoral vaccinia injections as vector for gene transfer, *Vaccine Res* 4:58, 1995.

Nicholas GL: Antisense oligodeoxynucleotides as therapeutic agents for chronic myelogenous leukemia, *Antisense Res Develop* 5:67, 1995.

Robinson A: Gene therapy— the future touches down, *Can Med Assoc J* 150:377, 1960.

Rosenberg SA: Gene therapy for cancer, *JAMA* 268:2416, 1992.

Tahara H et al: Effective eradication of established murine tumors with IL-12 gene therapy using a polycistronic retroviral vector, *J Immunol* 154:6466, 1995.

Apoptosis

Agoff SN et al: Regulation of the human hsp 70 promoter by p53, *Science* 259:84, 1993.

Caron de Fromentel C, Soussi T: TP53 tumor suppressor gene: a model for investigating human mutagenesis, *Genes Chromosome Cancer*, 4:1, 1992.

Cohen JJ, Duke RC: Apoptosis and programmed cell death in immunity, *Annu Rev Immunolo* 10:267, 1992.

Collins MKL et al: Interleukin 3 protects murine bone marrow cells from apoptosis induced by DNA damaging agents, *J Exp Med* 176:1043, 1992.

Dive C, Hickman JA: Drug target interactions: only the first step in the commitment to a programmed cell death? *Br J Cancer* 64:192, 1991.

Donehower LA et al: Mice deficient for p53 are developmentally normal but susceptible to spontaneous tumours, *Nature* 356:215, 1992.

Evan GE et al: Induction of apoptosis in fibroblasts by c-myc protein, *Cell* 69:119, 1992.

Hollstein M et al: P 53 mutations in human cancers, *Science* 253:49, 1991.

Kerr JFR, Winterford CM, Harmon BV: Apoptosis, *Cancer* 73(8):2013, 1994.

Lane DP: A death in the life of p53, *Nature* 362:786, 1993.

Lane DP: P53, guardian of the genome, *Nature* 358:15, 1992.

Marx J: Cell death studies yield cancer clues, *Science* 259:760, 1993.

Meyn RE, Milas L, Stephens C: Programmed cell death in normal development and disease, *The Cancer Bulletin* 46, No 2, 1994.

Sellins KS, Cohen JJ: Hyperthermia induces apoptosis in thymocytes, *Radiat Res* 126:88, 1991.

Wyllie AH: Apoptosis and the regulation of cell numbers in normal and neoplastic tissues: an overview, *Cancer Metastasis Rev* 11:95, 1992.

Wyllie AH: The biology of cell death in tumours, *Anticancer Res* 5:131, 1985.

Yanagihara K, Tsumuraya M. Transforming growth factor b$_1$ induces apoptotic cell death in cultured human gastric carcinoma cells, *Cancer Res* 52:4042, 1992.

Yonish-Rouach E et al: P53-mediated cell death: relationship to cell cycle control, *Mol Cell Biol*, 13:1415, 1993.

Genetic studies in gynecologic malignancies

Amos CI et al: Age at onset for familial epithelial ovarian cancer, *JAMA* 268:1896, 1992.

Arca MJ, Mule JJ, Chang AE: Genetic approaches to adoptive cellular therapy for malignancy: *Semin Oncol* 23(1):108, 1996.

Baker VV, et al: C-myc amplification in ovarian cancer, *Gynecol Oncol* 38:340, 1990.

Barbosa MS, Schelegel R: The E6 and E7 genes of HPV-18 are sufficient for inducing two-stage in vitro transformation of human keratinocytes, *Oncogene* 4:1529, 1989.

Breast Cancer Linkage Consortium: An evaluation of genetic heterogenicity in 145 breast ovarian cancer families, *Am J Hum Genetics* 56:254, 1995.

Cullen AP et al: Analysis of the physical state of different human papillomavirus DNAs in intraepithelial and invasive cervical neoplasm, *J Virol* 65:606, 1991.

Ezzell C: BRCA1 shock: breast cancer gene encodes a secreted protein, *J NIH Research* 8:1996.

Holt JT et al: Growth retardation and tumour inhibition by BRCA1, *Nature Genetics* 12:298, 1996.

Kacinski BM et al: Ovarian adenocarcinomas express fms-complementary transcripts and fms antigen, often with co-expression of CSF-1, *Am J Pathol* 137:135, 1990.

Kacinski BM et al: Neu protein overexpression in benign, border-line, and malignant ovarian neoplasms, *Gynecol Oncol* 44:245, 1992.

Kastan MB et al: Participation of p53 protein in the cellular response to DNA damage, *Cancer Res* 51:6304, 1991.

Kessis T et al: Human papillomavirus 16 E6 disrupts the p53 mediated cellular response to DNA damage, *Proc Natl Acad Sci USA* 90:3988, 1993.

Kuerbitz S et al: Wild-type p53 is a cell cycle checkpoint determinant following irradiation, *Proc Natl Acad Sci USA* 51:7491, 1992.

Lynch HT et al: Hereditary ovarian cancer: heterogeneity in age at a diagnosis, *Cancer* 67:1460, 1991.

Marks JR et al: Over-expression and mutation of p53 in epithelial ovarian cancer, *Can Res* 51:2979, 1991.

Mazars R et al: P53 mutations in ovarian cancer: a late event? *Oncogene* 6:1685, 1991.

Mok CH et al: Unifocal origin of advanced human epithelial ovarian cancers, *Cancer Res* 52:5119, 1992.

Münger K et al: Biochemical and biological differences between E7 oncoproteins of the high- and low-risk human papillomavirus types are determined by amino-terminal sequences, *J Virol* 65:3943, 1991.

Okamoto A et al: Allelic loss on chromosome 17p and p53 mutations in human endometrial carcinoma of the uterus, *Cancer Res* 51:5632, 1991.

Okamoto A et al: Frequent allelic losses and mutations of the p53 gene in human ovarian cancer, *Cancer Res* 51:5171, 1991.

Risinger JL et al: P53 gene mutations in human endometrial carcinoma, *Mol Carcino* 5:250, 1992.

Sasano H et al: An analysis of abnormalities of the retinoblastoma gene in human ovarian and endometrial carcinoma, *Cancer* 66:2150, 1990.

Sasano H et al: Protooncogene amplification and tumor ploidy in human ovarian neoplasms, *Hum Pathol* 21:382, 1990.

Sato T et al: Allelotype of human ovarian cancer, *Cancer Res* 51:5118, 1991.

Slamon DJ et al: Studies of the HER-2/neu proto-oncogene in human breast and ovarian cancer, *Science* 244:707, 1989.

Tsao S et al: Molecular genetic evidence of a unifocal origin for human serous ovarian carcinomas, *Gynecol Oncol* 48:5, 1993.

Tsao SW et al: Involvement of p53 gene in the allelic deletion of chromosome 17p in human ovarian tumors, *Anticancer Res* 11:1975, 1991.

Worsham MJ et al: Consistent chromosome abnormalities in squamous cell carcinomas of the vulva, *Genes Chrom Cancer* 3:420, 1991.

Zheng JP et al: Distinction of low grade from high grade human ovarian carcinomas on the basis of losses of heterozygosity on chromosomes 3, 6, and 11 and HER-2/neu gene amplification, *Cancer Res* 51:4045, 1991.

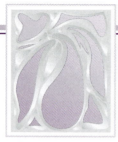

APPENDIX

A

Staging

STAGING OF CANCER AT GYNECOLOGIC SITES

Cervix Uteri, Corpus Uteri, Ovary, Vagina, Vulva, Gestational Trophoblastic Tumors, and Fallopian Tube

In 1976 the American Joint Committee adopted the classification of the International Federation of Gynecology and Obstetrics (FIGO), which is the format used in the "Annual Report on the Results of Treatment in Carcinoma of the Uterus, Vagina and Ovary." Published every 3 years, this report has used the FIGO classification with periodic modifications since 1937. Numerous institutions throughout the world contribute their statistics for inclusion in this voluntary collaborative presentation of data.

The cervix and corpus uteri were among the first anatomical sites to be classified by the TNM system. This utilizes extent of primary tumor (T), nodal metastasis (N), and distant metastasis status (M) to stage cancers. This system has been approved by the American Joint Committee on Cancer (AJCC) and the International Union Against Cancer (UICC). FIGO has worked closely for many years with the AJCC and UICC in the classification of cancer at gynecologic sites. Staging of malignant tumors is essentially the same and stages are comparable in the two (FIGO and TNM) systems regarding categories and details.

Anatomy and Classification by Sites of Malignant Tumors of the Female Pelvis

Cervix uteri

1.0 Anatomy
1. *Primary site:* The cervix is the lower third of the uterus. It is roughly cylindrical in shape, projects through the upper anterior vaginal wall, and communicates with the vagina through an orifice

called the external os. Cancer of the cervix may originate on the vaginal surface or in the canal.
2. *Nodal stations*: The cervix is drained by preureteral, postureteral, and uterosacral routes into the following first station nodes: parametrial, hypogastric (obturator), external iliac, presacral, and common iliac. Para-aortic nodes are second station and are considered metastases.
3. *Metastatic sites:* The most common sites of distant spread include the aortic and mediastinal nodes, the lungs, and the skeleton.

2.0 Rules for classification
1. *Clinical-diagnostic staging:* Staging of cervical cancer is based on clinical evaluation; therefore, careful clinical examination should be performed in all cases by an experienced examiner, preferably with the patient under anesthesia. The clinical staging must not be changed because of subsequent findings. When there is doubt as to which stage a particular cancer should be allocated, the earlier stage is mandatory. The following examinations are permitted: palpation, inspection, colposcopy, endocervical curettage, hysteroscopy, cystoscopy, proctoscopy, intravenous urography, and x-ray examination of the lungs and skeleton. Suspected bladder or rectal involvement should be confirmed by biopsy and histologic evidence. Findings of optional examinations, e.g., lymphangiography, arteriography, venography, laparoscopy, CT scan, and MRI are of value for planning therapy but because these are not generally available and the interpretation of results is variable, the findings of such studies should not be the basis for changing the clinical staging.
2. *Surgical-evaluative staging:* Surgical evaluation is applicable only after laparotomy or laparoscopy and examination of tumor and nodes. Fine needle

aspiration (FNA) of scan-detected suspicious lymph nodes may be helpful in treatment planning. Conization or amputation of the cervix is regarded as a clinical examination. Invasive cancers so identified are to be included in the reports (see 4).

3. *Postsurgical treatment—pathologic staging:* In cases treated by surgical procedures, the pathologist's findings in the removed tissues can be the basis for extremely accurate statements on the extent of disease. The findings should not be allowed to change the clinical staging but should be recorded in the manner described for the pathologic staging of disease. The TNM nomenclature is appropriate for this purpose. Infrequently it happens that hysterectomy is carried out in the presence of unsuspected extensive invasive cervical carcinoma. Such cases cannot be clinically staged or included in therapeutic statistics, but it is desirable that they be reported separately. Only if the rules for clinical staging are strictly observed will it be possible to present comparable results between clinics and by differing modes of therapy.

4. *Retreatment staging:* Complete examination using the procedures cited in Number 2 above, including a search for distant metastases, is recommended in cases known or suspected to have recurrence. Biopsy and histologic confirmation are particularly desirable when induration and fibrosis from previously treated disease are present.

5. Only if the rules for clinical staging are strictly observed will it be possible to compare results among clinics and by differing modes of therapy.

3.0 Staging classification

FIGO nomenclature

Stage 0	Carcinoma in situ, cervical intraepithelia neoplasia grade III
Stage I	The carcinoma is strictly confined to the cervix (extension to the corpus would be disregarded).
Stage Ia:	Invasive carcinoma that can be diagnosed only by microscopy. All macroscopically visible lesions—even with superficial invasion—are allotted stage Ib carcinomas. Invasion is limited to a measured stromal invasion with a maximal depth of 5.0 mm and a horizontal extension of not more than 7.0. Depth of invasion should not be more than 5.0 mm related to the basis of the epithelium of the original tissue —superficial or glandular. The involvement of vascular spaces—venous or lymphatic—should not change the stage allotment.
Stage Ia1:	Measured stromal invasion of not more than 3.0 mm in depth and extension of not more than 7.0 mm
Stage Ia2:	Measured stromal invasion of more than 3.0 mm and not more than 5.0 mm with an extension of not more than 7.0 mm
Stage Ib:	Clinically visible lesions limited to the cervix, uteri, or subclinical cancers greater than stage Ia
Stage Ib1:	Clinically visible lesions not larger than 4.0 cm
Stage Ib2:	Clinically visible lesions larger than 4.0 cm
Stage II	The carcinoma extends beyond the cervix but has not extended to the pelvic wall. The carcinoma involves the vagina but not as far as the lower third.
Stage IIa:	No obvious parametrial involvement
Stage IIb:	Obvious parametrial involvement
Stage III	The carcinoma has extended to the pelvic wall. On rectal examination, there is no cancer-free space between the tumor and the pelvic wall. The tumor involves the lower third of the vagina. All cases with hydronephrosis or nonfunctioning kidney are included, unless they are known to be due to other causes
Stage IIIa:	No extension to the pelvic wall
Stage IIIb:	Extension to the pelvic wall and/or hydronephrosis or nonfunctioning kidney.
Stage IV	The carcinoma has extended beyond the true pelvis or has clinically involved the mucosa of the bladder or rectum. A bullous edema as such does not permit a case to be allotted to stage IV
Stage IVa:	Spread of the growth to adjacent organs
Stage IVb:	Spread to distant organs

Notes about the staging

Stage 0 comprises those cases with full-thickness involvement of the epithelium with atypical cells but with no signs of invasion into the stroma.

The diagnosis of stages Ia1 and Ia2 should be based on microscopic examination of removed tissue, preferably a cone, which must include the entire lesion. The depth of invasion should not be more than 5 mm, taken from the base of the epithelium, either surface or glandular, from which it originates. The second dimension, the horizontal spread, must not exceed 7 mm. Vascular space involvement, either venous or lymphatic, should not alter the staging but should be specifically recorded because it may affect treatment decisions in the future.

Larger lesions should be staged as Ib.

As a rule, it is impossible to estimate clinically if a cancer of the cervix has extended to the corpus. Extension to the corpus should therefore be disregarded.

A patient with a growth fixed to the pelvic wall by a short and indurated but not nodular parametrium should be allotted to stage IIb. It is impossible at clinical examination to decide whether a smooth and indurated parametrium is truly cancerous or only inflammatory. Therefore the case should be placed in stage III only if the parametrium is nodular to the pelvic wall or if the growth itself extends to the pelvic wall.

The presence of hydronephrosis or nonfunctioning kidney resulting from stenosis of the ureter by cancer permits a case to be allotted to stage III, even if according to the other findings the case should be allotted to stage I or stage II.

The presence of bullous edema, as such, should not permit a case to be allotted to stage IV. Ridges and furrows into the bladder wall should be interpreted as signs of submucous involvement of the bladder if they remain fixed to the growth at palposcopy (i.e., examination from the vagina or the rectum during cystoscopy). Finding malignant cells in cytologic washings from the urinary bladder requires further examination and a biopsy from the wall of the bladder.

Histopathology

Cases should be classified as carcinomas of the cervix if the primary growth is in the cervix. All histologic types must be included. Grading by any of several methods is encouraged but is not a basis for modifying the stage groupings. When surgery is the primary treatment, the histologic findings permit the case to have pathologic staging as described in 2.0 Rules for Classification, 2. Surgical-evaluative staging, p. 594; in this the TNM nomenclature is to be used. All tumors are to be microscopically verified.

Histopathologic Types

Cervical intraepithelial neoplasia, grade III
Squamous cell carcinoma in situ
Squamous cell carcinoma
    Keratinizing
    Nonkeratinizing
    Verrucous
Adenocarcinoma in situ
Adenocarcinoma in situ, endocervical type
Endometrioid adenocarcinoma
Clear cell adenocarcinoma
Adenosquamous carcinoma
Adenoid cystic carcinoma
Small cell carcinoma
Undifferentiated carcinoma

Histopathologic Grade

G1 Well differentiated
G2 Moderately differentiated
G3 Poorly differentiated
G4 Undifferentiated

Stage Grouping for Cervix

FIGO/AJCC/UICC	T	N	M
0	Tis	N0	M0
Ia1	T1a1	N0	M0
Ia2	T1a2	N0	M0
Ib1	T1b1	N0	M0
Ib2	T1b2	N0	M0
IIa	T2a	N0	M0
IIb	T2b	N0	M0
IIIa	T3a	N0	M0
IIIb	T1	N1	M0
	T2	N1	M0
	T3	N1	M0
	T3b	any N	M0
IVa	T4	any N	M0
IVb	any T	any N	M1

Corpus

1.0 Anatomy

1.1 *Primary site:* The upper two thirds of the uterus above the level of the internal cervical os is called the corpus. The fallopian tubes enter at the upper lateral corners of a pear-shaped body. The portion of the muscular organ that is above a line joining the tubouterine orifices is often referred to as the fundus.

1.2 *Nodal stations:* The major lymphatic trunks are the utero-ovarian (infundibulo-pelvic), parametrial, and presacral, which drain into the hypogastric, external iliac, common iliac, presacral, and para-aortic nodes.

1.3 *Metastatic sites:* The vagina and lung are the common metastatic sites.

2.0 Rules for classification

The FIGO committee on gynecologic oncology agreed on the system for surgical staging for carcinoma of the corpus uteri at the meeting in Rio de Janeiro in October 1988.

3.0 Surgical staging classification

FIGO nomenclature

Stage Ia G123	Tumor limited to endometrium
Stage Ib G123	Invasion to less than half the myometrium
Stage Ic G123	Invasion to more than half the myometrium
Stage IIa G123	Endocervical glandular involvement only
Stage IIb G123	Cervical stromal invasion
Stage IIIa G123	Tumor invades serosa and/or adnexae and/or positive cytologic findings
Stage IIIb G123	Vaginal metastases
Stage IIIc G123	Metastases to pelvic and/or para-aortic lymph nodes
Stage IVa G123	Tumor invasion of bladder and/or bowel mucosa
Stage IVb	Distant metastases, including intra-abdominal and/or inguinal lymph nodes

4.0 Notes about the staging
Histopathology—degree of differentiation

Cases of carcinoma of the corpus should be grouped with regard to the degree of differentiation of the adenocarcinoma as follows:

G1:   5% or less of a nonsquamous or nonmorular solid growth pattern

G2:   6%-50% of a nonsquamous or nonmorular solid growth pattern

G3:   more than 50% of a nonsquamous or nonmorular solid growth pattern

Notes on pathologic grading

1. Notable nuclear atypia, inappropriate for the architectural grade, raises the grade of a grade 1 or grade 2 tumor by 1.
2. In serous and clear cell adenocarcinomas, nuclear grading takes precedent.
3. Adenocarcinomas with squamous differentiation are graded according to the nuclear grade of the glandular component.

Rules related to staging

1. Because corpus cancer is now surgically staged, procedures previously used for determination of stages are no longer applicable, such as the finding of fractional D&C to differentiate between stage I and stage II.
2. It is understood that there may be a small number of patients with corpus cancer who will be treated primarily with radiation therapy. If that is the case, the clinical staging adopted by FIGO in 1971 would still apply, but designation of that staging system would be noted.
3. Ideally, width of the myometrium should be measured along with the width of tumor invasion.

5.0 Histopathology

The histopathologic types are:

Endometrioid carcinoma
    Adenocarcinoma
    Adenocanthoma (adenocarcinoma with squamous metaplasia)
    Adenosquamous carcinoma (mixed adenocarcinoma and squamous cell carcinoma)
Mucinous adenocarcinoma
Serous adenocarcinoma
Clear cell adenocarcinoma
Squamous cell adenocarcinoma
Undifferentiated adenocarcinoma

Stage Grouping for Uterus

FIGO/AJCC/UICC	LDDLT	N	M
0	Tis	N0	M0
Ia	T1a	N0	M0
Ib	T1b	N0	M0
Ic	T1c	N0	M0
IIa	T2a	N0	M0
IIb	T2b	N0	M0
IIIa	T3a	N0	M0
IIIb	T3b	N0	M0
IIIc	T1	N1	M0
	T2	N1	M0
	T3a	N1	M0
	T3b	N1	M0
IVa	T4	any N	M0
IVb	any T	any N	M1

Ovary

1.0 Anatomy

1.1 *Primary site:* Ovaries are a pair of solid bodies, flattened ovoids 2-4 cm in diameter, that are connected by a peritoneal fold to the broad ligament and by the infundibulo-pelvic ligament to the lateral wall of the pelvis.

1.2 *Nodal stations:* The lymphatic drainage occurs by the utero-ovarian and round ligament trunks and an external iliac accessory route into the following regional nodes: external iliac, common iliac, hypogastric, lateral sacral, and para-aortic nodes, and rarely, to inguinal nodes.

1.3 *Metastatic sites:* The peritoneum, including the omentum and pelvic and abdominal viscera are common sites for seeding. Diaphragmatic involvement and liver metastases are common. Pulmonary and pleural involvements are frequently seen.

2.0 Rules for classification

Ovarian cancer is surgically staged. Operative findings prior to tumor debulking determine the stage, which may be modified by histopathologic as well as clinical or radiologic evaluation. Laparotomy and resection of the ovarian mass, as well as hysterectomy, form the basis for staging. Biopsies of all suspicious sites such as omentum, mesentery, liver, diaphragm, pelvic, and para-aortic nodes are required. The final histologic findings after surgery (and cytologic ones when available) are to be considered in the staging. Clinical studies, if carcinoma of the ovary is diagnosed, include routine radiology of the chest. CT may be helpful in initial staging and follow-up of tumors.

1. *Clinical-diagnostic staging:* Although clinical studies similar to those for other sites may be used, the establishment of a diagnosis most often requires a laparotomy, which is most widely accepted in surgical-pathologic staging. Clinical studies, if carcinoma of the ovary is diagnosed, include routine radiography of chest and abdomen, liver studies, and hemograms.

2. *Surgical-evaluative staging:* Laparotomy and biopsy of all suspected sites of involvement provide the basis for this type of staging; this staging is often identical to postsurgical staging. Histologic and cytologic data are required.

3. *Post-surgical treatment—pathologic staging:* This should include laparotomy and resection of ovarian masses, as well as hysterectomy. Biopsies of all suspicious sites, such as the omentum, mesentery, liver, diaphragm, and pelvic and para-aortic nodes, are required. Pleural effusions should be documented by cytology.

4. *Retreatment staging:* Second-look laparotomies and laparoscopy are being evaluated because of the limitation of routine pelvic and abdominal examinations in detecting early recurrence. Other optional and investigative procedures include ultrasound and computed tomography. All suspected recurrences need biopsy confirmation.

3.0 Staging classification

Staging is based mainly on findings seen at surgical exploration. Clinical evaluation and imaging studies should be done as appropriate. These findings may affect final staging. The histology is to be considered in the staging, as is cytology as far as effusions are concerned. It is desirable that a biopsy be taken from suspicious areas outside of the pelvis.

Stage I	Growth limited to the ovaries
Stage Ia:	Growth limited to one ovary; no ascites present containing malignant cells. No tumor on the external surface; capsule intact
Stage Ib:	Growth limited to both ovaries; no ascites present containing malignant cells; no tumor on the external surfaces; capsules intact
Stage Ic*:	Tumor stage Ia or Ib but with tumor on surface of one or both ovaries; or with capsule ruptured; or with ascites present containing malignant cells or with positive peritoneal washings
Stage II	Growth involving one or both ovaries with pelvic extension
Stage IIa:	Extension and/or metastases to the uterus and/or tubes
Stage IIb:	Extension to other pelvic tissues
Stage IIc*:	Tumor stage IIa or IIb but with tumor on surface of one or both ovaries; or with capsule(s) ruptured; or with ascites present containing malignant cells or with positive peritoneal washings

---

* To evaluate the impact on prognosis of the different criteria for allotting cases to stage Ic or IIc, it would be of value to know if rupture of the capsule was (1) spontaneous or (2) caused by the surgeon and if the source of malignant cells detected was (1) peritoneal washings or (2) ascites.

Stage III	Tumor involving one or both ovaries with peritoneal implants outside the pelvis and/or positive retroperitoneal or inguinal nodes; superficial liver metastases equals stage III. Tumor is limited to the true pelvis but with histologically proven malignant extension to small bowel or omentum
Stage IIIa:	Tumor grossly limited to the true pelvis with negative nodes but with histologically confirmed microscopic seeding of abdominal peritoneal surfaces
Stage IIIb:	Tumor of one or both ovaries with histologically confirmed implants of abdominal peritoneal surfaces, none exceeding 2 cm in diameter; nodes are negative
Stage IIIc:	Abdominal implants greater than 2 cm in diameter and/or positive retroperitoneal or inguinal nodes
Stage IV	Growth involving one or both ovaries with distant metastases. If pleural effusion is present, there must be positive cytology to allot a case to stage IV. Parenchymal liver metastasis equals stage IV

4.0 Histopathology

The task force of the AJC endorses the histologic typing of ovarian tumors as presented in the WHO publication no. 9, 1973, and recommends that all ovarian epithelial tumors be subdivided according to a simplified version. The types recommended are as follows: serous tumors, mucinous tumors, endometrioid tumors, clear cell (mesonephroid) tumors, undifferentiated tumors, and unclassified tumors.

  A. Serous tumors
    1. Benign serous cystadenomas
    2. Of borderline malignancy: Serous cystadenomas with proliferating activity of the epithelial cells and nuclear abnormalities but with no infiltrative destructive growth (carcinomas of low potential malignancy)
    3. Serous cystadenocarcinomas
  B. Mucinous tumors
    1. Benign mucinous cystadenomas Of boderline malignancy: Mucinous cystadenomas with proliferating activity of the epithelial cells and nuclear abnormalities but with no infiltrative destructive growth (carcinomas of low potential malignancy) Mucinous cystadenocarcinomas
  C. Endometrioid tumors
    1. Benign endometrioid cystadenomas
    2. Endometrioid tumors with proliferating activity of the epithelial cells and nuclear abnormalities but with no infiltrative destructive growth (carcinomas of low potential malignancy)
    3. Endometrioid adenocarcinomas
  D. Clear cell tumors
    1. Benign clear cell tumors
    2. Clear cell tumors with proliferating activity of

the epithelial cells and nuclear abnormalities but with no infiltrative destructive growth (low potential malignancy)

3. Clear cell cystadenocarcinomas

E. Brenner
   1. Benign Brenner
   2. Borderline malignancy
   3. Malignant
   4. Transitional cell

F. Undifferentiated carcinomas

A malignant tumor of epithelial structure that is too poorly differentiated to get placed in any other group.

G. Mixed epithelial tumors

These tumors are composed of two or more of the five major cell types of common epithelial tumors (types should be specified).

H. Cases with intraperitoneal carcinoma in which the ovaries appear to be incidentally involved and not the primary origin should be labeled as extra-ovarian peritoneal carcinoma.

Stage Grouping for Ovary

FIGO/AJCC/UICC	T	N	M
Ia	T1a	N0	M0
Ib	T1b	N0	M0
Ic	T1c	N0	M0
IIa	T2a	N0	M0
IIb	T2b	N0	M0
IIc	T2c	N0	
IIIa	T3a	N0	M0
IIIb	T3b	N0	M0
IIIc	T3c	N1	M0
	any T	N1	M0
IV	any T	any N	M1

Histopathologic Grade (G)
Borderline
Well differentiated
Moderately differentiated
Poorly differentiated or undifferentiated

Vagina

Classification by site

Cases should be classified as carcinoma of the vagina when the primary site of the growth is in the vagina. Tumors present in the vagina as secondary growths from genital or extragenital sites should be excluded. A growth that has extended to the portio and reached the area of the external os should always be allotted to carcinoma of the cervix. A growth limited to the urethra should be classified as carcinoma of the urethra. There should be histologic verification of the disease. The vagina is drained by lymphatics, toward the pelvic nodes in its upper two thirds and toward the inguinal nodes in the lower third. The rules for staging are similar to those for carcinoma of the cervix.

1.0 Staging classification
FIGO nomenclature

Stage 0	Carcinoma in situ; intra-epithelial carcinoma
Stage I	The carcinoma is limited to the vaginal wall
Stage II	The carcinoma has involved the subvaginal tissue but has not extended to the pelvic wall
Stage III	The carcinoma has extended to the pelvic wall
Stage IV	The carcinoma has extended beyond the true pelvis or has involved the mucosa of the bladder or rectum; bullous edema as such does not permit a case to be allotted to stage IV
Stage IVa	Spread of the growth to adjacent organs and/or direct extension beyond the true pelvis
Stage IVb	Spread to distant organs

Stage Grouping for Vagina

FIGO/AJCC/UICC	T	N	M
0	Tis	N0	M0
I	T1	N0	M0
II	T2	N0	M0
III	T1	N1	M0
	T2	N1	M0
	T3	N0	M0
	T3	N1	M0
IVa	T1	N2	M0
	T2	N2	M0
	T3	N2	M0
	T4	any N	M0
IVb	any T	any N	M1

Vulva

Cases should be classified as carcinoma of the vulva when the primary site of growth is in the vulva. Tumors present in the vulva as secondary growths from a genital or extragenital site should be excluded. Malignant melanoma should be separately reported. A carcinoma of the vulva that extends into the vagina should be considered as a carcinoma of the vulva. There should be histologic confirmation of the cancer. The femoral, inguinal, external iliac, and hypogastric nodes are the sites of regional spread. Involvement of pelvic lymph nodes (external, internal, and common iliac) are considered distant metastasis.

1.0 Staging classification
Definitions of the clinical stages in carcinoma of the vulva

Stage 0	Carcinoma in situ, intraepithelial carcinoma
Stage I	Lesions 2 cm or less in size confined to vulva or perineum. No nodal metastasis.
Stage Ia:	Lesions 2 cm or less in size confined to the vulva or perineum and with stromal invasion no greater than 1.0 mm.* No nodal metastasis.

---

*The depth of invasion is defined as the measurement of the tumor from the epithelial-stromal junction of the adjacent most superficial dermal papilla to the deepest point of invasion.

Stage Ib: Lesions 2 cm or less in size confined to the vulva or perineum and with stromal invasion greater than 1.0 mm.* No nodal metastasis.

Stage II Tumor confined to the vulva and/or perineum; more than 2 cm in greatest dimension; no nodal metastasis

Stage III Tumor of any size with adjacent spread of the lower urethra and/or the vagina, or the anus, and/or unilateral regional lymph node metastasis

Stage IVa Tumor invades any of the following:
Upper urethra, bladder mucosa, rectal mucosa, pelvic bone, and/or bilateral regional nodal metastasis

Stage IVb Any distant metastasis, including pelvic lymph nodes

Rules for staging

	Primary tumor
T	Tis Preinvasive carcinoma (carcinoma in situ)

T1	Tumor confined to the vulva and/or perineum; 2 cm or less in greatest dimension
	T1a and with stromal invasion no greater than 1.0 mm
	T1b and with stromal invasion greater than 1.0 mm
T2	Tumor confined to the vulva and/or perineum; more than 2 cm in greatest dimension
T3	Tumor of any size with adjacent spread to the urethra and/or vagina and/or the anus
T4	Tumor of any size infiltrating the bladder mucosa and/or the rectal mucosa, including the upper part of the urethral mucosa and/or fixed to the bone

N	Regional lymph nodes

N0	No lymph node metastasis
N1	Unilateral regional lymph node metastasis
N2	Bilateral regional lymph node metastasis

M	Distant metastasis; no clinical metastasis (MO)

M0	No distant metastasis
M1	Distant metastasis (including pelvic lymph node metastasis)

Stage Grouping for Vulva

FIGO/AJCC/UICC	T	N	M
0	Tis	N0	M0
Ia	T1a	N0	M0
Ib	T1b	N0	M0
II	T2	N0	M0
III	T1	N1	M0
	T2	N1	M0
	T3	N0	M0
	T3	N1	M0
IVa	T1	N2	M0
	T2	N2	M0
	T3	N2	M0
	T4	any N	M0
IVb	any T	any N	M1

Gestational trophoblastic tumors

In 1991, FIGO added non-surgical-pathologic prognostic risk factors to the classic anatomical staging system. These include beta-hCG levels of greater than 10^5 and the duration of an antecedent pregnancy greater than 6 months.

Since gestational trophoblastic tumors have a very high cure rate in virtually all patients, the ultimate goal of staging is to identify patients who are likely to respond to less intensive chemotherapeutic protocols from those who will require more intensive chemotherapy in order to achieve remission.

Staging should be based on history, clinical examination. and appropriate laboratory and radiologic studies. Since βhCG titers accurately reflect clinical disease, histologic verification is not required for diagnosis, although it may aid in therapy.

FIGO staging for trophoblastic tumors

Stage I	Disease confined to the uterus
Stage Ia	Disease confined to the uterus with no risk factors
Stage Ib	Disease confined to the uterus with one risk factor
Stage Ic	Disease confined to the uterus with two risk factors
Stage II	GTT extends outside of the uterus but is limited to the genital structures (adnexa, vagina, broad ligament)
Stage IIa	GTT involving genital structures without risk factors
Stage IIb	GTT extends outside of the uterus but limited to genital structures with one risk factor
Stage IIc	GTT extends outside of the uterus but limited to the genital structures with two risk factors
Stage III	GTT extends to the lungs, with or without known genital tract involvement
Stage IIIa	GTT extends to the lungs, with or without genital tract involvement and with no risk factors
Stage IIIb	GTT extends to the lungs, with or without genital tract involvement and with one risk factor
Stage IIIc	GTT extends to the lungs, with or without genital tract involvement and with two risk factors
Stage IV	All other metastatic sites
Stage IVa	All other metastatic sites, without risk factors
Stage IVb	All other metastatic sites, with one risk factor
Stage IVc	All other metastatic sites, with two risk factors

1. hCG >100,000 U/ml
2. Duration of disease >6 months from termination of the antecedent pregnancy

The following factors should be considered and noted in reporting:

1. 1. Prior chemotherapy for known GTT
2. Placental site tumors should be reported separately
3. Histologic verification of disease is not required

Fallopian tube

The fallopian tube extends from the posterior superior aspect of the uterine fundus laterally and anteriorly to the ovary. Its length is approximately 10 cm. The lateral end opens to the peritoneal cavity. Carcinoma of the oviduct can metastasize to the regional lymph nodes, including the para-aortic nodes. Direct extension to surrounding organs, as well as intraperitoneal seeding, occurs frequently. Peritoneal implants may occur with an intact tube.

1. Carcinoma in situ of the fallopian tube is a defined entity; therefore it is included in the staging under stage 0.
2. Because the fallopian tube is a hollow viscus and because extension into the submucosa or muscularis and to and beyond the serosa can be defined (a concept similar to that of Dukes' classification for colon cancer), these are taken into consideration in stage Ia, Ib, and Ic in addition to laterality, as well as the presence or absence of ascites. As in ovarian carcinoma, peritoneal washings positive for malignant cells or malignant ascites is placed into stage Ic.
3. It should be noted that in stage III the classification of the tumor is based on the size of the findings at the time of entry into the abdominal cavity, *not* on the residual at the end of the debulking. In addition, surface involvement of the liver is in stage III, as is inguinal node metastasis. As in ovarian cancer, pleural effusion must have malignant cells to be called stage IV.

Laparotomy and resection of tubal masses, as well as hysterectomy, form the basis for staging. Biopsies of all suspicious sites, such as the omentum, mesentery, liver, diaphragm, and pelvic and para-aortic nodes, are required.

The final histologic findings after surgery (and cytologic ones when available) are to be considered in the staging.

Clinical studies, if carcinoma of the tube is diagnosed, include routine radiography of chest. CT may be helpful in initial staging and follow-up of tumors.

FIGO staging for fallopian tube carcinoma

Staging for fallopian tube is by the surgical pathologic system. Operative findings prior to tumor debulking may be modified by histopathologic as well as clinical or radiologic evaluation.

Stage 0	Carcinoma in situ (limited to tubal mucosa)
Stage I	Growth limited to the fallopian tubes
Stage Ia:	Growth is limited to one tube, with extension into the submucosa and/or muscularis but not penetrating the serosal surface; no ascites
Stage Ib	Growth is limited to both tubes, with extension into the submucosa and/or muscularis but not penetrating the serosal surface; no ascites
Stage Ic	Tumor either stage Ia or Ib, but with tumor extension through or onto the tubal serosa or with ascites present containing malignant cells or with positive peritoneal washings
Stage II	Growth involving one or both fallopian tubes with pelvic extension
Stage IIa:	Extension and/or metastasis to the uterus and/or ovaries
Stage IIb:	Extension to other pelvic tissues
Stage IIc:	Tumor either stage IIa or IIb and with ascites present containing malignant cells or with positive peritoneal washings
Stage III	Tumor involves one or both fallopian tubes, with peritoneal implants outside the pelvis and/or positive retroperitoneal or inguinal nodes. Superficial liver metastasis equals stage III. Tumor appears limited to the true pelvis but with histologically proven malignant extension to the small bowel or omentum.
Stage IIIa:	Tumor is grossly limited to the true pelvis with negative nodes but with histologically confirmed microscopic seeding of abdominal peritoneal surfaces.
Stage IIIb:	Tumor involving one or both tubes with histologically confirmed implants of abdominal peritoneal surfaces, none exceeding 2 cm in diameter. Lymph nodes are negative.
Stage IIIc:	Abdominal implants greater than 2 cm in diameter and/or positive retroperitoneal or inguinal nodes.
Stage IV	Growth involving one or both fallopian tubes with distant metastases. If pleural effusion is present, there must be positive cytology to be stage IV. Parenchymal liver metastases equals stage IV.

Gynecologic Oncology Group Common Toxicity Criteria Grade— October 1988

Toxicity	0	1	2	3	4
Blood and bone marrow					
WBC	³4.0	3.0-3.9	2.0-2.9	1.0-1.9	|Ld1.0
PLT	WNL	75.0-normal	50.0-74.9	25.0-49.9	|Ld25.0
Hgb	WNL	10.0-normal	8.0-10.0	6.5-7.9	|Ld6.5
Granulocytes/bands	³2.0	1.5-1.9	1.0-1.4	0.5-0.9	|Ld0.5
Lymphocytes	³2.0	1.5-1.9	1.0-1.4	0.5-0.9	|Ld0.5
Hemorrhage (clinical, including operative)	None	Mild, no transfusion	Gross; 1-2 units transfusion per episode	Gross, 3-4 units transfusion per episode	Massive |Lf4 units transfusion per episode
Infection	None	Mild	Moderate	Severe	Life-threatening
Gastrointestinal					
Nausea	None	Able to eat reasonable intake	Intake significantly decreased but can eat	No significant intake	
Vomiting	None	1 episode in 24 hours	2-5 episodes in 24 hrs	6-10 episodes in 24 hrs	|Lf10 episodes in 24 hrs or requiring parenteral support
Diarrhea	None	Increase of 2-3 stools/day over pre-Rx	Increase of 4-6 stools/day or nocturnal stools or moderate cramping	Increase of 7-9 stools/day or incontinence or severe cramping	Increase of ³10 stools/day or grossly bloody diarrhea or need for parenteral support

	Grade 0	Grade 1	Grade 2	Grade 3	Grade 4
Stomatitis	None	Painless ulcers, ulcers, erythema, or mild soreness	Painful erythema, edema, or ulcers, but can eat	Painful erythema, edema, or ulcers and cannot eat	Requires parenteral or enteral support
Mechanical problems	None	Temporary ileus of 3 days or less duration	Ileus requiring tube decompression; narrowing of intestinal segment on x-ray or moderate mucosal edema on proctoscopy	Surgically correctable defect—no stoma	Fistula, perforation, chronic bleeding requiring division
Operative	None	Repair of mucosal disruption	Resection for enterotomy	Temporary diversion	Permanent diversion
Liver					
Bilirubin	WNL	$<1.6 \times N$		$1.6-3.0 \times N$	$>3.0 \times N$
Transaminase (SGOT, SGPT)	WNL	$\leq 2.5-N$	$2.6-5.0 \times N$	$5.1-20.0 \times N$	$>20.0 \times N$
Alk Phos or 5 nucleotidase	WNL	$\leq 2.5 \times N$	$2.6-5.0 \times N$	$5.1-20.0 \times N$	$>20.0 \times N$
Liver—clinical	No change from baseline			Precoma	Hepatic coma
Kidney and bladder					
Creatinine	WNL	$<1.5 \times N$	$1.5-3.0 \times N$	$3.1-6.0 \times N$	$>6.0 \times N$
Proteinuria	No change	1+ or <0.3 g%, or <3 g/l	2-3+ 0.3-1.0 g% or 3-10 g/l	4+ or >1.0 g% or >10 g/l	Nephrotic syndrome
Hematuria	Neg	Micro only	Gross, no clots	Gross + clots	Requires transfusion
Bladder and ureter acute	No problems	Dysuria: frequency and/or microscopic hematuria; injury of bladder with primary repair	Bacterial infection Infection gross hematuria not requiring transfusion (<2 gm% in HGB); injury requiring reanastomosis or reimplantation	Gross hematuria requiring transfusion (>2 gm% in HGB); sepsis, fistula or obstruction requiring secondary operation; loss of one kidney	Life-threatening hematuria or septic obstruction of both kidneys or vesicovaginal fistula requiring diversion
Chronic	None	Dysuria; frequency minimal telangiectasia with edema cytoscopy	Superficial ulceration; moderate telangiectasia; gross hematuria (<2 gm% in HGB); bladder volume less than 150 cc	Deep ulceration, severe pain; gross hematuria requiring transfusion (>2 gm% HgB); permanent unilateral loss of kidney	Decreased bladder volume requiring diversion or catheter drainage; fistula; necrosis; permanent bilateral obstruction or loss of renal function requiring dialysis
Operative	None	Bladder atony immediately postoperative	Bladder atony >6 weeks but transient	Bladder atony requiring intermittent catheterization	

Continued.

Toxicity	0	1	2	3	4
Alopecia					
Alopecia	No loss	Mild hair loss	Pronounced or total hair loss		
Heart					
Pulmonary	None or no change	Asymptomatic, with abnormality in PFTs	Dyspnea on significant exertion	Dyspnea at normal level of activity	Dyspnea at rest
Cardiac dysrhythmias	None	Asymptomatic, transient, requiring no therapy	Recurrent or persistent, no therapy required	Requires treatment	Requires monitoring or hypotension or ventricular tachycardia or fibrillation
Cardiac function	None	Asymptomatic, decline of resting ejection fraction by less than 20% of baseline value	Asymptomatic, decline of resting ejection fraction by more than 20% of baseline value	Mild CHF responsive to therapy	Severe or refractory CHF
Cardiac-ischemia	None	Nonspecific T-wave flattening	Asymptomatic ST and T wave changes suggesting ischemia	Angina without evidence for infarction	Acute myocardial infarction
Cardiac-pericardial	None	Asymptomatic effusion, no intervention required	Pericarditis (rub, chest pain, ECG changes)	Symptomatic effusion; drainage required	Tamponade; drainage urgently required
Blood pressure					
Hypertension	None or no change	Asymptomatic, transient increase by greater than 20 mm Hg (D) or to >150/100 if previously WNL. No treatment required	Recurrent or persistent increase by >20 mm Hg (D) or >150/100 if previously WNL. No treatment required	Requires therapy	Hypertensive crisis
Hypotension	None or no change	Changes requiring no therapy (including transient orthostatic hypotension)	Requires fluid replacement or other therapy but not hospitalization	Requires therapy and hospitalization resolves within 48 hrs of stopping the agent	Requires therapy and hospitalization for >48 hrs after stopping the agent
Venous problems	None	Superficial phlebitis; primary suture repair for injury with grade 0 or 1 blood loss	Pelvic or deep vein thrombophlebitis; primary suture repair for injury with grade 2 or greater blood loss	Pulmonary embolus; bypass for injury	Pulmonary embolus requiring embolectomy or caval ligation.
Arterial problems	None	Spasm, primary suture repair for injury with grade 0 or 1 blood loss	Ischemia not requiring surgical treatment; primary suture repair for injury with grade 2 or greater blood loss	Vascular thrombosis requiring resection with anastomosis; vascular occlusion requiring surgery; bypass for injury	Myocardial infarction; resection of organ (bowel, limb, etc.)

Neurologic

	0	1	2	3	4
Neurosensory	None or no change	Mild paresthesias, loss of deep-tendon reflexes	Mild or moderate objective sensory loss; moderate paresthesias	Severe objective sensory loss or paresthesias that interfere with function	
Neuromotor	None or no change	Subjective weakness; no objective findings	Mild objective weakness without significant impairment	Objective weakness with impairment	Paralysis
Neurocortical	None	Mild somnolence or agitation	Moderate somnolence or agitation	Severe somnolence agitation, confusion, disorientation, hallucination	Coma, seizures, toxic psychosis
Neurocerebellar	None	Slight incoordination, dysdiadochokinesis	Intention tremor, dysmetria, slurred speech, nystagmus	Locomotor ataxia	Cerebellar necrosis
Neuro-mood	No change	Mild anxiety or depression	Moderate anxiety or depression	Severe anxiety or depression	Suicidal ideation
Neuro-headache	None	Mild	Moderate or severe but transient	Unrelenting and severe	
Neuro-constipation	None or no change	Mild	Moderate	Severe	Ileus >96 hrs
Neuro-hearing	None or no change	Asymptomatic, hearing loss on audiometry only	Tinnitus	Hearing loss interfering with function but correctable with hearing aid	Deafness not correctable
Neuro-vision	None or no change			Symptomatic subtotal loss of vision	Blindness

Skin

	0	1	2	3	4
Skin	None or no change	Scattered macular or papular eruption or erythema that is asymptomatic	Scattered macular or papular eruption or erythema with pruritis or other associated symptoms	General symptomatic macular, papular, or vasicular eruption	Exfolliative dermatitis or ulcerating dermatitis
Wound—infectious	None	Cellulitis	Superficial infection	Abscess	Necrotizing fasciitis
Wound—noninfectious	None	Incisional separation	Incisional hernia	Fascial disruption without evisceration	
Allergy	None	Transient rash, drug fever <38° C, 100.4° F	Urticaria, drug fever 38° C, 100.4° F; Mild bronchospasm	Serum sickness, bronchospasm requiring parenteral medication	Anaphylaxis
Fever in absence of infection	None	37.1-38.0° C; 98.7-100.4° F	38.1-40.0° C; 100.5-104.0° F	>40.0° C; >104.0° F for less than 24 hrs	>40.0° C (104.0° F) for more than 24 hrs or fever accompanied by hypotension
Local	None	Pain	Pain and swelling, with inflammation or phlebitis	Ulceration	Plastic surgery indicated
Lymphatics	None	Mild lymphedema	Moderate lymphedema requiring compression; lymphocyst	Severe lymphedema limiting function; lymphocyst requiring surgery	Severe edema limiting function with ulceration

Continued.

Toxicity	0	1	2	3	4
Metabolic					
Weight gain/loss	<5.0%	5.0-9.9%	10.0-19.9%	>20.0%	
Hyperglycemia	<116	116-160	161-250	251-500	>500 or ketoacidosis
Hypoglycemia	>64	55-64	40-54	30-39	>30
Amylase	WNL	$<1.5 \times N$	$1.5\text{-}2.0 \times N$	$2.1 \times 5.0 \times N$	$>5.1 \times N$
Hypercalcemia	<10.6	10.6-11.5	11.6-12.5	12.6-13.5	>13.5
Hypocalcemia	>8.4	8.4-7.8	7.7-7.0	6.9-6.1	≤6.0
Hypomagnesemia	>1.4	1.4-1.2	1.1-0.9	0.8-0.6	≤0.5
Coagulation					
Fibrinogen	WNL	$0.99\text{-}0.75 \times N$	$0.74\text{-}0.50 \times N$	$0.49\text{-}0.25 \times N$	$\leq 0.24 \times N$
Prothrombin time	WNL	$1.01\text{-}1.25 \times N$	$1.26\text{-}1.50 \times N$	$1.51\text{-}2.00 \times N$	$>2.00 \times N$
Partial thromboplastin time	WNL	$1.01\text{-}1.66 \times N$	$1.67\text{-}2.33 \times N$	$2.34\text{-}3.00 \times N$	$>3.00 \times N$

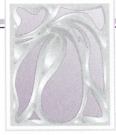

Blood Component Therapy

1. Blood component—a portion of blood that is separated by physical and mechanical means, such as differential centrifugation.
   a. Packed erythrocytes: prepared from whole blood by centrifugation and subsequent removal of plasma
      (1) Hematocrit: 60%-80%
      (2) Indications
         (a) Replacement of hemoglobin-containing cells in anemic patient with heart failure, renal failure, burns, bone marrow failure
         (b) Debilitated patients
         (c) Elderly patients
         (d) Patients with liver disease
      (3) Recommend to use packed erythrocytes for losses of blood less than 1000-1500 ml/70 kg; with losses greater than that, whole blood probably should be used
   b. Frozen red cells: long-term preservation of frozen red cells without damage can be accomplished by addition of glycerol; before transfusion, it should be thawed and washed to remove glycerol
      (1) Advantages:
         (a) Blood of rare types can be stored for long periods
         (b) 2, 3-diphosphoglycerol and adenosine triphosphate levels remain the same as they were on the day the blood was frozen
         (c) Free of plasma protein, platelets, white blood cells, and fibrin
         (d) Has been claimed to reduce the incidence of transfusion hepatitis
      (2) Disadvantages
         (a) Expensive
         (b) Outdated in 24 hours
         (c) Takes time to thaw and deglycerolize

   c. Buffy coat—poor erythrocytes; would reduce the incidence of febrile transfusion reaction
      (1) Indication
         (a) Patients with repeated febrile non-hemolytic transfusion reaction caused by leukocyte antibody
   d. Platelet concentrates
      (1) One unit of platelet concentrate contains 5.5×10^{10} platelets suspended in 30-50 ml of plasma
      (2) Shelf life: 72 hours at room temperature
      (3) Thrombocytopenia does not usually produce serious bleeding unless platelet count is less than 20,000 except if there is a platelet function defect, a coagulation defect, or local cause of hemorrhage (trauma, surgery)
      (4) Patient who has undergone trauma or requires surgery probably needs platelet count of $100,000/mm^3$ to maintain adequate hemostasis
      (5) One unit of platelet concentrate will increase platelet count by $7000-10,000/mm^3$
      (6) Repeated platelet transfusion can lead to immunization to HLA antigen and a refractory state
      (7) Should be administered through a 170 μm filter
   e. Fresh frozen plasma
      (1) Contains albumin, globulin, active coagulation factors, complement, and electrolytes
      (2) Should be type specific
      (3) Shelf life: 12 months at -20° C to -30° C; should be used within 2 hours after thawing
      (4) Indications
         (a) Deficiency in coagulation factors
         (b) Situation with plasma loss
         (c) Rapid reversal of oral anticoagulant therapy

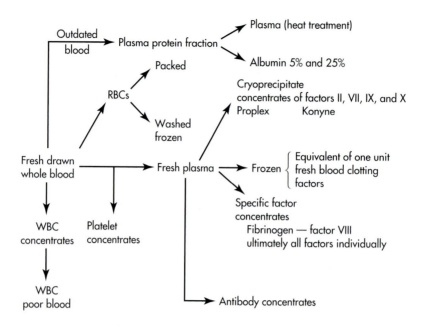

f. Cryoprecipitate—cold insoluble precipitate remaining when fresh frozen plasma is allowed to thaw at 4° C; contain factor VIII with fibrinogen, factor XIII
   (1) Indications
       (a) von Willebrand disease
       (b) Replacement of fibrinogen, factor XIII
2. Plasma fraction—derivatives of plasma obtained by chemical process, such as alcohol precipitation
   a. Coagulation factor concentrates
       (1) Factor VIII concentrates
       (2) Factor IX concentrates
       (3) Prothrombin complex (factor II, VII, IX, X concentrates)
       (4) Fibrinogen concentrates
   b. Immunoglobulin concentrates
   c. Albumin—filtered and pasteurized by heating for 10 hours at 60° C to eliminate the risks of viral hepatitis
       (1) 5% albumin: isosmotic, sodium 145 mEq/L; for rapid expansion of vascular volume

   (2) 25% albumin: sodium 145mEq/L; given IV, one volume of 25% albumin will draw about 4 volumes of additional fluid from extravascular space into circulation; for treatment of hypoalbuminemia
   d. Plasma protein factor—5% solution of selected human plasma protein in buffered saline solution; heat-treated to eliminate the risks of hepatitis; indicated for rapid expansion of vascular volume
3. Stroma-free hemoglobin solution
   a. a. Advantages
       (1) No necessity of blood typing
       (2) Longer storability
       (3) Maintains better microcirculation
       (4) Potentially improved oxygenation of ischemic myocardium
       (5) No antigenicity

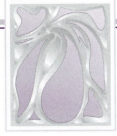

Commonly Used Statistical Terms

Null hypothesis. This hypothesis states there is no association between two variables. Testing for statistical significance allows one to reject or not reject a null hypothesis. It does not prove a null hypothesis. Failure to reject a null hypothesis may imply that the evidence is not strong enough to reject the assumption that a difference exists. The p value is the main statistic tool used to test the hypothesis. The point of significance has traditionally been placed at the 5% level. If $p < 0.05$, this is considered significant and the null hypothesis is rejected, whereas a $p > 0.05$ is considered not significant, in which case the null hypothesis is not rejected.

Type I (alpha) error. This is present when the null hypothesis is erroneously rejected and the study results are falsely accepted. There may be no association even when statistical significance is demonstrated. It may occur by chance alone.

Type II (beta) error. This is the opposite of type I error. The failure to reject the null hypothesis does not always mean no true difference exists. This may result from chance, a too small sample size, a small effect, or combination thereof.

Mean. The average of a sample of observations.

Median. Median is the middle value when they are arranged in the order of the smallest to the largest.

Sensitivity. Notes the number of patients with the disease who are correctly identified by the test.

Specificity. Measures the number of patients without disease who are correctly identified as disease free by the test.

Predictive value of a positive test. The proportion of patients with a positive test who are diseased.

Predictive value of a negative test. Proportion of patients with a negative test who are disease free.

These values, unlike sensitivity and specificity, indicate reliability of the test in the determination of presence/absence of disease.

$$\text{Sensitivity} = \frac{a}{a + c}$$

$$\text{Specificity} = \frac{d}{b + d}$$

$$\text{Positive predictive value} = \frac{a}{a + b}$$

$$\text{Negative predictive value} = \frac{d}{c + d}$$

Where

a = number of individuals with disease and test positive (true positive)

b = number of individuals disease free and test positive (false positive)

c = number of individuals with disease and test negative (false negative)

d = number of individuals disease free and test negative (true negative)

Incidence rate. Measures the new cases of a specific disease that develop over a defined period of time; the approximation of the risk for developing the disease. Focuses on events. Incidence measures probability of developing a disease.

$$\text{Incidence rate} = \frac{\text{number of disease onset}}{\text{sum of the time period of observation}}$$

Prevalence rate. Measures the proportion of a population affected by disease at a given point in time; the risk of having the disease at a point in time. Focuses on disease status. Prevalence measures the probability of having the disease at a specific time.

$$\text{Prevalence rate} = \frac{\text{number of disease at a point in time}}{\text{population at risk at a point in time}}$$

Chi square (χ^2). The primary statistical test used for studying the relationship between variables.

$$\chi^2 = \frac{(\text{observed number} - \text{expected number})^2}{\text{expected number}}$$

To compare two proportions, it is most common to tabulate the data in a 2×2 table.

p value. This tests the level of statistical significance. It indicates the probability of getting the observed difference in the sample population if there is no true difference in the comparison population. A p value of 0.01 indicates a 1% chance of achieving an observed difference if there is no true difference. Traditionally a p value of 0.05 is the highest p value to be considered statistically significant.

One-tail test. A test to determine a difference in only one direction; for example, if drug A is better than drug B.

Two-tail test. A test to determine any difference between the variable; for example, if either drug A or drug B is superior to the other. It is usually considered that in a two-tail test more trust can be placed in the statistically significant results than with a one-tail test. When in doubt, the two-tail test is preferred.

Standard deviation. A measure of the variability within each group. If there is a normal (bell-shaped curve) distribution, about 95% of the values are within two standard deviations on both sides of the average.

Relative risk. Measures the probability of the outcome if a certain variable is present vs the probability if the variable is not present.

$$RR =$$

$$\frac{\text{risk of the outcome if risk variable is present}}{\text{risk of the outcome if the risk variable is not present}}$$

Multivariate analysis. A technique of analysis of data that factors many variables. A mathematical model is constructed that simultaneously determines the effect of one variable while evaluating the effect of other factors that may have an influence on the variable being tested. The two most common algorithms developed to accomplish this task are the step-up and step-down procedure. Variables are added to an initial small set or deleted from an initial large set while testing repeatedly to see which new factor makes a statistical contribution to the overall model.

Actuarial (life table) survival. This technique uses grouped information to estimate the survival curve. The data grouped into fixed time periods (e.g., months, years) that include the maximum follow-up. The survival curve is estimated as a continuous curve. It gives an estimate of the proportions of a group of patients who will be alive at different times after initial observation. It includes patients with incomplete follow-up.

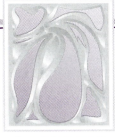

Suggested Recommendations for Routine Cancer Screening

Suggested Cancer Screening Guidelines

Cervical cancer. All women who are or have been sexually active or who have reached 18 should undergo an annual Pap test and pelvic examination. After a woman has had three or more consecutive, satisfactory annual examinations with normal findings, the Pap test may be performed less frequently at the discretion of her physician.

It is estimated that in the United States more than 90% of women 16 years of age or older have had at least one Pap test, and more than 60% have had a Pap test within 3 years. Because (1) cervical cancer has not been eradicated, (2) the incidence of CIN appears to have increased over the past decade, (3) the Pap test has an appreciable false negative rate, and (4) women have a tendency to extend screening intervals, the proposed screening guidelines of annual cervical cytology for most women are prudent and warranted if early precursors to cervical cancer are to be detected and successfully treated.

Breast cancer. A baseline mammogram should be obtained from a woman between the ages of 35 and 40. Thereafter, mammography is suggested every 1 or 2 years for women aged 40-50 years and annually for women over 50.

Evidence from several studies indicates that there is a decrease in mortality for all women when appropriate screening by mammography is instituted and performed by qualified personnel. The efficacy of mammography is not in doubt. The question that remains is the optimal screening frequency, and the answer may be provided by data now being compiled. Safety is no longer a concern but it is recognized that mammography is the most costly of all screening modalities. Dedicated equipment is essential, and considerable skill and experience are required to interpret the films. It is important, therefore, to determine the most prudent utilization of resources.

Until the optimal screening frequency is determined, it appears reasonable to follow recommendations of the American Cancer Society and the National Cancer Institute.

Endometrial cancer. Total population screening for endometrial cancer and its precursors is neither cost effective nor warranted. High-risk patients may require endometrial sampling.

The cost effectiveness of screening asymptomatic women for endometrial cancer and its precursors is very low and therefore the practice is unwarranted. On the other hand, perimenopausal and postmenopausal women with a history or evidence of abnormal vaginal hemorrhage are at high risk for endometrial cancer, and their symptoms should be investigated by endometrial biopsy or curettage. Dilation and curettage are recommended when endometrial hyperplasia or questionable endometrial carcinoma are present and when there is insufficient tissue for diagnosis by endometrial biopsy.

If estrogen-progestin therapy is instituted, endometrial biopsy is not required before treatment is begun unless there are reasons (such as abnormal bleeding) to place the patient at high risk for endometrial neoplasia. If unexpected breakthrough bleeding occurs during therapy, endometrial biopsy is recommended to rule out the development of abnormal endometrial histology. Endometrial biopsy by aspiration curettage performed in the office is diagnostically reliable and cost effective in symptomatic patients. The timing of further biopsies, if needed, is a clinical decision that should be based on previous histologic results and the patient's history.

Ovarian cancer. No available techniques are currently suitable for routine screening.

Many different techniques, including peritoneal fluid profiles, investigation of tumor-associated antigens, and ultrasonography, have been or are being investigated as possible screening tools for ovarian cancer. To date, none of these techniques has proved practical or effective.

Colorectal cancer. Women age 40-49 should undergo a digital rectal examination annually; thereafter, annual digital examination, annual fecal occult blood test, and sigmoidoscopy every 3-5 years after two consecutive annual negative examinations is recommended.

Available data do not substantiate the cost effectiveness of various screening recommendations. Because colorectal cancer is a significant risk to women, the task force suggests that the recommendations of the American Cancer Society and the National Cancer Institute be used as a guide.

Lung cancer. No available techniques are currently suitable for routine screening.

The only effective way to reduce mortality from lung cancer is to promote a "stop smoking" message to the public. Although some support is evolving for annual x-ray screening for those at risk, (i.e., women 50 years and older who smoke more than a pack of cigarettes daily) neither the American Cancer Society nor the National Cancer Institute has adopted this guideline.

Based on ACOG Committee Opinion, number 68, April 1989.

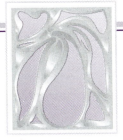

Nutritional Therapy

In the cancer patient, malnutrition may appear simultaneously with the disease. Such an individual frequently exhibits anorexia because of decreased nutritional intake with resultant weight loss. There may be an increased nutritional requirement because of the increased demands of the patient and her tumor. Resting metabolic rates can be extremely variable, but in as many as 60% of patients it may be elevated. The in stage of malnutrition in the cancer patient can lead to cachexia with weakness and tissue wasting. The extent of the malnutrition in the patient may be greater than can be explained by decreased nutritional intake. Metabolic abnormalities include abnormal response to glucose tolerance testing, increased gluconeogenesis, (which can result in decreased muscle protein synthesis), and abnormalities in protein and fat metabolism. A patient with a malignancy may need additional nutritional support as she undergoes intensive treatment, which can include surgery and chemotherapy. It appears that parenteral nutrition improves a patient's tolerance of treatment and improves her nutritional state, yet it has not been shown to improve survival.

Dietary nutrients required for good health include water, protein, fat, carbohydrates, vitamins, and minerals. Energy is required for normal body function, growth, and repair. Protein is necessary for growth and development to maintain body structures and function. It is the source of the essential amino acids and nitrogen needed for the synthesis of nonessential amino acids. Dietary protein replaces the essential amino acids and nitrogen lost through protein turnover and normal body functions. During illness, protein requirements increase. Nitrogen balance is essential for good health and requires intake of protein and energy. At higher energy intakes, less protein is needed to achieve nitrogen balance. Nitrogen is continuously lost in the body through normal body functions. Fat, of course, is the food substance with the highest concentration of calories.

Linoleic acid is the only essential fatty acid required in the diet; it is necessary for the synthesis of arachidonic acid, which is a major precursor of prostaglandin. Linoleic acid comes mainly from polyunsaturated vegetable oils. A deficiency of essential fatty acids results in poor wound healing, hair loss, and dermatitis. Fatty acids and cholesterol make up most of the fat in our diets. Carbohydrates include sugar, starch, and fibers. When carbohydrates are not in the diet, ketosis begins to take place, and there is excessive breakdown of protein as amino acids are used for gluconeogenesis. Vitamins, water soluble and fat soluble, cannot be synthesized in adequate amounts by the body. Fat-soluble vitamins are required for absorption, transport, metabolism, and storage. They are not excreted in the urine like the water-soluble vitamins, and an excess accumulation can lead to well-known toxic conditions. Major minerals, as well as trace elements, are important in human nutrition.

Dudrick suggests that patients who have a 10-pound weight loss or a 10% decrease in body weight 2 months prior to assessment, serum albumin less than 3.4 gm%, anergy to 4 of 5 standard skin test antigens, low total lymphocyte count, and who cannot or will not eat enough are candidates for nutritional assessment. Nutritional history, with a 24-hour dietary recall, can be used to assess nutritional intake. Anthropometric measurements are useful in assessing the nutritional status. Relative body weight is probably the most useful of these measurements since rapid weight loss is usually an indication of protein calorie undernutrition. The triceps skinfold test assesses fat stores, and mid-arm circumference tends to assess protein status. Edema, which is frequently seen with protein calorie deficiency, can mask true weight loss and muscle wasting. Serum albumin is probably the single most important test for determining protein calorie undernutrition. Albumin is the main plasma protein necessary to maintain plasma osmotic pressure as well as other functions. In a patient with low albumin, morbidity and mortality are increased. It must be remembered that albumin can be influenced by conditions other than malnutrition and may be affected by hydration status. Transferrin binds and transports iron in the plasma and is a good indicator of protein nutritional status.

The extent of malnutrition depends on the type and site of the cancer. Cancers, such as ovarian cancer with its potential effect on the GI tract appear to contribute to malnutrition to a greater degree than cervical cancer. Malnutrition becomes worse, as expected, as the cancer progresses. The mechanism of cancer-related malnutrition is unknown. There are probably multiple contributing factors. Decreased food intake because of anorexia, early satiety, nausea, and vomiting certainly can play a role. Poor absorption of nutrients can also be a contributing factor. Food aversion, particularly in patients undergoing chemotherapy or irradiation, is well known. Change of taste and smell can contribute to decreased intake. Generalized weakness also may contribute to decreased food intake.

Decrease in total lymphocyte count (less than 1200) is also suggestive of malnutrition. Creatinine height index (CHI) may be helpful, in that urinary creatinine excretion is proportional to total body muscle mass. As muscles become depleted, creatinine excretion falls. A CHI of ≥80% usually indicates a normal lean body mass. A CHI of 60%-80% notes moderate depletion; CHI of <60% indicates severe depletion.

The role of total parenteral nutrition (TPN) in the patient with cancer has yet to be determined. TPN can certainly correct nutritional deficits that commonly occur in the cancer patient. TPN can improve nitrogen balance and decrease catabolism; glucose turnover and clearance rates are increased, gluconeogenesis is suppressed, and free fatty acid oxidation is increased. TPN can increase body weight and reverse serum markers of malnutrition; yet as an adjuvant to cancer therapy the results have not been encouraging. TPN has not added to lean body mass or eliminated the GI or hematologic toxicity associated with chemotherapy. In patients treated with chemotherapy, response rates and survival have not been increased with TPN. Although irradiation can contribute to poor nutrition (diarrhea, enteritis and malabsorption), particularly to the GI tract when gynecologic cancers are treated, TPN has not shown a significant improvement regarding treatment response, tolerance to treatment, local control, survival, or decreased complications of therapy.

Nutritional support for the cancer patient requiring surgery is also ill defined. Certainly malnourished patients undergoing surgery have a higher postoperative morbidity and mortality compared to well nourished patients. Whether or not TPN can affect morbidity and mortality in the cancer patient is undetermined. The concern that TPN may stimulate tumor growth is unfounded. It does appear that although routine use of TPN in the cancer patient is not warranted, it may be indicated in severely malnourished patients undergoing surgery or those with postoperative complications.

Nutritional supports are of two main types: enteric and parenteral. For the patient with a functional GI tract, enteric nutrition may be considered through the use of a nasoenteric tube. A gastrostomy or jejunostomy tube may also be used. Obviously, GI dysfunction is a contraindication to this method. Nevertheless this method appears to be cost effective, probably maintains the GI mucosa integrity, provides a normal sequence of intestinal and hepatic metabolism prior to systemic distribution, appears to preserve normal hormonal patterns, and avoids the risk of sepsis. Enteric solutions differ in composition, calorie content, and multiple other factors. They are usually complete in that they contain a full supplement of nutrient requirements, or incomplete, when they are designated to contain a specific macronutrient such as fat, protein, or carbohydrate. Most solutions contain 1000 calories and 37-45 gm of protein per liter. Elemental diets are mainly amino acids and simple sugars. They are extremely hypertonic and may induce diarrhea. GI complications include diarrhea, which may be corrected with a formula of lower osmolarity. Electrolyte imbalance and glucose intolerance can also occur.

Many cancer patients who require nutritional supplementation will need parenteral administration (TPN). In some instances, this can be administered through a peripheral vein, particularly if only a short duration of TPN is anticipated. Although adequate protein can usually be infused peripherally, high caloric supplementation is usually given centrally. Fat solutions, which can account for a high caloric intake, can be given peripherally. A major complication of peripheral TPN is thrombophlebitis and infiltration. Most TPN is given through a central vein, via either the subclavian vein or major neck vessels. The catheter can be inserted in the superior vena cava, and this allows rapid infusion of hypertonic solutions without difficulty. Infusion of parenteral solution should be started slowly to prevent hyperglycemia. If glucose intolerance develops, a small amount of insulin is used to control blood sugars. Meticulous care for the central catheter must be carried out, as this can be a major source of infection. Frequent changing of IV tubing and

---

TPN INDICATIONS

- Severely malnourished patients undergoing surgery
- Patients with postoperative complications that require nutritional support
- Therapy induced complications that require nutritional support

Note: Routine use of TPN in patients with cancer is *not* indicated.

filters, as well as the catheter, is required routinely. TPN is usually managed as a team endeavor, with the attending physician, someone with a special interest in nutrition, nurse, pharmacist, and dietitian. Daily requirements must be standardized regarding calories, proteins, fat, minerals, vitamins, and trace elements. These should be varied as the situation demands. Metabolic complications may include hyper- or hypoglycemia, hyperosmolarity, azotemia, hypercholoremic metabolic acidosis, mineral electrolyte disorder, liver enzyme elevations, and anemias

---

NUTRITIONAL GUIDELINES FOR THE ADULT PATIENT

I. Daily Protein Needs
   Maintenance   0.8-1 g/kg
   Mild-moderate stress   1-1.5 g/kg
   Moderate-severe stress   1.5-2 g/kg
   Very high stress/burns   >2 g/kg

II. Daily Caloric Needs (Consider initiating HAL with 50%-75% of estimated patient needs on day 1)
   Maintenance, mild stress 20-25 kcal/kg (15-20 NPC/kg)
   Mild-moderate stress *(routine surgery, minor infection)*   25-30 kcal/kg (20-25 NPC/kg)
   Moderate-severe stress *(major surgery, sepsis, tumor tx)*   30-35 kcal/kg (25-30 NPC/kg)

III. Body Weight Calculations
   Total body weight (TBW) = pt weight (kg)
   Ideal body weight (IBW) male = 50 kg + (2.3 × # inches >5 ft)
                          female = 45 kg + (2.3 × # inches >5 ft)
   Adjusted body weight (ABW) for the obese patient = IBW + 0.3 × (TBW — IBW)

IV. Suggested Laboratory Tests
   Baseline and weekly: Chem 10, Chem 13
   Daily: Chem 10 x 3d or until stabilized prealbumin as clinically indicated

V. Formula
   A. Standard Formula

	Central	Peripheral ($D^{10}A_{3,6}$)
Amino acids (gm)	55 mg/L	30 g/L
Dextrose (kcal)	555 kcal/L	280 kcal/L
Lipids (kcal)	400 kcal/L	350 kcal/L
NPC	955 NPC/L	630 NPC/L
Total kcal	1175 kcal/L	750 kcal/L
Desired total volume/d	_____ ml*	_____ ml*

   B. Modified Central Formula
      1. Protein:
         Daily protein needs × Body weight calculations = _____ g protein/d
      2. Non-protein calories (NPC):
         Daily caloric needs × Body weight calculations = _____ NPC/d
      3. Percentages of NPC:
         Usually 50%-70% of daily NPC as CHO + usually 30%-50% of daily NPC as fat = 100%
      4. Infusion rate (see HAL bag for exact infusion rate)
         □ maximally concentrated† or □ infusion rate _____ mg/hr

VI. Electrolytes   □ Standard   □ Modified   Acetate/Chloride
   Sodium   80 mEq/L   ____ mEq/L   ____ balance
   Potassium   40 mEq/L   ____ mEq/L   ____ maximum acetate
   Calcium   5 mEq/L   ____ mEq/L   ____ maximum chloride
   Magnesium   8 mEq/L   ____ mEq/L   __:__ chloride : acetate

*See HAL bag for exact infusion rate
†Calculation of volume of maximally concentrated HAL:
  1. Amino acid (AA): ____ protein/d x 10 ml/g AA = ____ ml 10% AA solution
  2. Dextrose: ____ NPC/d x ____% as CHO = ____ kcal CHO ÷ 3.4 kcal/g CHO = ____ g CHO x 1.43 ml/g = ____ ml D70
  3. Lipid: ____ NPC/d x ____% as fat = ____kcal fat ÷ 2 kcal/ml = ____ ml 20% lipids
  4. Maximally concentrated volume = ____ (from 1 above) ml 10% AA + ____ (from 2 above) ml D70 + ____ (from 3 above) ml 20% lipids = ____ ml/d
  5. Approximate infusion rate = ____ (from 4 above) ml/d ÷ 24 hr/d = ____ ml/hr *(Actual infusion rate may be altered by volume of additives; see HAL bag for exact infusion rate.)*
Courtesy of the nutritional and pharmacy divisions of the Medical University of South Carolina.

Continued.

NUTRITIONAL GUIDELINES FOR THE ADULT PATIENT—cont'd

VII. Vitamins and Trace Elements (MV1-12 and standard trace elements will automatically be added unless otherwise specified)

____ Vitamin K 1 mg/d   ____ No vitamin K

A. Content of MV1-12

vitamin A	3300 IU	vitamin B_5	15 mg
vitamin D	200 IU	vitamin B_6	4 mg
vitamin E	10 mg	vitamin B_{12}	5 mcg
vitamin B_1	3 mg	vitamin C	100 mg
vitamin B_2	3.6 mg	biotin	60 mcg
vitamin B_3	40 mg	folic acid	0.4 mg

B. Content of standard trace elements

chromium chloride	12 mcg
copper sulfate	1.2 mg
manganese sulfate	0.3 mg
zinc sulfate	3 mg

VIII. Other Additives

____ Humulin regular insulin _____ units/d

____ H_2 antagonist _____ m/d

____ Other (specify)

IX. Hyperalimentation Access:

____ Central ____ Peripheral

X. Special Instructions

In many hospitals, standard hyperalimentation solutions with appropriate nutrients have been formulated, with adjustments made for specific needs. Intense metabolic monitoring is required in these patients, and established hospital protocols are available in many institutions today.

Today both enteric and parenteral nutritional support can be implemented successfully on an outpatient basis. Indications are not uniformly agreed on for this method of nutrition. In the cancer patient it may be indicated to help satisfy nutritional needs while toxicity of treatment is abating. Most authorities do not feel that home nutritional support is indicated for the terminally ill cancer patient.

A typical nutritional guideline for the adult patient follows. Many institutions have nutritional protocols in place and, although there may be variations on the theme, these guidelines have become relatively standardized.

BIBLIOGRAPHY

Arbeit JM, Lees DE, Corsey R, Brennan MF: Resting energy expenditure in controls and cancer patients with localized and diffuse disease, *An Surg* 199:292, 1984.

Baker JP, Detsky AS, Wesson DE et al: Nutritional assessment: a comparison of clinical judgement and objective measurements, *N Engl J Med* 306:969, 1982.

Bernstein LH, Leukardt-Fairfield CJ, Pleban W, Rudolph R: Usefulness of data on albumin and prealbumin concentrations in determining effectiveness of nutritional support, *Clin Chem* 35:271, 1989.

Brennan MF: Total parenteral nutrition in the cancer patient, *N. Engl J Med* 305:375, 1981.

Flowers JF, Ryan JA, Gough JA: Catheter-related complications of total parenteral nutrition. In Fischer JE, ed: *Total parenteral Nutrition,* Boston: Little, Brown and Company, 1991.

Grant JP: *Handbook of Total Parenteral Nutrition,* Philadelphia, W.B. Saunders, 1980.

Grant JP, Cuter PB, Thurlow JT: Current techniques of nutritional assessment, *Surg Clin North Am* 61:437, 1981.

Harrison LE, Brennan MF: The role of total parenteral nutrition in the patient with cancer, *Current Problems in Surgery* 10:833, 1995.

Kern KA, Norton JA: Cancer cachexia, *JPEN J Parentr Enteral Nutr* 12:286, 1988.

McGeer AJ, Detsky AS, O'Rourke K: Parenteral nutrition in patients receiving cancer chemotherapy, *An Intern Med* 110:734, 1989.

Nelson KA, Walsh D, Sheehan FA: The cancer anorexia-cachexia syndrome, *J Clin Oncol* 12:213, 1994.

Sclafani LM, Brennan MF: Nutritional support in the cancer patient. In Fischer JE, ed: *Total Parenteral Nutrition,* Boston: Little, Brown and Company 1994.

Smale BF, Mullen JL, Buzby GP, Rosato EF: The efficacy of nutritional assessment and support in cancer surgery, *Cancer* 47:2375, 1981.

Torosian MH, Mullen JL: Nutritional assessment. In Kaminski I, Mitchell V, eds: *Hyperalimentation: A Guide for Clinicians,* New York: Marcel Dekker, Inc., 1985.

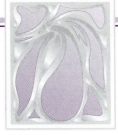

Basic Principles in Gynecologic Radiotherapy

All life on this planet evolved in a milieu in which the major source of all energy essential for biologic processes has been in the form of radiant energy, or radiation. Various forms of irradiation influence living material in a variety of ways. Sunlight provides heat, light, and energy for plant photosynthesis, whereas radio waves provide a means of communication (Table G-1). In general, most radiations are not harmful in ordinary quantities but actually are helpful to life processes. However, certain types of high energy, or "ionizing," radiation are not entirely harmless but provide useful tools in gynecology, both for diagnostic and therapeutic purposes. These high energy radiations are injurious to biologic material, and their use in oncology depends on the ability of these energy sources to provide an injury from which normal tissue may recover more effectively than malignant tissue. They can produce deleterious effects in all forms of life, from the relatively simple one-cell plants and animals to the complex higher organisms.

The change produced by these radiations may be grossly apparent soon after exposure of the living organism, but more often the radiation changes do not appear (on cursory examination) to have affected the organism at all. At this time there may be small cellular changes that can be detected only by careful chemical or microscopic study and may not be apparent for many years or indeed may manifest only in the offspring of the irradiated organism. The attitude concerning radiation exposure should always be that diagnostic tests, therapeutic radiation, and radiation acquired incidentally from the environment can all be detrimental. Although in many instances the chance of injury from diagnostic or environmental radiation is slight, the possibility of damage from a known exposure must always be weighed against the importance of the information to be gained or the effect desired. Certainly, incidental exposure must be avoided through control of environmental hazards wherever possible.

Table G-1   Electromagnetic spectrum

X-ray	124 eV-124 meV	Wavelength 100 Å-0.001 Å
Ultraviolet	3-124 eV	Wavelength 4000 Å-100 Å
Visible	2-3 eV	Wavelength 7000 Å-4000 Å
Infrared	0.01-1 eV	Wavelength 0.01 cm-10^4 cm
Radio waves	10^{10}-10^4 eV	Wavelength 3×10^5-1 cm

Table G-2   Modalities of external radiation

Modality	Voltage	Source
Low voltage (superficial)	85-150 kV	X-ray
Medium voltage (ortho-voltage)	180-400 kV	X-ray
Supervoltage	500 kv-8 mV	X-ray (linear accelerator) ^{60}Co ^{137}Cs ^{226}Ra
Megavoltage	Above supervoltage energy	Betatron Synchrotron Linear accelerator

The radiation emission of isotopes such as radium, iridium, and cesium is now used for therapeutic purposes in the treatment of many human malignancies. In addition, over the past four decades various machines capable of producing radiant energy of high intensity have become available and are also used extensively in the treatment of human malignancies. Machines that emit energies greater than 1 million electron volts (1 meV) are the most commonly used at present and constitute the so-called supravoltage-megavoltage era; among these pieces of equipment are cobalt generators, betatron, and linear accelerators (Table G-2).

Physical and Chemical Nature of Radiation

The physical forces of concern are termed *ionizing radiations* because of their characteristic ability to transfer their energy to matter by separating orbital electrons from their atoms, thus forming physical ion pairs. The term is an inclusive one, since the phenomenon may be caused by particulate radiations as well as electromagnetic waves (photons). Radiations that originate from decay of an atomic nucleus are termed *gamma rays*; those that originate outside the atomic nucleus are termed *x-rays* and are emitted when high-energy charged particles (electrons) bombard a suitable target such as tungsten. When these fast-moving electrons approach the fields around the nuclei of the atoms of the target material they are deflected from their path and energy is emitted in the form of electromagnetic radiation (photons). These emitted x-rays may have any energy from zero to a maximum that is determined by the kinetic energy of the bombarding electrons. Machines such as the betatron and linear accelerator can generate electrons at high accelerations and thus the x-rays generated by these machines

are quite high in energy. A continuous spectrum of x-rays of various energies can be produced when a large number of impinging electrons are involved. Other x-rays are produced when a high-speed electron impinging on a target material knocks out an orbital electron (ionization) from a target atom. When this electron is from an outer shell and comes to rest in another orbit, it is during this latter transition that an x-ray is given off. The photon energy of that x-ray represents the difference in energies of the inner and outer orbital electron levels. Remember that gamma rays and x-rays can be collectively termed *photons*, and what is of medical importance is the energy of the photon and not the source.

The interaction of photons with matter is accomplished through three mechanisms: the photoelectric effect, Compton scattering, and pair production. The Compton effect is the major interaction of photons in tissue used in modern radiotherapy (Figure G-1). The first step is to transform the energy of the photon into kinetic energy of the photon. The photon comes into contact with the electron and, in a "billiard-ball" effect, photon energy is

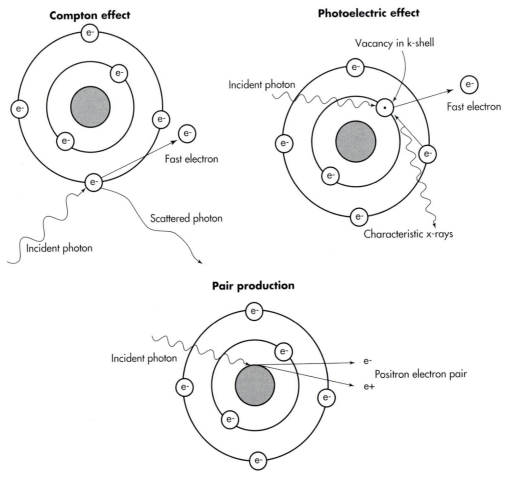

Figure G-1 See text for details.

given to the electron as kinetic energy. The photon is deflected with reduced energy. The electrons are propelled in a forward fashion. As a result, megavoltage photon beams have skin sparing effect. In the photoelectric effect, at lower energies, the incident photon is completely absorbed by the inner shell electrons with the electron being produced with kinetic energy equal to the incident photon energy less the electron binding energy. The vacancy left by the electron is replaced by an electron dropping from the outer orbit, producing a photon of characteristic radiation. In pair production, photon energies greater than 1.02 MeV may interact near the nucleus with its strong electric field and create a positron electron pair. This increases with increasing energy and atomic number. High energy beams have less scatter than low energy beams and are the choice for deep tumors such as seen in the pelvis. All of these processes result in ionization of molecules within the target or possible free radical formation. Free hydrogen atoms and free hydroxyl radicals are frequent products of the bombardment of water by high energy photons. About half of the H atoms encounter OH radicals and reform stable H_2O molecules. The other half encounter other hydrogen atoms and form H_2. The OH radicals may react in a similar way, meeting other OH radicals and forming H_2O_2 in about half the instances. In reality, the irradiation of pure water by electrons or photons results in very few H atoms before they diffuse away. The addition of soluble O_2, however, causes the H atoms to react so as to form the radical HO_2. This is less reactive than the OH radical and permits the decomposition of water to H_2O_2 to proceed. These excited and ionized molecules are very unstable and react with proteins and other key substances within the cell. Many other events may occur with photon bombardment: long-chained molecules may be split and regrouped, aggregates may be produced, and ring forms may be disrupted indiscriminately. Certainly, chemical bonds may be vulnerable to inactivation by oxidation, resulting in loss of functional capacity. All of the chemical changes may ultimately be translated into biologic injury at a cellular level.

Table G-3   Conventional radiation units, SI radiation units, and conversion factors

Quantity	Conventional unit	SI unit	Conversion factor
Exposure	R	C/kg	2.58×10^{-4} C/kg/R
Absorbed dose	rad	gray (Gy)	10^{-2} Gy/rad
Dose equivalent	rem	seivert (Sv)	10^{-2} Sv/rem
Activity	curie (Ci)	becquerel (Bq)	3.7×10^{10} Bq/Ci

RADIATION UNITS*

Those in training and in practice at this time must become familiar with a new set of special radiation units derived from the international system of weights and measures (SI). The SI units associated with classical radiation units and the appropriate conversions are shown in Table G-3.

When a radiation exposure occurs, the resulting ionizations deposit energy in the air. If an object such as a patient is present at the point of exposure, energy will be deposited by ionization in the patient. This deposition of energy by radiation exposure is called radiation absorbed dose, or simply absorbed dose, and it is measured in rads. One rad is equivalent to depositing 100 ergs of energy in each gram of the irradiated object. The SI unit of absorbed dose is the gray (Gy), and 1 Gy = 100 rads = 1 joule/kg. The erg and joule are units of energy.

BIOLOGIC EFFECTS OF RADIATION

The selective destruction of tissues forms the basis of therapeutic radiology. Neoplastic cells are usually more easily killed by radiation than are their parent cells in the surrounding normal tissues. The magnitude of the differences in radiovulnerability between normal and cancerous tissues determines in large part whether the particular neoplasm considered for radiation can be eradicated. This relative difference in local radiovulnerability is referred to as a difference in radiosensitivity, or the therapeutic ratio. It is essential that it be understood that radiosensitivity and radiocurability are not identical in meaning. Relatively radioresistant tumors accessible to high dose local radiation therapy are curable, whereas radiosensitive tumors that are widely metastasized at the beginning of therapy, or shortly thereafter, can be controlled locally only. An excellent example of a relatively radioresistant tumor is squamous cell carcinoma of the cervix, and yet this malignancy remains one of the most curable tumors of humans because of its accessibility to high dose irradiation and the relatively radioresistant nature of the hosting normal tissues (e.g., cervix and vagina). The ability to place radium or cesium in juxtaposition to the malignancy within dose ranges tolerable to the surrounding normal tissue is the key to success.

As a result of the chemical changes that have just been described, very large molecules (common in biologic systems) will undergo various structural changes that may lead to altered function. *Degradation*, or breaking into smaller units, has been shown to occur when large molecules are radiated. *Cross-linking* is another common structural change. A long molecule that is somewhat flexible in structure can undergo intramolecule cross-linking when a chemically active locus is produced on it

* From Ballenger PW, editor: *Merrill's atlas of radiographic positions and radiologic procedures,* ed 7, St. Louis, Mosby-Year Book, 1991.

and when this spot can come in contact with another reactive area. If the cross-linking is extensive, not only are the molecules incapable of normal function but they may no longer be soluble in the system. Many macromolecules are held in a rigid configuration by intramolecular cross-linking bonds, that is, by a specific chemical dimensional structure. The hydrogen bonds are among the weakest in the molecule and thus are the first to be broken by radiation. Such structural changes can lead to severe alterations in the biochemical properties of the molecule.

In this manner radiation effects on molecules such as proteins, enzymes, nucleic acids, and certain lipids can have profound effects on the cell that, in turn, can alter the organ and the organism. The initial chemical change occurs in a fraction of a second and is rarely detected directly. Some of these chemical changes are repaired almost immediately, and others that occur within less important structures may result in alterations that are rarely recognizable. The majority follow the pattern in which transition between a chemical change in a system and the biologic manifestation of this change is complicated and often obscure. Absorption and use of energy by a cell entail a complex chain of events in which multiple proteins are involved; radiation damage to these vital proteins can result in loss of cell membrane integrity and even cell death.

Although a variety of morphologic and functional changes have been described that occur in irradiated cells, the bulk of direct and indirect evidence suggests that cell nuclei are the major sites of radiation damage leading to cell death. For example, it has been calculated that 1 million cGy is required to inactivate certain cytoplasmic enzyme systems in the cell, and doses of 1000 cGy or more are usually required to damage cell membranes. In contrast, chromosomal aberrations and mutations can be produced by very low radiation doses. Because only a few hundred cGy are needed to produce a high degree of lethality in most proliferating cells in tissue culture, it seems most logical that nuclear changes produced by the low doses are responsible for the cell death.

Radiocurability and Radiosensitivity

Radiocurability and radiosensitivity have sometimes been used interchangeably. Radiocurability is the elimination of tumor at the primary or metastatic site that is due to a direct effect of radiation. Radiocurability is not necessarily similar to a patient's ultimate outcome.

On the other hand, radiosensitivity is the response of the tumor to irradiation that can be measured by the extent and length of time of regression. Radiosensitivity depends on several factors. These include hypoxia, in that it is felt that the higher the hypoxic fraction of cells the less responsive the tumor will be to the radiation. Clinical experience has noted that exophytic friable lesions on the cervix that hemorrhage easily on contact appear to respond much quicker and to a greater degree than

infiltrative lesions. It appears that the blood supply, and therefore oxygenization to the tumor cells, varies considerably between these two lesions. On the other hand, questions have been raised concerning this particular item, since the use of hyperbaric oxygen and radiosensitizers have been less than optimal to date. Another factor thought to be important in radiosensitivity is the proportion of clonogenic cells present in the radiation therapy fields. Proliferating cells are very radiosensitive. It also appears there are some tumor cells that have an adherent radiosensitivity. This involves the steepness of the initial slope of the cell survival curve and their response to radiation. It is well known clinically that certain tumors such as dysgerminomas are highly curable with relatively low doses of radiation (20-30 Gy) compared to cervical cancer, which may require >70 Gy to obtain cure. Finally, it is appreciated that there is a cellular repair of sublethal irradiation damage to tumor cell line. So-called potential lethal damage varies considerably from one tumor to another.

Clinicians have attempted to correlate tumor response to radiation and local tumor control. Generally, the faster and more complete the tumor response in relationship to the completion of the therapy, the greater the chance of curability, assuming that there is no distant metastasis. Although this is not uniformly true, it has been shown in cervical cancer that there is a good correlation between local tumor control and complete or partial regression of the cancer at the completion of radiation.

Many attempts have been made to develop assays to predict tumor radiosensitivity. Certain inherent cellular characteristics such as mitotic counts have been shown to correlate with prognosis in many tumors. No assay yet developed can predict the eventual outcome in a given tumor. This is probably due to the fact that it is accepted that most, if not all, tumors contain mixed cell populations with differing sensitivities to chemotherapeutic agents as well as radiation therapy. It appears that the therapy is selective in that certain cell populations that are sensitive can be eliminated, whereas those that are resistant eventually are responsible for the tumor being noncurable. This probably explains the fact that some tumors appear to initially respond to the therapy but are noncurable. It has been postulated that tumor cell resistance can be overcome with higher doses of radiation or increased doses of chemotherapy. Dose response curves for a variety of tumors have been developed. Probably one of the most important concepts in attempts to control and eradicate tumor cells is the volume of the tumor at the time of the initial therapy. Generally, the smaller the tumor volume, the less radiation required to destroy all cells. As the volume increases, the dose to obtain local control is increased. The concept of shrinking fields is to reduce the size of the radiation portals to give a higher dose of radiation therapy to the central portion of the tumor where presumably more hypoxic cells are present, in contrast to lesser doses that are required at the periphery and presumably better oxygenated tumor cells are present.

The limiting factor in regard to obtaining curability is the inherent toxicity to normal tissue by increasing radiation therapy doses. These effects depend on total dose, fractionation, and tumor volume. Certainly substantial injuries to the normal tissue within the treatment field can be significant. The ultimate goal is to obtain as high curability possible with the least possible side effects. Other than total dose, fractionation, and volume treated, there is a different susceptibility to ionizing radiation that depends on the organ being treated. Combining radiation therapy with surgery or chemotherapeutic agents also may decrease the tolerance of normal tissue to a given dose of radiation. Many of these factors have been well identified and quantified for many tumor sites—carcinoma of the cervix is the gynecologic cancer most investigated. Well-established port size, total dose, and fractionation have been identified. Variations are being investigated to increase curability as well as decrease complications.

Cellular radiosensitivity is generally measured as a loss of reproductive capacity of cells, which can usually be plotted in the form of a survival curve (Figure G-2). Survival curves are often variously characterized by parameters that describe both the slope of the curve and the size of the shoulder (Dq). The existence of a shoulder on survival curves indicates the ability of cells to accumulate sublethal radiation injury. From the perspective of radiation therapy, the existence of the shoulder on

cell survival curves is of great significance because it represents the ability of cells to accumulate sublethal injury capable of repair. Reirradiation results in an accumulation of sublethal injury and eventual loss of reproductive capacity. This repair of sublethal injury takes several hours (up to 6) for completion. The ability of cells to accumulate and repair sublethal injury forms the basis for the use of fractionated doses in clinical radiation therapy, in which differential capacities between normal tissue and tumor to accumulate and repair a sublethal injury can be exploited (Figure G-3). Reproductive cell death is primarily caused by damage to DNA, especially critical lesions such as double-strand breaks. The capacity of a particular cell to repair DNA damage of this type has marked influence on that cell's radiosensitivity. This DNA damage is most manifest when cells attempt to divide. Therefore rapidly dividing normal tissues (e.g., intestinal tract mucosa and bone marrow) or certain malignancies (e.g., lymphomas or squamous cell carcinomas) respond quickly to the effects of radiation, whereas the opposite is true for more slowly dividing tissues or tumors. This concept also explains why rapid response is not necessarily indicative of the level of cell kill or the magnitude of tumor control, which depends on cellular radiosensitivity rather than the particular cell kinetics of the tissue involved. The level of cell kill determines the probability of tumor control, and at times a slow response to radiation is associated with excellent tumor control.

Radiosensitivity is also a function of oxygen tension and blood supply. Tumor cells have potentially unlimited capacity for growth, and often they outgrow their blood

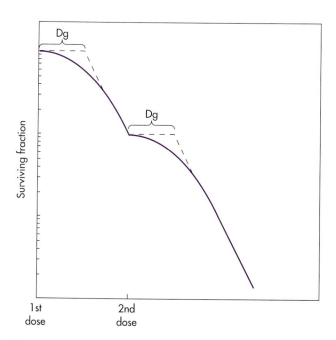

Figure G-2 Two-dose radiation survival curves for Chinese hamster cells demonstrating the return of the shoulder. Survival curves can also be characterized by the size of the shoulder *(Dg)*.

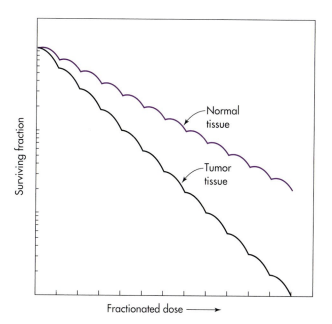

Figure G-3 Different capacities between normal tissue and tumor to accumulate and repair sublethal injury from fractionated doses results in contrasting survival.

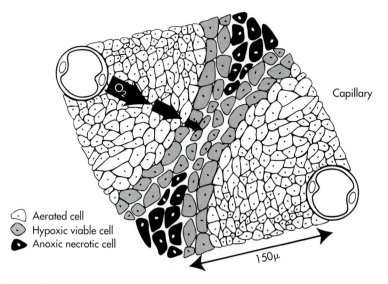

Figure G-4 As distance from blood supply increases, cells become hypoxic and even anoxic. Hypoxic cells are more radioresistant and therefore harder to sterilize. Oxygen diffuses about 150μ from the capillary.

supply. When this happens, certain regions of the tumor become deficient in certain nutrients, including oxygen. Under these conditions, the cells can enter a noncycling condition where oxygen is depleted and the cells are hypoxic or even anoxic and necrotic. This is very important from a radiobiologic standpoint because non-cycling cells can exhibit a greater capacity to repair radiation injury, and hypoxic cells are approximately three times more resistant to the effects of radiation than oxic cells. Thus, large tumors can be difficult to control with radiation therapy, not only because there is a greater number of cells to sterilize but also because a proportion of these cells are relatively hypoxic and radioresistant. (Figure G-4)

The radiosensitivity of cells varies with their position in the cell cycle, mitotic cells being most radiosensitive and late S-phase cells most radioresistant (Figure G-5). Thus, the cell-cycle distribution of cells in a particular tumor or in normal tissue has great impact on the overall radiosensitivity of that tumor or tissue.

GENETIC EFFECTS OF RADIATION

It is not possible to generalize and assign a specific mutation rate to a specific dose of radiation. Gene loci differ markedly in their mutability, and the rather random damage exerted by irradiation on any particular chromosome makes predictability exceedingly difficult. Certainly the mitotic stage, cell type, sex, species, and dose rate influence the rate of mutation production as studied in lower animals and bacteria. Data accumulated in lower animals are difficult to extrapolate to humans, and therefore prediction of mutation rates cannot be expected from the evidence that has been accumulated from various types of radiation exposure; direct evidence of radiation-

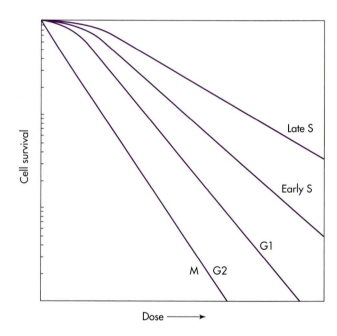

Figure G-5 The survival curve for cells in mitosis and G2 is steep and has no shoulder. The curve for cells late in S phase is shallower and has a large shoulder. G1 and early S are intermediate in sensitivity.

induced mutation in humans is lacking. The largest group of humans available for study are descendents of those exposed to radiation in Hiroshima and Nagasaki, and although there has been no detectable effect on the frequency of prenatal or neonatal deaths or on the frequency of malformations in subsequent generations, this does not mean that no hereditary effects were produced by the irradiation. The number of exposed parents was small, and for many the dosages were so low

Table G-4   Average radiation dose to fetus and to maternal gonads from various diagnostic examinations (first trimester)

Examination	Dose to fetus and maternal gonads (mcGy)
Lower extremity roentgenography	1
Cervical spine roentgenography	2
Skull roentgenography	4
Chest roentgenography	8
Pelvimetry	750
Chest fluoroscopy	70
Cholecystography	300
Lumbar spinal roentgenography	275
Abdominal roentgenography	185/film
Hip roentgenography	100
Intravenous or retrograde pyelography	585
Upper gastrointestinal roentgenography	330
Lower gastrointestinal roentgenography	465

Adapted from DiSaia PJ: *Basic principles in gynecologic radiotherapy.* In Scott JR, DiSaia PJ, Hammond CB, Spellacy WN, editors: *Danforth's obstetrics and gynecology,* ed 6, Philadelphia, 1990, JB Lippincott.

that it would have been surprising if an increase in mutation had been detected in such a brief period. There just has not been sufficient time for the several generations needed to reveal recessive damage.

It is perfectly logical to expect that radiation exposure will increase the mutation rate in humans. This is based largely on experiments in mice, where it is estimated that the doubling dose (that which will double the spontaneous mutation rate) for humans probably lies between 10 and 100 cGy. For an acute exposure to irradiation the probable value is between 15 and 30 cGy; for chronic irradiation it is probably around 100 cGy. The Committee on Genetics of the Nuclear Regulatory Commission has recommended that no individual from conception to the age of 30 years be subjected to more than 10 cGy of man-made irradiation to the gonads. Cosmic radiation, estimated to total approximately 4 cGy in this same span of years, is not included in this 10-cGy permissible dose. With the use of image intensifiers, improved x-ray film, and appropriate shielding to prevent scatter, it is possible to attain satisfactory x-ray visualization of internal structures with reduced exposure. The average dose of irradiation to the gonads of some common diagnostic techniques is given in Table G-4.

EFFECTS OF RADIATION ON THE FETUS

The classical effects of radiation on the mammalian embryo are (1) intrauterine and extrauterine growth retardation, (2) embryonic, fetal, or neonatal death, and

(3) gross congenital malformations. The structure most readily and consistently affected by radiation is the central nervous system. If the acute in utero exposure is below 25 cGy, these classic effects of radiation are never observed in experimental animals or, in all likelihood, in humans. Not only are the absorbed dose and the stage of gestation important in interpreting the effect of irradiation of a mammalian embryo but also the dose rate must be taken into consideration. Most embryonic pathologic effects are reduced significantly by decreasing the dose rate to allow a recovery process to function. The peak incidence of gross malformations occurs when the fetus is irradiated during the early organogenesis period (10 to 40 days of gestation in the human), although cellular, tissue, and organ hypoplasia can be produced by radiation throughout organogenetic, fetal, and neonatal periods if the dose is high enough. There is no stage of gestation during which an exposure of 50 cGy is not associated with a significant probability of an observable embryonic pathologic effect: increased incidence of death during the preimplantation period, malformations during the early organogenetic stage, and cell deletions and tissue hypoplasia during the fetal stages. Animal experiments indicate that all embryos exposed to 100 cGy or more after implantation will exhibit some degree of growth retardation. Finding and recognizing radiation-induced deleterious effects in offspring irradiated in utero becomes increasingly difficult with decreasing doses (less than 10 cGy) because of their low probability of occurrence and the high natural incidence of defects. From the clinical point of view, an absorbed dose of 10 cGy to the fetus at any time during gestation can be considered a practical threshold for the induction of congenital defects, below which the probability of producing adverse effects becomes exceedingly small. Diagnostic x-ray procedures (see Table G-4) should be avoided in the pregnant woman unless there is overwhelming urgency. In women of childbearing age possible damage to an early conceptus can be prevented by performing such tests immediately after the commencement of a menstrual period.

Some concrete information is available from the Japanese survivors of the A-bomb attacks in 1945. Plumer reported on 205 children, aged 4½ years, who were exposed at Hiroshima during the first half of intrauterine life. Of the 11 who were within 1200 meters of the hypocenter, 7 had microcephaly with mental retardation, a diagnosis not made in any of the 194 children exposed at greater distances. At Nagasaki, 30 mothers were exposed within 2000 meters of the hypocenter and showed major signs of having received large radiation doses, such as alopecia, purpura, oral pharyngeal lesions, or petechiae. There were 7 fetal deaths, 6 neonatal or infant deaths, and 4 instances of mental retardation among the 16 surviving children. Hall reached the following conclusions:

1. Moderately large doses of radiation (greater than 200 cGy) delivered to the human embryo before 2 to 3 weeks gestation is not likely to produce severe abnormalities in most children born, although a considerable number of embryos may be resorbed or aborted (all or none phenomenon).
2. Irradiation between 4 and 11 weeks gestation leads to severe abnormality of many organs in most or all children.
3. Irradiation between 11 and 16 weeks gestation may produce few eye, skeletal, and genital organ abnormalities but stunted growth, microcephaly, and mental retardation are frequently present.
4. Irradiation of the fetus between 16 and 30 weeks gestation may lead to a mild degree of microcephaly, mental retardation, and stunting of growth.
5. Irradiation after 30 weeks gestation is not likely to produce gross structural abnormalities leading to a serious handicap in early life but could cause functional disabilities.

Benjamin studied the effects of relatively low levels of ionizing radiation delivered during prenatal or postnatal development. The Collaborative Radiological Health Laboratory at Colorado State University has been conducting long-term animal experiments for the purpose of determining the lifetime hazards associated with prenatal and early postnatal exposure to ionizing radiation. These are life span studies of a moderately large and long-lived mammal, the beagle dog, exposed one of six times during development to discrete doses of external ^{60}Co gamma radiation. In the major long-term experiment, 1680 dogs received either a single, whole-body exposure to ^{60}Co gamma radiation or a sham radiation. The results of this study are preliminary, but it appears that there is an increased rate of malignancy occurring before the age of 2, especially malignant lymphomas, but the increased incidence does not persist as the dogs age. Decrements in skeletal growth and abnormalities of dental development have been identified in these dogs exposed to irradiation. Exposure to at least 10 cGy appears to be necessary before significant differences are seen. Additional information should be available as these studies mature.

GENERAL CONCEPTS OF CLINICAL RADIATION THERAPY

The technical modalities used in modern radiation therapy may be divided into two major categories:

1. External irradiation. This applies to irradiation from sources at a distance from the body (e.g., teletherapy with ^{60}Co, linear accelerator, betatron, or standard orthovoltage x-ray machines).
2. Local irradiation (brachytherapy). This applies to irradiation from sources in direct proximity to the tumor.
   a. Intracavitary irradiation with applicators loaded with radioactive materials such as radium or cesium (e.g., vaginal ovoids, vaginal cylinder, intrauterine tandem, or Heyman capsules).
   b. Interstitial irradiation (endocurie therapy) usually delivered in the form of removable needles containing radium, cesium, or iridium. Also applies to permanent isotope implants, such as ^{125}I seeds.
   c. Direct therapy usually delivered by means of cones from an orthovoltage machine (e.g., transvaginal).
   d. Intraperitoneal or intrapleural instillation of radioactive colloids, such as ^{32}P.

External Irradiation

The energy and penetrating power of ionizing radiation increase as the photon wavelength decreases (see Table G-1). Thus differences in the physical characteristics of the radiation used are of great importance in therapeutic radiology. The clinically important changes occur with radiation generated in the range of 400-800 kV (kilovolts). Above this energy, the advantages are reduced absorption of radiation in bone, less damage to the skin at the portal of entry, better tolerance of the vasculoconnective tissue, greater radiation at the depth relative to the surface dose, and reduced lateral scatter of radiation in the tissues (Figure G-6).

The reduced skin effect of supervoltage radiation, as compared with orthovoltage radiation, is based on the physical fact that with higher energy radiation, forward scattering (in the direction of the primary beam) of radiation in the absorber is greater and lateral scattering less. With supervoltage radiation the maximal ionization occurs below the level of the epidermis. For example, with ^{60}Co teletherapy, maximal ionization occurs about 5 mm below the surface, although the surface dose may be only 40% of this maximum. As the energy of irradiation increases, it becomes more penetrating; as photons and resultant electrons become more energetic, they travel a greater distance into absorbing material. Therefore the percentage of irradiation at any specific depth, compared with the surface dose, increases as the energy increases. This advantage of supervoltage and megavoltage is of clinical importance in the treatment of tumors that are located deep within the human organism (e.g, carcinomas of the bladder and endometrium), where the introduction of a sufficiently high dose with medium voltage radiation is difficult or impossible.

In the supervoltage range, absorption of radiation in bone approximates that in water or soft tissue per unit density, with medium voltage, radiation absorption is considerably greater in bone than in soft tissue. The vasculoconnective tissue immediately adjacent to the bone around the haversian channels receives a sufficiently higher dose because of static irradiation. This higher dose increases the risk of bone necrosis by destruction of the osteoblastic elements and damage to the vascular system. Furthermore, preferential bone absorption leads to a reduction in the dose at the point of interest when thick bone must be traversed by the radiation. In addition, it has

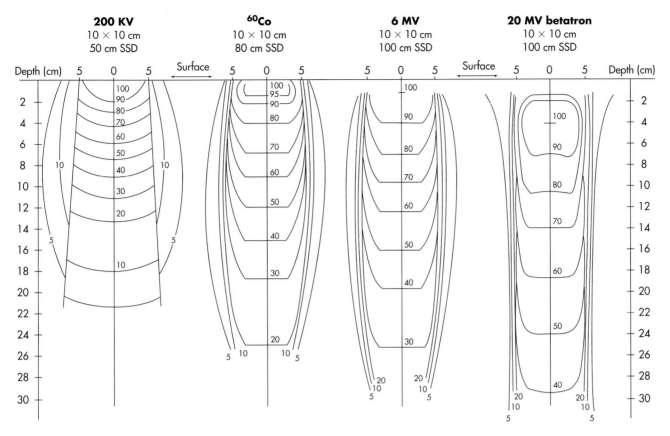

Figure G-6 Comparison isodose curves and depth-dose distribution through single field of varying machines delivering photons for medical use. Note that higher energy machines deliver radiation to a greater depth for same surface dose, and indeed there is considerable skin sparing with 6 mV and 20 mV equipment.

been observed clinically that as irradiation energy increases, similar tumor effects can be produced with less damage to important adjacent normal structures. The incidence of severe mucosal and skin reactions is reduced, and apparently there is less damage to the vasculoconnective tissue. This greater tolerance of vasculoconnective tissue to a higher dose of properly protracted supervoltage radiation therapy is one of the factors that permits the planned combination of radical preoperative radiation with surgery without appreciably increasing the surgical risks beyond those associated with surgery alone.

Local Irradiation (Brachytherapy)

Local application of radiation (also known as brachytherapy) permits very high doses to restricted tissue volumes. It is in this situation that the physical principle (inverse square law) that the intensity of irradiation rapidly decreases with distance from the radiation source is used to advantage. One needs a small tumor with well-defined limits and a clinical situation where it is desirable to restrict the volume of tissue irradiated. Larger volumes of tissue that need radiation therapy are best treated with external irradiation. Radium has been the most common element used for local application—in the form of tubes and needles. In recent times other materials

Table G-5   Isotopes commonly used in radiation therapy

Isotope	Energy (Mev)	Half-life
^{137}Cs	0.662	30 years
^{60}Co	1.173, 1.332	5.3 years
^{198}Au	0.411	2.69 days
^{192}Ir	0.47	74 days
^{226}Ra	0.8	1620 years
^{222}Rn	0.8	3.83 days
^{182}Ta	1.18	115 days
^{125}I	0.027-0.035	60 days
^{251}Cf	0.8 (photons)	
^{252}Cf	2.09 and 2.35 (neutrons)	265 days

From DiSaia PJ, Nolan JD, Ameson AP: *Gynecological radiotherapy.* In Danforth DN, editor: *Obstetrics and gynecology,* ed 3, New York, 1977, HarperCollins.

(^{60}Co, ^{137}Cs, ^{192}Ir, ^{182}Ta) have been available for local application (Table G-5). The major disadvantage of these materials compared with radium is the appreciably shorter half-life. Several of these materials have advantages over radium in that they may be incorporated in solid materials such as ceramics and need not be used in the form of a powder-gas substance as is the case with radium. Radium tubes and needles contain radium powder, and many of its decay products are in gas form within the same container. Other substances that have been used as implants in the

tumor are gold (^{196}Au) and iodine (^{125}I) seeds; these are permanent implantations and are difficult and awkward because of the difficulty of preparation, the rather rapid radioactive decay, and the difficulty in obtaining homogeneity of dosimetry.

The term *dosimetry* is applied to the measurement and calculation of dose that the patient receives. If the radiation intensity decreases rapidly with increasing depth in tissue, as is the case with local irradiation (Figure G-7), that tissue adjacent to the radiation source may theoretically be treated adequately without harmful irradiation to the underlying structures. The effectiveness of this distribution of irradiation depends, of course, on careful application of these sources. Interstitial application of radioactive sources is much more difficult than intracavitary application. A system of multiple discrete sources often results in a less homogeneous isodose pattern than irradiation from external sources or from a well-placed intracavitary source (Figure G-8).

Some of the high cure rates obtained by gynecologic oncologists are a result of the accessibility of vaginal and uterine cancer to local irradiation. This accessibility allows relatively high doses of irradiation to be delivered to the neoplasm with relatively safe amounts of normal tissue exposure. Indeed, meticulously applied local irradiation is often the factor that distinguishes institutions with low morbidity and high cure rates.

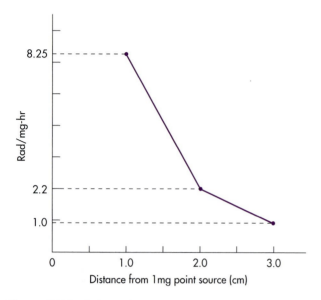

Figure G-7 Radiation effects at various distances from 1 mg point source of radium. (From Danforth DN, editor: *Obstetrics and gynecology,* ed 3, New York, 1977, HarperCollins.)

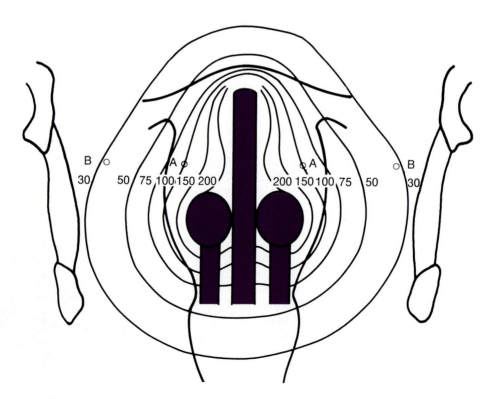

Figure G-8 Isodose curves surrounding typical Fletcher-Suit intracavitary application (tandem plus ovoids) for cervical cancer. Note location of points *A* and *B* and relative dose rates at distances from system.

TOLERANCE OF PELVIC ORGANS

The tolerance of any tissue (normal or tumor) to irradiation therapy depends on several characteristics of radiation, including (1) the fractionation technique, (2) the total dose given, (3) the dose rate, and (4) the volume irradiated. Fractionation is a function of the number of treatments. With external irradiation, the patient is usually treated 4 to 5 days per week. Fractionation is closely tied to dose rate, which is the quantity of irradiation given in each of these sessions, usually expressed as dose per week. Pelvic radiation delivered to a patient for a total dose of 5000 cGy given in five daily fractions each week for 5 weeks is well tolerated in most instances. However, if that same total dose of 5000 cGy were given in five fractions of 1000 cGy each and every Monday for 5 consecutive weeks, very few, if any, of the patients would tolerate that kind of fractionation or dose rate. The lower the dose rate and the higher the fractionation, the better the normal tissue tolerance of the irradiation given. Obviously there is a need for balance because excessive fractionation or very low dose rates will not accomplish tumor kill. The volume of tissue irradiated becomes an integral factor in tolerance and is difficult to separate from dose rate or fractionation. For example, a 1 cm circular field of skin would easily tolerate the fractionation and dose rate of 1000 cGy each Monday for 5 consecutive weeks. However, for a larger volume, such as whole-pelvis radiation, such a treatment plan could not be tolerated. The greater the volume of tissue irradiated, the more difficult the normal tolerance.

Previous surgery may have an effect on the morbidity of radiation therapy. In both cervix and corpus cancer, surgery may identify adverse surgical pathologic findings that may indicate the need of radiation therapy and enlarging ports. In cervical cancer, surgical evaluation of possible lymph node metastasis, particularly in advanced cancers, is frequently done. Transpertioneal evaluation followed by radiation to the pelvis and possibly para-aortic areas noted increased radiation-induced complications, particularly on both large and small bowel. These may be severe, including fistula formation, bowel obstruction and perforation. The retroperitoneal approach has decreased this complication rate and is the preferred method of surgically evaluating lymph node status in cervical cancer.

Irradiation tolerance of the normal organs of the pelvis varies slightly from patient to patient and is, of course, subject to the factors previously mentioned, such as volume, fractionation, and energy of irradiation received. The administration of brachytherapy by one technique or another may also result in different dose distributions and considerably affect tolerance. As is illustrated in many areas of oncology, the more advanced the lesion, the greater the radiation dose necessary for possible eradication and the greater the incidence of morbidity (Table G-6). With advanced disease, higher risks of injury are not

Table G-6   Squamous carcinoma dose–tumor volume relationships (90% control)

Subclinical disease	5000 cGy
<2 cm	6000 cGy
2-4 cm	6800 cGy
4-6 cm	7300 cGy
>6 cm	7890 cGy

From Wharton JT et al: *Obstet Gynecol* 49:333, 1977.

only present but justified. This, coupled with the fact that advanced cancer is often already compromising the integrity of the bladder and rectum, means that serious sequelae often develop in patients with advanced cervical, vaginal, and corpus lesions.

The normal tissues of the cervix and the corpus of the uterus can tolerate very high doses of radiation. In fact, they withstand higher doses better than any other comparable volume of tissue in the body; doses of 20,000-30,000 cGy in about 2 weeks are tolerated. This remarkable tolerance level permits a large tumor dose and allows a very high percentage of central control of cervical cancer. It is the unusual radiation tolerance of the uterus, as well as the vagina, that accounts for the success of brachytherapy in the treatment of cervical lesions. It appears that the epithelium of the uterus and vagina have unusual ability to recover from radiation injury.

In contrast, the sigmoid, rectosigmoid, and rectum are more susceptible to radiation injury than other pelvic organs. The frequency of injury to the large bowel often depends on the total dose administered by both the external beam and the intracavitary radium systems. With external beam alone, the large bowel is the most sensitive of pelvic structures to irradiation. The bladder tolerates slightly more radiation than the rectosigmoid according to most authorities. Fletcher proposed a rule of thumb that gives the upper limits of pelvic irradiation and indirectly gives the tolerance of the bladder and rectum. The rule is that the sum of the central dose by external beam plus the number of milligram-hours of radium or cesium administered by intracavitary techniques should never exceed 10,000. This rule of thumb may not be valid unless the Fletcher-Suit brachytherapy systems are used. Most of this is applicable to therapy for the uterus, cervix, and vagina. In general, if a heavy dose of intracavitary irradiation is applied centrally for a small lesion, the amount of external beam applied centrally must be kept to a minimum. Conversely, if a lesion is large and the vaginal geometry poor, a minimal intracavitary dose can be given, and the dose administered centrally by external beam may be quite high (6000-7000 cGy).

Pelvic radiation usually spares the small bowel, because that structure is normally in episodic motion. This tends to prevent any one segment from receiving an excessive dose. However, if loops of small bowel are immobilized as a result of adhesions caused by previous surgery, they may be held directly in the path of the radiation beam and thus be injured. The result of such an injury is usually not manifested for at least a year or longer after completion of radiation and is accomplished by narrowing of the lumen associated with mucosal ulceration of that segment of bowel.

It is extremely important that students of this subject comprehend the concept of injury to normal tissue as a function of dose (Figure G-9), as well as the permanent nature of that injury. When any area of the body is subjected to tumoricidal doses of radiation, the normal tissues of that area suffer an injury that is only partially repaired. The tumor tissue will disappear but the normal tissue bed remains, and the injury that is only partially repaired must be seriously considered should other disease processes affect that area in subsequent decades. Radiobiologists estimate that in the case of injury to normal tissues, only 5%-20% of the damage is repaired. Thus, the normal tissue in the irradiated area can suffer a considerable handicap. If a second malignant neoplasm should arise in that same area many years later, additional tumoricidal radiation is not possible because of the lingering injury. In addition, any surgical procedures performed within a previously irradiated field will be associated with a higher risk for poor healing, fistula formation, and so on.

Because of the potential of radiation-induced complications, attempts to reduce these problems have been addressed. The damage, at least in part, that is done by radiation is the production of free radicals, which causes cell death. These free radicals can be modified by reacting to oxygen or with sulfhydryl compounds or thiols that can prevent or repair damage caused by free radicals. Several decades ago, it was shown that sulfhydryl amino acid cysterine given before radiation therapy protected the bone marrow in rats against lethal irradiation. Subsequently, the importance of the sulfhydryl-containing compounds have been investigated. These protective agents also appear to be effective in protecting the bone marrow in patients receiving chemotherapy. WR-2721 (amifostine) has recently been evaluated by investigators in the hope of decreasing morbidity both from radiation and from chemotherapy. This drug appears to be radio-protective in small and large bowel, lung, and bone marrow. Studies in rectal cancer noted in a randomized study that radiation plus WR-2721 compound to radiation alone had significantly lower incidence of moderate or severe late toxicities in bladder and GI tract in the WR-2721 arm. The addition of WR-2721 did not appear to compromise tumor response to radiation. Complete response and survival was better in the WR-2721 arm. Side effects of WR-2721 include nausea and vomiting, which is dose related and can be controlled with antiemetics. Hypotension is easily reversed by stopping the drug

Radiation-induced soft tissue necrosis can be a significant complication. This is usually due to a progressive obliterative end arteritis that leads to decreased blood

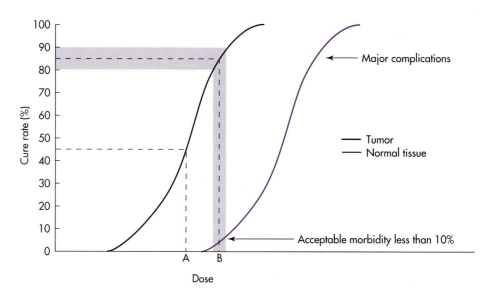

Figure G-9 Diagrammatic representation of parallel tumor response and normal tissue tolerance curves demonstrating relationship between increasing dose, increasing cure rate, and increasing morbidity. Under ideal circumstance *(B)*, 80%-90% cure rate can be achieved with 5%-10% morbidity. Pushing the cure rate carries with it an increase in morbidity. On the other hand, attempts to avoid all morbidity *(A)* significantly reduce ability to cure. Although shape of these curves will vary for various tumor types and dose rates, general concepts are valid whenever radiotherapy is used to treat malignant lesions.

flow, hypovasculation, and hypoxic tissue bed. This can lead to increased fibrosis and non-healing. Local conservative management (hydrogen peroxide douche, estrogen therapy) will resolve the problem in many instances. There is a small group of patients who have significant tissue breakdown that may be painful and may lead to fistula formation. Because of the high dose that can be given to the cervix and vagina, tissue breakdown with resultant non-healing can occur. The use of hyperbaric oxygen has been shown to enhance healing in these radiation-induced injuries. Hyperbaric oxygen has also been successfully used in osteoradionecrosis, particularly of the mandible.

NEW RADIATION MODALITIES

Hypoxic cells are more resistant to gamma ray and x-ray than oxygenated cells. Although the cells in most normal tissues are well oxygenated, most solid tumors have regions of hypoxic cells. To get adequate coverage of the tumor, radiation portals must include adjacent normal, well-oxygenated tissue. Therefore during treatment a point may be reached when all the well-oxygenated cells in the surrounding tissues have received a tolerance dose of radiation beyond which severe damage would result, yet the hypoxic cells in the tumor are still viable and will subsequently cause regrowth of the tumor.

Conventional radiation (x-rays or gamma rays) deposits its energy in tissues via electrons that lose their energy slowly, resulting in a low linear energy density along the electron track, or low linear energy transfer (LET). High LET radiations (fast neutrons or negative p mesons) are more effective against hypoxic cells than low LET radiations. This means that for the same reaction produced in the healthy cells by all radiation modalities, the high LET types have a higher probability (1.5 to 2.5 times that of x-rays) of killing the hypoxic tumor cells.

Fast Neutrons

Although the rationale for neutron radiotherapy is well established, treatment considerations are currently limited by the availability of suitable neutron sources. There are two practical sources of a fast-neutron beam for radiotherapy: the cyclotron and the D-T generator. The D-T generator derives its name from the fact that a deuteron beam (D) is accelerated into a tritium target (T), resulting in the release of a neutron and helium. The neutron is emitted with an energy of 14 meV, which results in a depth-dose distribution similar to that of ^{60}Co gamma rays. In the cyclotron the neutrons are generally produced by bombarding deuterons onto a beryllium target. In general, the average neutron energy will be a little less than half the deuteron energy, and with some of the larger machines this is approximately 15-16 meV.

Low dose rate neutron radiotherapy using fast neutrons emitted by the radionuclide ^{252}Cf can also be used as another source of neutron irradiation. ^{252}Cf allows the use of low dose rate neutrons for intracavitary brachytherapy of certain advanced cervical squamous cell cancers. Because many of these large cervical cancers undoubtedly contain many areas of hypoxic tumor cells where neutrons are effective, the potential definitely exists. Pilot studies are now under way using this new radionuclide in conjuction with conventional external irradiation therapy.

Negative π Mesons

Negative π mesons, or pions, are negatively charged particles that have a mass 273 times that of an electron. Pions can be produced in any nuclear interaction if the energy of the primary particle is sufficient to create the rest mass of the pion. For radiotherapy, pions with energies between 40-70 meV are of interest, because these particles have a depth range in tissue of approximately 6-13 cm. The production of pions involves a large and expensive accelerator facility. The dose delivered by a beam of negative pions to a tissue-like medium increases very slowly with depth in the beginning but gives rise to a sharply defined maximum near the end of the range. This is known as the Bragg peak and is a property that pions have in common with all other heavy charged particles. The unique characteristic of negative pions is that when they come to rest they are captured by the nuclei of the medium, which causes these nuclei to disintegrate, or to explode, into short-range and heavily ionizing fragments; this has been called the "star" effect. Thus, this radiation has a high biologic effectiveness and a low dependence on oxygen.

Hypoxic Cell Sensitizers and Radiopotentiators

Awareness of the importance of oxygen in tissue response to radiation has been known since 1921, when Holthusen noted that larger doses of radiation were needed to inactivate sea urchin eggs rendered hypoxic by liquid nitrogen. It has been demonstrated repeatedly in vitro that to achieve the same proportion of cell kill, hypoxic cells require about three times the radiation dose needed for well-oxygenated cells. The ratio of the dose required for a given level of cell killing under hypoxic conditions compared to the dose needed in air is called the oxygen enhancement ratio (OER).

Hypoxic cells can be sensitized to ionizing radiation by chemical compounds with electrophilic properties. The precise mechanism of sensitization is not known, although a great deal of basic chemical and biophysical research is ongoing. Current interest in hypoxic cell sensitizers centers on the nitroimidazole compounds (Table G-7). Encouraging in vitro studies demonstrate hypoxic cell sensitization at a nontoxic concentration of sensitizers; in vivo application with currently available agents is hindered by normal tissue toxic effects, particularly peripheral nerve injury. Nevertheless, hypoxic cell sensitizers have considerable theoretical appeal

Table G-7 Radiopotentiators	
Chemotherapeutic agents	**Nonchemotherapeutic agents**
Bleomycin	Hypoxic cell radiosensitizers
Chlorambucil	Vitroimidazoles
Cisplatin	Misonidazole
Cyclophosphamide	SR-2508
Doxorubicin	RO-03-8799
Hydroxyurea	Biologic response modifiers
6-mercaptopurine	Tumor necrosis factor
Methotrexate	Interferon
Mitomycin	Antiviral agents
Procarbazine	Acyclovir
Vincristine	

because they can be made widely available and are easily administered. Although several drugs have been identified as effective, radiation sensitizers in in vitro, experience clinically is limited. In gynecology, the most experience has been in advanced cervical cancer. The GOG has shown in a prospective randomized study that the addition of hydroxyurea to radiation therapy increases survival compared with radiation alone. Misonidazole, which has been shown to improve local control and survival in some cancers, did not improve survival in cervical cancer compared to hydroxyurea and radiation. A combination of 5-FU and cisplatin combined with radiation has been shown to be beneficial in head and neck, as well as anal, cancers when combined with radiation therapy. A prospective randomized study by the GOG compared 5-FU infusion and cisplatin plus radiation with hydroxyurea and radiation in advanced cervical cancer. This study is now closed but the follow up to data has not shown an improved survival for the 5-FU cisplatin arm over hydroxyurea. Taxol has shown a significant radiosensitizing effect on ovarian cell lines. This unique drug appears to have its main action on the microtubes and cells seem to accumulate in the G2/M phase of the cell cycle and as such may make the cells more radiosensitive. At the present time, the role of radiation therapy seems to be rather limited in ovarian cancer and clinical studies taking advantage of taxol as a chemotherapeutic agent, as well as a radiosensitizer, has not been done.

Intraoperative Radiation

Several centers throughout the world are attesting to the efficacy of large-fraction intraoperative external irradiation. Patients are subjected to operative procedures in which the area of involvement is carefully defined and radiation fractions of 1500-2500 cGy are delivered directly to the area identified. One application of this technique in gynecologic oncology has been in the treatment of biopsy-proven positive periaortic nodes at the time of staging laparotomy for cervical carcinoma.

Periaortic irradiation is delivered with a 2000-3000 cGy fraction with the bowel packed to the side, thereby minimizing the probability of visceral injuries. Experience in both primary and recurrent tumors has been reported. Although the results are encouraging, criteria for this therapy is strict and review of current literature in gynecologic cancers is limited. It appears the role of intraoperative radiation in gynecology is not wide spread and is limited to a handful of institutions capable of this specialized therapy.

Hyperbaric Oxygen

The recognition that hypoxic cells are relatively resistant to radiation and that oxygen, expecially under high pressure, is effective in increasing radiosensitivity has been one of the milestones in radiation therapy during the last 30 years. Numerous trials have been conducted over the past 30 years but with mixed results. Because of the cumbersome nature of a hyperbaric oxygen tank, higher daily doses were used in these trials. It appears that the sensitivity of hypoxic tumor cells to irradiation, as well as normal tissue reactions, increases as the daily dose is increased. Trials by the British Medical Research Council have shown improvement in local control and survival using hyperbaric oxygen treatments with a 5-year follow-up in stage III cervical cancer and a 5-year follow-up in advanced head and neck cancer. However, other trials in cervical cancer and in bladder cancer show no benefit of hyperbaric oxygen use over air breathing. Major limitations to using hyperbaric oxygen are that the technique is cumbersome, it requires departure from established time dose fraction agent experience, and it may increase the risk of complications.

Hyperthermia

Interest and experience with hyperthermia as a primary modality and as an adjunct to a cytotoxic drug or radiation sensitizer for the treatment of cancer continues to grow. Most major cancer research centers are developing programs to evaluate hyperthermia in laboratory and clinical investigations. Much of this interest stems from the possibility that hyperthermia may be useful for the treatment of lesions that have previously frustrated our treatment methods. Solid tumor masses often have hypovascular centers, which are poorly penetrated by antineoplastic drugs and have hypoxic cell fractions causing relative radioresistance. These same lesions have the greatest potential for response to the hyperthermia treatment modality.

Modern investigators of hyperthermia often note that the antitumor effects of heat have been reported for more than a century. Several earlier reports using heat in various ways documented tumor responses. Although there have been several anecdotal clinical observations, current interest in hyperthermia is principally based on the results of careful biologic studies on cells and transplantable tumors performed over the last 20 years. This work, based on increasing general understanding of cancer biology and increasing cancer laboratory technology, has, in turn, stimulated an extensive engineering effort to develop new technologies for providing practical hyperthermia treatment methods. Although the mechanism of action of hyperthermia is not well understood, it may involve damage to the plasma membrane, destruction of the cytoskeleton, protein damage, and inhibition of protein synthesis. Although there is no evidence that tumor cells are consistently more sensitive to heat than normal cells, several factors may contribute to a therapeutic gain. Tumors are likely to have hypoxic cell populations at low pH that will be preferentially killed and also radiosensitized by heat. Therapeutic gain may also be derived partially from the selective heating of the tumor. The hypoxic center core is likely to be heated more than the well-vascularized normal tissues, which are more efficient at removing heat. The abnormal vasculature of the tumor, with reduced capacity to increase blood flow in response to heating, may also render the neoplasm more vulnerable. Substantial clinical evidence now exists showing hyperthermia to be an active antineoplastic agent and a significant radiosensitizer, and its routine use in at least recurrent neoplasms has recently been advocated. The first notable use of hyperthermia in gynecologic oncology has been with interstitial hyperthermia for deep tumors of the pelvis. Interstitial source guides were used to introduce radio frequency heat fields with temperatures of 43°-44°C for 30-40 minutes and were loaded with radioactive sources 1-3 hours later. One study shows that complete responses were achieved in 21 of 33 patients so treated. Further studies are under way.

GLOSSARY

brachytherapy   Treatment of malignant tumors by radioactive sources that are implanted close to (intracavitary) or within (interstitial) the tumor.

central axis depth dose   The plot of the dose along the central axis from the point of beam entry into the patient.

dosimetry   The term applied to the measurement and calculation of dose that the patient receives.

electron volt (eV)   The energy of motion acquired by an electron accelerated through a potential difference of 1 volt.

excitation   The moving of an electron to a more distant orbit within the same atom.

gamma rays   (originate inside the nucleus) Electromagnetic irradiation emitted by excited nuclei. The gamma rays from an isotope will have one or several sharply defined energies.

Gray (Gy)   The special name for the unit of absorbed dose and specific energy impacted; 1 Gy = 1 joule/kg = 100 rads.

half-life   The time in which half the atoms of a radioactive species disintegrate.

HVL   Half-value layer: of a beam of x-rays or gamma rays this is the thickness of a given material that will reduce the radiation intensity to one half.

inverse square law   The intensity of radiation from a point varies inversely as the square of the distance from the source. Thus the dose rate at 2 cm from a source is one fourth that at 1 cm. At 3 cm the dose rate is one ninth that at 1 cm.

ionization   The removal of an electron from an atom, leaving a positively charged ion.

ionizing radiation   Radiation capable of causing ionization.

isotope   Nuclides having an equal number of protons but a different number of neutrons (excitable situation).

keV   1000 eV.

linear energy transfer (LET)   The energy lost by the particle or photon per micron of path depth. High LET radiations are more effective against hypoxic cells.

maximal permissible dose   The dose of whole-body irradiation that has been calculated as being within the limits of safety and expressed as 5(n-18) cGy, where n is the age in years of the individual.

meV   1,000,000 eV.

oxygen enhancement ratio (OER)   The ratio of the dose required for a given level of cell killing under hypoxic conditions compared to the dose needed in air.

penumbra The radiation outside the full beam. Often caused by scatter or incomplete collimation.

rad   A unit-absorbed dose of ionizing radiation equivalent to the absorption of 100 erg per gram of irradiated material.

roentgen (R)   An internationally accepted unit of radiation quantity: that quantity of "x-ray or gamma irradiation such that the associated corpuscular emission per 0.001293 grams of air produces, in air, ions carrying 1 esu of quantity of electricity of either sign." x-rays (originate outside the nucleus)

x-rays   emitted by a particular generator will emit a spectrum of energies.

BIBLIOGRAPHY

Ballenger PW, editor: *Merrill's atlas of radiographic positions and radiologic procedures*, ed 7, St Louis, 1991, Mosby-Year Book.

Beard CJ, Coleman CN: *Current therapeutic strategies toward hypoxic tumor cells: principles and practice of oncology*, ed 3, Philadelphia, 1991, JB Lippincott.

Danforth DN, editor: *Obstetrics and gynecology*, New York, 1977, HarperCollins.

Deacon J, Pecken MA, Steel GG: The radio responsiveness of human tumors in the initial slope of the cell survival curve, *Radiation Therapeutic Oncol* 2:317, 1984.

Elkin DMN: DNA damage and cell killing: cause and effect, *Cancer* 45:2123, 1985

Fletcher GH: *Textbook of radiotherapy,* ed 3, Philadelphia, 1980, Lea & Febiger.

Glicksman AS, Leith JT: Radiobiological considerations of brachytherapy, *Oncology* 2(1):25, 1988.

Hall EJ: *Radiobiology for the radiologist,* ed 3, Philadelphia, 1988, JB Lippincott.

Hellman S: *Principles of radiation therapy.* In Devita V Jr, Hellman S, Rosenberg SA, editors: *Cancer: principles and practice of oncology,* ed 3, Philadelphia, 1989, JB Lippincott.

Holthusen H: Beitrage zur biologie der Strahlen wirkung: unter such ungen an Ascarideneien, *Arch Ges Phys* 187:1, 1921.

Jacobs AJ, Faris C, Perez CA et al: Short term persistence of carcinoma of the uterine cervix following radiation: an indicator of long-term prognosis, *Cancer* 57:944, 1986.

Meyer JL, Kapp DS, Fessender P et al: Hyperthermic oncology: current biology, physics and clinical results, *Pharmacol Ther* 42:251, 1989.

Perez CA, Brady LW: *Priniciples and practice of radiation oncology,* ed 2, Philadelphia, JB Lippincott Company, l992.

Plumer C: Anomalies occurring in children exposed in utero to the atomic bomb in Hiroshima, *Pediatrics* 10:687, 1952.

Scott JR, DiSaia PJ, Hammond CB et al, editors: *Danforth's textbook of obstetrics and gynecology,* ed 6, Philadelphia, 1990, JB Lippincott.

Travis EL: *Primer of Medical Radio Biology,* ed 2, Chicago, Yearbook Medical Publishers, 1989

Index